THORACIC IMAGING

PULMONARY AND CARDIOVASCULAR RADIOLOGY

THORACIC IMAGING

PULMONARY AND CARDIOVASCULAR RADIOLOGY

W. RICHARD WEBB, M.D.

Professor of Radiology
Chief, Thoracic Imaging
Department of Radiology
University of California, San Francisco
San Francisco, California

CHARLES B. HIGGINS, M.D.

Professor of Radiology
Department of Radiology
University of California, San Francisco
San Francisco, California

LIPPINCOTT WILLIAMS & WILKINS
A **Wolters Kluwer** Company

Philadelphia • Baltimore • New York • London
Buenos Aires • Hong Kong • Sydney • Tokyo

Acquisitions Editor: Lisa McAllister
Developmental Editor: Scott Scheidt
Production Editors: Emily Lerman and Grace Caputo, Dovetail Content Solutions
Manufacturing Manager: Benjamin Rivera
Cover Designer: Christine Jenny
Compositor: Maryland Composition
Printer: Maple Press

Library of Congress Cataloging-in-Publication Data

Webb, W. Richard
    Thoracic imaging : pulmonary and cardiovascular radiology / W. Richard Webb, Charles B. Higgins.
        p. ; cm.
    Includes bibliographical references and index.
    ISBN-13 978-0-7817-4119-4
    ISBN 0-7817-4119-X
    1. Chest—Radiography. 2. Cardiopulmonary system—Diseases—Diagnosis. 3. Cardiopulmonary system--Radiography. I. Webb, W. Richard (Wayne Richard), 1945-
II. Title.
    [DNLM: 1. Cardiovascular Diseases—diagnosis. 2. Lung Diseases—diagnosis. 3. Diagnostic Imaging—methods. 4. Radiography, Thoracic—methods. WF 975 H636t 2005]
RC941.H497 2005
617.5'407'57—dc22

                                                                                    2004006191

10 9 8 7

To Emma and Brett, in the sincere hope I won't have to answer
so many questions after this book is published
—W.R.W.

To the many fellows who have contributed to our progress
in developing new cardiovascular imaging techniques
—C.B.H.

CONTENTS

CONTRIBUTING AUTHORS

William G. Berger, M.D.   Assistant Professor, Department of Radiology, University of Arizona, Tucson, Arizona

Douglas P. Boyd, Ph.D.   Adjunct Professor, Department of Radiology, University of California, San Francisco, San Francisco, California

Gary R. Caputo, M.D.   Associate Professor, Department of Radiology, University of California, San Francisco, San Francisco, California

Samuel K. Dawn, M.D.   Assistant Clinical Professor, Department of Radiology, University of California, San Francisco, San Francisco, California

Michael B. Gotway, M.D.   Assistant Professor in Residence, Director, Radiology Residency Training Program, University of California, San Francisco; Director, Thoracic Imaging, San Francisco General Hospital, San Francisco, California

Gabriele A. Krombach, M.D.   Department of Diagnostic Radiology, University Hospital, RWTH-Aachen, Aachen, Germany

Jessica W.T. Leung, M.D.   Assistant Professor, Department of Radiology, University of California, San Francisco, San Francisco, California

Gautham P. Reddy, M.D., M.P.H.   Professor of Radiology, Thoracic Imaging Section, University of California, San Francisco, San Francisco, California

Akhilesh Sista, M.D.   Medical Student, Johns Hopkins University Medical School, Baltimore, Maryland

PREFACE

Our goal in writing *Thoracic Imaging: Pulmonary and Cardiovascular Radiology* was to provide, in a single volume, a comprehensive but easy-to-digest discussion of the title topic and to review the use and interpretation of chest radiographs and advanced imaging techniques (e.g., spiral computed tomography [CT], high-resolution CT, magnetic resonance imaging [MRI], and magnetic resonance angiography).

We have tried to be thorough without being exhaustive. Rather than referencing specific studies, we have summarized what we consider to be the most important and pertinent information and have provided numerous tables to make key facts easily available to the reader. More than 1700 illustrations demonstrate important radiographic findings and the typical appearances of the various disease entities one might encounter in current clinical practice.

Imaging of the lungs and mediastinum requires an understanding of both plain radiography and CT. Although in many situations CT has assumed a preeminent role, knowledge of chest radiographs and their utility is essential to the radiographic assessment of patients with suspected pulmonary disease. We have attempted to review and illustrate both the plain radiographic and the CT findings of most abnormalities and disorders. Other imaging modalities, such as MRI and radionuclide imaging, are also discussed in situations in which they play a significant role.

Chapters in the pulmonary radiology section of this book are organized according to important radiographic findings, anatomic regions, clinical problems, or disease states, as is appropriate to an approach to diagnosis and differential diagnosis. Radiographic and CT techniques are not described in detail (e.g., there is no chapter specifically on techniques), but these are reviewed in context in various chapters. In most cases, normal radiographic and CT findings are reviewed where appropriate to the understanding of specific abnormal findings or diseases.

Cardiovascular imaging has transitioned nearly completely in the past two decades from dependence on x-ray angiography for definitive diagnosis to noninvasive tomographic imaging techniques. Therefore, *Thoracic Imaging* emphasizes the use of tomographic imaging for the evaluation of cardiovascular morphology and function. The currently employed tomographic techniques are echocardiography, MRI, and CT. Although echocardiography is the most frequently used imaging modality for the evaluation of cardiac disease, it is not included in this volume. Many books encompassing all aspects of echocardiography already exist, so inclusion of it would be not only repetitious but also incomplete because of the intended size of this book. Another practical consideration is that echocardiography is rarely practiced by radiologists.

Frequently, the initial radiographic study used in patients with cardiovascular disease is the thoracic radiograph. Two chapters describe a systematic approach to the evaluation of the thoracic radiograph in acquired and congenital heart disease. The major tomographic imaging technique employed by radiologists in the evaluation of cardiac disease is MRI. The use and interpretation of MRI is described in several chapters covering the various categories of cardiovascular diseases. The roles of MRI and CT in ischemic heart disease are under rapid evolution and are not fully predictable at this time. Individual chapters describe the current capabilities of MRI and CT in ischemic heart disease.

W. Richard Webb, M.D.
Charles B. Higgins, M.D.

CONGENITAL BRONCHOPULMONARY LESIONS

W. RICHARD WEBB

Congenital bronchopulmonary lesions represent a variety of vascular and nonvascular abnormalities of the lung and mediastinum. They often have characteristic plain film and computed tomography (CT) findings. Congenital abnormalities of the aorta and great vessels are reviewed in Chapter 35.

BRONCHIAL ANOMALIES

Anomalies of bronchial anatomy include abnormal origin, absent branches, and supernumerary branches (Table 1-1). Minor variation in subsegmental bronchial anatomy is common but clinically insignificant; a detailed knowledge of subsegmental bronchial anatomy is not necessary for clinical practice. Segmental bronchial anomalies are less frequent and not often of significance.

Tracheal Bronchus

Tracheal bronchi are common anomalies, present in about 0.1% of the population. A tracheal bronchus usually arises from the right tracheal wall, at or within 2 cm of the tracheal bifurcation. It supplies a variable portion of the medial or apical right upper lobe, most often the apical segment (Fig. 1-1); in occasional cases, the entire right upper lobe bronchus arises from the trachea (Fig. 1-2). When a tracheal bronchus is present, the azygos arch is seen above the tracheal bronchus. Tracheal bronchus is sometimes referred to as a "pig bronchus" or "bronchus suis" as it is common in pigs and other cloven-hoofed animals.

In most cases, this anomaly is insignificant. However, recurrent infection or bronchiectasis may result, since the tracheal bronchus is often slightly narrowed at its origin. A left tracheal bronchus, supplying the apical posterior segment of the left upper lobe, is rarely present; it is much less common than right-sided tracheal bronchi.

Accessory Cardiac Bronchus

Accessory cardiac bronchus is a supernumerary bronchus with an incidence of about 0.1%. It arises from the medial wall of the bronchus intermedius or right lower lobe bronchus and extends inferiorly and medially toward the mediastinum or heart. It may terminate within the mediastinum (Fig. 1-3). In some cases, the cardiac bronchus is a short, blind-ending bronchial stump without associated alveolar tissue; in others, a longer branching bronchus is present, associated with rudimentary lung tissue. In most cases, this anomaly is an incidental finding; occasionally, chronic infection or hemoptysis is associated.

Bronchial Isomerism

Bronchial isomerism refers to bilateral symmetry of the bronchi and associated pulmonary lobes. It may be isolated or associated with a variety of anomalies, particularly congenital heart disease. Bronchial anatomy may be bilaterally

TABLE 1-1. BRONCHIAL ANOMALIES

Subsegmental anomalies
Common but insignificant
Tracheal bronchus
Incidence 0.1%
Arises from right tracheal wall; rare on left
Usually supplies apical segment of right upper lobe; rarely entire right upper lobe
Increased incidence of infection or bronchiectasis
Accessory cardiac bronchus
Incidence 0.1%
Arises from medial wall of bronchus intermedius
Usually blind ending or supplies rudimentary lung
May terminate in the mediastinum
Increased incidence of infection or hemoptysis
Bronchial isomerism
Symmetrical bronchial anatomy
Bilateral right of left-sided bronchial anatomy
Associated with congenital heart disease, other anomalies

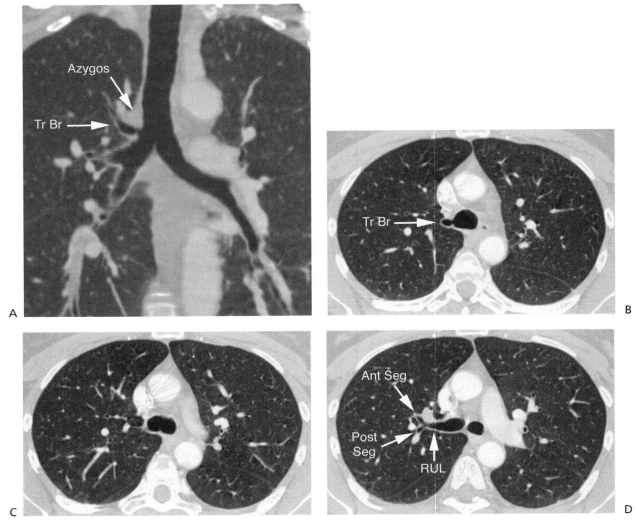

FIG. 1-1. Tracheal bronchus. **A.** Coronal CT reconstruction shows a tracheal bronchus *(Tr Br)* arising from the right tracheal wall just above the carina. **B.** The azygos arch *(Azygos)* is visible above the bronchus. CT (1.25-mm detectors) shows the origin of the tracheal bronchus. As in this case, slight narrowing at the origin of the bronchus is typical. The bronchus supplies the apical segment of the right upper lobe. **C.** The tracheal carina is seen slightly below **B**. **D.** Below **C**, the main right upper lobe bronchus *(RUL)* gives rise to the anterior *(Ant Seg)* and posterior *(Post Seg)* segmental bronchi.

right sided (associated with asplenia) or left sided (associated with polysplenia).

BRONCHIAL ATRESIA

Bronchial atresia is a developmental defect characterized by local narrowing or obliteration of a lobar, segmental, or subsegmental bronchus (Table 1-2). It is most common in the left upper lobe, followed by the right upper, and right middle lobes; it may occur in the lower lobes but is less common. This entity is usually detected incidentally in adults and is undoubtedly etiologically related to congenital lobar emphysema (CLE). Patients usually have no symptoms, but lung distal to the obstruction may occasionally become infected. In patients with chronic infection, resection may be necessary.

The lobe or segment distal to the bronchial obstruction usually remains aerated because of collateral ventilation (Figs. 1-4 and 1-5). Air trapping and decreased perfusion in the distal lung cause it to be hyperlucent and hypovascular in 90% of cases. Affected lung is often increased in vol-

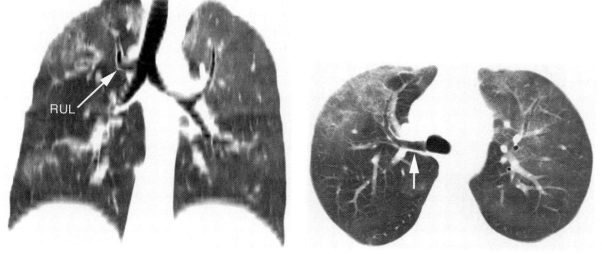

FIG. 1-2. Tracheal bronchus in a patient with pneumonia. **A.** Coronal reconstruction shows the entire right upper lobe bronchus *(RUL)* arising from the right tracheal wall above the carina. The apical segmental bronchus extends superiorly. **B.** Transaxial CT shows the right upper lobe bronchus *(arrow)* giving rise to anterior and posterior segments. Patchy areas of increased lung opacity reflect the presence of pneumonia.

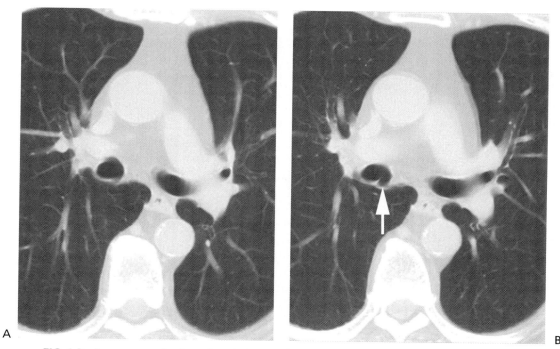

FIG. 1-3. Accessory cardiac bronchus. **A.** Scan at the level of the bronchus intermedius. **B.** Slightly below **A,** a bronchus arises from the medial wall of the bronchus intermedius *(arrow).* This represents the origin of a cardiac bronchus. *(Figure continues.)*

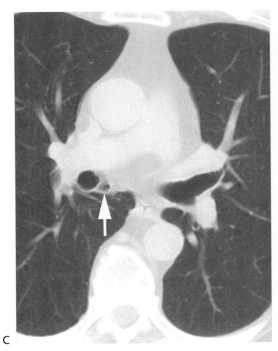
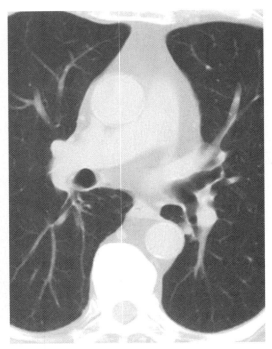

C   D

FIG. 1-3. *(Continued.)* **C.** Slightly below **B**, the cardiac bronchus *(arrow)* is seen extending into the mediastinum medial to the hilum. **D.** Below **C**, the bronchus is no longer seen.

ume, resulting in mediastinal shift or shift of a fissure. In 80% of cases, mucus accumulates within dilated bronchi distal to the obstruction, resulting in a tubular, branching, or ovoid density (mucous plug or *mucocele*). CT shows the affected lung to be lucent, hypovascular, and increased in volume. Mucus within dilated bronchi appears low in attenuation. Expiratory radiographs or CT scans show air trapping (see Fig. 1-5B).

The combination of these typical radiographic findings in a young patient is strongly suggestive of the diagnosis. Bronchoscopy may be warranted to rule out another cause of bronchial obstruction, such as tumor.

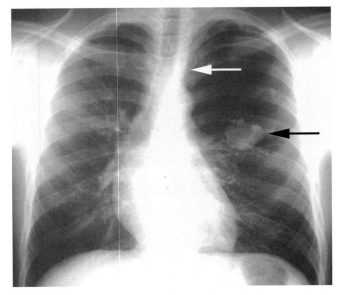

FIG. 1-4. Bronchial atresia. Chest radiograph shows a classic bronchial atresia involving the left upper lobe. The upper lobe is increased in volume, with mediastinal shift toward the opposite side *(white arrow)*. The lobe is lucent, and vascularity is decreased. A large, oval mucous plug *(black arrow)* is visible distal to the site of bronchial obstruction.

TABLE 1-2. BRONCHIAL ATRESIA

Narrowing or obliteration of a lobar, segmental, or subsegmental bronchus
Left upper lobe > right upper lobe > right middle lobe > lower lobes
Detected incidentally in adults
Infection may occur
Mucous plug distal to obstructed bronchial segment
Distal lung
   Lucent
   Increased in volume
   Decreased vessel size
   Air trapping on expiration
Rule out obstructing tumor

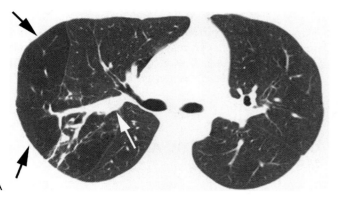
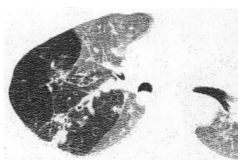
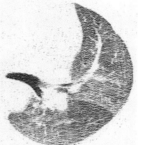

A   B

FIG. 1-5. Bronchial atresia. **A.** CT shows a branching mucous plug *(white arrow)* in the location of the posterior segment of the right upper lobe. Lung distal to the bronchus *(black arrows)* is hyperlucent and hypovascular. Slight mediastinal shift to the left side is present. **B.** Expiratory CT shows air trapping in the lung distal to the obstructed bronchus. Normal lung increases significantly in attenuation relative to **A.**

CONGENITAL LOBAR EMPHYSEMA

CLE is characterized by marked overinflation of a lobe (Table 1-3). Most cases present within the first month of life; symptoms of respiratory distress are typical. Presentation after the first month may occur.

Most cases of CLE are associated with partial or complete bronchial obstruction occurring as a result of (1) deficient cartilage; (2) external compression, usually by an anomalous vessel or bronchogenic cyst; or (3) luminal abnormalities such as mucosal folds. Some cases may not be associated with bronchial obstruction.

CLE is most common in the left upper lobe, followed by the right middle lobe and right upper lobe. Only a few percent occur in the lower lobes. Radiographs show marked overinflation and air trapping in the affected lobe, but the lobe may sometimes appear opaque because of retained fetal lung fluid. Mediastinal shift away from the abnormal lobe often occurs, and normal lobes are reduced in volume. Resection is often necessary.

It is reasonable to assume that cases of CLE that go unrecognized at birth may be diagnosed years later as bronchial atresia.

PULMONARY BRONCHOGENIC CYST

Bronchogenic cysts are foregut duplication cysts and result from abnormal development of the lung bud. They are lined by pseudostratified ciliated columnar epithelium, typical of bronchi. The cyst wall may also contain smooth muscle, mucous glands, or cartilage. Bronchogenic cysts are filled with fluid, which can be serous, hemorrhagic, or highly viscous and gelatinous because of its high protein content.

Bronchogenic cysts may be mediastinal or pulmonary. Mediastinal bronchogenic cysts are much more common than pulmonary cysts. They are discussed along with mediastinal masses in Chapter 8.

Pulmonary bronchogenic cysts are most common in the medial lung and the lower lobes (Table 1-4). They are

---

TABLE 1-3. CONGENITAL LOBAR EMPHYSEMA

Partial or complete bronchial obstruction caused by:
  Deficient cartilage
  External compression
  Luminal abnormalities
Some cases unassociated with bronchial obstruction
Left upper lobe > right middle lobe > right upper lobe > lower
  lobes
Respiratory distress in neonates
Presentation after 1st month uncommon
Marked overinflation of lobe
Air trapping
Sometimes the abnormal lobe retains fetal lung fluid
Resection often necessary

TABLE 1-4. PULMONARY BRONCHOGENIC CYST

Foregut duplication cyst
Lined by bronchial epithelium
Fluid contents can be serous, hemorrhagic, or viscous
Less common than mediastinal bronchogenic cysts
Most commonly in medial lung and lower lobes
Sharply circumscribed and round or oval
Thin wall; occasionally calcifies
Contents 0–20 HU in half; often 20–80 HU; milk of calcium rare
Infection occurs in 75%
  Rapid increase in size
  Blurring of outer edge
  Air-fluid level
  Air in cyst may remain after infection

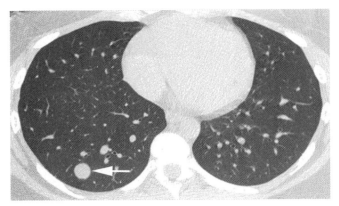

FIG. 1-6. Pulmonary bronchogenic cyst. A sharply marginated round nodular opacity *(arrow)* is visible in the right lower lobe. This measured 0 HU in attenuation. This appearance is typical of a fluid-filled bronchogenic cyst.

sharply circumscribed and round or oval. The cyst wall may calcify. Rarely, the cyst may contain milk of calcium and appear dense. Little change in size is typically seen over time unless infection occurs.

About half of fluid-filled bronchogenic cysts appear to be low in attenuation on CT (0 to 20 HU) (Fig. 1-6). However, as with mediastinal bronchogenic cysts, the CT attenuation of a pulmonary bronchogenic cyst is variable. High CT numbers (40 to 80 HU), suggesting a solid mass, can be seen. Such cysts contain blood or thick, proteinaceous fluid. Typically, the cyst wall appears very thin on CT or is invisible. They may be related to a small bronchus or may be isolated.

Infection eventually occurs in 75% of cases. In the presence of acute infection, a rapid increase in size of the cyst

may be seen. Also, the outer cyst wall may become less well defined because of surrounding lung inflammation. During or after infection, a cyst may contain air (Fig. 1-7; see also Fig. 9-29 in Chapter 9) or a combination of air and fluid (with an air-fluid level). When the cyst contains air, its wall appears very thin.

CONGENITAL CYSTIC ADENOMATOID MALFORMATION

Congenital cystic adenomatoid malformation (CCAM) consists of a multicystic, intralobar mass of disorganized lung tissue, derived primarily from bronchioles. About 70% present during the first week of life, but 10% are diagnosed after the first year, and rare cases in adults have been reported.

CCAMs can involve an entire lobe. Lower lobes are most often involved, but any lobe can be affected. The CCAM communicates with the bronchial tree and is supplied by the pulmonary artery; systemic arterial supply is rarely present.

CCAMs are often classified into three types, which have different histology, gross pathologic findings, radiographic appearance, and prognosis (Table 1-5).

Type I CCAMs (55% of cases) contain one or more cysts more than 2 cm in diameter (Fig. 1-8). They usually present as a large, air-filled multicystic lesion, sometimes with air-fluid levels, which may occupy the entire hemithorax.

Type II CCAMs (40% of cases) contain multiple cysts less than 2 cm in diameter. They present as an air-filled

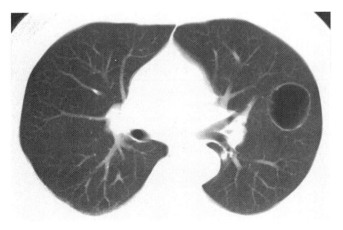

FIG. 1-7. Pulmonary bronchogenic cyst. A thin-walled, sharply marginated, air-filled bronchogenic cyst is visible in the left lung. The presence of air within the cyst indicates prior infection.

TABLE 1-5. CONGENITAL CYSTIC ADENOMATOID MALFORMATION

Multicystic, intralobar mass of disorganized lung tissue
70% present in 1st week; 10% after 1st year
Respiratory distress in neonates; recurrent infection in adults
Most common in lower lobe
Three types
   Type I (55%)
      One or more cysts, >2 cm in diameter
      May appear initially as solid mass
      Large air-filled multicystic lesion
      Sometimes with air-fluid levels
      May occupy the entire hemithorax
   Type II (40%)
      Multiple cysts <2 cm in diameter
      May appear initially as solid mass
      Air-filled multicystic mass or focal consolidation
      Associated renal and cardiac abnormalities
      Often a poor prognosis
   Type III (5%)
      Microscopic (<3–5 mm) cysts
      Solid mass

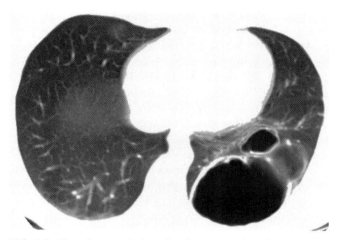

FIG. 1-8. Type I congenital cystic adenomatoid malformation. A multicystic lesion is visible in the left lower lobe. This is a typical appearance of type I in an adult.

multicystic mass or a solid mass or area of consolidation (see Fig. 1-9). This type may be associated with a poor prognosis because of associated renal and cardiac abnormalities.

Type III CCAMs (5% of cases) contain microscopic (less than 3 to 5 mm) cysts and present radiographically as a solid mass.

Sonography can be used for prenatal diagnosis. Findings include polyhydramnios, fetal hydrops, and a solid or cystic mass in the fetal thorax. Fetal surgery may be attempted.

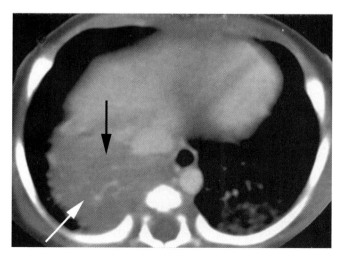

FIG. 1-9. Type II congenital cystic adenomatoid malformation. A solid mass *(arrows)* is visible in the right lower lobe, containing an opacified vessel. Type II may present as an air-filled or fluid-filled mass.

In infancy, CCAMs present as a space-occupying lesion. Symptoms of respiratory distress are common. In neonates, CCAMs usually present as a solid mass regardless of its type. Types I and II may become air filled over a period of days to weeks. They are often associated with progressive air trapping and mediastinal shift to the opposite side.

The treatment of choice is excision of the affected lobe. The prognosis of neonates with CCAMs is adversely affected by large CCAM size, underdevelopment of uninvolved lung (i.e., the presence of associated lung hypoplasia), and the presence of associated fetal hydrops or other congenital anomalies.

In adults, CCAMs usually present as an air-filled or air- and fluid-filled cystic or multicystic mass. Most adults present with recurrent pneumonia, although recurrent pneumothorax has also been associated. Occasionally, bronchioloalveolar carcinoma may arise in relation to a CCAM.

PULMONARY ARTERIOVENOUS MALFORMATION

Congenital arteriovenous malformations (AVMs), also known as arteriovenous fistula, likely result from deficient formation or abnormal dilation of pulmonary capillaries due to a developmental defect in the capillary wall. From 35% to 67% of cases are associated with Osler-Weber-Rendu syndrome (*hereditary hemorrhagic telangiectasia*), in which AVMs are found in the skin, mucous membranes, and viscera (Table 1-6). Also, AVMs may rarely occur in patients with hepatopulmonary syndrome or as a result of trauma.

Pulmonary arteriovenous fistulas slowly enlarge over time and are usually first diagnosed in adulthood. More than two thirds of AVMs are found in the lower lobes, and they are typically subpleural in location. Fistulas are multiple in 35% of patients and bilateral in 10%.

TABLE 1-6. PULMONARY ARTERIOVENOUS MALFORMATION (AVM)

35%–67% associated with Osler-Weber-Rendu syndrome
Multiple in 35%
Bilateral in 10%
Single AVM less often symptomatic than multiple AVMs (35% vs. 60%)
Symptoms: cyanosis, dyspnea, hemoptysis
Complications: rupture, paradoxical embolization
Simple AVM: 1 feeding artery and 1 draining vein
Complex AVM: multiple supplying vessels
Most common in lower lobes, subpleural
Diagnosis by morphology at CT
Treatment by embolization

Simple and Complex Arteriovenous Malformations

A *simple AVM* is a single, dilated vascular sac connecting one artery and one vein (Figs. 1-10 and 1-11). It is most frequent and accounts for the bulk of cases of AVM. *Complex AVMs,* which have more than one feeding artery, are rare.

Radiographically, a simple fistula appears as a peripheral, well-defined round, oval, lobulated, or serpentine density. Large vessels (feeders) extending centrally toward the hilum are usually visible (see Figs. 1-11C, 1-12, and 1-13). Enlargement of fistulas over a period of months or years is common and rapid increase in size can occur.

At CT, a simple AVM is visible as a smooth, sharply defined, round or elliptical nodule, almost always in a subpleural location (see Figs. 1-12 and 1-13). Arteriovenous fistulas characterized by a tangle of tortuous, dilated vessels are seen as lobulated, serpiginous masses and can often be suspected as being vascular simply by their morphology. In both instances, the feeding pulmonary artery branch and draining pulmonary vein are dilated, and with fistulas of significant size (larger than 1 to 2 cm), the feeders are easily recognizable. In general, the feeders are about half the diameter of the fistula.

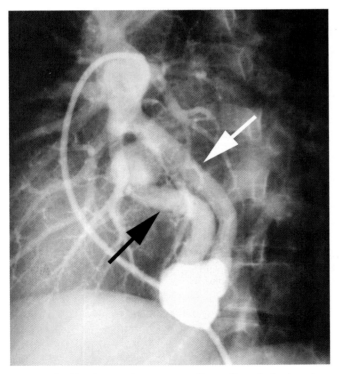

FIG. 1-10. Simple arteriovenous malformation. A single artery *(white arrow)* supplies a simple malformation drained by a single vein *(black arrow).* As is typical, the fistula is subpleural in location.

Spiral CT without contrast infusion is highly accurate in demonstrating AVMs and their architecture (see Figs. 1-11C, 1-12, and 1-13). In most cases, morphologic findings are sufficient for diagnosis of AVM (see Figs. 1-12B and E), but contrast infusion may be used for confirmation (see Fig. 1-12C). Following the bolus injection of contrast, pulmonary AVMs show rapid contrast opacification and washout, occurring in phase with opacification and washout of the main pulmonary artery and the right ventricle.

In general, AVMs appearing less than 2 cm in diameter on chest radiographs are asymptomatic. Single fistulas are less commonly symptomatic (35%) or associated with positive physical findings (70%) than are multiple fistulas (60% and 85%, respectively). An AVM results in a right to left shunt, and cyanosis is common, depending on the size of the shunt. The most frequent symptoms occurring in patients with AVMs are dyspnea, palpitation, hemoptysis, and chest pain. Cerebrovascular accidents (see Fig. 1-12H) associated with polycythemia or paradoxical embolization through the AVM from systemic veins are serious and potentially fatal complications. Rupture can result in pulmonary hemorrhage (Fig. 1-14) or hemothorax (Fig. 1-15). Without treatment, approximately 25% of patients with AVMs experience worsening of symptoms, and 50% of these will eventually die as a result of complications.

Pulmonary arteriography is advisable if embolization or surgical excision of the fistula is planned (see Fig. 1-12F and G). Transcatheter occlusion of fistulas using wire coils is the treatment of choice for simple AVMs. Recanalization of an AVF may occasionally occur after coil embolization. Complex AVMs (Fig. 1-16) are more often symptomatic that simple fistulas, because of a larger shunt. They are more difficult to treat because many feeders may be present, but wire coil embolization may be successful.

Pulmonary Telangiectasia

Pulmonary telangiectasia is an uncommon form of AVM characterized by innumerable very small fistulas scattered throughout both lungs. Symptoms are common and progressive, and cyanosis is present in all patients. Unlike simple AVMs, pulmonary telangiectasia is typically discovered by 10 years of age. Radiographs can be normal. If abnormal, radiographic findings are often limited to an abnormal pattern of pulmonary vessels, including (1) a coarse spidery appearance of pulmonary vessels, (2) vascular tortuosity, and (3) areas of hypervascularity. On angiograms, beaded or tortuous vessels, small aneurysmal sacs, or multiple ill-defined areas of vascular blush are visible. Treatment of this condition is difficult and prognosis is poor. Surgery is not possible because of the multiplicity of lesions.

(Text continues on page 15)

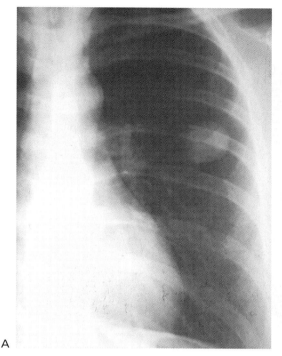

A

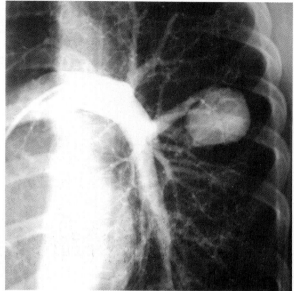

B

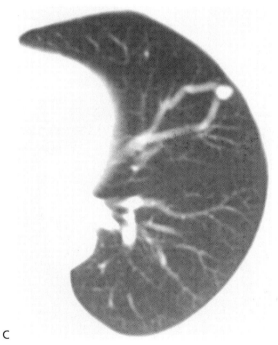

C

FIG. 1-11. Simple arteriovenous malformation (AVM). **A.** A well-defined, smooth, round, 3-cm nodule is visible on chest radiograph. **B.** Pulmonary arteriogram shows a simple AVM. The feeding artery is opacified. **C.** Simple AVM shown on CT in a different patient. A subpleural AVM is supplied a large artery and vein branch. The feeders are about half the diameter of the fistula.

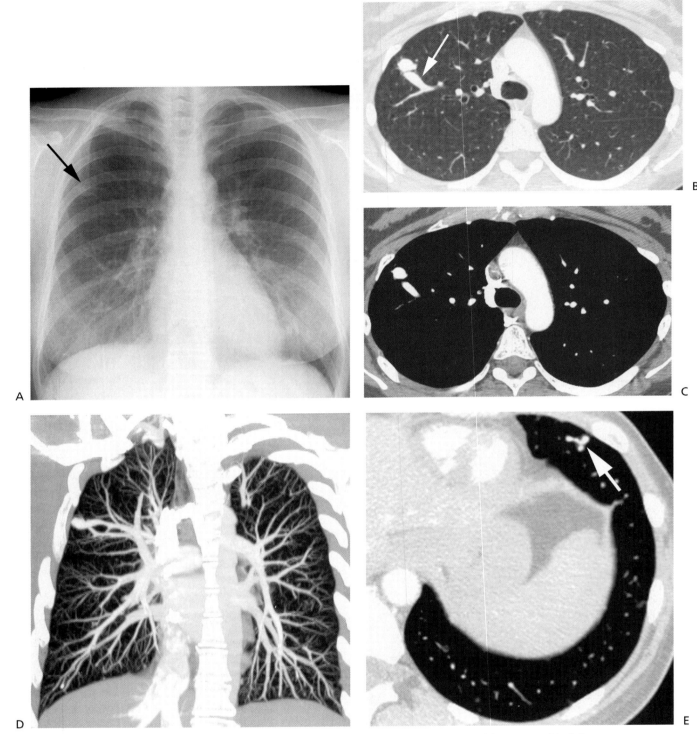

FIG. 1-12. Multiple arteriovenous malformations (AVMs) in a 30-year-old woman with Osler-Weber-Rendu syndrome. **A.** Chest radiograph shows a nodule in the right upper lobe *(arrow)*. **B.** Spiral CT with 1.25-mm detectors shows a well-defined subpleural nodule with a feeding vessel *(arrow)*, representing a vein. This appearance is typical of AVMs. **C.** With contrast injection, dense opacification of the fistula and feeding vein is seen. **D.** Coronal reconstruction shows the subpleural fistula and feeding artery and draining vein. **E.** Multiple other fistulas were visible. A small fistula *(arrow)* in the lower lobe may be diagnosed based on its morphology. *(Figure continues.)*

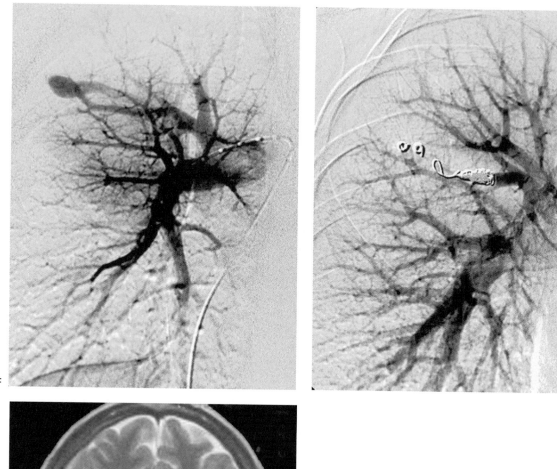

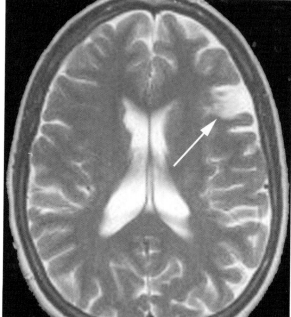

FIG. 1-12. *(Continued.)* **F.** Arteriogram performed at the time of embolization shows the fistula in **C** to **G**. The fistula shown in **F** has been occluded by wire coils. **H.** T2-weighted MRI of the brain shows findings of infarction. This is a common complication of AVMs.

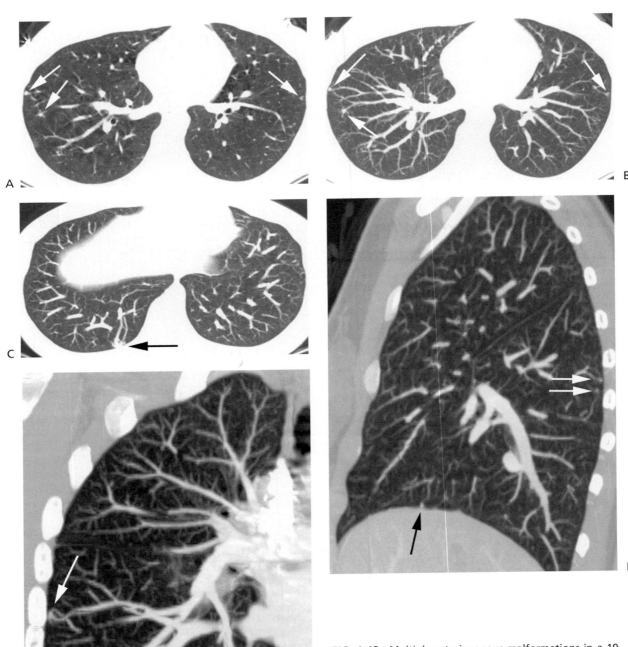

FIG. 1-13. Multiple arteriovenous malformations in a 19-year-old woman with Osler-Weber-Rendu syndrome. **A.** Multidetector spiral HRCT obtained with 1.25-mm detectors shows three small subpleural nodules *(arrows)*. **B.** A maximum intensity projection image (MIP) of a stack of HRCT images at the same level shows a small arteriovenous malformation *(arrows)* with feeding vessels. **C–E.** Transaxial (**C**), coronal (**D**), and sagittal (**E**) MIP reconstruction images show other subpleural fistulas *(arrows)*.

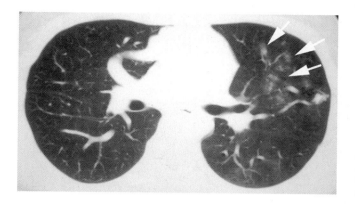

FIG. 1-14. Osler-Weber-Rendu syndrome with multiple arteriovenous malformations shown on CT and pulmonary hemorrhage. Patchy areas of ground-glass opacity *(arrows)* in the left lung represent blood due to rupture of an arteriovenous malformation.

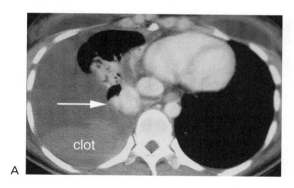

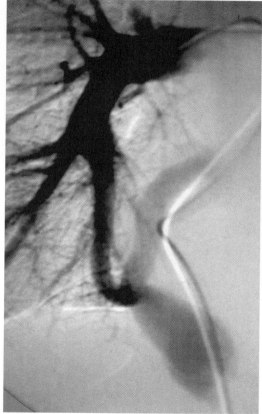

FIG. 1-15. Arteriovenous malformation (AVM) and hemothorax in a young woman with acute chest pain and shortness of breath. **A.** CT shows a right pleural effusion with a region of high attenuation indicating clot. A rounded lesion opacified by contrast is visible in the lung periphery *(arrow)*. This appearance suggests AVM. **B.** Arteriogram shows a simple AVM in the lung periphery. Wire-coil embolization was performed, with resolution of the symptoms.

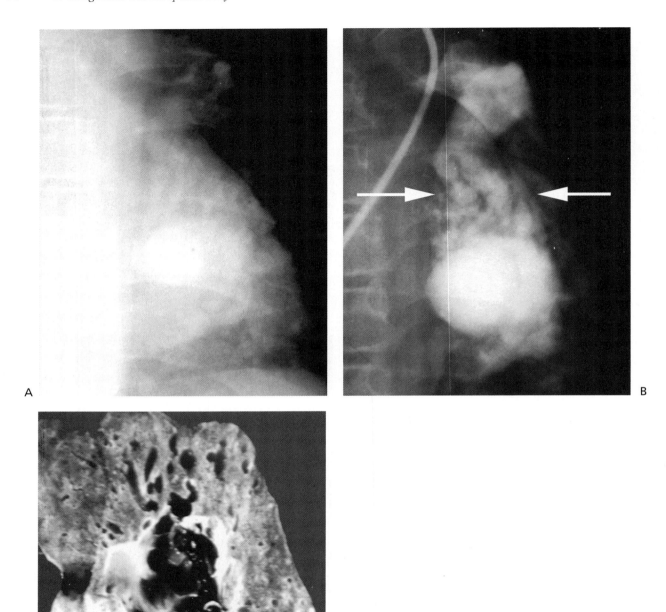

FIG. 1-16. Complex arteriovenous malformation in a patient with cyanosis. **A.** An ill-defined opacity is visible in the retrocardiac left lower lobe. **B.** Arteriogram shows a malformation with multiple feeding arteries *(arrows)*. **C.** The pathologic specimen following lower lobectomy shows the fistula and its complex arterial supply.

PULMONARY AGENESIS, APLASIA, AND HYPOPLASIA

Agenesis and Aplasia

Pulmonary agenesis and aplasia are nearly the same, and a distinction is not usually necessary. *Pulmonary agenesis* represents complete absence of a lung, its bronchi, and its vascular supply. *Pulmonary aplasia* is characterized by complete absence of a lung and its vascular supply, but a rudimentary bronchus is present (Fig. 1-17), ending in a blind pouch (Table 1-7). Either side may be affected. Associated congenital anomalies are often present.

Radiographically, pulmonary agenesis and aplasia result in opacification of a hemithorax and marked mediastinal shift (see Fig. 1-17). The heart is displaced into the posterior hemithorax on the side of agenesis or aplasia, along with other mediastinal structures. On lateral radiographs, the anterior chest appears abnormally lucent because of herniation of the remaining lung into the opposite hemithorax. CT demonstrates absence of the lung and pulmonary artery with marked mediastinal shift. In patients with agenesis, bronchi are also absent.

Hypoplasia

Pulmonary hypoplasia represents abnormal lung development associated with a reduction in lung volume and often

TABLE 1-7. PULMONARY AGENESIS, APLASIA, AND HYPOPLASIA

Agenesis: absence of a lung and its bronchi and vascular supply
Aplasia: absence of a lung and its vascular supply; rudimentary bronchus is present
  Occurs on either side
  Mediastinal herniation into affected hemithorax
  Congenital anomalies associated
  Poor prognosis
Hypoplasia
  Abnormal lung development
  Decreased alveoli and bronchial divisions
  Deficient lobes or segments may be present
  Causes:
    Hypogenetic lung syndrome
    Proximal interruption of pulmonary artery
    Lung compression during development

a decrease in the number of alveoli and bronchial divisions (see Table 1-7). There may also be anomalous lobes or segments, or they may be reduced in number. Hypoplasia is associated with other anomalies in *hypogenetic lung (scimitar) syndrome*. It may also result from abnormal lung development due to deficient vascular supply (e.g., *proximal interruption of the pulmonary artery*) or lung compression during gestation (e.g., congenital diaphragmatic hernia [Fig. 1-18],

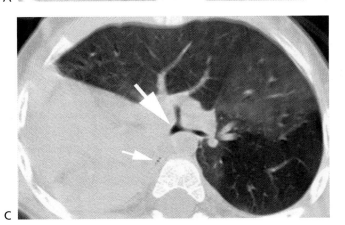

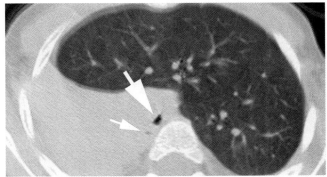

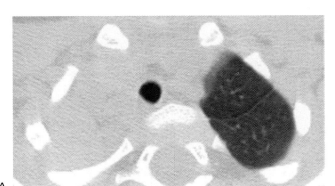

FIG. 1-17. Pulmonary aplasia in a child. **A.** CT through the upper chest shows opacification of the right hemithorax and shift of the trachea to the right side. **B.** Just distal to the tracheal carina, the left main bronchus *(large arrow)* and a small right-sided bronchus *(small arrow)* are visible. There is marked shift of the mediastinum to the right, with left lung herniating across the midline. **C.** At a lower level, the bronchi to the left lung *(large arrow)* and the small right-sided bronchus *(small arrow)* are both visible. The heart is displaced into the posterior right hemithorax.

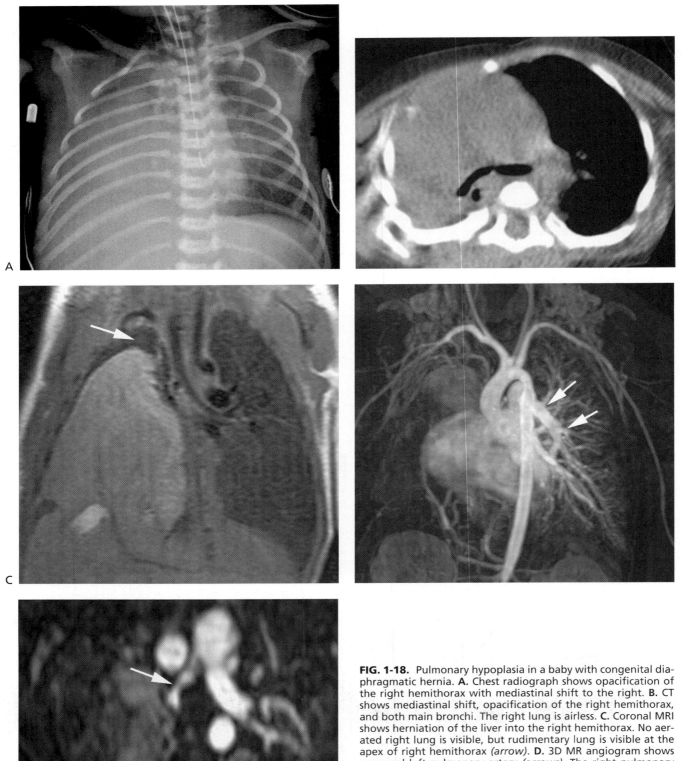

FIG. 1-18. Pulmonary hypoplasia in a baby with congenital dia-phragmatic hernia. **A.** Chest radiograph shows opacification of the right hemithorax with mediastinal shift to the right. **B.** CT shows mediastinal shift, opacification of the right hemithorax, and both main bronchi. The right lung is airless. **C.** Coronal MRI shows herniation of the liver into the right hemithorax. No aer-ated right lung is visible, but rudimentary lung is visible at the apex of right hemithorax *(arrow)*. **D.** 3D MR angiogram shows a normal left pulmonary artery *(arrows)*. The right pulmonary artery is not clearly seen. **E.** Transaxial MR shows a small right pulmonary artery.

space-occupying lesions, cystic adenomatoid malformation, sequestration, thoracic deformity, or oligohydramnios). The pulmonary artery supplying the lung is reduced in size or absent (see Fig. 1-18E), and the size of pulmonary vessels is reduced on the affected side. Mediastinal shift toward the hypoplastic lung occurs with hypogenetic lung syndrome and proximal interruption of the pulmonary artery. Mediastinal shift may or may not be present when hypoplasia results from an ipsilateral space-occupying lesion.

Pulmonary agenesis and aplasia are usually associated with a poor prognosis, with few patients surviving to adulthood. In patients with lung hypoplasia, the prognosis depends on the degree of abnormality and associated anomalies.

HYPOGENETIC LUNG (SCIMITAR) SYNDROME

A rare anomaly, almost always occurring on the right side, hypogenetic lung syndrome is characterized by (1) hypoplasia of the lung with abnormal segmental or lobar anatomy, (2) hypoplasia of the ipsilateral pulmonary artery, (3) anomalous pulmonary venous return to the inferior vena cava (or right atrium, hepatic veins, etc.), and (4) anomalous systemic arterial supply to a portion of the hypoplastic lung, usually the lower lobe (Table 1-8). Although these four features often coexist, hypogenetic lung syndrome shows considerable variation in the degree to which each feature is expressed. Patients may exhibit some features of this syndrome but not others.

This syndrome is usually diagnosed in patients less than

TABLE 1-8. HYPOGENETIC LUNG (SCIMITAR) SYNDROME

Four features typical (although each not always present):
 Hypoplasia of the lung with abnormal segmental or lobar anatomy
 Hypoplasia of the ipsilateral pulmonary artery
 Anomalous pulmonary venous return (scimitar vein)
 Anomalous systemic arterial supply to lower lobe
Almost always on the right side
Mediastinal shift toward the hypoplastic lung
Reduced size of ispilateral pulmonary artery
Anomalous (scimitar) vein usually paralleling right heart border
Congenital heart disease in 25% (atrial septal defect, patent ductus arteriosus)
Symptoms: recurrent infection, dyspnea

30 years of age, and more than half have symptoms. Recurrent respiratory infections and dyspnea on exertion are most common. Congenital heart lesions, most commonly septal defects and patent ductus arteriosus, are associated in 25%. Surgical treatment involves implantation of the anomalous vein into the left atrium.

Radiographically, the appearance of scimitar syndrome is often characteristic (Fig. 1-19). The hypoplastic lung is recognizable because of dextroposition of the heart, mediastinal shift to the right side, and right diaphragmatic elevation. CT may show abnormal bronchial anatomy on the side of the hypoplastic lung.

Hypoplasia of the pulmonary artery is usually recognizable by the decreased size of vessels within the hypoplastic lung (see Fig. 1-19A). Because most of the pulmonary blood

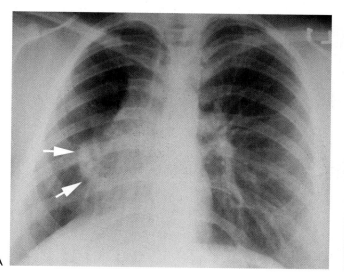
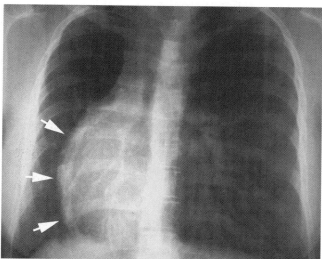

A B

FIG. 1-19. Scimitar syndrome in two different patients. Plain radiographs usually show displacement of the mediastinum toward the right side, reduction in size of pulmonary artery branches in the right lung (best shown in **A**), and the anomalous pulmonary vein paralleling the right heart border *(arrows)*.

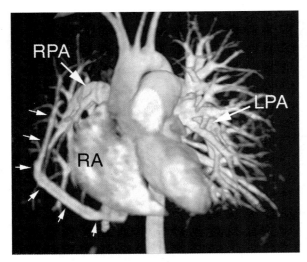

FIG. 1-20. 3D MR angiogram in scimitar syndrome. The right pulmonary artery *(RPA)* is smaller than the left *(LPA)*. The scimitar vein *(small arrows)* parallels the border of the right atrium *(RA)* and drains into the inferior vena cava.

TABLE 1-9. PROXIMAL INTERRUPTION OF THE PULMONARY ARTERY

Congenital absence of a main pulmonary artery
Almost always on the side opposite the aortic arch (i.e., usually the right)
Hypoplastic ipsilateral lung
Reduced size of ipsilateral pulmonary vessels
Lung vascular supply derived from bronchial arteries
Mediastinal shift toward the hypoplastic lung
Congenital heart disease common (tetralogy of Fallot, septal defects)

flow must traverse the normal artery on the side opposite the hypoplastic lung, the opposite pulmonary artery appears enlarged, further increasing the contrast between the right and left vasculature.

When the anomalous vein is visible radiographically, it appears as a broad arcuate band at the right lung base, paralleling the right heart border and extending to the diaphragmatic surface (see Figs. 1-19 to 1-21). This venous shadow often resembles a scimitar (see Figs 1-20 and 1-21D), hence the nickname of this syndrome. In nearly two thirds of patients, the scimitar vein drains the entire right lung. On CT, the scimitar vein is located in close relation to the major fissure. Left-sided scimitar syndrome, with the anomalous vein entering the coronary sinus, is rarely seen.

Systemic arteries, usually multiple and usually arising below the diaphragm, typically supply the lower lobe. These may be visible using CT (see Fig. 1-21C and E).

In some patients, findings of the scimitar syndrome may be associated with "horseshoe lung." Horseshoe lung is a rare congenital malformation in which an isthmus of pulmonary parenchyma extends from the right lung base across the midline behind the pericardium and fuses with the base of the left lung. Horseshoe lung may occur in the absence of scimitar syndrome.

PROXIMAL INTERRUPTION OF THE PULMONARY ARTERY

This anomaly can closely resemble hypogenetic lung syndrome. In proximal interruption of the pulmonary artery, the proximal portion of a main pulmonary artery, usually the right, fails to develop (Table 1-9). The ipsilateral lung is hypoplastic because of deficient growth but has a normal number of lobes and segments, and bronchial anatomy is normal. Vessels within the lung appear small (Fig. 1-22), whereas those on the opposite side are much larger. The

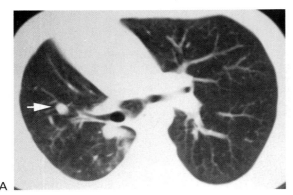
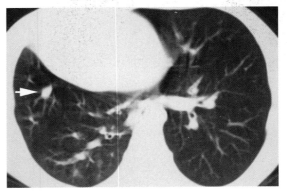

FIG. 1-21. CT in scimitar syndrome. **A–C.** Lung window scans show typical CT findings of scimitar syndrome, with hypoplasia of the right lung, evidenced by mediastinal shift to the right, relatively small arteries in the right lung, and the scimitar vein *(white arrows)*, seen in cross section. The scimitar vein drains into the inferior vena cava *(IVC)*. *(Figure continues.)*

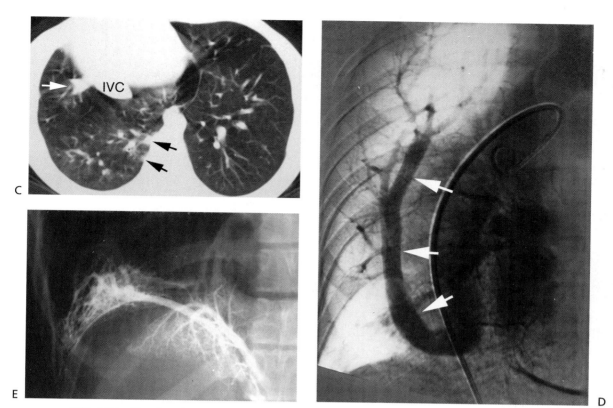

FIG. 1-21. *(Continued.)* Small vessels seen posteriorly *(black arrows* in **C**) are systemic arteries supplying the lung base. **D.** Right pulmonary arteriogram shows opacification of the scimitar vein *(arrows)*. **E.** Arteriogram shows anomalous systemic arteries supplying the right lung base.

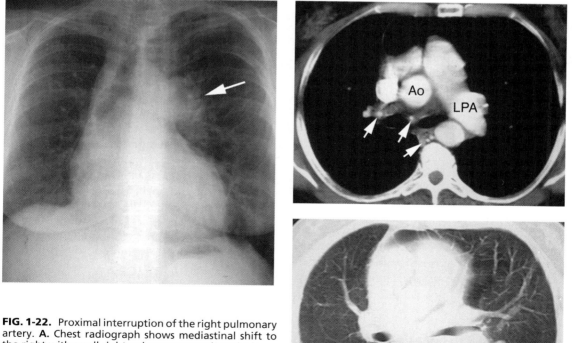

FIG. 1-22. Proximal interruption of the right pulmonary artery. **A.** Chest radiograph shows mediastinal shift to the right with small right pulmonary vessels and a large left pulmonary artery *(arrow)*. **B.** Contrast-enhanced CT shows the ascending aorta *(Ao)* and a large left pulmonary artery *(LPA)*, but the right pulmonary artery is absent. Large bronchial arteries *(arrows)* supply the right lung. **C.** Lung window scan shows hypoplasia of the right lung and small right lung vessels.

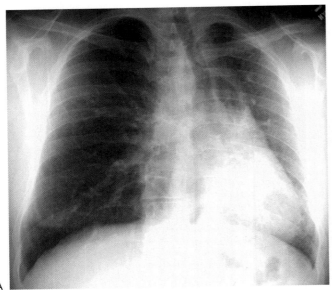
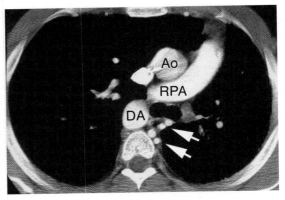

FIG. 1-23. Proximal interruption of the left pulmonary artery in a patient with right aortic arch. **A.** Chest radiograph shows mediastinal shift to the left. **B.** Contrast-enhanced CT shows the ascending aorta *(Ao)*, a right-sided descending aorta *(DA)*, and a large right pulmonary artery *(RPA)*, but the left pulmonary artery is absent. Large bronchial arteries *(arrows)* supply the hypoplastic left lung.

lung vascular supply is derived from hypertrophied bronchial arteries (see Fig. 1-22B). This entity is often associated with congenital heart disease, most typically tetralogy of Fallot and septal defects. This anomaly usually occurs on the side opposite the aortic arch (Fig. 1-23). When the interrupted pulmonary artery and aorta are ipsilateral, the incidence of congenital heart disease is higher than when they are not.

UNILATERAL PULMONARY VEIN ATRESIA

In unilateral pulmonary vein atresia, another rare entity, long segments of the pulmonary veins of one lung are congenitally atretic (Table 1-10). The involved lung can be normal in size or hypoplastic, and it often shows increased interstitial densities because of venous stasis, edema, and fibrosis. The ipsilateral pulmonary artery may appear small. Radionuclide imaging shows decreased perfusion. Angiography shows decreased size of the ipsilateral pulmonary artery,

peripheral pruning, contrast stasis, and nonvisualization of the pulmonary veins. Symptoms include hemoptysis and infection.

PULMONARY VEIN VARIX

Dilation of a pulmonary vein branch (pulmonary vein varix) can be congenital or acquired (Table 1-11). One or more veins appear dilated or tortuous near the point they enter the left atrium. With congenital varices, symptoms are usually absent, although rupture rarely occurs.

Acquired varies are associated with chronically elevated left atrial pressure, as in mitral stenosis. These most commonly involve the right inferior pulmonary vein. On plain radiographs, these are visible through the right part of the heart shadow and often appear rounded and sharply defined. They may mimic the appearance of a lung nodule, leading to further evaluation. CT is diagnostic.

TABLE 1-10. PULMONARY VEIN ATRESIA

Pulmonary veins of one lung atretic
Lung hypoplastic or normal in volume
Reduced size of ispilateral pulmonary artery
Increased interstitial opacity in lung

TABLE 1-11. PULMONARY VEIN VARIX

Congenital
Usually asymptomatic
Acquired
Associated with elevated left atrial pressure (e.g., mitral stenosis)
Usually on the right
Mimics a lung nodule

TABLE 1-12. ANOMALOUS PULMONARY VENOUS DRAINAGE

Pulmonary vein drainage into the right atrium, coronary sinus, or systemic vein
Left-to-right shunt
Partial: 0.5%, usually asymptomatic

ANOMALOUS PULMONARY VEIN DRAINAGE

Anomalous pulmonary vein drainage involves drainage of a pulmonary vein branch into the right atrium, coronary sinus, or systemic vein, producing a left-to-right shunt (Table 1-12).

Partial anomalous pulmonary venous drainage is present in about 0.5% of the population and is usually asymptomatic. The anomalous vein may drain into various vascular structures. On the right, the most common are the superior vena cava (Fig. 1-24), azygos vein, inferior vena cava, and right atrium. On the left, drainage may be through the left brachiocephalic vein, persistent left superior vena cava (vertical vein; Fig. 1-25), or coronary sinus. Drainage may also be below the diaphragm.

Total anomalous pulmonary venous drainage must be associated with a septal defect and is best considered to be a type of congenital heart disease.

BRONCHOPULMONARY SEQUESTRATION

Bronchopulmonary sequestration is a congenital malformation resulting from abnormal budding of the foregut and its associated structures during the period that lung, bronchi, and pulmonary vessels are developing. Pathologically, sequestration represents an area of disorganized pulmonary parenchyma without normal pulmonary arterial or bronchial communications (i.e., it is sequestered from bronchi and pulmonary arteries). Sequestration usually receives its blood supply from branches of the thoracic or abdominal aorta, and aortography is usually necessary before surgical excision in order to visualize these arterial branches. Fatal hemorrhage can occur if these systemic arteries are accidentally cut during surgery. There are two forms of sequestration—intralobar and extralobar. Although they share some features, they differ significantly in several important clinical and radiographic characteristics.

Intralobar Sequestration

Intralobar sequestration is the more common of these two malformations. In this anomaly, sequestered lung lies within the visceral pleura of one of the lobes. It occurs most often on the left side, and approximately two thirds are found adjacent to the diaphragm in relation to the posterior basal segment of the left lower lobe (Table 1-13). In almost 75% of cases, the arterial supply of an intralobar sequestration is from the descending thoracic aorta; others receive supply from branches of the abdominal aorta or from intercostal arteries. These systemic arteries often enter the lung via the inferior pulmonary ligament. Usually venous drainage is by pulmonary veins, but drainage into the azygos or hemiazygos system is not uncommon.

Intralobar sequestration usually presents in adults or older children. Acute or recurrent infection is most common as a presenting complaint (Fig. 1-26). Hemoptysis may occur. The systemic arterial to pulmonary venous shunt produced by interlobar sequestration is usually small and clinically insignificant. However, cases resulting in congestive heart failure have been reported. Bilateral sequestrations

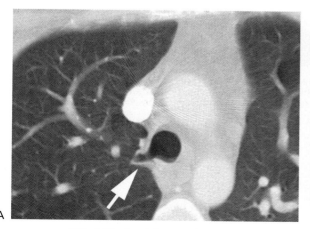 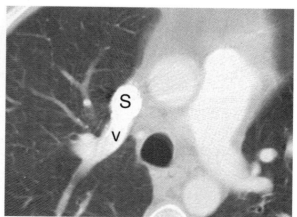

FIG. 1-24. Partial anomalous pulmonary vein drainage in a patient with a tracheal bronchus. **A.** The tracheal bronchus is visible arising from the right tracheal wall *(arrow).* **B.** At a lower level, a right superior pulmonary vein *(v)* branch enters the superior vena cava *(S).*

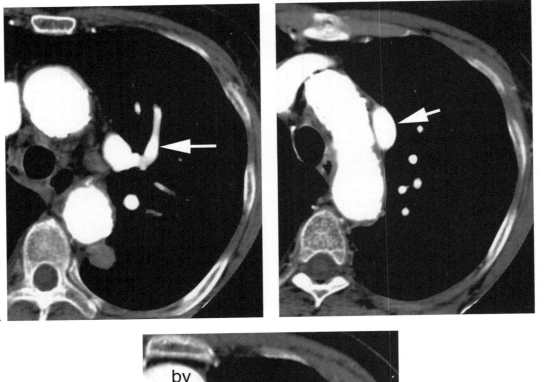

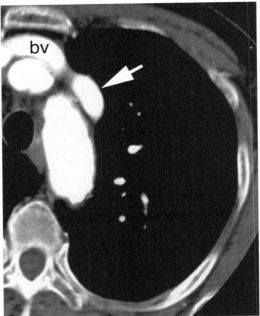

FIG. 1-25. Partial anomalous pulmonary vein drainage. **A.** A left pulmonary vein *(arrow)* enters a left superior vena cava (vertical vein). **B.** At a higher level, the left superior vena cava *(arrow)* is visible lateral to the aortic arch. **C.** The left superior vena cava *(arrow)* drains into the left brachiocephalic vein *(bv)*.

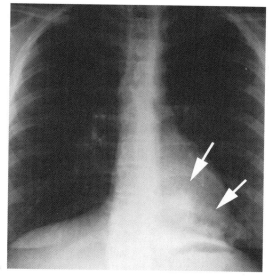

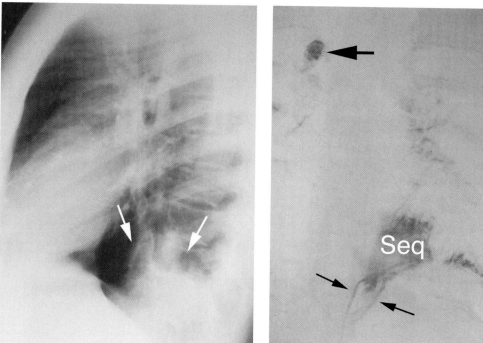

FIG. 1-26. Intralobar sequestration in a young woman with recurrent left lower lobe pneumonia. **A** and **B**. Patchy consolidation is visible in the left lower lobe *(arrows)*. **C**. Angiogram shows several branches *(small arrows)* of the descending aorta resulting in opacification of the sequestration *(Seq)*. Drainage is into the azygos vein *(large arrow)*.

TABLE 1-13. INTRALOBAR SEQUESTRATION

More common than extralobar sequestration
Within visceral pleural of lobe
65% at left base
No pulmonary artery or bronchial supply
Arterial supply from thoracic aorta in 75%
Drainage via pulmonary veins in most
Presentation in older children or adults
Recurrent infection
Imaging appearances:
    Homogeneous and well-defined mass lesion
    Cystic or multicystic air- and fluid-filled lesion
    Hyperlucent and hypovascular region of lung
    Combination of these

TABLE 1-14. EXTRALOBAR SEQUESTRATION

Within it own pleural envelope
90% at left base
No pulmonary artery or bronchial supply
Arterial supply from abdominal aorta in most
Drainage via systemic (e.g., azygos or hemiazygos) veins in
    most
Presentation in infancy in most
Presents as mass lesion; infection is rare
Imaging appearances:
    Homogeneous and well-defined mass lesion
    May contain fluid-filled cystic areas
    Rarely contains air

may occur. Connection to the esophagus is rarely seen. Association with other anomalies is uncommon.

Uncomplicated intralobar sequestration can have a variety of appearances. It may appear as (1) a homogeneous and well-defined mass lesion (Fig. 1-27), (2) a cystic or multicystic air and fluid-filled lesion, (3) a hyperlucent and hypovascular region of lung (Fig. 1-28), or (4) a combination of these. Hyperlucency is common in uncomplicated sequestration due to air trapping; this may be difficult to recognize on chest radiographs but is commonly seen at CT (see Fig. 1-28). The presence of mucous or fluid-filled cysts with air-fluid levels can be seen with or without infection. In such cases, a sequestration can closely mimic lung abscess. Rarely, bilateral sequestrations may be seen. These often are supplied by a single artery (Fig. 1-29).

On CT, bronchi or normal pulmonary arteries can be shown draped over the lesion (see Fig. 1-28) but do not enter a sequestration. With contrast-enhanced spiral CT, the supplying systemic arteries are often visible (see Figs. 1-27 and 1-28). If not, aortography can be used to confirm the diagnosis. The draining veins can also be identified following contrast infusion.

Extralobar Sequestration

Extralobar sequestration represents an anomaly in which the sequestered tissue is enclosed within its only pleural envelope; it is less common than intralobar sequestration. Approximately 90% of cases are visible at the left lung base, contiguous with the left hemidiaphragm (Table 1-14). Arterial supply is usually from the abdominal aorta and drainage is almost always by means of systemic veins (inferior vena cava, azygos, hemiazygos, or portal veins), producing a left-to-right shunt. Rarely, they may be located within the dia-

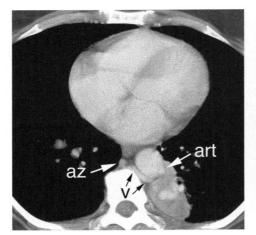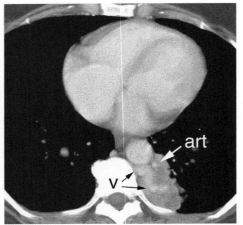

FIG. 1-27. Intralobar sequestration presenting as a mass. Contrast-enhanced CTs show a mass lesion posterior to the descending aorta. Large vessels are visible within the mass. An artery *(art)* can be seen arising from the aorta, supplying the sequestration. Venous drainage *(v)* is into the azygos vein *(az)*.

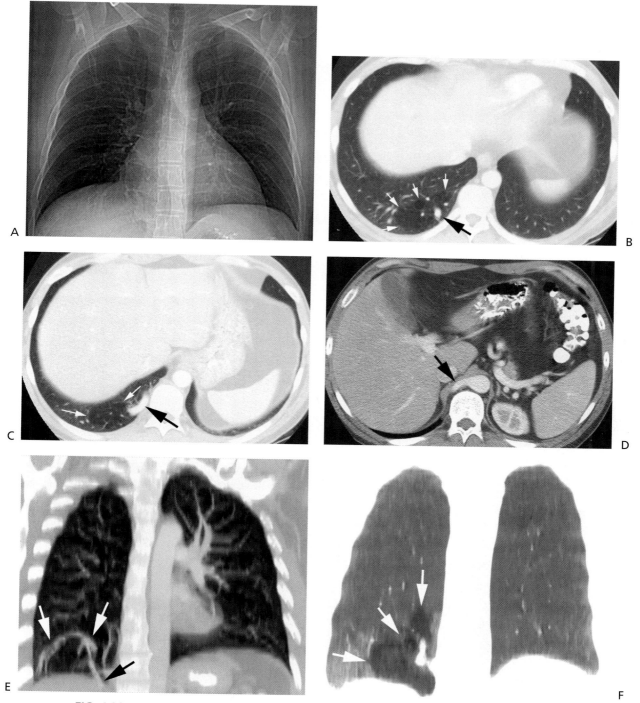

FIG. 1-28. Intralobar sequestration presenting as a hyperlucent lesion. **A.** Digital radiograph shows normal-appearing lungs. **B.** CT shows a lucent lesion *(white arrows)* at the right lung base. Pulmonary artery branches are draped over the surface of the lucency. A large, abnormal vessel *(black arrow)* is visible with the region of lucency, but fewer vessels are seen in the lesion than the surrounding lower lobe. **C.** At a lower level, the lucent lesion *(white arrows)* and abnormal vessel *(black arrow)* are visible. **D.** Contrast-enhanced scan at a lower level shows the abnormal vessel *(arrow)* arising from the descending aorta. **E.** Maximum intensity coronal reconstruction shows the abnormal aortic branch supplying the right lung base. **F.** Minimum intensity coronal reconstruction shows the hyperlucency intralobar sequestration *(arrows)* and its supplying vessel.

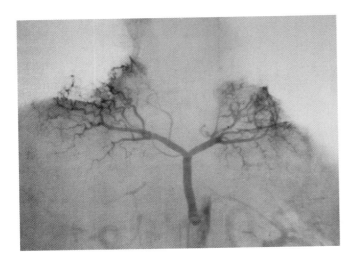

FIG. 1-29. Bilateral intralobar sequestrations supplied by a single anomalous branch of the descending aorta (subtracted arteriogram).

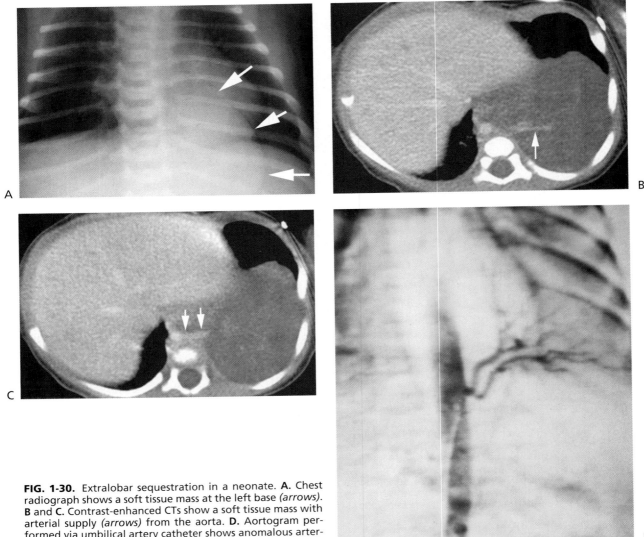

FIG. 1-30. Extralobar sequestration in a neonate. **A.** Chest radiograph shows a soft tissue mass at the left base *(arrows)*. **B** and **C.** Contrast-enhanced CTs show a soft tissue mass with arterial supply *(arrows)* from the aorta. **D.** Aortogram performed via umbilical artery catheter shows anomalous arteries supplying the left base.

TABLE 1-15. COMPARISON OF INTRALOBAR AND EXTRALOBAR SEQUESTRATION

	Intralobar sequestration	Extralobar sequestration
Patient age	Adult or older child	Infant or child
Symptoms	Infection common	Infection rare
Morphology	Within a lobe	Within its own pleural envelope
Location	65% at left base	90% at left base
Arterial supply	Thoracic or abdominal aorta	Usually abdominal aorta
Venous drainage	Usually pulmonary veins	Usually systemic veins
Appearance	Commonly contains air	Rarely contains air

phragm or immediately below the diaphragm in the upper abdomen.

Extralobar sequestration is often diagnosed in infancy (unlike intralobar sequestration) (Table 1-15). It is detected incidentally or presents as a mass lesion (Fig. 1-30). Unlike intralobar sequestration, infection is rare. Associated congenital anomalies, particularly diaphragmatic abnormalities and ipsilateral lung hypoplasia, are common. Because of its complete pleural envelope, extralobar sequestration rarely becomes infected.

Radiographically and on CT, extralobar sequestration appears as a sharply marginated mass lesion, which does not contain air (unlike intralobar sequestration) (see Figs. 1-30 and 1-31). It is usually homogeneous in appearance but may contain cystic areas. Its supplying artery may be seen on CT. If not, aortography may be need for diagnosis.

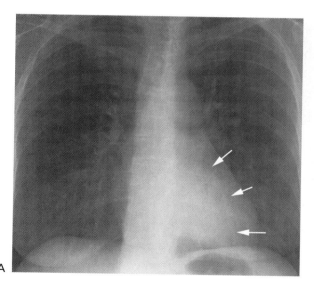

A

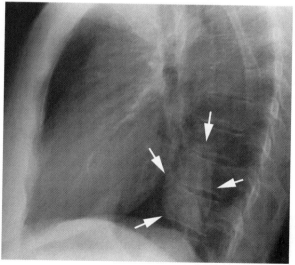

B

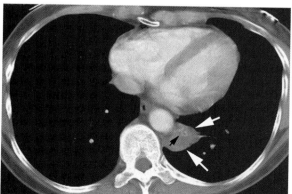

C

FIG. 1-31. Extralobar sequestration in an adult. PA (**A**) and lateral (**B**) chest radiographs show a mass *(arrows)* at the left base. **C.** Contrast-enhanced CT shows opacified vessels *(black arrow)* within the mass *(white arrows)*.

ANOMALOUS SYSTEMIC ARTERIES WITHOUT SEQUESTRATION (SYSTEMIC ARTERIAL MALFORMATION)

Systemic arteries may supply normal basal segments of lung (Table 1-16). Although these lesions can be thought of as representing systemic AVMs, they are unassociated with the large, dilated vascular sac typically seen with pulmonary

TABLE 1-16. SYSTEMIC ARTERY MALFORMATION

Arterial supply to lung from thoracic or abdominal aorta
Lung normal
Bronchi normal
Pulmonary artery normal or absent in affected region
Pulmonary vein drainage normal
Congestive heart failure or hemoptysis

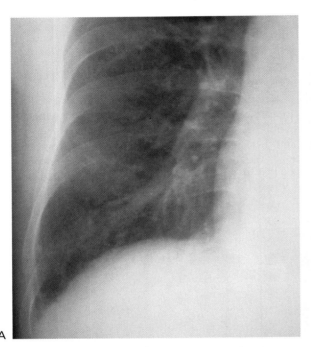

A

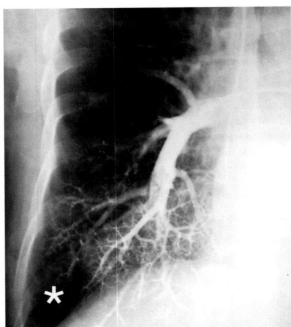

B

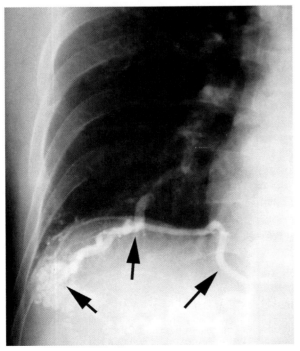

C

FIG. 1-32. Anomalous systemic arteries without sequestration in a patient with hemoptysis. **A.** Radiograph of the right lower lobe appears normal. **B.** Pulmonary arteriogram shows an area of lung (*) without pulmonary artery supply. **C.** An abnormal arterial branch *(arrows)* from the descending aorta supplies this region of lung.

AVMs. Rather, the arteriovenous communications in patients with systemic arterial malformations usually represent normal capillaries.

This lesion is probably best thought of as anomalous systemic arterial supply to an area of lung due to persistence of an embryonic aortic branch. The pulmonary parenchyma in the region supplied by the anomalous artery is normal, as are bronchial communications (Fig. 1-32). The pulmonary artery supply to these areas can be normal or absent.

A relationship may exist between systemic arterial malformations and pulmonary sequestration, and both these lesions represent different points on the spectrum of anomalies affecting the pulmonary artery, systemic arteries, and bronchial development. Some cases have been reported in which intralobar sequestration on one side coexists with systemic arterial malformation on the other. In such cases, both lesions are typically supplied by the same aortic branch.

Because systemic arterial malformation results in a left-to-left arterial shunt, left ventricular enlargement and congestive heart failure can occur. Hemoptysis may also occur. However, most patients have no symptoms. If the anomalous vessel supplies an area of lung also supplied by the pulmonary artery, treatment involves ligation or embolization of the anomalous vessel.

SELECTED READING

Dines DE, Arms RA, Bernatz PE, Gomes MR. Pulmonary arteriovenous fistulas. Mayo Clin Proc 1974; 49:460–465.

Do KH, Goo JM, Im JG, et al. Systemic arterial supply to the lungs in adults: spiral CT findings. Radiographics 2001; 21:387–402.

Fitch SJ, Tonkin ILD, Tonkin AK. Imaging of foregut cysts. Radiographics 1986; 6:189–201.

Ghaye B, Szapiro D, Fanchamps JM, Dondelinger RF. Congenital bronchial abnormalities revisited. Radiographics 2001; 21: 105–119.

Ikezoe J, Murayama S, Godwin JD, et al. Bronchopulmonary sequestration: CT assessment. Radiology 1990; 176:375–379.

Mata JM, Caceres J, Lucaya J, Garcia-Conesa JA. CT of congenital malformations of the lung. Radiographics 1990; 10:651–674.

McAdams HP, Kirejczyk WM, Rosado-de-Christenson ML, Matsumoto S. Bronchogenic cyst: imaging features with clinical and histopathologic correlation. Radiology 2000; 217:441–446.

Patz EF Jr, Müller NL, Swensen SJ, Dodd LG. Congenital cystic adenomatoid malformation in adults: CT findings. J Comput Assist Tomogr 1995; 19:361–364.

Rappaport DC, Herman SJ, Weisbrod GL. Congenital bronchopulmonary diseases in adults: CT findings. AJR Am J Roentgenol 1994; 162:1295–1299.

Remy J, Remy-Jardin M, Wattinne L, Deffontaines C. Pulmonary arteriovenous malformations: evaluation with CT of the chest before and after treatment. Radiology 1992; 182:809–816.

Roehm JOF, Jue KL, Amplatz K. Radiographic features of the scimitar syndrome. Radiology 1966; 86:856–859.

Rosado-de-Christenson ML, Stocker JT. Congenital cystic adenomatoid malformation. Radiographics 1991; 11:865–886.

Sener RN, Tugran C, Savas R, Alper H. CT findings in scimitar syndrome. AJR Am J Roentgenol 1993; 160:1361.

Shenoy SS, Culver GJ, Pirson HS. Agenesis of lung in an adult. AJR Am J Roentgenol 1979; 133:755–757.

Yamanaka A, Hirai T, Fujimoto T, et al. Anomalous systemic arterial supply to normal basal segments of the left lower lobe. Ann Thorac Surg 1999; 68:332–338.

2

CONSOLIDATION AND ATELECTASIS

W. RICHARD WEBB

Recognizing consolidation and atelectasis is fundamental to an understanding of pulmonary radiology.

AIR-SPACE CONSOLIDATION

Air-space consolidation represents replacement of alveolar air by fluid, blood, pus, cells, or other substances. *Alveolar consolidation* and *parenchymal consolidation* are synonyms for air-space consolidation.

Radiographic Findings

Radiographic and CT abnormalities indicating the presence of air-space consolidation include the following:

- Homogeneous opacity obscuring vessels
- Air bronchograms
- Ill-defined or fluffy opacities
- "Air alveolograms"
- Patchy opacities
- "Acinar" or air-space nodules
- Preserved lung volume
- Extension to pleural surface
- "CT angiogram" sign

Homogeneous Opacity Obscuring Vessels

With complete replacement of alveolar air, homogeneous opacification of lung results. Vessels within the consolidated lung are invisible (Fig. 2-1A).

Air Bronchograms

In patients with consolidation, air-filled bronchi are often visible on plain radiographs or CT, appearing lucent compared with opacified lung parenchyma (see Fig. 2-1). This is termed an *air bronchogram.*

With some causes of consolidation, air bronchograms may not be visible. This usually occurs because of central bronchial obstruction (e.g., by cancer or mucus) or filling of bronchi in association with the underlying pathologic process. For example, pulmonary infarction often results in consolidation without air bronchograms because of blood filling the bronchi. In patients with bronchopneumonia, bronchi may be filled with mucus or pus.

If air bronchograms are visible within an area of consolidation, bronchial obstruction is unlikely (but not ruled out) as its cause. Although air bronchograms are considered a classic sign of air-space consolidation, they may also be seen in the presence of confluent interstitial disease.

Ill-defined or Fluffy Opacities

Consolidation often results in opacities with ill-defined margins (Figs. 2-2 and 2-3), in contrast to the relatively sharp margins of a lung mass. This results from patchy local spread of disease with variable involvement of alveoli at the edges of the pathologic process.

Air Alveolograms

If lung consolidation is not confluent, small focal lucencies representing uninvolved lung may be visible (see Fig. 2-2). These have been termed "air alveolograms," but this is a misnomer as alveoli are too small to see radiographically. Nonetheless, these lucencies reflect incomplete lung consolidation.

Patchy Opacities

Variable consolidation of alveoli in different lung regions results in patchy areas of increased opacity (see Fig. 2-3). Pulmonary vessels may be obscured or poorly defined.

Patchy consolidation visible on chest radiographs sometimes appears to be lobular or multilobular on CT (i.e., involving individual pulmonary lobules; Fig. 2-4). Some lobules appear abnormally dense while adjacent lobules appear normally aerated.

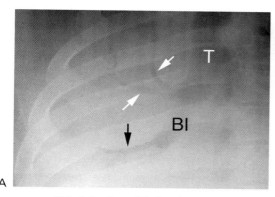

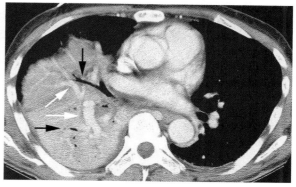

FIG. 2-1. Consolidation: homogeneous opacity obscuring vessels, air bronchograms, and the CT angiogram sign. **A.** Right lung consolidation due to retained secretions and atelectasis (i.e., drowned lung). Air bronchograms are visible within the consolidated lung. The trachea *(T)*, right upper lobe bronchi *(white arrows)*, bronchus intermedius *(BI)*, and right middle lobe bronchi *(black arrow)* are visible. **B.** Enhanced CT in a patient with right middle and lower lobe pneumonia shows homogeneous consolidation, preserved lung volume, air bronchograms *(black arrows)*, and opacified vessels *(white arrow)*, appearing denser than surrounding consolidated lung (i.e., the "CT angiogram" sign).

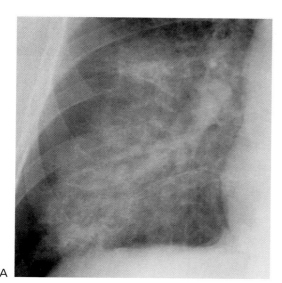

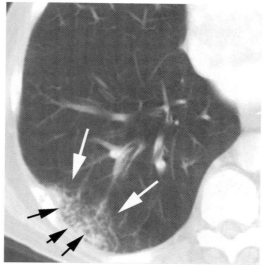

FIG. 2-2. Consolidation: ill-defined, fluffy opacities with "air alveolograms." **A.** Incomplete right lower lobe consolidation resulting in fluffy, ill-defined opacity containing small rounded lucencies. These lucencies have been termed air alveolograms, although they do not correspond to alveoli. **B.** Ill-defined fluffy consolidation *(white arrows)* is visible on CT in a patient with right lower lobe pneumonia. Small focal lucencies *(black arrows)* within the area of consolidation are "air alveolograms."

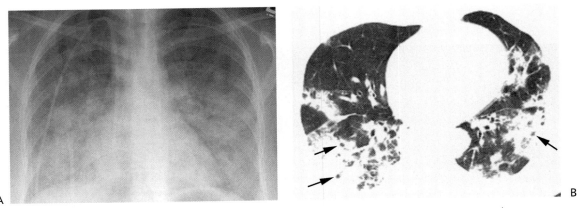

FIG. 2-3. Consolidation: patchy opacities. **A.** Chest radiograph in a patient with pulmonary edema due to renal failure shows patchy perihilar consolidation. **B.** Patchy areas of fluffy consolidation *(arrows)* are seen on CT. The fluffy margins are due to variable involvement of alveoli at the edges of the pathologic process.

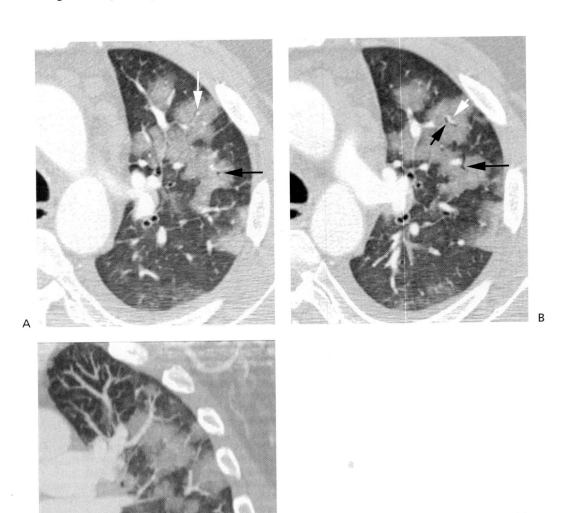

FIG. 2-4. Consolidation: patchy opacities with lobular consolidation. **A** and **B.** Contrast-enhanced HRCT in a patient with bronchopneumonia and lobular consolidation. Individual lobules are consolidated while others appear normal. Centrilobular arteries *(white arrow)* and bronchi *(black arrows)* are visible within consolidated lobules. **C.** Coronal reconstruction also shows the lobular distribution of the patchy lung opacities.

"Acinar" or Air-space Nodules

An acinus is the largest unit of lung structure in which all airways participate in gas exchange. Anatomically, it is located distal to a terminal bronchiole and is supplied by a first-order respiratory bronchiole. Acini average 7 to 8 mm in diameter.

The terms *acinar nodule* and *air-space nodule* are used to describe poorly marginated rounded opacities, usually 5 to 10 mm in diameter, that occur due to focal consolidation (Fig. 2-5). Although these nodules approximate the size of acini and look like they should be acinar, anatomically they tend to be centrilobular and peribronchiolar rather than acinar. These may be seen as the only finding of consolidation or may be seen in association with dense consolidation, usually at the edges of more abnormal lung.

These nodular opacities are more easily seen on high-resolution CT (HRCT) than on chest radiographs. On HRCT, their centrilobular location is usually visible. This appearance is described further in Chapter 10.

Preserved Lung Volume

In the presence of consolidation, because alveolar air is replaced by something else (e.g., fluid), the volume of affected lung tends to be preserved (see Fig. 2-1B). Although some volume loss may be seen in patients with consolidation, it is usually of a minor degree. Alternatively, in some patients with consolidation, the lobe is expanded.

Extension to Pleural Surfaces

Pathologic processes resulting in consolidation often spread from alveolus to alveolus until reaching a fissure or pleural surface (see Fig. 2-5B). The pleural surface prevents further

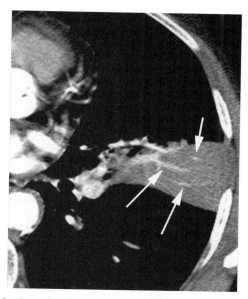

FIG. 2-6. Consolidation: the CT angiogram sign. Contrast-enhanced CT in a patient with pneumonia shows focal consolidation. Opacified arteries *(arrows)* appear denser than consolidated lung (i.e., the CT angiogram sign). The consolidation borders on the major fissure posteriorly and appears segmental.

spread. When extension to a pleural surface occurs, the process may appear lobar, as in lobar pneumonia.

CT Angiogram Sign

A unique finding seen on CT in patients with consolidation is the "CT angiogram" sign. This sign is present if normal-appearing opacified vessels are visible within the consolidated lung following the infusion of intravenous contrast (see Figs. 2-1B and 2-6). Although opacified vessels are

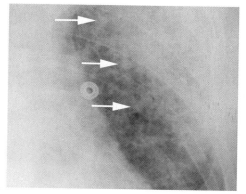
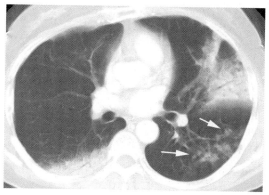

FIG. 2-5. Consolidation: acinar or air-space nodules. **A.** Chest radiograph shows a patchy left upper lobe pneumonia. Ill-defined nodular opacities less than 1 cm in diameter *(arrows)* are visible on the edge of the area of denser consolidation. These represent air-space or acinar nodules. **B.** CT (5-mm slice thickness) in a patient with bilateral consolidation. Air bronchograms are visible in the lingula and left lower lobe. Patchy consolidation with air-space nodules *(arrows)* is visible in the left lower lobe. These nodules are ill defined, 5 to 10 mm in diameter, and centrilobular in distribution. The lingular consolidation borders posteriorly on the major fissure.

sometimes seen within a lung mass, they usually appear compressed or distorted.

Differential Diagnosis

In general, the differential diagnosis of air-space consolidation may be considered in regard to the substance that is replacing alveolar air:

1. Water (e.g., types of pulmonary edema)
2. Blood (e.g., pulmonary hemorrhage)
3. Pus (e.g., pneumonia)
4. Cells (e.g., bronchioloalveolar carcinoma, lymphoma, eosinophilic pneumonia, bronchiolitis obliterans orga-

nizing pneumonia [BOOP], hypersensitivity pneumonitis, interstitial pneumonia)
5. Other substances (e.g., lipoprotein in alveolar proteinosis, lipid in lipoid pneumonia).

Patients with consolidation may be divided into two primary groups for the purposes of diagnosis: those with diffuse or bilateral consolidation and those with focal consolidation.

Diffuse Consolidation

Diffuse consolidation has a number of possible causes (Table 2-1), and the clinical history is often more important than the radiographic findings in making the diagnosis.

TABLE 2-1. DIFFERENTIAL DIAGNOSIS OF DIFFUSE CONSOLIDATION

Water (edema) (see Chapter 11)
Hydrostatic (cardiogenic) pulmonary edema
  Heart failure
  Left atrial or pulmonary venous obstruction
  Volume overload
  Low intravascular oncotic pressure
  Hypoalbuminemia
  Liver disease
  Renal failure
Increased permeability (noncardiogenic) pulmonary edema
  With diffuse alveolar damage (acute respiratory distress syndrome)
    Acute interstitial pneumonia
    Aspiration of gastric acid
    Drugs
    Fat embolism
    Infection and sepsis
    Near-drowning
    Pneumonia
    Radiation
    Shock
    Toxic fumes or gases
    Trauma
  Without diffuse alveolar damage
    Any cause of acute respiratory distress syndrome, in a mild form
    Drug reactions
    Hantavirus pulmonary syndrome
    Transfusion reaction
Mixed types of edema
  Air embolism
  High-altitude pulmonary edema
  Neurogenic pulmonary edema
  Posttransplantation edema
  Postpneumonectomy
  Reexpansion edema
  Reperfusion edema
  Tocolytic therapy
  Hydrostatic and permeability edema
Blood (hemorrhage) (see Chapter 19)
Aspiration of blood

Bleeding diathesis
  Anticoagulation
  Chemotherapy
  Leukemia
  Low platelets
Collagen-vascular disease and immune complex vasculitis
  Systemic lupus erythematosus most common
  Behçet's syndrome
  Henoch-Schönlein purpura
  Antiphospholipid syndrome
Goodpasture's syndrome
Idiopathic pulmonary hemosiderosis
Trauma
Vasculitis
  Wegener's granulomatosis
  Churg-Strauss granulomatosis
  Microscopic polyangiitis
Pus (pneumonia)
Bacterial bronchopneumonia (staphylococcal, gram-negative most common)
Pneumonia in an immunosuppressed patient
Tuberculosis
Fungal pneumonia (histoplasmosis, aspergillosis most common)
Atypical organisms
  Virus
  Pneumocystis
  Nontuberculous mycobacteria
Cells
Neoplasm
  Bronchioloalveolar carcinoma
  Lymphoma and other lymphoproliferative diseases
Eosinophilic pneumonia or other eosinophilic diseases
Bronchiolitis obliterans organizing pneumonia
Hypersensitivity pneumonitis
Idiopathic interstitial pneumonias
  Usual interstitial pneumonia
  Nonspecific interstitial pneumonia
  Desquamative interstitial pneumonia
Sarcoidosis
Other substances
Alveolar proteinosis (lipoprotein)
Lipoid pneumonia (lipid)

Pattern and Differential Diagnosis

The pattern or distribution of diffuse consolidation may be helpful in the differential diagnosis.

Perihilar "bat-wing" consolidation shows perihilar consolidation with sparing of the lung periphery (Figs. 2-7 and 2-8). It is most typical of pulmonary edema (hydrostatic or permeability). This pattern also may be seen with pulmonary hemorrhage, pneumonias (including bacteria and atypical pneumonias such as *Pneumocystis jiroveci (P. carinii)* pneumonia [PCP] and viral pneumonia), and inhalational lung injury. In patients with pulmonary edema, a perihilar distribution is most often present when rapid accumulation of fluid has occurred. Relative sparing of the lung periphery has been attributed to better lymphatic clearance of edema fluid in this region, although the exact mechanism is unclear and undoubtedly varies with the disease.

Peripheral subpleural consolidation is the opposite of a bat-wing pattern (i.e., a reverse bat-wing pattern). Consolidation is seen adjacent to the chest wall, with sparing of the perihilar regions. It is most often seen in patients with chronic diseases (also the reverse of what is true of a bat-wing pattern). It is classically seen with eosinophilic lung diseases, particularly eosinophilic pneumonia (Fig. 2-9A), but may occur with BOOP (see Fig. 2-9B), sarcoidosis, radiation pneumonitis, lung contusion, or bronchioloalveolar carcinoma. Peripheral consolidations need not always appear peripheral on the frontal (posteroanterior [PA] or

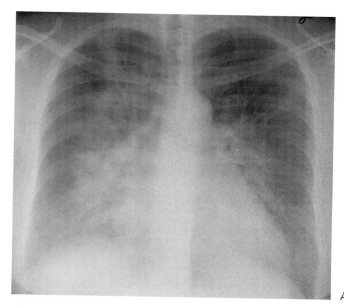

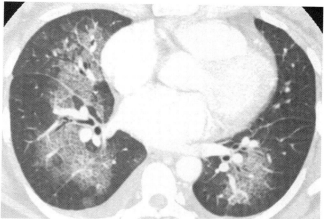

FIG. 2-8. Perihilar "bat-wing" consolidation in pulmonary edema. **A.** Chest radiograph shows a distinct perihilar predominance of consolidation. The heart is enlarged. **B.** CT shows sparing of the lung periphery.

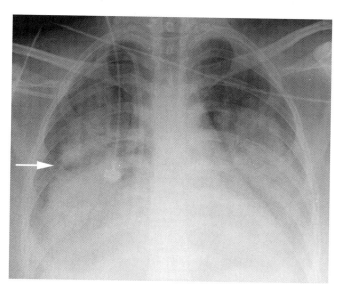

FIG. 2-7. Perihilar "bat-wing" consolidation in pulmonary edema. Chest radiograph in a patient with pulmonary edema due to renal failure (note the dialysis catheter in the right atrium) shows a distinct perihilar bat-wing pattern of consolidation. The lung periphery is spared. Note the lucency at the level of the minor fissure *(arrow)* because of sparing of peripheral lung adjacent to the fissure.

anteroposterior [AP]) radiograph; they may be peripheral in the anterior or posterior lung and overlie the parahilar regions.

Diffuse patchy consolidation (Fig. 2-10) may be seen with any pneumonia (bacterial, mycobacterial, fungal, viral, PCP); pulmonary edema (see Fig. 2-3A) (hydrostatic and permeability); acute respiratory distress syndrome (ARDS); pulmonary hemorrhage syndromes; aspiration; inhalational diseases; eosinophilic diseases; and diffuse bronchioloalveolar carcinoma. The patchy opacities may correspond to consolidation of lobules, subsegments, or segments.

Diffuse air-space nodules as a prominent feature of consolidation are typical of endobronchial spread of disease

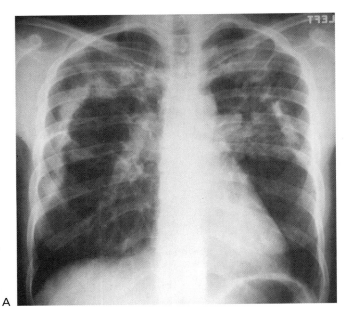

A

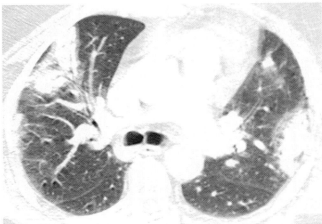

B

FIG. 2-9. Peripheral subpleural (reverse bat-wing) consolidation. **A.** Chest radiograph in a patient with chronic eosinophilic pneumonia shows areas of consolidation in the subpleural lung. The perihilar regions are spared. **B.** CT in a patient with BOOP shows patchy areas of consolidation in the subpleural lung.

(Fig. 2-11). They are seen in patients with endobronchial spread of infection such as tuberculosis (TB) or *Mycobacterium avium* complex (MAC), bacterial bronchopneumonia, viral pneumonia (cytomegalovirus [CMV], measles), endobronchial spread of bronchioloalveolar carcinoma, pulmonary hemorrhage, or sometimes aspiration.

Diffuse homogeneous consolidation is most typical in patients with pulmonary edema, ARDS, pulmonary hemorrhage, pneumonias (including viral and PCP), alveolar proteinosis, and extensive atelectasis.

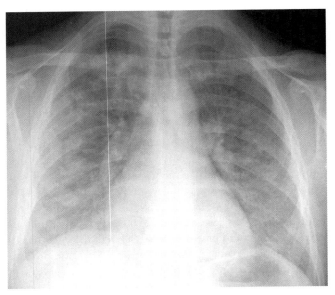

FIG. 2-10. Diffuse patchy consolidation in a patient with viral pneumonia.

Focal Consolidation

Although the differential diagnosis of abnormalities resulting in focal consolidation also includes water, blood, pus, cells, and other substances, the most likely causes of this pattern (Table 2-2) are different from those most likely to cause diffuse consolidation. Pneumonia, atelectasis with or without bronchial obstruction, and neoplasm are common causes of focal consolidation, while pulmonary edema and

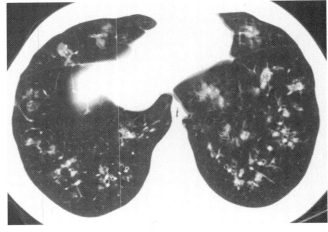

FIG. 2-11. Diffuse air-space nodules in bronchopneumonia. Multiple small nodular opacities are typical of spread of infection through the airways. This represented a bacterial bronchopneumonia, but other organisms such as TB, MAC, fungus, or viruses may be involved.

TABLE 2-2. DIFFERENTIAL DIAGNOSIS OF FOCAL CONSOLIDATION

Water (edema) (uncommon)
Papillary muscle rupture with mitral prolapse (right upper lobe)
Edema in a patient with:
   Pulmonary artery obstruction (e.g., pulmonary embolism)
   Hypoplastic pulmonary artery
   Swyer-James syndrome
Decubitus position
Reexpansion edema
Pulmonary vein occlusion
Systemic to pulmonary artery shunt (congenital or acquired)
Bland aspiration
Atelectasis with drowned lung
Blood (hemorrhage)
Contusion
Infarction
Aspiration of blood
Vasculitis
Pus (pneumonia)
Bacterial
Tuberculosis or nontuberculous mycobacterial
Fungal
Virus (uncommon)
Pneumocystis (uncommon)
Aspiration pneumonia
Atelectasis with postobstructive pneumonia
Cells
Neoplasm
   Bronchioloalveolar carcinoma
   Lymphoma and other lymphoproliferative diseases
Eosinophilic pneumonia or other eosinophilic diseases
Bronchiolitis obliterans organizing pneumonia
Sarcoidosis
Other substances
Lipoid pneumonia (lipid)

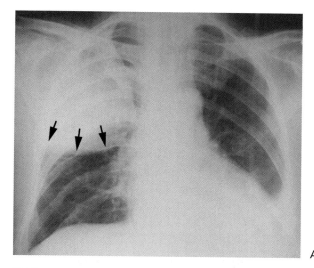

FIG. 2-12. Lobar consolidation with expansion. **A.** A patient with right upper lobe consolidation due to *Klebsiella* pneumonia shows downward bowing of the minor fissure *(arrows)* because of lobar expansion. **B.** Bronchioloalveolar carcinoma involving the left upper lobe with posterior bulging *(arrows)* of the left major fissure.

hemorrhage are much less likely than in patients with diffuse abnormalities.

Pattern and Differential Diagnosis

Focal consolidation involving a lobe or less may represent pneumonia (*Streptococcus pneumoniae, Klebsiella, Legionella,* TB, fungal pneumonias); postobstructive pneumonia; aspiration; bronchioloalveolar carcinoma; lymphoma or other lymphoproliferative disease; infarction; hemorrhage due to trauma, pulmonary embolism, or diseases such as Wegener's granulomatosis; pulmonary infarction; radiation pneumonitis; BOOP; eosinophilic pneumonia; atelectasis; or rarely focal edema. Focal consolidation may also occur because of confluent interstitial disease, as in patients with sarcoidosis. The appearance or pattern of focal or multifocal consolidation may be helpful in differential diagnosis.

Lobar consolidation is most typical of pneumonia (including *S. pneumoniae, Klebsiella* [Fig. 2-12A], *Legionella,*

and TB) and bronchial obstruction with postobstructive pneumonia or atelectasis. It may also be seen in patients with local spread of neoplasm, such as bronchioloalveolar carcinoma (see Fig. 2-12B) or lymphoma. It is uncommon with pulmonary embolism and pulmonary edema.

Lobar consolidation may occur by several mechanisms:

Bronchial obstruction. Postobstructive pneumonia or atelectasis occurring because of obstruction of a lobar bronchus is common.

Vascular abnormalities. Right upper lobe consolidation representing pulmonary edema may occur in patients with acute myocardial infarction resulting in papillary muscle rupture and mitral valve prolapse; it occurs because a jet of regurgitant blood is directed into the right superior pulmonary vein. Focal pulmonary hemorrhage may lead to a lobar consolidation. Lobar consolidation is uncommon with pulmonary embolism.

Interalveolar spread of disease. Some diseases produce lobar consolidation by progressively spreading from alveoli to adjacent alveoli via the *pores of Kohn* (small holes in alveolar walls). This type of spread continues until a fissure or pleural surface is reached.

Interalveolar spread is typical of lobar pneumonia. Organisms associated with spread of pneumonia via the pores of Kohn are characterized by thin secretions (thus passing easily through the pores). The presence of an incomplete fissure may lead to a lobar pneumonia becoming bilobar (or trilobar) (see Fig. 2-1B).

This type of spread may also be seen with lymphoma and local spread of bronchioloalveolar carcinoma. The term *lepidic growth* is used to describe the local interalveolar spread of a carcinoma, such as bronchioloalveolar carcinoma, using alveolar walls as a scaffold.

Consolidation of a specific lobe or lobes may be diagnosed by using the "silhouette" sign, described below, and by noting the relationship of consolidation to the interlobar fissures. Patterns of lobar consolidation are illustrated below.

Lobar expansion in association with lobar consolidation suggests infection, particularly by *Klebsiella* (see Fig. 2-12A)

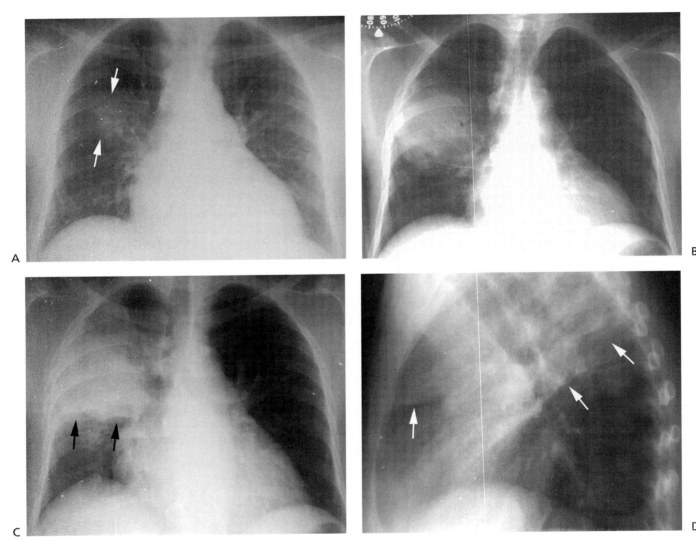

FIG. 2-13. Spherical consolidation due to pneumonia. **A.** On the initial radiograph, a patient with *Legionella* pneumonia shows a poorly defined area of consolidation *(arrows)* in the right upper lobe. This may be termed "round pneumonia." **B.** Over the next several days, the spherical consolidation increases in size because of local interalveolar spread. This appearance may be seen in the early stages of lobar pneumonias. **C.** Further progression results in consolidation of the right upper lobe, marginated by the minor fissure *(arrows)*. **D.** A lateral view at the same time as **C** shows upper lobe consolidation marginated by the major and minor fissures *(arrows)*. Partial right middle lobe consolidation is also present.

or *Pneumococcus*, TB, bronchial obstruction with postobstructive pneumonia, or consolidation associated with neoplasm (see Fig. 2-12B).

Round or spherical consolidation suggests bronchioloalveolar carcinoma, lymphoma or lymphoproliferative disease, or pneumonia (i.e., *round pneumonia*). A round or spherical pneumonia is typical of organisms that spread via the pores of Kohn and progress to being lobar, such as *S. pneumoniae, Klebsiella, Legionella,* or TB (Fig. 2-13). Such diseases begin in at a single site and result in an enlarging ill-defined sphere of consolidation as more and more alveoli become involved. As the growing sphere reaches a pleural surface or fissure and cannot spread further, it becomes lobar.

Segmental (or subsegmental) consolidation may be diagnosed if a wedge-shaped opacity of more than a few centimeters in size is visible with the apex of the wedge pointing toward the hilum (see Figs. 2-6 and 2-14). This finding suggests an abnormality related to a segmental (or subsegmental) bronchus or artery, such as bronchial obstruction due to mucus or tumor, bronchopneumonia, focal aspiration, or pulmonary embolism with infarction.

Focal patchy consolidation is typical of pneumonias, endobronchial spread of TB, or endobronchial spread of tumor such as bronchioloalveolar carcinoma (see Fig. 2-2). CT may show a pattern of lobular consolidation. Centrilobular nodules are seen in some cases (see Fig. 2-4).

Patchy consolidation is typical of bronchopneumonia. Pneumonias associated with this pattern (e.g., *Staphylococcus, Haemophilus, Pseudomonas*) are characterized by thick and tenacious secretions and spread via airways rather than the pores of Kohn. Infected secretions are typically present within the bronchi. Bronchopneumonia is also known as

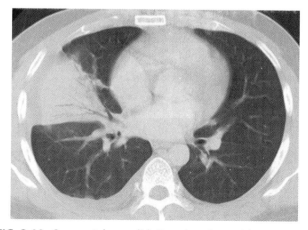

FIG. 2-14. Segmental consolidation. A patient with pneumonia shows consolidation of the lateral segment of the right middle lobe. The segmental bronchus is seen within the consolidated lung as an air bronchogram. The medial segment, adjacent to the right heart border, is normally aerated. The consolidated segment borders posteriorly on the major fissure.

lobular pneumonia because of its tendency to involve an individual lobule. Mycoplasmal pneumonia often results in this pattern.

Time Course in Diagnosis

Rapidly appearing consolidation (a few hours) suggests atelectasis with drowned lung, aspiration, pulmonary edema, pulmonary hemorrhage, infarction, or rapidly progressing pneumonia, particularly in an immunocompromised host. Of these, only pulmonary edema and drowned lung may clear quickly. Occasionally, a lymphoproliferative neoplasm progresses within hours.

Longstanding (chronic) consolidation (4 to 6 weeks) with little change suggests eosinophilic pneumonia, BOOP, bronchioloalveolar carcinoma, lymphoma, lipoid pneumonia, or some indolent pneumonias such as fungal infections. Recurrent processes (e.g., recurrent pulmonary edema, pulmonary hemorrhage, or aspiration) may appear to be chronic if radiographs are obtained only during the acute episodes.

SILHOUETTE SIGN

The borders of soft tissue structures such as the mediastinum, hila, and hemidiaphragms are visible on chest radiographs because they are outlined by adjacent air-containing lung. When consolidated lung (or a soft tissue mass) contacts one of these structures, its border becomes invisible or is poorly marginated. This is termed the "silhouette" sign. The silhouette sign is used to diagnose the presence of lung abnormality (i.e., consolidation, atelectasis, mass) and localize it to a specific lobe or lung region (Figs. 2-15 to 2-20).

On the frontal (PA or AP) radiograph, obscuration (in radiologic parlance, "silhouetting") of specific contours may been related to abnormalities in specific lobes. Specific contours and their corresponding lobes are listed below:

Right superior mediastinum (i.e., superior vena cava [SVC]) = right upper lobe (see Fig. 2-15)

Right heart border = right middle lobe (common; see Fig. 2-16) or medial right lower lobe (less common). This appearance may be mimicked by pectus excavatum.

Right hemidiaphragm = right lower lobe (see Figs. 2-17 and 2-18)

Left superior mediastinum (e.g., aortic arch) = left upper lobe (see Fig. 2-19)

Left heart border = lingular segments of left upper lobe (see Fig. 2-19)

Left hemidiaphragm or descending aorta = left lower lobe (see Fig. 2-20)

(Text continues on page 44)

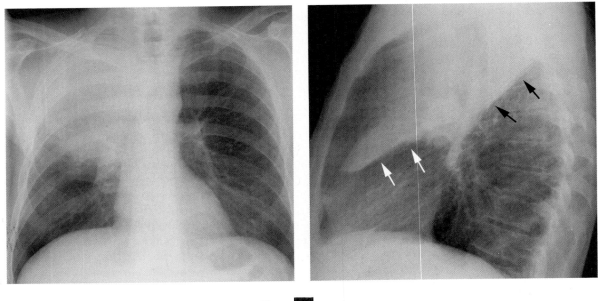

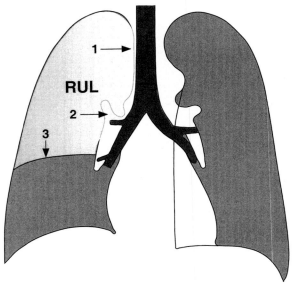

FIG. 2-15. The silhouette sign in right upper lobe pneumonia. **A.** Consolidation of the right upper lobe obscures (i.e., silhouettes) the border of the right superior mediastinum and superior vena cava. The upper part of the right hilum is also invisible. **B.** On the lateral view, the consolidated upper lobe is outlined superiorly by the upper aspect of the major fissure *(black arrows)*. Inferiorly, it is outlined by the minor fissure *(white arrows)*. **C.** Typical findings of right upper lobe consolidation: *(1)* obscuration of the right superior mediastinum, *(2)* obscuration of the superior right hilum, and *(3)* opacity marginated inferiorly by the minor fissure.

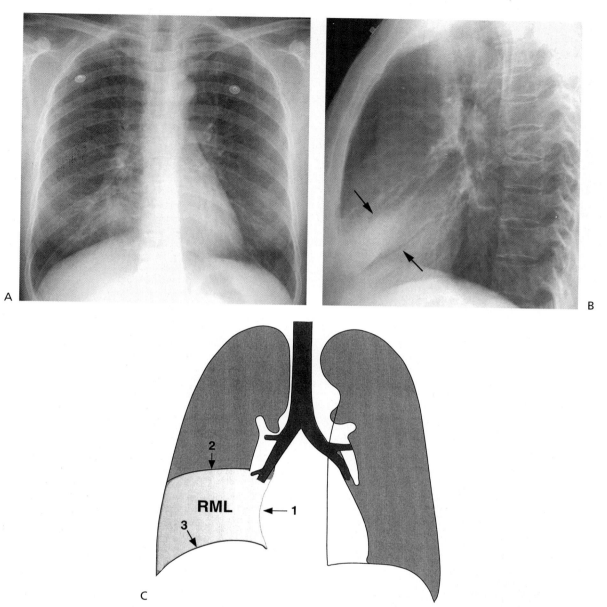

FIG. 2-16. The silhouette sign in right middle lobe pneumonia. **A.** Consolidation of the medial right middle lobe obscures ("silhouettes") the right heart border (i.e., it is not clearly seen). In contrast, the left heart border is sharply marginated. The diaphragm appears sharply marginated. **B.** On the lateral view, focal middle lobe consolidation is visible *(arrows)*. **C.** Typical findings of right middle lobe consolidation: *(1)* the right heart border is obscured, *(2)* the opacity is marginated superiorly by the minor fissure, and *(3)* the right diaphragm remains visible.

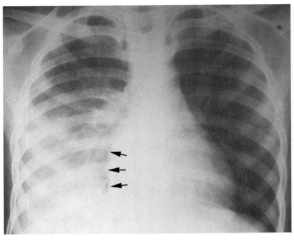
A

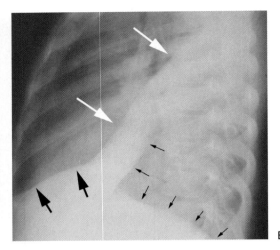
B

FIG. 2-17. The silhouette sign in right lower lobe pneumonia. **A.** The frontal view shows right lower lobe consolidation with obscuration of the diaphragm. The right heart border *(arrows)* remains visible as an edge. **B.** On the lateral view, complete right lower lobe consolidation is visible, outlined anteriorly by the major fissure *(white arrows)*. The right hemidiaphragm *(large black arrows)* is sharply marginated anterior to the consolidated lobe but is invisible posteriorly. The posterior left heart border and left hemidiaphragm are sharply marginated *(small black arrows)*. **C.** Typical findings of right lower lobe consolidation: *(1)* the superior mediastinum is well seen; *(2)* the inferior right hilum is obscured; *(3)* the right heart border remains visible; *(4)* the right hemidiaphragm is obscured; and *(5)* the right minor fissure remains visible as a line.

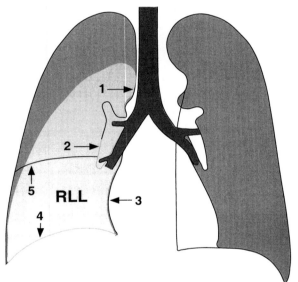
C

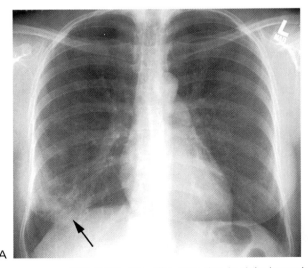
A

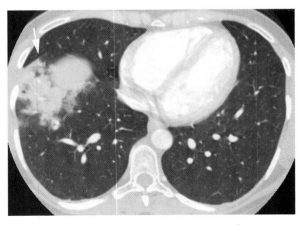
B

FIG. 2-18. The silhouette sign in right lower lobe pneumonia. **A.** There is focal obscuration of the midportion of the right hemidiaphragm *(arrow)* indicating partial right lower lobe consolidation. **B.** CT shows patchy consolidation of the lateral right lower lobe near the surface of the diaphragm, marginated anteriorly by the major fissure *(arrow)*.

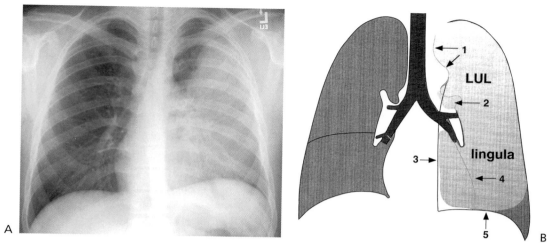

A

B

FIG. 2-19. The silhouette sign in left upper lobe pneumonia. **A.** The left heart border is obscured because of lingular consolidation. The left superior mediastinum remains sharply marginated because the medial portions of the anterior and apical segments of the left upper lobe remain aerated. **B.** Typical findings of left upper lobe (and lingular) consolidation: *(1)* the left superior mediastinum and aortic arch are obscured; *(2)* the superior left hilum is obscured; *(3)* the descending aorta remains visible; *(4)* the left heart border is obscured; and *(5)* the left hemidiaphragm remains visible.

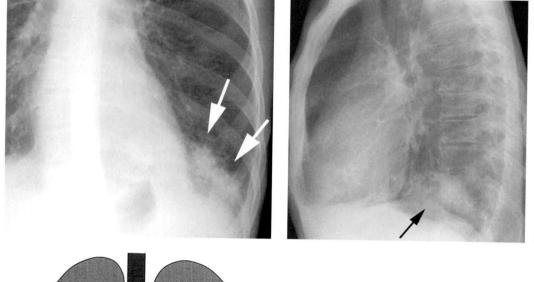

A

B

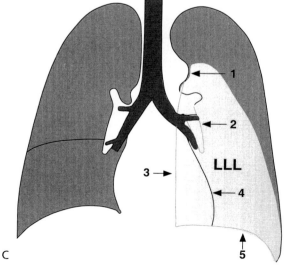

C

FIG. 2-20. The silhouette sign in left lower lobe pneumonia. **A.** The left hemidiaphragm is partially obscured by left lower lobe consolidation *(arrows).* **B.** On the lateral view, a portion of the left hemidiaphragm *(arrow)* also is obscured. **C.** Typical findings of left lower lobe consolidation: *(1)* the left superior mediastinum and aortic arch remain visible; *(2)* the inferior left hilum is obscured; *(3)* the descending aorta is obscured; *(4)* the left heart border remains visible; and *(5)* the left hemidiaphragm is obscured.

The silhouette sign is also used on the lateral projection:

Posterior margin of the heart or posterior left hemidiaphragm = left lower lobe (hiatal hernia may mimic this; see Fig. 2-20)

Anterior right hemidiaphragm = right middle lobe
Posterior right hemidiaphragm = right lower lobe (see Figs. 2-17 and 2-21)

The diaphragmatic contour seen on the frontal (PA or AP) radiograph represents the dome of the diaphragm. The diaphragmatic dome is relatively anterior, and lower lobe consolidation may be posterior to it (see Fig. 2-21).

If the border of a specific structure remains visible, absence of the silhouette sign may be used to indicate that an abnormality is *not* in that location. For example, if a lung abnormality is visible at the medial right base but the right heart border remains visible, the lesion is not likely to be in the middle lobe.

There are two caveats regarding the silhouette sign:

1. The silhouette sign does not always work. Correlate it with other findings.
2. The presence of volume loss (i.e., atelectasis) may alter these specific relationships.

ATELECTASIS

The term *atelectasis* means "incomplete stretching" in Greek. It is used to indicate loss of volume of lung tissue associated with a decrease in the amount of air it contains. It is synonymous with collapse.

Types

Four different types or mechanisms of atelectasis are recognized (Table 2-3).

Resorption (Obstructive) Atelectasis

Resorption atelectasis occurs when alveolar gas is absorbed by circulating blood and not replaced by inspired air. It occurs in the presence of airway obstruction. The obstructed airway may be the trachea, main bronchi, lobar bronchi, or multiple small bronchi or bronchioles. Small bronchial or bronchiolar obstruction by mucus resulting in resorption atelectasis is common after surgery and general anesthesia.

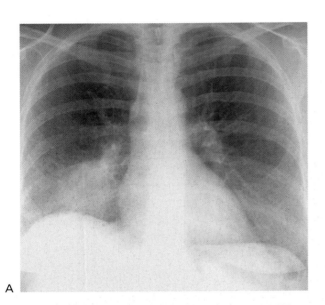

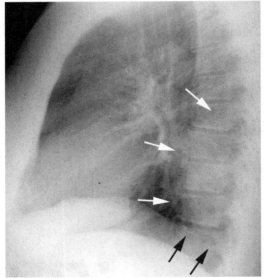

FIG. 2-21. The silhouette sign (lateral radiograph) in right lower lobe pneumonia. **A.** There is focal right lower lobe consolidation, which appears to be segmental. The right hemidiaphragm is sharply defined because the consolidated lung is located posterior to the dome of the diaphragm. **B.** The lateral view shows consolidation *(white arrows)* that obscures the posterior aspect of the right hemidiaphragm *(black arrows)*. The dome of the right diaphragm (seen on the frontal projection) is sharply marginated.

TABLE 2-3. TYPES OF ATELECTASIS

Resorption (obstructive) atelectasis
Caused by airway obstruction and resorption of alveolar gas
Occurs within 24 hours
More rapid when breathing oxygen
May result in drowned lung with little volume loss
Collateral ventilation may prevent collapse.
With large airway obstruction, air bronchograms are often absent.
Relaxation (passive) atelectasis
Atelectasis due to pleural effusion, pneumothorax, or mass
Lung decreases in volume to its inherent size.
Lung density need not be increased.
Adhesive atelectasis
Atelectasis caused by loss of lung surfactant
Typical of respiratory distress syndrome of the newborn, acute respiratory distress syndrome, radiation pneumonitis
Cicatricial atelectasis
Atelectasis caused by lung fibrosis

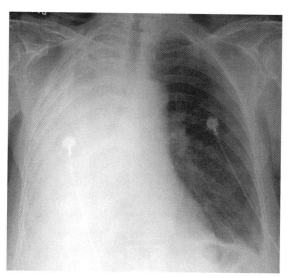

FIG. 2-22. Drowned lung in acute bronchial obstruction by mucus. The right lung is nearly airless, but volume loss is minimal. Slight shift of the trachea and mediastinum to the right is visible. Air bronchograms are invisible because of central bronchial obstruction.

Bronchial obstruction will result in lung becoming airless within 24 hours. Since oxygen is absorbed from the alveoli more rapidly than other inspired gases, resorption atelectasis occurs much more quickly when the patient is breathing pure oxygen; it may occur within minutes. Rapid resorption atelectasis may also occur in the presence of an endobronchial lesion acting as a one-way valve.

In the presence of bronchial obstruction, resorption of gas may be accompanied by rapid transudation of fluid from the circulating blood into the interstitium and alveoli (because of reduced interstitial and alveolar pressure). When this happens, lung becomes airless (consolidated) without with a minor reduction in lung volume (see Figs. 2-1A and 2-22). This occurrence is termed *drowned lung*. If the bronchial obstruction is relieved, the lung rapidly returns to normal density in most cases. This occurrence is common in ICU patients with mucous plugging or retention of secretions.

Obstruction of a main bronchus will cause atelectasis of a lung. Air bronchograms are often absent in an obstructed and collapsed lung (see Fig. 2-22). In a patient with a collapsed lung resulting from obstruction of small peripheral bronchi by secretions, air bronchograms are usually visible (see Fig. 2-1A).

Obstruction of a lobar or smaller bronchus may or may not result in atelectasis, depending on the absence or presence of *collateral ventilation* or collateral air drift. Collateral ventilation is aeration of a lung lobe or segment from adjacent alveoli (usually via the pores of Kohn) rather than from its supplying bronchus. Collateral ventilation between adjacent lobes may occur in the presence of incomplete fissures. Collateral ventilation between smaller lung units (e.g., segments) occurs more readily. The presence of lung disease, such as pneumonia, may prevent collateral ventilation.

Relaxation (Passive) and Compression Atelectasis

When contained within the chest, the volume of a lung is larger than its natural or inherent volume. The lung is elastic and stretches to fill the thoracic cavity because of negative intrapleural pressure.

The presence of pneumothorax, pleural effusion, or a mass lesion within the thoracic cavity allows the lung to decrease in volume or *relax* to its natural size. This is termed *relaxation atelectasis* or *passive atelectasis* (Fig. 2-23). The

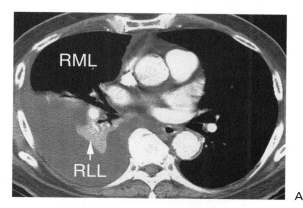

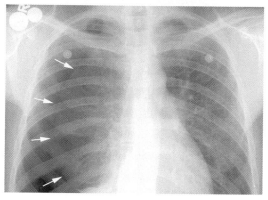

FIG. 2-23. Relaxation (compression) atelectasis. **A.** Contrast-enhanced CT in a patient with a right pleural effusion shows right lower lobe *(RLL)* atelectasis. The right lower lobe is airless. Fluid in the major fissure allows the aerated right middle lobe *(RML)* to float anteriorly. Little if any mediastinal shift is present because the increased volume of the effusion is compensated for by the decreased volume of the lower lobe. **B.** Right pneumothorax with relaxation atelectasis of the right lung. Despite its reduction in volume *(arrows)*, the right lung is not abnormally dense. Vessels in the right lung appear reduced in size compared to those on the left. This reflects reduced lung perfusion. The right lower lobe maintains its contact with the mediastinum because of the inferior pulmonary ligament. Air is seen within the minor fissure, separating the lobes.

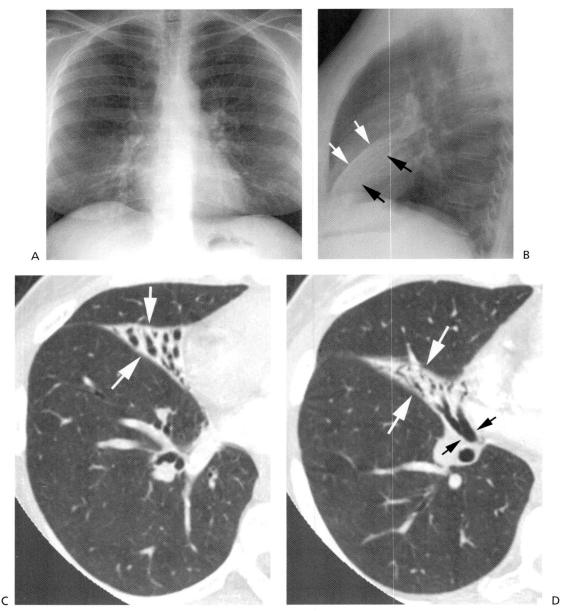

FIG. 2-24. Cicatricial atelectasis in a patient with chronic right middle lobe collapse (right middle lobe syndrome) leading to fibrosis. **A.** Frontal chest radiograph shows poor definition of the right heart border, typical of right middle lobe consolidation. There is little increase in opacity at the right base. **B.** Lateral view shows volume loss in the right middle lobe with downward bowing of the minor fissure *(white arrows)* and anterior displacement of the major fissure *(black arrows)*. Crowded air bronchograms are visible within the collapsed lobe. **C** and **D.** CT scans at two levels show a typical appearance for right middle lobe collapse, having a triangular configuration *(white arrows)*. The right middle lobe bronchus *(black arrows)* is patent, and air bronchograms are visible within the collapsed lobe. Collapse in the absence of bronchial obstruction is typical of right middle lobe syndrome. The dilated air bronchograms may indicate reversible bronchiectasis.

term *compressive atelectasis* can also be used to describe this occurrence, although it implies a reduction in lung volume beyond its normal resting state.

Approximately half of the density of lung is blood, and when lung collapses in the presence of pneumothorax, a significant increase in lung density need not be visible (see Fig. 2-23B). Reduction in lung volume also results in a reduction in lung perfusion. However, until the lung become very small, its density does not significantly increase.

Adhesive Atelectasis

Surfactant reduces the surface tension of alveolar fluid and tends to prevent collapse as the alveoli decrease in volume. Deficiency of surfactant causes adhesive atelectasis. The lung is generally reduced in volume. This is most typical of respiratory distress syndrome of the newborn but is also seen in patients with ARDS, acute radiation pneumonitis, or hypoxemia, and in the postoperative period.

Cicatricial Atelectasis

This term refers to loss of lung volume occurring in the presence of lung fibrosis. It may be focal, lobar (Fig. 2-24), or diffuse, depending on the disease responsible. Findings of fibrosis are typically present.

Radiographic Findings of Atelectasis

Radiographic findings of atelectasis are usually considered as direct or indirect (Table 2-4). For practical purposes, the diagnosis is based on a combination of these findings.

Direct Signs

Direct signs of atelectasis indicate loss of volume in the abnormal lobe.

TABLE 2-4. RADIOGRAPHIC SIGNS OF ATELECTASIS

Direct signs: due to lobar volume loss
Displacement of fissures
Crowding of vessels
Indirect signs: secondary to volume loss
Diaphragmatic elevation
Mediastinal shift
Compensatory overinflation
Hilar displacement
Reorientation of the hilum or bronchi
Approximation of the ribs
Increased lung opacity
Absence of air bronchograms
Shifting granuloma sign

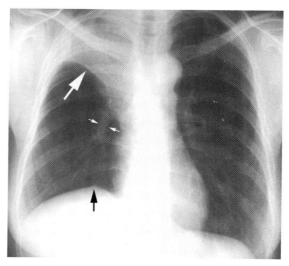

FIG. 2-25. Signs of atelectasis in right upper lobe collapse. The right hemidiaphragm is elevated. The minor fissure is displaced and bowed upward *(large white arrow)*. The right hilum is elevated compared to the left, and the descending pulmonary artery is rotated outward *(small white arrows)*, being more easily seen than normal. The thin triangular opacity at the dome of the right hemidiaphragm *(black arrow)* is a so-called juxtaphrenic peak, which may be seen in upper lobe atelectasis.

Displacement of Interlobar Fissures
Displacement of interlobar fissures is the best sign of atelectasis (see Figs. 2-24 to 2-26) but is not always visible. The appearance of fissure displacement reflects the specific lobe involved. Specific patterns of lobar atelectasis are described below.

Crowding of Vessels or Bronchi
Crowding of vessels or bronchi in a given lobe reflects volume loss and is useful in diagnosis if a shift of fissures is not visible. Crowded air bronchograms may be seen in the presence of collapsed and consolidated lung (see Fig. 2-24B–D). Crowded vessels are visible on radiographs if volume loss is present without consolidation. Vascular crowding in collapsed and consolidated lung is commonly seen on CT following contrast infusion.

Indirect Signs

Indirect signs of atelectasis are those not directly due to lobar volume loss but occurring secondary to it.

Diaphragmatic Elevation
Diaphragmatic elevation occurs because of ipsilateral volume loss (see Figs. 2-25 to 2-27). It is more common with lower lobe atelectasis than upper lobe atelectasis, although it may be difficult to see if the lower lobe is consolidated. Diagnosis is based on knowledge of normal diaphragmatic position or comparison to prior radiographs.

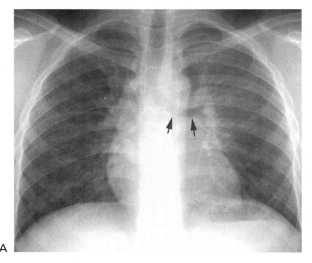

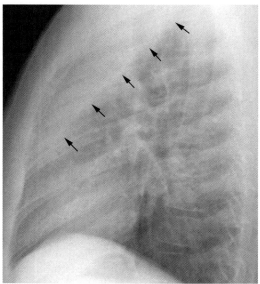

FIG. 2-26. Signs of atelectasis in left upper lobe collapse. **A.** The left hilum is elevated. The left main and left upper lobe bronchi *(arrows)* are elevated and appear more horizontal than normal. The left hemidiaphragm is higher than the right and a slight increase in opacity is seen in the left upper lung. **B.** Lateral radiograph in the same patient as **A** shows marked anterior displacement of the major fissure *(arrows)*. As the left upper lobe loses more volume, it appears thinner on the lateral view and less dense on the frontal radiograph.

The right hemidiaphragm is up to 2 cm higher than the left in 90% of normal persons. In about 10% of normal persons, the right hemidiaphragm is more than 3 cm higher than the left, the hemidiaphragms are at the same level, or the left hemidiaphragm is higher than the right.

Mediastinal Shift

Mediastinal shift occurs with atelectasis (see Figs. 2-27 and 2-28A). Shift of the upper mediastinum usually occurs with

upper lobe collapse (see Fig. 2-27A) and is most easily recognized by shift of the trachea. Shift of the heart and lower mediastinum is most predominant with lower lobe atelectasis (see Fig. 2-28A). This may be manifested as shift of the anterior junction line, posterior junction line, or azygoesophageal interface, so-called lung herniation.

Compensatory Overinflation

Compensatory overinflation of normal lung on the same side as atelectasis appears as increased volume and decreased density of lung, associated with splaying of vessels. Decreased lung density is easiest to see on CT.

Hilar Displacement

Hilar displacement may occur in the presence of upper or lower lobe atelectasis (see Figs. 2-25 and 2-26). The hilum

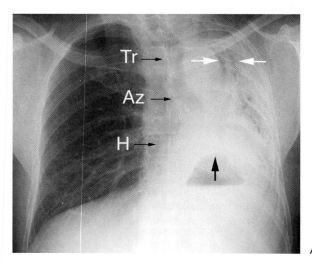

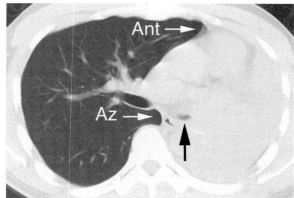

FIG. 2-27. Left lung atelectasis due to TB with bronchostenosis. **A.** The position of the superior aspect of the stomach bubble *(large black arrow)* indicates elevation of the left hemidiaphragm. Marked leftward shift of the trachea *(Tr)*, azygoesophageal recess *(Az)*, and right heart border *(H)* is present. Air bronchograms *(white arrow)* are visible in the left upper lobe. **B.** CT shows narrowing of the left main bronchus *(black arrow)*. The anterior mediastinum *(Ant)* and azygoesophageal recess *(Az)* are shifted to the left. Air bronchograms are not visible at this level.

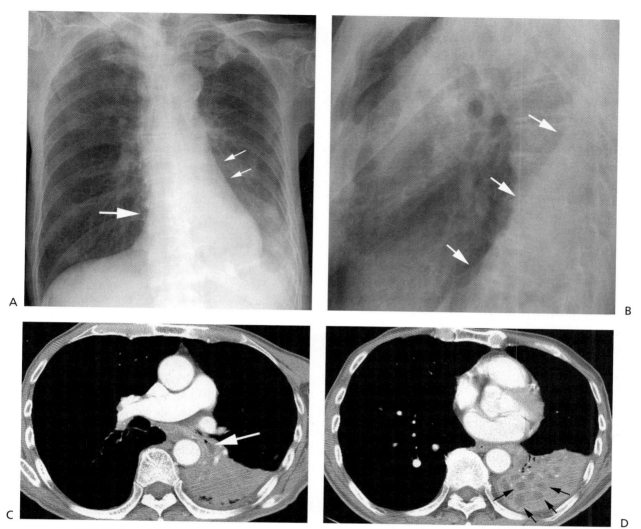

FIG. 2-28. Left lower lobe atelectasis due to mucous plugging. **A.** Chest radiograph shows consolidation at the left base with obscuration of the left hemidiaphragm. The heart is displaced to the left *(large arrow)*. The left interlobar pulmonary artery is poorly defined, as is typical in left lower lobe atelectasis. There is flattening of the left heart border *(white arrows)* due to leftward rotation of the heart and great vessels, termed the "flat waist" sign. The left ribs appear closer together than the right. **B.** Lateral view shows left lower lobe atelectasis with posterior displacement of the major fissure *(arrows)*. **C.** Obstruction of the left lower lobe bronchus *(arrow)* is due to mucus. Mucus in the obstructed bronchus appears lower in attenuation than surrounding consolidated lung. Consolidation borders on the major fissure, which is displaced posteriorly. The mediastinum is shifted to the left. **D.** At a lower level, mucous bronchograms *(arrows)* are visible. The mucus-filled bronchi are dilated, but this represents "reversible bronchiectasis."

is elevated in the presence of upper lobe collapse and depressed if lower lobe collapse in present. The left hilum is higher than the right in most normals. If the hila appear to be at the same level, right upper lobe collapse or left lower lobe collapse may be present.

Reorientation of the Hilum or Bronchi
Reorientation of the hilum or bronchi occurs in association with hilar displacement. With upper lobe collapse, the hilum rotates outward and the descending pulmonary artery

and bronchi are less vertical than normal and more easily seen (see Fig. 2-25). The left main bronchus may appear elevated and more horizontal than normal in the presence of left upper lobe collapse (see Fig. 2-26A). With lower lobe collapse, the hila are depressed and the bronchi appear more vertical than normal.

Approximation of the Ribs
The ipsilateral ribs may appear closer together in the presence of ipsilateral volume loss (see Fig. 2-28A). Although

this finding may be seen in patients with collapse, other findings of atelectasis will always be seen; never base a diagnosis on this sign alone. Rotation of the patient may mimic this appearance.

Increased Lung Opacity

An increase in lung opacity or attenuation may be seen, but this is nonspecific. It may reflect replacement of alveolar air by fluid (i.e., drowned lung) or, when extreme, compressed and airless lung tissue (see Figs. 2-24 to 2-28).

Absence of Air Bronchograms

In a patient with lung consolidation, the absence of air bronchograms suggests central bronchial obstruction (see Figs. 2-22 and 2-28). However, air bronchograms are sometimes seen in the presence of a (partially) obstructing central bronchial lesion (see Fig. 2-27A) or resorption atelectasis resulting from small peripheral mucous plugs (see Fig. 2-1A).

In patients with atelectasis and air bronchograms, the air-filled bronchi may appear dilated on plain radiographs or CT because of the collapse, simulating bronchiectasis. This is termed *reversible bronchiectasis* (an oxymoron) as it disappears following reexpansion of the lobe. Bronchiectasis is defined as irreversible bronchial dilatation.

Mucous Bronchograms

In the presence of bronchial obstruction, CT may show low-attenuation mucus within obstructed bronchi (see Fig. 2-28D). Mucus-filled bronchi may appear dilated. This may be due to large mucous plugs or reversible bronchiectasis.

Shifting Granuloma Sign

Shift in the location of a parenchymal lesion visible on prior films may be seen in the presence of atelectasis.

Indirect Signs Seen With Specific Types of Atelectasis

Other indirect signs of atelectasis associated with specific types of atelectasis include the following:

Golden's S sign: right upper lobe atelectasis
Juxtaphrenic peak: upper lobe atelectasis
Luftsichel sign: left upper lobe atelectasis
Flat waist sign: left lower lobe atelectasis
Comet-tail sign: rounded atelectasis

These are described below.

Appearances of Atelectasis

Specific appearances occur with lung collapse and collapse of an individual lobe or lobes in combination. These appearances may be modified by the degree of volume loss, the degree of lung consolidation occurring in association with volume loss, and the presence of pleural effusion or pneumothorax.

Atelectasis of an Entire Lung

Lung atelectasis usually results from obstruction of a main bronchus by an endobronchial lesion (or intubation of the opposite main bronchus), obstruction of small peripheral bronchi by secretions, or large ipsilateral pneumothorax or pleural effusion.

Bronchial Obstruction With Lung Collapse

With bronchial obstruction, the ipsilateral diaphragm is elevated, shift of both the upper and lower mediastinum to the side of atelectasis is present, the ipsilateral ribs appear too close together, and the lung is increased in density in comparison to the opposite side (see Fig. 2-27). The cause of bronchial obstruction may be evident.

In the presence of bronchial obstruction with acute collapse, alveoli may rapidly fill with fluid, resulting in drowned lung. In this case, little mediastinal shift may be seen (see Fig. 2-22). If complete opacification of a hemithorax occurs acutely with significant mediastinal shift to the opposite side, pleural effusion is the likely diagnosis; if complete opacification of a hemithorax occurs acutely without significant mediastinal shift to the opposite side, drowned lung is the likely diagnosis. Absence of air bronchograms suggests a central obstruction; visible air bronchograms suggest peripheral small airway obstruction.

Pneumothorax With Lung Collapse

Pneumothorax causes the lung to collapse centrally toward the hilum and mediastinum. The shape of the collapsed lung usually is maintained (see Fig. 2-23B). Because of the inferior pulmonary ligament, the lower lobe usually maintains its contact with the paracardiac mediastinum and diaphragm.

Until collapse is complete and the lung becomes airless, it may appear normal in density or relatively lucent despite its small size (see Fig. 2-23B). This occurs because of reduced perfusion associated with volume loss. Some shift of the mediastinum to the opposite side is typical in patients with a sizable pneumothorax regardless of the presence of tension.

Pleural Effusion With Lung Collapse

Massive pleural effusion results in relaxation or compressive atelectasis of the lung, a variable degree of mediastinal shift to the opposite side (depending on the size of the effusion and the degree of collapse), and variable opacification of the hemithorax (depending on the extent of residual aerated lung).

Large pleural effusion may result in loss of lung volume without complete lung opacification. Because a free effusion in an upright patient predominantly occupies the inferior hemithorax, the lower lobe is usually more compressed, contains less air, and appears denser than the upper lobe.

Collapsed lung is tethered at the hilum, and the lower lobe maintains its relationship to the mediastinum because of the inferior pulmonary ligament (see Fig. 2-23A). However, fluid often separates the peripheral part of the lobe from the chest wall and enters the major fissure or major and minor fissures, allowing adjacent lobes to float apart. These findings are difficult to recognize on chest radiographs unless the lung remains partially aerated. On CT obtained with contrast infusion, collapsed lobes opacify and appear denser than fluid in the pleural space. On unenhanced CT, the collapsed lung appears slightly denser than fluid.

Lobar Atelectasis

Lobar collapse usually results from bronchial obstruction (resorption atelectasis). Lobar cicatricial atelectasis is less common but may be associated with chronic infection. Several general rules apply to lobar atelectasis:

1. Atelectasis usually results in bowing of a fissure toward the collapsing lobe.
2. An atelectatic lobe generally assumes the shape of a triangle or pyramid, with the apex of the triangle or pyramid at the hilum.
3. Unless atelectasis is severe or pleural effusion or pneumothorax is present, a collapsed upper or lower lobe maintains its contact with the costal (peripheral) pleural surface. The middle lobe, on the other hand, commonly loses its costal pleural contact with atelectasis.

4. Because atelectasis is associated with decreased lung perfusion and blood volume, collapse does not result in increased lung density unless the lobe is moderately reduced in volume or air-space consolidation is associated with volume loss.
5. With total lobar collapse, and in the absence of consolidation or drowned lung, collapsed lobes are very thin and may be difficult to recognize en face as an area of increased density.
6. Collapsed lung often appears densely opacified on CT following contrast infusion.
7. Hilar masses causing collapse usually appear less dense than collapsed lung on contrast-enhanced CT.

Interlobar Fissures

Recognition of lobar collapse is fundamentally based on knowledge of the normal positions of the fissures. They are described in greater detail in Chapter 26.

Major (Oblique) Fissure. On the right, the major fissure separates the upper and middle lobes from the lower lobe. On the left, it separates the upper lobe from the lower lobe. The major fissures originate posteriorly above the level of the aortic arch, near the level of the fifth thoracic vertebra, and angle anteriorly and inferiorly, nearly parallel to the sixth rib (Fig. 2-29). Posteriorly, the superior aspect of the left major fissure is cephalad to the right in 75%. They

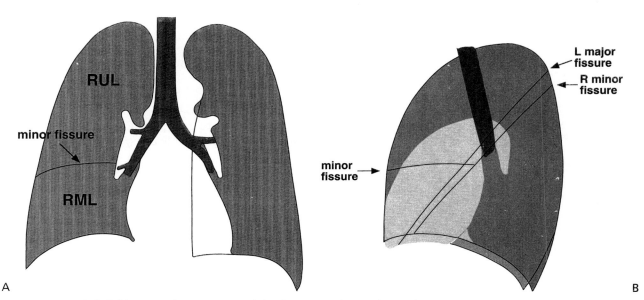

FIG. 2-29. Normal appearances of the fissures on chest radiographs. **A.** Frontal projection. The major fissures are not normally visible. The minor fissure is visible in 50% to 80% of cases, appearing as a roughly horizontal line, generally at or near the level of the anterior fourth rib. Medially, it arises at the level of the interlobar pulmonary artery, and its lateral part is often inferior to its medial part. **B.** Lateral projection. The major fissures originate posteriorly above the level of the aortic arch, near the level of the fifth thoracic vertebra. Posteriorly, the superior aspect of the left major fissure is cephalad to the right in 75%. They terminate along the anterior diaphragmatic pleural surface of each lung, several centimeters posterior to the anterior chest wall.

terminate along the anterior diaphragmatic pleural surface of each lung, several centimeters posterior to the anterior chest wall. The right and left fissures may be identified by noting their relationships to the right or left hemidiaphragms or posterior ribs. The major fissures are not clearly seen on frontal (PA or AP) radiographs unless there is lower lobe volume loss.

On CT, the orientation of the major fissures varies at different levels. In the upper thorax, the major fissures angle posterolaterally from the mediastinum. Within the lower thorax, the major fissures angle anterolaterally from the mediastinum (Fig. 2-30A). The fissure may be seen as a linear opacity on scans obtained with thin collimation. Alterna-

tively, its position may be localized by recognizing a 1- to 2-cm avascular band within the lung (i.e., lung adjacent to the fissure containing only small vessels) having a typical orientation.

Minor (Horizontal) Fissure. The minor or horizontal fissure separates the superior aspect of the right middle lobe from the right upper lobe. On frontal (PA or AP) radiographs, the minor fissure or a portion is visible in 50% to 80% of cases, appearing as a roughly horizontal line, generally at or near the level of the anterior fourth rib (see Fig. 2-29). Its contour is variable, but its lateral part is often visible inferior to its medial part. Medially, the fissure usu-

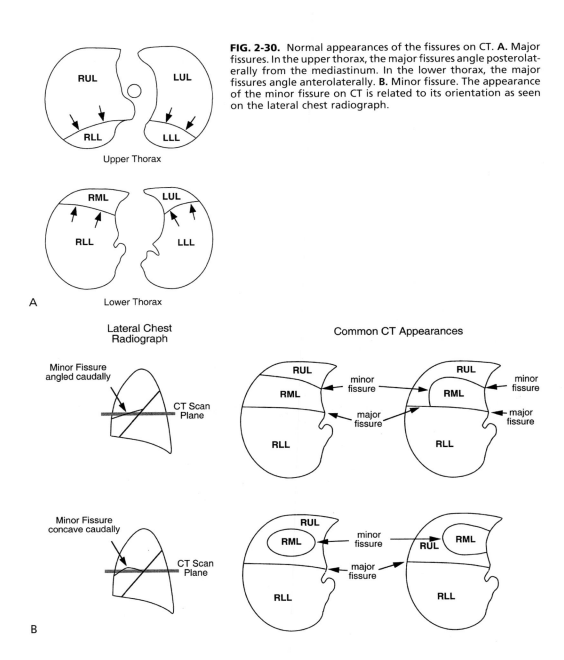

FIG. 2-30. Normal appearances of the fissures on CT. **A.** Major fissures. In the upper thorax, the major fissures angle posterolaterally from the mediastinum. In the lower thorax, the major fissures angle anterolaterally. **B.** Minor fissure. The appearance of the minor fissure on CT is related to its orientation as seen on the lateral chest radiograph.

ally appears to arise at the level of the right hilum and interlobar pulmonary artery.

On the lateral radiograph, the anterior part of the fissure often appears inferior to its posterior part. The posterior part of the fissure may be seen to end at the major fissure or may extend posterior to it due to variation in the location in the parts of these fissures imaged on the lateral view.

On CT, the minor fissure tends to parallel the scan plane and is usually difficult to see. Characteristically, the position of the minor fissure can be inferred because of a broad avascular region in the anterior portion of the right lung, anterior to the major fissure, at the level of the bronchus intermedius. The minor fissure may be seen as a discrete line, similar to the appearance of the major fissure, when scans are obtained with thin collimation.

When visible, the minor fissure is variable in appearance, depending on its orientation. Because the minor fissure often angles caudally, the lower lobe, middle lobe, and upper lobe may all be seen on a single CT scan (see Fig. 2-30B). If this is the case, the major and minor fissures can have a similar appearance, with the major fissure being posterior and the minor fissure anterior; in this situation, the lower lobe is most posterior, the upper lobe is most anterior, and the middle lobe is in the middle.

If the minor fissure is concave caudally, it can sometimes be seen in two locations or can appear ring-shaped, with the middle lobe between the fissure lines or in the center of the ring and the upper lobe anterior to the most anterior part of the fissure.

Right Upper Lobe Atelectasis
Frontal (PA or AP) Radiograph. On the frontal radiograph, the minor fissure bows upward (Table 2-5; see Figs. 2-25 and 2-31A). The medial aspect of the lobe maintains its relationship to the hilum, and its lateral aspect (marginated by the minor fissure) rotates toward the upper mediastinum in a clockwise fashion. Collapsed and consolidated lung obscures superior mediastinal contours.

TABLE 2-5. RADIOGRAPHIC FINDINGS OF RIGHT UPPER LOBE ATELECTASIS

Frontal radiograph
Ill-defined increase in opacity in the upper thorax
Apparent right mediastinal widening
Silhouetting of the right upper mediastinum
Tracheal shift to the right
Upward bowing and displacement of the minor fissure
Golden's S sign
Elevation of the hilum
Outward rotation of the hilum or bronchus
Right-sided juxtaphrenic peak
Lateral radiograph
Upward displacement and bowing of the minor fissure
Anterior displacement and bowing of the upper major fissure

With complete collapse, the upper lobe appears pancaked against the upper mediastinum. It may have a concave margin laterally, representing the displaced minor fissure, or may have a convex lateral edge, mimicking the appearance of mediastinal widening.

In patients with right upper lobe collapse associated with bronchogenic carcinoma (the right upper lobe is the most common site for lung cancer) or other mass lesion producing bronchial obstruction, a characteristic appearance may be seen, termed *Golden's S sign*. This sign refers to a combination of upward bowing of the lateral aspect of the minor fissure due to volume loss, with downward bulging of the medial fissure due to the presence of a hilar mass (see Fig. 2-31A). This combination results in a shallow reverse-S appearance. Although described as a sign of right upper lobe collapse, a similar appearance may be seen in any lobe if the fissure bordering it is visible in profile.

Shift of the trachea toward the right may be seen as a result of right upper lobe volume loss. The hilum is typically elevated, the bronchus intermedius rotates outward, appearing less vertical than normal, and the upper lobe region may appear abnormally dense (see Fig. 2-25).

With upper lobe atelectasis, a finding termed the *juxtaphrenic peak* may be seen on the frontal (PA or AP) radiograph (see Fig. 2-25). This appears as a small sharp triangular opacity near the dome of the ipsilateral hemidiaphragm. It is related to stretching of an inferior accessory fissure or folds or septa on the undersurface of the lung adjacent to the phrenic nerves or inferior pulmonary ligament.

Lateral Radiograph. On the lateral radiograph, the minor fissure bows upward and rotates superiorly, being anchored at the hilum (see Fig. 2-31B). The superior portion of the major fissure bows anteriorly in a similar fashion, and the lobe assumes the shape of a progressively thinner wedge as it loses volume. The collapsed upper lobe maintains its contact with the anterior chest wall. With marked upper lobe volume loss, a very thin dense wedge may be seen, associated with anterior displacement of the entire major fissure.

CT. On CT, the minor fissure rotates anteriorly and medially as the upper lobe progressively flattens against the mediastinum, marginating its lateral aspect (see Fig. 2-31C). The collapsed lobe appears thinner near the hilum than in the apex unless a hilar mass is present. The lobe usually appears triangular in cross section. The major fissure outlines the posterior margin of the collapsed lobe and may be bowed anteriorly (see Fig. 2-31D and E). In the presence of a hilar mass, an appearance similar to Golden's S sign is visible with posterior bulging of the fissure.

Left Upper Lobe Collapse
Frontal (PA or AP) Radiograph. On the frontal radiograph, an ill-defined increase in lung density is typically visible, being most obvious in the upper portion of the

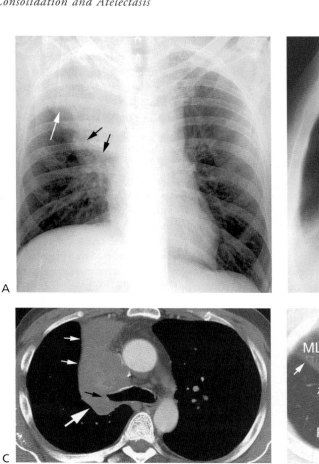

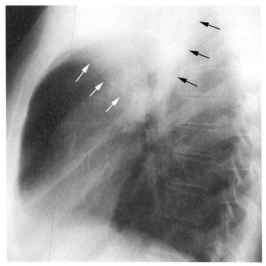

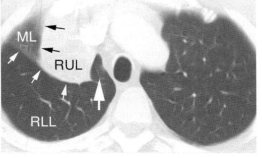

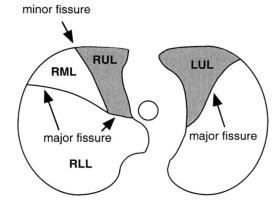

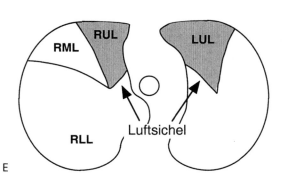

FIG. 2-31. Right upper lobe collapse with Golden's S sign. **A.** PA chest radiograph in a patient with a right hilar carcinoma shows elevation of the lateral aspect of the minor fissure *(white arrow)* due to atelectasis and downward convexity of the medial fissure *(black arrows)* due to the hilar mass. Right upper mediastinal contours are obscured because of adjacent consolidation. The right hemidiaphragm is also elevated. **B.** The lateral view shows upward bowing of the minor fissure *(white arrows)*, with the anterior aspect of the fissure being most displaced. There is anterior displacement of the upper portion of the major fissure *(black arrows)*. The right upper lobe assumes the shape of a wedge as it loses volume. The collapsed upper lobe maintains its contact with the hilum and anterior chest wall. **C.** CT shows anterior rotation and bowing of the minor fissure *(small white arrows)* outlining the collapsed right upper lobe. The hilar mass results in bulging of the posterior aspect of the major fissure *(large white arrow)*, resulting in the CT equivalent of the S sign. The right upper lobe bronchus is obstructed *(black arrow)*. **D.** CT with a lung window setting at a higher level shows the collapsed and consolidated upper lobe *(RUL)* outlined laterally by the minor fissure *(black arrows)* and posteriorly by the anteriorly displaced major fissure *(small white arrows)*. A tongue of lung extending medial to the collapsed lobe represents a portion of superior segment of lower lobe. This may result in a luftsichel sign visible on a plain radiograph. *ML,* middle lobe; *RLL,* right lower lobe. **E.** Diagram of right and left upper lobe collapse on CT. In some cases, lung extending medial to the collapse lobe may result in a luftsichel sign, as seen on a chest radiograph.

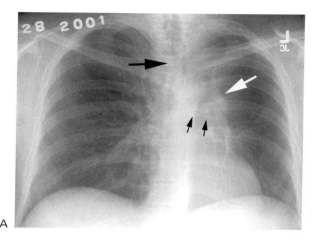

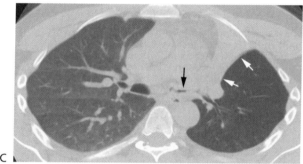

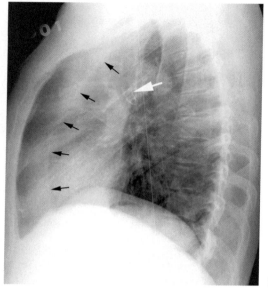

FIG. 2-32. Left upper lobe atelectasis associated with bronchostenosis. **A.** The frontal radiograph shows tracheal shift to the left *(large black arrow)*, elevation of the left hilum *(white arrow)*, an ill-defined increase in lung density, and obscuration of the left superior mediastinum and cardiac border. The edge of the aortic arch, a relatively posterior structure, remains well defined. The left main bronchus *(small black arrows)*, faintly outlined by a stent in its lumen, is elevated and appears more horizontal than is normal. The inferior left heart border remains sharply defined because of marked volume loss. **B.** On the lateral view, the left upper lobe is dense and there is anterior displacement of the major fissure *(black arrows)* paralleling the anterior chest wall. The stent within the left main bronchus *(white arrow)* is visible. **C.** CT shows anterior bowing and anteromedial displacement of the major fissure *(white arrows)*. The left main bronchus *(black arrow)* is narrowed. A relative decrease in the density of the left lower lobe is due to compensatory hyperexpansion.

hemithorax (Table 2-6). Increased lung opacity is usually associated with obscuration of the left superior mediastinum and left cardiac margin (because of the silhouette sign; Figs. 2-32A and 2-33A). However, with marked collapse, the left upper lobe may become very thin and may be difficult to recognize as abnormally dense, and the silhouette sign may not be clearly seen (see Fig. 2-26A and B). If the lingular segments of the left upper lobe remain aerated, the left heart border may remain well defined. On the other hand, if lingular collapse is unassociated with collapse of the apical posterior and anterior segments of the upper lobe, only the left heart border is obscured.

In the presence of upper lobe atelectasis and anterior shift of the major fissure, the superior segment of the lower lobe expands to occupy the apex of the hemithorax. On the frontal radiograph, the superior segment may insinuate itself between the upper lobe and the mediastinum, resulting in

TABLE 2-6. RADIOGRAPHIC FINDINGS OF LEFT UPPER LOBE ATELECTASIS

Frontal radiograph
Ill-defined increase in opacity in the upper thorax (decreasing with increased collapse)
Silhouetting of the left upper mediastinum
Tracheal shift to the left
Luftsichel sign
Apical cap
Elevation of the hilum
Outward rotation of the hilum or bronchus
Juxtaphrenic peak
Lateral radiograph
Anterior bowing and displacement of the major fissure

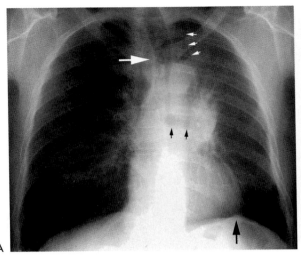
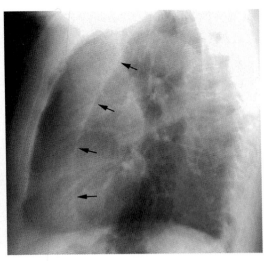

FIG. 2-33. Left upper lobe collapse due to bronchogenic carcinoma. **A.** Frontal chest radiograph shows increased density in the left upper lobe region, but a crescentic lucency *(small white arrows)* in the medial aspect of the left lung apex represents insinuation of the aerated superior segment of the lower lobe, the so-called luftsichel sign. Other findings of left upper lobe collapse include tracheal shift *(large white arrow)*, elevation of the left main bronchus *(small black arrows)*, and a juxtaphrenic peak *(large black arrow)*. A left hilar mass represents the carcinoma. **B.** Anterior displacement and bowing of the major fissure are visible on the lateral view.

an interface where lucent lung contacts collapsed lung. This interface is often crescentic in appearance and has been termed the "luftsichel" sign (*luftsichel* means "air crescent" in German; see Fig. 2-33A). The luftsichel sign is uncommon with right upper lobe collapse but may be seen.

If the expanded superior segment does not reach the apex of the hemithorax (usually because upper lobe volume loss is not marked), the airless upper lobe may result in the appearance of a crescentic soft tissue–density shadow over the lung apex (termed an *apical cap*), mimicking apical pleural thickening or effusion, Pancoast tumor, or an extrapleural fluid collection (Fig. 2-34). This appearance has been termed *peripheral* upper lobe atelectasis. It may also be seen on the right.

As on the right, left upper lobe collapse may be associated with a left-sided juxtaphrenic peak (see Fig. 2-33A). Elevation of the left hilum may be seen; the left main bronchus may appear elevated and more horizontal than normal; and leftward shift of the upper mediastinum and trachea is typically present.

Lateral Radiograph. On the lateral radiograph, left upper lobe atelectasis results in progressive anterior displacement of the major fissure along a line paralleling the anterior chest wall (see Figs. 2-26B, 2-32B, and 2-33B). Lung anterior to the displaced fissure appears abnormally dense. With complete collapse, a very thin dense band may be seen along the anterior chest wall. The left hilum and bronchi may be displaced anteriorly.

CT. On CT, the major fissure rotates anteromedially with upper lobe collapse (see Fig. 2-32C). If lingular segments remain aerated, the appearance closely mimics that of right upper lobe collapse. The luftsichel sign is associated with a V-shaped appearance at the posterior margin of the collapsed lobe, with the superior segment of the lower lobe

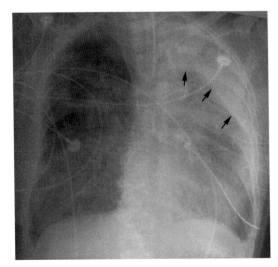

FIG. 2-34. Left upper lobe collapse mimicking apical pleural thickening. A crescentic soft tissue opacity at the left apex represents collapsed upper lobe outlined inferiorly by the aerated superior segment of the lower lobe *(arrows)*. This appearance is sometimes termed *peripheral* atelectasis.

TABLE 2-7. RADIOGRAPHIC FINDINGS OF MIDDLE LOBE ATELECTASIS

Frontal radiograph
Minor fissure is invisible.
Increased lung opacity (decreasing with increased collapse)
Silhouetting of the right heart border
Lateral radiograph
Downward bowing and displacement of the minor fissure
Anterior bowing and displacement of the inferior major fissure
Wedge of consolidated lung anchored at the hilum

extending medial to the collapsed lobe (see Fig. 2-31D and E).

Right Middle Lobe Collapse

Frontal (PA or AP) Radiograph. On the frontal radiograph, the minor fissure is usually invisible in the presence of middle lobe atelectasis; it rotates downward (as shown on the lateral view) and is no longer tangent to the x-ray beam (Table 2-7). Depending on the amount of consolidation and the degree of volume loss, increased lung opacity may be seen, obscuring the right heart border (see Figs. 2-24A and 2-35A). With marked volume loss, increased density may not be visible (see Fig. 2-24A), or the right heart border may appear normal. A lordotic radiograph may be helpful in showing the displaced minor fissure and area of increased density, but this is uncommonly used in clinical practice for this diagnosis.

With middle lobe collapse, volume loss may not be sufficient to cause hilar displacement or mediastinal shift.

Chronic right middle lobe atelectasis may not resolve even if its original cause is alleviated. The presence of chronic inflammation or infection, bronchiectasis, and fibrosis may prevent reexpansion (i.e., cicatricial atelectasis). The occurrence of chronic nonobstructive middle lobe collapse is often termed *right middle lobe syndrome* (see Fig. 2-24). It was originally described as occurring in association with tuberculous hilar lymph node enlargement resulting in transient bronchial obstruction. Typically the right middle lobe bronchus appears patent, and dilated air bronchograms may be visible in the collapsed lobe.

Lateral Radiograph. On the lateral radiograph, middle lobe collapse results in upward bowing and displacement of the inferior major fissure and downward displacement of the minor fissure, resulting in a thin wedge-shaped opacity with its apex at the hilum (see Fig. 2-35B).

The appearance of right middle lobe collapse on the lateral view may mimic fluid within the major fissure. However, with fissural fluid the lower edge of the opacity is often convex downward instead of concave downward, as is typical of middle lobe collapse. If a minor fissure is seen as separate from a similar wedge-shaped opacity, occurring in a normal position, fissural fluid may be diagnosed.

CT. On CT, as the middle lobe loses volume, the minor fissure, which normally is difficult to see because it lies in the plane of scan, rotates downward and medially and becomes

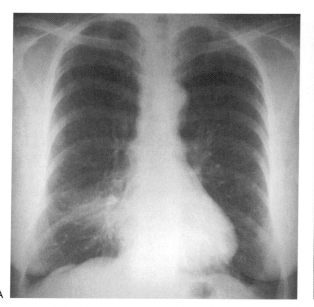
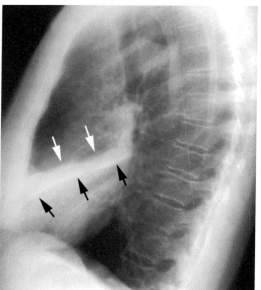

A   B

FIG. 2-35. Right middle lobe collapse. **A.** On the frontal radiograph, ill-defined middle lobe consolidation obscures the right heart border. **B.** The lateral view shows downward displacement of the minor fissure *(white arrows)* and anterior displacement of the major fissure *(black arrows)*. The collapsed middle lobe appears to be a thin wedge-shaped opacity with its apex at the hilum.

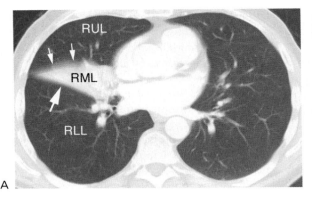

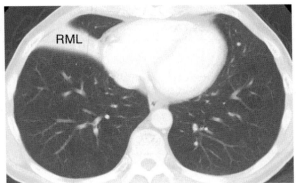

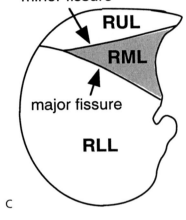

FIG. 2-36. CT of right middle lobe collapse. **A.** CT through the inferior right hilum shows anterior displacement of the major fissure *(large arrow)* and downward displacement of the minor fissure *(small arrows)*. The minor fissure is less well defined because of its greater obliquity relative to the scan plane. The collapsed and consolidated middle lobe *(RML)* has a typical triangular configuration. *RUL*, right upper lobe; *RLL*, right lower lobe. **B.** At a lower level the collapsed lobe appears bandlike, outlined by the upper and lower lobes. **C.** Diagram of right middle lobe collapse on CT.

visible on CT. The collapsed lobe assumes a triangular shape, with one side of the triangle abutting the mediastinum and anchored at the hilum (Fig. 2-36). The apex of the triangle is directed laterally. The upper lobe is anterolateral to the collapsed lobe, and the lower lobe borders it posterolaterally (i.e., the middle lobe is in the middle). These aerated lobes usually contact each other lateral to the collapsed middle lobe and separate it from the lateral chest wall.

Lower Lobe Collapse

Findings of lower lobe collapse are identical on the right and left.

Frontal (PA or AP) Radiograph. With moderate atelectasis, the major fissure may not be visible on the frontal radiograph (see Fig. 2-28A). With further volume loss, the major fissure rotates toward the mediastinum, resulting in the typical triangular or wedge-shaped opacity of lower lobe collapse (Table 2-8; Fig. 2-37A). Often the upper portion of the major fissure is best seen. The apex of the triangle is at the hilum, and its base is at the diaphragm. Because of the inferior pulmonary ligament, the medial surface of the lower lobe maintains its contact with the mediastinum. With total

atelectasis, a thin wedge of consolidated lung may be seen adjacent to the thoracic spine (Fig. 2-38A).

Lower lobe collapse usually results in downward displacement of the hilum (see Figs. 2-37A and 2-38A). The interlobar pulmonary artery is commonly invisible or poorly defined because of adjacent lower lobe consolidation. Obscuration of the diaphragm may be present on frontal or lateral radiographs.

TABLE 2-8. RADIOGRAPHIC FINDINGS OF LOWER LOBE ATELECTASIS
Frontal radiograph
Major fissure becomes visible (upper portion best seen).
Triangular opacity
Downward bowing of the minor fissure (right lower lobe atelectasis)
Downward displacement of the hilum
Invisibility of the interlobar pulmonary artery
Obscuration of the diaphragm
Shift of the heart
Flat-waist sign (left lower lobe atelectasis)
Lateral radiograph
Obscuration of the posterior diaphragm
Posterior bowing of the major fissure (lateral radiograph)

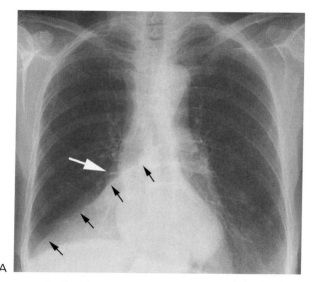

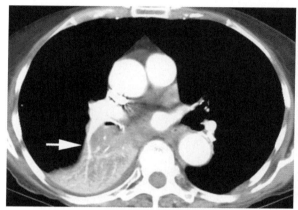

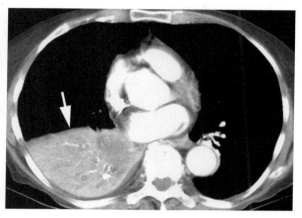

FIG. 2-37. Right lower lobe atelectasis secondary to bronchogenic carcinoma. **A.** Frontal radiograph shows the typical triangular appearance of right lower lobe atelectasis marginated by the major fissure *(black arrows).* The upper portion of the major fissure is most sharply defined. The right hilum *(white arrow)* is displaced downward, and the interlobar pulmonary artery is poorly seen. **B.** There is narrowing of the bronchus intermedius. Opacified arteries are visible within the collapsed right lower lobe. Posterior rotation of the major fissure *(arrow)* causes it to be well seen on the frontal radiograph. **C.** At a lower level, the major fissure *(arrow)* is displaced posteriorly.

Mediastinal shift is commonly present. Leftward shift and rotation of the heart may result in a straightening of the left mediastinal border, including the left heart margin, aorta, and pulmonary artery. This has been termed the "flat waist" sign (see Fig. 2-28A).

Right lower lobe atelectasis may result in downward displacement of the minor fissure seen on the frontal radiograph.

Lateral Radiograph. In its early stages, lower lobe collapse results in posterior and downward displacement of the major fissure seen on the lateral view (see Fig. 2-28B). However, with more severe atelectasis, the lateral aspect of the major fissure rotates posterior and medially, and the fissure may become invisible on the lateral view (see Fig. 2-38B). Increased density overlying the lower spine may be the only visible finding (normally the thoracic spine appears less dense in the inferior chest than at higher levels; this may not be true in the presence of lower lobe atelectasis or consolidation). On the lateral view, the hilum and bronchi may be displaced posteriorly.

CT. On CT, the major fissure rotates posteromedially from the hilum with collapse, it may be displaced posteriorly, or both (see Figs. 2-28, 2-37, and 2-38). The collapsed lobe contacts the posterior mediastinum and posteromedial chest wall and maintains contact with the medial diaphragm.

Combined Collapse of Right Middle and Lower Lobes
This occurs in patients with obstruction of the bronchus intermedius. On the frontal and lateral radiographs, both the displaced major and minor fissures may be variably visible, outlining the consolidated lung. On the frontal view, both the right heart border and diaphragm often appear obscured (Fig. 2-39). This appearance may closely mimic that of right lower lobe collapse associated with an elevated hemidiaphragm or subpulmonic pleural effusion. Absence of a visible minor fissure at a higher level and obscuration of the right heart border favors combined collapse.

Combined Collapse of Right Middle and Upper Lobes
This combination cannot be explained by a single bronchial lesion, an occurrence termed the "double lesion" sign. This

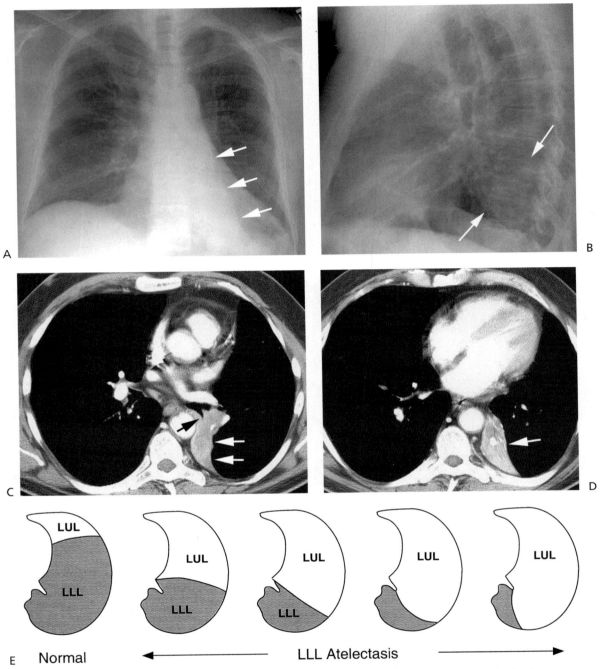

FIG. 2-38. Marked left lower lobe atelectasis secondary to bronchogenic carcinoma. **A.** On the frontal radiograph, a thin wedge of consolidated lung *(arrows)* is seen adjacent to the spine. This represents the collapsed lower lobe. The heart is displaced to the left. **B.** Lateral view shows a vague opacity in the region of the lower lobe. **C** and **D.** CT shows obstruction of the lower lobe bronchus *(black arrow)* and marked posteromedial rotation of the major fissure *(white arrows)*. **E.** Diagram of CT appearances of lower lobe atelectasis. With progressive atelectasis *(left to right)*, the major fissure rotates posteriorly.

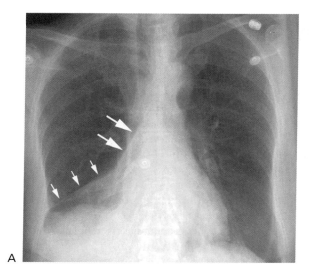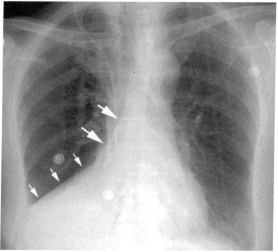

A   B

FIG. 2-39. Combined right middle and right lower lobe atelectasis. **A.** The superior aspect of the major fissure *(large arrows)* is visible, marginating the collapsed lower lobe. The major fissure merges inferiorly with the minor fissure *(small arrows)*, which is displaced inferiorly. The right middle and lower lobes remain partially aerated. **B.** One day later, both the middle and lower lobes are consolidated (drowned lung). The major *(large arrows)* and minor *(small arrows)* fissures sharply marginate consolidated (drowned) lung. Both the right heart border and diaphragm are obscured.

most commonly occurs when lung cancer involves the hilum, with invasion of the upper and middle lobe bronchi while the lower lobe bronchus remains patent, but it may also be seen with multiple isolated bronchial lesions, as in a patient with mucous plugging.

On the frontal radiograph, right upper lobe opacification obscures the right superior mediastinum while right middle lobe opacification obscures the right heart border (Fig. 2-40A). Since both lobes anterior to the major fissure are collapsed, the appearance of combined middle and upper lobe collapse on the lateral radiograph is identical to that of left upper lobe atelectasis (see Fig. 2-40B).

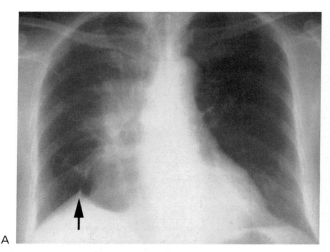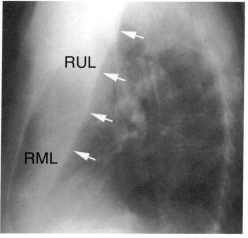

A   B

FIG. 2-40. Combined right middle and right upper lobe atelectasis in a patient with right hilar bronchogenic carcinoma. **A.** Right-sided volume loss is present with mediastinal shift to the right. The upper mediastinal contour and right heart border are partially obscured and poorly defined. The right hemidiaphragm is elevated and a juxtaphrenic peak is visible *(arrow)*. **B.** The lateral view shows anterior displacement of the major fissure *(arrows)* because of collapse of both right upper *(RUL)* and middle *(RML)* lobes. Both lobes are homogeneously consolidated. This appearance mimics that of left upper lobe collapse.

Segmental Atelectasis

Segmental (or subsegmental) atelectasis may occur secondary to obstruction of segmental (or subsegmental) bronchi by tumor, mucus, inflammatory lesions, and so forth. Typically wedge-shaped opacities are seen radiating outward from the hilum or involving the peripheral lung, with the base of the wedge touching the pleural surface. Indirect findings of volume loss are typically absent because of the small amount of lung tissue involved.

Platelike or Discoid Atelectasis

Linear areas of atelectasis, a few millimeters to 1 cm thick and at least several centimeters in length, commonly occur in patients with decreased depth of breathing or diminished diaphragmatic excursions. They tend to occur at the lung bases, several centimeters above and parallel to the diaphragm (Fig. 2-41). They cross segmental boundaries. They may also occur in the medial infrahilar regions, typically angled upward from the mediastinum at about a 45-degree angle. They are thought to occur because of decreased ventilation of lung associated with retained secretions. Bronchial obstruction is not a cause. They are of little clinical significance but serve as a marker of poor ventilatory function.

Rounded Atelectasis

The term "rounded atelectasis" refers to the presence of focal rounded lung collapse. In some patients, it is associated with invagination of the visceral pleura with folding or rolling of the collapsed lung. It usually occurs in the presence of pleural thickening or effusion, and likely results from local constriction of lung expansion. It is most commonly associated with asbestos exposure, empyema, tuberculous effusions, renal failure, and pleural neoplasm but may occur with pleural effusion of any cause. On plain radiographs, rounded atelectasis may mimic neoplasm, but its CT appearance is often characteristic.

To suggest the diagnosis of rounded atelectasis on the basis of chest radiographs or CT, the opacity should be (1) round or elliptical; (2) associated with an ipsilateral pleural

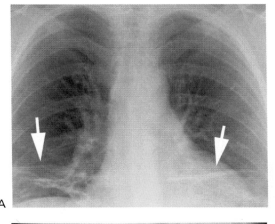
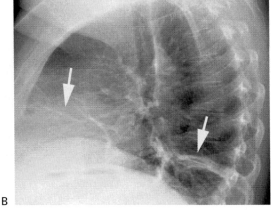
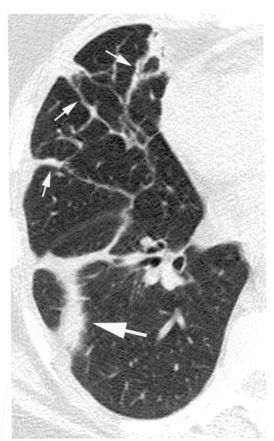

FIG. 2-41. Disk atelectasis. Frontal **(A)** and lateral **(B)** radiographs show disk atelectasis *(arrows)* at the lung bases, roughly paralleling the hemidiaphragms. **C.** HRCT at the right base shows linear areas of atelectasis *(small arrows)*. When these are oriented parallel to the plane of scan, large areas of opacity may be seen *(large arrow)*.

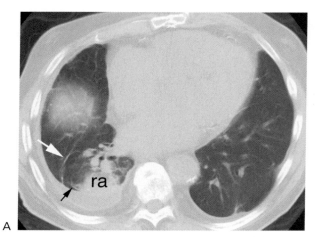
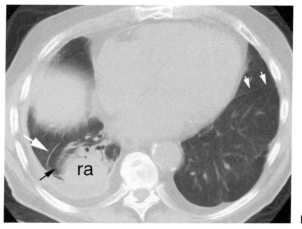

A   B

FIG. 2-42. Typical rounded atelectasis associated with pleural effusion. CT scans at two adjacent levels show characteristic findings of rounded atelectasis. An elliptical opacity is visible *(ra)*, which is peripheral in location and has significant contact with the pleural surface in contiguity with a right pleural effusion. Vessels *(small black arrows)* curve into the edge of the lesion (i.e., the so-called comet-tail sign). Posterior displacement of the major fissure *(large white arrows)* indicates volume loss in the right lower lobe. For comparison, note the location of the normal left major fissure *(small white arrows)*. Because these findings are typical, follow-up should be sufficient.

abnormality, either effusion or pleural thickening; (3) peripheral in location, having significant contact with the abnormal pleural surface; (4) associated with curving of pulmonary vessels or bronchi into the edge of the lesion (the so-called "comet-tail" sign); and (5) associated with volume loss in the affected lobe (Figs. 2-42 and 2-43; Table 2-9).

If each of these criteria for rounded atelectasis is met, a confident diagnosis can usually be made, and radiographic follow-up should be sufficient.

Rounded atelectasis is most common in the posterior lower lobes; this location is typical of patients with free pleural effusion (see Figs. 2-42 and 2-43). In patients with

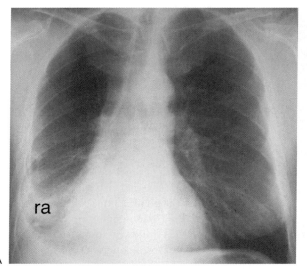
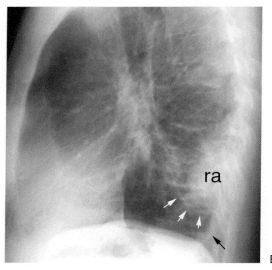

A   B

FIG. 2-43. Typical rounded atelectasis associated with pleural effusion. **A.** Frontal chest radiograph shows blunting of the right costophrenic angle due to pleural effusion. An ill-defined opacity *(ra)* at the right base represents rounded atelectasis. Note the presence of mediastinal shift to the right. **B.** On the lateral view, a well-defined elliptical opacity *(ra)* is seen posteriorly, having extensive pleural contact. This location, several centimeters above the blunted posterior costophrenic angle *(black arrow)*, is characteristic of rounded atelectasis in patients with effusion. Curving of vessels *(white arrows)* into the inferior aspect of the opacity reflects the comet-tail sign. The appearance in this case is sufficiently characteristic to allow follow-up.

TABLE 2-9. CT AND RADIOGRAPHIC FINDINGS OF ROUNDED ATELECTASIS

Round or elliptical opacity
Associated with an ipsilateral pleural abnormality
Peripheral in location
Extensive contact with the abnormal pleural surface
Comet-tail sign
Volume loss
Posterior, paravertebral lower lobe in patients with effusion
Atypical appearances when associated with pleural fibrosis
Dense opacification on CT after contrast infusion

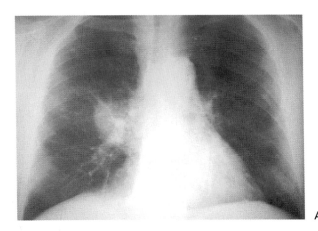

bilateral effusions, it may be bilateral or symmetrical. Rounded atelectasis in patients with pleural fibrosis may be anterior in location (Figs. 2-44 to 2-46).

On chest radiographs, posteriorly located rounded atelectasis usually appears ill defined on the frontal projection

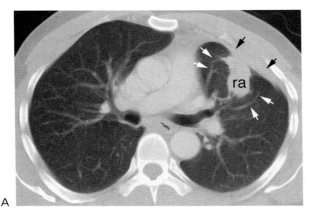

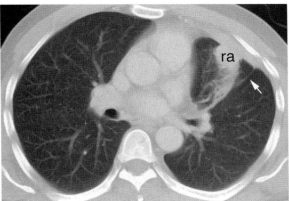

FIG. 2-44. Anterior rounded atelectasis associated with pleural fibrosis in a patient with prior tuberculosis. **A.** CT shows left pleural thickening anteriorly *(black arrows)*. The area of rounded atelectasis *(ra)* is irregular in shape but contacts the pleural surface and is associated with the comet-tail sign *(white arrows)*. **B.** At a lower level, anterior displacement of the major fissure *(white arrow)* indicates volume loss in the upper lobe.

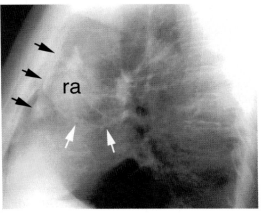

FIG. 2-45. Anterior rounded atelectasis in a patient with asbestos-related pleural thickening. **A.** Frontal chest radiograph shows a mass overlying the right hilum. This appearance suggests bronchogenic carcinoma. **B.** Lateral chest radiograph shows anterior pleural thickening and calcification *(black arrows)*. A comet-tail sign *(white arrows)* is seen adjacent to the area of rounded atelectasis *(ra)*. The area of rounded atelectasis does not appear to contact the anterior chest wall.

and well defined and elliptical on the lateral view, having extensive pleural contact. It is most often seen several centimeters above a blunted posterior costophrenic angle (see Fig. 2-43). Vessels may be seen curving into its inferior edge, representing the comet-tail sign.

Rounded atelectasis may have acute or obtuse angles where it contacts the pleura. Since rounded atelectasis represents collapsed lung parenchyma, it can show significant enhancement on CT following the intravenous injection of contrast agents. Air bronchograms may be visible within the collapsed lung.

Atypical examples of rounded atelectasis are often encountered in patients who have pleural thickening and fibrosis rather than pleural effusion (see Fig. 2-45). Such cases may show rounded atelectasis that is irregular in shape, unassociated with the comet-tail sign, separated from the pleural surface, or anterior in location.

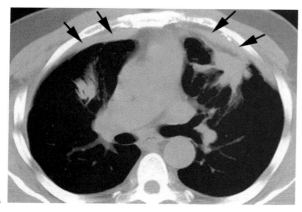 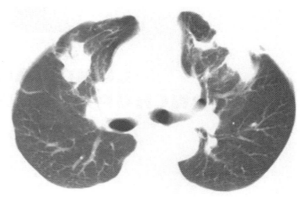

FIG. 2-46. Atypical rounded atelectasis in a patient with asbestos-related pleural thickening. **A.** CT using a soft tissue window shows anterior pleural thickening with calcification *(arrows).* Irregular lung masses are also visible. **B.** CT with a lung window setting shows bilateral masses. Although there is some evidence of the comet-tail sign on each side, the right-sided mass does not contact the pleural surface, and the left-sided mass is very irregular in contour. Biopsy of each mass was negative, and follow-up CT showed no change.

Specifically, rounded atelectasis is seen in as many as 10% of patients with asbestos exposure, usually due to visceral or parietal pleural thickening or plaques, diffuse pleural thickening, or sometimes exudative effusion, and it often appears atypical. Atypical cases of rounded atelectasis may represent a diagnostic problem because lung cancer has an increased incidence in asbestos-exposed individuals. Needle biopsy may be necessary to exclude carcinoma.

SELECTED READING

Batra P, Brown K, Hayashi K, Mori M. Rounded atelectasis. J Thorac Imag 1996; 11:187–197.

Blankenbaker DG. The luftsichel sign. Radiology 1998; 208: 319–320.

Davis SD, Yankelevitz DF, Wand A, Chiarella DA. Juxtaphrenic peak in upper and middle lobe volume loss: assessment with CT. Radiology 1996; 198:143–149.

Felson B. The roentgen diagnosis of disseminated pulmonary alveolar diseases. Semin Roentgenol 1967; 2:3–21.

Genereux GP. Pattern recognition in diffuse lung disease: a review of theory and practice. Med Radiogr Photogr 1985; 61:2–31.

Kattan KR, Wlot JF. Cardiac rotation in left lower lobe collapse: "the flat waist sign." Radiology 1976; 118:275–279.

Naidich DP, Ettinger N, Leitman BS, McCauley DI. CT of lobar collapse. Semin Roentgenol 1984; 19:222–235.

Reed JC, Madewell JE. The air bronchogram in interstitial disease of the lungs: a radiological-pathological correlation. Radiology 1975; 116:1–9.

Rohlfing BM. The shifting granuloma: an internal marker of atelectasis. Radiology 1977; 123:283–285.

Shah RM, Friedman AC. CT angiogram sign: incidence and significance in lobar consolidations evaluated by contrast-enhanced CT. AJR Am J Roentgenol 1998; 170:719–721.

Westcott JL, Cole S. Plate atelectasis. Radiology 1985; 155:1–9.

Woodring JH. The computed tomography mucous bronchogram sign. J Comput Tomogr 1988; 12:165–168.

Woodring JH, Reed JC. Types and mechanisms of pulmonary atelectasis. J Thorac Imag 1996; 11:92–108.

Woodring JH, Reed JC. Radiographic manifestations of lobar atelectasis. J Thorac Imag 1996; 11:109–144.

3

LUNG CANCER AND BRONCHOPULMONARY NEOPLASMS

W. RICHARD WEBB

LUNG CARCINOMA

Lung carcinoma is the most common fatal malignancy in both men and women. Its incidence in the United States has continued to rise since the early 1900s, and approximately 175,000 new cases of lung cancer occur yearly. The incidence of lung carcinoma is higher in men than women, but at present the incidence is decreasing in men and increasing in women.

RISK FACTORS FOR LUNG CANCER

Tobacco smoking accounts for 80% to 90% of lung cancers. In smokers, the risk of lung cancer correlates with younger age at the onset of smoking, the duration and cumulative amount of exposure, and the depth of inhalation. Heavy smoking is associated with a 20- to 30-fold increase in lung cancer risk compared to nonsmokers. A decrease in risk following smoking cessation has also been demonstrated. Well-differentiated squamous cell carcinoma, small cell carcinoma, large cell carcinoma, and to a lesser extent adenocarcinoma all demonstrate an increased incidence with increasing cigarette consumption. About 25% of lung cancers in nonsmokers have been attributed to second-hand smoke.

Increasing age is associated with an increased risk of lung cancer. Lung cancers are rare in patients under age 30.

Occupational exposures to various substances have been linked to lung cancer; as many as 10% of lung cancer cases may be due to occupational exposure. Agents associated with occupational lung cancer include arsenic, nickel, chromium, asbestos, beryllium, cadmium, chromium, mustard gas, pesticides, and radon or uranium.

Asbestos exposure is the best-recognized occupational risk for lung cancer and is the most frequent exposure in the general population (Fig. 3-1). A dose–response relationship between the severity and duration of asbestos exposure and the likelihood of developing lung cancer is well established,

although the risk of exposure depends not only on the amount of asbestos to which one is exposed but also the fiber type (increased risk with amphibole fibers), the industrial use of asbestos, the conditions of exposure, and the presence of asbestosis. The risk of lung cancer in a heavily exposed asbestos worker is about five times that of a nonexposed subject. Also, smoking is a synergistic risk in asbestos-exposed subjects: the risk of lung cancer in an asbestos worker who is a heavy smoker is about 20 times that of a nonsmoking asbestos worker and 100 times that of a nonexposed nonsmoker (Table 3-1).

Diffuse pulmonary fibrosis has been associated with a 10-fold increase in the risk of lung cancer. In addition, patients with focal lung scarring, particularly as a result of tuberculosis, can develop a carcinoma in association with areas of fibrosis or scarring. Although this is infrequent, cases of carcinoma arising in areas of scarring, so-called scar carcinoma, are encountered in clinical practice.

Chronic obstructive lung disease (chronic bronchitis and emphysema) is a risk factor for developing lung cancer, independent of cigarette smoking. In both chronic obstructive pulmonary disease (COPD) and diffuse pulmonary fibrosis, proposed mechanisms of increased cancer risk include decreased clearance of inhaled carcinogens and epithelial metaplasia.

Genetic predisposition plays a role in the development of lung cancer. In general, relatives of subjects with lung cancer have a higher risk of developing lung cancer (about twofold) than the general population. An increased risk of lung cancer has been associated with specific oncogenes, chromosome defects, specific HLA antigens, enzyme defects, and defects in proteins normally produced by tumor suppressor genes.

CELL TYPES OF LUNG CANCER

Lung carcinomas have been classified by the World Health Organization (WHO) based on their light-microscopic ap-

TABLE 3-1. INCREASED RISK OF LUNG CANCER ASSOCIATED WITH SMOKING AND ASBESTOS EXPOSURE

Risk factor	Comparison group	Relative risk
Heavy asbestos exposure	No asbestos exposure	5:1
Heavy smoking	Nonsmoker	20:1
Heavy smoking and heavy asbestos exposure	No smoking history and no asbestos exposure	100:1

pearances (Table 3-2). The large majority of lung cancers are classified by WHO criteria as one of four major histologic types: squamous cell carcinoma, adenocarcinoma, small cell carcinoma, and large cell carcinoma. Numerous subtypes of these four major tumors have also been defined, but most of these are unimportant from a radiologic or clinical standpoint.

These cell types are not absolutely distinct. As many as 50% of lung tumors have mixed appearances, and the most differentiated feature of the carcinoma is used to define its cell type. Many tumors classified as one histologic type (e.g., large cell carcinoma) using light microscopy and the WHO system would be reclassified if electron microscopy were used. Cytologic examination uncommonly allows a specific cell type to be determined; cytologic diagnosis of lung cancer is usually limited to the designation non–small cell bronchogenic carcinoma or small cell carcinoma.

Preinvasive Lesions

These lesions are dysplastic or localized and include atypical adenomatous hyperplasia, squamous dysplasia and carcinoma in situ, and diffuse idiopathic pulmonary neuroendocrine cell hyperplasia (described below along with carcinoid tumors).

Atypical adenomatous hyperplasia (AAH) represents a

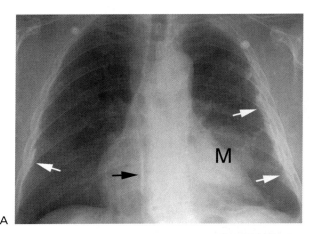

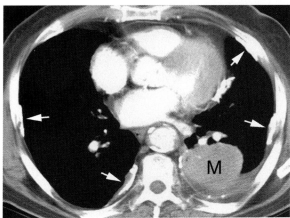

FIG. 3-1. Lung cancer associated with asbestos exposure. **A.** Chest radiograph shows a large left lung mass *(M)* representing lung cancer. Bilateral pleural thickening with calcification is also visible *(arrows)*. **B.** CT shows a left lung mass *(M)* and bilateral localized calcified pleural plaques *(arrows)* typical of asbestos exposure.

TABLE 3-2. CLASSIFICATION OF LUNG CARCINOMA AND IMPORTANT SUBTYPES FROM THE 1999 WHO CLASSIFICATION

Preinvasive lesions
   Atypical adenomatous hyperplasia
Squamous cell carcinoma
Adenocarcinoma
Bronchioloalveolar carcinoma
     Nonmucinous
     Mucinous
Small cell carcinoma
Large cell carcinoma
   Large cell neuroendocrine carcinoma
Adenosquamous carcinoma
Carcinoma with pleomorphic, sarcomatoid, or sarcomatous elements
Carcinoid tumor
   Typical carcinoid tumor
   Atypical carcinoid tumor
Carcinomas of salivary gland type
   Adenoid cystic carcinoma
   Mucoepidermoid carcinoma

(Modified from Travis WD. Pathology of lung cancer. Clin Chest Med 2002;23:65–81).

TABLE 3-3. SQUAMOUS CELL CARCINOMA

30% of lung cancer cases
Strongly associated with cigarette smoking
65% arise in main, lobar, or segmental bronchi:
  Endobronchial mass
  Bronchial obstruction
  Infiltration of bronchial wall
  Local invasion
  Hilar mass
  Atelectasis and consolidation common
30% present as solitary nodule or mass:
  Cavitation relatively common
Metastasizes late
Relatively good prognosis

benign bronchioloalveolar proliferation that resembles but does not meet the criteria for bronchioloalveolar carcinoma. Its incidence ranges from 5% to 20%. Most lesions are 5 mm or less in diameter, and lesions are often multiple. AAH is most often found incidentally in pathologic specimens but may mimic lung carcinoma radiographically (particularly on CT), leading to resection.

Squamous Cell Carcinoma

Until recently, squamous cell carcinoma was the most common cell type of lung carcinoma; it currently accounts for about 30% of cases. It is strongly associated with cigarette smoking (Table 3-3).

Squamous cell carcinoma frequently (65%) arises in main, lobar, or segmental bronchi. In this location, tumor growth results in obstruction of the bronchial lumen, infiltration of the bronchial wall, and invasion of the adjacent lung or vessels. This tumor tends to cause symptoms early in its course because of its proximal and endobronchial location and may be detected using sputum cytology before being radiographically visible. Early metastasis is uncommon, and it has a relatively good 5-year survival rate.

A polypoid endobronchial mass or bronchial obstruction is frequent (Fig. 3-2A). Hilar mass is also common due to the central location of the tumor, with local invasion and involvement of hilar lymph nodes (see Fig. 3-2B). Atelectasis (Fig. 3-3), consolidation, mucoid impaction, and bronchiectasis are common radiographic findings, reflecting the presence of bronchial obstruction (see Table 3-3). Only about 30% of squamous cell carcinomas present in the lung

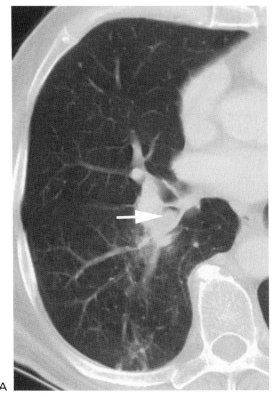
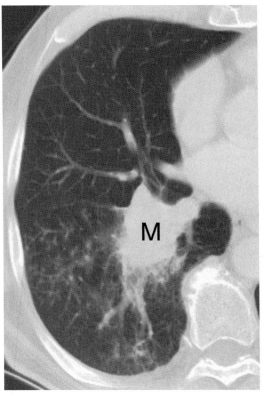

A   B

FIG. 3-2. Squamous cell carcinoma with an endobronchial and hilar mass. **A.** CT shows a polypoid mass *(arrows)* within the right lower lobe bronchus, typical of squamous cell carcinoma. **B.** At a slightly lower level, the bronchial lumen appears obstructed and local invasion has resulted in a hilar mass *(M).*

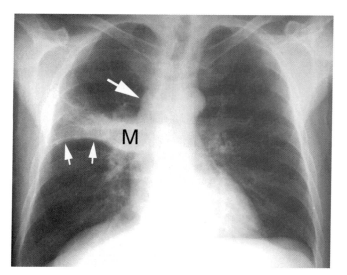

FIG. 3-3. Squamous cell carcinoma with bronchial obstruction and atelectasis. Chest radiograph shows a right hilar mass *(M)* with upward bowing of the minor fissure *(small arrows)*. This combination results in Golden's S sign. Mediastinal lymph node enlargement is also present *(large arrow)*.

periphery as a lung nodule. Central necrosis and cavitation (Fig. 3-4) are more common than with other cell types.

Adenocarcinoma

Adenocarcinoma is the most common cell type of lung cancer and accounts for 30% to 35% of lung cancer cases (Table 3-4). As with squamous cell cancer, it is related to cigarette smoking, although its association with smoking is relatively weak. Adenocarcinoma is thought to arise from bronchiolar

TABLE 3-4. ADENOCARCINOMA

30%–35% of lung cancer cases (most common cell type)
Weak association with smoking
Early metastases common
75% present as peripheral lung nodule
Common in the upper lobes
Associated with lung fibrosis
Often appear spiculated

or alveolar epithelium and is characterized by glandular differentiation. Early metastasis is more common than with squamous cell carcinoma, particularly to the central nervous system and adrenal glands. Seventy-five percent originate in the lung periphery, presenting as a solitary pulmonary nodule (Fig. 3-5). In a few cases, adenocarcinoma originates within large airways. It is most common in the upper lobes. It is often associated with fibrosis; it may arise in relation to preexisting lung fibrosis (i.e., a scar carcinoma) or may result in a desmoplastic reaction in surrounding lung.

Adenocarcinomas often appear ill defined on chest radiographs because of their irregular margin (see Fig. 3-5A). On high-resolution CT, adenocarcinoma presenting as a solitary nodule may appear round or lobulated. They frequently have an irregular and spiculated margin because of associated lung fibrosis (see Fig. 3-5B). When occurring in a subpleural location, this may result in thin linear extensions to the pleural surface (i.e., a *pleural tail*; see Fig. 3-5C). Air bronchograms may be visible within the nodule using CT; although central necrosis is common, cavitation visible on radiographs or CT is uncommon. When adenocarcinoma arises from the wall of a central bronchus, it is radiographically indistinguishable from squamous cell carcinoma.

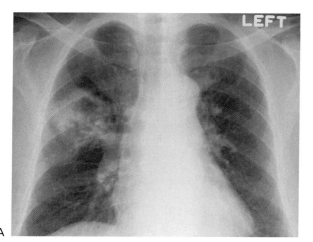

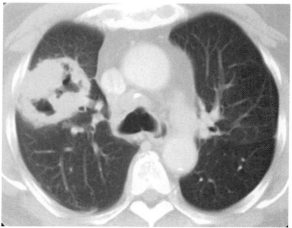

A   B

FIG. 3-4. Squamous cell carcinoma with a cavitary lung mass. **A.** On a chest radiograph, a large, thick-walled cavitary mass is visible in the right upper lobe. **B.** CT shows the cavity to have a thick and nodular wall. This is typical of cavitary carcinoma. This would be considered a T2 carcinoma.

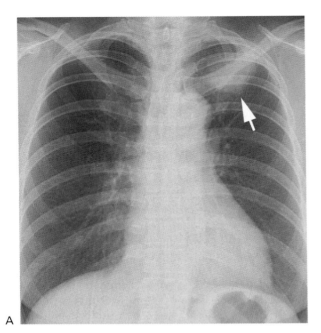

A

FIG. 3-5. Typical appearances of adenocarcinoma. **A.** Chest radiograph in a patient with adenocarcinoma shows an ill-defined nodule in the left lung apex *(arrow)*. Adenocarcinomas often appear ill defined on radiographs because of their irregular and spiculated edge. **B.** High-resolution CT in a patient with adenocarcinoma in the left upper lobe shows a solitary lung nodule with an irregular and spiculated edge. Spiculation usually results from lung fibrosis associated with the tumor. This tumor would be classified as a T1 carcinoma in the lung cancer staging system. **C.** High-resolution CT in a patient with adenocarcinoma presenting as a solitary nodule in the posterior right upper lobe. The nodule appears lobulated and spiculated. Extensions to the pleural surface *(arrows)* are termed *pleural tails*. They result from fibrosis with a puckering of the visceral pleural surface.

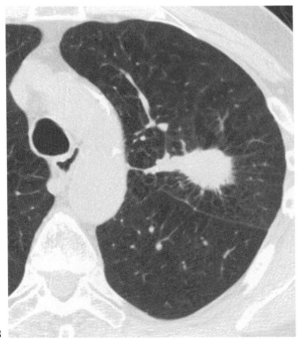

B

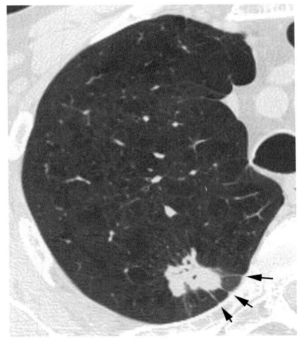

C

Bronchioloalveolar Carcinoma

Bronchioloalveolar carcinoma (BAC) is a well-differentiated subtype of adenocarcinoma that also tends to occur in the lung periphery (Table 3-5). In the current WHO classification, BAC is defined as unassociated with invasion of pleura, vessels, or lung stroma. Using this restrictive definition, BAC is relatively uncommon, accounting for fewer than 5% of lung malignancies. It has a very good prognosis when localized, with a 5-year survival rate approaching 100%.

BAC spreads as a thin layer of cells, using the alveolar or bronchiolar walls as a framework or scaffold. This pattern of growth is termed *lepidic*. Other types of adenocarcinoma usually invade and destroy lung parenchyma as they grow, a pattern termed *hilic*.

TABLE 3-5. BRONCHIOLOALVEOLAR CARCINOMA

Subtype of adenocarcinoma
Noninvasive tumor characterized by lepidic growth
60% present as a solitary nodule
   Usually nonmucinous cell type
   Ill-defined nodule of ground-glass opacity
   Air bronchograms and cystic areas (pseudocavitation)
   Excellent prognosis
40% appear as diffuse or patchy consolidation and/or nodules
   Mucinous cell type
   Lung consolidation due to mucus filling alveoli
   CT angiogram sign
   Poor prognosis

Nonmucinous and **mucinous** subtypes of BAC occur in about equal numbers. These cell types correlate with radiographic appearance.

BAC most commonly presents as solitary nodule (60%) and radiographically may be indistinguishable from adenocarcinoma. BAC presenting as a solitary nodule is usually the nonmucinous subtype of BAC. Because of its lepidic growth pattern, radiographs and CT usually show a very ill-defined nodule (Fig. 3-6), often of ground-glass opacity (Fig. 3-7), containing air bronchograms or bubbly lucencies. The bubbly lucencies represent cystic air-filled areas within the tumor termed pseudocavitation (see Fig. 3-6B).

In 40% of cases, BAC presents with diffuse or multifocal lung involvement having the appearance of lung consolidation or multiple ill-defined nodules (Figs. 3-8 and 3-9; see Fig. 3-22). This appearance is typical of the mucinous subtype of BAC. It is unclear whether this pattern results from multicentric origin of the tumor or endobronchial spread of the neoplasm. Although lepidic growth is present in such patients, with tumor cells lining alveolar walls, mucin produced by the tumor fills the alveoli, resulting in the radiographic appearance of consolidation. The CT angiogram sign, in which opacified vessels are visible within consolidated lung, is often seen if CT is obtained with contrast infusion (see Chapter 2). Such patients can present with profuse watery sputum production, termed *bronchorrhea,* as a result of extensive mucin production. Diffuse bronchioloalveolar carcinoma has a poor prognosis.

Small Cell Carcinoma

Small cell carcinoma is the third most common histologic variety of primary lung cancer (15% to 20% of cases) and is made up of small cells, similar in size to lymphocytes, that have scanty cytoplasm (Table 3-6). It is thought to originate from neuroendocrine cells, and electron microscopy shows neurosecretory granules in many cases of small cell carcinoma. Along with carcinoid tumor and atypical carcinoid tumor, small cell carcinoma is considered to be a

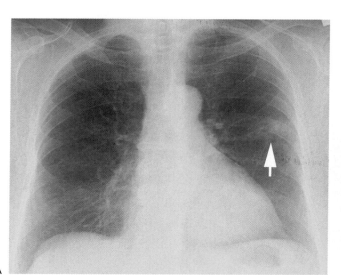
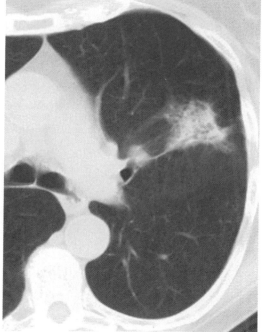

FIG. 3-6. Focal bronchioloalveolar carcinoma (BAC). **A.** Chest radiograph shows a very ill-defined nodule *(arrow)* in the left lung. **B.** CT with 5-mm slice thickness shows an ill-defined, irregular, spiculated nodule, containing both air bronchograms and bubbly lucencies. This appearance is typical of focal BAC.

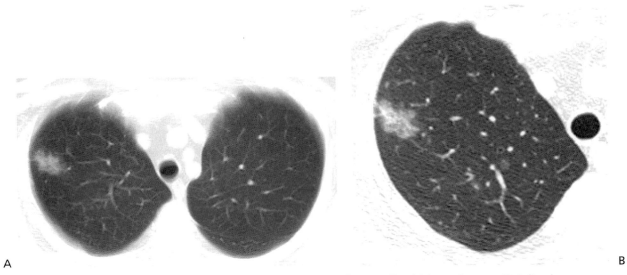

A   B

FIG. 3-7. Focal bronchioloalveolar carcinoma. **A.** CT with 5-mm slice thickness shows an ill-defined nodule. **B.** High-resolution CT shows the nodule to be largely of ground-glass opacity. This appearance is typical of carcinoma having lepidic growth.

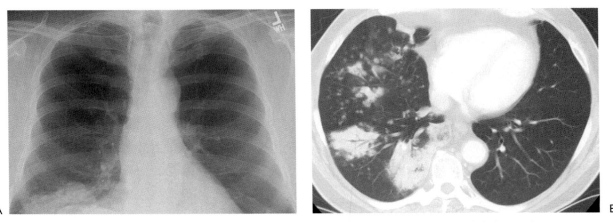

A   B

FIG. 3-8. Diffuse bronchioloalveolar carcinoma. **A.** Chest radiograph shows consolidation at the right lung base. **B.** CT with 5-mm slice thickness shows multiple areas of consolidation, with air bronchograms, and numerous ill-defined nodules. These nodules are typically centrilobular; they represent air-space or acinar nodules and are common with diffuse bronchioloaveolar carcinoma.

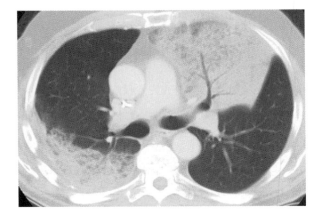

FIG. 3-9. Diffuse bronchioloalveolar carcinoma involving both upper lobes, with air-space consolidation and air bronchograms.

TABLE 3-6. SMALL CELL CARCINOMA

15%–20% of lung cancers
Strongly associated with smoking
Neuroendocrine carcinoma
Paraneoplastic syndromes commonly associated
Most occur in main or lobar bronchi
Extensive peribronchial invasion
Large hilar or parahilar mass
Bronchial narrowing
Lymph node enlargement
Metastases at diagnosis in >90%
Prognosis very poor

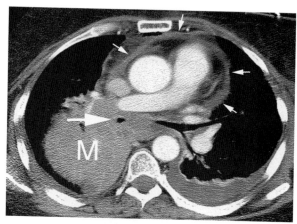

FIG. 3-11. Small cell carcinoma. Contrast-enhanced CT shows a large hilar mass *(M)*. Tumor surrounds and narrows the bronchus intermedius *(large arrow)* and extends into the subcarinal space. Pericardial thickening *(small arrows)* is likely due to local invasion. A left pleural effusion is also present.

type of *neuroendocrine carcinoma* and is described further below. It is a common cause of paraneoplastic syndromes. It is strongly associated with smoking.

Small cell carcinoma tends to occur in the main or lobar bronchi and is associated with extensive peribronchial invasion and a large hilar or parahilar mass (Fig. 3-10). Endobronchial tumor masses are less common than with squamous cell carcinoma, but the large tumor mass frequently compresses bronchi (Fig. 3-11). Atelectasis may be associated. This tumor is commonly associated with marked mediastinal lymph node enlargement (Fig. 3-12). It is a common cause of superior vena cava (SVC) syndrome. Presentation as a lung nodule is very uncommon, accounting for less than 5% of cases.

Although the tumor is relatively radiosensitive, its prognosis is very poor because of the frequent presence of distant metastases at the time of diagnosis. Small cell lung cancer is not generally considered amenable to surgical treatment. Over 90% of cases are stage IV at diagnosis. Reported cases of small cell carcinoma that present as lung nodules or masses, and that have been cured at surgery, may in fact represent misclassified cases of atypical carcinoid.

Large Cell Carcinoma

The term large cell carcinoma is used to describe tumors that do not show squamous or adenomatous differentiation or have typical features of small cell carcinoma. Distinction from poorly differentiated squamous cell or adenocarcinoma can be difficult, and in fact many cases classified as large cell carcinoma on the basis of light microscopy are reclassified as other cell types if electron microscopy is used.

Large cell carcinoma accounts for 10% of lung cancers (Table 3-7). It tends to present as a large peripheral mass; more than 60% are larger than 4 cm at presentation (Fig. 3-13). It is similar to adenocarcinoma in its radiologic characteristics (except for its large size), histologic ultrastructure, and survival statistics. As with adenocarcinoma, it tends to

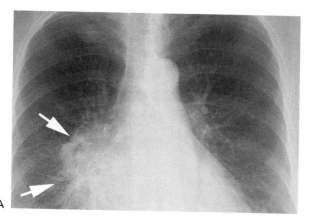

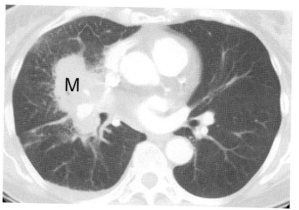

FIG. 3-10. Small cell carcinoma. **A.** Chest radiograph show a large right hilar mass *(arrows)*. **B.** CT shows the large mass *(M)*. Interstitial thickening characterized by interlobular septal thickening in the middle lobe indicates local lymphangitic spread of tumor.

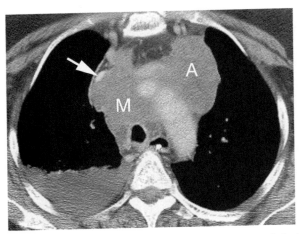

FIG. 3-12. Small cell carcinoma. CT following contrast infusion shows extensive mediastinal lymph node enlargement typical of small cell carcinoma. The superior vena cava *(arrow)* is displaced anteriorly and markedly narrowed by lymph node mass *(M)* in the pretracheal space. A large anterior mediastinal lymph node mass *(A)* is also visible. A right pleural effusion is also present.

metastasize early and has a poor prognosis. It is strongly associated with smoking.

Large cell neuroendocrine carcinoma is an important subtype of large cell carcinoma, differing histologically from other neuroendocrine tumors such as small cell carcinoma and atypical carcinoid tumor. As with small cell carcinoma, it has a very poor prognosis.

Adenosquamous Carcinoma

Adenosquamous carcinoma has mixed histologic characteristics of both adenocarcinoma and squamous cell carcinoma.

TABLE 3-7. LARGE CELL CARCINOMA

10% of lung cancers
Strongly associated with smoking
Overlap with other cell types
Usually present as a large peripheral mass (>4 cm)
Metastasizes early
Prognosis poor

If light microscopy is used for classification, adenosquamous carcinoma accounts for a few percent of lung cancers at most. If electron microscopy is used, as many as one third of all lung cancers have mixed characteristics. These tumors usually present as masses in the lung periphery and are indistinguishable from adenocarcinoma or large cell carcinoma. Metastases are common. Adenosquamous carcinomas are aggressive and have a poor prognosis.

Carcinoma With Pleomorphic, Sarcomatoid, or Sarcomatous Features

This disparate group of tumors includes those characterized pathologically by a combination of epithelial and mesenchymal tissues (e.g., giant cell carcinoma, carcinosarcoma, pulmonary blastoma). These tumors are rare and may present as polypoid endobronchial masses or large lung masses. Their prognosis is poor.

Carcinoid Tumor

Carcinoid tumor originates from neuroendocrine cells in the bronchial wall. It is classified as typical or atypical carci-

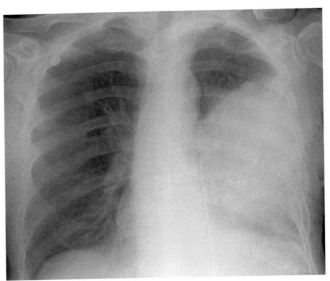

A

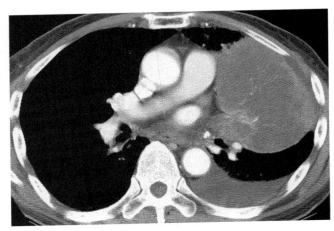

B

FIG. 3-13. Large cell carcinoma. **A.** Chest radiograph shows a large left lung mass. **B.** On contrast-enhanced CT, a large mass occupies the left lung. A left pleural effusion is also present.

noid tumor. *Typical carcinoid tumor* is a low-grade malignancy and accounts for a few percent of all primary lung malignancies. This tumor most often occurs in the central bronchi, resulting in an endobronchial mass, and is locally invasive. Metastases are relatively uncommon. *Atypical carcinoid tumor* is a more aggressive variant and has a poorer prognosis. Typical carcinoid tumor, atypical carcinoid tumor, large cell neuroendocrine carcinoma, and small cell carcinoma are considered to be different types of neuroendocrine carcinoma. Carcinoid tumors are discussed in detail below because of their distinct clinical and radiographic appearances.

Carcinomas of Salivary Gland Type

Salivary gland type carcinomas, also referred to as bronchial gland carcinomas, include adenoid cystic carcinoma (cylindroma) and mucoepidermoid carcinoma. These are similar to salivary gland tumors in their histologic characteristics and arise from glands in the tracheal or bronchial wall. These tumors account for much less than 1% of tracheobronchial malignancies. As with carcinoid tumors, they are locally invasive and uncommonly metastasize, and are discussed in detail below.

RADIOGRAPHIC APPEARANCES OF LUNG CANCER

In most patients with lung cancer, the findings on chest radiographs are sufficiently characteristic to suggest the diagnosis and lead to appropriate clinical and imaging evaluation. Although lung cancer can manifest in a variety of ways, a short list of radiographic abnormalities is commonly seen. These abnormalities reflect the location and manner in which lung cancer arises and the sites to which it most commonly spreads. Such abnormalities include the presence of a lung nodule, evidence of bronchial obstruction with collapse or consolidation of a lobe or lung, a hilar or mediastinal mass, and benign or malignant pleural effusion.

Although the frequency of these findings varies according to the cell type of the tumor (Table 3-8), each of the four major cell types of lung carcinoma (squamous cell carcinoma, adenocarcinoma, small cell carcinoma, large cell carcinoma) can show similar findings. Radiographic findings associated with carcinoid tumor and the bronchial gland carcinomas are discussed later in this chapter because of their somewhat different biological behavior and x-ray appearances.

Solitary Pulmonary Nodule or Mass

Approximately one third of lung cancers present radiographically as a solitary pulmonary nodule or lung mass.

A solitary pulmonary nodule (see Figs. 3-5 to 3-7) is usually defined as being visible as a focal opacity on chest radiographs or CT and is:

1. Relatively well defined
2. At least partially surrounded by lung
3. Roughly spherical
4. 3 cm or less in diameter

Similar lesions larger than 3 cm in diameter are usually referred to using the term *mass* (see Figs. 3-1, 3-4, and 3-13). This measurement is also used to distinguish a T1 carcinoma (3 cm or less in diameter) from a T2 carcinoma (larger than 3 cm).

Among lung cancers presenting as a solitary nodule or mass, the most common cell types are adenocarcinoma (40% of cases), squamous cell carcinoma (20%), large cell carcinoma (15%), and bronchioloalveolar carcinoma (10%). Since bronchioloalveolar carcinoma is considered to be a subtype of adenocarcinoma, adenocarcinomas account for half of cases (see Figs. 3-5 to 3-7). Large cell carcinoma typically results in a mass (see Fig. 3-13) that at diagnosis is larger than that seen with other cell types, averaging nearly twice the diameter of adenocarcinoma or bronchioloalveolar carcinoma. Small cell carcinoma uncommonly results in a solitary nodule.

Lung cancers presenting as a solitary pulmonary nodule may have specific radiographic appearances that suggest the

---

TABLE 3-8. PLAIN RADIOLOGIC FINDINGS IN LUNG CANCER BY CELL TYPE[a]

Finding	Squamous	Adenocarcinoma	Small cell	Large cell
Peripheral nodule or mass	30%	**75%**	15%	**65%**
Atelectasis	**40%**	10%	20%	15%
Consolidation	20%	15%	20%	25%
Hilar enlargement	**40%**	20%	**80%**	30%
Mediastinal mass	<5%	<5%	**15%**	**10%**
Pleural effusions	5%	5%	5%	5%
No abnormalities	5%	<5%	0%	0%
Multiple abnormalities	35%	30%	65%	45%

[a] Boldface findings are those most helpful in differentiating cell types. Percentages are approximate.

TABLE 3-9. RADIOGRAPHIC CHARACTERISTICS OF LUNG CANCER PRESENTING AS A SOLITARY PULMONARY NODULE

Diameter >2 cm
Most common in the upper lobes
Ill-defined, irregular, or spiculated margin
Lobulated or irregular in shape
Containing air bronchograms or bubbly lucencies
    (pseudocavitation)
Cavitation with a thick (>15 mm) and nodular wall
Cavitation without an air-fluid level
Satellite nodules absent
Calcification absent or not typical of benign disease
Enhancement of ≥15 HU following contrast infusion
Doubling time of 30–200 days

diagnosis (Table 3-9); if a combination of radiologic, clinical, and laboratory information is used, malignant pulmonary nodules can be diagnosed in over 90% of patients. The radiographic assessment of a solitary pulmonary nodule is a common and important problem; this topic is discussed

in greater detail in Chapter 9. The differential diagnosis of a solitary nodule is reviewed in Table 9-1 in Chapter 9.

Superior Sulcus (Pancoast) Tumor

Tumors arising at or near the lung apex are termed *superior sulcus carcinoma, thoracic inlet carcinoma,* or simply *apical carcinoma.* The term **Pancoast tumor** is best reserved for patients with some (although not necessarily all) manifestations of the Pancoast syndrome. Approximately 5% of lung cancers occur in the superior sulcus; any cell type may be responsible.

Superior sulcus tumors are commonly associated with symptoms because of their propensity to invade structures in the thoracic inlet, including the brachial plexus, cervicothoracic sympathetic ganglia, subclavian artery and vein (Fig. 3-14), and vertebral column. Pancoast syndrome results from involvement of the brachial plexus and sympathetic ganglia and consists of the combination of:

1. Pain in the shoulder
2. Radicular pain along the distribution of the eighth cervi-

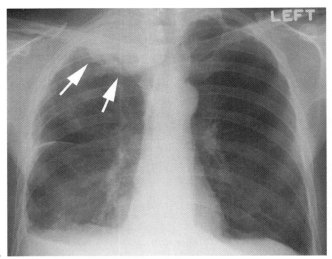

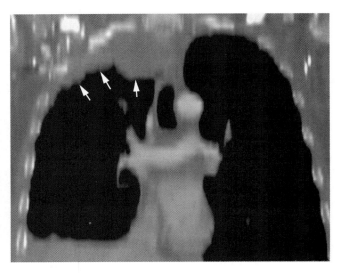

FIG. 3-14. Superior sulcus tumor. **A.** Chest radiograph shows a mass *(arrows)* at the right lung apex. **B.** CT following contrast injection via the right arm shows the tumor *(T)* occupying the lung apex. Obstruction of the right subclavian vein *(arrow)* is associated with numerous venous collaterals in the chest wall. **C.** Coronal CT reformation shows the apical mass *(arrows)* extending along the chest wall.

cal and first and second thoracic nerves, sometimes associated with wasting of the small muscles of the hand
3. Horner's syndrome, consisting of ptosis, miosis, and hemifacial anhidrosis

Classic Pancoast syndrome is uncommon. Most superior sulcus tumors present with shoulder or scapular pain that radiates down the arm and may be associated with ulnar neuropathy. Horner's syndrome is present in only about 25% of patients; atrophy or weakness of the hand muscles is uncommon. Rib or vertebral body invasion is common in patients with superior sulcus tumors.

Radiographic findings include an apical mass (60%; see Fig. 3-14), unilateral or asymmetrical apical pleural thickening ("apical cap," 40%; Fig. 3-15), and bone destruction (25%). Asymmetry in the thickness of an apical cap exceeding 5 mm is considered suggestive. The presence of an apical cap may reflect diseases other than carcinoma (Table 3-10).

Superior sulcus carcinomas, even if invasive, can be treated using a combination of radiation and en bloc resection of the tumor and adjacent chest wall; 5-year survival rates as high as 30% have been reported using this approach. Contraindications to this combined therapy generally include (1) tumor involvement of the great vessels above the lung apex, principally the subclavian artery or vein; (2) extensive brachial plexus invasion; (3) extensive vertebral body or spinal canal invasion; (4) clinical evidence of recurrent laryngeal nerve or phrenic nerve involvement; (5) involvement of the mediastinum, including the trachea or esophagus; and (6) distant metastases. Some patients may have restaging of such an extensive tumor following chemotherapy to determine whether resection is possible.

MRI in the sagittal or coronal planes is advantageous in imaging apical tumors. It is more accurate than CT in diagnosing apical chest wall invasion and its extent. MRI is often obtained preoperatively in patients with superior

sulcus carcinoma to define the relationship of the tumor to great vessels and the brachial plexus (Fig. 3-16). The radiographic assessment of chest wall invasion and superior sulcus tumor is discussed in detail in the section on lung cancer staging below.

Airway Abnormalities

Airway abnormalities are common in lung cancer. The segmental bronchi are most often involved by the primary tumor, followed in frequency by the lobar bronchi and the main bronchi. The trachea is rarely involved as the site of origin.

Radiographs or CT can show evidence of bronchial narrowing or obstruction, or abnormalities that produce secondary bronchial obstruction, such as mucous plugging, air trapping, atelectasis, or obstructive pneumonia. Although lung cancer is a common cause of bronchial obstruction, the differential diagnosis is long and should be kept in mind (Table 3-11).

TABLE 3-10. DIFFERENTIAL DIAGNOSIS: APICAL CAP/APICAL MASS

Normal apical cap: Unilateral or bilateral apical caps, usually <5 mm in thickness, are each seen in 10% of normals on chest radiographs. These represent apical lung scars unassociated with tuberculosis, although their etiology is unclear.

Extrapleural fat: Extrapleural fat deposition can result in smooth, symmetrical apical caps. This can be seen in normals, obese patients, and patients with Cushing's syndrome or those receiving steroids.

Inflammatory disease (tuberculosis): Apical caps associated with inflammatory disease (particularly TB) are rarely the only abnormality visible. Associated upper lobe fibrosis, volume loss, lung destruction, or other evidence of inflammatory disease is usually present. The cap is often quite irregular in appearance because of adjacent lung abnormalities and in one study ranged from 5 to 27 mm in thickness (mean 16.5 mm). In patients with TB, thickened extrapleural fat accounts for most of the apical cap, variably associated with thickening of the pleura and atelectatic lung.

Superior sulcus carcinoma

Neural tumor or other posterior mediastinal mass: These are typically localized masses.

Mesothelioma: Diffuse pleural thickening is often seen.

Mediastinal hemorrhage: Mediastinal blood can dissect laterally in the extrapleural space over the lung apex, resulting in a smooth apical cap. This can be seen with traumatic aortic rupture and is more common on the left.

Radiation fibrosis: Radiation therapy can result in apical lung fibrosis mimicking an apical cap. This is most common following head and neck or supraclavicular node radiation.

Peripheral upper lobe collapse: Peripheral upper lobe collapse is said to be present when the peripheral part of a collapsed upper lobe is pancaked against the apical pleural surface (see Fig. 2–34). It has been reported in a variety of conditions, including inflammatory diseases and bronchial obstruction.

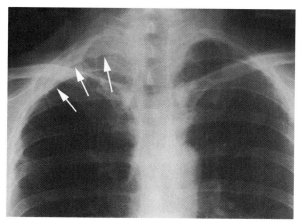

FIG. 3-15. Superior sulcus tumor appearing as an apical cap. A right apical Pancoast tumor *(arrows)* mimics pleural thickening. The underlying second rib is partially destroyed.

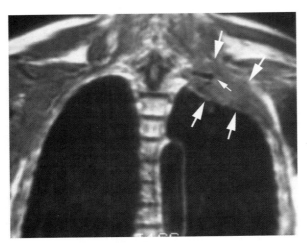

FIG. 3-16. MRI of superior sulcus tumor. Coronal T1-weighted image shows an apical mass with extension into the chest wall *(large arrows)*. The mass surrounds the left subclavian artery *(small arrow)*.

Bronchial Abnormalities

Bronchial abnormalities sometimes can be recognized on chest radiographs in patients with lung cancer, but CT is much more sensitive. Abnormalities include:

1. Narrowing or tapering of the bronchial lumen, a finding that reflects the tendency of lung carcinomas to infiltrate

---

TABLE 3-11. DIFFERENTIAL DIAGNOSIS OF BRONCHIAL NARROWING OR OBSTRUCTION

Congenital (bronchial atresia, bronchogenic cyst, cartilage deficiency)
Primary malignant tumor
  Lung carcinoma
  Carcinoid and atypical carcinoid
  Salivary gland type carcinoma
  Sarcoma
Metastatic tumor
Lymphoma
Benign bronchial tumor (e.g., hamartoma)
Papilloma or papillomatosis
Granulomas
  Infectious (e.g., tuberculosis, fungal infection)
  Noninfectious (e.g., sarcoidosis, Wegener's granulomatosis)
Inflammatory stricture (many causes)
Malacia
  Postinflammatory
Polychondritis
Foreign body
Mucous plug
Infiltrative diseases (e.g., amyloidosis)
Compression by enlarged lymph nodes (many causes)
Broncholithiasis
Traumatic hematoma or bronchial fracture
Postoperative (e.g., lung transplantation)

---

along the bronchial wall (Fig. 3-17A); a tapered narrowing, or "rat-tail," appearance of the bronchial lumen is highly suggestive of carcinoma.
2. Sharp cutoff of the bronchial lumen (see Fig. 3-17B)
3. An endobronchial mass, sessile, irregular, or polypoid in appearance (see Figs. 3-2A and 3-17C)
4. Bronchial wall thickening, most easily seen involving the posterior wall of the right upper lobe bronchus or bronchus intermedius (see Figs. 3-17D and 3-24B)
5. Smooth luminal narrowing caused by bronchial wall infiltration or bronchial compression by an extrinsic mass (see Figs. 3-17E and 3-24B).

CT is commonly used to identify bronchial abnormalities in patients with lung cancer, in conjunction with bronchoscopy. CT can serve to identify the bronchi involved by the mass, thus guiding bronchoscopy, and can better assess the presence and degree of tumor extension outside the bronchus.

Generally speaking, the CT findings of an endobronchial lesion, an abrupt bronchial occlusion, or bronchial wall irregularities correlate closely with what is seen at bronchoscopy, but the appearances of smooth luminal narrowing or tapered bronchial occlusion can be seen with either endobronchial disease or extrinsic mass.

Mucous Plugging

Rarely, an obstructing or partially obstructing tumor causes retention of mucus distal to the obstruction, while the lobe remains aerated because of collateral ventilation. This can result in a mucous plug or plugs visible on radiographs or CT (Fig. 3-18). It can be recognized on plain film or CT by its typical branching, "finger-in-a-glove," or clustered-grape appearance. On CT, mucous plugs appear low in attenuation.

More common causes of mucous plugging include asthma, allergic bronchopulmonary aspergillosis, and cystic fibrosis. In patients with these diseases, however, mucous plugs are usually multiple and bilateral. In a patient with focal mucous plugging, bronchoscopy is advisable to rule out an obstructing lesion. In addition to lung cancer, focal mucous plugging can result from benign tumors, strictures, or congenital bronchial atresia.

Air Trapping

An obstructing or partially obstructing carcinoma rarely causes air trapping within the lung distal to the tumor. If a lobar bronchus is involved, the volume of the lobe may be increased. If the lesion involves a main bronchus, the distal lung is of normal or slightly decreased volume on inspiration, but on expiration air trapping will be recognized. In some patients, air trapping can be detected because of hypovascularity of the involved lobe or lung; poorly ventilated lung tends to be poorly perfused.

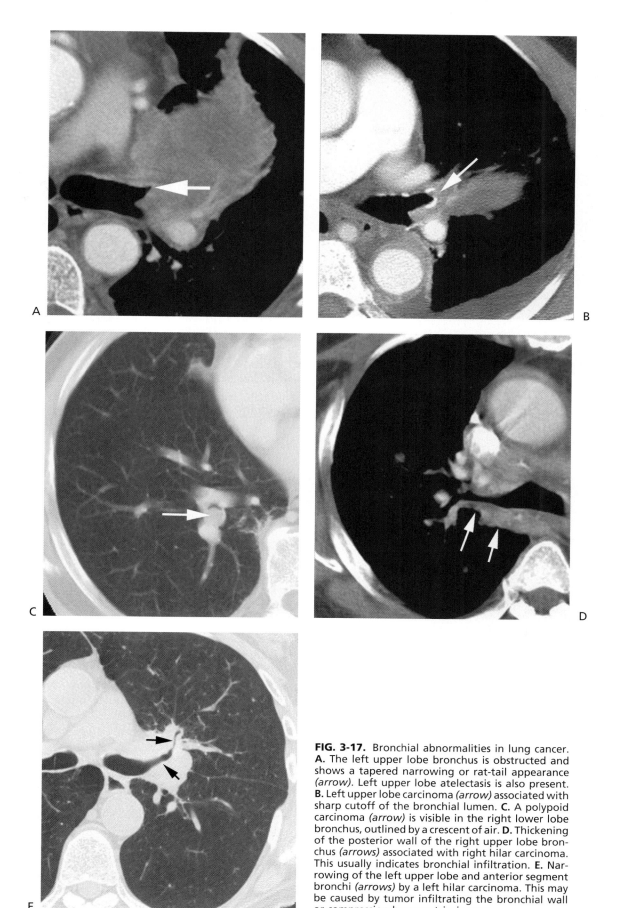

FIG. 3-17. Bronchial abnormalities in lung cancer. **A.** The left upper lobe bronchus is obstructed and shows a tapered narrowing or rat-tail appearance *(arrow)*. Left upper lobe atelectasis is also present. **B.** Left upper lobe carcinoma *(arrow)* associated with sharp cutoff of the bronchial lumen. **C.** A polypoid carcinoma *(arrow)* is visible in the right lower lobe bronchus, outlined by a crescent of air. **D.** Thickening of the posterior wall of the right upper lobe bronchus *(arrows)* associated with right hilar carcinoma. This usually indicates bronchial infiltration. **E.** Narrowing of the left upper lobe and anterior segment bronchi *(arrows)* by a left hilar carcinoma. This may be caused by tumor infiltrating the bronchial wall or compression by an extrinsic mass.

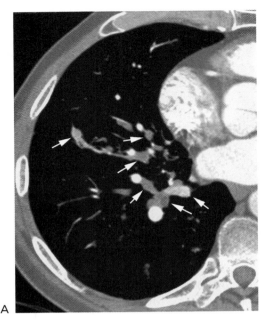

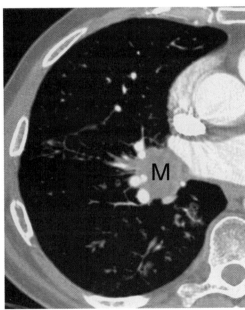

FIG. 3-18. Mucous plugs in a patient with carcinoma and bronchial obstruction. **A.** Mucous plugs *(arrows)* fill lower lobe bronchi. Note that the mucus-filled bronchi lie adjacent to opacified pulmonary arteries. The distal lung remains aerated. **B.** At a higher level, a hilar mass *(M)* is associated with obstruction of the right lower lobe bronchus.

Tracheal Carcinoma

Less than 1% of lung carcinomas arise in the trachea. Squamous cell carcinoma and carcinomas of mucous gland origin (adenoid cystic carcinoma) occur in nearly equal numbers. Squamous cell carcinomas arise most commonly in the distal trachea (Fig. 3-19), near the carina, and may cause ob-

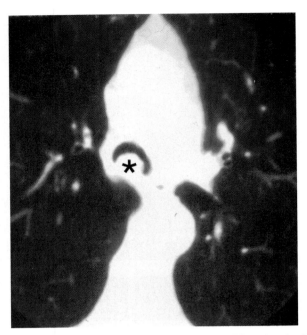

FIG. 3-19. Polypoid squamous cell carcinoma *(*)* arising in the distal trachea.

struction of a main bronchus; adenoid cystic carcinoma is most common in the proximal trachea and often arises from the posterior or lateral tracheal wall.

Radiographic studies may be important in suggesting the diagnosis, because symptoms are often late and nonspecific. Radiographic findings are similar to those seen with tumors affecting the bronchi. However, findings of obstructive pneumonitis or air trapping are not seen unless there is secondary involvement of a main bronchus. Focal tracheal narrowing associated with thickening of the right paratracheal stripe, a focal endotracheal lesion, or mediastinal mass are most commonly seen (Fig. 3-20A). Invasion of the mediastinum may occur. If the mass extends posteriorly, esophageal obstruction can result (see Fig. 3-20B). If a tracheal lesion is suspected on plain radiographs, evaluation using CT and bronchoscopy is appropriate. Surgery can be curative if the diagnosis is made prior to mediastinal invasion. Tracheal tumors are also discussed on pages in Chapter 22.

Atelectasis, Consolidation, and Diffuse Parenchymal Involvement

Atelectasis and Consolidation. Almost half of all lung cancers demonstrate atelectasis and/or consolidation as a result of obstruction of the lobar, main, or segmental bronchi. Atelectasis is common; a segment, lobe, or entire lung may be involved (see Fig. 3-3). Infection with pneumonia or lung abscess can also result.

The degree of volume loss associated with obstructive

bronchial obstruction in lung cancer and is visible in about 35% of patients with squamous cell carcinoma. This term refers to the presence of obstructive atelectasis, bronchial dilatation and mucous plugging, fibrosis, and parenchymal consolidation by lipid-filled macrophages and inflammatory cells. This entity is sometimes referred to as *endogenous lipoid pneumonia* or *golden pneumonia* because of its yellow color at gross pathology. Infection need not be present. On chest radiographs, lung consolidation and volume loss are typically present. On CT, bronchial obstruction by tumor, lung consolidation, and dilated fluid- or mucus-filled bronchi within the consolidated lung ("mucous bronchograms") are commonly seen, particularly when contrast infusion is used (Fig. 3-21). Air bronchograms are usually absent. However, air bronchograms are sometimes seen in the presence of a partially obstructing central bronchial lesion associated with collapse and consolidation. Air bronchograms can also be seen in patients with bronchioloalveolar carcinoma who show consolidation. Areas of necrosis within the tumor mass or lung are sometimes visible using CT.

Typically, a lung carcinoma involves a single bronchus, resulting in collapse of the segment, lobe, or lung distal to the lesion. It has been suggested that the collapse of two segments or lobes that cannot be explained by the presence of a single endobronchial lesion (e.g., the right upper and middle lobes, with the lower lobe being normal) indicates that a benign process is much more likely than lung cancer. This association of two or more endobronchial lesion with

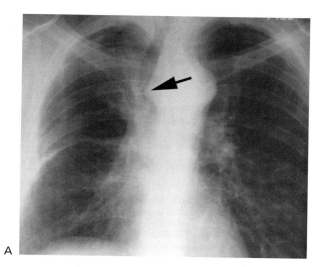
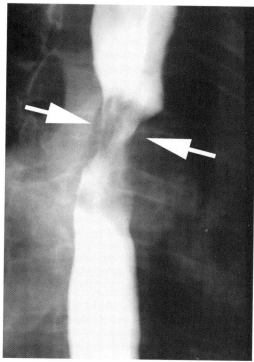

FIG. 3-20. Squamous cell carcinoma of the trachea with mediastinal invasion and esophageal involvement. **A.** Plain radiograph shows tracheal displacement to the right by a large mediastinal mass *(arrow)*. Focal tracheal narrowing by an endobronchial mass is present. **B.** Esophagogram shows esophageal compression and narrowing *(arrows)* because of invasion by the tumor.

atelectasis is variable. The affected lung may be completely airless and reduced to its minimum volume. Alternatively, the obstructed lobe or lung may become filled with desquamated material, mucus, and fluid and lose little of its volume. In both instances the absence of air bronchograms is suggestive of obstruction (see Chapter 2).

Obstructive pneumonia is a common manifestation of

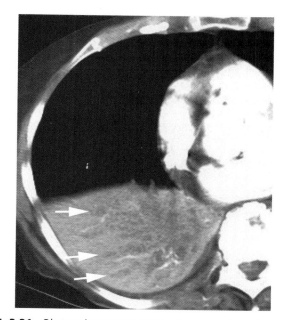

FIG. 3-21. Obstructive pneumonia with mucous bronchograms. In a patient with a right hilar carcinoma, right lower lobe consolidation is associated with minimal volume loss. This is typical of obstructive pneumonia. Mucous bronchograms *(arrows)* are visible.

benign disease has been termed the double-lesion sign (see Fig. 1-40 in Chapter 1). Rarely, a hilar lung carcinoma produces a double-lesion sign by arising in one bronchus and invading or compressing another. In any patient with persisting bronchial obstruction, regardless of what segments or lobes are involved, CT and bronchoscopy are advisable.

Consolidation in Bronchioloalveolar Carcinoma

Forty percent of patients with BAC show radiographic findings of diffuse lung involvement by tumor; these are typically the mucinous subtype of BAC. Although most patients show a combination of findings, the predominant radiographic pattern of diffuse BAC is:

1. Patchy, lobar, or diffuse consolidation, with air bronchograms (60%; see Figs. 3-8, 3-9, 3-22A)

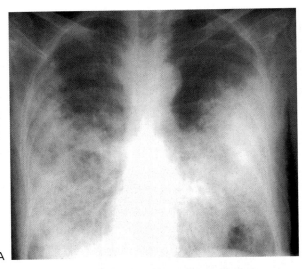

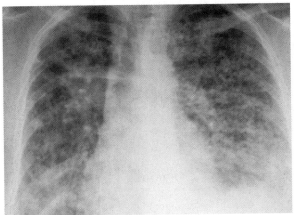

FIG. 3-22. Diffuse bronchioloalveolar carcinoma (BAC). **A.** BAC with bilateral lung consolidation. **B.** BAC with multiple bilateral ill-defined nodules.

2. Multiple ill-defined nodules (30%; see Figs. 3-8B and 3-22B)
3. Patchy, lobar, or diffuse ground-glass opacity (10%)

Consolidation in patients with BAC is usually indistinguishable from pneumonia on plain films. However, in some patients, consolidation is associated with adjacent linear opacities or a spiculated margin, reflecting the same type of fibrotic response seen in patients with BAC who present with a solitary nodule.

On CT, the consolidation seen in patients with BAC is typically low in attenuation; this largely reflects the presence of watery fluid and mucus produced by the tumor. If a contrast agent is infused, enhancing pulmonary vessels can be seen within areas of consolidation; this has been termed the CT angiogram sign and reflects the low density of the consolidated lung (see Fig. 2-6 in Chapter 2). The CT angiogram sign is typical of BAC and should suggest this diagnosis, but it can also be seen with any other cause of consolidation, particularly when rapid contrast infusion is used. In BAC, lung consolidation is not associated with bronchial obstruction; however, air bronchograms may be absent because of fluid within the bronchi.

Ill-defined nodules associated with BAC reflect focal areas of consolidation and have characteristics typical of airspace nodules (see Figs. 3-8B and 3-22B). They usually measure from 5 mm to 1 cm in diameter but can be larger. On CT, they are usually centrilobular in location.

Lymphangitic Spread of Tumor

Lung carcinoma commonly spreads via the lymphatic system. Diffuse involvement of the pulmonary lymphatics results in the appearance of lymphangitic spread of carcinoma, often in association with hilar node enlargement and pleural effusion. The classic appearance is a unilateral or asymmetrical increase in pulmonary interstitial markings, which may be associated with Kerley's B lines; however, atypical appearances are common. High-resolution CT typically shows interlobular septal thickening (Fig. 3-23), thickening of the peribronchovascular interstitium, and thickening of fissures.

Hilar and Mediastinal Mass or Lymph Node Enlargement

Hilar and mediastinal node enlargement is detected radiographically in up to 35% of lung cancers at diagnosis, although 50% have evidence of node metastasis at surgery. The diagnosis of hilar and mediastinal mass and lymph node enlargement is discussed in detail in other chapters.

Hilar enlargement can reflect the primary tumor arising in a central location (usually this results in a poorly marginated hilar mass that may be large; Fig. 3-24) or metastases to hilar lymph nodes from a peripheral lung primary (usually a well-defined hilar mass; Fig. 3-25). Hilar mass is common

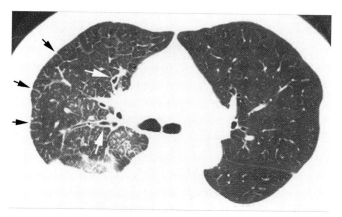

FIG. 3-23. Lymphangitic spread of lung carcinoma. High-resolution CT shows typical findings of unilateral interlobular septal thickening *(black arrows)* and thickening of the peribronchovascular interstitium *(white arrows)*. A right pleural effusion is also present.

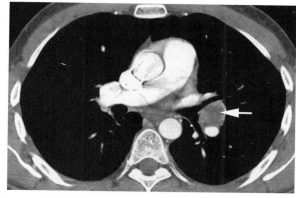

FIG. 3-25. Left hilar lymph node enlargement *(arrow)* due to metastasis from a peripheral cancer. The hilar mass is sharply marginated.

in squamous cell carcinoma. Enlargement of hilar lymph nodes in association with a central mass is characteristic of small cell carcinoma (see Table 3-8). Hilar enlargement is the first detectable radiographic finding in 10% to 15% of cases of lung cancer. Airway abnormalities (narrowing or obstruction) are commonly, but not invariably, seen in patients with a hilar mass or lymph node enlargement.

Mediastinal lymph node metastases are common in patients with lung carcinoma, occurring in up to 40% of patients at diagnosis, depending on the size, location, and cell type of the primary tumor. In patients with a small lung nodule as the only presenting finding, mediastinal metastases are found in approximately 20%.

However, mediastinal lymph node enlargement is an uncommon plain film abnormality at initial presentation (see Table 3-8). When visible radiographically, lymph node enlargement is usually limited to the middle mediastinum and is associated with a visible lung or hilar mass. The most common sites of mediastinal node enlargement seen on plain radiographs are the right paratracheal mediastinum for right-sided tumors and the aorticopulmonary window for left-sided tumors. The subcarinal lymph nodes are also commonly involved but are difficult to recognize on plain radiographs unless they are quite large. It is unusual for mediastinal lymph nodes to be involved radiographically without involvement of the hilum.

In some patients with lung carcinoma, a mediastinal mass may be the first and only presenting abnormality, occurring

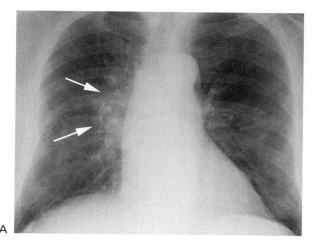

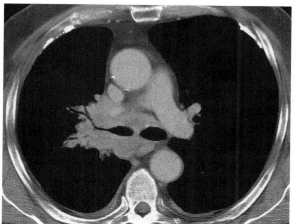

FIG. 3-24. Right hilar carcinoma in a patient with asbestos exposure. **A.** Chest radiograph shows an ill-defined right hilar mass *(arrows)*. This is typical of carcinoma originating in the hilum. Pleural thickening and calcification typical of asbestos exposure are visible. **B.** A large, poorly marginated right hilar mass surrounds and narrows the right upper lobe bronchus. This appearance is most typical of small cell carcinoma.

in the absence of a visible lung mass. These mediastinal masses may be middle mediastinal, involving the pretracheal lymph node group, or may be more atypical in location, often occurring in the anterior mediastinum rather than middle mediastinum, and are usually small cell carcinoma or poorly differentiated carcinoma.

Pleural Abnormalities

Pleural Effusions or Masses

Small pleural effusions are common in patients with lung cancer; pleural effusion occurs in 5% to 15% of patients. They can result from pleural metastases, lymphatic obstruction in the hilum or mediastinum, or inflammatory lung disease associated with bronchial obstruction. The term *malignant effusion* should be reserved for effusions containing malignant cells. The presence of a pleural effusion, particularly when bloody, indicates a poor prognosis in lung cancer, but only a malignant effusion rules out surgical treatment.

Decubitus radiographs, ultrasound, and CT are sensitive methods of detecting pleural effusion. On CT, the presence of pleural thickening or nodularity in association with effusion should be considered highly suspicious for malignancy. However, malignant effusions typically occur without visible pleural thickening. Extensive involvement of the pleural space mimicking malignant mesothelioma is sometimes seen, particularly in patients with adenocarcinoma.

Pneumothorax

Spontaneous pneumothorax is rare with bronchogenic carcinoma and usually results from direct invasion of the visceral pleura or cavitation (Fig. 3-26). Occasionally airway obstruction due to a proximal endobronchial lesion causes rupture of a subpleural bulla, producing a pneumothorax.

Pneumothorax ex vacuo is an unusual occurrence in lung cancer. It occurs in the presence of acute lobar collapse due to bronchial obstruction. A sudden decrease in intrapleural pressure around the collapsed lobe results in gas being drawn from blood and tissues into the pleural space. Radiographs or CT scans show a crescentic gas collection localized to the pleural space surrounding the collapsed lobe (Fig. 3-27). It is most common in the right upper lobe and resolves with alleviation of the obstruction.

Missed Lung Cancer

Lung cancers presenting as a solitary nodule may be difficult to see on chest radiographs. The *conspicuity* of a lesion is determined by (1) the sharpness of its edge, (2) the visual complexity of the region in which it is seen, (3) its size, and (4) its density. Cancers are usually missed on chest radiographs because of their poor conspicuity, being ill de-

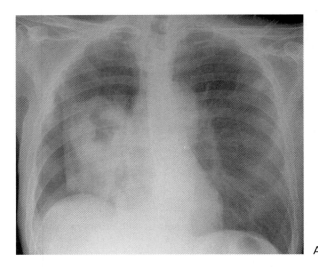

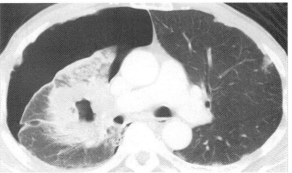

FIG. 3-26. Cavitary squamous cell carcinoma with pneumothorax shown on chest radiograph **(A)** and CT **(B)**.

fined, located in areas that are complex and difficult to evaluate (e.g., in the lung apex, in the perihilar lung regions, in the posterior costophrenic angle and projected below the dome of the diaphragm), or small.

Lung cancers smaller than 5 mm are very difficult to see, but many missed cancers are not small. Missed cancers average about 1.5 cm in diameter but may be more than 3 cm. On chest radiographs, most (80%) missed cancers are in an upper lobe, with the right upper lobe being the most common site (50% of missed cancers). Lung cancers are more commonly missed in women than in men. Lateral radiographs may show the lesion better than frontal films.

Cancers may be missed when films are interpreted prospectively, but visible in retrospect. This does not imply malpractice. The detection rate for nodules 1 cm in diameter ranges from 40% to 90%. In patients with inconspicuous lesions, as many as 25% of visible lung cancers are missed by experienced observers, even if they know a cancer is present.

Cancers may also be missed using CT, even when the purpose of the scan is lung cancer screening and the reader's

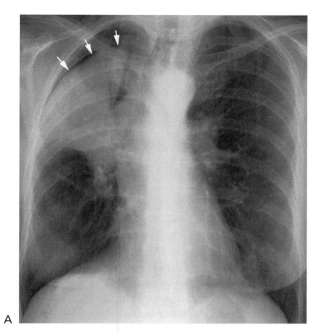

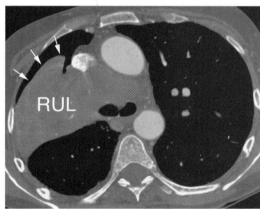

FIG. 3-27. Pneumothorax ex vacuo in small cell carcinoma obstructing the right upper lobe bronchus. **A.** Chest radiograph shows a right hilar mass and right upper lobe collapse associated with an apical pneumothorax *(arrows)*. **B.** CT shows right upper lobe collapse *(RUL)* capped by a pneumothorax *(arrows)*. The right upper lobe bronchus is obstructed and invisible. This appearance is typical of pneumothorax ex vacuo.

suspicion is high. Missed cancers may be small and endobronchial or may present as solitary nodules. Missed solitary nodules are usually small (often less than 3 mm), indistinguishable from adjacent vessels or other lung disease (e.g., old tuberculosis), poorly defined and of ground-glass opacity, or may mimic air space consolidation or pleural thickening. Cancers missed on CT are often present in a lower lobe. The presence of other significant abnormalities on the CT scan may distract the observer. Missing something because the reader sees something else that is more obvious is termed *satisfaction of search.*

CLINICAL MANIFESTATIONS OF LUNG CANCER

Lung cancer is more common in men and most frequently presents in patients in their 50s and 60s. It is uncommon in patients less than 30 years of age. The clinical manifestations of lung carcinoma result from the following:

1. Local tumor growth
2. Intrathoracic metastases
3. Extrathoracic metastases
4. Presence of a paraneoplastic syndrome

Local Tumor Growth and Intrathoracic Metastases

Symptoms associated with lung cancer are largely nonspecific and are present in a minority of patients when the tumor is first detected radiographically (Table 3-12). Most patients with cancer are smokers and have a history of chronic cough; any change in their pattern of cough or sputum production should be considered significant.

Symptoms are most common in patients with central carcinomas involving large bronchi or mediastinal structures, and in patients with tumors metastatic to hilar or mediastinal lymph nodes. Symptoms of central carcinoma can include the following:

1. Bronchial obstruction with cough, hemoptysis, wheezing, dyspnea, or fever due to postobstructive pneumonia
2. Hoarseness from involvement of the recurrent laryngeal nerve
3. SVC syndrome resulting from mediastinal invasion or metastases
4. Dysphagia from esophageal invasion or compression
5. Chylothorax from involvement of the thoracic duct
6. Diaphragmatic paralysis from involvement of the phrenic nerve

Peripheral lung cancers can be associated with pleural or chest wall invasion, resulting in chest pain, dyspnea, or

TABLE 3-12. SYMPTOMS IN PATIENTS WITH LUNG CANCER

Symptom	Patients with symptom
Cough	75%
Dyspnea	60%
Chest pain	45%
Hemoptysis	35%
Hypertrophic pulmonary osteoarthropathy	10%
Hoarseness	10%
Wheezing	2%

cough. At autopsy, about 10% of patients with lung cancer have chest wall involvement by direct extension. Peripheral carcinomas in the superior sulcus can produce Pancoast syndrome.

Superior Vena Cava Syndrome

Obstruction or narrowing of mediastinal vessels as a result of mediastinal invasion or lymph node metastases is a relatively common manifestation of lung cancer. Because of its location and relatively thin wall, the SVC is particularly susceptible to involvement by tumor, and 65% to 85% of cases of SVC syndrome are caused by lung carcinoma. Symptoms and signs of SVC syndrome include the following:

1. Facial fullness, flushing, and cyanosis
2. Headache
3. Edema of the upper extremities
4. Prominent veins on the face and upper chest

Other common causes of SVC syndrome include granulomatous diseases such as histoplasmosis or tuberculosis involving the mediastinum (granulomatous mediastinitis), and venous thrombosis.

Extrathoracic Metastases

Small cell carcinoma grows rapidly and tends to metastasize early. Adenocarcinoma may grow slowly but metastasizes early. Squamous cell carcinoma may grow rapidly but tends to metastasize late.

Hematogenous spread to many sites has been reported with lung cancer, but the central nervous system, bones, liver, and adrenal glands are most commonly involved. Such metastases preclude successful surgical resection. The use of imaging studies to detect distant metastases in lung cancer patients is discussed below.

Paraneoplastic Syndromes

Paraneoplastic syndromes are disorders associated with malignant neoplasms but not directly related to the physical effects of the primary tumor. Such syndromes are present in 10% of patients with lung carcinoma (20% of those with small cell carcinoma) and result from the production of hormones or peptides by the tumor, antigen–antibody interactions resulting from tumor products, or neurovascular mechanisms. They may precede pulmonary findings by months or even years. A large variety of manifestations have been reported.

Hypertrophic Pulmonary Osteoarthropathy

Digital clubbing and hypertrophic pulmonary osteoarthropathy (HPO) are the most common cutaneous disorders. Eighty percent of cases of HPO in adults are due to lung cancer. Squamous cell carcinoma is most commonly associated with HPO; HPO is uncommon with small cell carcinoma. Relief of symptoms commonly follows resection of the primary neoplasm. Pulmonary osteoarthropathy may precede discovery of the lung neoplasm by up to 2 years.

Vascular Disorders

Thrombophlebitis has an increased incidence in lung cancer patients and is most common with adenocarcinoma.

Endocrine Disorders

Cushing's syndrome, resulting from tumor secretion of ectopic adrenocorticotrophic hormone (ACTH), consists of weakness, hyperglycemia, polyuria, and hypokalemic alkalosis; in patients with lung cancer it is typically of rapid onset and progression. It can be associated with any cell type of tumor. Cushing's syndrome is most common in patients with carcinoid tumor, and approximately 30% of patients with an ectopic cause of this syndrome have a bronchial carcinoid tumor. Small cell carcinoma is associated with Cushing's syndrome in less than 5% of cases, at least partially because of the relatively short life expectancy of patients with this tumor.

Hypercalcemia associated with lung cancer is most common with squamous cell carcinoma. Occasionally it is associated with bone metastases, but it is more often due to production of a peptide similar to parathyroid hormone. Other mediators such as prostaglandin have also been implicated in hypercalcemia.

Inappropriate antidiuretic hormone secretion, resulting in hyponatremia, is usually associated with small cell carcinoma. Although 50% of patients with small cell carcinoma have elevated levels of antidiuretic hormone, only 10% to 15% have hyponatremia, and less than 5% of patients have symptoms attributable to this syndrome.

Neuromuscular Syndromes

Neuromuscular syndromes associated with lung cancer may result from immunologic mechanisms. Small cell carcinoma is most commonly responsible. Symptoms may precede the diagnosis of the tumor or may be the first sign of recurrence.

Eaton-Lambert syndrome is characterized by proximal muscle weakness similar to myasthenia gravis, with the exception that muscle strength increases (rather than decreases) with use. Hyporeflexia and autonomic dysfunction are also parts of this syndrome. Small cell carcinoma is the most common malignant tumor associated with Eaton-Lambert syndrome; it can also be seen with extrathoracic tumors, and approximately 50% of cases are not associated with a detectable tumor. This syndrome apparently results from the production of anti–calcium channel antibodies, which impairs the release of acetylcholine.

Peripheral neuropathy is associated with small cell carcinoma and less often with squamous cell carcinoma and adenocarcinoma. Antineuronal nuclear antibodies are likely involved. Chronic intestinal pseudoobstruction, limbic encephalitis, necrotizing myelopathy, and visual paraneoplastic syndrome also occur with small cell carcinoma and are associated with antineuronal nuclear antibodies. Symptoms from the neuropathy may precede the discovery of the carcinoma by years; however, in most cases, advanced disease is present.

Other neuromuscular manifestations include subacute cerebellar degeneration (ataxia, vertigo, uncoordination) and dementia.

STAGING OF LUNG CANCER

In patients with lung cancer, both the cell type of the tumor and the tumor extent affect the prognosis and survival following treatment. However, the anatomic extent of the tumor at diagnosis is usually most important in determining what therapeutic approach will be chosen. Imaging studies play a prominent role in determining the extent of tumor, or in other words its anatomic stage.

Lung cancer is staged using a TNM classification, which is based on a combination of findings: the location and morphologic characteristics of the primary tumor (T), the presence or absence of hilar, mediastinal, or other lymphadenopathy (N), and the presence or absence of distant metastases (M). This staging system is shown in detail in Tables 3-13 and 3-14 and in Figure 3-28A. Using this classification, excellent correlations can be made between tumor stage and survival after treatment (see Fig. 3-28B).

Small cell carcinomas have a very poor prognosis regardless of tumor stage and are usually assumed to be associated with metastases at diagnosis. Because of this, anatomic lung cancer staging using the TNM classification is generally limited to non–small cell bronchogenic carcinoma (NSCBC).

The manner in which NSCBC is treated is fundamentally based on the tumor stage, although treatment may vary in individual cases. Stage I and II tumors are usually treated by resection; stage IIIA tumors are often treated by radiation or chemotherapy followed by resection (if anatomically possible); stage IIIB by radiation, chemotherapy, or both; and stage IV by chemotherapy (Table 3-15).

In radiologic lung cancer staging, it is most important to determine which patients have localized disease and are likely to benefit from surgical resection, and alternatively which patients have extensive disease not amenable to surgical treatment. Generally speaking, tumors are considered to be unresectable if they are classified as T4, N3, or M1.

Different surgeons have different anatomic criteria for considering a tumor to be unresectable, and a careful and detailed discussion of the radiographic findings with the surgeon is necessary. Generally, you should be reluctant to

TABLE 3-13. TNM STAGING OF LUNG CANCER[a]

T (primary tumor)

T0 No evidence of a primary tumor

Tis Carcinoma in situ

T1 A tumor that is:
  a. 3 cm or less in greatest diameter
  b. Surrounded by lung or visceral pleura
  c. Without invasion proximal to a lobar bronchus (i.e., involving main bronchus)

T2 A tumor with any of the following features:
  a. Larger than 3 cm in greatest diameter
  b. Involving a main bronchus ≥2 cm distal to the carina
  c. Invading the visceral pleura
  d. Producing atelectasis or obstructive pneumonia, extending to the hilum, but involving less than the entire lung

T3 A tumor of any size that either:
  a. Invades chest wall, diaphragm, mediastinal pleura, or parietal pericardium
  or
  b. Is located <2 cm distal to the carina without involvement of the carina or associated with atelectasis or obstructive pneumonia of an entire lung

T4 A tumor of any size with any of the following features:
  a. *Invading the mediastinum, heart, great vessels, trachea, esophagus, vertebral body, or carina*
  b. *Producing malignant pleural or pericardial effusion* (pleural effusion not obviously associated with metastases has no effect of stage)
  c. Associated with satellite tumor nodules in the same lobe as the primary tumor (nodules in a different lobe are considered metastases or M1)

N (nodal involvement)

N0 No regional node metastases

N1 Metastases to ipsilateral peribronchial, hilar, or intrapulmonary nodes

N2 Metastases to ipsilateral mediastinal nodes or subcarinal nodes

N3 *Metastases to contralateral hilar or mediastinal lymph nodes, or scalene or supraclavicular lymph node*

M (distant metastases)

M0 Metastases absent

M1 *Metastases present*

[a] Italics used for findings that indicate unresectability in most situations.
(Modified from Mountain CF. Revisions in the international system for staging lung cancer. Chest 1997; 111:1710–1717.)

make a dogmatic statement about resectability solely on the basis of the radiographic findings (which in themselves may be nonspecific). The results of imaging studies must be considered in the framework of what diagnostic or therapeutic options are available.

Primary Tumor

T1 Carcinoma

A T1 carcinoma usually presents as a small peripheral nodule (3 cm or less) surrounded by lung (see Fig. 3-5B). Endo-

TABLE 3-14. LUNG CANCER STAGING GROUPS

Stage	TNM criteria
IA	T1,N0,M0
IB	T2,N0,M0
IIA	T1,N1,M0
IIB	T2,N1,M0
	T3,N0,M0
IIIA	T1,N2,M0
	T2,N2,M0
	T3,N1,M0
	T3,N2,M0
IIIB	T1,N3,M0
	T2,N3,M0
	T3,N3,M0
IV	M1

TABLE 3-15. LUNG CANCER TREATMENT RELATED TO STAGE

Stage	Common treatment
I	Resection
II	Resection
IIIA	Radiation or chemotherapy followed by resection
IIIB	Radiation and/or chemotherapy
IV	Chemotherapy

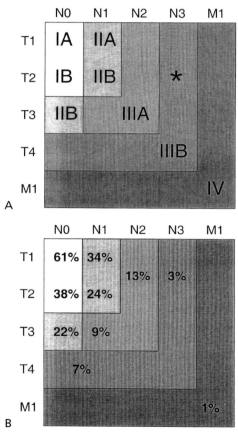

FIG. 3-28. Lung cancer staging classifications. **A.** Lung cancer stage related to combinations of T, N, and M. To determine the stage, find the correct T class and go across the square until reaching the appropriate N class. For example, the asterisk corresponds to a T2-N3 lesion and is classified as IIIB. M1 indicates stage IV regardless of T or N. **B.** Five-year survival rates according to combinations of T, N, and M determined clinically (rather than pathologically). Survival decreases from the top left to bottom right of the diagram. Also, slightly different survival rates have been reported for stages IIIA and IIIB, depending on whether it is based on an advanced T or an advanced N.

bronchial T1 carcinoma, limited to a lobar bronchus and not associated with atelectasis extending to the hilum, is an uncommon radiographic presentation (see Fig. 3-17C). These tumors are easily resectable.

T2 Carcinoma

T2 carcinomas may present either as a lung mass larger than 3 cm in diameter (see Fig. 3-4) or as an endobronchial tumor involving a main bronchus 2 cm or more from the carina or associated with atelectasis or obstructive pneumonia extending to the hilum. Both presentations are common. These tumors are easily resectable.

T3 Carcinoma

T3 carcinomas may present as a lung nodule or mass invading the chest wall (Fig. 3-29), diaphragm, mediastinal pleura, or parietal pericardium, without invasion of important structures (listed under T4). A T3 carcinoma may also be one involving a main bronchus less than 2 cm from the carina or associated with atelectasis or obstructive pneumonia of an entire lung. These tumors are resectable with difficulty in many cases.

T4 Carcinoma

T4 carcinomas may present as a lung nodule, mass, or bronchial lesion resulting in the following:

1. Invasion of the chest wall with involvement of great vessels or vertebral body
2. Invasion of the mediastinum with involvement of the heart, great vessels, trachea, or esophagus
3. Invasion the tracheal carina
4. Malignant pleural or pericardial effusion
5. Satellite nodules in the same lobe as the primary tumor

With the exception of tumors associated with satellite nodules, these tumors are uncommonly resectable.

Resectability of the Primary Tumor: Radiographic Assessment

When determining the primary tumor extent and T classification, several key observations need to be made, including

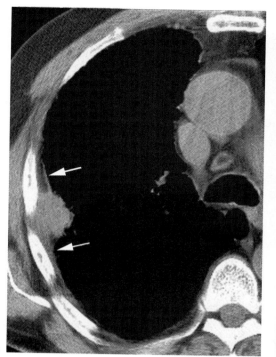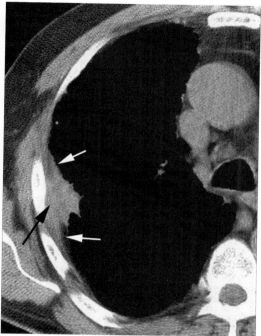

A B

FIG. 3-29. Chest wall invasion classified as T3 in the lung cancer staging system. A small peripheral carcinoma is associated with pleural thickening *(white arrows)*. The tumor has an obtuse angle at the point it contacts the pleura. These findings suggest chest wall invasion, but their specificity is limited. Also, tumor can be seen invading and thickening extrapleural soft tissues *(black arrow in* **B***)*.

the size of the tumor, its location within a bronchus, and its association with atelectasis or consolidation. However, of most importance in determining respectability is assessment of the specific features of a T4 lesion.

Chest Wall Invasion

Direct invasion of the pleura and chest wall by a peripheral lung carcinoma may or may not indicate that the tumor is unresectable. Only extensive chest wall invasion rules out surgery.

Unless obvious rib destruction is present, the diagnosis of chest wall invasion on plain radiographs is difficult. Pleural thickening adjacent to a lung mass is nonspecific and need not indicate chest wall invasion. Tumors with extensive contact with the pleural surface are more likely invasive than those with minimal contact. A tumor that appears to flatten out against the pleura (i.e., it appears sessile, lenticular, or crescentic in profile) may be invasive.

The accuracy of CT in diagnosing chest wall invasion is 70% to 80%, although sensitivity and specificity values vary from 40% to 90% in different studies. CT findings of value in the diagnosis of chest wall invasion (Figs. 3-30 and 3-31) include the presence of the following:

1. Obtuse angles or pleural thickening at the point of contact between tumor and pleura
2. More than 3 cm of contact between tumor and the pleural surface (5 cm of contact is more specific but less sensitive)
3. A ratio of the tumor diameter to the length of pleural contact by the tumor exceeding 0.5 (the higher this ratio, the more specific this finding)
4. Invisibility of extrapleural (chest wall) fat planes at the point tumor contacts chest wall
5. A mass involving the chest wall
6. Rib destruction

The only definite findings include rib destruction or chest wall mass. Otherwise, invisibility of the extrapleural fat plane (sensitivity 85%, specificity 85%) and a ratio of tumor diameter to pleura contact exceeding 0.9 (sensitivity 85%, specificity 80%) are most accurate in predicting invasion (Table 3-16; see Fig. 3-31).

The demonstration of motion of the tumor relative to the chest wall during respiration indicates that no invasion is present; alternatively, the absence of motion during respiration suggests that invasion is present. This may be assessed using fluoroscopy, sonography, or dynamic spiral CT.

The extent of chest wall invasion adjacent to a lung

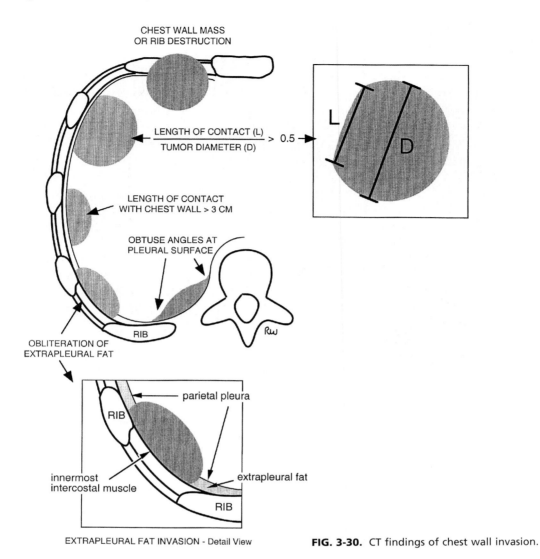

FIG. 3-30. CT findings of chest wall invasion.

TABLE 3-16. ACCURACY OF CT FINDINGS FOR DIAGNOSING CHEST WALL INVASION

CT finding	Sensitivity (%)	Specificity (%)
Obtuse angles at pleural surface	60	75
Length of contact with chest wall		
>3 cm	95	40
>4 cm	90	55
>5 cm	75	70
Ratio of:		
Length of contact/tumor diameter		
>0.5	100	35
>0.7	90	60
>0.9	85	80
Obliteration of chest wall fat plane	85	85
Chest wall mass	33	100
Rib destruction	16	100

(Modified from Ratto GB, Piacenza G, Frola C, et al. Chest wall involvement by lung cancer: computed tomographic detection and results of operation. Ann Thorac Surg 1991; 51:182–188.)

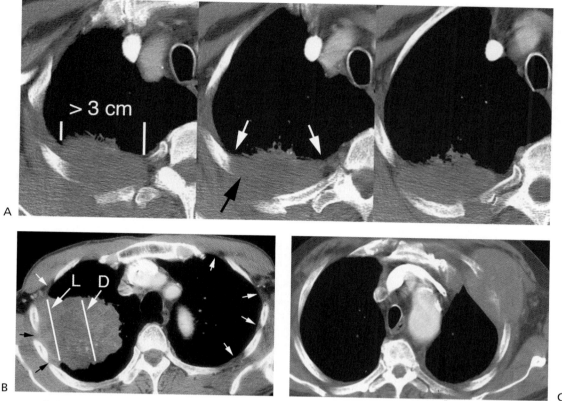

FIG. 3-31. CT findings of chest wall invasion in three patients. **A.** CT at three adjacent levels shows a lenticular mass having more than 3 cm of contact with the chest wall, obtuse angles at the point it contacts the chest wall *(white arrows)*, and rib destruction *(black arrow)*. **B.** There is extensive pleural contact, with the length of contact *(L)* being 5 cm. The tumor diameter *(D)* equals the length of pleural contact (i.e., their ratio is 1). Normal fat is seen in intercostal spaces *(small white arrows)*, while these fat planes are invisible where the tumor contacts the chest wall *(small black arrows)*. **C.** Chest wall invasion by lung cancer with rib destruction and a large chest wall mass.

tumor may be better shown using MRI than CT because of the better contrast between tumor and chest wall fat and muscle that can be obtained using MRI.

In patients with superior sulcus tumors, vertebral body invasion (Fig. 3-32A) and invasion of the great vessels above the lung apex (see Fig. 3-16) prevent surgical resection. MRI in the sagittal or coronal planes can be advantageous in imaging apical tumors and is more accurate than CT in diagnosing chest wall invasion and its extent in the lung apex. In patients with a superior sulcus tumor who are being considered for resection, MRI is recommended to determine the extent of chest wall invasion and possible involvement of the subclavian artery or brachial plexus (see Fig. 3-32B).

Mediastinal Invasion

Contiguous invasion of the mediastinum by tumor, with involvement of the heart, great vessels, trachea, or esophagus, precludes resection, as does significant invasion of me-

diastinal fat. Invasion of the mediastinal pleura or parietal pericardium does not prevent resection.

On plain radiographs, findings that suggest mediastinal invasion include the presence of a mediastinal mass, extensive contact of tumor with the mediastinum (Fig. 3-33A), or diaphragmatic paralysis, which in turn implies involvement of the phrenic nerve.

CT is more accurate than plain radiographs in assessing mediastinal invasion. However, some caution in interpreting the CT is necessary. Contiguity of tumor mass with the mediastinal pleura or thickening of the mediastinal pleura does not necessarily indicate mediastinal invasion. Also, not all findings indicative of mediastinal invasion indicate unresectability.

CT findings (Fig. 3-34A) usually regarded as indicating "definite" or "gross" mediastinal invasion and unresectability (although they are not 100% accurate) include the following:

1. Extensive replacement of mediastinal fat by soft-tissue mass (see Figs. 3-33B and 3-35)

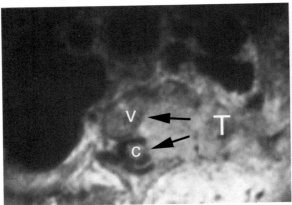
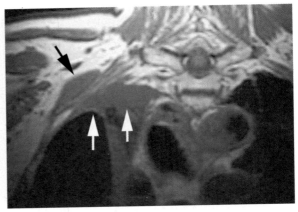

FIG. 3-32. MRI diagnosis of chest wall invasion. **A.** Vertebral invasion by a superior sulcus tumor shown using T1-weighted MRI. Tumor *(T)* invades *(arrows)* the vertebral body *(V)*. *c*, spinal cord. **B.** A superior sulcus tumor *(white arrows)* invades the chest wall *(black arrow)*, surrounding the brachial plexus.

2. Mass surrounding mediastinal vessels, trachea, or esophagus
3. Mass resulting in obvious invasion of one of these structures (see Fig. 3-35)

In lung cancer patients who do not have gross mediastinal invasion, additional CT findings may be of value in predicting that invasion of the mediastinum and mediastinal structures is present. These CT findings (see Figs. 3-34B and 3-36) include the following:

1. Tumor contact of more than 3 cm with the mediastinum

2. Tumor contact with more than one fourth (90°) of the circumference of the aorta or other mediastinal structures
3. Obliteration of the fat planes that are normally seen adjacent to the aorta or other mediastinal structures
4. Compression of mediastinal structures by a mass
5. Mediastinal pleural or pericardial thickening

The first three findings are highly sensitive but have poor specificity (Table 3-17). Because of the high sensitivity of these three findings, if they are all absent, the tumor will likely be resectable, even if mediastinal invasion is present.

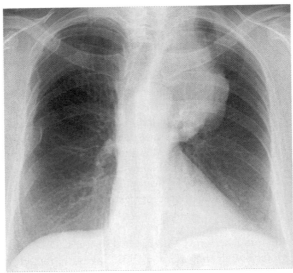
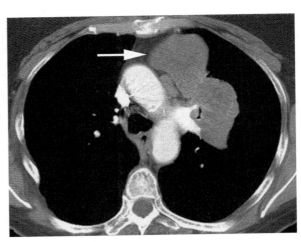

FIG. 3-33. Mediastinal invasion by lung cancer. **A.** Chest radiograph shows extensive contact of tumor with mediastinum. **B.** CT shows extensive contact of tumor with mediastinum and a mediastinal mass *(arrow)* contiguous with the lung tumor, with soft tissue replacing mediastinal fat.

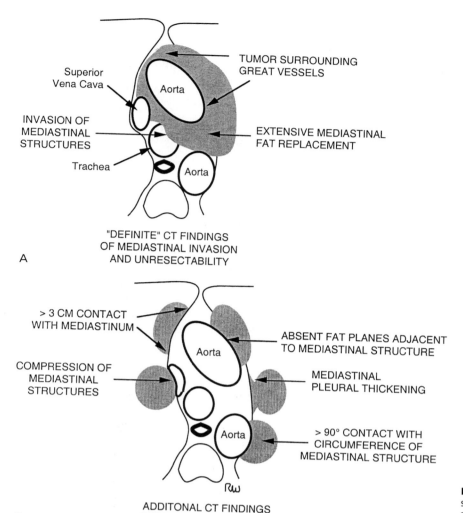

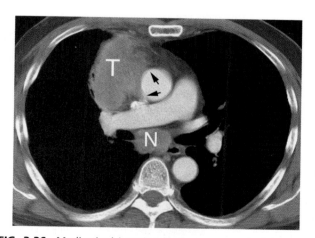

FIG. 3-34. CT findings of mediastinal invasion. **A.** Definite findings of mediastinal invasion. **B.** Additional findings of mediastinal invasion.

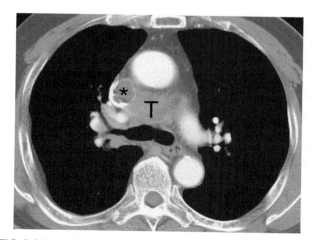

FIG. 3-35. Mediastinal and superior vena cava invasion by lung cancer. Tumor *(T)* has invaded mediastinal fat anterior to the carina. Invasion of the superior vena cava with a tumor thrombus *(*)* in its lumen is also visible.

FIG. 3-36. Mediastinal invasion by lung cancer. A right upper lobe tumor *(T)* shows more than 3 cm of contact with the mediastinum, replaces mediastinal fat, obliterates the fat plane adjacent to the aorta, and contacts more than one fourth of its circumference *(arrows)*. An enlarged subcarinal lymph node *(N)* is also seen.

TABLE 3-17. ACCURACY OF CT FINDINGS FOR DIAGNOSING MEDIASTINAL INVASION

CT finding	Sensitivity (%)	Specificity (%)
Contact with mediastinum >3 cm	80	55
Contact with aorta >1/4 circumference	85	75
Absent mediastinal fat plane	90	10
Compression of mediastinal structure	35	75
Mediastinal pleural or pericardial thickening	40	80

(Modified from Glazer HS, Kaiser LR, Anderson DJ, et al. Indeterminate mediastinal invasion in bronchogenic carcinoma: CT evaluation. Radiology 1989; 173:37–42.)

MRI does not have a great advantage in the diagnosis of mediastinal invasion unless the patient cannot have contrast-enhanced CT.

Tracheal and Central Bronchial Lesions

Although tumor masses that cause total lung collapse or consolidation or involve the proximal bronchus may be difficult to treat surgically, they are not generally considered unresectable unless they involve the tracheal carina or trachea (Fig. 3-37). In this situation, it is difficult to perform a pneumonectomy, resect the tumor, and surgically close the remaining airway. However, some surgeons may excise tumors that involve the carina or even the distal trachea, reanastomosing the tracheal stump to the remaining bronchus or bronchi.

In some patients, plain radiographs or CT can demonstrate the relationship of a proximal tumor mass to the main bronchus, carina, or trachea. CT findings that suggest carinal involvement include bronchial wall thickening that extends to the carina, or carinal thickening, blunting, or nodularity. However, bronchoscopy is more accurate in making

this diagnosis. On bronchoscopy, minimal mucosal involvement by tumor can be diagnosed, while on CT or plain radiographs, only discrete masses are visible. Bronchoscopic confirmation of an apparent carinal or tracheal tumor is usually necessary unless the findings are gross.

Malignant Pleural Effusion

In a patient with lung carcinoma, pleural effusion can occur for a variety of reasons, including pleural invasion, obstructive pneumonia, and lymphatic or pulmonary venous obstruction by the tumor. Although the presence of effusion indicates a poor prognosis, only patients who have tumor cells in the pleural fluid or pleural biopsy are considered to have unresectable disease. Patients with other causes of effusion are considered to have resectable lesions despite their poor prognosis; nonmalignant effusion has no effect on stage classification. Usually plain radiographs are sufficient for the diagnosis of pleural effusion, leading to thoracentesis or pleural biopsy.

On CT, the presence of pleural thickening or nodularity in association with effusion should be considered highly suspicious for malignancy (see Chapter 26). However, malignant effusions can occur without pleural thickening (Fig. 3-38), and pleural thickening can be seen in many cases of transudative pleural effusion. Small nodules at the pleural surface or within a fissure may also indicate pleural dissemination of tumor.

Satellite Nodules

The presence of a satellite nodule or nodules (small nodules in association with but separate from a larger lesion) in the same lobe as a primary tumor (Fig. 3-39) is associated with a poorer survival than a nodule not accompanied by a satellite. Although this finding indicates T4 in the current staging system, such lesions are easily resected.

Lymph Node Metastases

Hilar Lymph Node Metastases

The presence of a hilar mass on radiographs or CT may reflect a primary bronchial tumor with local extension

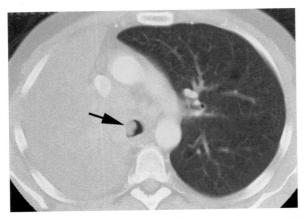

FIG. 3-37. Tracheal invasion by a right hilar carcinoma. Right lung atelectasis is due to a carcinoma arising in the right main bronchus. Tumor invades the trachea *(arrow)*, precluding resection.

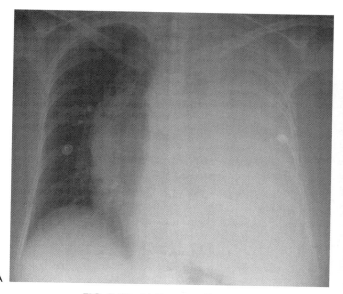

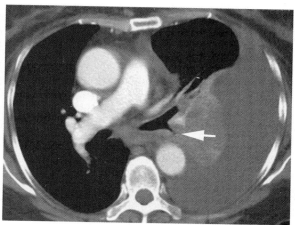

FIG. 3-38. Malignant effusion in lung cancer. **A.** Chest radiograph shows a large left pleural effusion with mediastinal shift to the right. **B.** CT shows a tapered obstruction (rat-tail appearance) of the left lower lobe bronchus associated with left lower lobe collapse. There is no evidence of pleural thickening.

(T1–T3 depending on its location) or hilar lymph node metastases (N1; see Fig. 3-25). Hilar involvement by a carcinoma does not generally affect resectability. However, the presence of hilar tumor often means that a pneumonectomy rather than lobectomy needs to be performed. In patients with poor respiratory function who cannot tolerate a pneumonectomy, the presence of hilar metastases may make them inoperable despite the fact that the tumor itself is technically resectable.

CT is superior to plain radiographs in evaluating the pulmonary hila. CT findings of bronchial obstruction or narrowing correlate closely with bronchoscopic findings (see Fig. 3-17). Spiral CT is quite accurate is showing hilar lymph enlargement; generally a least lymph node diameter of 1 cm is used to distinguish normal from abnormal lymph nodes. However, as with the CT diagnosis of mediastinal lymph node metastases, the sensitivity and specificity of CT are limited, respectively, by the presence of microscopic metastases and benign hyperplastic lymph nodes. Large (more than 2 cm) hilar lymph nodes in a lung cancer patient usually are associated with metastases.

Assessment of Mediastinal Lymph Nodes

Because large or bulky mediastinal masses in patients with lung cancer are considered unresectable by virtually all surgeons, a patient who has a mediastinal mass visible on plain radiographs (indicating its large size) is not likely a surgical candidate. In such patients, CT followed by mediastinoscopy or biopsy should be performed to confirm the presence of mediastinal disease.

CT is helpful in detecting lymph node enlargement in patients with lung carcinoma who have normal plain radiographs. By convention, a short axis (least diameter) lymph node diameter of 1 cm is commonly used on CT to distinguish normal from abnormal nodes. The short axis of a mediastinal lymph node rather than its long axis correlates most closely with the actual lymph node diameter and volume measured pathologically. However, normal lymph node size varies with the lymph node group being assessed

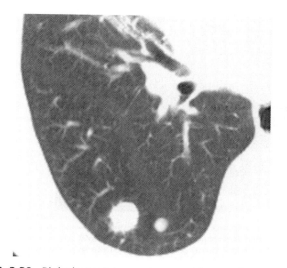

FIG. 3-39. Right lower lobe carcinoma with a satellite nodule.

(see Chapter 8). An upper limit of 1.5 cm is usually used for the nodes in the subcarinal space (see Fig. 3-37). Lymph nodes containing metastases are quite variable in size, although those larger than 2 cm are nearly always involved by tumor (Fig. 3-40).

The accuracy of CT in predicting the presence or absence of mediastinal node metastases on the basis of node diameter is limited by two factors. On the one hand, the sensitivity of CT in diagnosing lymph node metastases is reduced by the common occurrence of microscopic lymph node metastases not resulting in increased lymph node size; on the other hand, specificity is reduced by the presence of enlarged benign hyperplastic lymph nodes, particularly in patients with squamous cell carcinoma.

A number of studies evaluating the accuracy of CT in diagnosing mediastinal node metastases from lung carcinoma have been performed. An assessment of the accuracy of CT in diagnosing mediastinal metastases must be based on a correlation of CT findings with surgical exploration (total nodal sampling) and histologic analysis. When total nodal sampling is performed, the average accuracy of CT ranges from about 67% to 79%, with a sensitivity of 60% to 79%. Improvements in CT technology and attempts to refine the criteria for determining nodes to be normal or abnormal have had little effect on accuracy.

Furthermore, in patients who have enlarged mediastinal nodes on CT, the nodal metastases found at surgery are not always in the nodes that appear large on CT. Thus, the sensitivity of CT in diagnosing mediastinal node metastases on a patient-by-patient basis is higher than its sensitivity in

detecting metastases in a specific node or node group (about 40%). In general, MR is similar to CT in its ability to detect and define mediastinal lymph nodes, and its accuracy in diagnosing mediastinal metastases is similar to that of CT.

Stage and Resectability

Ipsilateral mediastinal or subcarinal node metastases are classified N2 and are considered potentially resectable, usually following preoperative chemotherapy, but this remains controversial. Contralateral hilar or mediastinal node metastases or supraclavicular or scalene lymph node metastases are considered N3 and unresectable (see Fig. 3-40). Treatment usually includes chemotherapy.

The American Joint Committee on Cancer (AJCC) and the Union Internationale Contre le Cancer (UICC) have recently proposed a numeric system for localizing intrathoracic lymph nodes for the purpose of lung cancer staging (described in detail in Chapter 8); this represents a modification of the system devised by the American Thoracic Society. According to the AJCC/UICC system of lymph node localization ("lymph node stations") in patients with lung cancer, the tracheal midline is used to distinguish ipsilateral nodes from contralateral nodes, although this is somewhat arbitrary and does not necessarily correlate with pathways of lymphatic spread or ease of resection of the abnormal lymph nodes.

Other factors that also affect the prognosis associated with mediastinal lymph node metastases include the following:

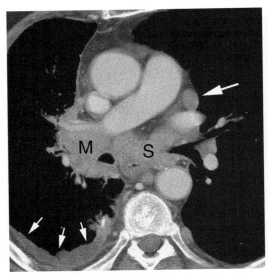
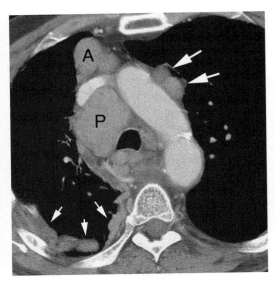

FIG. 3-40. Mediastinal lymph node metastases from small cell carcinoma. A large right hilar mass (*M*) is associated with lymph node enlargement in the subcarinal space (*S*), pretracheal space (*P*), anterior mediastinum (*A*), and the contralateral mediastinum (*large arrows*). Right pleural thickening and effusion (*small arrows*) are due to pleural metastases. The large bulky mediastinal nodes and contralateral nodes (N3) preclude resection.

1. Mediastinal nodal metastases detected at mediastinoscopy are associated with a poor prognosis (5-year survival rate of 10%) compared to those not found at mediastinoscopy and resected surgically (5-year survival rate of 20%).
2. Lymph nodes in the superior mediastinum are associated with a poor prognosis.
3. The presence of gross or bulky mediastinal node metastases (see Fig. 3-40), numerous abnormal lymph nodes, and node metastases that have invaded through the node capsule are associated with a poor survival after surgery.

CT and Mediastinoscopy

CT is helpful in determining which patients should have mediastinoscopy prior to surgery. In general, patients who have enlarged mediastinal lymph nodes seen on CT have mediastinoscopy prior to surgery; patients with normal-sized mediastinal lymph nodes on CT often have surgery without mediastinoscopy. This approach, however, varies among surgeons, and some perform mediastinoscopy routinely.

CT is also used as a guide for invasive procedures performed before an attempt at curative resection. Although mediastinoscopy is generally regarded as the gold standard of preoperative mediastinal evaluation, routine mediastinoscopy through a suprasternal incision does not evaluate all mediastinal compartments or lymph node groups. A significant percentage (up to 30%) of patients with lung carcinoma who have a negative mediastinoscopy prove to have mediastinal nodal metastases at surgery.

Routine mediastinoscopy can evaluate pretracheal lymph nodes, nodes in the anterior subcarinal space, and lymph nodes extending anterior to the right main bronchus (Fig. 3-41A). Lymph nodes in the anterior mediastinum (prevascular space), aortopulmonary window, and posterior portions of the mediastinum (e.g., posterior subcarinal space, azygoesophageal recess) are generally inaccessible using this technique (see Fig. 3-41B), although some of these can be evaluated using a left parasternal mediastinoscopy (Chamberlain procedure). CT can serve to guide the mediastinoscopist to the most suspicious lymph nodes. It may also suggest that needle aspiration biopsy, transbronchoscopic needle aspiration biopsy, or parasternal mediastinotomy would be appropriate.

Positron Emission Tomography

The use of positron emission tomography (PET) following injection of 2-[fluorine-18]-fluoro-2-deoxy-D-glucose (FDG) is becoming routine for lung cancer staging where available. PET is significantly more sensitive and specific

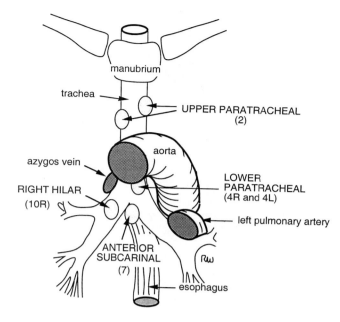

ACCESSIBLE LYMPH NODE STATIONS

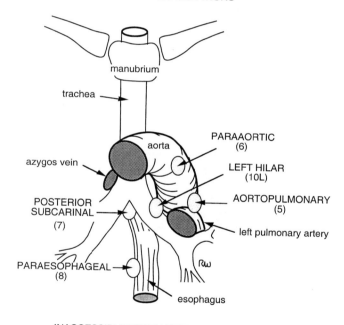

INACCESSIBLE LYMPH NODE STATIONS

FIG. 3-41. Mediastinal nodes accessible and inaccessible at routine mediastinoscopy performed through a suprasternal incision, as viewed from the front. Numbers indicate the corresponding AJCC/UICC lymph node stations (see Chapter 8).

(80% to 95%) in diagnosing mediastinal lymph node metastases in lung cancer than is CT (60% to 70% sensitivity and specificity; Fig. 3-42). Lymph node metastases may be diagnosed using PET when lymph nodes appear normal on CT.

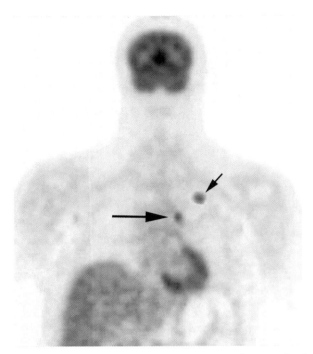

FIG. 3-42. Mediastinal lymph node metastasis diagnosed using FDG-PET. A metabolically active left upper lobe carcinoma *(small arrow)* is associated with a lymph node metastasis *(large arrow)* in the aortopulmonary window. High activity is also seen in the myocardium and brain.

PET may also be used to diagnose a lung nodule as malignant, with similar sensitivity and specificity (see Chapter 9). Scans are evaluated quantitatively using the *standardized uptake ratio* (SUR), which compares the activity of a lesion to that of other tissues. A SUR of more than 2.5 is usually used to diagnose lung cancer or metastases; benign lesions have a lower SUR. Because of the high sensitivity of PET, mediastinoscopy can be reserved for patients with a positive scan. However, the anatomic resolution of PET is quite limited, and it should be combined with CT when staging the mediastinum.

Distant Metastases

Distant metastases (M1) are present at diagnosis in 10% to 35% of patients with NSCBC; they are most common with adenocarcinoma or large cell carcinoma. Approximately 60% to 65% of patients with small cell carcinoma have detectable M1 disease at diagnosis, and many of the rest have microscopic metastases. Distant metastases rule out surgery; patients are treated with chemotherapy and have a poor prognosis.

Common sites of extrathoracic spread in patients with NSCBC include the adrenal glands, liver, bone, and brain. Satellite nodules involving a lobe other than that of the primary tumor are considered M1, as are nodules in the opposite lung.

History, physical examination (including a detailed neurologic evaluation), and blood tests (including liver function tests and serum calcium and alkaline phosphatase determinations) are used to suggest possible metastatic sites but are limited in accuracy. Imaging studies including radionuclide bone scanning with technetium 99m-methylene diphosphonate, contrast-enhanced brain and abdominal CT, brain and abdominal MRI, abdominal ultrasound, and FDG-PET are used to confirm organ-specific involvement as suggested by the clinical findings, although recommendations vary. Whole-body PET scanning is particularly useful in assessing distant metastases, except for those involving the brain (because of the high background activity of brain).

Adrenal metastases are present in up to 20% of patients with NSCBC at diagnosis and are often the only site of extrathoracic spread. Because of this, a chest CT in patients with lung cancer should be extended to encompass the upper abdomen. However, adrenal adenomas are common (3% to 5%) in the general population, and as many as 65% of small (less than 3 cm) adrenal masses in patients with lung cancer represent an adrenal adenoma rather than a metastasis. Although CT without contrast infusion and enhanced CT with delayed images can be helpful in distinguishing benign and malignant adrenal lesions, they may be nonspecific. Other methods of evaluating an adrenal mass include FDG-PET (which is highly accurate), chemical-shift MRI, and biopsy.

Liver metastases are present in 5% to 15% of cases. Their appearance on routine staging CT is often nonspecific and difficult to distinguish from cysts, hemangiomas, or other lesions without further imaging. However, isolated liver metastases are uncommon. CT, MRI, or FDG-PET may be used for diagnosing liver metastases.

Skeletal metastases are present at diagnosis in 5% to 20% of patients with lung carcinoma; they are present at autopsy in up to 30%. Squamous cell carcinoma and large cell carcinoma tend to cause osteolytic lesions, while small cell carcinoma and adenocarcinoma produce osteolytic or osteoblastic metastases. The bones most commonly involved are the vertebrae, pelvic bones, and proximal long bones. Metastases to the distal extremities are unusual, but lung carcinoma is the most common cause of distal metastases. Radionuclide imaging should be reserved for patients with symptoms or biochemical abnormalities and has a high false-positive rate (40%). FDG-PET scanning also allows detection of metastases and has a lower false-positive rate.

Central nervous system metastases are common and are often symptomatic (although the symptoms may be vague). However, asymptomatic brain metastases occur in up to 15% of patients with NSCBC and have a higher incidence with adenocarcinoma and large cell carcinoma than with other cell types. Consequently, routine brain CT or MRI is recommended in asymptomatic patients with these tumors.

With other cell types, imaging is usually limited to patients with symptoms. PET is less valuable.

CARCINOID TUMOR

About 25% of all primary lung tumors can be considered to be neuroectodermal carcinomas in that they arise from neuroectodermal cells, contain secretory granules, and can produce active peptides; this group includes typical carcinoid tumor, atypical carcinoid tumor, small cell carcinoma, and large cell neuroendocrine carcinoma. These tumors reflect a spectrum of abnormalities ranging from typical carcinoid tumor (which has a good prognosis) to small cell carcinoma (which has a poor prognosis; Table 3-18).

Typical Carcinoid Tumor

Carcinoid tumors account for 1% to 2% of tracheobronchial neoplasms. They are considered the best-differentiated type of neuroectodermal carcinoma.

Typical carcinoid tumors are slowly growing and locally invasive. They metastasize to regional lymph nodes in 5% to 15% of cases, and a lesser number of patients have distant metastases.

Typical carcinoid tumors occur most commonly in patients 40 to 60 years of age (mean age, 45 to 55). However, they are not uncommon in patients younger than 20 years, and this tumor tends to occur in a younger population than other lung carcinomas. It is slightly more common in women. There is no association with smoking.

Approximately 80% of typical carcinoid tumors occur centrally, in the main, lobar, or segmental bronchi; 1% are intratracheal. Involvement of lobar bronchi (75% of those with airway lesions) is most common (Fig. 3-43). Because of associated bronchial obstruction, symptoms are common, occurring in approximately 75% of cases; they include cough, fever, and wheezing. These tumors are highly vascular, and hemoptysis is a common presenting complaint. Pe-

ripheral carcinoid tumors may be asymptomatic. Patients who have central carcinoid tumors associated with bronchial obstruction tend to present at a younger age than patients with peripheral lesions.

Nearly half of typical carcinoid tumors are associated with radiographic findings of bronchial obstruction, primarily atelectasis or consolidation, typically limited to a lobe or segment (see Fig. 3-43A). Atelectasis and consolidation are often intermittent, and recurrent episodes of infection can result in bronchiectasis or lung abscess. Bronchiectasis is present pathologically in more than one third of patients but is less often visible on radiographs. Air trapping related to bronchial obstruction is sometimes seen.

Central tumors, with or without findings of obstruction, may be visible as discrete mass lesions in or near the hila. These masses, which are usually less than 4 cm in diameter, can be difficult to recognize without CT. In many cases, these tumors have a large endobronchial component and appear on CT as intraluminal masses (see Fig. 3-43B and C) with a convex margin pointing toward the hilum. Also, lesions that are largely endobronchial can expand the bronchus as they grow, typically resulting in a flaring of the bronchial lumen at the point of obstruction. Because they are highly vascular, dense enhancement may be seen on CT (see Fig. 3-43D).

A peripheral nodule or mass, not associated with findings of obstruction, is present in approximately 20% of patients (Fig. 3-44). These nodules are often well defined, round or oval, and slightly lobulated.

Rarely, calcification and ossification are seen on plain films in a patient with carcinoid tumor. On CT, calcification of central carcinoid tumors is seen in nearly 40%. Calcifications may be large.

Radionuclide imaging with somatostatin analogs (e.g., octreotide) may be used to localize an occult carcinoid tumor in a patient with Cushing's syndrome or carcinoid syndrome or to diagnose metastases (Fig. 3-45).

Local extension of typical carcinoid tumors beyond the bronchial wall is common, and endoscopic removal of visi-

TABLE 3-18. FEATURES DISTINGUISHING THE NEUROENDOCRINE CARCINOMAS

	Typical carcinoid	Atypical carcinoid	Small cell carcinoma
Mean age (yr)	45–50	60	>60
Male:female ratio	0.8:1	2:1	4:1
Smoking history	Uncommon	Common	Very common
Symptoms	75%	50%	90%
Regional metastases	5%–15%	40%–60%	>90%
Distant metastases	Rare	20%	>90%
5-year survival	90%–95%	50%–70%	<5%
Endobronchial mass	80%	10%	20%
Lung nodule or mass	20%	90%	20%
Large hilar mass	50%	10%	80%

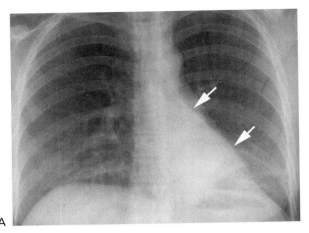

FIG. 3-43. Typical carcinoid tumor presenting as an endobronchial mass in a 30-year-old patient with recurrent left lower lobe pneumonia. **A.** Chest radiograph shows left lower lobe atelectasis *(arrows)*. **B.** CT at a later date shows a lobulated endobronchial mass *(*)* associated with obstruction of the left lower lobe bronchus. **C.** Contrast-enhanced CT at the same level shows enhancement of the tumor *(large arrow)* and its relationship to the left upper lobe bronchus *(LUL)* and the interlobar left pulmonary artery *(LPa)*. **D.** Coronal reformation shows the mass *(*)* obstructing the proximal left lower lobe bronchus *(LLL)*. The left upper lobe bronchus *(LUL)* is normal. **E.** Bronchoscopic photograph shows the endobronchial mass *(M)* protruding from the left lower lobe bronchus. This mass appeared highly vascular and bled easily.

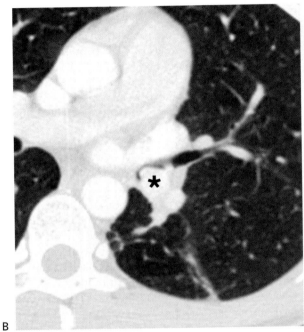

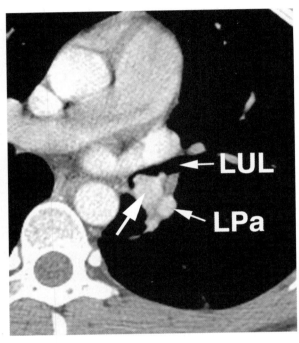

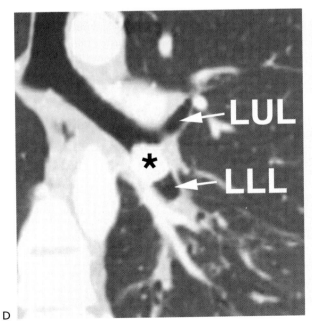

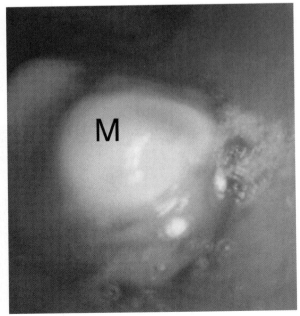

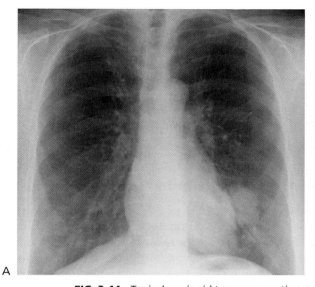
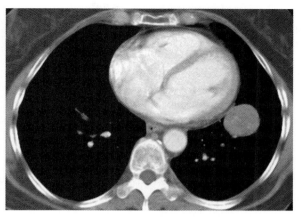

A   B

FIG. 3-44. Typical carcinoid tumor presenting as a lung mass. A well-defined and sharply margin-ated rounded mass is visible in the left lower lobe on the chest radiograph (**A**) and CT (**B**).

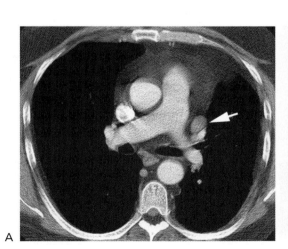
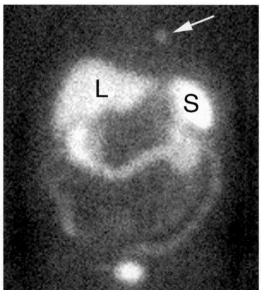

A   B

FIG. 3-45. Lymph node metastasis in a patient following resection of a carcinoid tumor. **A.** Chest CT shows an enlarged left mediastinal lymph node *(arrow)*. **B.** Octreotide radionuclide scan shows increased activity in the lymph node *(arrow)*. The liver *(L)* and spleen *(S)* are indicated for orientation.

ble tumor is not usually curative. Surgical resection is the treatment of choice. Peripheral carcinoid tumors can be excised using wedge resection or segmentectomy. For central endobronchial lesions, a sleeve resection may be performed to avoid pneumonectomy or lobectomy. In this procedure, a segment of bronchus containing the tumor is resected and the two bronchial stumps are sutured together.

For patients treated surgically, the prognosis is good. The 10-year survival rate of patients treated by surgery is as high as 90%. Following resection, distant metastasis is more common than local recurrence at the primary site. Bone metastases, either lytic or blastic, can occur.

Clinical Syndromes Associated With Carcinoid Tumor

Carcinoid tumors are capable of producing a number of active neuroendocrine peptides, and several clinical syndromes have been associated with this tumor. Typically, metastases are present before these syndromes become manifest; it is unusual for a small localized tumor to produce a sufficient amount of active peptides to result in clinical manifestations.

Carcinoid syndrome occurs in 2% to 5% of patients with pulmonary carcinoid tumor. It is most common in the presence of liver metastases. The carcinoid syndrome consists of flushing, fever, nausea, diarrhea, hypotension, and wheezing; it results from secretion of 5-hydroxytryptamine and other active agents such as bradykinin and prostaglandins. Cardiac valvular lesions and heart murmurs associated with this syndrome may be limited to the left side of the heart because of high concentrations of active substances in the pulmonary venous blood; cardiac valvular abnormalities associated with gastrointestinal carcinoid tumors usually involve the right side of the heart. Some other symptoms are said to help distinguish bronchial carcinoid syndrome from that resulting from intestinal tumors; these include

severe flushing, facial edema, lacrimation, salivation, rhinorrhea, and diaphoresis.

Cushing's syndrome can result from production of ACTH or ACTH-releasing hormone by the tumor. It is uncommon, being seen in about 2% of cases (Fig. 3-46). Approximately 1% of cases of Cushing's syndrome are produced by bronchial carcinoid. Other syndromes associated with bronchial carcinoid tumor include Zollinger-Ellison syndrome, hyperinsulinemia, and acromegaly.

Atypical Carcinoid Tumor

Approximately 10% to 25% of carcinoid tumors can be classified as atypical carcinoid tumor because of histologic features suggesting a more aggressive behavior, including an increased frequency of mitoses and the presence of necrosis. These tumors are considered to be intermediate between typical carcinoid tumor and small cell carcinoma in differentiation, the incidence of metastases, and mortality. Lymph node metastases are present in approximately 50% of patients. Patients with atypical carcinoid tend to be slightly older than those with typical carcinoid, and men outnumber women. There is an association with smoking.

Atypical carcinoid tumors tend to present as a lung nodule or mass, round or ovoid, lobulated, and somewhat larger than those seen with typical carcinoid tumor (10 cm or smaller). An endobronchial mass resulting in obstruction and atelectasis is less common that with typical carcinoid tumor, occurring in about 10%.

These tumors have a worse prognosis than typical pulmonary carcinoids, and a more aggressive surgical approach is usually employed (lobectomy, sometimes with radiation or chemotherapy). Surgical cures have been reported, and 5-year survival rates range from 50% to 70%. As with typical carcinoid tumor, they can be associated with various clinical syndromes.

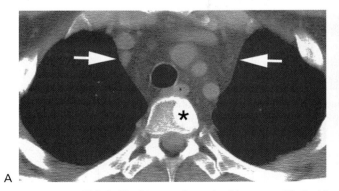
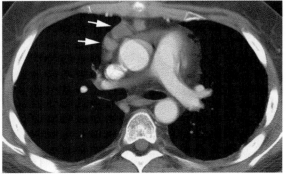

FIG. 3-46. Metastatic carcinoid tumor with Cushing's syndrome. **A.** CT shows mediastinal widening and fat deposition (lipomatosis; *arrows*) secondary to Cushing's syndrome. A sclerotic vertebral metastasis (*) is visible. **B.** At a lower level, enlarged mediastinal lymph nodes *(arrows)* reflect metastatic tumor.

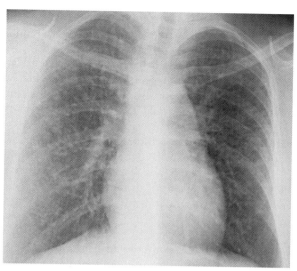

FIG. 3-47. Multiple carcinoid tumorlets visible as small lung nodules.

Neuroendocrine (Carcinoid) Tumorlets

Very small nodular collections or tumorlets of neuroendocrine cells may be seen in the walls of small airways in patients with chronic lung diseases such as bronchiectasis or lung fibrosis (termed *diffuse idiopathic pulmonary neuroendocrine cell hyperplasia* in the WHO system). In many cases these are hyperplastic. In other cases they are precursors to, or associated with, carcinoid tumors. They may be asymptomatic or associated with airway obstruction because of their relationship to the walls of small airways; Cushing's syndrome is rarely associated. In occasional cases, they are visible as small lung nodules (Fig. 3-47). There is a distinct predominance in women.

SALIVARY GLAND TYPE TUMORS

Tumors referred to as "salivary gland type" because of histologic similarities to lesions originating in the salivary glands arise from mucous glands in the walls of the trachea and bronchi; they may also be termed "bronchial gland neoplasms." They are subdivided into several cell types; adenoid cystic carcinoma (cylindroma) and mucoepidermoid carcinoma are the most common. Bronchial gland tumors account for 0.1% to 0.2% of all lung and bronchial tumors and are one-tenth as common as carcinoid tumor.

Adenoid Cystic Carcinoma (Cylindroma)

Adenoid cystic carcinoma is the most common bronchial gland tumor, accounting for 75% of cases. The mean age at diagnosis is 50; it has not been associated with smoking.

Approximately 50% of adenoid cystic carcinomas originate in the main or lobar bronchi (Fig. 3-48), 40% originate in the trachea, and 10% present as peripheral lung nodules. Although adenoid cystic carcinoma is an uncommon neoplasm, it is responsible for as many as 30% to 35% of tracheal malignancies. Although carcinoid is much more common among central bronchial tumors, adenoid cystic carcinoma outnumbers carcinoid in the trachea by 20 to 1.

When it occurs in an endobronchial location, adenoid cystic carcinoma presents with symptoms and radiographic findings similar to carcinoid. The tumor usually protrudes into the airway lumen and may be polypoid or sessile.

When it is endotracheal, this lesion most commonly appears as a sessile mass, with obtuse angles where it contacts the tracheal wall; in some patients it is polypoid. It tends to originate from the posterior or posterolateral tracheal wall (see Figs. 22-4 and 22-5B in Chapter 22). Although CT can be helpful in assessing endotracheal adenoid cystic carcinoma, it tends to underestimate the longitudinal extent of the tumor because of partial volume averaging and the tendency of adenoid cystic carcinoma to grow submucosally. CT, however, accurately demonstrates extratracheal extension of tumor, which is helpful in planning the surgical approach.

Adenoid cystic carcinoma has a much better prognosis than more common forms of lung carcinoma. However, it behaves in a more malignant fashion than carcinoid tumor, tends to be more infiltrative than carcinoid tumor (see Fig. 3-48), and metastasizes more frequently.

These tumors are treated using surgical excision but tend to recur locally. Recent advances in tracheal resection and carinal reconstruction have made many tracheal lesions resectable. The 5-year survival rate is about 75%.

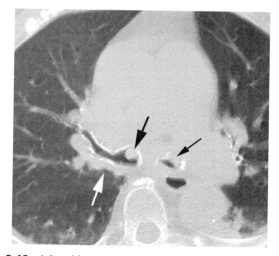

FIG. 3-48. Adenoid cystic carcinoma. A polypoid lesion is visible in the right main bronchus *(large black arrow)*. Thickening of the right upper lobe bronchial wall *(white arrow)* is due to local infiltration. Infiltration of the left main bronchus is associated with narrowing of its lumen *(small black arrow)*.

Mucoepidermoid Carcinoma

Mucoepidermoid carcinoma is a rare tumor. The average age at diagnosis is 35 to 45 years. It usually occurs in the main or lobar bronchi; tracheal or peripheral lesions are uncommon. It tends to exhibit a more benign course than adenoid cystic carcinoma or carcinoid tumor, but it may be locally invasive. High-grade mucoepidermoid carcinoma has been reported to have a poor prognosis.

Presentation and radiographic findings are similar to those of adenoid cystic carcinoma. These tumors arise in the trachea or central bronchi and result in symptoms and radiographic findings of obstruction. Surgery is usually curative.

Bronchial Adenoma

True "bronchial adenomas" are rare. The most common cell type of bronchial adenoma is *mucous gland adenoma*. Rarer cell types include pleomorphic adenoma and oncocytoma.

These tumors are benign tumors originating from glands in the tracheal or bronchial wall. As with bronchial gland carcinomas, they are similar histologically to tumors arising in the salivary glands. Bronchial adenomas occur in patients of all ages. These tumors usually originate in the main, lobar, or segmental bronchi and are associated with findings of bronchial obstruction. Radiographically, they typically appear as smooth, sessile or rounded endobronchial masses. Presentation as a solitary nodule is much less frequent. Excision is usually curative.

HAMARTOMA

Hamartoma is the most common mesenchymal tumor of the respiratory tract, and it accounts for more than 75% of benign lung tumors (Table 3-19). Hamartomas contain the various connective-tissue elements that are normally found in the lung and bronchi, but in a disorganized state. This tumor almost always contains cartilage and is sometimes referred to as chondromatous hamartoma. Also found in varying amounts are fat, fibrous tissue, smooth muscle, myxomatous tissue, and epithelial tissue. Hamartomas most likely originate within embryonic rests in the bronchial wall, but it has also been hypothesized that they derive from undifferentiated mesenchymal tissues and represent true neoplasms.

Hamartomas are most commonly diagnosed in patients older than 50 and are twice as common in men as in women. They are rare in children, and less than 10% occur in patients younger than 40. Prior to the advent of CT (which greatly assists in their preoperative diagnosis), hamartomas accounted for as many as 6% to 8% of resected lung nodules.

Despite their origin from bronchial tissues, only 5% to 15% of hamartomas present as endobronchial (Fig. 3-49). In more than 85% of cases, hamartomas appear radiographically as a solitary pulmonary nodule. Peripheral hamartomas are usually 1 to 4 cm in diameter, well defined, sharply circumscribed, and often lobulated. Calcification of cartilage is reported to be visible on plain radiographs in approximately 30% of hamartomas, and the frequency of calcification increases with the tumor's size. Calcification is seen in less than 10% of hamartomas less than 3 cm in diameter but is present in 75% of those 5 cm or larger.

Calcification of hamartomas can be stippled or conglomerate. Conglomerate or "popcorn" calcification is characteristic of hamartomas and is rarely seen with other lesions; it occurs because of calcification of nodules of cartilage (Fig.

TABLE 3-19. HAMARTOMAS

75% of benign lung tumors
Patients >50 yr
Twice as common in men
5%–15% endobronchial
≥85% present as solitary nodule
   Usually 1–4 cm
   Sharply circumscribed
   Round or lobulated
Calcification in 25%
   Popcorn calcification
Fat visible on CT in 60%
Slow growth

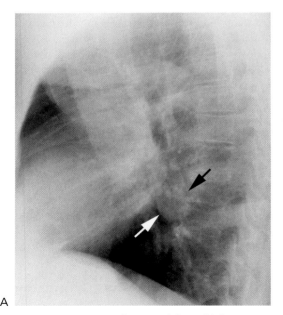

A

FIG. 3-49. Hamartoma with an endobronchial component. **A.** Lateral chest radiograph shows a well-defined hilar nodule (*arrows*). (*Figure continues.*)

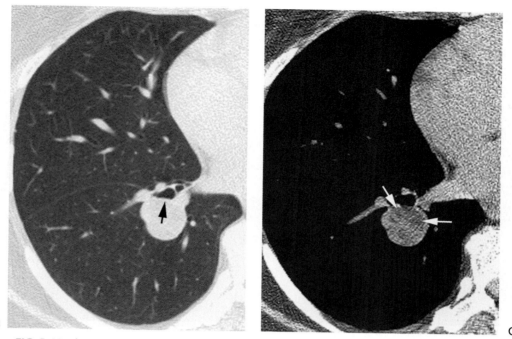

B

C

FIG. 3-49. *(Continued.)* **B.** High-resolution CT with a lung window shows a sharply marginated lobulated nodule narrowing the right lower lobe bronchus *(arrow).* **C.** High-resolution with a soft-tissue window shows areas of fat attenuation (−80 HU; *arrows*), common in hamartoma.

3-50). Accumulations of fat can produce lucent or low-attenuation areas within the tumor, usually visible only on CT. Rarely, cystic, air-filled hamartomas have been reported.

High-resolution CT is valuable in diagnosing pulmonary hamartoma. Nearly 65% of hamartomas may be diagnosed using high-resolution CT because of visible fat (see Figs. 3-49 and 3-51), either focal or diffuse (CT numbers ranging from −40 to −120 HU) or a combination of fat and calcium. Thin collimation (i.e., 1 mm) must be used to

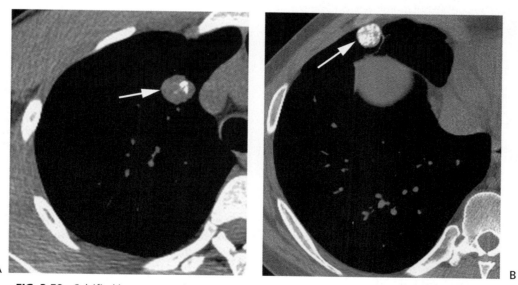

A

B

FIG. 3-50. Calcified hamartomas in two patients. **A.** Hamartoma *(arrow)* with focal calcification. The nodule is round and sharply defined. **B.** Hamartoma *(arrow)* with popcorn calcification. This appearance results from calcification of nodules of cartilage in the tumor.

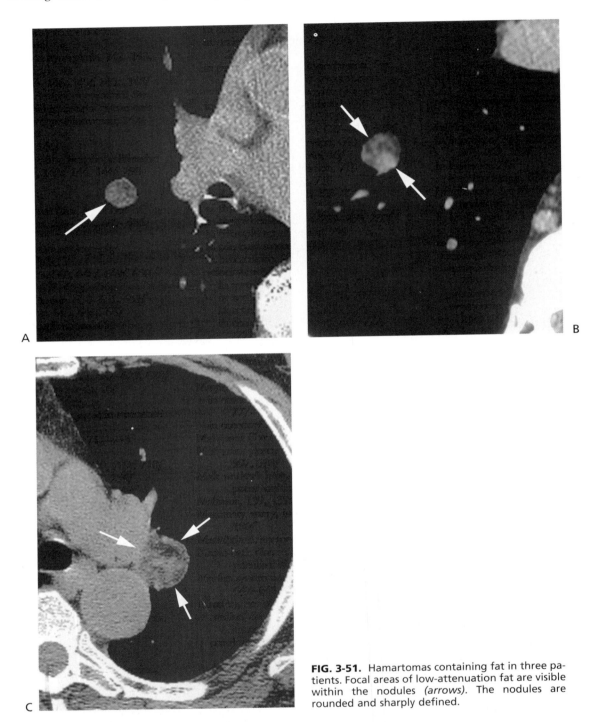

FIG. 3-51. Hamartomas containing fat in three patients. Focal areas of low-attenuation fat are visible within the nodules *(arrows)*. The nodules are rounded and sharply defined.

make the diagnosis of fat within a nodule; otherwise, volume averaging may simulate this appearance. A nodule containing fat has a very limited differential diagnosis; lipoid pneumonia is another but much less common cause of this finding. Pulmonary teratoma could also show fat, but this is extremely rare.

In most cases, hamartomas grow slowly, increasing in diameter from 0.5 to 5 mm per year (Fig. 3-52). Rapid growth can occur, however, causing hamartomas to be confused with lung carcinoma. Endobronchial lesions can be resected bronchoscopically unless infection has caused destruction of the distal lung. Needle biopsy can be diagnostic in some cases, but peripheral tumors may require excision for diagnosis.

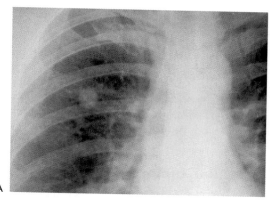
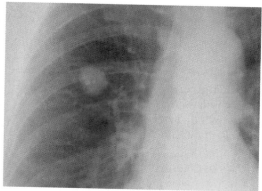

FIG. 3-52. Hamartomas with growth. **A.** Chest radiograph shows a well-defined upper lobe nodule measuring 1 cm. **B.** Radiograph 3 years later. The nodule now measures 2 cm in diameter. Several foci of calcification are visible within the nodule. The doubling time of this nodule is 1 year.

RARE LUNG TUMORS

Mesenchymal Tumors

Except for hamartoma, mesenchymal tumors of the lung are rare. Benign mesenchymal tumors are much more common than malignant neoplasms.

Mesenchymal tumors may present as (1) an endobronchial lesion, often rounded or sessile, and associated with symptoms of bronchial obstruction or (2) a nodule or mass in the lung periphery, usually detected incidentally on chest radiographs or CT, or when malignant, associated with chest wall invasion.

Lipoma and Liposarcoma

Lipoma and liposarcoma originate in collections of fat found in the walls of cartilage-containing airways. Lipoma overlaps with fatty hamartoma; liposarcoma is rare. They may occur in patients of any age, usually ranging from 30 to 65, and nearly 90% occur in men.

Lipomas are most common in the main or lobar bronchi and typically are found in the bronchial lumen. Endobronchial lesions are usually oval, measuring several centimeters in length. They uncommonly occur in the peripheral lung. Symptoms and radiographic findings of bronchial obstruction are common, and obstructive pneumonitis and bronchiectasis are often present. Occasionally a lipoma extends in a dumbbell fashion to lie primarily outside the bronchus. CT can be diagnostic, showing uniform low attenuation indistinguishable from a fat-containing hamartoma.

Chondroma and Chondrosarcoma

True chondromas, containing only cartilage, are exceedingly rare, and their relationship to hamartomas is uncertain. They may occur as an endobronchial lesion or a well-defined solitary nodule. Calcification occurs in about 30%.

Pulmonary chondroma may occur as part of *Carney's triad*. This unusual entity is characterized by the combination of multiple pulmonary chondromas, gastric epithelioid leiomyosarcoma, and extraadrenal paraganglioma. In some cases, only two of the three manifestations are present. This syndrome is most common in young women less than 30; only 10% of cases occur in men.

Chondrosarcoma is rare. This tumor occurs much more commonly as a pulmonary mass lesion than as a mass within the trachea or bronchial lumen. In general, pulmonary lesions have a very poor prognosis.

Leiomyoma and Leiomyosarcoma

Leiomyoma is thought to arise from smooth muscle found in the walls of the bronchi or perhaps blood vessels. The average age at diagnosis is 50, but it occurs in patients ranging from 5 to 65; women are more frequently affected. Leiomyoma may occur as a lung nodule (slightly more common) or an endobronchial lesion. Pulmonary parenchymal leiomyomas are usually asymptomatic and detected incidentally. They appear radiographically as well-defined, lobulated, peripheral mass lesions and range up to 20 cm in diameter. Calcification is rare and cavitation does not occur. Endobronchial lesions usually occur in the main or lobar bronchi. Symptoms are common and often due to obstructive pneumonia. In such patients, radiographic findings are usually limited to signs of airway obstruction. CT may show an endobronchial mass.

Leiomyosarcoma is more common than leiomyoma. Leiomyosarcoma is more common in men than women with a ratio of 2 to 1. Patients are usually symptomatic. Radiographs demonstrate a pulmonary mass in most cases, and in general tumors are larger than leiomyomas. Cavitation may occur. Endobronchial obstruction with atelectasis occurs in about a third of patients.

Multiple pulmonary "leiomyomas" associated with smooth muscle tumors of the uterus in women ("benign metastasizing leiomyoma") represent pulmonary metastases from a low-grade uterine leiomyosarcoma. Single or multiple lung masses are usually seen. They may be quite large, may calcify, and grow slowly (Fig. 3-53).

Fibroma and Fibrosarcoma

Fibroma can involve the lung or tracheobronchial tree and is rare. Pulmonary parenchymal lesions are most common and are usually asymptomatic. Tracheal or bronchial lesions produce symptoms and signs of obstruction.

Fibrosarcomas, regardless of their location, are usually symptomatic. They more often appear as a nodule or mass rather than as an endobronchial lesion. Endobronchial lesions are most common in children and young adults, while pulmonary masses are found in patients of middle age. Pul-

monary lesions are usually round and well defined, measuring up to 20 cm in diameter.

Malignant Fibrous Histiocytoma

Primary involvement of the lung is uncommon with this tumor. The average age at diagnosis is about 50. Most appear as smooth or lobulated lung masses.

Vascular Tumors

Vascular tumors of the lung and bronchi are rare. Although vessels are present within the tumors, they are solid masses and rarely exhibit significant opacification during angiography or CT.

Glomus tumor is derived from smooth muscle cells of the glomus body and consists of irregular vascular channels. It most often occurs as a polypoid mass arising from the tracheal or bronchial wall. Hemoptysis or bronchial obstruction may be present.

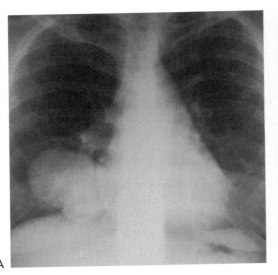

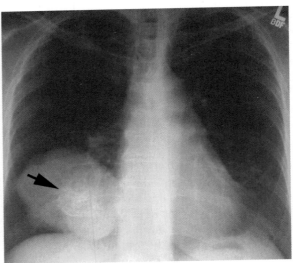

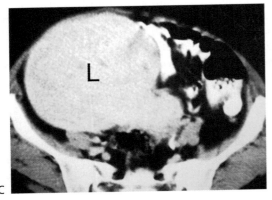

FIG. 3-53. Benign metastasizing leiomyoma. **A.** Chest radiograph shows a large right lower lobe mass. **B.** Ten years later, the mass has increased in size. Some central calcification is visible *(arrow)*. **C.** CT at the time of prior hysterectomy shows a large uterine mass, representing a low-grade leiomyosarcoma *(L)*.

Hemangiopericytoma is characterized by profuse proliferation of capillaries surrounded by neoplastic accumulations of pericytes. Tumors tend to be peripheral, appearing as a well-defined solitary nodule or mass, and ranging in size from 2 to 15 cm. Hemangiopericytoma can be benign or malignant, and excision is the treatment of choice.

Epithelioid hemangioendothelioma is a rare multifocal pulmonary neoplasm. It is manifested by multiple well-defined lung nodules up to 2 cm in diameter, mimicking the appearance of metastases. Eighty percent of cases occur in women, often less than 40 years old. The tumors may be asymptomatic or associated with cough, hemoptysis, or systemic symptoms. This entity is thought to represent a low-grade sarcoma, and metastases may occur. Liver involvement may be associated, representing metastases or synchronous development in multiple sites.

Neural Tumors

Neurogenic tumors of the lung and tracheobronchial tree, both benign and malignant, are rare. They are thought to arise from sympathetic nerve fibers accompanying arterioles or bronchioles. Among benign tumors are neurofibroma, schwannoma, paraganglioma, meningioma, granular cell tumor (granular cell myoblastoma), and meningothelial-like nodules. Neurofibrosarcoma is less common. These most often present as well-defined solitary nodules within the lung parenchyma, but endobronchial lesions have been reported. Neurofibroma, schwannoma, and neurofibrosarcoma may be associated with neurofibromatosis, particularly when multiple.

Epithelial Tumors

Squamous Papilloma and Tracheobronchial Papillomatosis

Squamous papilloma represents an abnormal proliferation of stratified squamous, or sometimes ciliated columnar epithelium forming a polypoid mass within the airway lumen. These lesions are supported by a core of fibrovascular tissue connecting them to the tracheal or bronchial wall. They are benign and of viral origin, caused by the human papillomavirus. Malignant change sometimes occurs.

Papilloma is the most common laryngeal tumor of childhood, and laryngeal papillomas occasionally occur in adults. Laryngeal lesions are often multiple and spread locally. In children, papillomas are successfully treated by surgical excision or regress at puberty. In 2% to 5% of patients, however, the lesions spread distally to involve the tracheobronchial tree, a condition referred to as *tracheobronchial papillomatosis*; the trachea is almost always involved when distal spread occurs. Tracheobronchial spread is associated with instrumentation for resection of laryngeal lesions.

Involvement of the trachea often results in cough or hemoptysis. Hoarseness due to laryngeal lesions may also be present. In most cases, the lesions are multiple and small, ranging from a few millimeters to 1 cm in diameter, but they can be large, resulting in tracheal obstruction. Plain radiographs are rarely of value; CT is usually necessary for diagnosis (Fig. 3-54).

Extension of papillomas to the bronchi, bronchioles, and lung parenchyma is rare. The interval between the diagnosis of laryngeal lesions and bronchial spread ranges from 1 to 36 years. Although laryngeal lesions are most common in children younger than 5, the average age of patients with tumors involving the bronchial tree is 15. Bronchial obstruction results in wheezing, atelectasis, and recurrent pneumonia. Papillomas may be visible radiographically as nodular mass lesions within the lung, and they often cavitate. Eventually, cavitary lesions may progress to large thick- or thin-walled cysts. Nodules representing papillomas may be seen within cysts (Figs. 3-55 and 3-56).

Bronchoscopic excision of tracheal or bronchial papillomas has been the treatment of choice, but the lesions recur following resection in more than 90% of patients. Tracheostomy may be required for associated laryngeal lesions that produce airway obstruction. Cystic pulmonary lesions are not usually associated with symptoms, and unless they are infected no treatment is necessary. In recent studies, interferon has been of some value in treatment. Malignant degeneration of pulmonary lesions may occur, leading to squamous cell carcinoma (see Fig. 3-56C).

Solitary papillomas occasionally occur in adults, usually

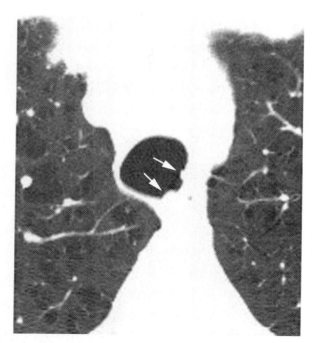

FIG. 3-54. Tracheal papillomas. Small nodules *(arrows)* are visible arising from the tracheal wall.

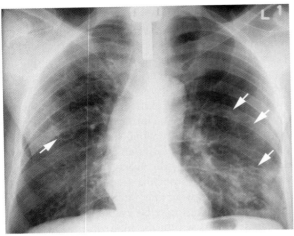

FIG. 3-55. Tracheobronchial papillomatosis. Tracheostomy is in place because of upper airway lesions. Multiple cystic pulmonary lesions are present bilaterally *(arrows)*.

Inflammatory Polyps

Inflammatory polyps of the tracheobronchial tree are characterized histologically by a loose connective-tissue core covered by normal bronchial epithelium; they lack the squamous overgrowth typical of papillomas and in general occur in older patients. These lesions may be polypoid or sessile and are larger than squamous papillomas. In most patients, polyps range from 0.5 to 2 cm in diameter (Fig. 3-57). Occasionally polyps are multiple, and findings of bronchial obstruction are common. Recurrence following excision does not occur.

Pulmonary Adenomas

Tracheobronchial adenomas occurring as endobronchial lesions are reviewed above (see Salivary Gland Type Tumors). Adenomas arising in the lung periphery, derived from bronchiolar or alveolar epithelium and usually presenting as a lung nodule, include mucinous cystadenoma, papillary and alveolar adenoma, and sclerosing hemangioma.

Miscellaneous Tumors

Other tumors rarely occurring in the lung or bronchial tree include thymoma, teratoma, seminoma, endometriosis, and lymphangioma. With exception of teratoma, which may

middle-aged men, in the absence of prior laryngeal lesions. They are usually less than 1.5 cm in diameter and are most commonly found in a lobar or segmental bronchus. They may result in bronchial obstruction, and symptoms include cough and hemoptysis. Histology is identical to that found in papillomatosis.

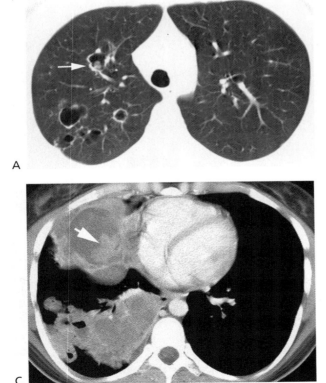

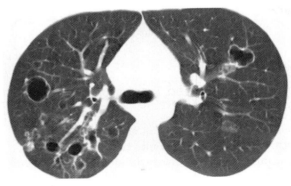

FIG. 3-56. Tracheobronchial papillomatosis. **A** and **B**. Multiple thick- and thin-walled cavities, cysts, and nodules are visible bilaterally. A cystic lesion *(arrow)* contains a nodule. **C**. Progression of abnormalities with large masses indicates development of squamous cell carcinoma. A nodule of tumor *(arrow)* is visible within a fluid-filled cyst.

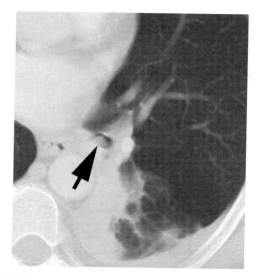

FIG. 3-57. Inflammatory polyp. A polypoid lesion is visible in the left lower lobe bronchus *(arrow)*.

mimic mediastinal teratoma, their appearances are nonspecific.

SELECTED READING

Bepler G. Lung cancer epidemiology and genetics. J Thorac Imaging 1999; 14:228–234.

Dales RE, Stark RM, Raman S. Computed tomography to stage lung cancer: approaching a controversy using meta-analysis. Am Rev Respir Dis 1990; 141:1096–1101.

Forster BB, Müller NL, Miller RR, et al. Neuroendocrine carcinomas of the lung: clinical, radiologic, and pathologic correlation. Radiology 1989; 170:441–445.

Glazer HS, Duncan MJ, Aronberg DJ, et al. Pleural and chest wall invasion in bronchogenic carcinoma: CT evaluation. Radiology 1985; 157:191–194.

Glazer HS, Kaiser LR, Anderson DJ, et al. Indeterminate mediastinal invasion in bronchogenic carcinoma: CT evaluation. Radiology 1989; 173:37–42.

Heelan RT, Demas BE, Caravelli JF, et al. Superior sulcus tumors: CT and MR imaging. Radiology 1989; 170:637–641.

Kakinuma R, Ohmatsu H, Kaneko M, et al. Detection failures in spiral CT screening for lung cancer: analysis of CT findings. Radiology 1999; 212:61–66.

McLoud TC, Bourgouin PM, Greenberg RW, et al. Bronchogenic carcinoma: analysis of staging in the mediastinum with CT by correlative lymph node mapping and sampling. Radiology 1992; 182:319–323.

Mountain CF. Revisions in the international system for staging lung cancer. Chest 1997; 111:1710–1717.

Patel AM, Peters SG. Clinical manifestations of lung cancer. Mayo Clin Proc 1993; 68:273–277.

Pennes DR, Glazer GM, Wimbish KJ, et al. Chest wall invasion by lung cancer: limitations of CT evaluation. AJR Am J Roentgenol 1985; 144:507–511.

Ratto GB, Piacenza G, Frola C, et al. Chest wall involvement by lung cancer: computed tomographic detection and results of operation. Ann Thorac Surg 1991; 51:182–188.

Rosado de Christenson ML, Abbott GF, Kirejczyk WM, Galvin JR, Travis WD. Thoracic carcinoids: radiologic-pathologic correlation. Radiographics 1999; 19:707–736.

Salvatierra A, Baamonde C, Llamas JM, et al. Extrathoracic staging of bronchogenic carcinoma. Chest 1990; 97:1052–1058.

Scott IR, Müller NL, Miller RR, et al. Resectable stage III lung cancer: CT, surgical, and pathologic correlation. Radiology 1988; 166:75–79.

Siegelman SS, Khouri NF, Scott WW, et al. Pulmonary hamartoma: CT findings. Radiology 1986; 160:313–317.

Staples CA, Müller NL, Miller RR, et al. Mediastinal nodes in bronchogenic carcinoma: comparison between CT and mediastinoscopy. Radiology 1988; 167:367–372.

Travis WD. Pathology of lung cancer. Clin Chest Med 2002; 23: 65–81.

Webb WR, Gatsonis C, Zerhouni EA, et al. CT and MR imaging in staging non–small cell bronchogenic carcinoma: report of the Radiologic Diagnostic Oncology Group. Radiology 1991; 178: 705–713.

Webb WR, Golden JA. Imaging strategies in the staging of lung cancer. Clin Chest Med 1991; 12:133–150.

White CS, Salis AI, Meyer CA. Missed lung cancer on chest radiography and computed tomography: imaging and medicolegal issues. J Thorac Imaging 1999; 14:63–68.

Whitesell PL, Drage CW. Occupational lung cancer. Mayo Clin Proc 1993; 68:183–188.

Zwiebel BR, Austin JHM, Grines MM. Bronchial carcinoid tumors: assessment with CT of location and intratumoral calcification in 31 patients. Radiology 1991; 179:483–486.

Zwirewich CV, Vedal S, Miller RR, Müller NL. Solitary pulmonary nodule: high-resolution CT and radiologic-pathologic correlation. Radiology 1991; 179:469–476.

4

METASTATIC TUMOR

W. RICHARD WEBB

Thoracic structures commonly are involved in patients with metastatic neoplasm, and the chest often is the first site in which metastases are detected.

MECHANISMS OF SPREAD

Metastatic tumor may involve thoracic structures in several ways.

Direct extension from the primary tumor with secondary involvement of the lung, pleura, or mediastinal structures. This mode of spread is most common with thyroid tumors, esophageal carcinoma, thymoma and thymic malignancies, lymphoma, and malignant germ cell tumors.

Hematogenous spread of tumor emboli to pulmonary or bronchial arteries. This usually results in the presence of lung nodules and is most common with primary tumors that have a good vascular supply.

Lymphatic spread to involve the lung, pleura, or mediastinal lymph nodes. The lung may be diffusely involved by tumor following lymphatic or lymphangitic spread of cells from hematogenous metastases, hilar lymph node metastases, or upper abdominal tumors. Lymphatic spread of extrathoracic tumors to mediastinal lymph nodes also may occur via the thoracic duct, with retrograde involvement of hilar lymph nodes and the lung parenchyma. Tumors that commonly metastasize in this fashion include carcinomas of the breast, stomach, pancreas, prostate, cervix, and thyroid.

Spread within the pleural space due to pleural invasion from a local tumor (e.g., thymoma) or lung carcinoma.

Endobronchial spread of cells from an airway tumor. This mechanism of metastasis is uncommon. It is most common in patients with bronchioloalveolar carcinoma (Fig. 4-1). but may be seen with other cell types of lung cancer (Fig. 4-2). It also is thought to occur in patients with tracheobronchial papillomatosis (see Figs. 3-55 and 3-56 in Chapter 3).

MANIFESTATIONS OF METASTATIC TUMOR

Lung Nodules

Lung nodules are the most common thoracic manifestation of metastasis. In most cases they are hematogenous in origin (Table 4-1). They tend to predominate in the lung bases, which receive more blood flow than the upper lobes.

Nodules tend to be sharply marginated in most cases and round or lobulated in contour (Fig. 4-3). Poorly marginated nodules may be seen in the presence of surrounding hemorrhage or local invasion of adjacent lung (Fig. 4-4). In some cases, individual metastases are seen to have a relationship to small vascular branches, suggesting a hematogenous origin. This is termed the "feeding vessel" sign (Fig. 4-5). Nodules may be small or large. Using computed tomography (CT), metastases as small as 1 to 2 mm may be visible.

Cavitation of metastases is not as common as with primary lung carcinoma, but it does occur in about 5% of cases. It may be seen even with small nodules (Fig. 4-6). The likelihood of cavitation varies with histology. Cavitation is most common with squamous cell tumors and transitional cell tumors, but also may be seen in adenocarcinomas, particularly from the colon, and in some sarcomas.

Calcification of metastases occurs most commonly with osteogenic sarcoma, chondrosarcoma, synovial sarcoma, thyroid carcinoma, and mucinous adenocarcinoma (Fig. 4-7). Calcification may be dense, particularly with osteogenic

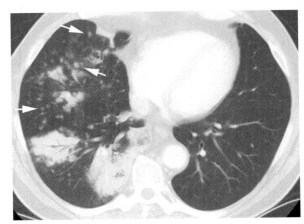

FIG. 4-1. Endobronchial spread of bronchioloalveolar carcinoma. Patchy areas of consolidation are visible. Centrilobular nodules *(arrows)* associated with bronchioloalveolar carcinoma are thought to be due to endobronchial spread.

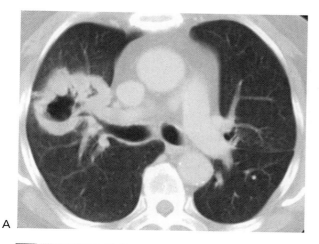

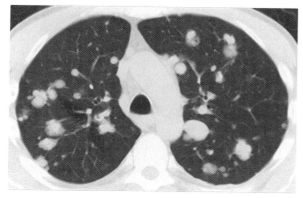

FIG. 4-2. Endobronchial spread of squamous cell carcinoma. **A.** CT shows a cavitary mass closely associated with the right upper lobe bronchus. **B.** Years later, extensive bilateral nodular and cavitary masses are visible. Extensive endobronchial tumor was present.

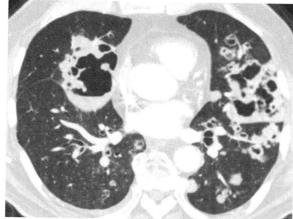

FIG. 4-3. Metastatic salivary gland carcinoma with rounded and lobulated metastases. Nodules vary in size; this is typical with metastatic tumor and is less common with benign diseases.

TABLE 4-1. NODULAR METASTASES

Hematogenous spread
Multiple nodules typically of different sizes
Basal predominance in size and number
Feeding vessel sign
Diffuse or "random" distribution
Poorly marginated nodules
  Hemorrhage or invasion
Small nodules
  Thyroid carcinoma
  Melanoma
  Adenocarcinoma
  Sarcomas
Cannonball metastases
  Renal cell carcinoma
  Testicular carcinoma
  Colon carcinoma
Cavitation
  Squamous cell
  Transitional cell
  Adenocarcioma (e.g., colon)
  Sarcomas
Calcification
  Osteogenic sarcoma
  Chondrosarcoma
  Synovial sarcoma
  Thyroid carcinoma
  Mucinous adenocarcinoma
Solitary metastases
  Colon carcinoma
  Renal cell carcinoma
  Testicular carcinoma
  Sarcomas
  Melanoma

following successful chemotherapy despite resolution of the nodules.

Computed tomography is considerably more sensitive than plain radiographs in detecting lung nodules, although the sensitivity of CT varies with the technique used. The sensitivity of chest radiographs for detecting nodules in patients with suspected metastases is about 40% to 45%. Using spiral CT with 5-mm collimation, a sensitivity of about 70% has been reported for detection of individual nodules 5 mm or less in diameter, with a sensitivity of 95% for those larger than 5 mm. Computed tomography has limited specificity in patients with suspected metastases, because small granulomas or intrapulmonary lymph nodes, measuring only a few millimeters in diameter, may mimic small metastases and are very common. If very small nodules are seen on CT in a patient with suspected metastases, CT follow-up at 6 weeks to 3 months is appropriate; nodules that are metastases should grow. In the absence of a history of neoplasm, the presence of small nodules most likely indicates benign disease. Between 80% and 85% of nodules detected by CT in patients with extrathoracic neoplasm are malignant.

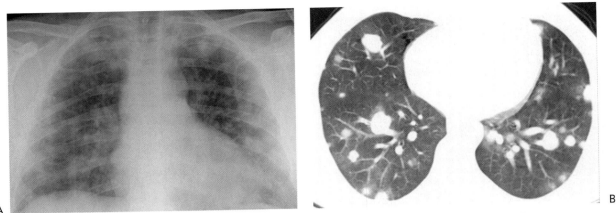

FIG. 4-4. Metastases from choriocarcinoma. **A.** Chest radiograph shows multiple ill-defined lung nodules with a preponderance at the lung bases. **B.** CT shows rounded and lobulated nodules, many of which are surrounded by ground-glass opacities (i.e., the halo sign). This appearance results from hemorrhage and is common with choriocarcinoma and other vascular tumors. It also may reflect invasion of adjacent lung.

Multiple Nodules

Nodular metastases usually are multiple. The nodules often vary in size, representing multiple episodes of tumor embolization or different growth rates (see Figs. 4-3, 4-4, and 4-8); this appearance is less common with benign nodular disease, such as sarcoidosis. Occasionally, all of the nodular metastases are of the same size. When there are numerous nodules, they tend to be distributed throughout the lung (Fig. 4-9). When the metastases are few in number, they may be predominantly subpleural (see Fig. 4-4B). On CT, numerous nodules tend to involve the lung in a diffuse fashion without regard for specific anatomic structures, a distribution termed "random" (see Figs. 4-3 and 4-9B). This pattern is described in detail in Chapter 10.

The size and number of nodules vary greatly. Nodules may be small (i.e., miliary) and very numerous (Fig. 4-10); this appearance often is seen with very vascular tumors (e.g., thyroid carcinoma, renal cell carcinoma, adenocarcinoma, sarcomas) and presumably reflects a single massive shower of tumor emboli. Fewer, larger metastases also may be seen; when these are well defined, they are referred to as "cannonball metastases" (see Figs. 4-8 and 4-11). This type of metastasis is seen most commonly with tumors of the gastrointestinal or genitourinary tract.

Most patients (80%–90%) with multiple metastases

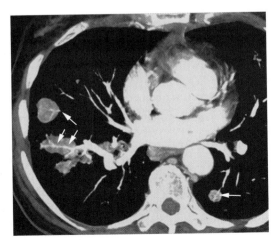

FIG. 4-5. The feeding vessel sign. Vascular supply of lung metastases *(arrows)* in a patient with bladder carcinoma is shown using a maximum-intensity projection image obtained with 1.25-mm slice thickness after contrast infusion.

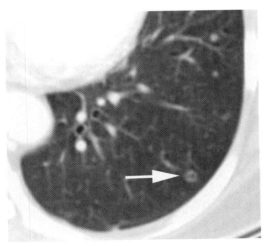

FIG. 4-6. Cavitary nodule in metastatic transitional cell carcinoma. Even though the nodule is very small *(arrow)*, a distinct cavity is visible.

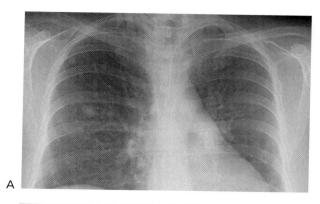

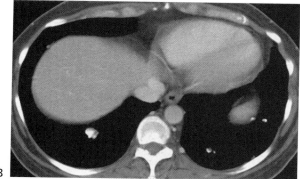

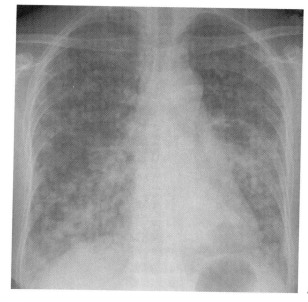

A

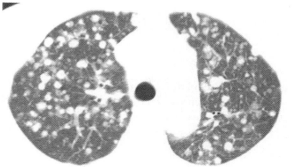

B

FIG. 4-7. Ossified metastases secondary to osteogenic carcinoma. **A.** Chest radiograph shows dense nodules. **B.** CT shows dense calcification, which is typical of this tumor.

FIG. 4-9. Metastatic adenocarcinoma. **A.** Chest radiograph shows numerous small, diffusely distributed nodules. Nodules appear more numerous and larger at the lung bases. **B.** CT shows a diffuse distribution of nodules. This pattern is termed "random," because it involves the lung randomly relative to lung structures. Some nodules typically are seen to involve the pleural surface with a random pattern.

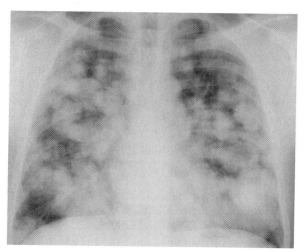

FIG. 4-8. Metastatic testicular carcinoma. Nodules vary in size and appear more numerous and larger at the lung bases. A basal preponderance is typical of metastases. Large nodular metastases are sometimes called "cannonball" metastases.

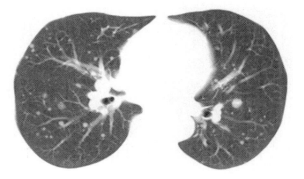

FIG. 4-10. Metastatic thyroid carcinoma. Numerous small metastases are visible, distributed throughout the lung.

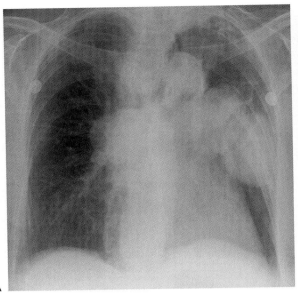
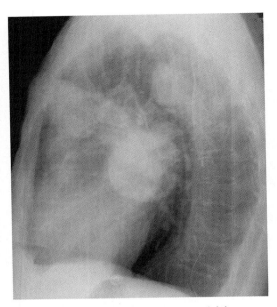

FIG. 4-11. Cannonball metastases in metastatic vaginal carcinoma. Frontal **(A)** and lateral **(B)** radiographs show several large, well-defined metastases.

have a history of neoplasm. In some patients, however, there is no history of a primary tumor at the time of diagnosis; in others, the primary tumor may never be found.

Solitary Nodules

A metastatic tumor occasionally presents as a solitary nodule (Fig. 4-12). About 5% to 10% of solitary nodules represent solitary metastases. It must be emphasized that many patients who appear to have a solitary metastasis on chest radiograph are discovered to have multiple pulmonary nodules on CT, with one nodule being dominant. Solitary me-

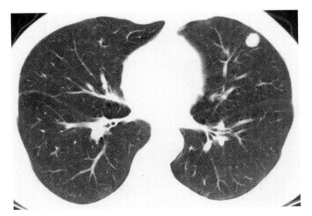

FIG. 4-12. Solitary metastasis shown on CT at the lung base. No other nodules were visible. This nodule is sharply marginated. Biopsy showed the same cell type as the primary tumor.

tastases are most common with carcinomas of the colon, kidney, and testis, and with sarcomas and melanoma.

A solitary metastasis is more likely to have a smooth margin than is primary lung carcinoma (see Fig. 4-12), but this finding on its own is not adequate to permit a reliable distinction between primary and metastatic tumors. Solitary metastases may appear spiculated, and primary carcinomas may be smooth. A solitary metastasis is more likely when the tumor is located at the lung base than is primary carcinoma, which tends to predominate in the upper lobes.

In a patient with a known extrathoracic tumor and a solitary nodule detected radiographically, the likelihood that the nodule is a metastasis (as opposed to primary lung cancer) varies with the cell type of the primary tumor.

Patients with carcinomas of the head and neck, bladder, breast, cervix, bile ducts, esophagus, ovary, prostate, or stomach are more likely to have primary lung carcinoma than lung metastasis (ratio, 8:1 for patients with head and neck cancers; 3:1 for patients with other types of cancer).

Patients with carcinomas of the salivary glands, adrenal gland, colon, parotid gland, kidney, thyroid gland, thymus, or uterus have fairly even odds (ratio, 1:1).

Patients with melanoma, sarcoma, or testicular carcinoma are more likely to have a solitary metastasis than a lung carcinoma (ratio, 2.5:1).

Lymphangitic Spread of Tumor

Lymphangitic spread of tumor refers to tumor growth in the lymphatic system of the lungs (Table 4-2). It

TABLE 4-2. LYMPHANGITIC SPREAD OF NEOPLASM

Results from:
  Hematogenous metastasis with lymphatic invasion
  Spread from hilar node metastases
  Direct spread from upper abdominal tumors
Findings:
  Interlobular septal thickening (i.e., Kerley's lines)
  Thickening of the peribronchovascular interstitium
  Thickening of the fissures
  Perilymphatic nodules
Abnormalities asymmetric or unilateral in 50%
Common causes:
  Breast carcinoma
  Lung carcinoma
  Stomach carcinoma
  Pancreas carcinoma
  Prostate carcinoma
  Cervical carcinoma
  Thyroid carcinoma
  Adenocarcinoma from an unknown site

occurs most commonly in patients with carcinomas of the breast, lung, stomach, pancreas, prostate, cervix, or thyroid, and in patients with metastatic adenocarcinoma from an unknown primary site; about 80% of cases are due to adenocarcinoma. It usually results from hematogenous spread to the lung, with subsequent interstitial and lymphatic invasion, but also can occur because of direct lymphatic spread of tumor from mediastinal and hilar lymph nodes. Symptoms of shortness of breath are common and can predate radiographic abnormalities.

The radiographic manifestations of pulmonary lymphangitic carcinomatosis include reticular or reticulonodular opacities, Kerley's lines, hilar and mediastinal lymphadenopathy, and pleural effusion (Fig. 4-13A and B). The appearance of unilateral or asymmetrical Kerley's lines is particularly suggestive. However, these findings are nonspecific. In some patients, the chest radiograph is normal.

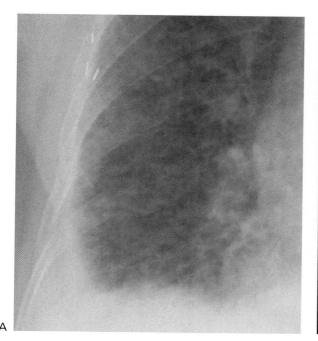

A

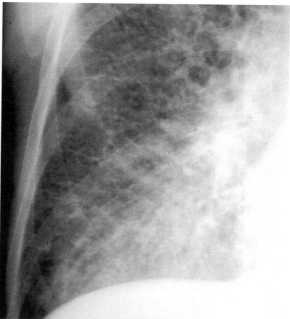

B

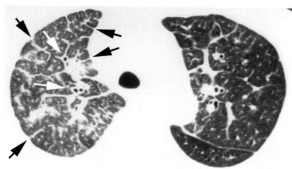

C

FIG. 4-13. Lymphangitic spread of breast carcinoma. **A.** Coned-down radiograph showing the right lower lobe demonstrates an abnormal reticular pattern. **B.** Coned-down radiograph in another patient shows distinct Kerley's B lines. **C.** HRCT in a different patient with breast carcinoma. There is asymmetric lung involvement characterized by smooth interlobular septal thickening *(black arrows)* and thickening of the peribronchovascular interstitium surrounding vessels and bronchi in the perihilar lung (i.e., "peribronchial cuffing"; *white arrows)*. Slight thickening of the left major fissure also is seen.

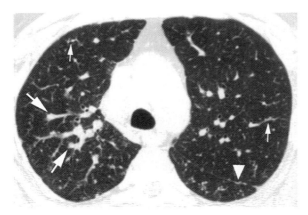

FIG. 4-14. Lymphangitic spread of thyroid carcinoma. HRCT shows nodular thickening of interlobular septa *(small arrows)*, the peribronchovascular interstitium *(large arrows)*, and the left major fissure *(arrowhead)*.

TABLE 4-3. AIRWAY METASTASES

Result from:
  Local spread from adjacent lung or lymph node metastases
  Hematogenous spread to bronchial wall
  Endobronchial spread
Mimics primary lung cancer
Bronchial narrowing or polypoid mass
Common causes:
  Melanoma
  Thyroid carcinoma
  Renal cell carcinoma
  Testicular carcinoma
  Breast carcinoma
  Sarcomas

On high-resolution CT (HRCT), lymphangitic spread of tumor typically shows (1) smooth thickening of the interlobular septa, (2) smooth thickening of the peribronchovascular interstitium surrounding vessels and bronchi in the perihilar lung (i.e., "peribronchial cuffing"), and (3) smooth subpleural interstitial thickening (i.e., thickening of the fissures; see Fig. 4-13C). Less often, nodular thickening of these structures is visible (Fig. 4-14). This pattern of nodules is termed "perilymphatic" (see Chapter 10).

In about 50% of patients, the abnormalities of lymphangitic spread appear focal, unilateral, or asymmetrical rather than diffuse on CT (see Fig. 4-13C). Hilar lymphadenopathy is visible on CT in only 50% of patients with lymphangitic spread. Mediastinal lymph node enlargement also can be seen. Lymph node enlargement can be symmetrical or asymmetrical. Pleural effusion is common.

Airway Metastases

Metastatic tumors may involve the tracheal or bronchial wall because of local spread from adjacent lung or lymph node metastases or because of hematogenous spread (Table 4-3). Oddly, involvement of the airway wall because of spread from other endobronchial tumors via the bronchial lumen is much less common. This pattern of metastasis occurs commonly with tracheobronchial papillomatosis (see Chapter 3).

Airway metastases may present with symptoms or findings of airway obstruction and atelectasis (Fig. 4-15). If this occurs in the presence of multiple nodular metastases, the diagnosis is not difficult. However, if no other findings are present, or if other findings include lymphangitic spread or hilar lymph node enlargement, it is difficult to distinguish

between metastases and primary lung cancer. In some patients, airway obstruction may be the first manifestation of the extrathoracic neoplasm.

Radiographs or CT may show a tapered narrowing of the airway lumen ("rat-tail" appearance), often due to local invasion, or a sessile or polypoid endobronchial mass (Fig. 4-16; see also Fig. 22-6 in Chapter 22), often due to hematogenous spread to the airway wall.

Airway metastases are most common in melanoma, thyroid carcinoma, renal cell carcinoma, testicular carcinoma, breast carcinoma, and sarcomas.

Vascular Metastases

Most tumor emboli associated with hematogenous metastasis are microscopic. In occasional patients, tumor emboli

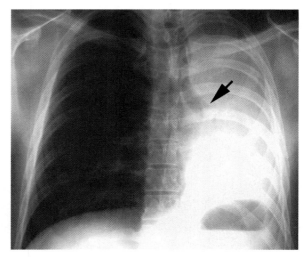

FIG. 4-15. Metastasis to the left main bronchus *(arrow)* from testicular carcinoma. There is obstruction of the left main bronchus with left lung atelectasis.

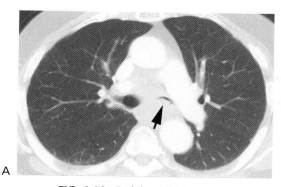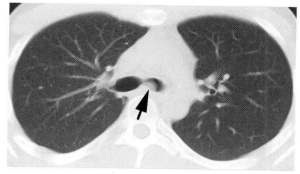

FIG. 4-16. Endobronchial metastases. **A.** Metastasis to the left main bronchus from a head and neck carcinoma. A polypoid mass is seen within the left main bronchus. **B.** Polypoid endobronchial mass in metastatic melanoma.

are large enough or numerous enough to result in symptoms or findings of vascular occlusion as a primary manifestation (Table 4-4). Vascular metastases may mimic pulmonary infarction (large tumor emboli) clinically and radiographically or pulmonary hypertension (large or numerous tumor emboli). Vascular metastases may occur with or without other findings of metastatic tumor.

Radiographic findings include (1) visible tumor emboli mimicking the appearance of pulmonary emboli on contrast-enhanced scans; (2) findings of pulmonary infarction; (3) a nodular or beaded appearance or peripheral pulmonary arteries due to smaller tumor emboli; and (4) pulmonary artery dilatation due to large tumor emboli or pulmonary hypertension.

Large tumor emboli are most common with tumors resulting in invasion of large systemic veins or the right heart, most often renal cell carcinoma, hepatoma, right atrial myxoma, and angiosarcoma. Numerous small emboli resulting in pulmonary hypertension and cor pulmonale may occur with very vascular primary tumors. In addition to those listed, these include choriocarcinoma and adenocarcinoma.

Lymph Node Metastases

Metastases to mediastinal or hilar lymph nodes from extrathoracic malignancies are uncommon, occurring in less than 3% of cases. The extrathoracic tumors most likely to metastasize to the mediastinum and hila are carcinomas of the head and neck (including thyroid tumors), genitourinary tract (e.g., renal and testicular carcinoma), breast, and melanoma (Table 4-5). Enlarged lymph nodes may be unilateral or bilateral and symmetrical or asymmetrical. In distinction to hilar masses occurring in lung cancer, which may be quite irregular and ill-defined due to local invasion, hilar node enlargement in patients with metastases are often sharply marginated (Figs. 4-17 and 4-18).

Most metastatic tumors result in lymph node enlargement without distinguishing characteristics. However, enhancing nodes may be seen secondary to metastatic renal cell carcinoma, papillary thyroid carcinoma, lung cancer, sarcomas, melanoma, and some other tumors (Fig. 4-19). Calcified lymph node metastases are most typical of thyroid carcinoma, mucinous adenocarcinoma, and sarcomas. Calcification of treated metastases also may occur (Figs. 4-20 and 4-21). Necrotic, rim-enhancing, or low-attenuation lymph nodes also may be seen (Fig. 4-22); these are common in testicular carcinoma, renal cell carcinoma, breast cancer, and lung cancer.

The location of enlarged nodes sometimes is suggestive of the primary tumor site.

Superior mediastinal lymph node involvement suggests a head and neck tumor (see Fig. 4-18).

Posterior mediastinal or paravertebral lymph node enlargement suggests an abdominal location for the primary tumor (see Fig. 4-19) or tumors metastasizing via retroperitoneal lymph nodes, such as testicular carcinoma. Retrocrural lymph node enlargement often is an associated finding.

Internal mammary lymph node metastases are most like due to breast carcinoma (Fig. 4-23). They may be associated with paracardiac node enlargement.

TABLE 4-4. VASCULAR METASTASES

Large tumor emboli uncommon
Findings:
    Vascular filling defects mimicking pulmonary embolism
    Pulmonary infarction
    Beaded vessels
    Pulmonary artery dilatation
Common causes:
    Renal cell carcinoma
    Hepatoma
    Right atrial myxoma
    Angiosarcoma

TABLE 4-5. LYMPH NODE METASTASES

Result from:
    Spread via the thoracic duct
    Spread to lymph nodes from hematogenous lung
      metastases
Unilateral or bilateral
Sharply marginated node masses
Common causes:
    Head and neck tumors
    Thyroid carcinoma
    Renal cell carcinoma
    Testicular carcinoma
    Breast carcinoma
    Melanoma
Enhancing lymph node metastases, common causes:
    Thyroid carcinoma
    Renal cell carcinoma
    Testicular carcinoma
    Breast carcinoma
    Melanoma
Calcified lymph node metastases, common causes:
    Thyroid carcinoma
    Mucinous adenocarcinoma
    Sarcomas
Superior mediastinal lymph nodes, common causes:
    Head and neck tumor
    Thyroid carcinoma
Internal mammary lymph node metastases, common
    causes:
    Breast carcinoma
Posterior mediastinal lymph node metastases, common
    causes:
    Abdominal tumors
Paracardiac lymph node metastases, common causes:
    Colon carcinoma
    Lung carcinoma
    Ovarian carcinoma
    Breast carcinoma

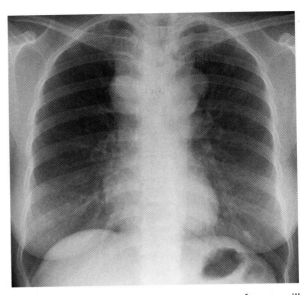

FIG. 4-18. Mediastinal lymph node metastases from papillary thyroid carcinoma. Bilateral superior mediastinal and paratracheal masses are visible. The hila appear normal.

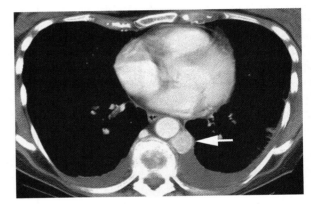

FIG. 4-19. Enhancing lymph node metastasis with metastatic paraganglioma. A left paraaortic lymph node *(arrow)* is densely enhancing.

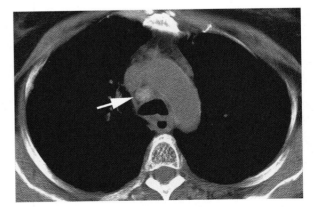

FIG. 4-20. Calcified lymph node metastasis in thyroid carcinoma. A faintly calcified and enlarged pretracheal lymph node *(arrow)* is visible. Lymph node calcification is characteristic of tumors that calcify at their primary site.

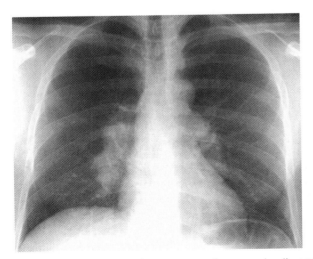

FIG. 4-17. Hilar lymph node metastases from renal cell carcinoma. Well-defined, lobulated hilar masses are visible bilaterally.

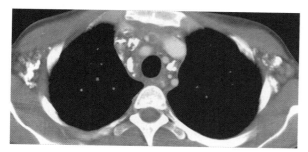

FIG. 4-21. Calcified lymph nodes following treatment of metastatic gastric cancer. Multiple densely calcified axillary and mediastinal nodes are visible.

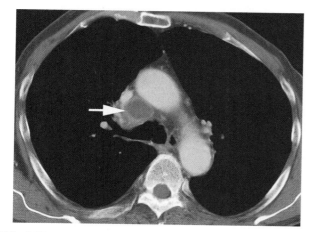

FIG. 4-22. Necrotic lymph node in metastatic renal cell carcinoma. An enlarged pretracheal lymph node *(arrow)* shows a low attenuation center and rim enhancement.

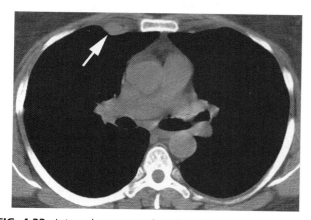

FIG. 4-23. Internal mammary lymph node metastasis in breast cancer. An enlarged node *(arrow)* is visible on the right.

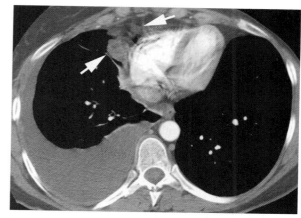

FIG. 4-24. Paracardiac lymph node metastases in breast cancer. Enlarged right paracardiac lymph nodes *(arrows)* are visible. A malignant pleural effusion is also present. No pleural thickening is visible.

Paracardiac lymph node enlargement may occur as a result of metastasis from abdominal or thoracic tumors, in approximately equal numbers; most common are carcinomas of the colon, lung, ovary, and breast (Figs. 4-24 and 4-25).

Pleural Metastases

The appearance of pleural metastases is discussed in detail in Chapter 26. Pleural metastasis may result from local spread, hematogenous spread, or lymphatic spread. It is most common with adenocarcinoma (Table 4-6).

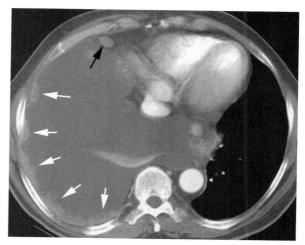

FIG. 4-25. Metastatic colon carcinoma with malignant effusion. Multiple pleural nodules *(white arrows)* are highly suggestive for metastases. Paracardiac lymph node enlargement *(black arrow)* is also present.

TABLE 4-6. PLEURAL METASTASES

Result from:
    Local spread
    Hematogenous spread
    Lymphatic spread
Pleural effusion nonspecific
Findings suggesting neoplasm:
    Nodular pleural thickening
    Concentric pleural thickening

TABLE 4-7. KAPOSI'S SARCOMA

Occurs in 15%–20% of AIDS patients
Caused by a herpes virus infection
Pulmonary involvement in 20%–50%
Usually preceded by cutaneous involvement
Airway lesions visible at bronchoscopy
Coarse reticular opacities at the lung bases
Ill-defined or spiculated (flame-shaped) nodules
Parahilar or peribronchovascular distribution
Interlobular septal thickening
Pleural effusion
Lymph node enlargement

In patients with pleural metastases, plain films usually show pleural effusion or pleural thickening, which may be lobulated, nodular, or concentric (i.e., surrounding the lung). The presence of pleural effusion in patients with neoplasm is nonspecific; it may result from lymphatic obstruction (i.e., lymphangitic spread of tumor, hilar or mediastinal node metastases, thoracic duct obstruction) rather than pleural metastases. CT may show pleural effusion with or without pleural thickening (see Fig. 4-24); pleural masses or nodular pleural thickening (see Fig. 4-25); or concentric pleural thickening.

Pneumothorax

Spontaneous pneumothorax may result from metastases involving the visceral pleural surface. The pleural metastases may appear necrotic or cavitary, or they may appear solid, with pneumothorax presumably resulting from other mechanisms of pleural disruption or airway obstruction with air trapping (Fig. 4-26). Pneumothorax is most typical of metastatic sarcoma, and may be the first symptom of metastasis.

KAPOSI'S SARCOMA

Kaposi's sarcoma (KS) is a tumor derived from primitive vascular tissues, occurring in (1) patients with AIDS, in

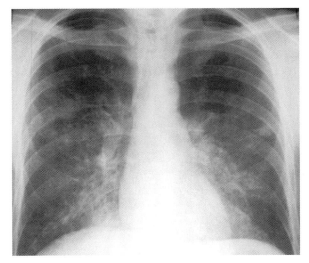

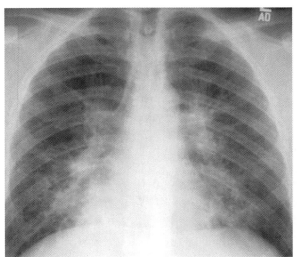

FIG. 4-27. Radiographic appearances of Kaposi's sarcoma in two AIDS patients. **A.** Coarse, ill-defined opacities and consolidation are visible in the perihilar regions and lower lobes. This is typical of Kaposi's sarcoma. Several nodules are also visible. **B.** Streaky opacities are visible in the lower lobes. Hilar lymph node enlargement is also visible.

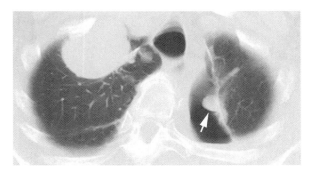

FIG. 4-26. Metastatic melanoma with pneumothorax. A solid-appearing metastasis *(arrow)* involving the visceral pleural surface of the left lung is associated with a pneumothorax. A large metastasis is also visible at the right apex.

whom lymph node and visceral organ involvement is common, and the prognosis is poor, and (2) in elderly individuals, in whom the disease primarily involves skin, and the prognosis is good. The former type is most common.

KS develops in about 15% to 20% of patients with AIDS (Table 4-7). KS is much more common among subjects who acquire AIDS through sexual contact. Almost all cases occur in homosexual or bisexual men, and KS occurs less frequently in intravenous drug users or patients exposed to HIV by different means. It is likely that KS results from infection by a herpes virus.

Pulmonary involvement occurs in 20% to 50% of AIDS patients with KS, and usually, but not always, is preceded by cutaneous or visceral involvement. Endobronchial lesions detected at bronchoscopy tend to predict the presence of pulmonary disease. Pathologically, pulmonary involvement

in KS is patchy, but it has a distinct relationship to the peribronchovascular interstitium in the perihilar regions and the pleura.

Chest radiographs typically show bilateral, diffuse abnormalities characterized by the presence of (1) coarse reticular opacities or ill-defined consolidation in the perihilar regions or lower lobes (90% of cases; Fig. 4-27), (2) poorly defined nodules up to several centimeters in diameter (Fig. 4-28A), and (3) focal ill-defined areas of consolidation. A basal predominance of abnormalities is common, and the earliest abnormalities recognized often include thickening of the peribronchovascular interstitium at the lung bases (see Fig. 4-27). Kerley's lines may be seen. Pleural effusions, usually bilateral, are seen in 30% of cases. Hilar or mediastinal lymph node enlargement is apparent on the chest radiograph in approximately 10% of patients (see Fig. 4-27B).

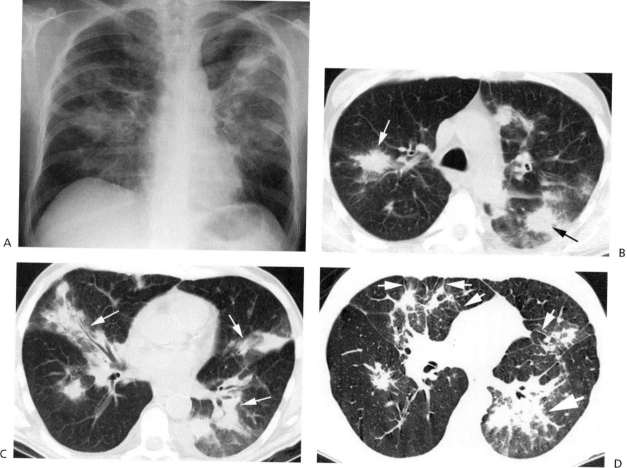

FIG. 4-28. Kaposi's sarcoma (KS) in an AIDS patient with a CD4 count of 41. **A.** Chest radiograph shows ill-defined nodular opacities and an increase in streaky opacity at the right base. **B.** CT with 5-mm slice thickness shows ill-defined and spiculated nodules *(arrows)*. These are typical of the later stages of KS. **C.** CT with 5-mm slice thickness at a lower level shows involvement of the peribronchovascular regions typical of KS. **D.** HRCT shows spiculated nodules, peribronchovascular infiltration *(large arrow)*, and interlobular septal thickening *(small arrows)*. Areas of ground-glass opacity may represent associated pulmonary hemorrhage.

The chest radiographic appearance is somewhat analogous to that of lymphangitic spread of carcinoma.

Early CT findings include thickening of the peribronchovascular interstitium, particularly at the lung bases, mimicking the appearance of infectious AIDS-related airways disease. Typical CT features of KS in more advanced cases include (1) irregular and ill-defined or spiculated (flame-shaped) nodules, often predominating in the peribronchovascular regions (see Fig. 4-28B–D); (2) peribronchovascular interstitial thickening (see Fig. 4-27D); (3) interlobular septal thickening (see Fig. 4-27D); (4) pleural effusion; and (5) lymphadenopathy. Although a number of infections and tumors in AIDS patients may present radiographically with lung nodules, CT findings of irregular nodules, larger than 1 cm, with a perihilar distribution usually allow KS to be distinguished from other thoracic complications.

SELECTED READING

Davis SD. CT evaluation for pulmonary metastases in patients with extrathoracic malignancy. Radiology 1991; 180:1–12.

Diederich S, Semik M, Lentschig MG, et al. Helical CT of pulmonary nodules in patients with extrathoracic malignancy: CT-surgical correlation. AJR Am J Roentgenol 1999; 172:353–360.

Edinburgh KJ, Jasmer RM, Huang L, et al. Multiple pulmonary nodules in AIDS: usefulness of CT in distinguishing among potential causes. Radiology 2000; 214:427–432.

Goldsmith SH, Bailey HD, Callahan EL, Beattie EJ. Pulmonary metastases from breast carcinoma. Arch Surg 1967; 94:483–488.

Gruden JF, Huang L, Webb WR, et al. AIDS-related Kaposi sarcoma

of the lung: radiographic findings and staging system with bronchoscopic correlation. Radiology 1995; 195:545–552.

Hartman TE, Primack SL, Müller NL, Staples CA. Diagnosis of thoracic complications in AIDS: accuracy of CT. AJR 1994; 162: 547–553.

Janower ML, Blennerhasset JB. Lymphangitic spread of metastatic tumor to lung. Radiology 1971; 101:267–273.

Johkoh T, Ikezoe J, Tomiyama N, et al. CT findings in lymphangitic carcinomatosis of the lung: correlation with histologic findings and pulmonary function tests. AJR 1992; 158:1217–1222.

McGuinness G, Gruden JF, Bhalla M, et al. AIDS-related airway disease. AJR Am J Roentgenol 1997; 168:67–77.

McLoud TC, Kalisher L, Stark P, Greene R. Intrathoracic lymph node metastases from extrathoracic neoplasms. AJR 1978; 131: 403–407.

Munden RF, Pugatch RD, Liptay MJ, et al. Small pulmonary lesions detected at CT: clinical importance. Radiology 1997; 202: 105–110.

Munk PL, Müller NL, Miller RR, Ostrow DN. Pulmonary lymphangitic carcinomatosis: CT and pathologic findings. Radiology 1988; 166:705–709.

Naidich DP, McGuinness G. Pulmonary manifestations of AIDS: CT and radiographic correlations. Radiol Clin North Am 1991; 29:999–1017.

Naidich DP, Tarras M, Garay SM, et al. Kaposi sarcoma: CT-radiographic correlation. Chest 1989; 96:723–728.

Peuchot M, Libshitz HI. Pulmonary metastatic disease: radiologic-surgical correlation. Radiology 1987; 164:719–722.

Quint LE, Park CH, Iannettoni MD. Solitary pulmonary nodules in patients with extrapulmonary neoplasms. Radiology 2000; 217: 257–261.

Ren H, Hruban RH, Kuhlman JE, et al. Computed tomography of inflation-fixed lungs: the beaded septum sign of pulmonary metastases. J Comput Assist Tomogr 1989; 13:411–416.

Stein MG, Mayo J, Müller N, et al. Pulmonary lymphangitic spread of carcinoma: appearance on CT scans. Radiology 1987; 162: 371–375.

5

LYMPHOMA AND LYMPHOPROLIFERATIVE DISEASE

W. RICHARD WEBB

Lymphoma accounts for about 4% of newly diagnosed malignancies. Although they are not primary thoracic neoplasms, lymphomas commonly involve the mediastinum, hila, and lung parenchyma.

Lymphomas are primary neoplasms of the lymphoreticular system and are classified in two main types: Hodgkin's disease (HD) and non-Hodgkin's lymphoma (NHL). Although HD is the less common of the two types, representing about 25% to 30% of cases, it is more common as a cause of mediastinal involvement.

HODGKIN'S DISEASE

HD occurs at all ages, but its peak incidence is in the third and eighth decades; it accounts for about 0.5% to 1% of all newly diagnosed malignancies (Table 5-1). It is more prevalent in males, with a male to female ratio of 1.4 to 1.9. Intrathoracic HD usually is associated with disease elsewhere; cervical lymph nodes commonly are involved. Constitutional symptoms may be present.

HD is characterized histologically by the presence of Reed-Sternberg cells. Four histologic types of HD are recognized in the Rye classification: nodular sclerosis (accounting for 50 to 80% of adult HD cases); lymphocyte predominance; mixed cellularity; and lymphocyte depletion.

HD has a predilection for thoracic involvement. Up to 85% of patients with HD have thoracic involvement at the time of diagnosis; nearly all of these have mediastinal lymph node enlargement.

Lymph Node Involvement

HD most often involves superior mediastinal (i.e., prevascular, paratracheal, and aortopulmonary) lymph nodes. These node groups are abnormal in as many as 85% of patients with HD and 98% of those with thoracic involvement (Figs. 5-1 and 5-2); if these nodes appear normal on CT, intrathoracic adenopathy is unlikely to represent HD.

Other sites of involvement in patients with thoracic disease are as follows: the hilar nodes, in about 35% of patients; the subcarinal nodes, in about 25% of patients; the paracardiac (cardiophrenic angle) lymph nodes, in 10% of patients; the internal mammary nodes, in 5% of patients; and the posterior mediastinal (i.e., paravertebral, paraaortic, and retrocrural) nodes, in 5% of patients (see Figs. 5-2 and 5-3).

Multiple node groups are involved in 85% of those HD patients who have thoracic node involvement. Enlargement of a single node group can be seen in some patients with HD, but it is uncommon, seen in only 15% of cases with node involvement. Anterior (prevascular) lymph nodes most often are involved as a single group (Fig. 5-4), and this appearance usually indicates the presence of nodular sclerosing HD.

On plain radiographs, anterior mediastinal lymph node enlargement may result in a unilateral or bilateral mediastinal abnormality (see Figs. 5-1A and 5-3A). Enlargement of paratracheal or aortopulmonary window nodes often results

TABLE 5-1. HODGKIN'S DISEASE

Peak incidence in the 3rd and 8th decades
Characterized by Reed-Sternberg cells
Nodular sclerosis cell type accounts for 50%–80% of adult cases
Staged using Ann Arbor system
Thoracic involvement in 85% of cases at diagnosis
Lymph node involvement in nearly all with thoracic involvement
    Superior mediastinal node enlargement in 98%
    Multiple node groups involved in 85%
    Nodes show low attenuation in 10%–20%
    Residual mediastinal masses common after treatment
    Calcification of lymph nodes common after treatment
Lung disease
    10% have lung involvement at diagnosis
    Nearly always associated with enlarged nodes
    Direct infiltration, lung nodules, or consolidation
    Air bronchograms and cavitation may be seen
    Lung recurrence may occur without enlarged nodes
Pleural effusion in 15%, usually due to lymphatic obstruction

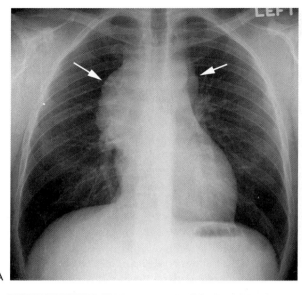

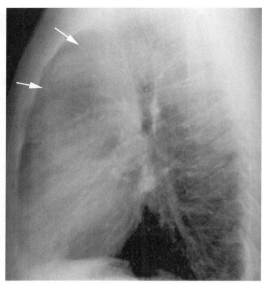

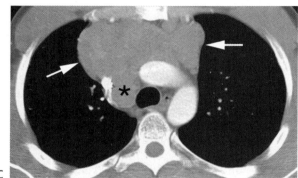

FIG. 5-1. Hodgkin's disease involving superior mediastinal lymph nodes. **A.** PA chest radiograph shows bilateral lobulated superior mediastinal masses *(arrows)*. **B.** The lateral view shows an anterior mediastinal mass *(arrows)*. **C.** Contrast-enhanced CT scan shows prevascular anterior mediastinal lymph node enlargement *(arrows)* and pretracheal lymph node enlargement *(*)*. Lymph node enlargement in these regions is typical of Hodgkin's disease.

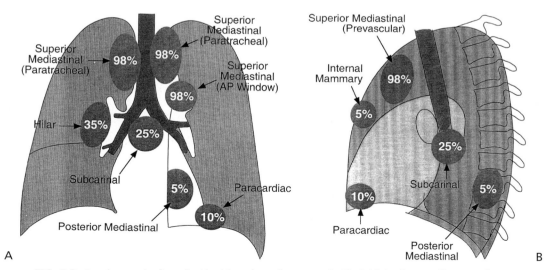

FIG. 5-2. Involvement of mediastinal lymph node groups in Hodgkin's disease, illustrated as a percentage of patients with thoracic disease. Lymph node groups as shown on the PA **(A)** and lateral **(B)** radiographs.

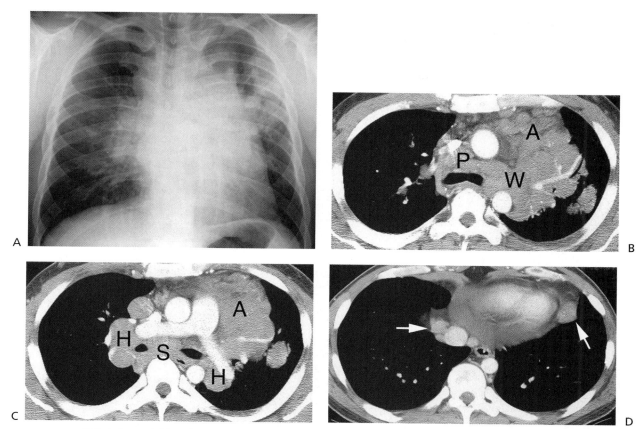

FIG. 5-3. Hodgkin's disease with involvement of multiple lymph node groups. **A.** PA chest radiograph shows superior mediastinal widening, hilar enlargement, and nodules in the left upper lobe. **B** and **C.** Large lymph nodes are visible in the prevascular anterior mediastinum *(A)*, pretracheal space *(P)*, aortopulmonary window *(W)*, subcarinal space *(S)*, and both hila *(H)*. Some discrete lymph nodes are visible, but other enlarged node masses appear matted together, with fat planes between them being invisible. **D.** Paracardiac lymph node enlargement *(arrows)* is visible at a lower level on CT.

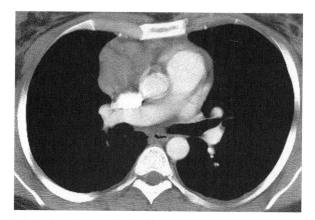

FIG. 5-4. Anterior mediastinal lymph node enlargement in nodular sclerosing Hodgkin's disease. CT shows lymphadenopathy localized to the anterior mediastinum, which is typical of nodular sclerosing Hodgkin's disease.

in a unilateral or asymmetrical abnormality. Because multiple lymph nodes are involved, mediastinal masses often appear elongated or lobulated in contour. Roughly spherical masses also can be seen (Fig. 5-5). Poor definition of the mass can indicate invasion or extension into adjacent lung. In the presence of thymic involvement, the mediastinal mass can project to both sides of the mediastinum.

Computed tomography (CT) is advantageous in showing abnormalities of the mediastinal lymph nodes in patients with HD. Although it is uncommon for CT to show evidence of mediastinal adenopathy if the chest radiograph is normal, in cases in which the radiograph shows lymph node enlargement, CT detects additional sites of adenopathy in many patients. Findings shown only on CT may change the treatment plan in as many as 10% of patients. CT is most helpful in diagnosing subcarinal, internal mammary, and aortopulmonary window node enlargement that is not visible on radiographs.

On CT, abnormal lymph nodes may appear well defined

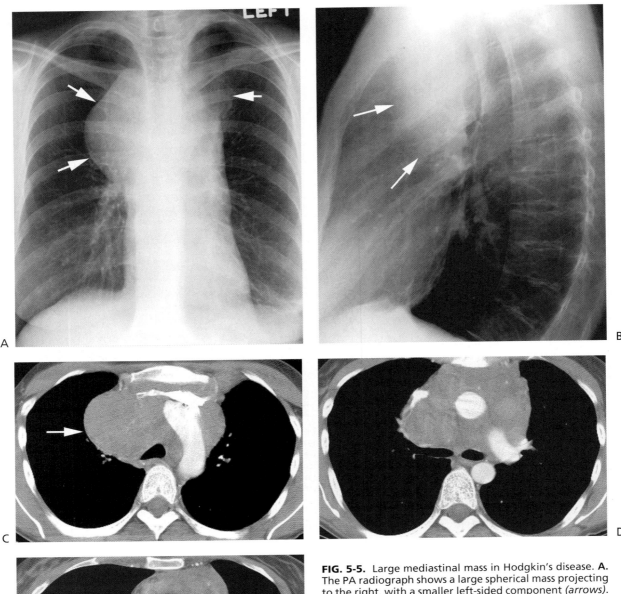

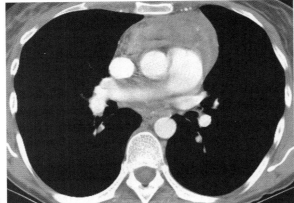

FIG. 5-5. Large mediastinal mass in Hodgkin's disease. **A.** The PA radiograph shows a large spherical mass projecting to the right, with a smaller left-sided component *(arrows)*. **B.** Lateral view shows the mass to be anterior *(arrows)*. **C.** At the level of the aortic arch, CT shows a large, rounded mass that largely involves the pretracheal mediastinum *(arrow)*. The opacified brachiocephalic veins are displaced anteriorly. Discrete nodal masses are not visible; the mediastinum appears infiltrated by tumor, and no mediastinal fat is visible. **D.** At the level of the left pulmonary artery, CT reveals that the mass occupies the prevascular anterior mediastinum and the precarinal space. The superior vena cava is displaced anteriorly and is compressed. At this level the mass appears somewhat inhomogenous in attenuation. Discrete, enlarged lymph nodes are not seen. **E.** At the level of the right pulmonary artery, anterior mediastinal mass appears to represent thymic involvement.

and discrete (Fig. 5-6); may appear matted (with fat planes between them being poorly seen) (see Fig. 5-3B and C); or may be associated with diffuse mediastinal infiltration (with individual lymph nodes being invisible; see Fig. 5-5C and D). Most often, enlarged lymph nodes are of homogeneous soft tissue attenuation, but in 10% to 20% of cases, lymph node masses show areas of low attenuation or necrosis following contrast enhancement (Fig. 5-7). Inhomogeneity without obvious necrosis also may be seen (see Fig. 5-5D). Invasion of mediastinal structures such as the superior vena cava, esophagus, or airways may occur.

Rarely, untreated patients show fine, stippled lymph node calcification (Fig. 5-8). Lymph node calcification is much more common following treatment, with a stippled, confluent, or, less often, "egg-shell" appearance. Calcification usually occurs after radiation; calcification after chemotherapy is less common.

HD also has a predilection for involvement of the thymus in association with mediastinal lymph node enlargement. Thymic enlargement is seen in 30% to 40% of cases, but

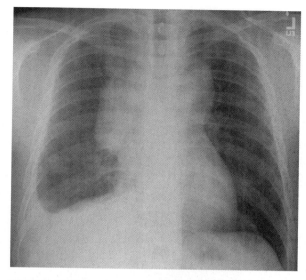

A

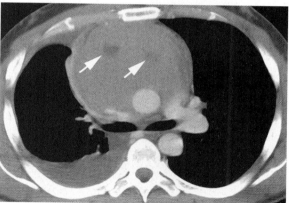

B

FIG. 5-7. Lymphoma with necrosis. **A.** Chest radiograph shows a large bilateral mediastinal mass and right pleural effusion, a portion of which is subpulmonic. **B.** Contrast-enhanced CT scan shows an anterior mediastinal mass containing a area of low attenuation *(arrows).* This finding is seen in 10% to 20% of patients with Hodgkin's disease.

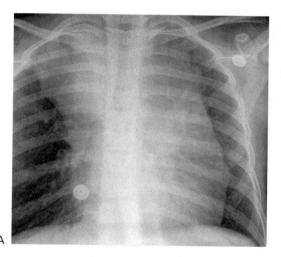

A

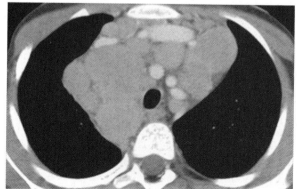

B

FIG. 5-6. Hodgkin's disease in a 9-year-old child. **A.** Chest radiograph shows bilateral superior mediastinal masses. **B.** On CT, multiple discrete enlarged lymph nodes are visible in the middle and anterior mediastinum.

may be difficult to distinguish from an anterior mediastinal lymph node mass unless the normal thymic shape is preserved (see Fig. 5-5E and 5-9).

HD is believed to be unifocal in origin, spreading to involve contiguous lymph nodes. It is unusual for HD to skip lymph node groups, and if nodes contiguous with the mediastinum, such as the lower neck or upper abdomen, are not involved by HD, it usually is not necessary to scan more distant regions, such as the pelvis.

However, in patients with mediastinal HD, scanning always should be extended to include the upper abdomen. Intra-abdominal paraaortic adenopathy can be found in 25% of patients with HD, and the spleen and liver are involved in 35% and 10% of patients, respectively.

The magnetic resonance imaging (MRI) appearance of lymph node masses in HD varies with the histology. In

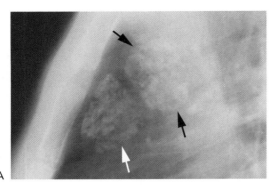

FIG. 5-8. Lymph node calcification following radiation treatment for Hodgkin's disease. **A.** Coned-down lateral radiograph shows stippled calcification of enlarged anterior mediastinal lymph nodes, typical of radiated Hodgkin's disease. Enlarged residual lymph nodes commonly are seen after treatment of Hodgkin's disease. **B** and **C.** Focal calcifications of enlarged anterior mediastinal lymph nodes shown on CT. Residual mediastinal lymph node masses following treatment of lymphoma are common, and most typical of nodular sclerosing Hodgkin's disease.

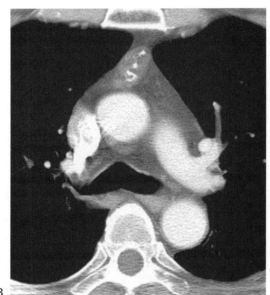

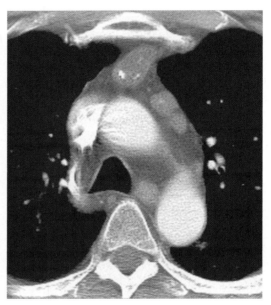

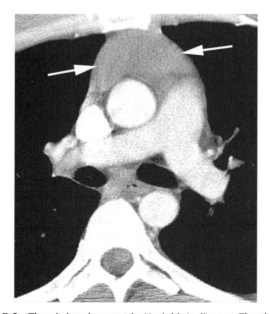

FIG. 5-9. Thymic involvement in Hodgkin's disease. The thymus is enlarged but maintains a normal shape *(arrows).*

nodular sclerosing HD, large amounts of fibrous tissue typically are interlaced with malignant cells. Typically, patients show a heterogeneous pattern with mixed high and low signal intensity on T2-weighted images. Low signal intensity areas on T2-weighted images are related to regions of fibrosis in the tumor, and high-intensity regions representing tumor tissue or cystic regions. HD also may demonstrate homogeneous high signal intensity similar to that of fat on T2-weighted images.

Lung Involvement

Lung involvement by HD is seen in 10% of patients at the time of presentation. It is almost always associated with mediastinal (and usually ipsilateral hilar) adenopathy (Fig. 5-10). A variety of manifestations of lung involvement may be seen, but the most common are (1) direct invasion of lung contiguous with abnormal nodes and (2) isolated single or multiple lung nodules, masses, or areas of consolidation. Direct invasion and the presence of nodules or masses occur with about equal frequency.

Direct extension from hilar or mediastinal nodes results

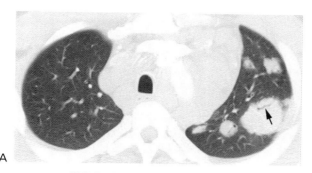

FIG. 5-10. Lung involvement in Hodgkin's disease in the same patient shown in Figure 5-3. Large lobulated nodules are visible in the left lung. Some are associated with small bronchi or contain air bronchograms *(arrow)*. Extensive mediastinal and hilar lymph node enlargement is present.

in coarse linear or streaky opacities radiating outward into the lung, corresponding on CT to thickening of the peribronchovascular interstitium. Kerley's lines and interlobular septal thickening may be associated. In some patients, the appearance may mimic that of lymphangitic spread of carcinoma.

When the lung is involved, discrete, single or multiple, well-defined or ill-defined, large or small nodules or mass-like lesions, or localized areas of air-space consolidation associated with air bronchograms may be seen (Figs. 5-10 and 5-11). These can cavitate, with thick or thin walls. Peripheral, subpleural masses are relatively common (Fig. 5-12).

HD occasionally involves bronchi with endobronchial masses or bronchial compression associated with atelectasis (Fig. 5-13).

In previously untreated patients, lung disease is uncommon in the absence of radiographically demonstrable lymph node enlargement; however, lung recurrence can be seen without node enlargement in patients with prior mediastinal radiation (see Fig. 5-11).

Pleural and Pericardial Effusion

Pleural effusion is present in about 15% of patients at diagnosis and usually reflects lymphatic or venous obstruction rather than pleural involvement by tumor (see Fig. 5-7). Effusions tend to resolve following local mediastinal or hilar radiation. However, about 20% to 25% of patients with HD who have effusion do have CT findings of pleural or extrapleural tumor or lymph node enlargement. Pericardial effusion, present in 5% of patients, usually indicates direct involvement of the pericardium.

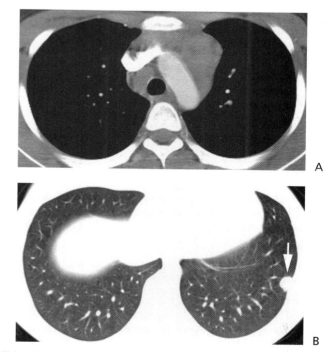

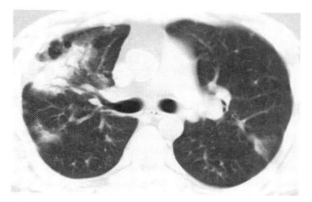

FIG. 5-11. Lung involvement in recurrent Hodgkin's disease. Poorly defined nodules and areas of consolidation are visible. The large area of consolidation on the right contains a number of air bronchograms. There is no obvious lymph node enlargement.

FIG. 5-12. Peripheral lung nodule in Hodgkin's disease. **A.** CT shows pretracheal and prevascular lymph node enlargement. **B.** A small, well-defined subpleural nodule is visible in the left lung. This was found at biopsy to represent Hodgkin's disease.

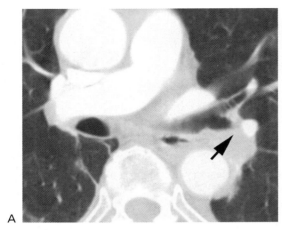
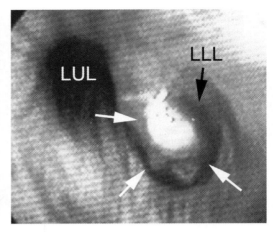

FIG. 5-13. Endobronchial Hodgkin's disease. **A.** The left lower lobe bronchus is narrowed *(arrow)* by a polypoid endobronchial mass. **B.** Endoscopic photograph showing the left upper lobe bronchus *(LUL)* and a polypoid mass *(white arrows)* filling the left lower lobe bronchus *(LLL).*

Chest Wall Involvement

Invasion of the chest wall contiguous with mediastinal or lung masses occurs in about 5% of cases. Tumor may involve ribs, sternum, or vertebral bodies and typically results in lytic bone destruction. Involvement of the skeleton because of dissemination often results in mixed lytic and blastic lesions (e.g., "ivory vertebra").

Staging

The Ann Arbor Staging Classification is used to describe the anatomic extent of disease at the time of diagnosis, and correlates well with prognosis (Table 5-2). Radiation is used for treatment of stages I and II. A combination of radiation and chemotherapy or chemotherapy alone is used in stages III and IV. There is a 75% to 80% cure rate for adult HD; in children, the cure rate is about 95%.

LYMPHOMA TREATMENT RESPONSE AND RELAPSE

Imaging studies commonly are obtained to judge the completeness of tumor response to treatment and to diagnose relapse.

Reduction of tumor bulk is always seen in patients with adequately treated tumor. Patients who show complete resolution of lymph node masses on CT usually are considered to have had a satisfactory response.

Residual mediastinal mass or lymph node enlargement often is seen in cured patients following treatment (see Figs. 5-8 and 5-14). This is particularly common in patients with treated nodular sclerosing HD; residual masses represent fibrous tissue components of the tumor itself, which change little with treatment, or post-treatment fibrosis. Residual mediastinal masses can be seen in as many as 88% of patients with HD and 40% of patients with NHL. In most patients, masses remain unchanged on follow-up. In some patients, residual masses continue to decrease in size or resolve over a period ranging from 3 to 11 months.

Most patients with thymic enlargement resulting from HD show a return to normal thymic size following treatment, although residual thymic enlargement may be seen in about 30% of cases.

Recurrent HD does not commonly involve previously irradiated (i.e., "in field") intrathoracic lymph nodes. However, so called in-field recurrence is seen in a small percentage of cases. Large masses and masses in the anterior medias-

TABLE 5-2. ANN ARBOR STAGING CLASSIFICATION FOR LYMPHOMA

Stage[a]	Definition
I	Involvement of a single lymph node region (I) or a single extralymphatic organ or site (I$_E$)
II	Involvement of two or more lymph node regions on the same side of the diaphragm (II) or localized involvement of an extralymphatic organ or site and of one or more lymph node regions of the same side of the diaphragm (II$_E$)
III	Involvement of lymph node regions on both sides of the diaphragm (III), which may also be accompanied by involvement of the spleen (III$_S$) or by localized involvement of an extralymphatic organ or site (III$_E$) or both (III$_{SE}$)
IV	Diffuse or disseminated involvement of one or more extralymphatic organs or tissues, with or without associated lymph node involvement

[a] The absence or presence of fever, night sweats, and/or unexplained loss of 10% or more of body weight in 6 months is denoted by the suffix A or B, respectively.

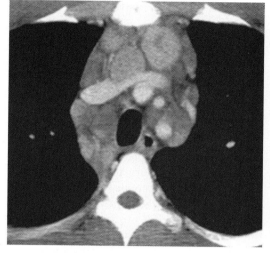

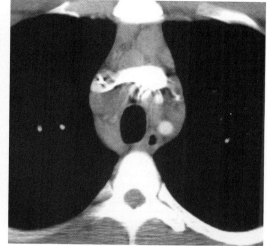

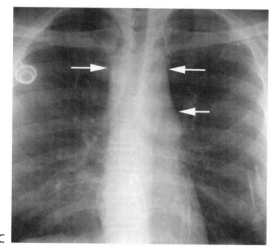

FIG. 5-14. Residual mediastinal mass in Hodgkin's disease. **A.** CT scan before treatment shows multiple enlarged mediastinal lymph nodes. **B.** CT performed 2 years after treatment shows a decrease in lymph node size, but lymph nodes remain enlarged. Persistent enlarged lymph nodes are common after treatment of Hodgkin's disease. **C.** Chest radiograph taken at the same time as the CT scan shown in **B** shows widening of the superior mediastinum and prominence of the aortopulmonary window *(arrows).*

tinum generally are considered to carry an increased risk of recurrence.

Common sites of recurrent HD include the upper mediastinum and lung, both seen in about half of cases with recurrence. Lymph node recurrence also may involve paracardiac lymph nodes, which usually are excluded from the treatment field because of their close relation to the heart (to avoid radiation pericarditis). Lung recurrence usually is associated with central or peripheral lung nodules, masses, or areas of focal consolidation, any of which may show cavitation. On chest radiographs, lung recurrence usually is not associated with visible lymph node enlargement, although it is visible on CT in about half of cases. Pleural effusions or masses and chest wall involvement also are common.

A homogenous hypointense pattern on both T1- and T2-weighted MRI images is characteristic of residual fibrotic masses in cured patients. Approximately 80% of cases show this pattern within 6 to 8 weeks of treatment. A heterogeneous appearance on T2-weighted imaging is seen after treatment in about 20% of cases, with regions of high signal intensity representing areas of necrosis or inflammation, or, in some patients, residual tumor. Thus, a high relative intensity with T2 weighting indicates the need for biopsy, follow-up, or further imaging. Gallium-67 or positron emission tomographic (PET) imaging can help in distinguishing active tumor from residual benign masses.

NON-HODGKIN'S LYMPHOMA

The term *non-Hodgkin's lymphoma* refers to a diverse group of neoplasms, varying in histology, clinical presentation, radiologic findings, course, and prognosis (Table 5-3). NHL accounts for about 3% of malignancies in adults.

The National Cancer Institute Working Formulation classifies NHL into low, intermediate, and high grades on the basis of histology, including 10 subtypes. The prognosis for low-grade NHL is better than that for high-grade NHL,

TABLE 5-3. NON-HODGKIN'S LYMPHOMA

Diverse group of neoplasms
More common than Hodgkin's disease (HD)
Mean age 55 years; more common than HD in children
Associated with immunodeficiency, HIV, immunosuppression
Classified as low-grade, intermediate-grade, high-grade, and
   miscellaneous
Prognosis related to grade and cell type
Staging less important than with HD
Thoracic involvement in 40%–50%
Lymphadenopathy in 75% with thoracic disease
   Superior mediastinal lymph nodes involved in nearly all
   Involvement of a single node group common (40%)
   Posterior mediastinal lymph nodes relatively common
Lung involvement (30%) more common than with HD

with intermediate grades having an intermediate prognosis. A miscellaneous group of NHL also includes mycosis fungoides, extramedullary plasmacytoma, histiocytic, and other cell types.

NHL usually occurs in older persons (40 to 70 years of age; mean, 55 years) than does HD. NHL also is more common than HD in children (Table 5-4).

The incidence of NHL, particularly of the intermediate and high grades, is significantly higher in immunodeficient patients. It is associated with congenital immunodeficiency syndromes, human immunodeficiency virus (HIV) infection, and immunosuppressive therapy. These tumors differ somewhat from those that occur spontaneously in immunocompetent patients: they usually are polyclonal rather than monoclonal and usually involve extranodal sites (e.g., central nervous system, lung, gastrointestinal tract).

Thoracic involvement is about half as common as with HD, occurring in 40% to 50% of cases.

Lymph Node Involvement

As with HD, mediastinal lymph node involvement is the most common thoracic abnormality in patients with NHL. It is present in more than 75% of patients with intrathoracic disease. Enlargement of pretracheal or anterior mediastinal (superior mediastinal) lymph nodes is the abnormality seen most often; 75% of patients with an intrathoracic abnormality (and 35% of all cases) have prevascular or pretracheal node involvement (Figs. 5-15 and 5-16). Subcarinal lymph node enlargement is present in about 30% of patients with an intrathoracic abnormality (15% of all cases; Fig. 5-17). Other sites of lymph node enlargement (expressed as a percentage of patients with intrathoracic disease) include the hila (20%); posterior mediastinal paraaortic, paravertebral, and retrocrural nodes (20%); and paracardiac nodes (10%).

The pattern of lymph node disease is different than that seen in HD. Involvement of a single node group is much more common in patients with NHL (see Figs. 5-17 and 5-18); 40% of patients with NHL and thoracic involvement have involvement of only one node group, whereas this is seen in only 15% of patients with HD. In addition, involvement of posterior mediastinal nodal groups is relatively more common with NHL than with HD; posterior lymph node masses often are contiguous with upper abdominal node enlargement (see Fig. 5-17).

Enlarged lymph nodes or mediastinal masses may appear low in attenuation due to necrosis, or may be cystic (Figs. 5-19 and 5-20). Calcification of nodes masses is rare.

As with HD, CT is more sensitive than chest radiographs in detecting lymph node enlargement in patients with NHL. It is most helpful in detecting subcarinal, posterior mediastinal, and paracardiac lymph nodes.

On MRI, lymph node masses in NHL appear homogeneous on T1-weighted images. They may demonstrate ho-

TABLE 5-4. COMPARISON OF HODGKIN'S DISEASE AND NON-HODGKIN'S LYMPHOMA

	Hodgkin's disease	Non-Hodgkin's lymphoma
Incidence	0.5%–1% malignancies	3% malignancies
Age at presentation	Peaks in 3rd and 8th decades	Peaks at age 40–70 years; more common than HD in children
Thoracic involvement	85% of cases	50% of cases
Node involvement		
Mediastinal nodes	Nearly all cases with thoracic involvement	75% of cases with thoracic involvement
Multiple node groups	85% of patients with lymph node disease	60% of patients with lymph node disease
Single node group	15% of patients with lymph node disease	40% of patients with lymph node disease
Superior mediastinal nodes	98% of cases with thoracic lymph node enlargement	75% of cases with thoracic lymph node enlargement
Posterior mediastinal nodes	5% of cases with thoracic lymph node enlargement	20% of cases with thoracic lymph node enlargement
Skips lymph node groups	Uncommon	Common
Lung involvement	10% of cases	30% of cases
Staging	Important (Ann Arbor Classification)	Less important (histology more valuable)

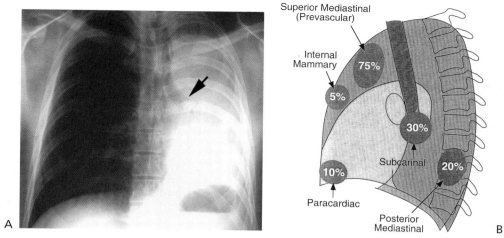

FIG. 5-15. Involvement of mediastinal lymph node groups in non-Hodgkin's lumphoma, as a percentage of patients with thoracic disease. Lymph node groups as seen on the PA **(A)** and lateral **(B)** radiographs.

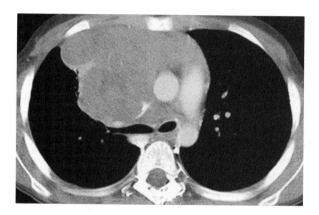

FIG. 5-16. Mediastinal lymph node enlargement with non-Hodgkin's lymphoma. Bulky lymphadenopathy is seen in the prevascular mediastinum with compression of the superior vena cava. Enlarged lymph nodes also are seen in the precarinal region. Nearly 75% of patients with non-Hodgkin's lymphoma and an intrathoracic abnormality have prevascular or pretracheal node involvement.

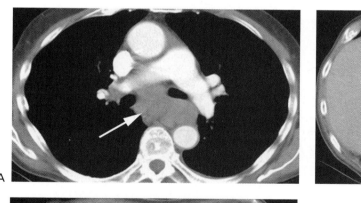

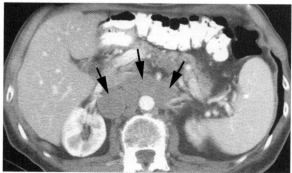

FIG. 5-17. Subcarinal and retrocrural lymph node enlargement with non-Hodgkin's lymphoma. **A.** Subcarinal and paraesophageal lymph node enlargement is visible *(arrow)*. **B.** At a lower level, retrocrural lymph node enlargement *(arrow)* also is seen. **C.** Multiple enlarged paraaortic lymph nodes *(arrows)* are visible in the upper abdomen.

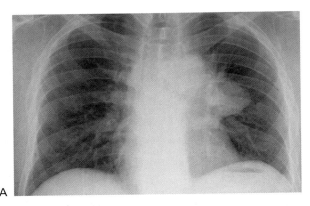

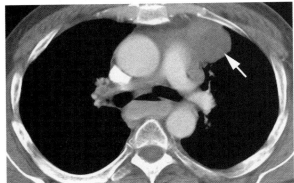

FIG. 5-18. Anterior mediastinal lymph node enlargement with non-Hodgkin's lymphoma. **A.** Left mediastinal mass is visible on the PA radiograph. Elevation of the left hemidiaphragm may reflect left diaphragmatic paralysis related to invasion or compression of the left phrenic nerve. **B.** Lymphadenopathy is limited to the prevascular mediastinum *(arrow)*. Involvement of a single lymph node group is much more common in patients with non-Hodgkin's lymphoma than in those with Hodgkin's disease.

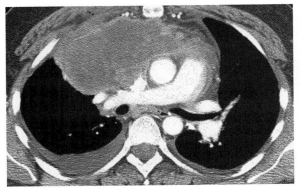

Fig. 5-19. Non-Hodgkin's lymphoma with a low-attenuation anterior mediastinal mass. The mass appears cystic due to necrosis. Bilateral pleural effusions also are present.

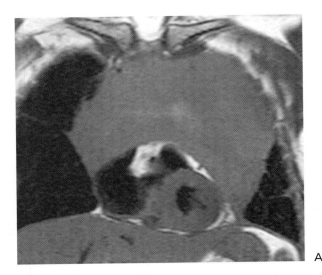

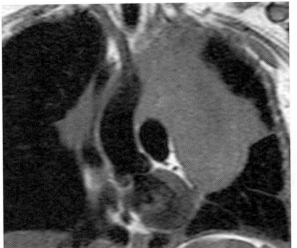

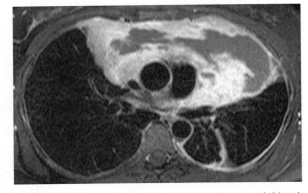

FIG. 5-20. MRI in a patient with mediastinal non-Hodgkin's lymphoma. **A** and **B.** A large anterior mediastinal mass is visible on T1-weighted coronal images. With this technique, the mass appears homogeneous in intensity **C.** An axial T1-weighted, gadolinium-enhanced, fat-saturated image shows enhancement of the large anterior mediastinal tumor. An irregular area of low intensity represents necrosis.

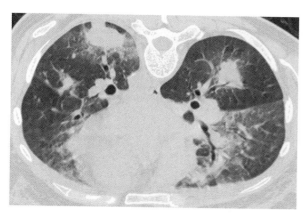

FIG. 5-21. Lung involvement with non-Hodgkin's lymphoma. HRCT in the prone position shows focal masses. This appearance is common when the lung is involved.

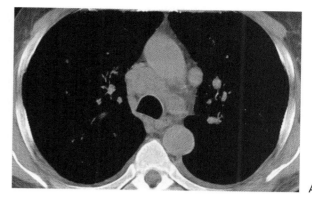

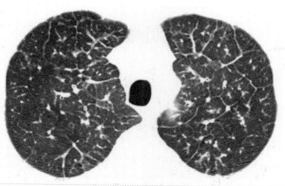

FIG. 5-23. Lymphangitic spread of non-Hodgkin's lymphoma. **A.** HRCT at a soft-tissue window shows enlarged mediastinal lymph nodes. **B.** HRCT shows diffuse lung infiltration with interlobular septal thickening and some nodularity closely mimicking the appearance of lymphangitic spread of carcinoma.

mogeneous high signal intensity similar to that of fat on T2-weighted images, because tumors may be composed almost entirely of malignant cells without significant fibrous tissue. However, areas of necrosis may be seen on T2-weighted images or with contrast enhancement (see Fig. 5-20).

Extranodal Disease

Extranodal involvement also is much more common with NHL. Extranodal disease seen in patients with a thoracic abnormality includes lung involvement in 30% of patients, pleural effusion or mass in 45% of patients, pericardial effusion or mass in 15% of patients, and chest wall involvement in 10% of patients.

Lung involvement may appear as discrete nodules or masses (Fig. 5-21), air-space consolidation, infiltration contiguous with enlarged lymph nodes or masses (Fig. 5-22), or interstitial thickening resembling lymphangitic spread of

carcinoma (Fig. 5-23). In some patients lung infiltration may be rapid, mimicking pneumonia. Bronchial narrowing or obstruction may occur because of compression by hilar mass (Fig. 5-24A) or bronchial involvement by tumor (see Fig. 5-24B).

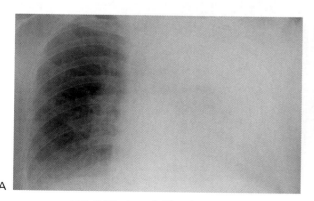

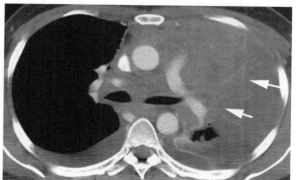

FIG. 5-22. Lung infiltration contiguous with mediastinal mass. **A.** Chest radiograph shows opacification of the left hemithorax. **B.** Enhanced CT shows invasion of lung *(arrows)* adjacent to a large mediastinal mass. Bilateral pleural effusions also are present.

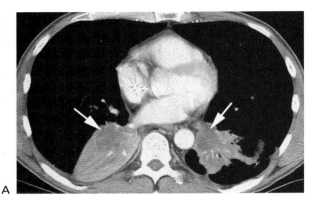

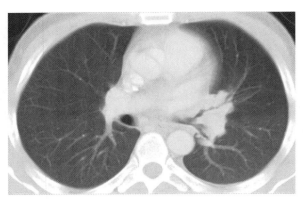

FIG. 5-24. Airway abnormalities in non-Hodgkin's lymphoma. **A.** Bilateral hilar masses with bronchial obstruction and atelectasis. The masses *(arrows)* appear lower in attenuation than the collapsed lung. **B.** Airway involvement by non-Hodgkin's lymphoma in a patient with AIDS. There is irregular narrowing of the left bronchi because of tumor involvement of the bronchial wall.

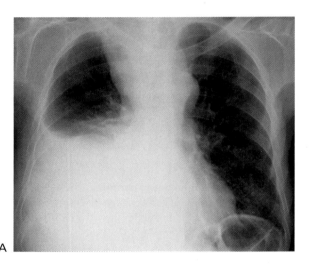

FIG. 5-25. Non-Hodgkin's lymphoma with pleural effusion and pleural and extrapleural tumor. **A.** Chest radiograph shows a right superior mediastinal mass and a large right pleural effusion. **B.** CT shows a large mass *(M)* posterior to the trachea and associated pleural or extrapleural masses *(arrows)*. **C.** At a lower level, a large pleural effusion is visible, with extensive infiltration of the parietal pleura or chest wall by tumor *(black arrows)*. A localized chest wall mass with rib destruction also is visible *(white arrows)*.

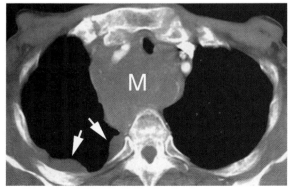

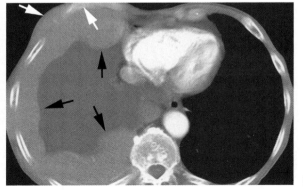

As with HD, pleural effusion most likely reflects lymphatic obstruction in many patients. Pleural effusion also may be associated with gross pleural or extrapleural (chest wall) tumor (Fig. 5-25).

Staging

In about 20% of patients with intrathoracic disease, CT can show abnormalities that are not recognized on plain radiographs. CT also shows more extensive intrathoracic disease in 75% of patients with abnormal chest radiographs. However, precise anatomic staging usually is less important in patients with NHL than in patients with HD. With HD, the anatomic extent of the tumor strongly predicts outcome; with NHL, the histopathologic classification is more predictive.

Patients with intermediate or high-grade NHL usually are treated with chemotherapy regardless of their anatomic stage, as are the majority of patients with low-grade lymphoma. The use of primary radiotherapy usually is limited to the 20% to 25% of patients with low-grade NHL who are Stage I or II at diagnosis (about 20% to 25%). In patients thought to have stage I or II low-grade NHL, CT is appropriate for determining whether intrathoracic disease is present and, if localized, in helping to plan the course of radiation; in patients with intermediate or high-grade NHL or stage III or IV disease, CT assessment of disease extent has little role.

In contrast to patients with HD, NHL is assumed to be multifocal in origin. The abdomen, pelvis, and neck must be scanned in patients with NHL, because noncontiguous spread is common. Abdominal involvement is more common than in patients with HD, and a variety of findings may be present: intra-abdominal paraaortic adenopathy is found in about 50% of patients with NHL (see Fig. 5-17C), the spleen is involved in 40% of patients, and the liver in 15% of patients. CT of the abdomen and pelvis results in an upgrading of the clinical stage in about 30% of patients with NHL and may detect unsuspected active disease in 40% of patients thought to be in remission.

Types

Primary Pulmonary Lymphoma

Pulmonary NHL is considered to be primary to the lung if it shows no evidence of extrathoracic dissemination for at least 3 months after the initial diagnosis (Table 5-5). Less than 1% of pulmonary lymphomas are primary. Primary pulmonary lymphoma is generally classified as a low-grade B-cell lymphoma or high-grade lymphoma.

Low-grade lymphoma (maltoma) accounts for more than 80% of primary pulmonary lymphomas. Most are derived from mucosa-associated lymphoid tissue (MALT), hence the term *maltoma*, which commonly is used to de-

---

TABLE 5-5. PRIMARY PULMONARY NON-HODGKIN'S LYMPHOMA

No evidence of extrathoracic dissemination for at least 3 months
<1% incidence of pulmonary lymphomas
Low-grade (maltoma)
Arises from mucosa-associated lymphoid tissue (MALT)
Solitary nodule or focal consolidation
Multiple nodules or areas of consolidation
Air bronchograms in 50%
Lymph node enlargement in 5%–30%
Good prognosis
High-grade
Solitary or multiple nodules
Air bronchograms common
Multifocal consolidation

---

scribe this entity. Patients with primary pulmonary low-grade B cell lymphoma have a good prognosis.

The most common radiologic manifestation of primary low-grade B-cell lymphoma is a solitary nodule or a focal area of consolidation, ranging in size from a few centimeters to an entire lobe. Multiple nodules or multifocal areas of consolidation also may be present. Air bronchograms are visible in 50% of cases. The parenchymal abnormalities typically show an indolent course with slow growth over months or years. On CT, the single or multiple masses or areas of consolidation may appear primarily peribronchial in location. Pleural effusion is present in approximately 10% of cases, usually in association with evidence of parenchymal involvement. Lymphadenopathy is evident radiographically in 5% to 30% of cases at presentation.

High-grade lymphoma is variable in histology. Some tumors occur in patients who have acquired immunodeficiency syndrome (AIDS) or organ transplants (posttransplant lymphoproliferative disorder). The most common radiographic presentation consists of solitary or multiple nodules (Fig. 5-26). As with maltoma, air bronchograms may be visible. Lymph node enlargement may be present. Other manifestations include bilateral consolidation or a diffuse reticulonodular pattern.

Primary Mediastinal Lymphoma

NHL may occur primarily in the mediastinum. The most common cell types presenting in this fashion are lymphoblastic lymphoma and large cell lymphoma (Table 5-6).

Lymphoblastic lymphoma accounts for about 60% of primary mediastinal NHL. If bone marrow and hematologic involvement are predominant features of this disease, it is termed *lymphoblastic leukemia*. Most patients are children or young adults. A large mediastinal mass representing thymic or lymph node enlargement typically is present (Fig. 5-27). Presenting symptoms usually are related to compression of mediastinal structures.

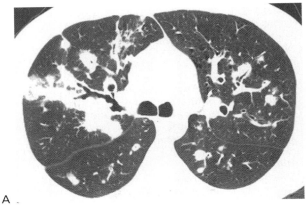
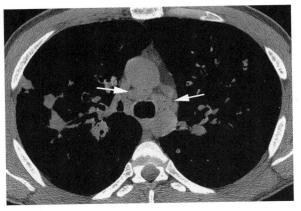

FIG. 5-26. High-grade primary pulmonary non-Hodgkin's lymphoma. **A.** HRCT shows multiple lung nodules and masses, some containing air bronchograms or arising in relation to bronchi. **B.** HRCT with a tissue window shows mildly enlarged mediastinal lymph nodes *(arrows)*.

Primary mediastinal large cell lymphoma is thought to arise from thymic medullary B cells. This entity is difficult to distinguish from HD, both clinically and radiographically. Affected patients usually are younger than other patients with NHL, with a median age of 35 years. A large, lobulated, anterior mediastinal mass averaging 10 cm in diameter is the predominant finding in nearly all patients (Fig. 5-28). Lymph node enlargement also may be seen in the subcarinal space and posterior mediastinum, but is less common. Low-attenuation areas of necrosis within the mass are seen in almost half of cases; calcification is uncommon. Pleural and pericardial effusions are present in about one third of cases.

AIDS-related Lymphoma

Lymphoma has an incidence of about 2% to 5% in patients with AIDS. In 90% of these patients, it is a B-cell NHL. AIDS-related lymphoma (ARL) typically is characterized by advanced clinical stage, high histologic grade, frequent posttreatment relapse, and poor survival. It originates predominantly in extranodal locations and often involves mul-

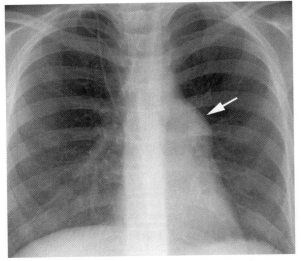
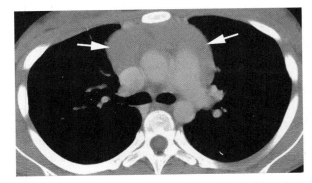

FIG. 5-27. Lymphoblastic lymphoma in a 14-year-old patient. **A.** Chest radiograph shows a left mediastinal mass *(arrow)*. **B.** CT shows an anterior mediastinal mass *(arrows)* that probably represents thymic enlargement. This appearance in a young patient is typical.

**TABLE 5-6. PRIMARY MEDIASTINAL
NON-HODGKIN'S LYMPHOMA (NHL)**

Lymphoblastic lymphoma
60% of primary mediastinal NHL
Termed *lymphoblastic leukemia* if bone marrow and
    hematologic abnormalities predominate
Children or young adults
Large anterior mediastinal mass
Primary mediastinal large cell lymphoma
Resembles Hodgkin's disease
Median age 35 years
Large anterior mediastinal mass

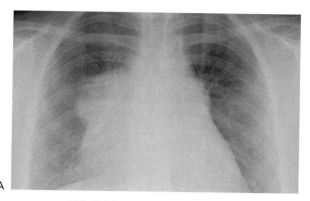
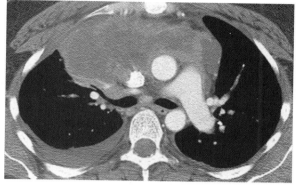

FIG. 5-28. Primary mediastinal large cell lymphoma in a 36-year-old man. **A.** Chest radiograph shows mediastinal widening. **B.** CT shows a large inhomogeneous anterior mediastinal mass with regions of low attenuation that probably are due to necrosis.

tiple sites, including bone marrow, central nervous system, lung, liver, and bowel. ARL is associated with advanced AIDS and low CD4 counts.

Thoracic involvement is present in 20% to 40% of patients with ARL (Table 5-7). Primary pulmonary ARL accounts for only 10% to 15% of cases.

Multiple pulmonary nodules and masses, ranging in size from 1 to 5 cm, are seen most commonly on radiographs or CT (Fig. 5-29). The nodules are usually well-defined. Cavitation may be present but is not common. Localized consolidation, mass lesions, or reticular opacities also may be seen. Mediastinal lymph node enlargement (30% to 50% of cases) is more common in patients with lung involvement associated with disseminated ARL than it is in patients with primary or localized pulmonary ARL. Pleural effusion is common, usually in combination with multiple nodules.

Waldenström's Macroglobulinemia

Waldenström's macroglobulinemia is an uncommon form of lymphoma characterized by malignant lymphoma plasmacytoid cells and a monoclonal IgM gammopathy. Bone marrow infiltration, hepatosplenomegaly, and peripheral lymph node enlargement are common manifestations. Lung or mediastinal involvement is very uncommon. Radiographs or CT may show lung consolidation or interstitial infiltration, mediastinal lymph node enlargement, or pleural effusion (Fig. 5-30).

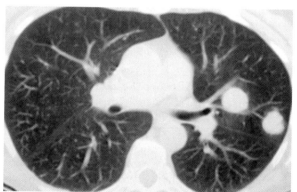

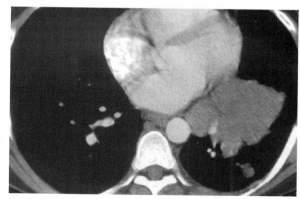

FIG. 5-29. AIDS-related lymphoma. **A.** A typical appearance of AIDS-related lymphoma is that of multiple well-defined nodules, without visible lymph node enlargement. **B.** In another patient with AIDS, a large mass represents pulmonary lymphoma.

TABLE 5-7. AIDS-RELATED LYMPHOMA

High histologic grade and poor survival
Thoracic involvement in 20%–40%
Multiple nodules or masses most common, usually well-defined
Cavitation in some
Consolidation or reticular opacities
Lymph node enlargement in 30%–50%, usually those with dissemination
Pulmonary AIDS-related lymphoma often unassociated with lymph node enlargement

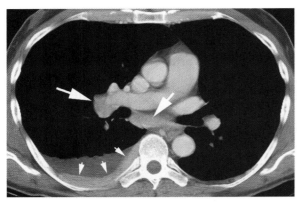

FIG. 5-30. Waldenström's macroglobulinemia. CT shows hilar and mediastinal lymph node enlargement *(large arrows)*, pleural effusion, and pleural or extrapleural tumor *(small arrows)*.

Mycosis Fungoides

Mycosis fungoides is a T-cell lymphoma that primarily affects the skin. Dissemination (Sézary syndrome) commonly is associated with lung involvement. Radiographic findings are similar to those of other lymphomas and include lung nodules, infiltration of the perihilar peribronchovascular interstitium, areas of lung consolidation, diffuse interstitial infiltration, pleural effusion, and hilar or mediastinal lymph node enlargement.

Plasmacytoma

Plasmacytoma is a focal neoplastic proliferation of plasma cells unassociated with a generalized plasma cell disorder, such as multiple myeloma. Plasmacytoma usually originates in bone, resulting in an expansile osteolytic lesion; extramedullary plasmacytoma, which arises in soft tissues, is much less common. Radiologic manifestations of extramedullary plasmacytoma include a tracheal or endobronchial mass or pulmonary nodules or mass lesions. The plasma cell tumor associated with myeloma can show similar findings.

LYMPHOPROLIFERATIVE DISEASES

In addition to HD and the NHLs, pulmonary lymphoproliferative diseases represent a spectrum of focal and diffuse lung abnormalities associated with either a benign or malignant course (Table 5-8). As with maltoma, described earlier, many of these diseases are related to abnormal proliferation of submucosal lymphoid follicles distributed along distal bronchi and bronchioles, termed *mucosa-associated lymphoid tissue* (MALT). Proliferations of MALT may be either hyperplastic or neoplastic. Polyclonal cellular proliferations usually are hyperplastic and benign, whereas most monoclonal cellular proliferations are malignant. However, in

TABLE 5-8. PULMONARY LYMPHOPROLIFERATIVE DISEASES

Focal lymphoid hyperplasia
Benign focal lesion
Formerly termed pseudolymphoma
Solitary nodule or a focal consolidation
Multiple nodules less common
Air bronchograms
No lymph node enlargement
Lymphocytic interstitial pneumonia
Benign
Diffuse interstitial infiltrate
Sjögren's syndrome and AIDS
Ground-glass opacity
Consolidation
Poorly defined centrilobular nodules
Small well-defined nodules
Interlobular septal thickening
Cystic airspaces
Angioimmunoblastic lymphadenopathy
Intrathoracic lymph node enlargement in 50%
Interstitial lung involvement in 35%
May progress to lymphoma
Fever and weight loss
Hepatomegaly and splenomegaly
Polyclonal hypergammopathy
Post-transplantation lymphoproliferative disorder
Bone marrow or solid organ transplantation
Occurs in the first year after transplantation
Ranges from benign to lymphoma
Associated with Epstein-Barr virus infection
85% show single or multiple lung nodules
5%–25% lymph node enlargement
Lymphomatoid granulomatosis
Angiocentric, angiodestructive lesions
May progress to lymphoma
Associated with Epstein-Barr virus
Lung commonly involved
Mimics Wegener's granulomatosis
   Bilateral, poorly defined nodules or masses
   Basal predominance
   Cavitation

some cases both hyperplasia and neoplasia may be present, and many lymphoproliferative diseases at least have malignant potential.

Focal Lymphoid Hyperplasia

Focal lymphoid hyperplasia is an uncommon benign condition characterized histologically by localized proliferation of benign mononuclear cells consisting of a mixture of polyclonal lymphocytes, plasma cells, and histiocytes. It has been referred to a "pseudolymphoma." The most commonly seen radiologic manifestation of focal lymphoid hyperplasia consists of a solitary nodule or a focal area of consolidation, but multiple nodules may be seen. The nodules or nodular areas of consolidation usually measure several centimeters in

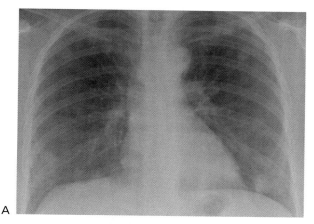
A

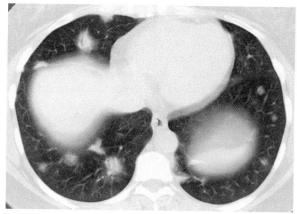
B

FIG. 5-31. Focal lymphoid hyperplasia in a patient with Sjögren's syndrome. **A.** Chest radiograph shows multiple nodular opacities. **B.** CT shows multiple ill-defined nodules, many of which contain air bronchograms.

diameter and contain air bronchograms (Fig. 5-31). There is no associated lymphadenopathy. It may occur in association with Sjögren's syndrome.

Lymphoid Interstitial Pneumonia

Lymphoid (lymphocytic) interstitial pneumonia (LIP) may be classified as a benign lymphoproliferative disorder or an interstitial pneumonia (see Chapter 13). It is characterized histologically by a diffuse interstitial infiltrate of mononuclear cells consisting predominantly of lymphocytes and plasma cells. LIP often occurs in association with Sjögren's syndrome and AIDS. In patients with AIDS, LIP usually occurs in children (Fig. 5-32); most other patients with LIP are adults (mean age, 50 years). The main clinical symptoms are cough and dyspnea.

The radiographic findings consist of a reticular or reticulonodular pattern involving mainly the lower lung zones. Less common abnormalities include a nodular pattern or air-space consolidation. On high-resolution CT (HRCT) typical findings include diffuse or patchy areas of ground-glass opacity or consolidation; poorly defined centrilobular nodules; small, well-defined nodules (see Fig. 5-32); and cystic airspaces (typical in Sjögren's syndrome; see Chapter 14). The appearance also may mimic lymphangitic spread of carcinoma, with interlobular septal thickening and nodules.

Angioimmunoblastic Lymphadenopathy

Angioimmunoblastic lymphadenopathy (AILD) is an uncommon systemic disease that commonly results in intrathoracic lymph node enlargement. In some cases, the lung and pleura also are involved. Histologically, abnormal lymph nodes show a proliferation of vessels and infiltration by a heterogeneous population of lymphocytes, plasma cells,

and immunoblasts. An association with drug treatment suggests that a hypersensitivity reaction also may be involved in the development of AILD. Progression to malignant lymphoma may occur, a condition termed *AILD-like T-cell lymphoma.* Patients usually are over 50 years of age. Constitutional symptoms are typical, with fever and weight loss; other findings include hepatomegaly, splenomegaly, rash,

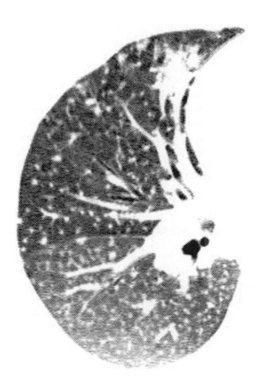

FIG. 5-32. Lymphoid (lymphocytic) interstitial pneumonia. An 11-year-old child with AIDS shows multiple small nodules and a focal area of consolidation.

generalized lymph node enlargement, polyclonal hypergam-mopathy, and Coombs'-positive anemia. The clinical course is variable, with three distinct patterns identified thus far. Fifty percent of patients have rapid progression to death; 25% have prolonged survival with corticosteroid and anti-neoplastic treatment; and 25% have prolonged survival without treatment.

The radiographic appearance of AILD is similar to that of lymphoma. Approximately 50% of cases show extensive mediastinal and hilar lymph node enlargement, and 35% of cases show lung involvement. Interstitial infiltration in the lower lobes associated with septal thickening or patchy consolidation is typical. Pleural effusion may be present. Enlarged lymph nodes may be seen to enhance if CT with contrast infusion is used.

Posttransplantation Lymphoproliferative Disorder

Several histologic patterns of lymphocyte proliferation, known collectively as *posttransplantation lymphoproliferative disorder* (PTLD), can occur after bone marrow or solid organ transplantation. The histologic patterns range from benign hyperplastic proliferation of lymphocytes to malig-nant lymphoma.

Most cases of PTLD have been associated with Epstein-Barr virus infection. PTLD affects up to 10% of transplant recipients. Most patients present in the first year after trans-plantation. PTLD can manifest as localized or disseminated disease and has a predilection for extranodal involvement. Lung involvement may occur as part of multiorgan disease or in isolation.

In 85% of cases, radiographs and CT show single or multiple pulmonary nodules, which may be small or large (0.3 to 5 cm), well- or ill-defined (Fig. 5-33). Other findings include patchy or focal consolidation or ground-glass opac-ity, a predominantly peribronchial and subpleural or diffuse distribution of parenchymal abnormalities, and hilar or me-diastinal lymphadenopathy (5% to 25%). Pleural effusion may be present.

Lymphomatoid Granulomatosis

The term *lymphomatoid granulomatosis* refers to a group of angiocentric, angiodestructive abnormalities characterized by a lymphoid infiltrate and a variable degree of cellular atypia. Three grades are thought to exist, based on the de-gree of cytologic abnormalities and necrosis and their re-sponse to treatment. Progression to histologically overt lym-phoma may occur. B cells appear to constitute the primary neoplastic proliferation in patients with lymphomatoid granulomatosis, although an exuberant T-cell reaction also is present. Epstein-Barr virus has been detected in most cases. The lung is the primary site of disease, although other

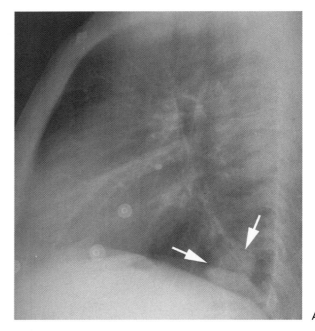

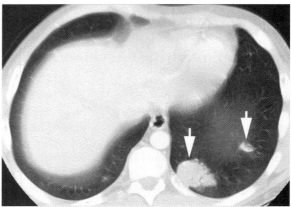

FIG. 5-33. Posttransplantation lymphoproliferative disorder. **A.** Lateral radiograph shows a nodule *(arrows)* in the posterior lower lobe. **B.** CT shows two irregular and poorly marginated nodules *(arrows)*.

organs—including skin, brain, kidneys, and heart—may be involved.

Radiographic and CT findings consist primarily of bilat-eral, poorly defined nodular lesions, ranging from 0.5 to 8 cm in diameter, with a basal predominance. Lesions may progress rapidly and cavitate, mimicking Wegener's granu-lomatosis. Pleural effusion may be present.

LEUKEMIA

Leukemia may result in lymph node enlargement, lung infil-tration, or pleural abnormalities (Table 5-9).

TABLE 5-9. LEUKEMIA

Mediastinal lymph node enlargement
25% of chronic lymphocytic leukemia
  Chronic, slowing progressive
10%–20% of acute lymphoblastic leukemia
  Large symptomatic anterior mediastinal mass
  Acute lymphoblastic lymphoma
5% of acute or chronic myeologenous leukemia
  Granulocytic sarcoma (chloroma)
Lung abnormalities
20%–40% lung infiltration at autopsy
Radiographic and CT abnormalities seldom due to leukemia
  alone
Pneumonia, hemorrhage, drug reactions, edema
Pulmonary leukostatis
  Acute myelogenous leukemia
  WBC count usually >200,000/mm³
  Pulmonary edema

Mediastinal Abnormalities

Mediastinal lymph nodes commonly are involved in patients with chronic lymphocytic leukemia (CLL) and acute lymphoblastic leukemia (ALL) (see section on lymphoblastic lymphoma earlier in this chapter). CLL typically occurs in adults older than 60 years; ALL is more common in children than in adults.

Mediastinal lymph node enlargement is visible radiographically in about 25% of patients with CLL (Fig. 5-34) and 10% to 20% of patients with ALL, although it is more common at autopsy, being present in more than half of cases. Hilar lymph node enlargement also may be seen but is less common. CLL typically presents with painless lymph node enlargement or hepatosplenomegaly; these abnormalities may be chronic and slowly progressive over a period of

years. ALL may present with a large, symptomatic anterior mediastinal mass (see Fig. 5-27).

In patients with acute or chronic myelogenous leukemia, masses of malignant myeloid precursor cells may be found in an extramedullary location, including lymph nodes; these masses are termed *granulocytic sarcoma* or *chloroma* (because of their green color). Granulocytic sarcoma occurs in about 5% of adults and 15% of children with myelogenous leukemia; the thorax is involved uncommonly. In about 50% of cases with thoracic involvement, it involves the mediastinum, either as a focal mass, lymph node enlargement, or generalized widening (Fig. 5-35). Less common sites of involvement include the lungs, pleura, the pericardium, and the hila.

Lung Abnormalities

Pulmonary infiltration is evident at autopsy in 20% to 40% of patients with leukemia. Radiographic findings of pulmonary leukemic infiltration consist of bilateral reticulation that resembles interstitial edema or lymphangitic carcinomatosis. HRCT abnormalities consist of interlobular septal thickening and thickening of the peribronchovascular interstitium. However, pulmonary abnormalities seen on radiographs or CT in patients with leukemia seldom are due to leukemic infiltration alone. In almost all patients, lung abnormalities are due to pneumonia, hemorrhage, drug-induced lung damage, or pulmonary edema.

Dyspnea in patients with leukemia is sometimes related to *pulmonary leukostasis*. Leukostasis is most common in acute myelogenous leukemia, and it occurs in patients with very high white blood cell counts (usually over 200,000/mm³). Symptoms result from vascular obstruction (in the lungs and other organs) by leukemic cells. Little if any invasion of the pulmonary interstitium occurs in patients with pulmonary leukostasis, and chest radiographs are often nor-

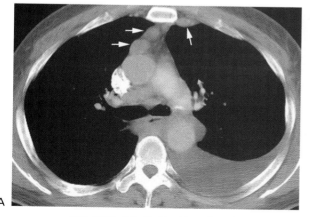
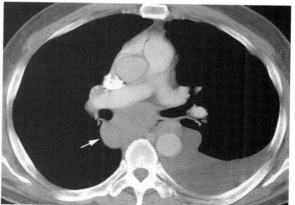

FIG. 5-34. Mediastinal lymph node enlargement in chronic lymphocytic leukemia. Enlarged lymph nodes are visible in the prevascular space and internal mammary chain (*arrows* in **A**) and subcarinal space (*arrow* in **B**). A left pleural effusion, which may reflect lymphatic obstruction, also is present.

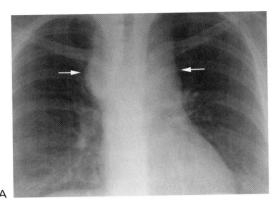

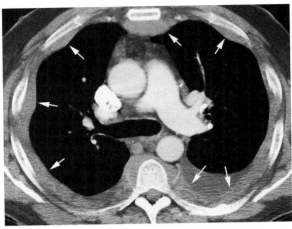

FIG. 5-37. Chronic lymphocytic leukemia with extrapleural involvement and pleural effusion. A number of masses *(arrows)* appear to be associated with the sternum and ribs. A left pleural effusion also is present. This appearance is similar to that in Figures 5-25 and 5-29.

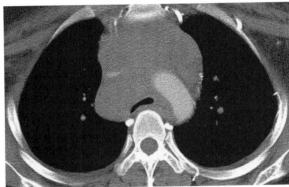

FIG. 5-35. Chronic granulocytic leukemia with involvement of mediastinal lymph nodes, so-called granulocytic sarcoma or "chloroma." **A.** Chest radiograph shows a lobulated mediastinal mass *(arrows)*. **B.** CT shows extensive lymph node enlargement in the pretracheal and prevascular mediastinum.

mal. In some cases, however, air-space consolidation is visible radiographically due to pulmonary edema (Fig. 5-36). Edema may be due to increased capillary permeability related to the presence of numerous white cells or cardiac failure related to coronary artery leukostasis. Leukostasis is considered an oncologic emergency.

Pleural Disease

As with lymphoma, pleural effusion may reflect lymphatic obstruction (see Fig. 5-34) or pleural involvement by tumor (Fig. 5-37).

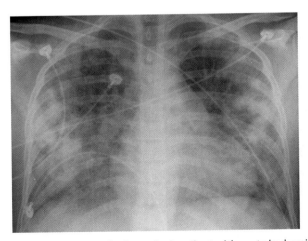

FIG. 5-36. Pulmonary leukostasis. A patient with acute leukemia, high white cell count, and leukostasis shows patchy areas of consolidation in the peripheral lung. These usually represent pulmonary edema.

SELECTED READING

Aquino SL, Chen MY, Kuo WT, Chiles C. The CT appearance of pleural and extrapleural disease in lymphoma. Clin Radiol 1999; 54:647–650.

Au V, Leung AN. Radiologic manifestations of lymphoma in the thorax. AJR Am J Roentgenol 1997; 168:93–98.

Blunt DM, Padley SP. Radiographic manifestations of AIDS related lymphoma in the thorax. Clin Radiol 1995; 50:607–612.

Bragg DG, Colby TV, Ward JH. New concepts in the non-Hodgkin lymphomas: radiologic implications. Radiology 1986; 159: 289–304.

Bragg DG, Chor PJ, Murray KA, Kjeldsberg CR. Lymphoproliferative disorders of the lung: histopathology, clinical manifestations, and imaging features. AJR Am J Roentgenol 1994; 163:273–281.

Carignan S, Staples CA, Müller NL. Intrathoracic lymphoproliferative disorders in the immunocompromised patient: CT findings. Radiology 1995; 197:53–58.

Castellino RA. Hodgkin disease: practical concepts for the diagnostic radiologist. Radiology 1986; 157:305–310.

Castellino RA. The non-Hodgkin lymphomas: practical concepts for the diagnostic radiologist. Radiology 1991; 178:315–321.

Castellino RA, Blank N, Hoppe RT, Cho C. Hodgkin disease: contributions of chest CT in the initial staging evaluation. Radiology 1986; 160:603–605.

Castellino RA, Hilton S, O'Brien JP, Portlock CS. Non-Hodgkin lymphoma: contribution of chest CT in the initial staging evaluation. Radiology 1996; 199:129–132.

Cobby M, Whipp E, Bullimore J, et al. CT appearances of relapse of lymphoma in the lung. Clin Radiol 1990; 41:232–238.

Collins J, Müller NL, Leung AN, et al. Epstein-Barr virus–associated lymphoproliferative disease of the lung: CT and histologic findings. Radiology 1998; 208:749–759.

Costello P, Mauch P. Radiographic features of recurrent intrathoracic Hodgkin's disease following radiation therapy. AJR Am J Roentgenol 1979; 133:201–206.

Dodd G, Ledesma-Medina J, Baron RL, Fuhrman CR. Posttransplant lymphoproliferative disorder: intrathoracic manifestations. Radiology 1992; 184:65–69.

Eisner MD, Kaplan LD, Herndier B, Stulbarg MS. The pulmonary manifestations of AIDS-related non-Hodgkin's lymphoma. Chest 1996; 110:729–736.

Filly R, Blank N, Castellino R. Radiographic distribution of intrathoracic disease in previously untreated patients with Hodgkin's disease and non-Hodgkin's lymphoma. Radiology 1976; 120:277.

Gibson M, Hansell DM. Lymphocytic disorders of the chest: pathology and imaging. Clin Radiol 1998; 53:469–480.

Heyneman LE, Johkoh T, Ward S, et al. Pulmonary leukemic infiltrates: high-resolution CT findings in 10 patients. AJR Am J Roentgenol 2000; 174:517–521.

Jochelson M, Mauch P, Balikian J, et al. The significance of the residual mediastinal mass in treated Hodgkin's disease. J Clin Oncol 1985; 3:637–640.

Johkoh T, Müller NL, Pickford HA, et al. Lymphocytic interstitial pneumonia: thin-section CT findings in 22 patients. Radiology 1999; 212:567–572.

Knisely BL, Mastey LA, Mergo PJ, et al. Pulmonary mucosa-associated lymphoid tissue lymphoma: CT and pathologic findings. AJR Am J Roentgenol 1999; 172:1321–1326.

Koss MN. Pulmonary lymphoid disorders. Semin Diagn Pathol 1995; 12:158–171.

Lee DK, Im JG, Lee KS, et al. B-cell lymphoma of bronchus-associated lymphoid tissue (BALT): CT features in 10 patients. J Comput Assist Tomogr 2000; 24:30–34.

Lee KS, Kim Y, Primack SL. Imaging of pulmonary lymphomas. AJR Am J Roentgenol 1997; 168:339–345.

Limpert J, MacMahon H, Variakojis D. Angioimmunoblastic lymphadenopathy: clinical and radiological features. Radiology 1984; 152:27–30.

O'Donnell PG, Jackson SA, Tung KT, et al. Radiological appearances of lymphomas arising from mucosa-associated lymphoid tissue (MALT) in the lung. Clin Radiol 1998; 53:258–263.

Rappaport DC, Chamberlain DW, Shepherd FA, Hutcheon MA. Lymphoproliferative disorders after lung transplantation: imaging features. Radiology 1998; 206:519–524.

Shaffer K, Smith D, Kirn D, et al. Primary mediastinal large–B-cell lymphoma: radiologic findings at presentation. AJR 1996; 167:425–430.

Sider L, Weiss AJ, Smith MD, et al. Varied appearance of AIDS-related lymphoma in the chest. Radiology 1989; 171:629–632.

Takasugi JE, Godwin JD, Marglin SI, Petersdorf SH. Intrathoracic granulocytic sarcomas. J Thorac Imaging 1996; 11:223–230.

Thompson GP, Utz JP, Rosenow EC, et al. Pulmonary lymphoproliferative disorders. Mayo Clin Proc 1993; 68:804–817.

6

THE PULMONARY HILA

W. RICHARD WEBB

Although plain radiographs play an important role in the diagnosis of hilar abnormalities, CT is used when specific information is required.

CHEST RADIOGRAPHS

In most cases, plain films are adequate for identifying large hilar masses. Small masses can be more difficult to detect because of the rather large variation in the appearances of the normal hila.

However, on chest radiographs, careful anatomic evaluation of the hila can often yield significant diagnostic information. Abnormalities may present as a change in hilar size or density, bronchial wall thickening or narrowing of the bronchial lumen, or as an alteration in the hilar contour.

Normal Hilar Contours

Frontal Radiograph

On a frontal (posteroanterior [PA] or anteroposterior [AP]) radiograph, the hilar shadows primarily represent the silhouettes of the hilar pulmonary arteries. The left pulmonary artery is situated higher than the right, and consequently the left hilum appears higher than the right in 97% of cases; in the remainder, they are at the same level.

Right Hilum

The superior portion of the right hilum is made up of the medially located truncus anterior, the artery supplying most of the upper lobe, and the right superior pulmonary vein, which forms the lateral margin of the upper hilum (Fig. 6-1). The anterior segment bronchus of the right upper lobe (RUL) is visible in 80% of patients as a 4- to 5-mm ring shadow in the lateral aspect of the hilum, accompanied by an artery of similar size. The RUL bronchus is sometimes visible.

The lower aspect of the right hilum is made up of the interlobar or descending pulmonary artery laterally and the bronchus intermedius medially. The pulmonary artery should measure 16 mm or less in thickness lateral to the bronchus (approximately the diameter of a dime) in men and 15 mm or less in women. The interlobar artery tapers inferiorly as it branches, with its lateral aspect appearing straight or slightly convex. Branches of the interlobar artery and segmental bronchi may be seen in the inferior hilum. Occasionally the lower part of the interlobar artery appears rounded, mimicking a mass or enlarged lymph node. This is most commonly seen when lung volumes are low.

A shallow angle is formed at the point the superior pulmonary vein crosses the interlobar pulmonary artery. This is termed the *hilar angle*.

The right inferior pulmonary vein is located inferior and medial to the hilar shadows and does not contribute significantly.

Left Hilum

The left pulmonary artery passes above the left main and upper lobe bronchus, gives off small upper lobe branches, and descends posterior and lateral to the left upper lobe (LUL) bronchus and lower lobe bronchus. The superior hilar shadow is made up of the superior aspect of the left pulmonary artery, superior pulmonary vein, and small arterial branches (Fig. 6-2). The anterior segmental bronchus of the LUL may be seen in the lateral hilum at this level. As on the right, the interlobar pulmonary artery tapers as it extends inferiorly, but it is less clearly seen and more difficult to measure than the right pulmonary artery. The left inferior pulmonary vein contributes little to the hilar shadow.

Lateral Radiograph

The right and left hilar shadows are superimposed on the lateral radiograph, but specific parts of the right and left hila can be seen (Figs. 6-3 and 6-4). Identification of the hilar bronchi should be the first step in analysis of the hila.

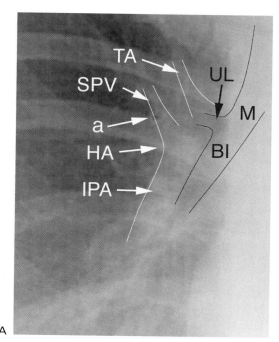

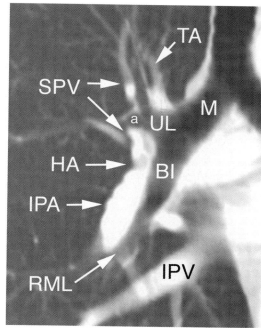

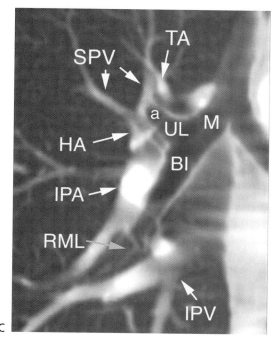

FIG. 6-1. Normal right hilum. **A.** Plain radiograph. The large bronchi (*M*, right main bronchus; *UL*, right upper lobe bronchus; *BI*, bronchus intermedius) are visible in the medial hilum. The anterior segment bronchus *(a)* is visible as a ring shadow lateral to the pulmonary arteries. Visible vascular structures include the apical branch of the truncus anterior *(TA)* in the medial superior hilum, and the superior pulmonary vein *(SPV)* in the lateral aspect of the superior hilum. The interlobar pulmonary artery *(IPA)* forms the lateral aspect of the inferior hilum and should measure 16 mm or less in men and 15 mm or less in women. A concavity is visible in the lateral hilum at the point the superior pulmonary vein crosses the interlobar pulmonary artery. This is termed the hilar angle *(HA)*. **B** and **C.** Coronal CT reformations through the right hilum in two patients. In addition to the structures visible in **A**, the right middle lobe bronchus *(RML)* is visible inferiorly. The inferior pulmonary vein *(IPV)* lies medial and below the hilar shadow and is difficult to recognize on the chest radiograph because of the heart shadow.

Right Hilum

The location of the tracheal carina and therefore the origins of the main bronchi can be determined by following the tracheal air column inferiorly. The carina is located at the point the air column begins to taper.

Below this level, a thin line, termed the *intermediate stem line,* is at least partially visible in 95% of patients (see Fig. 6-3). This line may be 5 cm or more in length and measures up to 3 mm in thickness. It corresponds superiorly to the posterior wall of the right main bronchus and more inferiorly to the posterior wall of the bronchus intermedius. The RUL bronchus is visible in 50% of patients as a rounded lucency anterior to the upper aspect of the intermediate stem line, but it is seldom seen well.

The anterior wall of the bronchus intermedius is visible as an edge, outlined by the right pulmonary artery and superior

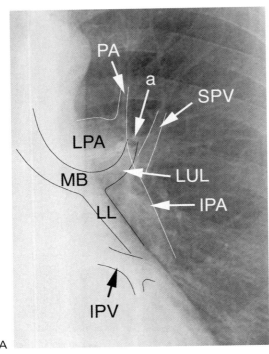
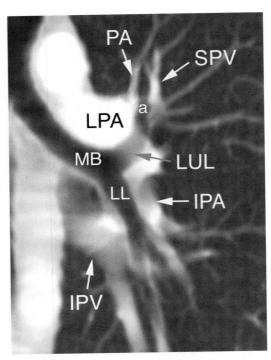

A

B

FIG. 6-2. Normal left hilum. **A.** PA radiograph. **B.** Coronal CT reformation. *MB*, left main bronchus; *LUL*, left upper lobe bronchus; *LL*, left lower lobe bronchus. The anterior segment bronchus *(a)* is visible as a ring shadow lateral to the main pulmonary artery, overlying the superior trunk of the left upper lobe bronchus. The left pulmonary artery *(LPA)* is visible as an oval opacity above the main and left upper lobe bronchus. The apical branch of the left pulmonary artery *(PA)* arises from the superior aspect of the pulmonary artery and as on the right is located medially. The superior pulmonary vein *(SPV)* forms the lateral aspect of the superior hilum. The interlobar pulmonary artery *(IPA)* forms the lateral aspect of the inferior hilum. The inferior pulmonary vein *(IPV)* may be visible inferiorly.

pulmonary vein. In combination, these vessels create an oval shadow making up the anterior portion of the combined hilar silhouette. The right middle lobe bronchus is sometimes seen curving anteriorly below the inferior edge of this oval shadow. In 15% of individuals, the anterior wall of the RLL bronchus is visible below this level as a thin straight line 1 to 2 cm long.

Left Hilum

Below the carina, the left main bronchus is superimposed on the right main bronchus (see Fig. 6-4). A well-defined rounded lucency representing the horizontal portion of the distal left main bronchus and LUL bronchus is visible in 80% of subjects several centimeters below the carina. This lucency is more clearly seen, is larger, and is better defined than the rounded lucency representing the RUL bronchus because vessels surround most of its circumference. Because the left main bronchus is longer than the right, the LUL bronchus is seen at a lower level than the RUL bronchus.

The anterior wall of the left lower lobe (LLL) bronchus is visible below the lucency of the LUL as a thin curved

line, convex anteriorly, in about 45% of cases. It arises tangential to the anterior wall of the LUL bronchus.

The left pulmonary artery forms a comma-shaped opacity seen above the lucency of the LUL bronchus and then passing posterior to it. Thus, while the right hilar vasculature largely accounts for the soft tissue in the anterior aspect of the combined hilar silhouette, the left pulmonary artery primarily accounts for its posterior aspect.

Plain Film Diagnosis of Hilar Mass or Lymphadenopathy

Frontal Radiograph

On a frontal radiograph, patients with a hilar mass or lymph node enlargement may show one of several findings:

- Hilar enlargement (Fig. 6-5A)
- A focal mass (see Fig. 6-5B)
- Increase in hilar density (see Fig. 6-5C)
- Hilar lobulation (see Fig. 6-5D)
- Convexity of the hilar angle (see Fig. 6-5E)

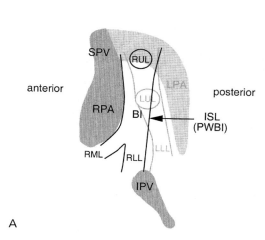

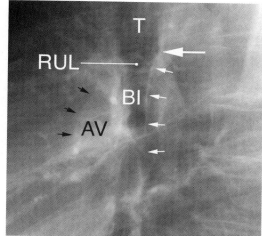

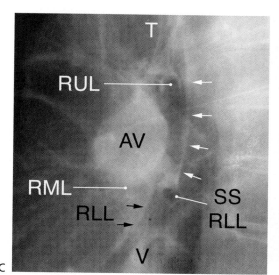

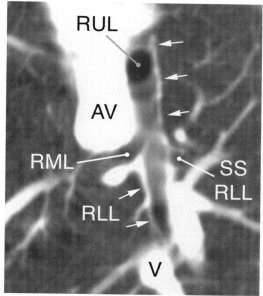

FIG. 6-3. Lateral chest radiograph; normal right hilar anatomy **A.** Diagram of hilar anatomy. Anterior is to the left and posterior to the right. Right hilar structures appear dark and left hilar structures are dimmed. *RUL,* right upper lobe bronchus; *BI,* bronchus intermedius; *RML,* right middle lobe bronchus; *RLL,* right lower lobe bronchus; *ISL,* intermediate stem line; *PWBI,* posterior wall of bronchus intermedius. The interlobar right pulmonary artery *(RPA)* results in an oval shadow anterior to the BI. The superior pulmonary vein *(SPV),* along with the truncus anterior, forms the superior part of the vascular shadow anterior to the bronchi. The inferior pulmonary veins are inferior. Left hilar structures are described in Figure 6-4A. **B.** Lateral radiograph showing right hilar anatomy. The trachea *(T)* is visible superiorly. The point at which the tracheal air column narrows *(large white arrow)* is the carina; the main and lobar bronchi are seen below this level. The right upper lobe bronchus *(RUL)* may be seen as a rounded lucency within the superior hilar shadow, slightly below the carina. Below the RUL, the bronchus intermedius *(BI)* is visible to the level of its bifurcation. The intermediate stem line or posterior wall of the bronchus intermedius is often visible as a thin white line *(small white arrows).* The oval shadow of the right hilar arteries and veins *(black arrows; AV)* is visible anterior to the bronchus intermedius. **C.** Lateral radiograph showing right hilar anatomy in a patient with left pneumonectomy. Only right hilar structures are visible. The trachea *(T)* is visible superiorly. Visible are the right upper lobe bronchus *(RUL),* intermediate stem line (posterior wall of the bronchus intermedius) *(white arrows),* right middle lobe bronchus *(RML),* superior segmental bronchus of the right lower lobe *(SS RLL),* and the anterior wall of the right lower lobe bronchus *(arrows; RLL).* Below the RUL, the bronchus intermedius *(BI)* is visible to the level of its bifurcation. The oval shadow of the right hilar arteries and veins *(AV)* is visible anterior to the bronchus intermedius, and the inferior pulmonary veins *(V)* are located inferiorly. **D.** CT reformation through the right hilum. *RUL,* right upper lobe bronchus; *white arrows,* intermediate stem line (posterior wall of the bronchus intermedius); *RML,* right middle lobe bronchus; *SS RLL,* superior segment bronchus of the right lower lobe; *RLL,* anterior wall of the right lower lobe bronchus; *AV,* right hilar arteries and veins; *V,* inferior pulmonary veins.

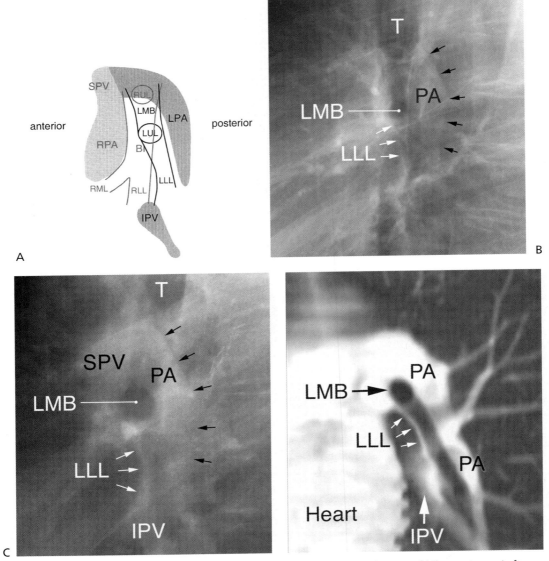

FIG. 6-4. Lateral chest radiograph; normal left hilar anatomy **A.** Diagram of hilar anatomy. Left hilar structures appear dark and right hilar structures are dimmed. *LMB,* left main bronchus; *LUL,* left upper lobe bronchus; *LLL,* left lower lobe bronchus; *LPA,* left pulmonary artery; *IPV,* inferior pulmonary veins. For right hilar structures see Figure 6-3A. **B.** Lateral radiograph showing left hilar anatomy; this is the same radiograph as in Figure 6-3B. The trachea *(T)* is visible superiorly. The horizontal portion of the left main and left upper lobe bronchus *(LMB)* results in an easily seen oval lucency. Above this level and superimposed on the bronchus intermedius, the left main portion of the left main bronchus may be seen. The anterior wall of the left lower lobe bronchus *(LLL)* is visible below the LMB as a thin white line and typically appears concave anteriorly. **C.** Lateral radiograph showing left hilar anatomy in a patient with a right pneumonectomy. Only left hilar structures are visible. The trachea *(T)* is visible superiorly. The oval lucency of the horizontal portion of the left main and left upper lobe bronchus *(LMB)* is easily seen. Below this level, the anterior wall of the left lower lobe bronchus *(LLL)* is visible as a thin white line, concave anteriorly. The left pulmonary artery *(PA)* is situated above and behind the LMB *(black arrows).* The left superior pulmonary veins are visible anterior and superior to the LMB, and the inferior pulmonary veins *(IPV)* are located inferiorly. **D.** CT reformation through the left hilum. LMB, left main and left upper lobe bronchus; LLL, anterior wall of the left lower lobe bronchus; PA, left pulmonary artery; IPV, inferior pulmonary veins.

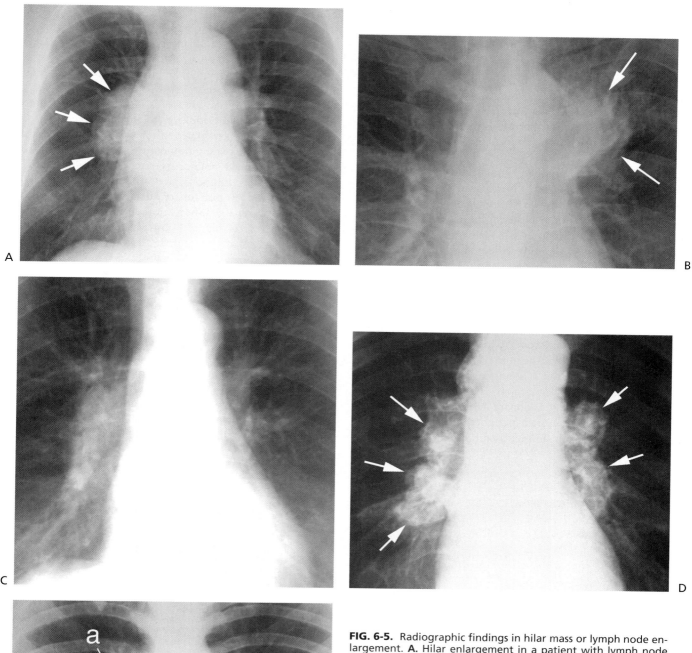

FIG. 6-5. Radiographic findings in hilar mass or lymph node enlargement. **A.** Hilar enlargement in a patient with lymph node enlargement due to metastatic renal cell carcinoma. The right hilum *(arrows)* is markedly enlarged and is rounded in contour, without its normal "vascular" shape. **B.** Focal hilar mass in bronchogenic carcinoma. A single, poorly marginated mass *(arrows)* obscures the upper left hilum. This appearance is typical of lung cancer originating in the hilum. **C.** Increase in hilar density due to right hilar carcinoma. The right hilum appears denser than the left. This is often due to mass or enlarged nodes anterior or posterior to the hilar shadow. The right hilum is also enlarged, with a subtle convexity in the hilar angle. **D.** Hilar lobulation due to sarcoidosis. The hila have distinct lobulated contours *(arrows)* typical of lymph node enlargement. Node calcification is also seen. **E.** Convexity of the hilar angle in a patient with Castleman's disease involving the right hilum. A mass *(arrow)* is visible in the region of the hilar angle. The mass projects lateral to the anterior segment bronchus *(a)* of the upper lobe.

Hilar enlargement is often present in patients with hilar lymph node enlargement (see Fig. 6-5A) or hilar mass (see Fig. 6-5B); it may be unilateral or bilateral. In the large majority of patients, the hila appear equal in size on frontal radiographs; comparison to the opposite side is helpful in patients with a unilateral abnormality. Measurement of the width of the right hilum lateral to the bronchus intermedius may also be valuable in diagnosis; as indicated above, this measurement should be 16 mm or less in men and 15 mm or less in women.

Masses sometimes produce a unilateral increase in hilar density on frontal radiographs (see Fig. 6-5A and C). This generally results when a mass or lymph node enlargement is located in the anterior or posterior hilum and is superimposed on the hilar shadow. In some patients, an increase in hilar density may be the only visible abnormality on the frontal radiograph; in such cases, the mass is often better seen on the lateral radiograph.

Hilar mass results in a focal alteration of the normal hilar contour. Lymph node enlargement may result in a focal abnormality or a more generalized lobulated appearance (see Fig. 6-5A and D). A common site for lymph node enlargement in the right hilum is the normally concave hilar angle; a convexity in this region is abnormal (see Fig. 6-5E).

The normal hila look vascular. The hilar shadows, primarily representing the pulmonary arteries, taper gradually with vessels arising from their periphery. Enlargement of a pulmonary artery results in increased hilar size and density,

but the hilum retains its "vascular" appearance (Fig. 6-6). The appearance of pulmonary vessels converging on the lateral aspect of the hilum is termed the "hilum convergence" sign and is indicative of vascular dilatation as the cause of hilar enlargement. The hilar angle typically retains its normal concave appearance.

Enlargement of hilar arteries is most typical of pulmonary hypertension. In addition to hilar enlargement, patients with pulmonary hypertension often show abnormal prominence of the main pulmonary artery on the PA radiograph and the main pulmonary artery and right ventricle on the lateral view. Pulmonic stenosis results in enlargement of the main and left pulmonary artery, while the right pulmonary artery usually appears normal in size.

Bronchial narrowing and obstruction associated with a hilar mass are usually difficult to diagnose on plain radiographs unless associated abnormalities such as mucous plugging, atelectasis, or obstructive pneumonia are visible (see Chapter 3).

Lateral Radiograph

Enlargement of the oval and comma-shaped shadows of the right and left pulmonary arteries indicates pulmonary artery dilatation (see Fig. 6-6B). As on the frontal radiograph, increased hilar size, focal mass, lobulation of hilar contours, or alternation in the normal oval and comma-shaped shadows can indicate a hilar mass or lymph node enlargement.

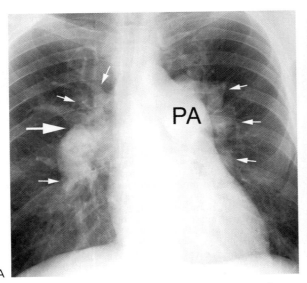
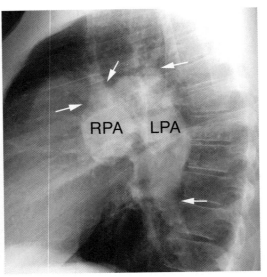

FIG. 6-6. Hilar enlargement in pulmonary hypertension. **A.** Enlargement of a pulmonary artery results in increased hilar size and density, but the hilum retains its "vascular" appearance. Vessels *(small arrows)* may be seen arising from the edges of the hilar shadow, the so-called hilum convergence sign, indicating the presence of vascular enlargement. The hilar angle *(large arrow)* remains concave. The main pulmonary artery *(PA)* is also enlarged. **B.** Lateral view. Although increased in size, the right *(RPA)* and left *(LPA)* pulmonary arteries retain their shape. Small branches arising from the edges of the arteries *(arrows)* result in the hilum convergence sign. *(Figure continues.)*

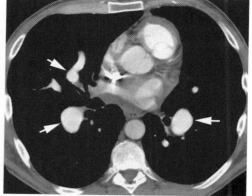

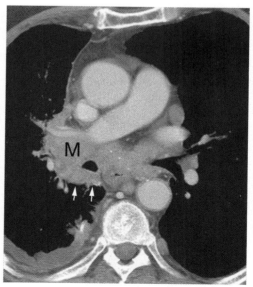

C

D

FIG. 6-6. Continued. **C** and **D**. CT shows enlargement of the main pulmonary artery *(PA)*, right *(RPA)* and left *(LPA)* pulmonary arteries, and the interlobar and middle lobe branches *(arrows)*.

Attention to several specific regions visible on the lateral radiograph may also be helpful in diagnosis, including the posterior wall of the bronchus intermedius (PWBI), the inferior hilar window, and the RUL bronchus (sign).

Posterior Wall of the Bronchus Intermedius

The PWBI is seen as a vertical or slightly oblique line or stripe in about 95% of patients (see Fig. 6-3). At its upper extent, the PWBI is contiguous with the posterior wall of the right main bronchus, forming the intermediate stem line described above. This stripe is normally 0.5 to 3 mm thick. Thickening of this stripe may be seen in patients with neoplasm involving the hilum (Fig. 6-7), hilar adenopathy, interstitial pulmonary edema (Fig. 6-8), or interstitial thickening of various causes. Obliteration of the posterior bronchial wall and the presence of soft-tissue densities behind it are virtually diagnostic of a mass in the hilum or adjacent lung.

Inferior Hilar Window

On the lateral radiograph, the oval soft-tissue shadow representing the right hilar vessels is visible in the anterior aspect of the composite hilar shadow, while the comma-shaped left pulmonary artery occupies its superior and posterior

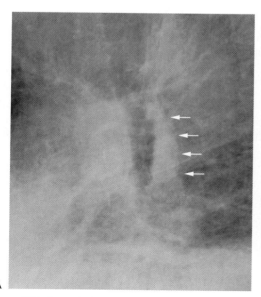

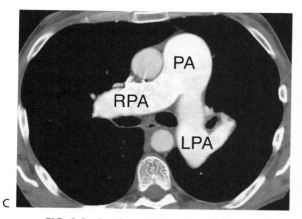

A

B

FIG. 6-7. Thickening of the posterior wall of the bronchus intermedius in right hilar carcinoma. **A.** Lateral chest radiograph shows marked thickening of the posterior wall of the bronchus intermedius *(arrows)*. **B.** CT in this patient shows a right hilar mass *(M)* with infiltration and thickening of the posterior bronchial wall *(arrows)*.

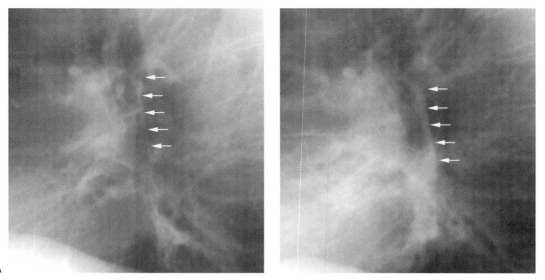

FIG. 6-8. Thickening of the posterior wall of the bronchus intermedius in pulmonary edema. **A.** A patient with longstanding renal failure shows a normal posterior bronchial wall *(arrows).* **B.** When the patient is in pulmonary edema, the posterior bronchial wall appears thickened *(arrows).*

aspect. The inferior hilar shadow contains no large vessels and consequently is termed the inferior hilar window (IHW). The IHW corresponds to an avascular region anterior to both lower lobe bronchi. It appears as a roughly triangular lucency in the anterior and inferior hilar shadow (Figs. 6-9 and 6-10).

In normal subjects, the inferior hilum appears radiolucent, and the composite hilar shadow appears as an incomplete oval. The presence of a soft-tissue opacity of more than 1 cm in the IHW is more than 90% accurate in diagnosing a hilar mass or adenopathy in this region. In abnormals, the addition of an opacity in the inferior hilum (IHW) results

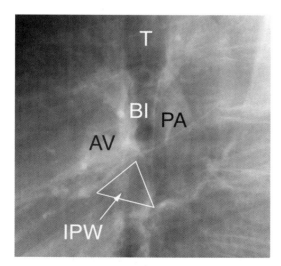

FIG. 6-9. The inferior hilar window. Lateral view. This image is the same as that in Figures 6-3B and 6-4B. The right hilar vessels *(AV)* occupy the anterior part of the hilar shadow. The left pulmonary artery *(PA)* is visible posteriorly and superiorly. The inferior hilar window is a roughly triangular lucency *(IPW)* in the anterior and inferior hilar shadow, below these major vascular branches. It represents an avascular region anterior to both lower lobe bronchi. *T,* trachea; *BI,* bronchus intermedius.

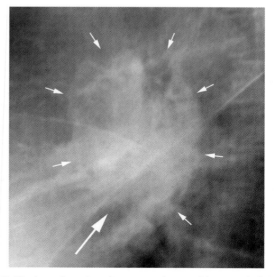

FIG. 6-10. Lymph node enlargement in sarcoidosis, with filling in of the inferior hilar window. Enlarged lymph nodes in the inferior hilar window *(large arrow),* when added to the shadows of the pulmonary arteries, result in a complete oval shadow on the lateral view *(small arrows).* This differs from the normal incomplete oval.

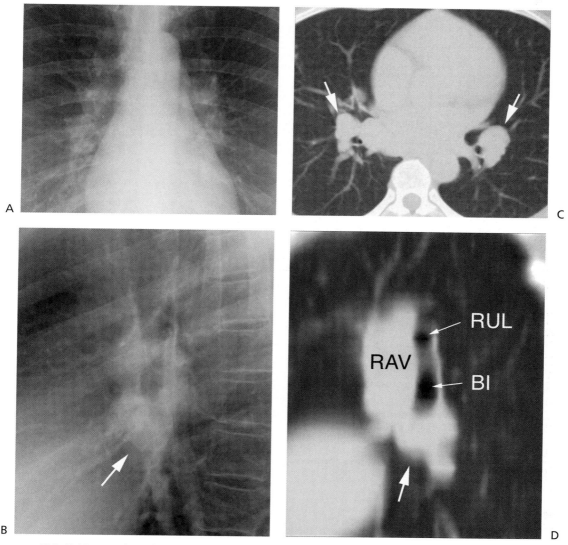

FIG. 6-11. Lymph node enlargement in sarcoidosis, with filling in of the inferior hilar window. **A.** PA chest radiograph shows subtle hilar lobulation. **B.** Lateral view shows lobulation of the hilar contours with filling in of the inferior hilar window *(arrow)*. The hilar silhouette forms a complete oval. **C.** CT shows lymph node enlargement in the anterior inferior hila, in the space anterior to the lower lobe bronchi. **D.** CT reformation through the right hilum shows lymph node enlargement in the inferior hilar window *(large arrow)*, inferior to the right hilar artery and vein *(RAV). RUL,* right upper lobe bronchus; *BI,* bronchus intermedius.

in the appearance of a complete oval shadow on lateral radiographs (Figs. 6-11 and 6-12). The side of the mass may be difficult to determine, although the frontal radiograph may help. Also, if a lower lobe bronchus is visible as a linear shadow, the mass must be on the opposite side.

Right Upper Lobe Bronchus (Sign)
Below the tracheal carina, two rounded radiolucencies are commonly seen, one above the other, in line with the tracheal air column and overlying the hilar bronchi. The lower of the two lucencies represents the horizontal por-

tion of the left main and upper lobe bronchus. The upper lucency represents the RUL bronchus (see Fig. 6-3). It is usually less well seen, as it is not surrounded by vascular structures.

If the RUL bronchus is sharply marginated throughout its circumference (and more importantly if this represents a change compared to prior radiographs), hilar mass or adenopathy (surrounding and outlining the bronchus) is likely present (see Fig. 6-12). This sign can also be helpful in distinguishing hilar vascular enlargement (which does not result in this sign) from hilar node enlargement.

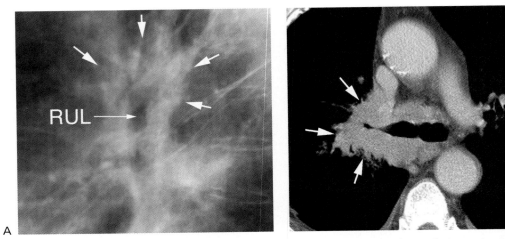

FIG. 6-12. Right upper lobe bronchus sign in lung cancer. **A.** Lateral radiograph shows the right upper lobe bronchus sign *(RUL)* as a lucency surrounded by mass *(arrows)*. Thickening of the posterior wall of the bronchus intermedius is also visible. **B.** CT shows a large mass *(arrows)* surrounding the upper lobe bronchus.

CT OF THE HILA

The pulmonary hila are complex structures containing the lobar and segmental bronchi, pulmonary arteries and veins, bronchial arteries and veins, soft tissue, and lymph nodes. The appearances of bronchi, vessels, and nodes and their consistent relationships at different hilar levels allow for reliable identification of these structures. Identification of specific bronchi is the first step in analysis of the hila. Bronchi are quite consistent in their branching pattern (Fig. 6-13).

CT of the Hilar Bronchi

Using a spiral CT technique and a slice thickness of 3 to 5 mm, all segmental bronchi should be visible. Their appearance depends on their orientation.

Bronchi oriented in or near the scan plane, and therefore seen along their axes as tubular structures, include the RUL bronchus (including both the anterior and posterior segmental bronchi), the LUL bronchus (including the anterior segmental bronchus), a portion of the middle lobe bronchus, and the superior segmental bronchi of both lower lobes.

Bronchi having a vertical course are seen in cross section and appear as circular lucencies. These include the apical segmental bronchus of the RUL, the apical-posterior segmental bronchus of the LUL, and proximal portions of both lower lobe bronchi (below the takeoff of the superior segmental bronchi), and the medial and posterior basal lower lobe segments.

The most difficult bronchi to visualize clearly are those oriented obliquely relative to the scan plane, including the

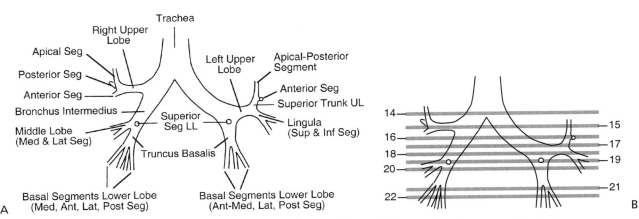

FIG. 6-13. Normal bronchial anatomy. **A.** Anatomy of bronchial segments as shown on a PA chest radiograph. **B.** Levels of CT slices shown in Figures 6-14 to 6-22.

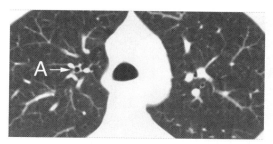

FIG. 6-14. Apical segment bronchus right upper lobe. The bronchus *(A)* is visible as a ring shadow at a level near the carina. A vessel of similar size and shape medial to the bronchus represents the artery to the apical segment. A vein characteristically lies lateral to the bronchus.

superior and inferior lingular bronchi, the lateral and medial segmental bronchi of the middle lobe, and the anterior and lateral basal lower lobe segments. Such bronchi appear elliptical on CT.

Right Bronchial Anatomy

The right main bronchus is relatively short, dividing into the RUL bronchus and bronchus intermedius. Often the carina, right main bronchus, and RUL bronchus are visible on a single scan.

Right Upper Lobe Bronchus

The RUL bronchus is always found at or just below the carina. The RUL bronchus courses laterally for 1 to 2 cm

before dividing into its three segmental branches (apical, anterior, and posterior; Figs. 6-14 and 6-15A). Characteristically, the posterior wall of the RUL bronchus is sharply outlined by lung and is seen as a thin line (see Fig. 6-15A). The upper limit of normal for the posterior wall of the RUL bronchus is 3 to 5 mm. However, the posterior part of the arch of the azygos vein can result in apparent bronchial wall thickening.

The precise branching pattern of the RUL bronchus is variable, primarily due to variation in the site of origin of the apical segmental bronchus.

Apical Segment

The apical segmental bronchus of the RUL is visible above the RUL bronchus itself, usually at or near the level of the distal trachea (see Fig. 6-14). It is seen in cross section as a circular lucency.

Anterior and Posterior Segments

The anterior and posterior segmental bronchi arise as a Y-shaped bifurcation of the RUL bronchus (see Fig. 6-15A). The anterior segment bronchus almost always lies in the plane of scan and is more easily seen. The posterior segmental bronchus may have a similar appearance but often angles slightly cephalad from its origin and is usually visible at progressively higher levels as it courses posteriorly.

In many patients a trifurcation of the RUL bronchus is present, with the origin of the apical segment bronchus seen as a rounded area of lucency superimposed on the distal portion of the RUL bronchus, at or just above the origins

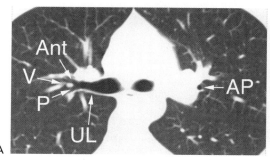
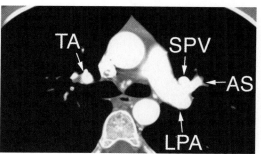

FIG. 6-15. Right upper lobe bronchus; apical posterior segment bronchus of left upper lobe. **A.** Lung window. On the right side, slightly below the carina, the right upper lobe bronchus *(UL)* is visible along its axis. Its posterior wall is visible as a thin white line. It branches in a Y shape into its anterior *(Ant)* and posterior *(P)* segments. On the left side, the apical posterior segment bronchus *(AP)* is visible as a ring shadow. **B.** Soft-tissue window scan following contrast enhancement. On the right, the truncus anterior *(TA)* lies anterior to the right upper lobe bronchus and appears similar in size to the main bronchus seen on the same scan. A vein lies between the anterior and posterior segmental bronchi. On the left, the left pulmonary artery *(LPA)* is posterior. The artery supplying the anterior segment *(AS)* of the left upper lobe is located medial to the apical posterior segment bronchus. The superior pulmonary vein *(SPV)* is anterior and medial to the anterior segment artery.

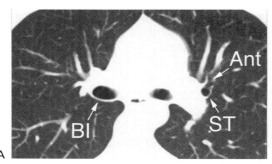
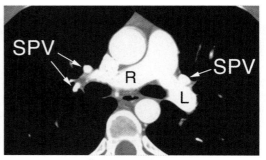

FIG. 6-16. Bronchus intermedius; anterior segment left upper lobe. **A.** On the right, the bronchus intermedius *(BI)* is visible as an oval lucency. Its posterior wall is sharply outlined by lung and appears a few millimeters thick. On the left, the anterior segment bronchus *(Ant)* of the left upper lobe is seen arising from the anterior aspect of the superior bronchial trunk *(ST)* of the left upper lobe. **B.** On the right, the right pulmonary artery *(R)* is visible medial to the bronchus, with the interlobar pulmonary artery passing anterior to the BI. Two branches of the superior pulmonary vein *(SPV)* are visible anterior and lateral to the artery and bronchus. Normal lymph nodes are visible lateral to the pulmonary artery and medial to the SPV. On the left, the left pulmonary artery is posterior. The SPV is anterior and medial to the superior trunk.

of the anterior and posterior segments. Major anatomic variants are unusual. Most frequent is tracheal bronchus, described in Chapter 1.

Bronchus Intermedius

The bronchus intermedius is 3 to 4 cm long, beginning at the level of the RUL bronchus. It gives rise to the middle lobe and lower lobe bronchi inferiorly. Because of its length, it is seen on a number of adjacent scans (Figs. 6-16 to 6-18).

The bronchus intermedius appears round or oval in cross section. The posterior wall of the bronchus intermedius is in contact with the superior segment of the RLL and is sharply outlined. It should appear thin and of uniform thickness, usually measuring no more than 3 mm. A portion of the medial bronchial wall also may be outlined by lung.

An anomalous bronchus termed the accessory cardiac bronchus may arise from the medial bronchus intermedius or lower lobe bronchus, extending medially toward the heart. It supplies a small area of aerated lung or rudimentary (nonaerated) lung tissue (see Fig. 1-3 in Chapter 1).

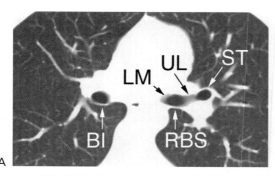
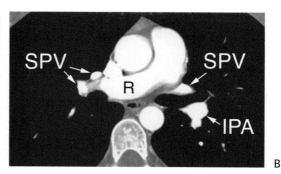

FIG. 6-17. Bronchus intermedius; left main bronchus and upper aspect of the left upper lobe bronchus. **A.** On the right, the bronchus intermedius *(BI)* appears as an oval lucency. On the left, the posterior wall of the left main bronchus *(LM)* is visible as a thin stripe, the left retrobronchial stripe *(RBS)*. The superior aspect of the left upper lobe bronchus *(UL)* is visible, giving rise laterally to the superior trunk *(ST)* of the left upper lobe. The posterior wall of the left upper lobe bronchus is slightly concave at this level. **B.** On the right, the anatomy of hilar vessels is similar to Figure 6-16B. The right pulmonary artery is medial, the interlobar pulmonary artery is anterior to the bronchus, and the superior pulmonary vein *(SPV)* branches are visible anterior and lateral to the artery and bronchus. On the left, the interlobar left pulmonary artery *(IPA)* produces a large convexity in the posterior hilum, and the superior pulmonary vein *(SPV)* results in an anterior convexity.

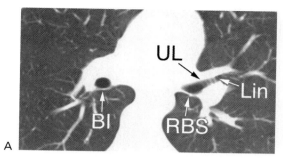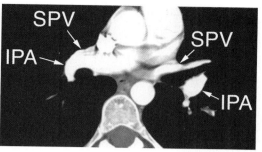

FIG. 6-18. Bronchus intermedius; lower aspect of the left upper lobe bronchus and lingular bronchus. **A.** On the right, the bronchus intermedius *(BI)* appears as an oval lucency. On the left, the left retrobronchial stripe *(RBS)* is again seen. The inferior aspect of the left upper lobe bronchus *(UL)* is visible, giving rise laterally to the lingular branch *(Lin)* of the left upper lobe. **B.** On the right, the interlobar pulmonary artery *(IPA)* passes anterior and lateral to the BI. Branches to the superior segment of the lower lobe are directed posteriorly. The combination of the IPA and superior segment branches resembles an elephant's head. The SPV is visible anteriorly. On the left, the left IPA is seen in cross section and lies lateral to the lower lobe bronchi, posterolateral to the lingular bronchus, and anterolateral to the superior segmental bronchus. It is round or oval. The SPV passes anterior and medial to the bronchi to enter the left atrium.

Right Middle Lobe Bronchus

The middle lobe bronchus arises from the anterolateral wall of the bronchus intermedius and extends anteriorly at an angle of about 45°. The origin of the middle lobe bronchus also marks the point of origin of the RLL bronchus (Fig. 6-19A). A thin carina may be seen separating the origins of the right middle lobe (RML) and RLL bronchi. The middle lobe bronchus lies oblique to the scan plane and appears as an oval lucency. Only a short segment of the RML bronchus may be visible on any one scan, depending

on its orientation, the scan thickness, and the degree of volume averaging.

Medial and Lateral Segments

The middle lobe bronchus extends for about 1 to 2 cm before dividing into its medial and lateral segmental branches. Because of its orientation, the main portion of the RML bronchus and the medial and lateral segments are often seen at a level 1 to 2 cm below the origin of the RML bronchus (Fig. 6-20A).

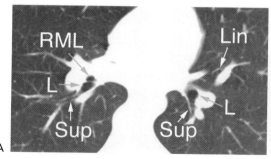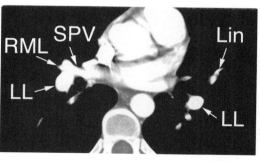

FIG. 6-19. Right middle lobe and superior segment right lower lobe; lingular bronchus and superior segment left lower lobe. **A.** On the right, the origin of the right middle lobe bronchus *(RML)* is visible. Posterior to it is the lower lobe bronchus *(L)* and the superior segment of the lower lobe *(Sup)*. A thin carina separates the middle and lower lobe bronchi. On the left, the lingular bronchus *(Lin)*, lower lobe bronchus *(L)*, and superior segment of the lower lobe *(Sup)* have a similar appearance to the right-sided bronchi. **B.** On the right, the lower lobe pulmonary artery *(LL)* lies lateral to the lateral borders of both the middle and lower lobe bronchi. The lower lobe artery at this point is oriented perpendicular to the scan plane and is thus seen in cross section as an elliptical structure. The right middle lobe artery *(RML)* is seen as an anterior branch. The right superior pulmonary vein *(SPV)* passes anterior and medial to the middle and lower lobe bronchi. On the left, the lower lobe artery *(LL)* lies lateral to the lower lobe bronchus. The lingular artery *(Lin)* is anterior.

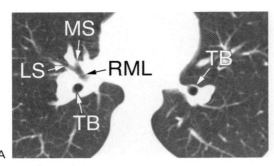 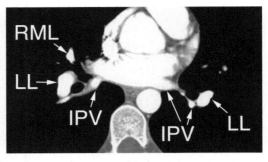

FIG. 6-20. Right middle lobe and its segments; basal lower lobe trunks. **A.** On the right, the right middle lobe bronchus *(RML)* and its medial *(MS)* and lateral segments *(LS)* are visible. The truncus basalis *(TB)* or basal lower lobe trunk is visible on both sides. The anterior wall of the left TB is outlined by lung. **B.** On the right, the lower lobe pulmonary artery *(LL)* lies lateral to the lateral border of the lower lobe bronchus. The right middle lobe artery *(RML)* is seen as an anterior branch. The right inferior pulmonary vein lies medial to the lower lobe bronchus. On the left, the lower lobe artery *(LL)* has a lobulated appearance as it begins to divide. Inferior pulmonary vein branches *(IPV)* are medial and posterior.

In 60% of cases, the middle lobe bronchus divides into medial and lateral segmental branches of equal size. In most of the remaining cases, the medial segmental bronchus appears larger. Although both middle lobe segmental bronchi are directed inferiorly, the lateral segmental bronchus lies closer to the scan plane and is imaged over a greater distance on each scan.

Right Lower Lobe Bronchus

The undivided lower lobe bronchus is very short. Near its origin, it gives rise to the superior segmental bronchus (see Fig. 6-19A). Distal to the origin of the superior segment, the basal bronchial trunk continues for a short distance (see Fig. 6-20A) before dividing into the four basal segmental branches of the RLL: the medial, anterior, lateral, and posterior segments (Fig. 6-21A).

Superior Segment

The superior segmental bronchus of the RLL bronchus may arise at the same level as or slightly caudal to the origin of the RML bronchus (see Fig. 6-19A). In some cases, the superior segmental bronchus arises at a level cephalad to the origin of the RML bronchus.

The superior segmental bronchus, which is about 1 cm in length, arises from the posterior wall of the RLL bronchus and courses posteriorly and laterally within the scan plane (see Fig. 6-19A). Lung often outlines the medial aspect of the superior segment bronchus.

Truncus Basalis and Basal Segments

Below the origin of the superior segmental bronchus, the lower lobe bronchus continues for about 5 to 10 mm as the truncus basalis or basal bronchial trunk, visible as a

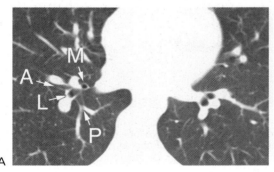 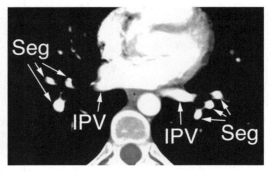

FIG. 6-21. Basal segments of the right lower lobe. **A.** On the right, the four basal segments are visible. In a counter-clockwise direction, these are the medial basal *(M)*, anterior basal *(A)*, lateral basal *(L)*, and posterior basal *(P)*, spelling MALP. On the left, two branches of the truncus basalis are visible at this level. **B.** On both sides, the segmental arteries *(Seg)* lie posterolateral to the proximal portions of the basilar segmental bronchi. The inferior pulmonary vein *(IPV)* passes posterior to the lower lobe bronchi and arteries before entering into the lower portion of the left atrium.

circular lucency (see Fig. 6-20A). The anterior wall of the truncus basalis is commonly outlined by lung.

The basal segments have a typical orientation of M-A-L-P, beginning medially and anteriorly and proceeding counterclockwise (see Fig. 6-21A). The medial basal segmental bronchus usually arises as the first branch of the basal trunk, lying just anterior to the inferior pulmonary vein. Although variable in appearance, the anterior, lateral, and posterior basilar bronchi may all be identified because of their positions relative to one another and because they each course toward the segments they supply. In general, the medial and posterior segmental bronchi are imaged more nearly in cross section than the anterior and lateral, which are more obliquely oriented (see Figs. 6-21A and 6-22A). Anatomic variation in the origins of these segments is common.

Left Bronchial Anatomy

The left main bronchus is much longer than the right and is typically seen on three or four contiguous slices below the carina (see Figs. 6-13 and 6-15 to 6-17). It divides into left upper and lower lobe branches.

Left Upper Lobe Bronchus

The LUL bronchus is 2 to 3 cm long (see Figs. 6-17 and 6-18). In about 75% of patients, the LUL branches into a superior trunk and the lingular bronchus. The superior trunk is about 1 cm in length, giving rise to the anterior and apical-posterior segmental bronchi (Figs. 6-16 to 6-18). In 25% of cases, the LUL bronchus trifurcates into the apical-posterior segment bronchus, anterior segment bronchus, and lingular bronchus.

At the level of the superior aspect of the LUL bronchus, its posterior wall is smooth and slightly concave (see Fig. 6-17A). At this level, the origin of the apical-posterior seg-

mental bronchus, or the superior bronchial trunk that gives rise to the apical posterior and anterior segmental bronchi, can be recognized as a rounded area of increased lucency superimposed on the distal portion of the LUL bronchus.

In 90% of cases, the superior segment of the LLL abuts the posterior wall of the left main or upper lobe bronchus, outlining the left "retrobronchial stripe" (see Figs. 6-17A and 6-18A). The bronchial wall should appear similar to that of the posterior bronchus intermedius.

Apical-Posterior and Anterior Segments

The anterior segment bronchus of the LUL bronchus is usually visible above the level of the LUL bronchus itself (see Fig. 6-16A). It lies roughly in the plane of scan and is oriented almost directly anteriorly; it is usually visible over several centimeters. It is the only LUL branch that has this course.

The apical-posterior segment bronchus is visible as a circular lucency at and above the origin of the anterior segment bronchus (see Fig. 6-15A). If a bronchus is seen in cross section below the anterior segment and above the LUL bronchus, it represents the short superior bronchial trunk; although similar in appearance to the apical-posterior segment and following the same course, it is larger.

Lingular Bronchus

The lingular bronchus arises from the undersurface of the distal portion of the LUL bronchus and courses obliquely downward, as does the RML bronchus (see Fig. 6-18A). It usually appears elliptical. The origin of the lingular bronchus may be identified as a lucency superimposed on the distal portion of the LUL bronchus. The origin of the lingular bronchus may be distinguished from the origin of the anterior segmental bronchus of the LUL bronchus by noting its relationship to the inferior aspect of the upper lobe bronchus or by identifying a thin carina or spur that is usually seen between the lingular bronchus and the LLL bronchus.

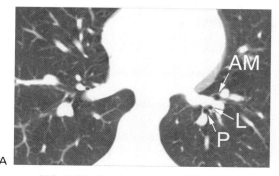
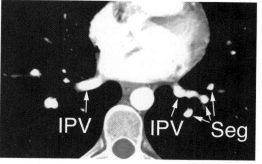

FIG. 6-22. Basal segments of the left lower lobe. **A.** On the left, the three basal segments are visible. In a clockwise direction, these are the anteromedial basal *(AM)*, lateral basal *(L)*, and posterior basal *(P)*. The four basal segments are again visible on the right. **B.** On both sides, the segmental arteries *(Seg)* lie posterolateral to the proximal portions of the basilar segmental bronchi. The inferior pulmonary vein *(IPV)* passes posterior and medial to the lower lobe bronchi.

Superior and Inferior Lingular Segments

The lingular bronchus extends anteriorly and inferiorly for 2 to 3 cm before dividing into its superior and inferior segmental branches. The superior segmental bronchus of the lingula is directed more laterally than the inferior segment and lies closer to the scan plane, analogous to the pattern of branching of the medial and lateral segments of the right middle lobe.

Left Lower Lobe Bronchus

The LLL bronchus usually conforms to the same general branching pattern as the RLL bronchus, although only three basal segments are generally present: the anteromedial, lateral, and posterior.

Superior Segment

The superior segmental bronchus of the LLL bronchus arises within 1 cm of the origin of the LLL bronchus and is identical in shape and configuration to the superior segment bronchus on the right side (see Fig. 6-19A).

Truncus Basalis and Basal Segments

The truncus basalis, the lower lobe bronchus giving rise to the basal lower lobe segments, is visible below the origin of the superior segment for a distance of 1 to 2 cm (see Fig. 6-20A). It is generally longer than the truncus basalis on the right. As on the right, the anterior wall of the basal trunk may be outlined by lung.

The basilar segmental bronchi are almost mirror images of the RLL basilar bronchi, except that on the left side the medial and anterior basilar bronchi characteristically originate together as a common trunk (see Fig. 6-22A). Again, the key to the identification of the basal segments is to note the general configuration and position of these bronchi as they course to their corresponding segments. In a clockwise fashion, the relative positions of the bronchi are M-A (in this case anteromedial)-L-P.

CT of the Hilar Vessels

Bronchi serve as an anatomic framework for the hila. Hilar vessels have a consistent relationship to bronchi, and identifying hilar bronchi is the first step to analyzing the hila. Despite some variation in the branching of segmental hilar arteries, most can be identified by noting their close association with specific segmental bronchi, by following their courses on sequential images, and by determining their sites of origin.

Evaluation of the vascular structures of the hila is simplified by the recognition of specific levels relative to the bronchi (see Figs. 6-15 to 6-22). At these levels, the hila have characteristic silhouettes.

Right side:
- Tracheal carina and apical segmental bronchus of the RUL
- RUL bronchus
- Bronchus intermedius
- Middle lobe bronchus
- Lower lobe basilar segmental bronchi

Left side:
- Apical posterior and anterior segmental bronchi of the LUL
- LUL bronchus
- Lingular bronchus
- Lower lobe basilar segmental bronchi

Vascular Anatomy of the Right Hilum

Tracheal Carina and Apical Segmental Bronchus

At or near the level of the carina, a branch or branches of the truncus anterior supplying the apical segment of the RUL and a branch or branches of the right superior pulmonary vein draining the apical segment are visible in cross section, adjacent to the apical segmental bronchus. Typically, the apical segmental artery lies medial to the bronchus and the veins lie lateral to it (see Fig. 6-14).

Right Upper Lobe Bronchus Level

At the level of the RUL bronchus, the undivided truncus anterior is usually identifiable (see Fig. 6-15B). This large vessel is the first major branch of the right main pulmonary artery, arising within the pericardium, and characteristically lies just anterior to the RUL bronchus. As a rule of thumb, the truncus anterior usually appears similar in size to the right main bronchus seen at the same level.

Typically, a large branch of the right superior pulmonary vein, the posterior vein, lies within the angle formed by the bifurcation of the RUL bronchus into anterior and posterior segmental bronchi (see Fig. 6-15A). Anterior and medial to the truncus anterior, a small convexity is frequently visible touching the mediastinum, representing another RUL vein, the apical-anterior vein, which is often identifiable without the injection of contrast agent.

Bronchus Intermedius Level

On scans showing the bronchus intermedius, the interlobar pulmonary artery lies anterior and lateral to the bronchus (see Figs. 6-16 to 6-18). The right superior pulmonary vein lies anterior to the right interlobar pulmonary artery. Frequently, two veins are visible in this location; these should not be mistaken for lymph node enlargement. Infrequently, a small vein branch draining a portion of the posterior segment of the upper lobe passes posterior to the bronchus intermedius; it can be seen to pass medially at successively lower levels to join the inferior pulmonary vein.

Once the interlobar pulmonary artery reaches the lateral

border of the bronchus intermedius and enters the major fissure, the artery often resembles an elephant's head (the main portion of the artery) and trunk (the superior segment artery; see Fig. 6-18).

Middle Lobe Bronchus Level

At the level of the origin of the middle lobe bronchus, the lower lobe pulmonary artery lies immediately lateral to the lateral borders of both the middle and lower lobe bronchi, and the right middle lobe artery parallels the RML bronchus (see Figs. 6-19 and 6-20). The lower lobe artery at this point is oriented perpendicular to the scan plane and is thus seen in cross section as an elliptical structure.

The right superior pulmonary vein passes anterior and medial to the middle and lower lobe bronchi and can be seen entering the upper portion of the left atrium. The middle lobe vein is sometimes seen joining the superior pulmonary vein at this level.

Level of the Basal Segmental Bronchi of the Right Lower Lobe

Below the level of the origin of the middle lobe bronchus, the lower lobe pulmonary artery often bifurcates into two short trunks, which in turn divide into the four basilar segmental pulmonary arteries. These have a characteristic, rounded configuration, lying posterolateral to the proximal portions of the basilar segmental bronchi (see Figs. 6-21 and 6-22). Unlike the basilar pulmonary arteries, which are imaged in cross section, the inferior pulmonary veins are oriented in the transverse plane. They join to form the inferior pulmonary vein, which passes posterior to the lower lobe bronchi and arteries before entering into the lower portion of the left atrium.

Vascular Anatomy of the Left Hilum

On the left side, although characteristic relationships between vessels and airways are also present, there is far more anatomic variation than on the right.

Level of the Apical-Posterior and Anterior Segments of the Left Upper Lobe

The apical-posterior segmental bronchus and associated arteries and veins have a similar appearance to the right apical segmental bronchus and associated vessels. The artery supplying the anterior segment of the LUL is seen medial to the anterior segment bronchus (see Fig. 6-15).

Left Upper Lobe Bronchus Level

At the level of the left upper bronchus, the interlobar left pulmonary artery produces a large convexity in the posterior

hilum, and the superior pulmonary vein results in an anterior convexity, medial to the ascending bronchial trunk or anterior segmental bronchus, if visible (see Fig. 6-17).

Lingular Bronchus Level

The lingular bronchus is usually visible at a level near the undersurface of the LUL bronchus. The appearance of the hilar vessels at this level is analogous to that of the right hilum at the level of the middle lobe bronchus. The left interlobar pulmonary artery is seen in cross section and lies lateral to the lower lobe bronchi, posterolateral to the lingular bronchus, and anterolateral to the superior segmental bronchus (see Fig. 6-18). It is round or oval. The superior pulmonary vein passes anterior and medial to the bronchi to enter the left atrium.

Level of the Basilar Segmental Bronchi of the Left Lower Lobe

At the level of the basilar segmental bronchi, the anatomy of the inferior portion of the left hilum is nearly a mirror image of that on the right (see Figs. 6-21 and 6-22). Branches of the pulmonary artery to the LLL lie lateral and posterior to the LLL basilar bronchi. The left inferior pulmonary vein passes anterolateral to descending aorta and posterior to the bronchi and arteries to enter the left atrium.

CT of the Hilar Lymph Nodes

The use of contrast enhancement usually allows the accurate differentiation of hilar lymph nodes from normal vessels. Hilar lymph nodes are not located randomly but are found in consistent locations. The most important groups are described below in relation to bronchial anatomy.

Right Upper Lobe Bronchus and Left Pulmonary Artery Level

Lymph nodes are common adjacent to the segmental branches of the RUL bronchus but tend to be small (Fig. 6-23). Lymph nodes are commonly seen both medial and lateral to the left pulmonary artery. Lateral nodes are medial to the superior bronchial trunk. These may be mistaken for pulmonary embolism.

Bronchus Intermedius and Left Upper Lobe Bronchus Level

On the right, slightly below the RUL bronchus, lateral to the bifurcation of the main pulmonary artery, anterolateral to the bronchus intermedius, and medial to superior pulmonary vein branches, it is very common in normal subjects

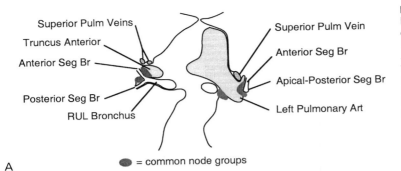

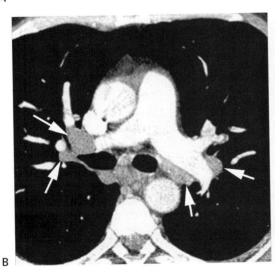

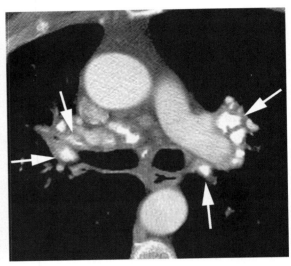

FIG. 6-23. Lymph node groups, level of the right upper lobe bronchus and left pulmonary artery. **A.** Diagram of common node groups. *Seg Br*, segment bronchus; *Art*, artery. **B.** Enlarged lymph nodes *(arrows)* in these groups in a patient with non-Hodgkin's lymphoma. **C.** Calcified lymph nodes *(arrows)* at this level in sarcoidosis.

to see a large area of unenhanced soft tissue comprising small nodes and fat (see Figs. 6-16B and 6-24). This can range up to 1.5 cm in diameter in some normals. Nodes in this region represent part of the "lymphatic sump" of the right lung. They can be easily mistaken for a hilar mass or thrombus in the right pulmonary artery. Lymph nodes tend to be medial and lateral to the posterior wall of the bronchus intermedius but not immediately posterior to it. Lymph nodes in this region are in the hilar angle.

At the level of the upper portion of the LUL bronchus, a rim of soft tissue largely representing normal nodes is always seen between the posterior bronchial wall and the pulmonary artery. Lymph nodes are common adjacent to the retrobronchial stripe but are not normally seen.

Right Middle Lobe Bronchus and Lingular Level

At the level of the right middle lobe bronchus and node group, lymph nodes are commonly seen (70%) lateral to the origin of the middle lobe or lower lobe bronchi and medial to the interlobar pulmonary artery (Fig. 6-25). These can be more than 5 mm in some normal patients. Normal

lymph nodes having a similar appearance are also commonly seen on the left, in relation to the lingular bronchus.

Lower Lobe Bronchi and the Inferior Hilar Window

At the level of the lower lobe bronchial segments, most nodes are interposed between bronchi and pulmonary arteries (Fig. 6-26). Lymph nodes anterior to the truncus basalis and basal lower lobe bronchi are also commonly present, visible in about 15% to 20% of normals. These nodes lie within the region termed the inferior hilar window.

Normal Hilar Lymph Node Size

In most regions, normal nodes measure only a few millimeters in size as shown on CT, with a short axis diameter of 3 mm or less. In three locations described above, however, larger conglomerates of nodes and soft tissue are often visible. These three regions are found at the levels of (1) the bronchus intermedius and bifurcation of the right pulmonary artery, (2) the right middle lobe bronchus, and (3) the

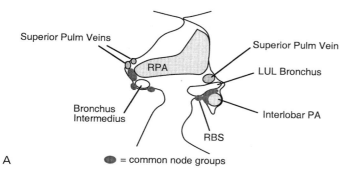

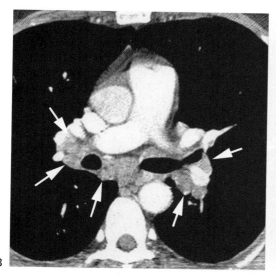

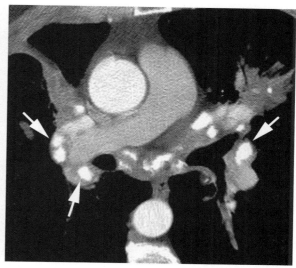

FIG. 6-24. Lymph node groups, level of the bronchus intermedius and left upper lobe bronchus. **A.** Diagram of common node groups. *Pulm*, pulmonary; *RBS*, retrobronchial stripe; *PA*, pulmonary artery. **B.** Enlarged lymph nodes *(arrows)* in these groups in a patient with non-Hodgkin's lymphoma. **C.** Calcified lymph nodes *(arrows)* at this level in sarcoidosis.

LUL and lingular and bronchus. In only the first of these, however, can unenhanced soft tissue exceeding 1 cm in least diameter be seen. Except in this one region, it would seem appropriate to use a least node diameter of 10 mm as the upper limit of normal.

CT DIAGNOSIS OF HILAR ABNORMALITIES

Bronchial Abnormalities

Generally speaking, scans viewed with a lung window setting (−700/1000 HU) are best for identifying normal bronchi and detecting bronchial abnormalities but may overestimate the degree of bronchial narrowing. Also, a normal bronchus slightly out of the plane of scan and being volume-averaged with adjacent soft tissue can appear narrowed on lung window scans. A soft-tissue window is often best for looking at narrowed or obstructed bronchi and associated mass or lymph node enlargement. A wide lung window (−600/1500 HU) is a good compromise, providing information about bronchi and soft-tissue masses.

Thin-collimation scans or high-resolution CT, particularly with spiral acquisition, can be of great value in identifying bronchial abnormalities. Although the use of 3D reconstruction techniques may be of some value in the diagnosis of bronchial lesions, their advantage appears to be minimal compared to careful review of the transaxial images and multiplanar reconstructions.

Accurate indicators of bronchial pathology include bronchial wall thickening, endobronchial mass, bronchial obstruction, and narrowing of the bronchial lumen. Other findings that may indicate the presence of a bronchial abnormality include mucous plugging, air trapping, atelectasis, or obstructive pneumonia. The differential diagnosis of an endobronchial mass or bronchial obstruction is listed in Table 3-11 in Chapter 3.

Bronchial Wall Thickening

Bronchial wall thickening is most easily assessed for bronchi partially outlined by lung. Specific bronchi assessed in this manner include the right main bronchus, RUL bronchus, bronchus intermedius, and left main and upper lobe bronchus (left retrobronchial stripe). Smooth bronchial wall thickening can be due to inflammation or tumor infiltration, while a localized or lobulated thickening usually indi-

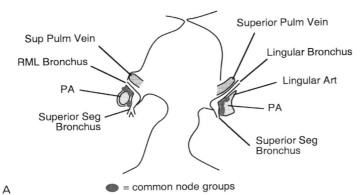

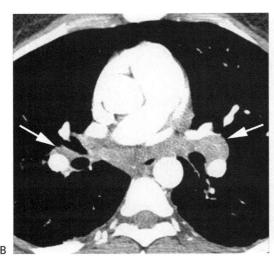

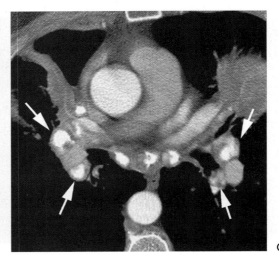

FIG. 6-25. Lymph node groups, level of the right middle lobe and lingular bronchi. **A.** Diagram of common node groups. *Pulm*, pulmonary; *Art*, artery; *PA*, pulmonary artery; *Seg*, segment. **B.** Enlarged lymph nodes *(arrows)* in these groups in a patient with sarcoidosis. **C.** Calcified lymph nodes *(arrows)* at this level in sarcoidosis.

cates localized tumor infiltration or lymph node enlargement.

Right Main and Right Upper Lobe Bronchus

The posterior walls of the RML and RUL bronchi are sharply outlined by lung in normal subjects and should appear quite thin. Generalized thickening suggests tumor infiltration (see Fig. 6-12B).

Posterior Wall of the Bronchus Intermedius

On CT, the PWBI is visible in all patients. Its upper extent is clearly definable by, and is contiguous with, the origin of the RUL bronchus. The inferior extent of the PWBI is obscured by a branch of the inferior pulmonary vein crossing behind the bronchus to enter the left atrium. This usually occurs at the level of the origin of the superior segmental bronchus of the RLL. Thickening or nodularity of the PWBI can be seen with tumor infiltration (see Fig. 6-7B), most commonly by bronchogenic carcinoma, or lymph node enlargement. Slight thickening may be seen in patients with pulmonary edema or interstitial lung disease. Obliteration of the posterior bronchial wall and the presence of soft-

tissue densities behind it are virtually diagnostic of a mass in the hilum or adjacent lung.

Left Retrobronchial Stripe

The left posterior bronchial wall is outlined by lung only at the level of the LUL bronchus. On CT, in approximately 90% of subjects, lung sharply outlines the posterior wall of the left main or upper lobe bronchus, medial to the descending pulmonary artery, termed the left retrobronchial stripe (see Fig. 6-17). Thickening of the left retrobronchial stripe, as seen on CT, indicates lymph node enlargement or bronchial wall thickening, analogous to thickening of the PWBI on the right (Fig. 6-27). In 10% of normal individuals, lung does not contact the bronchial wall because the descending pulmonary artery is positioned medially, contacting the lateral aorta.

Endobronchial Lesions and Bronchial Obstruction

Endobronchial lesions are sometimes diagnosed because a lesion is visible within the bronchus or focal bronchial ob-

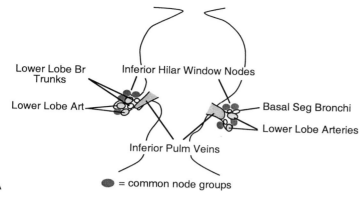

FIG. 6-26. Lymph node groups, level of the lower lobe bronchi. **A.** Diagram of common node groups. *Pulm,* pulmonary; *Art,* artery; *Br,* bronchus; *Seg,* segment. **B.** Enlarged lymph nodes *(arrows)* in a patient with sarcoidosis. The left-sided lymph nodes are in the region of the inferior hilar window. **C.** Calcified lymph nodes *(arrows)* at this level in sarcoidosis.

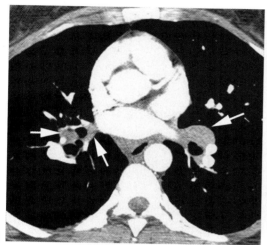

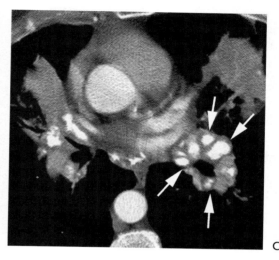

FIG. 6-27. Thickening of the left retrobronchial stripe due to metastatic nasopharyngeal carcinoma. Lymph node enlargement posterior to the left upper lobe bronchus *(arrow)* results in thickening of this stripe. Left hilar and subcarinal lymph node enlargement is also seen.

struction is present in the absence of hilar mass. The differential diagnosis of an endobronchial lesion includes primary malignant and benign bronchial tumors, metastases, lymphoma, stricture, granulomas (infectious or noninfectious), foreign body, broncholith, and mucus (see Table 3-11 in Chapter 3).

Caveats: In patients with a hilar mass, it is difficult to distinguish bronchial compression and obstruction from an endobronchial mass. Endobronchial abnormalities that are primarily mucosal can be missed using CT.

Narrowing of the Bronchial Lumen

Bronchial narrowing in the absence of obstruction may be caused by an infiltrating tumor, inflammation, stricture, or bronchomalacia. Carcinoma often produces a gradual or tapered bronchial narrowing, a so-called rat-tail appearance, because of bronchial wall infiltration by tumor (see Fig. 3-17 in Chapter 3). The presence of an associated mass is important in the differential diagnosis and strongly suggests carcinoma. It is important to look at adjacent scans to confirm that the apparent bronchial narrowing does not reflect an oblique bronchial course or volume averaging.

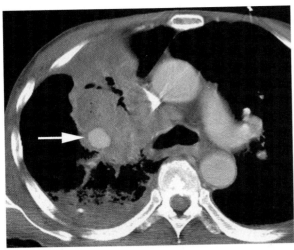

FIG. 6-28. False aneurysm in bronchogenic carcinoma. A right hilar carcinoma results in right upper lobe collapse. The right hilar mass is associated with pooling of contrast in a false aneurysm *(arrow).*

Vascular Abnormalities

CT is very useful in the diagnosis of pulmonary vascular abnormalities. Pulmonary embolism is discussed in Chapter 27.

Pulmonary Artery

Involvement of the pulmonary artery is common in patients with bronchogenic carcinoma involving the hilum. Usually artery narrowing or obstruction occurs. Rarely a false aneurysm is seen in relation to the tumor (Fig. 6-28).

Increased Artery Size

A variety of conditions may result in pulmonary artery enlargement (Table 6-1). Most common is pulmonary hyper-

tension with dilatation of the main and hilar pulmonary arteries (see Fig. 6-6). In normal subjects, the main pulmonary artery measures 22 to 36 mm in diameter. Dilatation of the main pulmonary artery (more than 29 mm) correlates with the presence of pulmonary hypertension. The main pulmonary artery may also be considered dilated if it appears larger than the adjacent ascending aorta on CT. Pulmonary artery dilatation also occurs with left-to-right shunt.

Enlargement of a hilar pulmonary artery may occur because of pulmonary embolism. This generally reflects the presence of a large clot impacted in the artery, but pulmonary hypertension associated with the embolus also may contribute to this appearance.

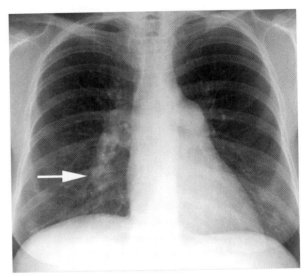

A

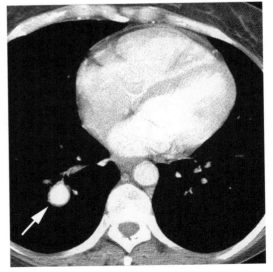

B

FIG. 6-29. Pulmonary artery aneurysm in pulmonary hypertension. **A.** Chest radiograph shows enlargement of the main pulmonary artery *(arrow)* due to pulmonary hypertension. A focal lesion is visible overlying the inferior hilum. **B.** Contrast-enhanced CT shows a focal aneurysm *(arrow)* of a segmental pulmonary artery.

TABLE 6-1. PULMONARY ARTERY ENLARGEMENT

Pulmonary hypertension
Left-to-right shunt
Pulmonary embolism
Pulmonic stenosis
Absent pulmonary valve
Pulmonary artery sarcoma
Pulmonary artery aneurysm
  Mycotic
  Catheter-related complications
  Takayasu's arteritis
  Williams syndrome
  Prenatal varicella
  Pulmonary hypertension
  Behcet's syndrome

TABLE 6-2. DECREASED PULMONARY ARTERY SIZE

Hypoplastic lung
Scimitar syndrome
Proximal interruption of the pulmonary artery
Pulmonary embolism
Atelectasis
Swyer-James syndrome
Ipsilateral lung disease

Enlargement of the main and left pulmonary arteries is seen in patients with pulmonic stenosis or absent pulmonary valve. The pulmonary outflow tract usually appears dilated as well. The right pulmonary artery usually appears normal.

Pulmonary artery sarcoma is a rare neoplasm resulting in an intravascular mass. This may result in dilatation of the main, right, or left pulmonary arteries.

Pulmonary artery aneurysms are rarely seen (Fig. 6-29); they may be (1) mycotic in origin; (2) due to catheter-related complications; (3) associated with multiple pulmonary artery stenoses or coarctations in patients with Takayasu's arteritis, Williams syndrome, and prenatal varicella; (4) associated with pulmonary hypertension; or (5) associated with Behçet's syndrome.

Decreased Artery Size

Decrease in size of a hilar pulmonary artery has a variety of causes (Table 6-2). It may represent artery or lung hypoplasia, proximal interruption of the pulmonary artery, or conditions resulting in decreased lung perfusion such as chronic pulmonary embolism (Fig. 6-30), chronic collapse, severe unilateral fibrosis or lung destruction, or Swyer-James syndrome. In some patients, enlargement of bronchial ar-

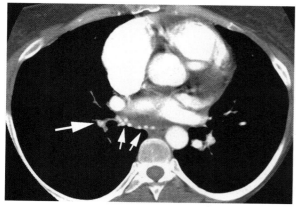

FIG. 6-30. Decreased size of pulmonary artery in chronic pulmonary embolism. The right interlobar pulmonary artery is markedly reduced in size *(large arrow)*. Bronchial arteries *(small arrows)* are enlarged.

teries is seen on the side of decreased perfusion (see Fig. 6-30). These are best seen with thin collimation and rapid contrast infusion.

Pulmonary Veins

Pulmonary vein abnormalities are uncommon. Pulmonary vein dilatation (i.e., vein varices) occurring in association with chronic elevation of left atrial pressure and anomalous pulmonary vein drainage is most common (see Fig. 9-47 in Chapter 9). In patients with lung cancer or metastatic neoplasm, tumor may invade the pulmonary vein, appearing as a filling defect on contrast-enhanced scans.

Hilar Lymph Node Enlargement and Hilar Masses

There is some value in attempting to distinguish hilar lymph node enlargement from hilar mass, although this is not always possible.

Hilar Lymph Node Enlargement

Hilar lymph node enlargement may be suggested if abnormal soft tissue is localized to node-bearing regions, particularly if more than one node group is involved (see Figs. 6-23 to 6-27). Nodes usually appear well defined, smooth, and rounded. Except at the level of the bronchus intermedius, nodes larger than 1 cm may be considered pathologic. Nodes larger than 5 mm are also usually abnormal, but these are commonly seen and are likely to be hyperplastic. Very large hilar nodes may result in smooth bronchial compression.

The presence of hilar lymph node enlargement, depending on the clinical situation, suggests hilar metastases from bronchogenic carcinoma, metastatic carcinoma, lymphoma, sarcoidosis, or infection. The differential diagnosis of hilar lymph node enlargement depends on whether it is unilateral or bilateral (Table 6-3).

Hilar Masses

Hilar masses usually are localized to one region, appear irregular in contour, and are often associated with an endobronchial mass or bronchial obstruction (Fig. 6-31). The presence of a mass suggests bronchogenic carcinoma or other primary tumor and makes lymph node diseases less likely. In patients with a hilar mass and bronchial obstruction, collapse or consolidation of distal lung can obscure the margins of the mass, making it more difficult to diagnose.

Common Causes of Hilar Node Enlargement or Masses

Bronchogenic Carcinoma

The most common cause of hilar mass or lymph node enlargement is bronchogenic carcinoma. The hilar mass can

TABLE 6-3. UNILATERAL AND BILATERAL LYMPH NODE ENLARGEMENT

Unilateral
  Bronchogenic carcinoma
  Lymph node metastases
    Head and neck
    Thyroid carcinoma
    Melanoma
    Renal
    Testicular
    Breast
  Lymphoma
  Tuberculosis
  Histoplasmosis
  Coccidioidomycosis
  Bacterial infection
  Viral infection
Bilateral
  Sarcoid or berylliosis
  Silicosis
  Amyloidosis
  Collagen-vascular diseases

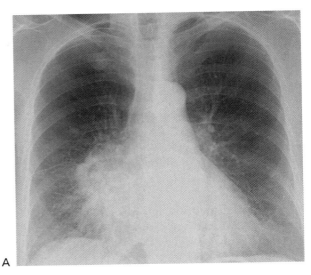

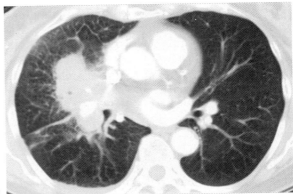

FIG. 6-31. Right hilar mass in small cell carcinoma. **A.** A large, ill-defined hilar enlargement is visible on the chest radiograph. This is more typical of hilar mass than lymph node enlargement. **B.** CT shows a large localized right hilar mass associated with obstruction of the right middle lobe bronchus and infiltration of adjacent lung.

appear irregular because of local infiltration of the lung parenchyma (see Figs. 6-5B, 6-7B, 6-28, and 6-31). In patients with tumors arising centrally (usually squamous cell carcinoma or small cell carcinoma), bronchial abnormalities are commonly visible on CT. When the carcinoma arises in the peripheral lung and the hila is abnormal because of node metastases, the hilar mass or masses may be smoother and more sharply defined than when the hilar mass represents the primary tumor. However, this distinction is not always easily made. Patients with a central mass and bronchial obstruction often show peripheral parenchymal abnormalities. In patients with hilar node metastases, a bronchial abnormality seen on CT usually reflects external compression by the enlarged hilar nodes, but bronchial invasion may also be present. Hilar node metastases are present at surgery in up to 40% of patients with lung cancer.

Other Primary Bronchial Tumors

Other primary bronchial tumors may be associated with a hilar mass. The most common of these is carcinoid tumor. This malignant tumor arises from the main, lobar, or segmental bronchi in 80% of cases. It tends to be slow-growing and locally invasive. A well-defined endobronchial mass is typical, but a large exobronchial, hilar mass is sometimes seen. Carcinoid tumors are very vascular and can enhance somewhat following contrast infusion. Carcinoid tumors occasionally calcify. Adenoid cystic carcinoma (cylindroma) can result in a similar appearance.

Benign bronchial tumors, such as fibroma, chondroma, or lipoma, usually appear focal and endobronchial on CT, rather than infiltrative, and do not commonly produce an

exobronchial mass. Obstruction is the primary finding on CT. They are relatively rare.

Lymphoma

Hilar adenopathy is present in 25% of patients with Hodgkin's and 10% of patients with non-Hodgkin's lymphoma (see Figs. 6-23B and 6-24B). Hilar involvement is usually asymmetrical. Multiple nodes in the hilum or mediastinum are usually involved. Endobronchial lesions can also be seen, or bronchi may be compressed by enlarged nodes, but this is much less common than with lung cancer. There are no specific features of the hilar abnormality seen in patients with lymphoma that allow a definite diagnosis.

Metastases

Metastases to hilar lymph nodes from an extrathoracic primary tumor are not uncommon. Hilar node metastases may

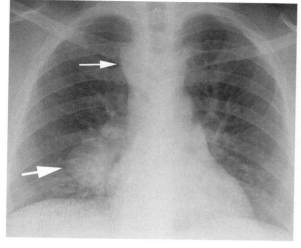

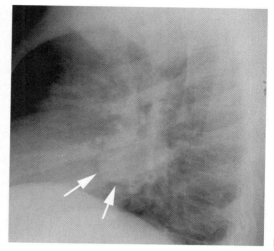

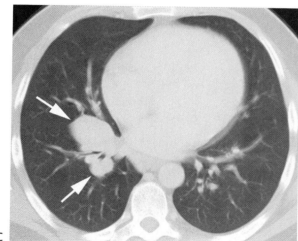

FIG. 6-32. Tuberculosis in an AIDS patient resulting in hilar and mediastinal lymph node enlargement. **A.** PA chest radiograph shows a right hilar mass *(large arrow)* and right paratracheal mediastinal lymph node enlargement *(small arrow)*. **B.** Lateral view shows enlarged lymph nodes *(arrows)* in the inferior hilar window. **C.** CT shows lymph node enlargement *(arrows)* in the inferior hilum.

be unilateral or bilateral (see Fig. 6-5A). Endobronchial metastases can also be seen without there being hilar node metastases; these may appear to be focal and endobronchial or infiltrative. Head and neck carcinomas, thyroid carcinoma, genitourinary tumors (particularly renal cell and testicular carcinoma), melanoma, and breast carcinomas are most commonly responsible for hilar or endobronchial metastases.

Inflammatory Disease

Unilateral or bilateral hilar lymphadenopathy can be seen in a number of infectious or inflammatory conditions. Primary tuberculosis usually causes unilateral hilar adenopathy (Fig. 6-32), and the presence of low-attenuation nodes on contrast-enhanced scans strongly suggests this diagnosis. Fungal infections, most notably histoplasmosis and coccidioidomycosis, cause unilateral or bilateral adenopathy. Sarcoidosis causes smooth, lobulated, bilateral, and symmetrical adenopathy in most patients (see Figs. 6-5D, 6-10, 6-11, and 6-23C).

SELECTED READING

Bankier AA, Fleischmann D, Mallek R, et al. Bronchial wall thickness: Appropriate window settings for thin-section CT and radiologic-anatomic correlation. Radiology 1996; 199:831–836.

Friedman PJ. Practical radiology of the hila and mediastinum. Postgrad Radiol 1981; 1:269–304.

Jardin M, Remy J. Segmental bronchovascular anatomy of the lower lobes: CT analysis. AJR Am J Roentgenol 1986; 147:457–468.

Lang EV, Friedman PJ. The anterior wall stripe of the left lower lobe bronchus on the lateral chest radiograph: CT correlative study. AJR Am J Roentgenol 1990; 154:33–39.

McGuinness G, Naidich DP, Garay SM, et al. Accessory cardiac bronchus: computed tomographic features and clinical significance. Radiology 1993; 189:563–566.

Müller NL, Webb WR. Radiographic imaging of the pulmonary hila. Invest Radiol 1985; 20:661–671.

Naidich DP, Khouri NF, Scott WJ, et al. Computed tomography of the pulmonary hila, 1: normal anatomy. J Comput Assist Tomogr 1981; 5:459–467.

Naidich DP, Khouri NF, Stitik FP, et al. Computed tomography of the pulmonary hila. 2. Abnormal anatomy. J Comput Assist Tomogr 1981; 5:468–475.

Naidich DP, Stitik FP, Khouri NF, et al. Computed tomography of the bronchi. 2. Pathology. J Comput Assist Tomogr 1980; 4: 754–762.

Naidich DP, Terry PB, Stitik FP, Siegelman SS. Computed tomography of the bronchi. 1. Normal anatomy. J Comput Assist Tomogr 1980; 4:746–753.

Naidich DP, Zinn WL, Ettenger NA, et al. Basilar segmental bronchi: thin-section CT evaluation. Radiology 1988; 169:11–16.

Ng CS, Wells AU, Padley SP. A CT sign of chronic pulmonary arterial hypertension: the ratio of main pulmonary artery to aortic diameter. J Thorac Imaging 1999; 14:270–278.

Park CK, Webb WR, Klein JS. Inferior hilar window. Radiology 1991; 178:163–168.

Proto AV, Speckman JM. The left lateral radiograph of the chest. Med Radiog Photog 1979; 55:30–74.

Quint LE, Whyte RI, Kazerooni EA, et al. Stenosis of the central airways: evaluation by using helical CT with multiplanar reconstructions. Radiology 1995; 194:871–877.

Remy-Jardin M, Duyck P, Remy J, et al. Hilar lymph nodes: identification with spiral CT and histologic correlation. Radiology 1995; 196:387–394.

Remy-Jardin M, Remy J, Artaud D, et al. Volume rendering of the tracheobronchial tree: clinical evaluation of bronchographic images. Radiology 1998; 208:761–770.

Schnur MJ, Winkler B, Austin JHM. Thickening of the posterior wall of the bronchus intermedius: a sign on lateral chest radiographs of congestive heart failure, lymph node enlargement, and neoplastic infiltration. Radiology 1981; 139:551–559.

Sone S, Higashihara T, Morimoto S, et al. CT anatomy of hilar lymphadenopathy. AJR Am J Roentgenol 1983; 140:887–892.

Vix VA, Klatte EC. The lateral chest radiograph in the diagnosis of hilar and mediastinal masses. Radiology 1970; 96:307–316.

Webb WR. Radiologic imaging of the pulmonary hila. Postgrad Radiol 1986; 6:145–168.

Webb WR, Gamsu G. Computed tomography of the left retrobronchial stripe. J Comput Assist Tomogr 1983; 7:65–69.

Webb WR, Gamsu G, Glazer G. Computed tomography of the abnormal pulmonary hilum. J Comput Assist Tomogr 1981; 5:485–490.

Webb WR, Glazer G, Gamsu G. Computed tomography of the normal pulmonary hilum. J Comput Assist Tomogr 1981; 5:476–484.

Webb WR, Hirji M, Gamsu G. Posterior wall of the bronchus intermedius: radiographic-CT correlation. AJR Am J Roentgenol 1984; 142:907–911.

7

THE NORMAL MEDIASTINUM

W. RICHARD WEBB

The mediastinum is defined as the tissue compartment located between the two lungs, posterior to the sternum, anterior to the vertebral column, and extending from the thoracic inlet to the diaphragm.

CT ANATOMY

The aorta and its branches, the great veins, the pulmonary arteries, and the trachea and main bronchi serve as reliable guides to localizing other important mediastinal structures. As an aid to understanding regional anatomy, the mediastinum can be divided into four compartments, respectively, from superior to inferior: (1) the superior or supraaortic mediastinum; (2) the region of the aortic arch and aortopulmonary window; (3) the pulmonary arteries, subcarinal space, and azygoesophageal recess; and (4) the heart and paracardiac mediastinum.

Supraaortic Mediastinum

Just below the thoracic inlet (Fig. 7-1A and B), the mediastinum is relatively narrow from anterior to posterior. The **trachea** is centrally located.

The **esophagus** lies posterior to the trachea but can be displaced to the left (more common) or right. It is often collapsed and appears as a flattened structure of soft-tissue attenuation. Small amounts of air or fluid may be seen in its lumen.

Other than the trachea and esophagus, the great arterial branches of the aorta and the brachiocephalic veins are the most apparent normal structures at this level. The **brachiocephalic veins** are the most anterior and lateral vessels visible, lying immediately behind the clavicular heads. Although they vary in size, their positions are relatively constant.

The **right brachiocephalic vein** has a nearly vertical course throughout its length. The **left brachiocephalic vein** is longer and courses horizontally as it crosses the mediastinum (see Fig. 7-1B). The precise cephalocaudal location of this vein is quite variable; although it is most frequently visible at this level, the horizontal portion of the left brachiocephalic vein also can be seen at the level of the aortic arch.

The **innominate, subclavian, and carotid arteries** lie posterior to the veins and adjacent to the anterior and lateral walls of the trachea. These can be reliably identified by their consistent positions. The **innominate (brachiocephalic) artery** is lo-

cated in close proximity to the anterior tracheal wall, near its midline or slightly to the right of midline in most normals; it is the most variable of all the great arteries. The **left common carotid artery** lies to the left and slightly posterior to the innominate artery; generally it has the smallest diameter of the three major arterial branches. The **left subclavian artery** is a relatively posterior structure throughout most of its course, lying to the left of the trachea or slightly posterior to its midline. The lateral border of the left subclavian artery typically indents the mediastinal surface of the left upper lobe. Small vascular branches, particularly the internal mammary veins and vertebral arteries, are often seen in this part of the mediastinum.

In some patients, the thyroid gland extends into the superior mediastinum, and the right and left thyroid lobes may be visible on each side of the trachea. On CT, the thyroid can be distinguished from other tissues or masses because of its iodine content, its attenuation greater than that of soft tissue.

Aortic Arch and Aortopulmonary Window

While the supraaortic region largely contains arterial and venous branches of the aorta and vena cava, this compartment contains the undivided mediastinal great vessels, the aorta and superior vena cava, and also several important mediastinal spaces and lymph node groups (Figs. 7-2 to 7-4).

The **aortic arch** has a characteristic but variable appearance (see Fig. 7-2A). The anterior aspect of the arch is located anterior and to the right of the trachea, with the arch passing to the left and posteriorly. The posterior arch usually lies anterior and lateral to the spine. The aortic arch tapers slightly along its length, from anterior to posterior.

The position of the anterior and posterior aspects of the arch can vary in the presence of atherosclerosis and aortic tortuosity; typically the anterior arch is located more anteriorly and to the right in patients with a tortuous aorta, while the posterior aorta lies more laterally and posteriorly, in a position to the left of the spine.

At this level, the **superior vena cava** is visible anterior and to the right of the trachea, usually being elliptical (see Fig. 7-2A).

The **esophagus** appears the same as at higher levels, being posterior to the trachea but variable in position. Often it lies somewhat to the left of the tracheal midline (see Fig. 7-2A).

The aortic arch on the left, the superior vena cava and me-

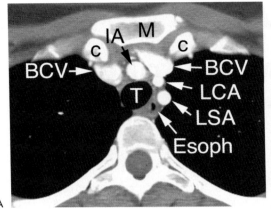
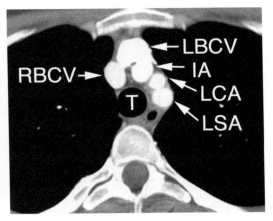

FIG. 7-1. Normal CT anatomy. Supraaortic mediastinum. **A.** *M,* manubrium; *c,* clavicular head; *T,* trachea; *Esoph,* esophagus; *BCV,* brachiocephalic vein; *IA,* innominate artery; *LCA,* left carotid artery; *LSA,* left subclavian artery. **B.** *T,* trachea; *RBCV,* right brachiocephalic vein; *LBCV,* left brachiocephalic vein; *IA,* innominate artery; *LCA,* left carotid artery; *LSA,* left subclavian artery

diastinal pleura on the right, and the trachea posteriorly serve to define a somewhat triangular space called the **pretracheal space** (see Figs. 7-2A and B). This fat-filled space contains mediastinal lymph nodes in the pretracheal or anterior paratracheal chain. Other mediastinal node groups are closely related to this group both spatially and in regard to lymphatic drainage. It is not uncommon to see a few normal-sized lymph nodes in the pretracheal space.

Anterior to the great vessels (aorta and superior vena cava) at this level is another triangular space called the **prevascular space** (see Figs. 7-2 and 7-3). The apex of this triangular space represents the anterior junction line (see Figs. 7-2A and 7-3A and B). This compartment, which is anterior mediastinal, primarily contains thymus (described in detail below), lymph nodes, and fat (see Figs. 7-2 and 7-3). The mediastinal pleural

reflections bordering the prevascular space may be concave or convex laterally, although a marked convexity suggests anterior mediastinal mass or thymic enlargement.

At a level slightly below the aortic arch, the ascending aorta and descending aorta are visible as separate structures (Figs. 7-3A and C). The average diameter of the proximal ascending aorta averages 3.6 cm (range, 2.4 to 4.7 cm), the ascending aorta just below the arch 3.5 cm (range, 2.2 to 4.6 cm), the proximal descending aorta 2.6 cm (range, 1.6 to 3.7 cm), the mid-descending aorta 2.5 cm (range, 1.6 to 3.7 cm), and the distal descending aorta 2.4 cm (range, 1.4 to 3.3 cm).

At or near this level, the **trachea** bifurcates into the right and left **main bronchi**. Near the carina, the trachea commonly assumes a somewhat triangular shape (see Fig. 7-2A). The carina is usually visible on CT (see Fig. 7-3A and B).

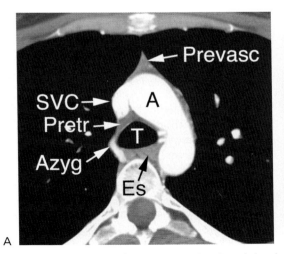
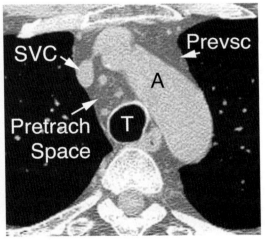

FIG. 7-2. Normal CT anatomy. Aortic arch level. **A.** Contrast-enhanced CT at a lower level in the same patient as in Figure 7-1. *T,* trachea; *Es,* esophagus; *A,* aortic arch; *SVC,* superior vena cava; *Azyg,* azygos arch; *Prevasc,* prevascular space containing thymus; *Pretr,* pretracheal space. **B.** Unenhanced high-resolution CT. *T,* trachea; *A,* aortic arch; *SVC,* superior vena cava; *Prevasc,* prevascular space; *Pretrach,* pretracheal space containing normal lymph nodes; *Prevsc,* prevascular space containing thymus replaced by fat.

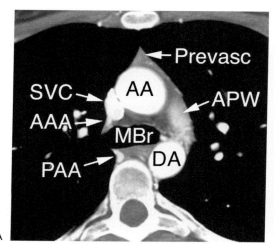
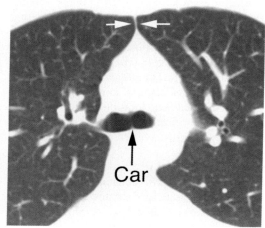

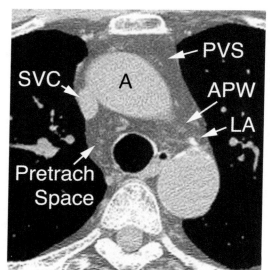

FIG. 7-3. Normal CT anatomy. Aortopulmonary window level. **A.** Contrast-enhanced CT at a lower level in the same patient as in Figures 7-1 and 7-2A. *MBr,* main bronchi at the level of the carina; *AA,* ascending aorta; *DA,* descending aorta; *SVC,* superior vena cava; *AAA,* anterior azygos arch; *PAA,* posterior azygos arch; *Prevasc,* prevascular space containing thymus; *APW,* aortopulmonary window with volume averaging of superior aspect of the left pulmonary artery. **B.** Lung window scan, same level as **A**. The tracheal carina *(carina)* is visible. The apex of the triangular prevascular space represents the anterior junction line *(white arrows)*. The mediastinal pleural reflections bordering the prevascular space are concave laterally. **C.** Unenhanced high-resolution CT at a lower level in the same patient as in Figure 7-2B. *A,* ascending aorta; *SVC,* superior vena cava; *PVS,* prevascular space containing thymus replaced by fat; *Pretrach Space,* pretracheal space containing normal lymph nodes; *APW,* aortopulmonary window containing normal lymph nodes; *LA,* ligamentum arteriosum.

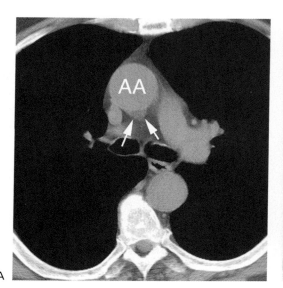
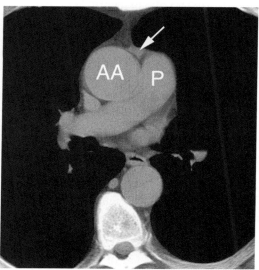

FIG. 7-4. Normal superior pericardial recess. Unenhanced CT. **A.** The superior pericardial recess *(arrows)* is visible posterior to the ascending aorta *(AA)* in the precarinal space. **B.** At a lower level, the anterior reflection of the superior pericardial recess *(arrow)* is visible in the groove between the ascending aorta *(AA)* and main pulmonary artery *(P)*.

On the right side, the **azygos arch** arises from the posterior wall of the superior vena cava, passes over the right main bronchus, and continues posteriorly along the mediastinum to lie to the right and anterior to the spine (see Figs. 7-2A and 7-3A). Below the level of the azygos arch, the **azygos vein** is consistently seen in this position. The azygos arch is often visible on one or two adjacent slices and sometimes appears nodular. However, its characteristic location is usually sufficient to allow its correct identification. When the azygos arch is visible, it marginates the right border of the pretracheal space.

The **aortopulmonary window** (APW) is located on the left side of the mediastinum, caudal to the aortic arch but cephalic to the main pulmonary artery (see Fig. 7-3A and C). The APW contains fat, lymph nodes, the recurrent laryngeal nerve, and the ligamentum arteriosum; the latter two are usually invisible. In some patients, the APW is not well seen, with the main pulmonary artery lying immediately below the aortic arch.

The **superior pericardial recess**, containing a small amount of pericardial fluid, is often visible in the pretracheal space immediately behind the ascending aorta (see Fig. 7-4A). Although it is sometimes confused with a lymph node, its typical location, contact with the aortic wall, oval or crescentic shape, and relatively low (water) attenuation allow it to be distinguished from an abnormality. The anterior recess of the pericardial space is sometimes seen anterior to the aortic arch, ascending aorta, and pulmonary artery (see Fig. 7-4B).

Pulmonary Arteries, Subcarinal Space, and Azygoesophageal Recess

At or near the level of the tracheal carina or main bronchi, the **main pulmonary artery** divides into its right and left branches (Fig. 7-5A–C). The **left pulmonary artery** is somewhat higher than the right, usually being seen 1 cm above it, and appears as the continuation of the main pulmonary artery, directed posterolaterally and to the left (see Fig. 7-5A and B). The **right pulmonary artery** arises at nearly a right angle to the main and left pulmonary and crosses the mediastinum from left to right, anterior to the carina or main bronchi (see Fig. 7-5B and C). The right pulmonary artery limits the most caudal extent of the pretracheal space and the anterior aspect of the subcarinal space.

The **azygos vein** parallels the esophagus along the right side of the mediastinum and laterally contacts the medial pleural reflections of the right lower lobe, defining the posterior border of the azygoesophageal recess (see Fig. 7-5A–C). On the left side, the hemiazygos vein parallels the descending aorta, lying posterior to it; it is not always visible (see Fig. 7-5C). The **hemiazygos vein** generally drains into the azygos vein via a branch that crosses the midline behind the aorta, near the level of the T8 vertebral body. This branch is sometimes seen on CT in normal individuals.

The **subcarinal space** is the region of the mediastinum immediately below the carina, marginated laterally by the main bronchi. It contains a number of lymph nodes and is closely related to the esophagus (see Fig. 7-5B and D).

Below the level of the tracheal carina and azygos arch, the medial aspect of the right lung contacts the mediastinum in close apposition to the azygos vein, esophagus, and subcarinal space. This region of the mediastinum is called the **azygoesophageal recess** (see Fig. 7-5C and D). The contour of the azygoesophageal recess is concave laterally in the large majority of normal subjects, and a convexity in this region should be regarded as suspicious of mass and the scan examined closely for a pathologic process. However, a convexity in this region may also be produced by a prominent normal esophagus or azygos vein and is particularly common in patients with a narrow mediastinum and in children.

Normal nodes are commonly visible in the subcarinal space, being larger than normal nodes in other parts of the mediastinum and up to 1.5 cm in short-axis diameter (see Fig. 7-5D). The esophagus usually is seen immediately posterior to the subcarinal space, and distinguishing nodes and esophagus may be difficult unless the esophagus contains air or contrast material, or its course is traced on adjacent scans.

Heart and Paracardiac Mediastinum

At the level of the heart, the prevascular mediastinum becomes thin or is obliterated by the heart contacting the anterior chest wall (Fig. 7-6). Little soft tissue is visible anterior and lateral to the cardiac chambers and origins of the main pulmonary artery and aorta. However, posterior to the heart, the azygoesophageal recess remains visible to the level of the diaphragm. As at higher levels, the contour of the azygoesophageal recess is concave laterally, closely opposed to the esophagus and azygos vein. Posterior to the descending aorta, fat, the hemiazygos vein and small lymph nodes occupy the left **paravertebral space**. The right paravertebral space is considerably thinner or invisible.

PLAIN RADIOGRAPHIC ANATOMY

On frontal (posteroanterior [PA] or anteroposterior [AP]) chest films, five important mediastinal structures should be easily identified (Fig. 7-7). In addition to their intrinsic importance in diagnosis, these structures serve to anchor a number of important mediastinal stripes, lines, and interfaces and orient the observer to specific mediastinal regions and compartments that are important in diagnosis. These structures are as follows:

- Trachea, tracheal carina, and main bronchi
- Aortic arch
- Main pulmonary artery
- Azygos vein
- Heart and its chambers

Trachea, Tracheal Carina, and Main Bronchi

The trachea extends from the inferior aspect of the cricoid cartilage to the tracheal carina. It is 10 to 12 cm in length in most individuals. It is divided into extrathoracic and intrathoracic portions at the point it passes posterior to the manubrium (see Fig. 7-7).

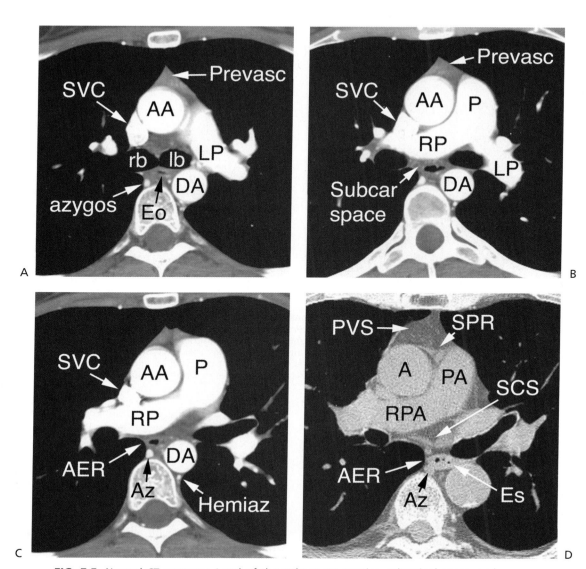

FIG. 7-5. Normal CT anatomy. Level of the pulmonary arteries, subcarinal space, and azygo-esophageal recess. **A.** Contrast-enhanced CT at a lower level in the same patient as in Figures 7-1, 7-2A, and 7-3A. *rb,* right main bronchus; *lb,* left main bronchus; *AA,* ascending aorta; *DA,* descending aorta; *SVC,* superior vena cava; *azygos,* azygos vein; *Eo,* esophagus; *Prevasc,* prevascular space containing thymus; *LP,* left pulmonary artery. **B.** Contrast-enhanced CT slightly below level shown in **A**. *AA,* ascending aorta; *P,* main pulmonary artery; *LP,* left pulmonary artery; *RP,* right pulmonary artery; *DA,* descending aorta; *SVC,* superior vena cava; *Prevasc,* prevascular space containing thymus; *Subcar space,* subcarinal space. **C.** Contrast-enhanced CT slightly below level shown in **B**. *AA,* ascending aorta; *P,* main pulmonary artery; *RP,* right pulmonary artery; *DA,* descending aorta; *SVC,* superior vena cava; *Az,* azygos vein; *Hemiaz,* hemiazygos vein; *AER,* azygo-esophageal recess. **D.** Unenhanced high-resolution CT at a lower level in the same patient as **B** and **C**. *A,* ascending aorta; *PA,* main pulmonary artery; *RPA,* right pulmonary artery; *PVS,* prevascular space containing thymus replaced by fat; *SPR,* anterior superior pericardial recess; *SCS,* subcarinal space containing normal lymph nodes; *AER,* azygoesophageal recess; *Az,* azygos, vein; *Es,* esophagus.

The trachea may appear to have a slightly serrated wall because of indentations on the tracheal air column adjacent to the tracheal rings. On the lateral view, serration is seen only along the anterior tracheal wall, as the posterior wall lacks cartilage. Calcification of tracheal cartilages is common in older patients, particularly women. Slight tracheal narrowing with an indentation on the left aortic wall is often seen at the level of the aortic arch.

The tracheal carina is visible at the bifurcation of the trachea into right and left main bronchi. The carina is usually seen near the level of the undersurface of the aortic arch. The right and left main bronchi are usually both visible, with the right main bronchus appearing more vertical than the left. The angle between the inferior walls of the main bronchi, the carinal angle, is variable, ranging from about 35 to 90 degrees.

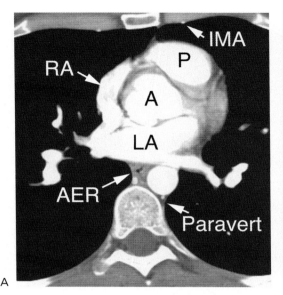
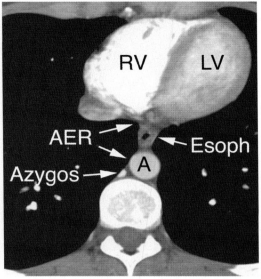

FIG. 7-6. Normal CT anatomy. Level of the heart and paracardiac mediastinum. **A.** Contrast-enhanced CT at a lower level in the same patient as in Figures 7-1, 7-2A, 7-3A, and 7-5A to C. *A,* aortic root; *P,* pulmonary outflow tract; *RA,* right atrium; *LA,* left atrium; *AER,* azygoesophageal recess; *Paravert,* left paravertebral space containing hemiazygos vein; *IMA,* internal mammary artery. **B.** Contrast-enhanced CT below the level of **A.** *RV,* right ventricle; *LV,* left ventricle; *AER,* azygoesophageal recess; *A,* descending aorta; *Azygos,* azygos vein; *Esoph,* esophagus.

Aortic Arch

The appearance of the aorta is characteristic, although it can vary in size and shape. The thoracic aorta is usually considered to consist of an ascending segment, a transverse segment or arch, and a descending segment.

The aortic arch begins at the innominate artery and consists of two segments. The proximal part of the arch is the longer and gives rise to the innominate, left carotid, and left subclavian arteries, although variations in the branching pattern of these vessels and their divisions are common. The distal part of the arch, between the origin of the left subclavian artery and the ligamentum arteriosum, is known as the aortic isthmus; it is relatively short, measuring 1 to 2 cm in length, and its lumen may be a few millimeters narrower in adults than the aorta immediately distal to the ligamentum. The descending thoracic aorta is distal to the ligamentum arteriosum.

On frontal radiographs, the lateral aspect of the aortic arch (the "aortic knob") is typically visible through about half of its circumference (see Fig. 7-7). The lateral edge of the aortic arch visible on radiographs usually represents the edge of the posterior arch. Although it is tempting to measure the aortic diameter as the distance between the edge of the tracheal air column medially and the interface between aorta and lung laterally, these lie in different planes and this measurement is not necessarily valid.

Main Pulmonary Artery

The main pulmonary artery arises at the base of the right ventricle and extends superiorly for a distance of approximately 5 cm before dividing into the right and left pulmonary arteries.

The main, right, and left pulmonary arteries are intrapericardial. The main pulmonary artery divides into right and left pulmonary arteries posterior to the ascending aorta and anterior to the main bronchi.

On frontal radiographs, the main pulmonary artery is identified below the aortic arch and above the left main bronchus at the point it appears relatively horizontal. It appears oval, oriented along the superior bronchial wall (see Fig. 7-7). In this location, the visible artery largely corresponds to main pulmonary artery.

Azygos Arch

The arch of the azygos vein is seen in the right tracheobronchial angle, to the right of the distal trachea, above and lateral to the origin of the right main bronchus (see Fig. 7-7). It results in an oval opacity, bordered by air in the trachea medially and air in the lung laterally, and is contiguous superiorly with the right paratracheal stripe. It usually measures 7 mm or less in transverse diameter in normal upright subjects but may be up to 10 mm. Enlargement (more than 10 mm) of this shadow may represent vein dilatation due to deep inspiration or a Mueller maneuver, supine position, pregnancy, increased blood volume, increased central venous pressure, collateral circulation via the azygos vein, or lymph node (i.e., azygos node) enlargement.

Heart

The appearance of the heart and its chambers is described in subsequent chapters.

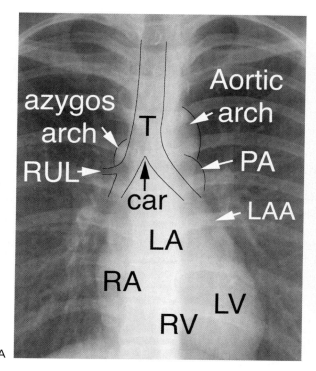

A

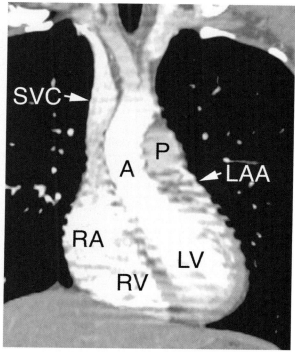

C

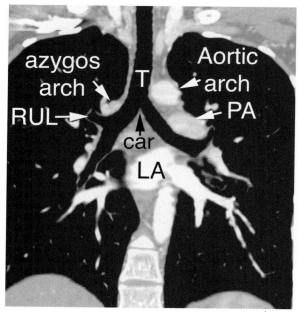

B

FIG. 7-7. Normal vascular structures. **A.** PA chest radiograph. *T,* intrathoracic trachea; *RUL,* right upper lobe bronchus; *car,* carina; *PA,* main pulmonary artery; *LA,* location of left atrium; *LAA,* left atrial appendage; *RA,* location of right atrium; *RV,* location of right ventricle; *LV,* location of left ventricle. **B.** Coronal CT reformation in the same patient through the plane of the trachea and main bronchi. *T,* intrathoracic trachea; *RUL,* right upper lobe bronchus; *car,* carina; *PA,* main and left pulmonary artery; *LA,* left atrium. **C.** Coronal reformation in the same patient at a more anterior level, through the heart. *SVA,* superior vena cava; *A,* ascending aorta; *P,* main pulmonary artery; *LAA,* left atrial appendage; *RA,* right atrium; *RV,* right ventricle; *LV,* left ventricle.

LINES, STRIPES, AND SPACES

A number of mediastinal lines, stripes, and spaces have been described as valuable in the assessment of specific mediastinal structures and compartments on plain radiographs. Their visibility and significance vary, and are detailed in Figures 7-8 to 7-22. The normal appearances of these lines, stripes, and interfaces is shown using CT reformations, for the large part from the same patient. In Figures 7-23 to 7-25 the lines and interfaces visible on the lateral radiograph are described. There are fewer than visible on the frontal radiograph.

ANTERIOR JUNCTION LINE

Location: Linear region of contact between the anterior portions of the right and left lungs, posterior to the sternum

Anatomy: Four layers of pleura (visceral pleura covering both lungs and two layers of mediastinal pleura) and a variable amount of retrosternal fat

Appearance: 1. A thin oblique line or sometimes a thicker stripe, beginning at the level of the inferior portion of the manubrium and extending inferiorly and usually slightly to the left, for a variable distance
2. It begins superiorly at the apex of an inverted triangular opacity, usually with concave sides, visible through the manubrium (termed the *anterior mediastinal triangle*)
3. Inferiorly, the line sometimes is seen to join with the apex of a triangular opacity in the "inferior recesses" of the anterior mediastinum

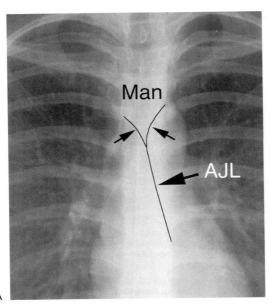

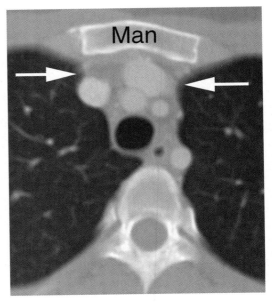

A   B

FIG. 7-8. Anterior junction line and anterior mediastinal triangle. **A.** PA chest radiograph. The anterior mediastinal triangle *(small black arrows)* is visible through the manubrium *(Man)*. *AJL*, anterior junction line. **B.** CT in the same patient at the level of the manubrium *(Man)*. Lung contacting the anterior mediastinum behind the manubrium *(arrows)* results in the anterior mediastinal triangle. *(Figure continues.)*

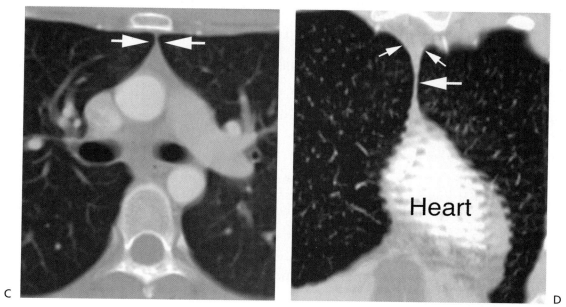

FIG. 7-8. *(Continued.)* **C.** CT in the same patient at a lower level. Contact between the lung results in the thin anterior junction line *(arrows).* **D.** CT reformation in the coronal plane shows the anterior mediastinal triangle *(small black arrows)* and anterior junction line *(large arrow)* anterior and superior to the heart.

ANTERIOR JUNCTION LINE

Visibility:	About 20% of cases; best seen in patients with emphysema because of lung hyperinflation
Significance:	1. May be displaced to the right or left in patients with atelectasis on the side to which it is displaced; usually associated with lower lobe volume loss
	2. In patients with upper lobe atelectasis and consolidation, the displaced anterior junction line is visible as an interface between the normal aerated upper lobe and the consolidated upper lobe; this occurrence is often referred to as "lung herniation"
	3. Uncommonly is recognized as focally or diffusely thickened in patients with an anterior mediastinal mass

CARDIOPHRENIC ANGLES (RIGHT AND LEFT)

Location:	Junction of the anterior hemidiaphragms with the right and left heart borders
Anatomy:	Inferior extent of the anterior mediastinum, containing fat and lymph nodes
Appearance:	Usually concave laterally on both sides; may be convex in the presence of increased mediastinal fat
Visibility:	Very common
Significance:	Convexity or mass may be seen in the presence of (1) large mediastinal fat pad, (2) lipoma, (3) pericardial cyst, (4) enlarged epicardiac lymph nodes, (5) thymic neoplasm or other anterior mediastinal mass, or (6) Morgagni hernia

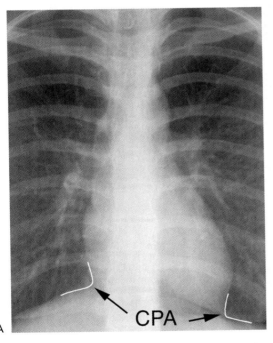

FIG. 7-9. Cardiophrenic angles. **A.** PA chest radiograph. The costophrenic angles *(CPA)* are seen at the junction of the anterior hemidiaphragms with the right and left heart borders. **B.** CT in the same patient at the level of the costophrenic angles. These represent contact of the lung with the fat-filled anterior mediastinum *(arrows)* anterior to the heart and liver. **C.** Coronal reformation in the same patient shows the concave costophrenic angles *(arrows)*.

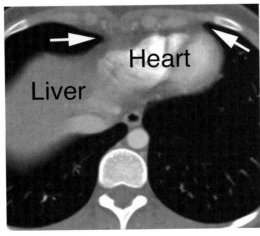

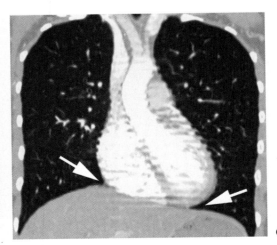

RIGHT PARATRACHEAL STRIPE

Location: Linear region of contact between the right lung and the right tracheal wall, below the thoracic inlet and above the azygos arch

Anatomy: Tracheal wall, a thin layer of mediastinal fat, two layers of pleura (visceral and parietal)

Appearance: A line or stripe, up to 4 mm thick in normal individuals, seen below the clavicles and blending with the superior aspect of the azygos arch

Visibility: Common, reported to be visible in up to 95% of normal individuals

Significance: Thickening (i.e., more than 4 mm) may be due to (1) tracheal wall abnormalities such as tumor or inflammatory disease; (2) pleural thickening adjacent to the trachea; (3) enlargement of pretracheal lymph nodes; (thickening of the paratracheal stripe occurs in about 30% of patients with pretracheal lymph node enlargement because these nodes are located anterior to the trachea); or (4) mediastinal infiltration (e.g., hemorrhage, infection, neoplasm)

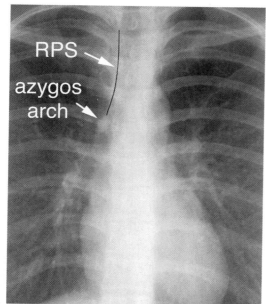

A

FIG. 7-10. Right paratracheal stripe. **A.** PA chest radiograph. The right paratracheal stripe *(RPS)* is a few millimeters thick and is seen from the level of the thoracic inlet to the azygos arch. **B.** CT shows lung contacting the trachea *(T)*, forming the right paratracheal stripe *(RPS)*. **C.** Coronal reformation in the same patient shows the right paratracheal stripe *(RPS)*, trachea *(T)*, and azygos arch.

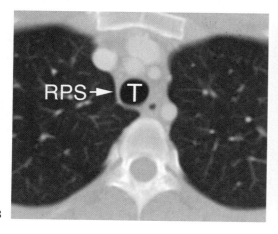

B

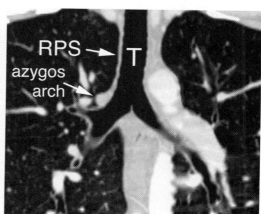

C

SUPERIOR VENA CAVA INTERFACE

Location/anatomy: Interface between the right lung and the right superior mediastinum, above the azygos arch and below the thoracic inlet, lateral to the superior vena cava and right brachiocephalic vein

Appearance: An interface between lung and mediastinum, slightly concave laterally, above the azygos arch and below the medial right clavicle

Visibility: Seen in almost all patients

Significance: Lateral convexity of the superior vena cava interface and increased density of the shadow of the superior vena cava may be seen with (1) dilatation of the superior vena cava (due to deep inspiration or Mueller maneuver [physiologic dilatation], supine position, pregnancy, increased blood volume, increased central venous pressure); (2) lymph node enlargement in the pretracheal space, (3) mediastinal mass, (4) mediastinal infiltration (blood, infection, tumor), or (5) a pleural abnormality

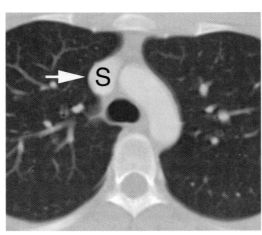

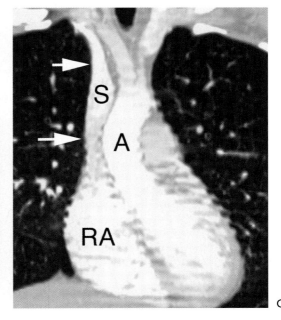

FIG. 7-11. Superior vena cava interface. **A.** PA chest radiograph. The right edge of the superior vena cava *(SVC)* is outlined by lung, forming an interface that is slightly concave laterally. It is seen from the thoracic inlet to the level of the azygos arch. **B.** CT in the same patient shows lung contacting the lateral wall of the superior vena cava *(S)*. This edge *(arrow)* forms the superior vena cava interface. **C.** Coronal reformation in the same patient shows the superior vena cava interface *(arrows)*. *S,* superior vena cava; *A,* aorta; *RA,* right atrium.

LEFT PARATRACHEAL STRIPE OR INTERFACE

Location:	Linear region of contact between the left lung and the left tracheal wall and adjacent mediastinal soft tissues, below the thoracic inlet and above the aorta
Anatomy:	Tracheal wall, mediastinal fat, two layers of pleura (visceral and parietal)
Appearance:	A line or stripe of variable thickness seen below the clavicles and above the aortic arch
Visibility:	Uncommonly visible as a thin stripe; in 90%, the left subclavian or carotid artery and mediastinal fat are interposed between the left tracheal wall and aerated lung; what is often perceived as the lateral aspect of the "left paratracheal stripe" usually represents the interface of left subclavian artery or mediastinal fat with lung
Significance:	Thickening is difficult to diagnose because of variability in appearance

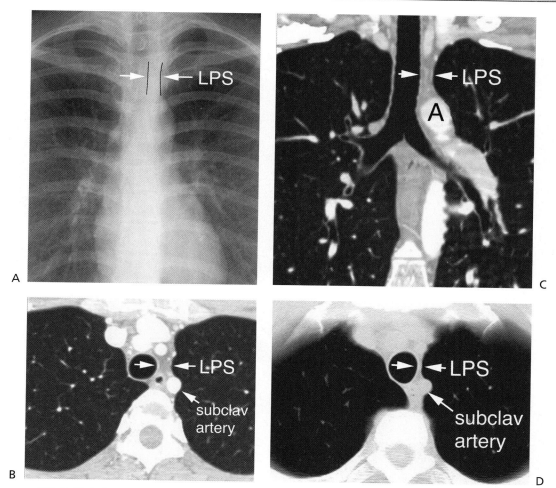

FIG. 7-12. Left paratracheal stripe. **A.** PA chest radiograph. The left paratracheal stripe *(LPS)* represents the linear region of contact between the left lung and the left tracheal wall and adjacent mediastinal soft tissues, below the thoracic inlet and above the aorta. It is usually much thicker than the right paratracheal stripe. **B.** CT in the same patient shows lung contacting the lateral wall of the left mediastinum anterior to the left subclavian artery *(subclav artery)*. Mediastinal soft tissues along with left tracheal wall make up the left paratracheal stripe *(LPS)*. **C.** Coronal reformation in the same patient shows the left paratracheal stripe above the aorta *(A)*. **D.** CT in a different patient shows a thin left paratracheal stripe corresponding to the left tracheal wall. It is anterior to the left subclavian artery *(subclav artery)*.

LEFT SUBCLAVIAN ARTERY INTERFACE

Location:	Interface between the left lung and the left superior mediastinum, above the aorta and below the thoracic inlet
Anatomy:	Pleura outlining the lateral aspect of the left subclavian artery or adjacent mediastinal fat
Appearance:	An interface, usually concave laterally, extending from the shadow of the aortic arch to the level of the medial left clavicle
Visibility:	Common
Significance:	Convexity of this interface indicates (1) subclavian artery dilatation or tortuosity, (2) mediastinal mass or lymph node enlargement, or (3) paramediastinal pleural abnormality

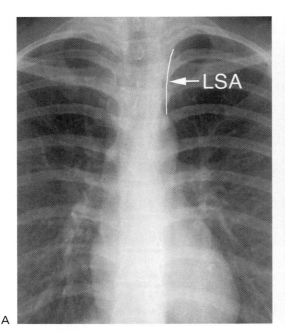

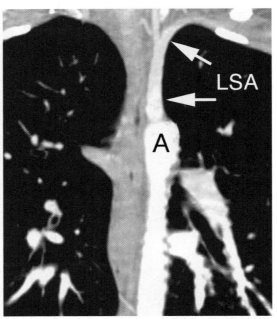

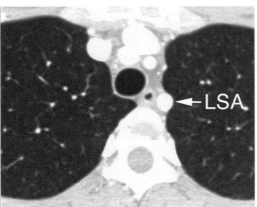

FIG. 7-13. Left subclavian artery interface. **A.** PA chest radiograph. Contact of the left lung with the left subclavian artery above the aortic arch results in an interface *(LSA)*, concave laterally, extending superiorly to the thoracic inlet. It is somewhat lateral to the left paratracheal stripe and more concave. **B.** CT in the same patient shows lung contacting the lateral wall of the left subclavian artery *(LSA)*. **C.** Coronal reformation in the same patient shows the left subclavian artery above the aorta *(A)*. It results in a concave edge.

VASCULAR PEDICLE

Location:	Transverse width of the upper mediastinum
Anatomy:	The overall shadow of the great systemic arteries and veins (i.e., the "vascular pedicle" of the heart); mediastinal contents
Appearance:	The width of the vascular pedicle is measured from the point the superior vena cava interface crosses the right main bronchus to a vertical line drawn inferiorly from the point the left subclavian artery arises from the aortic arch; width is variable but measures up to 58 mm in normal subjects
Visibility:	Common
Significance:	Widening may be due to (1) dilatation of the great vessels (due to deep inspiration or Mueller maneuver [physiologic dilatation], supine position, pregnancy, increased blood volume, increased central venous pressure); (2) lymph node enlargement in the pretracheal space; (3) mediastinal mass; (4) mediastinal infiltration (blood, infection, tumor); (5) a paramediastinal pleural abnormality

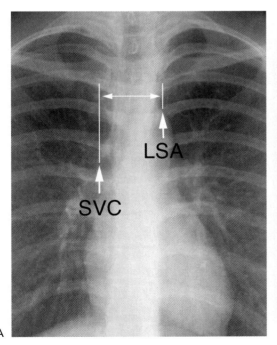
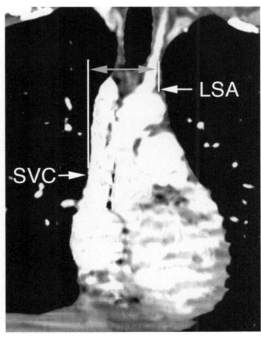

A   B

FIG. 7-14. Vascular pedicle. **A.** PA chest radiograph. The vascular pedicle *(arrows)* is measured from the point the superior vena cava *(SVC)* interface crosses the right main bronchus to a vertical line drawn inferiorly from the point the left subclavian artery *(LSA)* arises from the aortic arch. **B.** Coronal CT reformation shows the same sites of measurement.

POSTERIOR JUNCTION LINE OR STRIPE

Location: Linear region of contact between the posterior portions of the right and left lungs in the superior mediastinum, behind the esophagus, and anterior to the upper thoracic vertebral bodies

Anatomy: Four layers of pleura (visceral pleura covering both lungs and two layers of mediastinal pleura); a variable amount of fat; the esophagus may compose a portion of this line or stripe

Appearance: Usually seen through or adjacent to the tracheal air column; a straight line or variably concave laterally; it may be seen to reflect onto the superior aspect of the aortic arch or the "middle" portion of the azygos arch; it is of variable thickness depending on the amount of fat included or its relationship to the esophagus, ranging from a few millimeters to nearly 1 cm thick

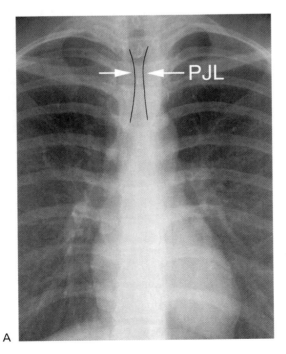

A

FIG. 7-15. Posterior junction line. **A.** PA chest radiograph. The posterior junction line *(PJL)* represents the region of contact between the posterior portions of the right and left lungs in the superior mediastinum, behind the esophagus, and anterior to the upper thoracic vertebral bodies. It is often seen through the tracheal air column and may be straight or variably concave. It is of variable thickness. *(Figure continues.)*

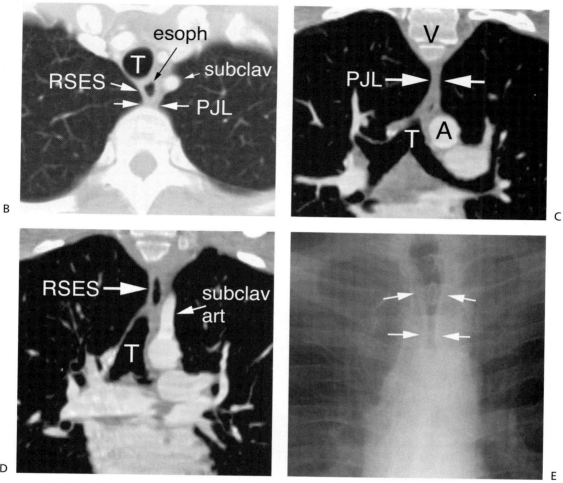

FIG. 7-15. *(Continued.)* **B.** CT shows lung contacting the right lateral wall of the esophagus. Because of air in the esophageal lumen, this may be seen as the right superior esophageal stripe *(RSES)*. The posterior junction line *(PJL)* represents contact of both lungs with the mediastinum. **C.** Coronal reformation in the same patient shows the posterior junction line anterior to the vertebral column *(V)* and cephalad to the aorta *(A)*. *T,* trachea. **D.** Coronal reformation slightly anterior to **C** shows the right superior esophageal stripe *(RSES)* outlined by air in the lung and esophageal lumen. *T,* trachea; *subclav art,* subclavian artery. **E.** Right and left superior esophageal stripes *(arrows)* are visible in a patient with intraesophageal air.

POSTERIOR JUNCTION LINE OR STRIPE	
Variant:	If air is present in the esophagus, two stripes may be visible, each principally representing the right or left esophageal walls; when this occurs, these stripes are referred to as the *right and left superior esophageal (or pleuroesophageal) stripes*
Visibility:	Common; posterior junction line and esophageal stripes each visible in about 40% of normal subjects
Significance:	Because of the variability in the appearance of this line or stripe, it is of limited utility in diagnosis; abnormalities are most typically associated with esophageal abnormalities or masses in this region

LEFT SUPERIOR INTERCOSTAL VEIN

Location:	Adjacent to or immediately above the aortic arch shadow
Anatomy:	Left superior intercostal vein drains the left second, third, and fourth intercostal veins into the left brachiocephalic vein; it communicates with the hemiazygos venous system in about 75%

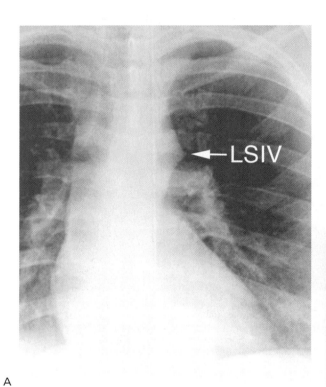

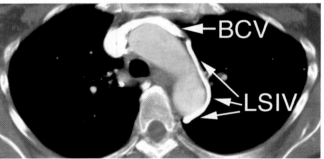

A   B

FIG. 7-16. Left superior intercostal vein (aortic nipple). **A.** Chest radiograph shows a normal left superior intercostal vein *(LSIV)*. **B.** CT in another normal patient shows contrast reflex into the left superior intercostal vein *(LSIV)*. It extends posteriorly from the left brachiocephalic vein *(BCV)*. *(Figure continues.)*

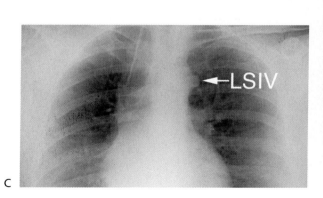

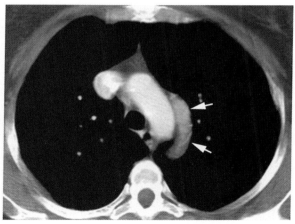

C

D

FIG. 7-16. *(Continued.)* **C.** Radiograph in another patient shows enlargement of the left superior intercostal vein *(LSIV)*. It serves as a collateral pathway. **D.** CT in the same patient as **C** shows enlargement of the left superior intercostal vein *(arrows)*.

LEFT SUPERIOR INTERCOSTAL VEIN	
Appearance:	A small round or triangular shadow ("aortic nipple") less than 5 mm in diameter
Visibility:	Uncommon; less than 5% of normal subjects
Significance:	Dilatation typically occurs as a result of collateral flow through this vein to the hemiazygos and azygos systems; most commonly due to obstruction of the superior vena cava or left brachiocephalic vein

AORTOPULMONARY WINDOW

Location: Aortopulmonary window is outlined by the left lung between the aortic arch and the left pulmonary artery

Anatomy: Lateral boundary of the aortopulmonary window is the parietal pleura forming the visible interface; the medial boundary of the aortopulmonary window is the ligamentum arteriosum; the aortopulmonary window largely contains fat and lymph nodes

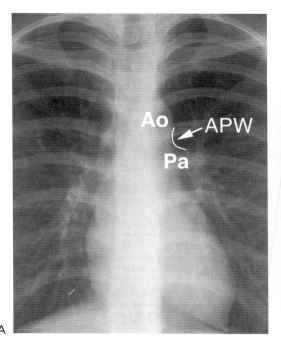

A

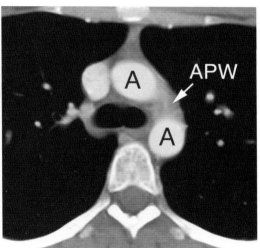

B

FIG. 7-17. Aortopulmonary window. **A.** The aortopulmonary window *(APW)* represents a concave interface between the aorta *(Ao)* and main pulmonary artery *(Pa)*. **B.** CT in the same patient shows fat in the aortopulmonary window *(APW)*, under the aortic arch *(A)*. *(Figure continues.)*

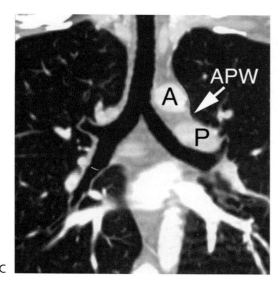
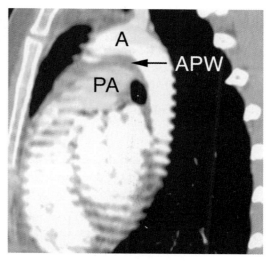

C

D

FIG. 7-17. *(Continued.)* **C.** Coronal reformation in the same patient shows the aortopulmonary window *(APW)* as an interface, concave laterally, between the aorta *(A)* and the pulmonary artery *(P)*. This space contains fat and lymph nodes. **D.** Sagittal reformation in the same patient. The aortopulmonary window *(APW)* is located under the aortic arch *(A)* and above the pulmonary artery *(PA)*.

AORTOPULMONARY WINDOW

Appearance: The aortopulmonary window interface is normally concave laterally or straight; it is more concave in the presence of emphysema. However, the appearance of the mediastinal interface in this region is variable, with two common patterns:

1. The interface may be localized to the region below the aorta and above the pulmonary artery
2. The interface may continue inferiorly, overlying the shadow of the left pulmonary artery, merging inferiorly with the left heart border

Visibility: Almost always visible

Significance: Convexity of this interface may indicate (1) lymph node enlargement (most common), (2) mediastinal mass, (3) enlargement of the ductus arteriosus, or (4) aortic aneurysm

AZYGOESOPHAGEAL RECESS

Location: Azygoesophageal recess is a portion of the retrocardiac mediastinum, outlined by the right lower lobe, from the level of the azygos arch above to the level of the diaphragm below

Anatomy: The azygoesophageal recess contains the posterior azygos vein, esophagus, thoracic duct, and lymph nodes; the superior aspect of the azygoesophageal recess is closely associated with the subcarinal space

Appearance: The interface between the azygoesophageal recess and the right lung begins at the level of the azygos arch and has a shallow reverse-C or reverse-S contour, ending at the diaphragm

In some patients, the superior aspect of the azygoesophageal interface is contiguous with the posterior junction line at the azygos arch, resulting in a shallow 3-shaped shadow

Variant: If air is present in the esophagus, a stripe is commonly visible at the point of contact of right lower lobe and the right esophageal wall; this is referred to as the *right inferior esophageal (or pleuroesophageal) stripe*; it is most commonly seen immediately under the aortic arch

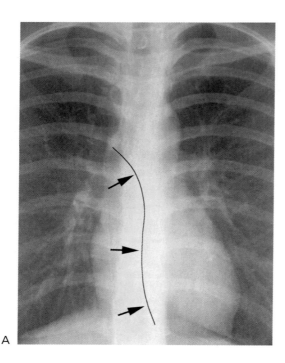

A

FIG. 7-18. Azygoesophageal recess. **A.** PA chest radiograph. The azygoesophageal recess *(arrows)* represents contact between the right lung with the retrocardiac mediastinum, closely related to the locations of the azygos vein and esophagus. It has a shallow reverse-C or reverse-S contour, ending at the diaphragm. *(Figure continues.)*

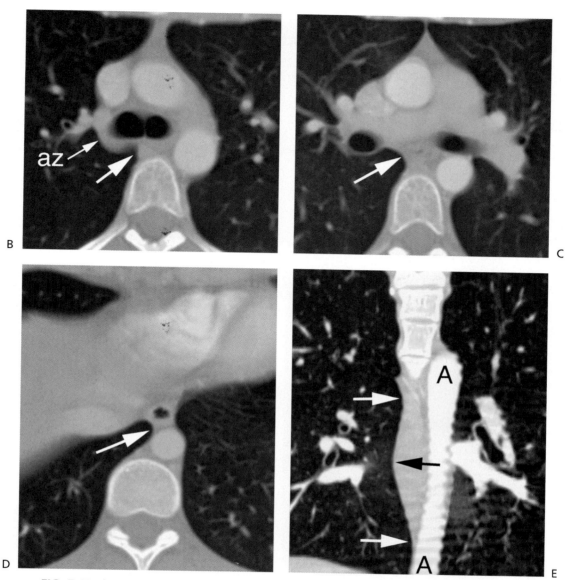

FIG. 7-18. *(Continued.)* **B–D.** CT at different levels in the same patient shows the azygoe-sophageal recess *(arrows)*. It begins at the level of the azygos arch *(az)* and ends at the diaphragm. **E.** Coronal reformation in the same patient shows the azygoesophageal recess *(arrows)*, with a typical contour. *A,* aorta.

AZYGOESOPHAGEAL RECESS

Visibility: Almost always visible on well-penetrated radiographs

Significance: Convexity of the superior aspect of the azygoesophageal recess is most common with (1) subcarinal lymph node enlargement, (2) subcarinal bronchogenic cyst, (3) left atrial dilatation, (4) dilatation of the azygos vein, (5) esophageal mass or di-latation. Convexity of the inferior aspect of the azygoesophageal stripe is most common with (1) esophageal mass or dilatation or (2) hiatal hernia

LEFT PARAAORTIC INTERFACE

Location:	Line of contact between descending aorta and medial left lung
Anatomy:	Descending aorta, adjacent fat, and two layers of pleura
Appearance:	A straight, concave, or convex interface below the aortic arch, parallel to the left paravertebral stripe

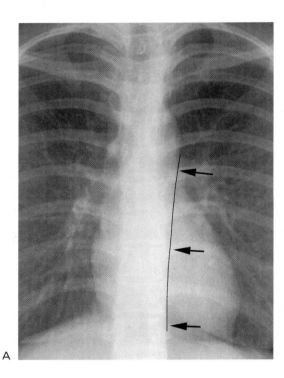

A

FIG. 7-19. Left paraaortic interface. **A.** PA chest radiograph. The line of contact between the descending aorta and medial left lung represents the paraaortic interface. This edge is straight, concave, or convex and is seen below the aortic arch and parallel but lateral to the left paravertebral stripe. *(Figure continues.)*

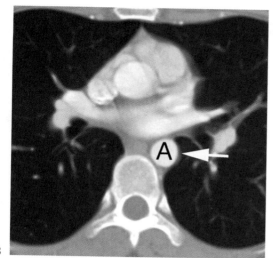

B

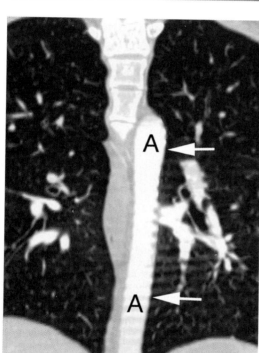

C

FIG. 7-19. B. *(Continued.)* CT in the same patient. Lung outlines the left lateral wall *(arrow)* of the aorta *(A).* **C.** Coronal reformation in the same patient shows the left paraaortic interface *(arrows).* Its contour is wavy because of pulsations. *A,* descending aorta.

LEFT PARAAORTIC INTERFACE	
Visibility:	Very common
Significance:	Increased convexity is related to tortuosity of the aorta or diffuse dilatation (e.g., aneurysm or dissection); focal convexity indicates aneurysm, lymph node enlargement, or paraaortic mediastinal mass

PREAORTIC RECESS

Location: Recess in the left mediastinum outlined by lung, behind the heart, below the aortic arch, and anterior to the descending aorta

Anatomy: The preaortic recess on the left is analogous to the azygoesophageal recess on the right but is usually thinner and less well seen; the esophagus is variably related to the preaortic recess

Appearance: This interface is most commonly seen immediately below the aortic arch as the *preaortic line*, which is usually straight

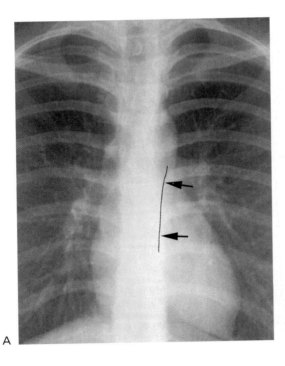

A

FIG. 7-20. Preaortic recess. **A.** PA chest radiograph. The preaortic recess *(arrows)* is outlined by lung, behind the heart, below the aortic arch, and anterior to the descending aorta. It is seen medial to the descending aorta. It is seen in the left mediastinum and is analogous to the azygoesophageal recess on the right, although it is less well seen. *(Figure continues.)*

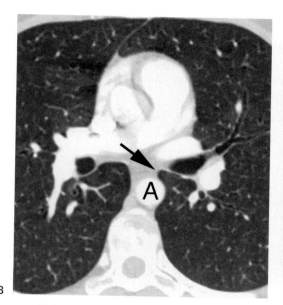

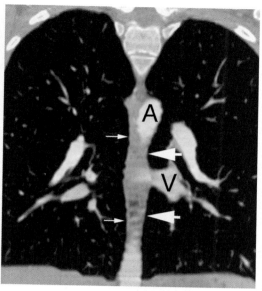

B

C

FIG. 7-20. *(Continued.)* **B.** CT shows the preaortic recess *(arrow)* outlined by lung, anterior to the aorta *(A)*. **C.** Coronal reformation in the same patient shows the preaortic recess *(large arrows).* Its contour is similar to that of the azygoesophageal recess on the right *(small arrows). A,* aortic arch; *V,* left pulmonary veins.

<table>
<tr><td colspan="2" align="center">PREAORTIC RECESS</td></tr>
<tr><td>Variant:</td><td>If air is present in the esophagus, a stripe is commonly visible representing the left esophageal wall; this is referred to as the left inferior esophageal (or pleuro-esophageal) stripe; it is most commonly seen immediately under the aortic arch.</td></tr>
<tr><td>Visibility:</td><td>Uncommon</td></tr>
<tr><td>Significance:</td><td>Most useful in diagnosing esophageal or aortic lesions; a lateral convexity in the inferior portion of this line is common with hiatal hernia in association with convexity in the inferior azygoesophageal recess</td></tr>
</table>

PARAVERTEBRAL STRIPES (LEFT AND RIGHT)

Location: Linear regions of contact between the posterior lower lobes and the paravertebral soft tissues adjacent to the spine

Anatomy: Pleural reflections over paravertebral fat, lymph nodes, and vessels; on the left, the pleural reflection is posterior to the descending aorta and closely related to the hemiazygos vein

Appearance: Left paravertebral stripe:

1. Commonly visible below the aortic arch, although in obese individuals it may be seen above the arch because of increased paravertebral fat
2. Inferiorly, is visible to below the level of the diaphragmatic dome, merging with the shadow of the diaphragmatic crus
3. Parallels the spine; often seen halfway between the spine and lateral margin of the aorta
4. Usually thin

Right paravertebral stripe:

1. Thinner and less often seen than the left paravertebral stripe
2. Visible only adjacent to the lower thoracic spine
3. Inferiorly, it merges with the shadow of the diaphragmatic crus

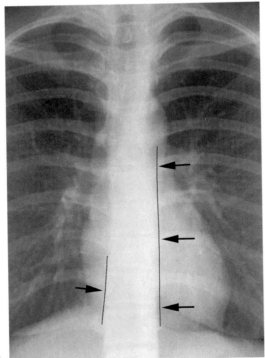

A

FIG. 7-21. Paravertebral stripes. **A.** PA chest radiograph. The paravertebral stripes *(arrows)* represent the linear regions of contact between the posterior lower lobes and the paravertebral soft tissues adjacent to the spine. They parallel the spine. On the left, this stripe is seen medial to the descending aorta. The left paravertebral stripe is usually better seen and seen over a longer course than the right. *(Figure continues.)*

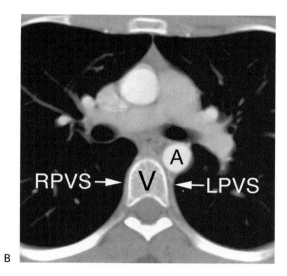

B

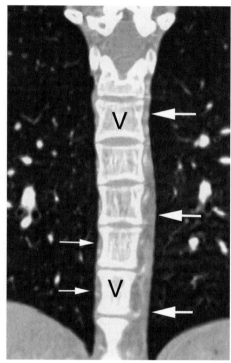

C

FIG. 7-21. *(Continued.)* **B.** CT in the same patient shows the left *(LPVS)* and right *(RPVS)* paravertebral stripes *(arrows)* outlined by lung, lateral to the vertebral body *(V)*. The LPVS is thicker and located posterior to the descending aorta *(A)* and medial to its lateral edge. **C.** Coronal reformation in the same patient shows the right *(small arrows)* and left paravertebral stripes *(large arrows)*. Their edges parallel the edges of the vertebral column *(V)*. Intercostal arteries and veins are visible within soft tissue of the paravertebral stripes.

PARAVERTEBRAL STRIPES (LEFT AND RIGHT)

Caveats: Left stripe increases in thickness with aortic tortuosity or supine position; right stripe increases in thickness in patients with osteophytes

Significance: Increased in thickness with (1) pleural effusion; (2) lymph node enlargement; (3) vertebral abnormalities (fracture, infection, neoplasm); (4) posterior mediastinal masses; (5) hemiazygos vein enlargement (left stripe); or (6) azygos vein enlargement (right stripe)

RETROSTERNAL STRIPE

Location:	The linear region of contact between the anterior lungs and the retrosternal soft tissues
Anatomy:	Retrosternal fat anterior to the lungs associated with the internal mammary lymph nodes and vessels
Appearance:	A smooth stripe of soft tissue, up to 7 mm in thickness in normal individuals, seen posterior to the sternum; inferiorly, the thickness of this stripe increases significantly in relation to the cardiac incisura and is variable in appearance; superiorly, the thickness increases in relation to the brachiocephalic veins and is variable

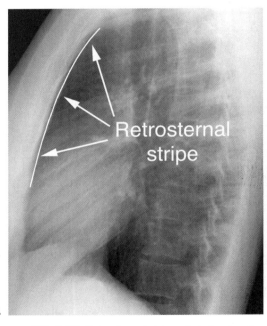

A

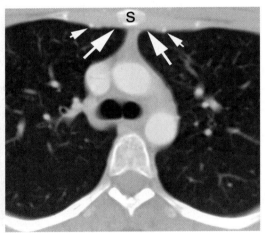

B

FIG. 7-22. Retrosternal stripe. **A.** Lateral radiograph in the same patient as shown in Figure 7-21. The retrosternal stripe is a linear region of contact between the anterior lungs and the retrosternal soft tissues and is visible as a thin line of soft tissue behind the sternum. **B.** CT in the same patient shows soft tissue posterior to the sternum *(s)* forming an interface with the anterior lung *(large arrows)*. The retrosternal stripe may also reflect contact of anterior lung with the region of the internal mammary vessels *(small arrows)* or nodes. *(Figure continues.)*

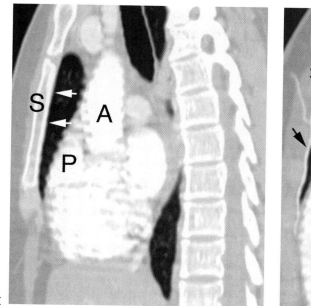
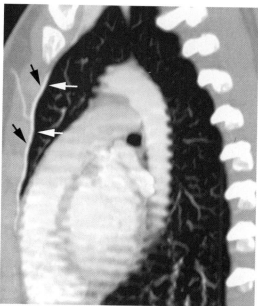

C

D

FIG. 7-22. *(Continued.)* **C.** Sagittal reformation in the same patient shows a very thin retrosternal stripe *(arrows)* posterior to the sternum *(S)*. *A,* ascending aorta; *P,* main pulmonary artery. **D.** Sagittal reformation in a more lateral location in the same patient shows a wavy contour of the soft-tissue stripe *(white arrows)*. This contour is typically seen with slight rotation. The wavy contour is related to the ribs or costal cartilage. The internal mammary artery *(black arrows)* is visible.

RETROSTERNAL STRIPE	
Caveat:	Slight rotation may project the right or left anterior chest wall posterior to the sternum, mimicking increased thickness of the retrosternal stripe; look for the location of the anterior ribs and costal cartilage before diagnosing an apparent thickening of the retrosternal stripe; a wavy contour of the soft tissue stripe (related to the ribs) often indicates it is due to rotation
Visibility:	Common
Significance:	Increases in thickness with (1) internal mammary lymph node enlargement, (2) tortuosity of internal mammary arteries (e.g., coarctation), (3) post–median sternotomy, or (4) sternal lesions

RETROSTERNAL CLEAR SPACE

Synonym:	Anterior clear space
Location:	Region posterior to the sternum; anterior and superior to the heart, main pulmonary artery, and ascending aorta; and anterior to the trachea and superior vena cava
Anatomy:	This space corresponds to the prevascular space seen on CT, largely representing thymus and retrosternal tissues
Appearance:	An area of lucency anterior to the heart and great vessels; the anterior margins of the heart and great vessels may or may not be clearly seen

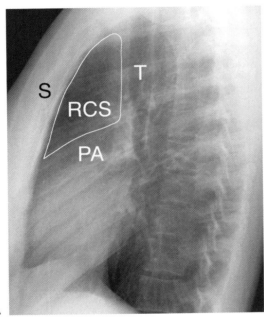

FIG. 7-23. Retrosternal clear space. **A.** Lateral radiograph shows an area of relative lucency (RCS) posterior to the sternum (S), superior to the main pulmonary artery (PA), and anterior to the trachea (T). (Figure continues.)

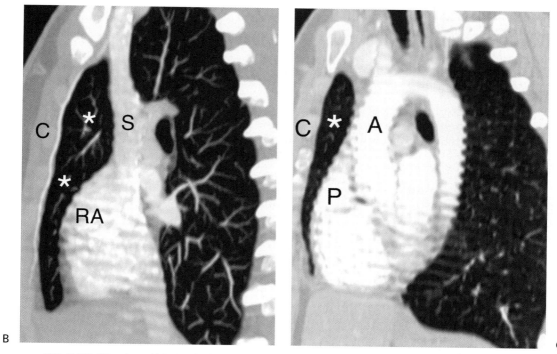

B

C

FIG. 7-23. *(Continued.)* **B.** Sagittal reformation in the same patient to the right of midline shows this area of lucency *(*)* posterior to costal cartilage *(C)*, anterior to the superior vena cava *(S)*, and anterior and superior to the right atrium *(RA)*. **C.** Sagittal reformation in the same patient to the left of midline shows the retrosternal lucency *(*)* posterior to the costal cartilage *(C)*, anterior to the aortic arch *(A)* and main pulmonary artery *(P)*.

RETROSTERNAL CLEAR SPACE	
Caveat:	In patients with a large amount of prevascular fat, lucency may be minimal
Visibility:	Common
Significance:	Increase in depth and lucency with emphysema; decrease in depth with right ventricular or main pulmonary artery dilatation; decrease in lucency in patients with anterior mediastinal mass

POSTERIOR TRACHEAL BAND OR STRIPE

Location: Linear region corresponding to the posterior tracheal wall and sometimes esophagus; below the thoracic inlet and above the tracheal bifurcation

Anatomy: Posterior tracheal wall, a small amount of mediastinal fat, and (variably) one or both esophageal walls, outlined posteriorly by air in lung or the esophageal lumen and outlined anteriorly by air in the tracheal lumen

Appearance: Variable appearance because of variable anatomy:

1. Posterior tracheal wall only: visible as a very thin line.
2. Posterior tracheal wall, esophagus with or without air in the esophageal lumen: a thicker stripe or band.

May be seen for the entire length of the trachea; because of variable anatomy, may measure 1 to 6 mm thick in normal individuals

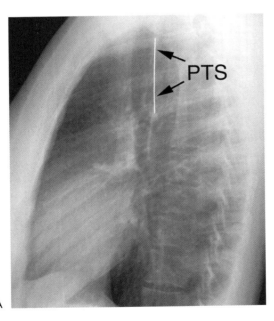

A

FIG. 7-24. Posterior tracheal stripe. **A.** Lateral radiograph. The posterior tracheal stripe *(PTS)* is a linear opacity corresponding to the posterior tracheal wall and sometimes the esophagus, seen below the thoracic inlet and above the tracheal bifurcation. It is of variable thickness. *(Figure continues.)*

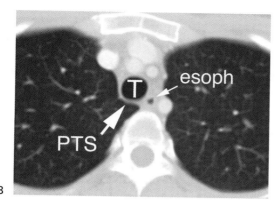

B

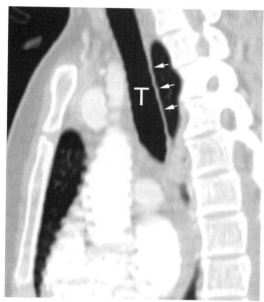

C

FIG. 7-24. *(Continued.)* **B.** CT in the same patient shows lung contacting posterior tracheal wall, outlining the posterior tracheal stripe *(PTS)*. *T,* trachea; *esoph,* esophagus. **C.** Sagittal reformation in the same patient shows lung outlining the posterior wall of the trachea *(T)*, forming the posterior tracheal stripe.

POSTERIOR TRACHEAL BAND OR STRIPE	
Variant:	If the stripe also includes anterior esophageal wall (with air in the esophageal lumen) or the entire esophagus, it is termed the *posterior tracheoesophageal stripe*
Visibility:	Common
Significance:	Variability in thickness limits usefulness; increased thickness usually indicates (1) esophageal carcinoma, (2) much less often, tracheal wall thickening, or (3) focal thickening with aberrant subclavian artery

RETROTRACHEAL TRIANGLE

Location:	Region posterior to the trachea, anterior to the spine, and above the posterior aortic arch
Anatomy:	Primarily esophagus with associated lymph nodes; it corresponds to the region of the posterior junction line seen on the frontal film
Appearance:	A relatively lucent region marginated anteriorly by the posterior tracheal stripe and posteriorly by the spine
Visibility:	Common
Significance:	Increased attenuation in this space most common with (1) esophageal lesions, (2) lymph node enlargement, (3) thyroid mass, (4) aberrant subclavian artery, (5) aneurysm, (6) bronchogenic cyst

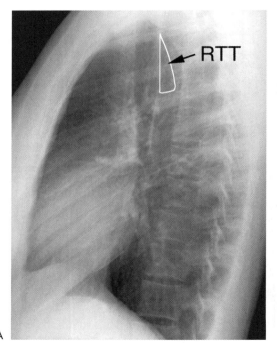

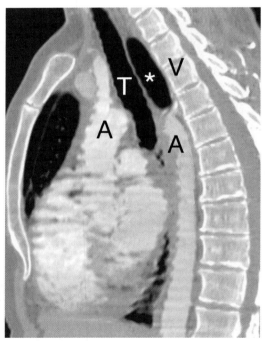

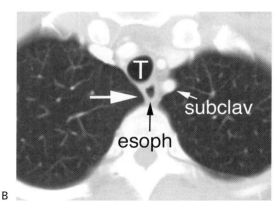

FIG. 7-25. Retrotracheal triangle. **A.** Lateral radiograph. The retrotracheal triangle *(RTT)* a relatively lucent region marginated anteriorly by the posterior tracheal stripe and posteriorly by the spine. **B.** CT in the same patient. The retrotracheal triangle corresponds to the region of the posterior junction line seen on the PA radiograph and reflects a narrowing of the mediastinum *(arrow)* behind the trachea *(T)* and left subclavian artery *(subclav)*, and in relation to the esophagus *(esoph)*. **C.** Sagittal reformation in the same patient shows the lucent retrotracheal triangle *(*)*, posterior to the trachea *(T)*, anterior to the vertebral column, and above the aortic arch *(A)*.

SELECTED READING

Aronberg DJ, Glazer HS, Madsen K, Sagel SS. Normal thoracic aortic diameters by computed tomography. J Comput Assist Tomogr 1984; 8:247–250.

Aronberg DJ, Peterson RR, Glazer HS, Sagel SS. The superior sinus of the pericardium: CT appearance. Radiology 1984; 153:489–492.

Baron RL, Lee JK, Sagel SS, Peterson RR. Computed tomography of the normal thymus. Radiology 1982; 142:121–125.

Blank N, Castellino RA. Patterns of pleural reflections of the left superior mediastinum. Normal anatomy and distortions produced by adenopathy. Radiology 1972; 102:585–589.

Breatnach E, Abbott GC, Fraser RG. Dimensions of the normal human trachea. AJR Am J Roentgenol 1984; 141:903.

de Geer G, Webb WR, Gamsu G. Normal thymus: assessment with MR and CT. Radiology 1986; 158:313–317.

Friedmand AC, Chambers E, Sprayregen S. The normal and abnormal left superior intercostal vein. AJR Am J Roentgenol 1978; 131:599–602.

Gamsu G, Webb WR. Computed tomography of the trachea and mainstem bronchi. Semin Roentgenol 1983; 18:51–60.

Genereux GP. The posterior pleural reflections. AJR Am J Roentgenol 1983; 141:141–149.

Glazer GM, Gross BH, Quint LE, et al. Normal mediastinal lymph nodes: number and size according to American Thoracic Society mapping. AJR Am J Roentgenol 1985; 144:261–265.

Heitzman ER, Lane EJ, Hammack DB, Rimmler LJ. Radiological evaluation of the aortic-pulmonic window. Radiology 1975; 116:513–518.

Heitzman ER, Scrivani JV, Martino J, Moro J. The azygos vein and its pleural reflections. I. Normal roentgen anatomy. Radiology 1971; 101:249–258.

Kiyono K, Sone S, Sakai F, et al. The number and size of normal mediastinal lymph nodes: a postmortem study. AJR Am J Roentgenol 1988; 150:771–776.

Landay MJ. Anterior clear space: how clear? How often? How come? Radiology 1994; 192:165–169.

Milne EN, Pistolesi M, Miniati M, Giuntini C. The vascular pedicle of the heart and the vena azygos. Part I: The normal subject. Radiology 1984; 152:1–8.

Palayew MJ. The tracheo-esophageal stripe and the posterior tracheal band. Radiology 1979; 132:11–13.

Proto AV. Mediastinal anatomy: emphasis on conventional images with anatomic and computed tomographic correlations. J Thorac Imaging 1987; 2:1–48.

Savoca CJ, Austin JH, Goldberg HI. The right paratracheal stripe. Radiology 1977; 122:295–301.

Smathers RL, Buschi AJ, Pope TL, et al. The azygos arch: normal and pathologic CT appearance. AJR Am J Roentgenol 1982; 139:477–483.

8

THE MEDIASTINUM: MEDIASTINAL MASSES

W. RICHARD WEBB

DIAGNOSIS OF MEDIASTINAL MASS

Although radiographs can show recognizable abnormalities in many patients with mediastinal pathology, they are limited in their sensitivity and ability to delineate the extent of mediastinal abnormalities and their relationship to specific mediastinal structures. CT is indispensable in the radiographic assessment of the mediastinum.

CT techniques vary somewhat according to the specific indications for the study and the type of scanner used, and various protocols are appropriate. In patients with a suspected mediastinal mass, an appropriate CT protocol would be as follows:

- Full inspiration
- Supine position
- 2.5- to 5-mm slice thickness
- Infusion of contrast agent at a rate appropriate for the scan sequence duration (usually about 2 to 2.5 ml/sec)

The differential diagnosis of a mediastinal mass on CT is usually based on several findings:

1. Location (anterior, middle, posterior mediastinum) or the identification of the specific structure from which it is arising
2. Nature
   a. Solitary lesion
   b. Multifocal (i.e., lymph nodes)
   c. Diffuse
3. Attenuation
   a. Fat
   b. Fluid
   c. Soft tissue
   d. Calcification
   e. Opacification following administration of contrast agents

Location

Anatomically, the mediastinum is divided into four compartments: anterior, middle, posterior, and superior.

Anatomic Divisions

Anterior

Extent: anterior to the pericardium, posterior to the sternum

Contents: fat, lymph vessels, and nodes

Middle

Extent: posterior to the anterior mediastinum, anterior to the posterior mediastinum; defined by its contents

Contents: the heart, pericardium, ascending aorta, superior vena cava, azygos arch, tracheal bifurcation, right and left pulmonary arteries and veins

Posterior

Extent: anterior to the spine, posterior to the heart and pericardium

Contents: descending aorta, azygos vein, superior intercostal vein, thoracic duct, esophagus, vagus nerves

Superior

Extent: below the root of the neck, above the pericardium

Contents: trachea, esophagus, thymus, and great vessels

Plain Radiographic Divisions

To allow an easier localization of mediastinal abnormalities on plain radiographs, the boundaries of the anterior, middle, and posterior mediastinal compartments were modified by Felson. In this classification, the superior mediastinum is not considered to be distinct, and its structures are assigned to the anterior, middle, or posterior compartment based on easily recognizable anatomic features (Fig. 8-1).

A more detailed analysis of the plain film, and localization of mediastinal abnormalities, may be based on identification of specific mediastinal lines, stripes, interfaces, and spaces, listed below and described in Chapter 7.

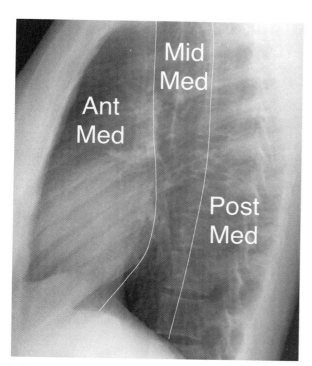

FIG. 8-1. Lateral chest radiograph showing Felson's mediastinal divisions. The anterior mediastinum *(Ant Med)* lies posterior to the sternum and anterior to a line drawn along the anterior tracheal wall in the upper mediastinum and the posterior border of the heart in the lower mediastinum. The posterior mediastinum *(Post Med)* lies posterior to a line 1 cm behind the anterior margin of the vertebral column and anterior to the chest wall. The middle mediastinum *(Mid Med)* lies between these.

Anterior

Extent: posterior to the sternum, anterior to a line drawn along the anterior tracheal wall in the upper mediastinum and the posterior border of the heart in the lower mediastinum

Contents: thymus, heart, ascending aorta and great vessels, anterior portion of the main pulmonary artery, pericardium, fat, lymph vessels, nodes

Corresponding plain film features: anterior junction line, cardiophrenic angles, retrosternal stripe, retrosternal space

Middle

Extent: between the anterior compartment in front and the posterior compartment behind

Contents: the trachea and main bronchi, superior vena cava, mid-portion of the aortic arch, azygos arch, lymph nodes, esophagus, descending aorta (sometimes)

Corresponding plain film features: right and left paratracheal stripes, superior vena cava interface, aortopulmonary window, left subclavian artery interface, azygoesophageal recess, preaortic interface

Posterior

Extent: posterior to a line 1 cm behind the anterior margin of the vertebral column, anterior to the chest wall

Contents: vertebral bodies, paravertebral tissues, descending aorta (sometimes), posterior azygos vein, hemiazygos vein, lymph nodes

Corresponding plain film features: paravertebral stripes

CT Divisions

On CT, it is most appropriate to base the differential diagnosis of a mediastinal mass on a direct observation of the tissue or structure from which the mass is arising (e.g., lymph nodes, veins and arteries, thymus, thyroid, trachea, esophagus, vertebral column). If this is not possible, then localizing the mass to specific regions of the mediastinum (e.g., prevascular space, pretracheal space, subcarinal space, aortopulmonary window, anterior cardiophrenic angle, paraspinal region) is valuable in differential diagnosis and more specific than considering only anterior, middle, and posterior divisions (Table 8-1). The anatomy of these regions is described in Chapter 7.

THE NORMAL THYMUS

The thymus has two lobes, the right and the left, which are fused superiorly near the thyroid gland and smoothly molded to the anterior aspect of the great vessels and anterior heart. It occupies the thyropericardic space. The thymus is rarely found in an ectopic location, usually the neck. The left thymic lobe usually is larger than the right.

The thymus weighs an average of about 25 g at birth and increases progressively to reach a maximum weight at puberty of approximately 35 to 50 g, although this is variable. The thymus begins to involute after puberty, and this process continues for a period of 5 to 15 years. During thymic involution, thymic follicles atrophy and are progressively replaced by fat. The relative proportion of fat to thymic tissue increases progressively until after age 60. At this age, little thymic tissue remains.

Plain Radiographs

In adults, the thymus is usually invisible on chest radiographs. In children, the thymus may be quite prominent, mimicking a mass (Fig. 8-2). However, radiographic findings may help in the correct identification of the thymus in children.

The thymus may project to one or both sides of the mediastinum, showing a sharply marginated undersurface, having the appearance of a sail (the "thymic sail" sign). The edge of the thymus may have a wavy appearance because of indentation by the anterior ribs or costal cartilage (the "thymic wave" sign).

TABLE 8-1. DIFFERENTIAL DIAGNOSIS OF MEDIASTINAL MASSES BASED ON COMMON SITES OF ORIGIN

Anterior mediastinum (prevascular space)
- Thymic masses
  - Hyperplasia
  - Thymoma
  - Thymic carcinoma
  - Thymic carcinoid tumor
  - Thymolipoma
  - Thymic cyst
  - Thymic lymphoma and metastases
- Germ cell tumors
  - Teratoma
  - Seminoma
  - Nonseminomatous germ cell tumors
- Thyroid abnormalities (goiter and neoplasm)
- Parathyroid tumor or hyperplasia
- Lymph node masses (particularly Hodgkin's lymphoma)
- Vascular abnormalities (aorta and great vessels)
- Mesenchymal abnormalities (e.g., lipomatosis, lipoma)
- Foregut cyst
- Lymphangioma and hemangioma

Anterior mediastinum (cardiophrenic angle)
- Lymph node masses (particularly lymphoma and metastases)
- Pericardial cyst
- Morgagni hernia
- Thymic masses
- Germ cell tumors

Middle mediastinum (pretracheal space)
- Lymph node masses
  - Lung carcinoma
  - Sarcoidosis
  - Lymphoma (particularly Hodgkin's disease)
  - Metastases
  - Infections (e.g., tuberculosis)
- Foregut cyst
- Tracheal tumor
- Mesenchymal masses (e.g., lipomatosis, lipoma)
- Thyroid abnormalities
- Vascular abnormalities (aorta and great vessels)
- Lymphangioma and hemangioma

Middle mediastinum (aortopulmonary window)
- Lymph node masses
  - Lung carcinoma

- Sarcoidosis
- Lymphoma
- Metastases
- Infections (e.g., tuberculosis)
- Mesenchymal masses (e.g., lipomatosis, lipoma)
- Vascular abnormalities (aorta or pulmonary artery)
- Chemodectoma
- Foregut cyst

Middle mediastinum (subcarinal space and azygoesophageal recess)
- Lymph node masses
  - Lung carcinoma
  - Sarcoidosis
  - Lymphoma
  - Metastases
  - Infections (e.g., tuberculosis)
- Foregut cyst
- Dilated azygos vein
- Esophageal masses
- Varices
- Hernia

Posterior mediastinum (paravertebral region)
- Neurogenic tumor
  - Nerve sheath tumors
  - Sympathetic ganglia tumors
  - Paraganglioma
- Foregut cyst
- Meningocele
- Extramedullary hematopoiesis
- Pseudocyst
- Thoracic spine abnormalities
- Hernias
- Esophageal masses
- Varices
- Mesenchymal masses (e.g., lipomatosis, lipoma)
- Lymph node masses
  - Lymphoma (particularly non-Hodgkin's)
  - Metastases
- Dilated azygos or hemiazygos vein
- Hernia
- Lymphangioma and hemangioma
- Thymic mass or germ cell tumor

CT

In children, the normal thymus fills the prevascular space, draping itself over the great vessels and cardiac margins (see Fig. 8-2B and C). Cephalad, the thymus extends above the innominate vein (see Fig. 8-2D). In infancy, the thymus is commonly seen to the level of the pulmonary arteries or below, but its inferior extent decreases with age.

In infants and young children, the thymus appears quadrilateral on CT. As the child grows, the thymus assumes a more triangular shape, often appearing arrowhead shaped or bilobed, with each of the two thymic lobes contacting the mediastinal pleura. Its margins are sharp, smooth, and convex in infants (see Fig. 8-2B) and often become straight in older children. Each lobe usually measures 1 to 2 cm in thickness (perpendicular to the pleura), but this is variable.

On unenhanced CT, the thymus is approximately the same attenuation as muscle. The mean attenuation of the thymus has been found to be 36 HU; the thymus shows homogeneous enhancement of 20 to 30 HU after bolus contrast injection.

From puberty to the age of about 25 years, the thymus appears triangular or bilobed, usually outlined by mediastinal fat (Fig. 8-3). The left lobe is usually larger, being seen lateral to the aortic arch; the right lobe may be inconspicuous. Typically the lateral borders of the thymus are flat or concave where they contact the pleura; uncommonly they are slightly convex. Its attenuation is usually less than that of muscle because of fatty replacement.

Over the age of 25 years, the thymus is no longer recognizable as a soft-tissue structure on CT because of progres-

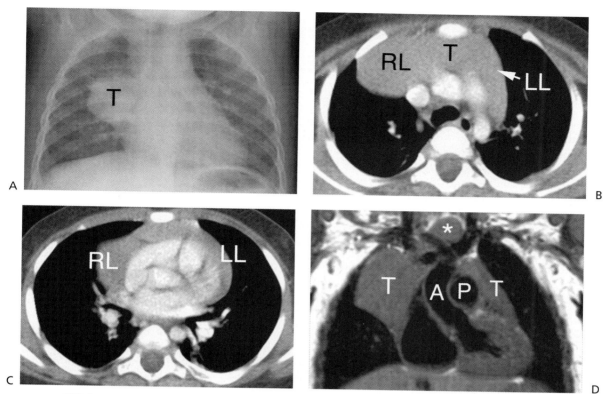

FIG. 8-2. Prominent normal thymus mimicking mass in a 1-year-old. **A.** PA chest radiograph shows an apparent right mediastinal mass representing thymus *(T)*. A slight wavy contour laterally is an example of the thymic wave sign. **B.** CT shows a prominent normal thymus *(T)* in the prevascular space. Both the right lobe *(RL)* and left lobe *(LL)* are visible. **C.** The right *(RL)* and left lobes *(LL)* lie lateral to the heart. **D.** T1-weighted coronal MRI showing intermediate-intensity thymus *(T)*, with some tissue extending above the innominate vein into the base of the neck *(*)*. Inferiorly, the thymus extends below the pulmonary artery *(P)*. A, aortic arch.

sive fatty involution. The thymus appears to be composed primarily of fat, containing islands or wisps of soft tissue (Fig. 8-4). The rapidity and degree of thymic involution are variable, and occasionally the thymus is still recognized as a discrete structure up to the age of 40. With complete

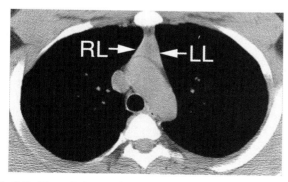

FIG. 8-3. Normal thymus in a 21-year-old patient. The thymus occupies the prevascular space and appears triangular and of soft-tissue attenuation, the left lobe *(LL)* being larger than the right *(RL)*.

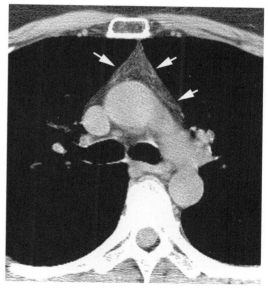

FIG. 8-4. Normal thymus in a 51-year-old patient. The thymus *(arrows)* appears to be composed primarily of fat, containing islands or wisps of soft tissue. The left thymic lobe extends more posteriorly than the right.

thymic involution, the anterior mediastinum appears to be entirely filled with fat; this fat represents the thymic remnant and may have a CT density slightly higher than that of subcutaneous fat.

Thymic Measurement

Thymic size can be quantitated using its length (measured in the cephalocaudal dimension), width (measured in the transverse dimension), and thickness (measured perpendicular to its length). On CT, the average thickness of the thymus is 1.4 cm in children aged 5 years or less. The maximum normal allowable thickness is 1.8 cm in patients under 20 and 1.3 cm in older adults.

MRI

On MRI, the normal thymus characteristically appears homogeneous and of intermediate signal intensity on T1-weighted images, being less intense than surrounding mediastinal fat but greater intensity than muscle (see Fig. 8-2D). However, because of progressive thymic involution, its appearance is dependent on the age of the patient. In patients over 30 years of age, differentiation between the thymus and adjacent mediastinal fat may be difficult because of thymic involution. The T2 relaxation times of the thymus are similar to fat at all ages.

THYMIC LYMPHOID FOLLICULAR HYPERPLASIA

The term thymic lymphoid follicular hyperplasia (LFH) is used to describe a condition characterized by the presence

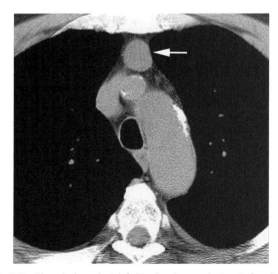

FIG. 8-5. Thymic lymphoid follicular hyperplasia. A focal mass *(arrow)* in the prevascular space represented follicular hyperplasia. Its appearance is nonspecific and cannot be distinguished from thymoma.

of hyperplastic lymphoid germinal centers in the thymic medulla, associated with a lymphocytic and plasma cell infiltrate. The presence of LFH is commonly associated with myasthenia gravis, connective tissue disease, pure red blood cell hypoplasia, and infection with HIV; it may also be seen in some normal young subjects.

Plain radiographs are usually normal. On CT, patients with LFH can have a normal-appearing thymus (45%), an enlarged thymus with a normal shape (35%), or a focal thymus mass (20%) (Fig. 8-5).

THYMIC HYPERPLASIA AND REBOUND

Thymic hyperplasia, as distinguished from LFH, is defined by an increase in size of the thymus associated with an otherwise normal gross and histologic appearance. It may be associated with hyperthyroidism (Graves' disease; Fig. 8-6), sarcoidosis, red blood cell aplasia, and other entities. It most commonly is seen in association with recovery from chemotherapy, stress, or burns, a phenomenon known as thymic rebound (described below).

Chest radiographs in adults are usually normal. In children, thymic enlargement may be seen. CT demonstrates increased thickness of the thymic lobes but an otherwise normal-appearing thymus.

Thymic Rebound

The thymus involutes during periods of stress (e.g., burns, chemotherapy) and may decrease significantly in size, depending on the age of the patient and the severity and duration of the stress. This is most marked in children, but it has also been observed in young adults (Fig. 8-7). A decrease in thymic volume of more than 40% may be seen. Following involution, the thymus will generally regrow to its original size within several months of the stressful episode. It may also exhibit "rebound," or growth to a size significantly larger than its original size; an increase in thymic volume of 50% in comparison to baseline may be seen. Thymic enlargement may be observed shortly after the stressful episode, or from 1 to 9 months afterward. The incidence of rebound following chemotherapy is 10% to 25%.

Increased thymic size may be seen on plain radiographs, particularly in children, but thymic rebound is detected with greater frequency when CT is used. In patients being treated for an extrathoracic malignancy, the appearance of thymic rebound should not pose a diagnostic problem; however, in patients with lymphoma, distinction from recurrent mediastinal tumor may be difficult. The presence of lymph node enlargement in association with thymic enlargement should suggest recurrent tumor, while isolated thymic enlargement should suggest thymic rebound. On MR, patients with thymic hyperplasia or thymic rebound may show en-

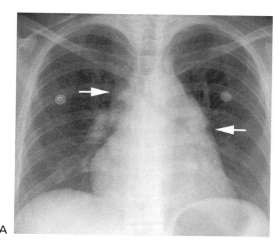

A

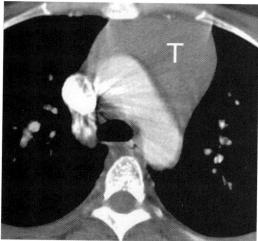

B

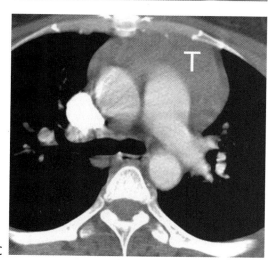

C

FIG. 8-6. Thymic hyperplasia in Graves' disease. **A.** Chest radiograph in a 40-year-old woman shows mediastinal widening *(arrows)*. **B and C.** CT shows enlargement of the thymus *(T)* in the prevascular space. The left thymic lobe is largest.

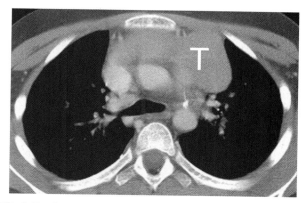

FIG. 8-7. Thymic rebound in a 10-year-old patient following chemotherapy for lymphoma. The thymus *(T)* is enlarged.

largement of the thymus, but its signal intensity is the same as for normal thymus.

THYMIC MASSES

A number of masses arise in relation to the thymus. Thymic masses and tumors include thymoma, thymic carcinoma, thymic carcinoid tumors, thymic cyst, thymolipoma, and lymphoma. Overall, they account for 20% to 25% of primary mediastinal tumors.

Thymoma

The term *thymoma* should be used to describe only neoplasms originating from the thymic epithelium, although they also contain a variable number of lymphocytes. Thymoma is the most common primary thymic tumor. It accounts for about 15% to 20% of primary mediastinal masses (Table 8-2).

TABLE 8-2. THYMOMA

Originates from thymic epithelium
Most common thymic tumor
15%–20% of mediastinal masses
Most common in patients 50–60 years old
Myasthenia gravis in 30%–50%
10%–30% of patients with myasthenia have thymoma
Invasive (30%) or noninvasive (70%), not benign and malignant
Metastases outside thorax in 3%–5%
Radiographic findings
  Sharply marginated, smooth or lobulated
  Usually project to one side of the mediastinum
  Retrosternal clear space or costophrenic angles
CT findings
  Focal or lobulated mass
  Homogeneous or cystic, may calcify
  Invasion difficult to diagnose with certainty

Thymomas are rare before age 20 and are most common in patients aged 50 to 60 years. No distinct sex predominance is present. Patients may be asymptomatic, but 20% to 30% have symptoms related to compression of mediastinal structures. Myasthenia gravis develops in 30% to 50% of patients with a thymoma. Hematologic abnormalities are also associated with thymoma and include pure red blood cell aplasia and hypogammaglobulinemia. Approximately 10% to 30% of patients with myasthenia or red cell aplasia have a thymoma. Autoimmune and collagen-vascular diseases such as systemic lupus erythematosus, rheumatoid arthritis, Graves' disease, and inflammatory bowel disease may also be associated with thymoma.

Thymomas are usually encapsulated and round or lobular. They may contain areas of calcification, necrosis, cysts, or hemorrhage. Most are slow-growing and behave in a benign fashion. Histologic appearances do not allow a reliable differentiation of benign and malignant thymomas; malignancy can be established only by the presence of tumor growth into or through the tumor capsule with invasion of local structures. Thus, thymomas are most appropriately referred to as *invasive* or *noninvasive* rather than malignant or benign.

About 30% of thymomas are locally aggressive and invasive, or recur following excision. Invasive thymomas infiltrate adjacent structures, including the pericardium, pleura, superior vena cava, great vessels, airways, and heart, and may cross the diaphragm to involve the retroperitoneum. Spread to involve one pleural cavity can result in a typical appearance of multiple lenticular pleural implants occurring in the absence of pleural effusion. Thymoma rarely (3% to 5%) metastasizes outside the thorax.

Thymomas can be staged at the time of surgery based on the presence and extent of invasion:

Stage 1: capsule is intact
Stage 2: pericapsular growth with invasion of mediastinal fat
Stage 3: invasion of surrounding organs or pleural implants at a distance from the primary tumor
Stage 4 (used in some systems): distant metastases or pleural implants

Resection is usually indicated, sometimes in association with radiation, or radiation or chemotherapy for stages 2 and 3. Although invasive thymomas may recur, they tend to grow slowly, and prolonged survival is usually possible.

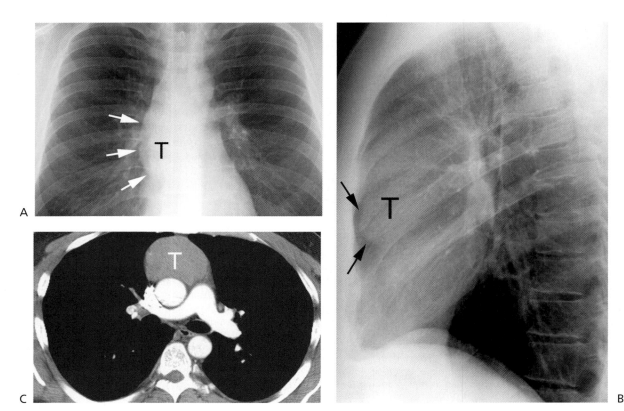

FIG. 8-8. Thymoma, invasive. **A.** PA chest radiograph shows prominence of the right mediastinum *(arrows)* due to a thymoma *(T)*. **B.** On the lateral radiograph, an opacity *(T)* is visible in the inferior aspect of the retrosternal clear space, with a well-defined edge inferiorly *(arrows)*. **C.** CT shows a homogeneous soft-tissue mass in the prevascular space. No fat plane is seen separating the thymoma *(T)* from the ascending aorta. Pericardial invasion was found at surgery.

The 5-year survival rate for noninvasive thymoma is 75% to 90%; for invasive thymoma, the 5-year survival rate is 50% to 60%.

Plain Radiographs

Most thymomas occur near the junction of the heart and great vessels, although they may be seen superiorly to the level of the clavicles and inferiorly to the level of the costophrenic angles. Their distribution on the frontal radiograph may be likened to an upside-down horseshoe embracing the heart. They may be subtle or invisible on chest radiographs.

Thymomas typically appear sharply marginated, smooth or lobulated in contour, and usually project to one side of the mediastinum (Figs. 8-8A and 8-9A). They usually range in size from 5 to 10 cm in diameter when visible on radiographs, and may obscure the right or left heart border, de-

pending on their location and size. Dense calcification may be seen in the periphery of the mass or throughout its substance.

On lateral radiographs, thymoma often produces a distinct opacity in the inferior aspect of the retrosternal clear space, the relatively lucent triangular region posterior to the sternum and anterior to the aortic arch, main pulmonary artery, and heart (see Figs. 8-8B and 8-9B). However, lack of lucency in this space or poor definition or obscuration of the anterior margin of the ascending aorta or pulmonary artery may be normal findings. A mass overlying the heart and region of the cardiophrenic angle may be seen, although this may be mimicked by fat pads and the normal cardiac incisura.

Invasive and noninvasive thymoma cannot usually be distinguished on plain radiographs; however, pleural involvement with invasive thymoma occasionally results in pleural thickening, nodularity, or pleural effusion.

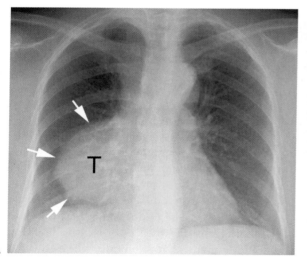

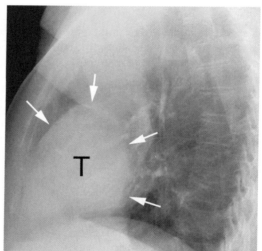

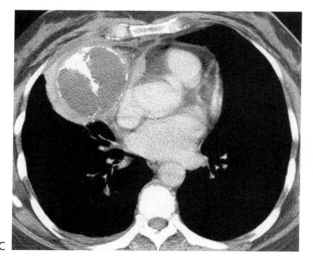

FIG. 8-9. Cystic thymoma, noninvasive. **A.** PA chest radiograph shows a large thymoma *(T, arrows)*, obscuring the right heart border, extending into the right cardiophrenic angle. **B.** On the lateral radiograph, the thymoma *(T)* is visible overlying the heart shadow *(arrows)*. **C.** CT shows a cystic (fluid attenuation) mass in the right cardiophrenic angle. The mass shows dense calcification, including calcification of its capsule. A noninvasive cystic thymoma was found at surgery.

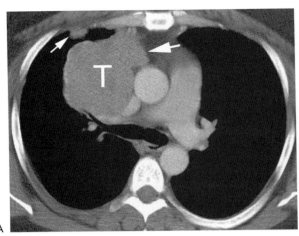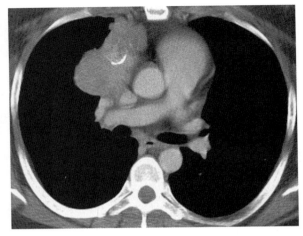

FIG. 8-10. Invasive thymoma with calcification in a patient with myasthenia gravis. **A.** CT shows a lobulated mass *(T)* in the prevascular space, typical of thymoma. Medially, the mass invades mediastinal fat *(large arrow)*. A small pleural nodule *(small arrow)* is also seen, resulting from pleural invasion. Compression of the superior vena cava is also present. **B.** At a lower level, calcification is visible.

CT

In nearly all cases, thymomas occur in the prevascular space and displace the great vessels (aorta and its branches, superior vena cava and its branches, and main pulmonary artery) posteriorly (see Figs. 8-8C and 8-9C).

Thymoma or other thymic neoplasm may be distinguished from thymic hyperplasia if enlargement of the thymus is grossly asymmetric, if the thymus has a lobular contour, or if a focal rounded lesion is visible (Fig. 8-10). However, follicular thymic hyperplasia can result in a focal thymic mass up to 5 cm in diameter (see Fig. 8-5).

Approximately 80% of thymomas occur at the base of the heart, as shown on CT (see Figs. 8-8C and 8-9C). They usually appear as homogeneous soft-tissue attenuation masses that are sharply demarcated and oval, round, or lobulated and do not conform to the normal shape of the thymus (see Figs. 8-8C, 8-9C, 8-10). Most often the tumor grows

asymmetrically to one side of the prevascular space. Because ectopic thymic tissue in the neck is found in up to 20% of subjects, thymoma can occur in the neck or at the thoracic inlet, thus mimicking a thyroid mass (Fig. 8-11), or rarely occurs in the posterior mediastinum.

Thymomas usually appear homogeneous in attenuation with or without contrast medium injection (see Figs. 8-8C and 8-10). However, some large thymomas appear cystic (see Fig. 8-9C) or contain areas of necrosis. Calcification may occur in the capsule (see Fig. 8-9C) or within the tumor (see Figs. 8-10B and 8-12).

It is often difficult to distinguish invasive and noninvasive thymoma on CT. The presence of clearly defined fat planes between the tumor and adjacent mediastinal structures suggests the absence of extensive local invasion (Fig. 8-13), but limited invasion cannot be excluded. Also, obliteration of fat planes between the tumor and mediastinum

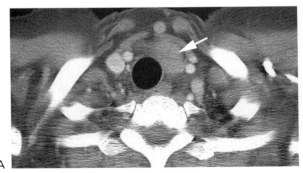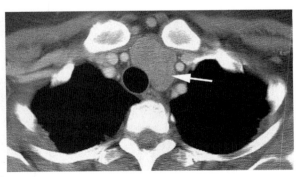

FIG. 8-11. Cervical thymoma. **A.** CT through the neck shows a left neck mass *(arrow)*, mimicking thyroid enlargement. **B.** The mass *(arrow)* extends into the upper mediastinum.

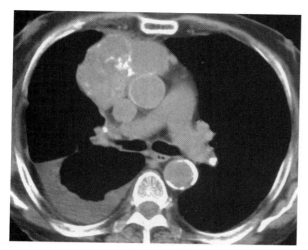

FIG. 8-12 . Invasive thymoma with calcification. CT shows a lobulated thymoma with multiple calcifications. The presence of pleural effusion strongly suggests invasion.

suggests the possibility of invasion, but this finding cannot be relied upon (see Fig. 8-8C). Findings highly suggestive of invasion include pericardial thickening contiguous with the tumor, pleural thickening, nodules, or effusion (see Figs. 8-10A, 8-12, and 8-14), encasement of mediastinal structures, fat infiltration (see Fig. 8-10A), and an irregular interface between the tumor and lung. Invasive thymomas may extend to involve the posterior mediastinum and by conti-

guity the retroperitoneum. Consequently, it has been recommended that CT staging of thymoma include the upper abdomen.

Myasthenia gravis is commonly associated with thymic pathology (see Fig. 8-10). Sixty-five percent of patients with myasthenia gravis have thymic hyperplasia, and 10% to 30% have thymoma. In patients with myasthenia, a normal-appearing thymus on CT may be associated with normal histology or focal lymphoid hyperplasia; an enlarged but otherwise normal-appearing thymus indicates focal lymphoid hyperplasia; and a focal nodule or mass may represent focal lymphoid hyperplasia or mass.

MR

The role of MR in diagnosing thymic masses is limited. On MR, thymomas typically have a low signal intensity on T1-weighted images, which increases with T2 weighting; they may appear homogeneous in intensity or inhomogeneous with or without cystic components, or may show nodules or lobules of tumor separated by relatively low-intensity septations. MR has proven valuable in identifying the presence or absence of vascular invasion in patients with thymoma, especially in patients to whom intravenous contrast cannot be administered.

Thymic Carcinoma

Thymic carcinoma, like thymoma, arises from thymic epithelial cells, but it is much less common. Thymic carcinoma

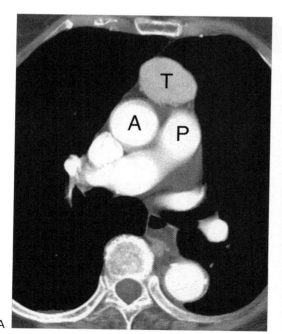
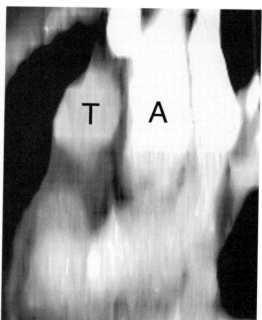

FIG. 8-13. Noninvasive thymoma. **A.** CT shows a homogeneous thymoma *(T)* separated from the aorta *(A)* and pulmonary artery *(P)* by a layer of fat. **B.** Oblique sagittal reconstruction shows separation of the thymoma *(T)* from the ascending aorta *(A)*.

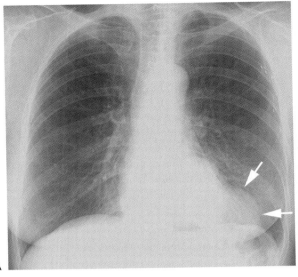

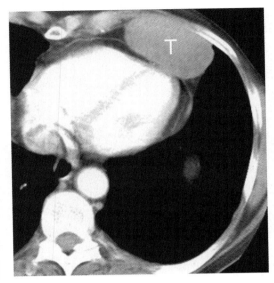

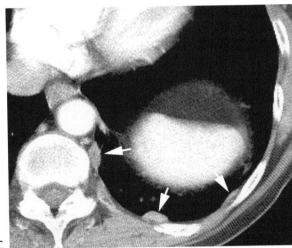

FIG. 8-14. Invasive thymoma with pleural metastases. **A.** PA chest radiograph shows a mass at the left cardiophrenic angle *(arrows)*. **B.** CT shows a homogeneous rounded mass *(T)* representing thymoma. **C.** At a lower level, CT shows focal pleural thickening or nodules *(arrows)*, typical of pleural metastases. Pleural nodules are usually unassociated with pleural effusion. This finding indicates invasion.

accounts for about 20% of thymic epithelial tumors (Table 8-3). Unlike thymoma, thymic carcinoma can be diagnosed as malignant on the basis of histologic criteria; however, the specific histologic pattern is variable. The tumor is aggressive and more likely to result in distant metastases than invasive thymoma; although distant metastases are present in only about 5% of patients with invasive thymoma, they are present at diagnosis in 50% to 65% of patients with thymic carcinoma. Frequent sites of metastasis include the lungs, liver, brain, and bone. It has a poor prognosis, with a 5-year survival rate of 30%. Average age at presentation is 50 years.

Symptoms are usually attributable to the mediastinal mass. Invasion of mediastinal structures is common, and superior vena cava syndrome may be present. Although paraneoplastic syndromes such as myasthenia gravis, pure red cell aplasia, and hypogammaglobulinemia are common with thymoma, they are rare with thymic carcinoma.

Thymic carcinoma usually results in a mass 5 to 15 cm in diameter. A large mass with or without areas of low attenuation is typical (Fig. 8-15). Calcification may be present (see Fig. 8-15). Thymic carcinoma cannot be distinguished from thymoma on CT unless enlarged lymph nodes are visible in the mediastinum or distant metastases are evident.

TABLE 8-3. THYMIC CARCINOMA

Originates from thymic epithelium
20% of thymic epithelial tumors
Average age 50
Unlike thymoma, appears malignant histologically
Invasion common, distant metastases in 50%–65%
Myasthenia rare
Appearance indistinguishable from thymoma unless metastases
    are visible

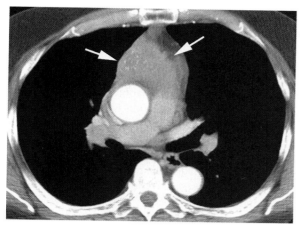

FIG. 8-15. Thymic carcinoma. A large mass *(arrows)* is visible in the prevascular space. Stippled calcifications are visible within the mass. This mass cannot be distinguished from thymoma.

Thymic carcinoma is less likely than thymoma to result in pleural implants.

On MR, thymic carcinoma appears higher in signal intensity than muscle on T1-weighted MR images, with an increase in signal on T2-weighted images. Heterogeneous signal may reflect the presence of necrosis, cystic regions within the tumor, or hemorrhage. Thymoma appears to have a greater tendency to show a multinodular appearance on MR than does thymic carcinoma.

Thymic Carcinoid Tumor

Thymic carcinoid tumors are believed to arise from thymic cells of neural crest origin (amine precursor uptake and decarboxylase cells; APUD); they are usually malignant, with a tendency for local recurrence following resection (Table 8-4). Average age at presentation is 45 years; men are more commonly involved.

Approximately 25% to 40% of patients have Cushing's syndrome as a result of tumor secretion of ACTH. Nearly 20% of cases have been associated with multiple endocrine neoplasia (MEN) syndromes I (more common) and II.

This lesion does not differ significantly from thymoma

TABLE 8-4. THYMIC CARCINOID TUMOR

Originates from neural crest cells (APUDoma)
Average age 45
Usually malignant
Cushing's syndrome in 25%–40%
MEN in 20%
Mimics thymoma radiographically
Dense enhancement possibly seen on CT

in its radiographic or CT appearance (Fig. 8-16). In some patients, a mediastinal mass is not visible on CT despite the presence of endocrine abnormalities. MR findings are nonspecific and identical to those of thymoma. Dense contrast enhancement may be seen on CT.

This tumor is more aggressive than thymoma, being malignant in most cases, and superior vena cava obstruction is much more common with thymic carcinoid than with thymoma. The 5-year survival rate is about 65%. Metastases may be visible.

Thymolipoma

Thymolipoma is a rare, benign, well-encapsulated thymic tumor consisting primarily of fat but also containing vari-

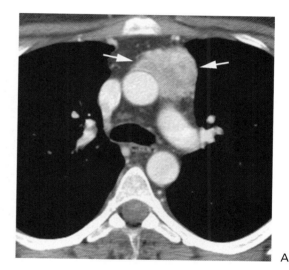

A

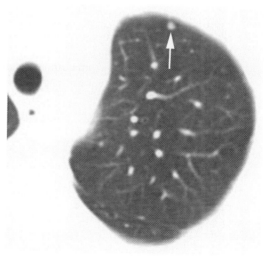

B

FIG. 8-16. Thymic carcinoid tumor in a patient with Cushing's syndrome. **A.** A prevascular space mass *(arrows)* shows significant enhancement following contrast infusion. This may be seen in carcinoid tumor. **B.** Lung window scans showed pulmonary metastases *(arrow)*.

TABLE 8-5. THYMOLIPOMA

Consists of fat and thymic tissue
5% of thymic tumors
Benign
Often young patients
Usually asymptomatic
Large droopy mediastinal mass containing fat and strands of tissue

able amounts of thymic tissue; it can arise within the thymus or be connected to the thymus by a pedicle. Eighty percent of patients present in the first four decades. It accounts for less than 5% of thymic tumors (Table 8-5).

In most cases, thymolipoma is unaccompanied by symptoms and is detected incidentally on chest radiographs. It is often large, averaging nearly 20 cm in diameter at diagnosis, and it may project into both hemithoraces. Because of its fatty content and pliability, thymolipoma tends to drape over the heart, extending inferiorly into the cardiophrenic angles. It can simulate cardiac enlargement, lower lobe collapse, or elevation of a hemidiaphragm (Figs. 8-17A and B). There is no known association with myasthenia gravis.

On CT, thymolipoma may appear to be predominantly fat but usually appears to contain wisps, whorls, or small nodules of soft tissue in combination with fat (see Fig. 8-17C). Uncommonly it appears to be primarily of soft-tissue attenuation. In all cases, CT shows a connection between the mass and the thymic bed.

As would be expected from its fat content, MR shows areas of high signal intensity on T1-weighted spin-echo images, similar to the intensity of subcutaneous fat, with areas of intermediate signal intensity reflecting the presence of

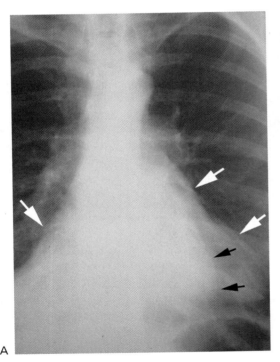

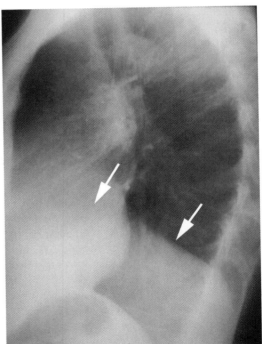

FIG. 8-17. Thymolipoma. **A.** PA chest radiograph shows a triangular mass *(white arrows)* overlying the heart shadow *(black arrows)* and projecting into both hemithoraces. **B.** On the lateral view, a portion of the mass mimics elevation of the right diaphragm *(white arrows)*. **C.** CT shows the large bilateral mass *(arrows)*. The mass extends posteriorly on the right side. It is largely of fat attenuation but contains wisps of soft tissue.

soft tissue. Despite attaining a large size, thymolipomas do not invade surrounding structures. However, some compression of mediastinal structures is visible in half of cases. They do not recur following resection.

Thymic Cyst

Thymic cysts are uncommon. They can be either congenital or acquired. Congenital thymic cysts are rare; acquired thymic cysts have been reported following radiation therapy, in association with thymic tumors, and following thoracotomy. Their attenuation is usually that of water but can be higher or lower depending on the presence of hemorrhage or fat.

One should be cautious in making the diagnosis of thymic cyst; cystic regions can be seen in a variety of thymic tumors, including thymoma and lymphoma. CT can suggest the diagnosis of thymic cyst if the lesion (1) appears thin-walled; (2) is unassociated with a mass lesion; (3) contains fluid with a density close to that of water; and (4) remains unopacified following contrast infusion. Calcification of the cyst wall can also be seen. MR characteristics are similar to those of other cystic lesions.

Thymic Lymphoma and Metastases

Hodgkin's disease (HD) has a predilection for involvement of the thymus in conjunction with involvement of mediastinal lymph nodes. Thymic enlargement may be seen in 30% of patients with intrathoracic HD. Non-Hodgkin's lymphoma (NHL) much less commonly involves the thymus.

Thymic lymphoma usually results in homogeneous thymic enlargement (Fig. 8-18). However, lobulation or a nodular appearance is seen in some patients, and cystic areas of necrosis are visible on CT in 20% of adults. Calcification uncommonly occurs in the absence of radiation or chemotherapy. Although its appearance is nonspecific, the combination of a thymic mass with mass or lymph node enlargement in other areas of the mediastinum is suggestive of this diagnosis. On MR, thymic lymphoma shows low intensity on T1-weighted images, with a variable change on T2-weighted images.

Metastatic tumors, particularly lung and breast carcinomas, can also involve the thymus. Involvement of mediastinal lymph nodes is also typically present. CT and MRI appearances of thymic metastases are nonspecific.

GERM CELL TUMORS

Germ cell tumors account for about 10% of primary mediastinal masses and arise from primitive germ cells that have arrested their embryologic migration in the mediastinum, frequently within the thymus. They are more common in the anterior mediastinum; only about 5% originate in the posterior mediastinum. Most germ cell tumors present during the second to fourth decades of life.

Germ cell tumors include benign and malignant teratoma, seminoma, embryonal carcinoma, endodermal sinus (yolk sac) tumor, choriocarcinoma, and mixed cell types.

Overall, more than 80% of germ cell tumors are benign, with the large majority of these being benign teratomas. Although the sex distribution of benign germ cell tumors is about equal, there is a strong preponderance of males among patients with malignant germ cell tumors. Among patients with malignant tumors, seminoma is most common, representing about 30% of cases, with embryonal carcinoma and malignant teratoma each responsible for about 10%, and choriocarcinoma and endodermal sinus tumor responsible for about 5% each; the remainder of malignancies, approximately 40% of cases, represent mixed tumors.

Benign tumors are often asymptomatic, while malignant tumors are more likely to cause symptoms. Confirmation that these lesions are primary to the mediastinum requires that there be no evidence of a testicular or retroperitoneal tumor.

Teratoma

Teratomas contain elements of all germinal layers. They are classified as mature, cystic (dermoid cyst), immature, and malignant (Table 8-6).

Mature teratomas are most common and are composed of well-differentiated tissues, with ectodermal elements such as skin and hair predominating, but they also contain cartilage, fat, and muscle. They are benign. They constitute 60% to 75% of mediastinal germ cell tumors. Sex incidence is equal, and they most commonly occur in children and

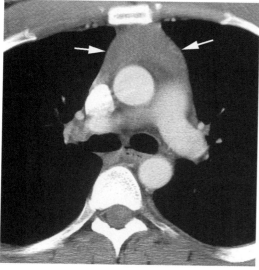

FIG. 8-18. Thymic enlargement in Hodgkin's disease. The thymus *(arrows)* is homogeneously enlarged.

TABLE 8-6. TERATOMA

Contains elements of all germinal layers
Mature teratomas (contain mature tissues)
  Benign
  60%–75% of mediastinal germ cell tumors
  Occur in children and young adults
  Dermoid cyst
Immature teratomas (contain immature tissue)
  Often have benign course in infants or young children
  Often aggressive and malignant in adults
Malignant teratoma (contains frankly malignant tissues)
  Poor prognosis
  Usually men
Anterior mediastinal mass; posterior in 5%
Smooth, rounded, or lobulated mass
Mature teratoma
  Well defined, smooth, cystic
  Teeth and bone rare
  Fluid in 90%; fat in 75%; calcification in 50%
Immature or malignant teratoma
  Nodular or poorly defined
  Fat in 40%
  Compression or invasion of mediastinal structures
  Enhancing capsule

young adults. They do not usually result in symptoms unless large.

Dermoid cysts are said to contain elements of only the ectodermal layer of germ cells, specifically skin and its appendages, but small rests of endodermal and mesodermal cells are often present; they are benign.

Immature teratomas contain less well-developed tissues more typical of those present during fetal development; in infancy or early childhood, these tumors often have a benign course, while in adults they usually behave in an aggressive and malignant fashion.

Malignant teratomas contain frankly malignant tissues in addition to immature or mature tissues and have a very poor prognosis; they are seen almost exclusively in men.

Plain Radiographs

Plain radiographs usually show an anterior mediastinal mass projecting to one side of the mediastinum (Fig. 8-19). Their distribution is similar to that of thymoma. Middle mediastinal or posterior masses are occasionally seen. Teratoma appears as a smooth, rounded, or lobulated mass. Mature teratoma is typically well defined and often large at diagnosis, averaging 8 to 10 cm in diameter. Calcification is visible in about 20% of mature teratomas. Teeth or bone are diagnostic but rarely seen.

CT

Teratomas are usually found in the prevascular space, although 5% occur in the posterior mediastinum. Regardless of their histology, CT often shows a combination of fluid-filled cysts, fat, soft tissue, and areas of calcification (Fig. 8-20). Calcification is visible in about 50% of cases, being focal or rimlike or rarely representing teeth or bone. In patients with mature teratoma, 90% contain fluid and 75%

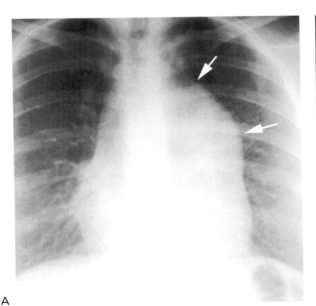
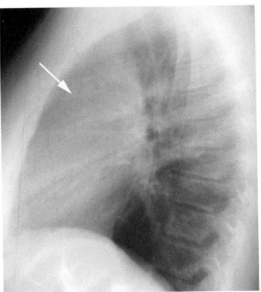

FIG. 8-19. Mature mediastinal teratoma. **A.** PA chest radiograph shows a smooth, sharply marginated left mediastinal mass *(arrows).* It obscures the left heart border, indicating its anterior location. **B.** Lateral view shows increased density of the retrosternal clear space *(arrow),* but a discrete mass is not visible.

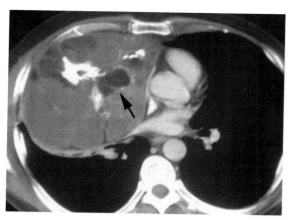

FIG. 8-20. Mature mediastinal teratoma. A large mass is compressing right cardiac structures. It contains calcifications, areas of fat *(arrow)*, and cystic or soft-tissue regions.

Plain radiographs typically show a large, lobulated, anterior mediastinal mass projecting to one or both sides of the mediastinum and often obscuring a portion of the heart border (Fig. 8-21). On CT, primary mediastinal seminomas present as large, smooth or lobulated, homogeneous soft-tissue masses, although small areas of low attenuation can be seen. Obliteration of fat planes is common, and pleural or pericardial effusion may be present. Seminomas are very radiosensitive, and the 5-year survival rate is 50% to 75%.

Nonseminomatous Germ Cell Tumors

Nonseminomatous germ cell tumors, namely embryonal carcinoma, endodermal sinus (yolk sac) tumor, choriocarcinoma and mixed types, are often grouped together because

contain fat. Common combinations include fluid, soft tissue, fat, and calcium (40% of cases); fluid, soft tissue, and fat (25% of cases); and fluid and soft tissue (15% of cases). A fat-fluid level within the mass is diagnostic and is present in about 10% of cases. The fluid within the cystic parts of the tumors also may vary in attenuation. Teratomas are typically encapsulated and well demarcated. Rim enhancement can be seen.

Various CT findings can help in differentiating benign and malignant lesions. Benign lesions are typically well defined, smooth, and cystic, and 90% contain fat. Malignant teratomas are nodular or poorly defined, they are more likely to appear solid, and a smaller proportion (40%) contains fat. Malignant teratoma has a greater tendency to compress surrounding structures. Following contrast infusion, malignant teratoma can show a thick enhancing capsule.

MR can show various appearances, depending on the composition of the tumor. They commonly contain fat, which is intense on T1-weighted images, and cystic areas, which are low in intensity on T1-weighted images but increase with T2 weighting.

Seminoma

Seminoma occurs almost entirely in men, with a mean age at presentation of 29 years. It is the most common malignant mediastinal germ cell tumor, accounting for 30% of cases (Table 8-7).

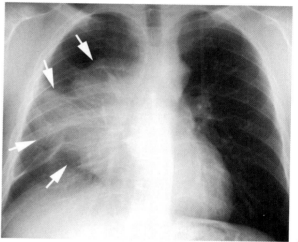

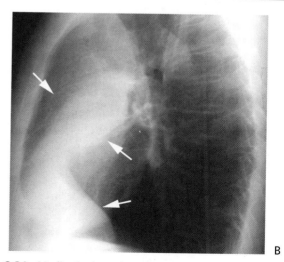

FIG. 8-21. Mediastinal seminoma. **A.** PA radiograph shows a large, lobulated, and poorly marginated mediastinal mass *(arrows)* obscuring the right heart border. A small right pleural effusion is also visible. **B.** Lateral view shows a large anterior mediastinal mass *(arrows)*.

TABLE 8-7. SEMINOMA

30% of germ cell tumors
Mean age 29
Large, lobulated, anterior mediastinal mass
Homogeneous in attenuation
Good prognosis; 5-year survival rate 50%–75%

TABLE 8-8. NONSEMINOMATOUS GERM CELL TUMOR

Cell types
  Embryonal carcinoma
  Endodermal sinus (yolk sac) tumor
  Choriocarcinoma
  Mixed types
Large, lobulated, anterior mediastinal mass
Inhomogeneous in attenuation
Poor prognosis

of their rarity, similar appearance, aggressive behavior, and poor prognosis (Table 8-8). The tumors are usually unresectable at diagnosis because of local invasion or distant metastasis. Unlike in seminoma, radiotherapy is of limited value.

Plain radiographs show large, lobulated, anterior mediastinal masses. They may be ill defined or associated with pleural effusion because of local invasion of lung and pleura.

On CT, these tumors often show heterogeneous opacity, including ill-defined areas of low attenuation secondary to necrosis and hemorrhage or cystic areas. They often appear infiltrative, with obliteration of fat planes, and may be spiculated. Calcification may be seen. MR findings also reflect the inhomogeneous nature of these lesions.

THYROID GLAND AND THYROID ENLARGEMENT

The thyroid gland is located in close approximation to the thoracic inlet, and thyroid enlargement is commonly associated with extension into the mediastinum. Multinodular goiter is the most common condition in which a mediastinal thyroid abnormality is detected; carcinoma and thyroiditis are relatively rare causes.

Intrathoracic extension of thyroid lesions is common, representing nearly 10% of mediastinal masses resected at thoracotomy (Table 8-9). Such lesions are almost always connected to the thyroid, being seen in the superior medias-

tinum. Truly ectopic mediastinal thyroid tissue, not showing a connection to the thyroid gland, is uncommon.

Thyroid masses are most often anterior in location. In 75% to 90% of cases, an enlarged thyroid extends into the thyropericardiac space anterior to the subclavian and innominate vessels. Posterior mediastinal goiters constitute approximately 10% to 25% of cases. Presumably arising from the posterolateral portion of the gland, posterior goiters descend behind the brachiocephalic vessels and are most commonly found on the right side, in close proximity to the trachea. Less often, thyroid tissue extends between the esophagus and trachea or posterior to the esophagus.

Plain Radiographs

Mediastinal thyroid abnormalities typically present as a sharply marginated, superior mediastinal mass, causing tracheal narrowing or displacement of the trachea to the contralateral side. The mass usually appears poorly marginated above the level of the clavicles (Figs. 8-22 and 8-23A).

CT

The appearance of normal thyroid tissue is characteristic. On noncontrast scans, thyroid tissue is high in attenuation

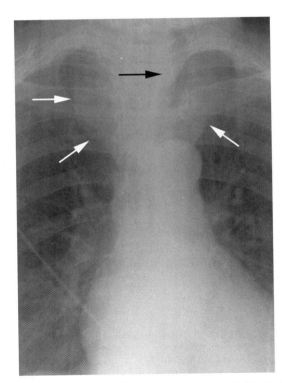

FIG. 8-22. Mediastinal goiter. A mass in the superior mediastinum *(white arrows)* is sharply defined inferiorly and poorly defined above the clavicles. The trachea is displaced to the left *(black arrow)*.

TABLE 8-9. MEDIASTINAL THYROID MASS

10% of mediastinal masses
Almost always connected to cervical thyroid
Anterior in 75%–90%; posterior in 10%–25%
Masses high in attenuation on CT; densely enhance with contrast
Cystic or inhomogeneous
Punctate calcifications
Distinguishing goiter and carcinoma difficult

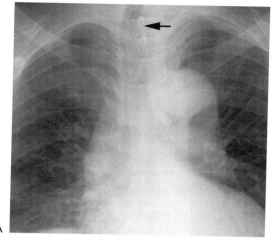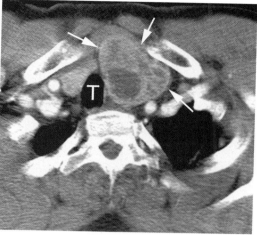

FIG. 8-23. Cystic cervical and mediastinal goiter. **A.** Chest radiograph shows displacement of the trachea to the right *(arrow)* and poorly defined superior mediastinal widening at the level of the thoracic inlet. **B.** CT shows an enhancing multicystic mass *(arrows)* at the level of the thoracic inlet. The trachea *(T)* is displaced to the right and slightly narrowed.

relative to adjacent soft tissues because of its high iodine content. Normal thyroid tissue measures around 100 HU, although in hypothyroid patients thyroid attenuation is only slightly greater than soft tissue. Following the administration of contrast, thyroid tissue significantly enhances (see Figs. 8-23B and 8-24).

Recognizing that a mediastinal mass originates from the thyroid gland depends on (1) demonstration of a communication with the cervical portion of the thyroid gland on contiguous slices (see Fig. 8-24); (2) high attenuation of at least a portion of the mass; (3) marked enhancement after contrast injection (see Figs. 8-24 and 25); and (4) prolonged enhancement (more than 2 minutes). Mediastinal thyroid masses commonly appear inhomogeneous and cystic (see

Figs. 8-23B and 8-25) on CT. Curvilinear, punctate, or ringlike calcifications can also be seen. The appearance of thyroid masses is usually nonspecific. Differentiation of goiter and thyroid carcinoma is difficult unless associated lymph node metastases are seen.

MR

Characteristically, on T1-weighted images, the signal intensity of the normal thyroid is equal to or slightly greater than that seen in the adjacent sternocleidomastoid muscle; on T2-weighted scans, the signal intensity of the thyroid gland is significantly greater (Fig. 8-26). Most focal pathologic processes, including adenomas, cysts, and cancer, are easily

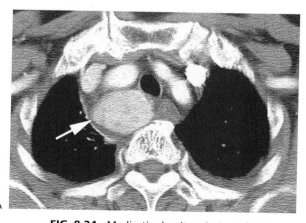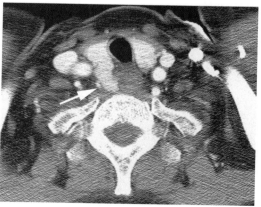

FIG. 8-24. Mediastinal goiter. **A.** An enhancing mass is visible in the right paratracheal mediastinum *(arrow)*. **B.** At a higher level, this mass is seen to arise from the inferior pole of the right thyroid lobe *(arrow)*. The thyroid also densely enhances.

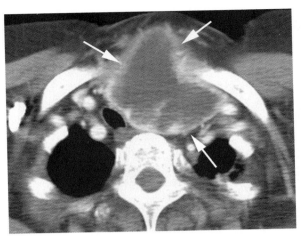

FIG. 8-25. Large cystic goiter. A large mass *(arrows)* at the thoracic inlet has a densely enhancing rim and a cystic center. The trachea is displaced to the right and narrowed. The mass protrudes anteriorly into the suprasternal notch.

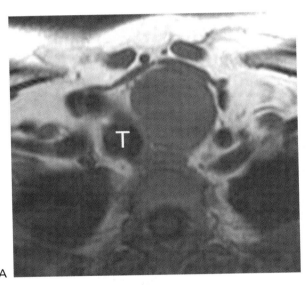

A

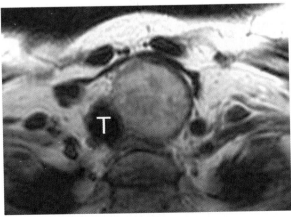

B

FIG. 8-26. MR of goiter. **A.** T1-weighted image shows a left thyroid mass to be slightly more intense than strap muscles. The trachea *(T)* is displaced to the right. **B.** With T2 weighting, the mass is more intense than muscle. *T*, trachea.

identified on T2-weighted sequences because of their markedly prolonged T2 values. Multinodular goiter has inhomogeneous signal characteristics.

PARATHYROID ADENOMA

Four parathyroid glands are usually present. The upper pair is typically located dorsal to the superior poles of the thyroid gland, while the lower pair lies just below the lower thyroid poles. However, the precise location of glands may vary, and the lower pair is most variable in location. Most parathyroid adenomas are found in the lower group of parathyroid glands.

Approximately 10% of parathyroid glands are ectopic (Table 8-10). About 60% of these are located in the anterior mediastinum; 30% are embedded within thyroid tissue; and 10% are found in the posterior-superior mediastinum, in the region of the tracheoesophageal groove. Anterior mediastinal parathyroid glands are thought to result from islands of parathyroid tissue that are carried into the anterior mediastinum by the descending thymus during embryologic development. Anterior mediastinal parathyroid adenomas are intimately connected with the thymus.

Primary hyperparathyroidism results from a solitary adenoma in approximately 85% of cases. Other causes include diffuse hyperplasia (10%), multiple adenomas (5%), and rarely carcinoma (1%). Various studies are available for detecting parathyroid abnormalities. These include high-resolution ultrasonography, radionuclide imaging using thallium or sestamibi, high-resolution contrast-enhanced CT, MRI, and selective venous catheterization.

Normal parathyroid glands cannot be identified on CT. Parathyroid adenomas and hyperplastic glands are usually small but vary in size from 0.3 to 3 cm; rarely are they large enough to be detected on plain radiographs. When visible on CT, they usually appear homogeneous in density. Rarely, parathyroid adenomas appear calcified. No CT criteria reliably differentiate an adenoma from hyperplasia or carcinoma.

In patients with primary hyperparathyroidism, surgical neck exploration with resection of parathyroid tissues is curative in about 90% to 95% of cases. As a consequence, imaging is not generally performed prior to surgery. However, the persistence of hyperparathyroidism following surgical resection of the cervical glands suggests the presence

TABLE 8-10. MEDIASTINAL PARATHYROID MASS

10% of parathyroid glands are ectopic
　60% in the anterior mediastinum
　10% in the posterior-superior mediastinum
Adenoma and hyperplastic gland usually small
Mediastinal parathyroid present in 40%–50% of patients with persistent hyperparathyroidism after surgery

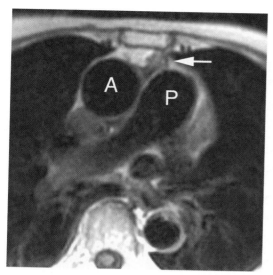

FIG. 8-27. Anterior mediastinal parathyroid adenoma on T1-weighted MRI in a patient with persistent hyperparathyroidism after parathyroid surgery. A small mass *(arrow)* is visible anterior to the ascending aorta *(A)* and main pulmonary artery *(P)*, in the region of the thymus.

of an ectopic parathyroid adenoma or ectopic hyperfunctioning gland. Forty to 50% of these patients will have mediastinal parathyroid glands. In the anterior mediastinum, ectopic adenomas are usually found in the expected location of the thymus and may be indistinguishable from small thymic remnants, small thymomas, or small lymph nodes (Fig. 8-27). Parathyroid adenomas are rarely found in the aortopulmonary window.

Similar to thyroid adenomas, most parathyroid adenomas, hyperplastic glands, and carcinomas appear intense on T2-weighted images, increasing significantly in intensity compared to T1-weighted images. Enhancement following gadolinium infusion is typical, and fat-suppression images can be valuable.

MEDIASTINAL LYMPH NODES AND LYMPH NODE MASSES

On average, more than 60 mediastinal lymph nodes are found at autopsy. Almost 80% of mediastinal lymph nodes are located in relation to the trachea and main bronchi and serve to drain the lungs.

Mediastinal lymph node abnormalities can be seen in any part of the mediastinum, although they most commonly involve middle mediastinal regions such as the pretracheal space, aortopulmonary window, and subcarinal space. Their detection and diagnosis are important in the evaluation of a number of thoracic diseases, including bronchogenic carcinoma, lymphoma, and granulomatous diseases. The assessment of mediastinal lymph nodes in patients with bronchogenic carcinoma is discussed in detail in Chapter 3.

Mediastinal lymph nodes are generally classified by location, and most descriptive systems are based on Rouvière's classification of lymph node groups. Thoracic lymph nodes are usually grouped into parietal and visceral, depending on their location and drainage. The parietal lymph nodes lie outside the parietal pleura, primarily drain structures of the chest wall, and are classified as internal mammary, diaphragmatic, paracardiac, and intercostal. Visceral node groups are located within the mediastinum or are related to the lung hila, and include intrapulmonary, bronchopulmonary, tracheobronchial, paratracheal, paraesophageal, and anterior mediastinal lymph nodes.

Lymph Node Groups

The following classification is based on a modification of well-recognized anatomic descriptions of lymphatic anatomy, although some terms have been modified to be consistent with current usage and emphasize the localization of lymph nodes on imaging studies.

Lymph nodes will be considered in anterior, tracheobronchial, and posterior node groups, generally corresponding to the plain radiographic divisions of anterior, middle, and posterior mediastinum.

Anterior Lymph Nodes

Internal mammary lymph nodes are located in a retrosternal position, in the anterior intercostal spaces, near the internal mammary artery and veins; they are considered to be part of the parietal lymph node group. They drain the anterior chest wall, anterior diaphragm, and medial breasts and freely communicate with prevascular lymph nodes and paracardiac or diaphragmatic lymph nodes. They are most often enlarged as a result of lymphoma or metastatic breast cancer (Figs. 8-28A and B and 8-29A and B).

Prevascular lymph nodes lie anterior to the aorta and in relation to the great vessels. These nodes drain most anterior mediastinal structures, including the pericardium, thymus, thyroid, pleura, and the anterior hila. They represent visceral nodes. They communicate with the internal mammary chain of nodes anteriorly and paratracheal and aortopulmonary lymph nodes posteriorly. They may be involved in a variety of diseases, notably lymphoma (see Figs. 5-3 and 5-4 in Chapter 5) and granulomatous diseases, but their involvement in lung cancer is relatively uncommon.

Paracardiac or cardiophrenic angle lymph nodes lie anterior to or lateral to the heart and pericardium, on the surface of the diaphragm. They communicate with the lower internal mammary chain and drain the lower intercostal spaces, pericardium, diaphragm, and liver. As with internal mammary nodes, paracardiac nodes are most commonly enlarged in patients with lymphoma (see Fig. 8-28C) and metastatic

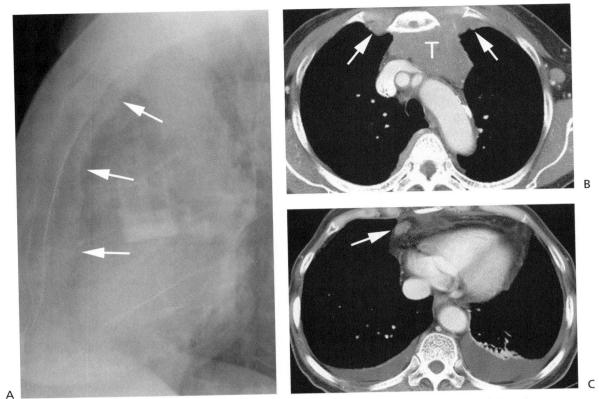

FIG. 8-28. Internal mammary and paracardiac lymph node enlargement. **A.** Lateral plain radiograph in a patient with non-Hodgkin's lymphoma shows thickening of the retrosternal stripe *(arrows)*. **B.** CT shows enlargement of internal mammary lymph nodes *(arrows)* bilaterally, in association with involvement of the thymus *(T)* in the anterior mediastinum, left axillary lymph node enlargement, and pleural effusions. **C.** At a lower level, a right paracardiac lymph node *(arrow)* is also enlarged.

carcinoma, particularly breast cancer. Paracardiac lymph nodes correspond to the anterior (prepericardiac) and middle (juxtaphrenic) subgroups of the diaphragmatic parietal lymph node group. Prepericardiac nodes are located posterior to the xiphoid process and slightly lateral to it. Juxtaphrenic lymph nodes are situated adjacent to the pericardium, where the phrenic nerves meet the diaphragm. From a clinical standpoint, there is little reason to distinguish between them.

Tracheobronchial Lymph Nodes

Tracheobronchial lymph nodes generally serve to drain the lungs. Lung diseases (e.g., lung cancer, sarcoidosis, tuberculosis, fungal infections) that secondarily involve lymph nodes typically involve the tracheobronchial lymph nodes. Tracheobronchial lymph nodes are subdivided into a number of important node groups, which are all closely related.

Paratracheal nodes lie anterior to, and on either side of, the trachea, thus occupying the pretracheal (or anterior

paratracheal) space (Figs. 8-30 and 8-31). Retrotracheal nodes may also be seen. The most inferior node in this region is the so-called azygos node, medial to the azygos arch. These nodes form the final pathway of lymphatic drainage from most of both lungs, excepting the left upper lobe. Because of this, they are commonly abnormal regardless of the location of lung disease.

Aortopulmonary nodes are grouped by Rouvière with prevascular nodes, but because they serve the same function on the left as paratracheal nodes on the right and freely communicate with paratracheal nodes, it is most appropriate to group them together. They lie in the aortopulmonary window, lateral to the left main bronchus and between the aorta and pulmonary artery. The left upper lobe drains via this node group.

Peribronchial nodes surround the main bronchi on each side and lie between the main bronchi in the subcarinal space. These drain the lungs. *Bronchopulmonary nodes* are located distal to the main bronchi and are usually considered to be hilar.

Subcarinal nodes represent peribronchial nodes lying be-

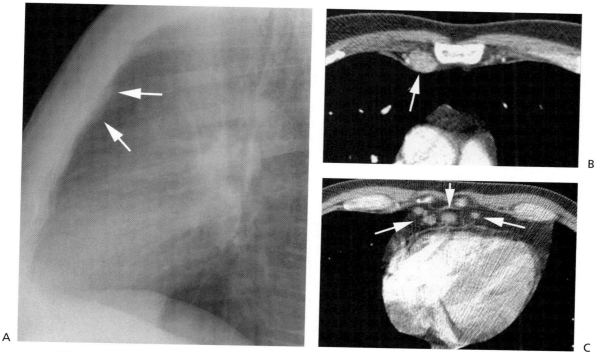

FIG. 8-29. Internal mammary and paracardiac lymph node enlargement. **A.** Lateral plain radiograph in a patient with non-Hodgkin's lymphoma shows lobulation of the retrosternal stripe *(arrows)*. **B.** CT shows enlargement of internal mammary lymph node *(arrow)* in association with the internal mammary vessels. **C.** At a lower level, a group of enlarged paracardiac lymph nodes *(arrows)* is also visible.

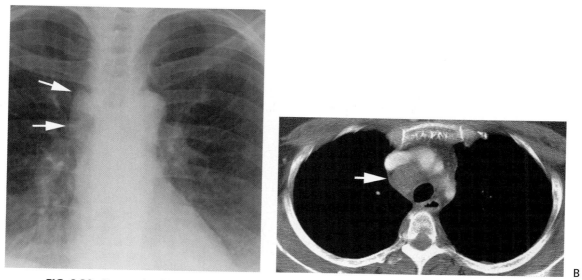

FIG. 8-30. Paratracheal lymph node enlargement in metastatic carcinoma. **A.** Chest radiographs shows abnormal convexity of the right superior mediastinum *(arrows)*. The right paratracheal stripe and the normal contour of the superior vena cava are not visible. **B.** CT shows lymph node enlargement in the pretracheal space *(arrow)*, corresponding to paratracheal lymph nodes. The superior vena cava is displaced laterally and anteriorly, and the normal right paratracheal stripe is obscured by the large nodes.

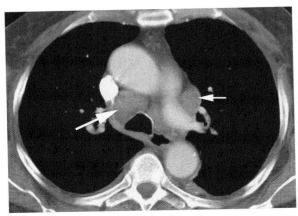

FIG. 8-31. Paratracheal and aortopulmonary window lymph node enlargement in non-Hodgkin's lymphoma. Enlarged nodes in the pretracheal space *(large arrow)* and aortopulmonary window *(small arrow)* are visible.

tween the main bronchi in the subcarinal space (Fig. 8-32). These nodes drain the inferior hila and lower lobes on both the right and left and communicate in turn with the right paratracheal chain.

Posterior Lymph Nodes

Paraesophageal and inferior pulmonary ligament nodes are associated with the esophagus and descending aorta and lie medial to the inferior pulmonary ligament (Figs. 8-33A and B). They represent visceral nodes and drain the medial lower lobes, esophagus, pericardium, and posterior diaphragm. On the right, they are impossible to distinguish from subcarinal nodes unless they are near the diaphragm.

Intercostal and paravertebral lymph nodes are found in the posterior intercostal spaces and adjacent to thoracic vertebral bodies (see Figs. 8-33B and C). These drain the posterior pleura, chest wall, and spine and communicate with other posterior mediastinal lymph nodes.

Retrocrural lymph nodes lie posterior to the diaphragmatic crura (Fig. 8-34). They communicate with lumbar nodes and posterior mediastinal lymph nodes, drain the diaphragm and liver, and represent the posterior group of diaphragmatic parietal lymph nodes.

Lymph Node Stations

In the 1970s, the American Joint Committee on Cancer (AJCC) and the Union Internationale Contre le Cancer (UICC) introduced a numeric system for localization of intrathoracic lymph nodes for the purpose of lung cancer staging. Lymph nodes were described relative to regions in the mediastinum termed "lymph node stations" (Table 8-11). The AJCC/UICC node mapping system was modified in 1983 by the American Thoracic Society (ATS) to more precisely define anatomic and CT criteria for each station, and the ATS classification system has been in common

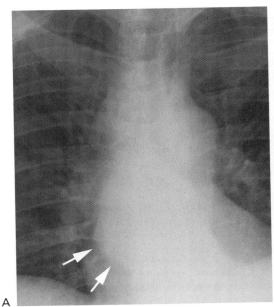

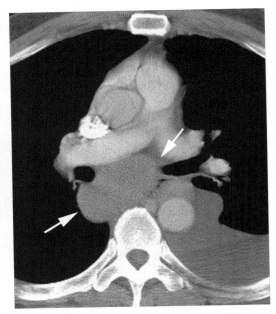

FIG. 8-32. Subcarinal lymph node enlargement in chronic lymphocytic leukemia. **A.** Chest radiographs show an abnormal convexity in the region of the azygoesophageal recess *(arrows)*, corresponding to subcarinal lymph node enlargement. **B.** CT shows abnormally enlarged subcarinal lymph nodes *(arrows)*.

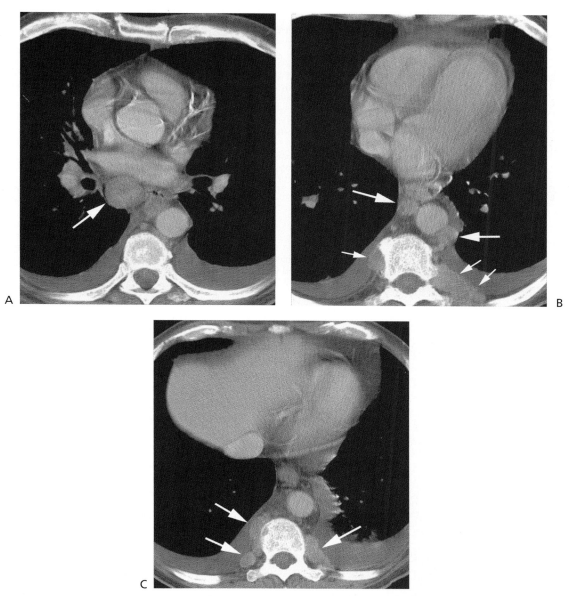

FIG. 8-33. Paraesophageal and paravertebral lymph node enlargement in metastatic carcinoma. **A.** An enlarged lymph node *(arrow)* is visible in the right paraesophageal region. Pleural effusions are also seen. **B.** At a lower level, paraesophageal and paraaortic lymph nodes *(large arrows)* and paravertebral lymph nodes *(small arrows)* are enlarged. **C.** At a level below **B**, enlarged paravertebral lymph nodes *(arrows)* are visible. They are higher in attenuation than the pleural fluid.

TABLE 8-11. COMPARISON OF ATS AND AJCC/UICC LYMPH NODE STATIONS

Node group	ATS node station	ATS designation	ATS anatomic criteria	AJCC/UICC station	AJCC/UICC designation	AJCC/UICC anatomic criteria
Paratracheal				1	Highest mediastinal	Cranial to the superior aspect of L brachiocephalic vein
Paratracheal	2R	R upper paratracheal	R of the tracheal midline, between the lung apex and the caudal margin of the innominate artery (or for radiologists, the superior aspect of the aortic arch as with 2L)	2	Upper paratracheal	Below station 1 and cranial to superior aspect of the aortic arch
	2L	L upper paratracheal	L of the tracheal midline, between the lung apex and the superior aortic arch			
Prevascular				3	Prevascular	Anterior to the great vessel branches and cranial to aortic arch
Paraesophageal					Retrotracheal	Posterior to the trachea and cranial to the inferior aspect of azygos arch
Paratracheal	4R	R lower paratracheal	R of the tracheal midline, below 2R and above the azygos arch	4R	R lower paratracheal	R of tracheal midline, below 2, and cranial to the RUL bronchus (this equals ATS 4R + 10R)
	4L	L lower paratracheal	L of the tracheal midline, below 2L, cephalad to the carina, and medial to the ligamentum arteriosum	4L	L lower paratracheal	L of the tracheal midline, below 2, and cranial to the LUL bronchus (this equals ATS 4L + 10L)
Aortopulmonary	5	Aortopulmonary	Subaortic and paraaortic nodes lateral to the ligamentum arteriosum, aorta, or LPA, proximal to the first branch of the LPA	5	Subaortic or aortopulmonary	Lateral to the ligamentum arteriosum, aorta, or LPA, proximal to the first branch of the LPA within the mediastinal pleural envelope
Prevascular	6	Anterior	Anterior to aortic arch or innominate artery (including some pretracheal and preaortic nodes)	6	Paraaortic (ascending aortic or phrenic)	Anterior and lateral to the ascending aorta and the aortic arch and innominate artery, caudal to the superior aspect of aortic arch
Subcarinal	7	Subcarinal	Caudal to the carina but not associated with the lower lobe bronchi or arteries within the lung	7	Subcarinal	Caudal to the carina but not associated with the lower lobe bronchi or pulmonary arteries within the lung
Paraesophageal	8	Paraesophageal	Dorsal to the posterior wall of trachea and on either side of the esophagus (not subcarinal nodes)	8	Paraesophageal	Adjacent to the wall of the esophagus and to the right of left of esophagus
Inferior pulmonary ligament	9	R or L pulmonary ligament	In relation to right or left inferior pulmonary ligaments	9	Pulmonary ligament	Within the pulmonary ligament, including those in the posterior wall and lower part of the inferior pulmonary vein
Peribronchial (hilar)	10R	Tracheobronchial	R of the tracheal midline, caudal to 4R and above the origin of the RUL bronchus	10R	R hilar	Caudal to the superior RUL bronchus, adjacent to the R main bronchus or proximal bronchus intermedius
	10L	Peribronchial	L of the tracheal midline, between the carina and the LUL bronchus, medial to the ligamentum arteriosum	10L	R hilar	Caudal to the superior LUL bronchus, adjacent to L main bronchus
Bronchopulmonary (hilar)	11	Intrapulmonary	Nodes removed at pneumonectomy or distal to the mainstem bronchi or secondary carina (includes interlobar, lobar, and segmental nodes)	11	Interlobar	Between lobar bronchi and adjacent to proximal lobar bronchi
Lobar	12		May be determined postthoracotomy	12	Lobar	Adjacent to distal lobar bronchi
Segmental	13		May be determined postthoracotomy	13	Segmental	Adjacent to segmental bronchi
				14	Subsegmental	Adjacent to subsegmental bronchi

L, left; R, right; LPA, left pulmonary artery; LUL, left upper lobe; RUL, right upper lobe.

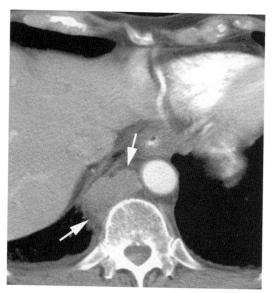

FIG. 8-34. Retrocrural lymph node enlargement in lymphoma. Enlarged nodes *(arrows)* are visible in a retrocrural, paraaortic location.

usage since then (Fig. 8-35). In 1997, the AJCC/UICC published a further revision intended to be a compromise between the AJCC and ATS classifications (Fig. 8-36). A detailed knowledge of lymph node stations is not necessary in clinical practice, but a passing familiarity with this classification is encouraged. Figures 8-35 and 8-36 and Table 8-11 may be used for reference and provide a comparison of ATS and AJCC/UICC criteria.

Lymph Node Enlargement

Radiographs

Normal lymph nodes are not visible on chest radiographs. Abnormally enlarged nodes may be recognized because of distortion of normal mediastinal contours or abnormalities of mediastinal lines, interfaces, or spaces (Table 8-12).

Enlarged right paratracheal (pretracheal lymph) nodes usually result in an abnormal convexity of the superior vena cava interface or thickening of the right paratracheal stripe (see Fig. 8-30A). Inferiorly, right paratracheal nodes are contiguous with the right tracheobronchial nodes, recognizable when enlarged as enlargement of the shadow of the azygos arch.

Enlarged left paratracheal lymph nodes are not commonly visible on chest radiographs but may result in an convexity in the region of the left paratracheal stripe or in relation to the left subclavian artery interface, above the aortic arch.

Enlargement of aortopulmonary nodes results in a convexity of the aortopulmonary window.

Enlarged subcarinal lymph nodes result in a convexity in the region of the superior aspect of the azygoesophageal recess (see Fig. 8-32A). Paraesophageal lymph node enlargement also may result in an abnormal convexity in the azygoesophageal recess or an abnormality of the retrotracheal band on the lateral film.

CT

On CT, lymph nodes are generally visible as round, elliptical, or triangular; discrete and surrounded by mediastinal

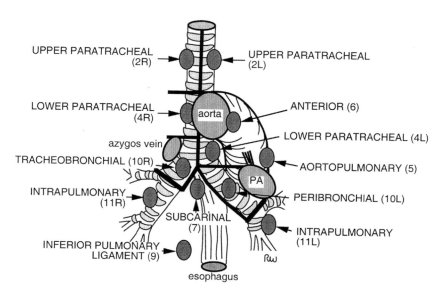

FIG. 8-35. ATS lymph node stations.

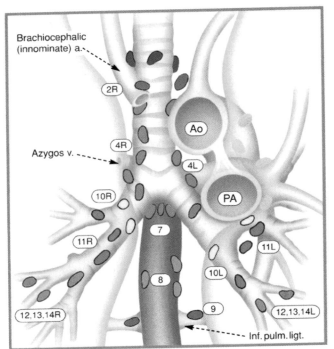

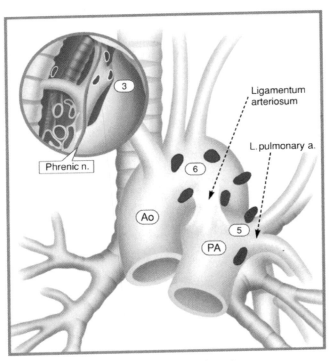

FIG. 8-36. AJCC/UICC lymph node stations. (From Mountain CF, Dresler CM. Regional lymph node classification for lung cancer staging. Chest 1997; 111:1718–1723.)

TABLE 8-12. PLAIN FILM FINDINGS OF LYMPH NODE ENLARGEMENT

Node group	ATS node station(s)	Plain film finding when nodes are enlarged
Right paratracheal	2R, 4R	1. Convexity of the superior vena cava interface 2. Thickening of the right paratracheal stripe
Left paratracheal	2L, 4L	1. Convexity of the left subclavian artery interface 2. Thickening of the left paratracheal stripe (uncommon)
Aortopulmonary	5	Convexity of the aortopulmonary window interface
Prevascular	6	1. Anterior mediastinal mass 2. Filling in of the retrosternal clear space (lateral film)
Subcarinal	7	Convexity in the superior aspect of the azygoesophageal recess
Paraesophageal	8	1. Thickening of the posterior tracheal band 2. Convexity of the azygoesophageal recess
Inferior pulmonary ligament	9	Convexity in the inferior aspect of the azygoesophageal recess
Peribronchial (hilar)	10R and L	Hilar enlargement and lobulation (see Chapter 6)
Bronchopulmonary (hilar)	11	Hilar enlargement and lobulation (see Chapter 6)
Paracardiac	14R and L	Convexity in the cardiophrenic angles
Internal mammary	—	Lobulation of the retrosternal stripe
Retrocrural	8R and L	Convexity of the paravertebral stripes
Intercostal or paravertebral	—	Convexity of the paravertebral stripes

fat; and of soft-tissue attenuation (see Figs. 8-28 to 8-34). The node hilum is sometimes seen to contain a small quantity of fat.

Lymph nodes can usually be distinguished from vessels by their location. However, the ability to recognize and correctly identify lymph nodes is directly related to the amount of mediastinal fat surrounding them; in patients having little mediastinal fat, lymph nodes can be difficult to distinguish from vessels without contrast infusion. In many parts of the mediastinum, lymph nodes often occur in clusters of a few nodes of similar size.

The short axis or least diameter (i.e., the smallest diameter seen in cross section) of a lymph node should generally be used when measuring its size. This measurement more closely reflects the actual node diameter when nodes are obliquely oriented relative to the scan plane and shows less variation among normal subjects than does the long axis or greatest diameter.

There are significant variations in normal node size, depending on the location of the node (Table 8-13). However, by convention, the upper limit of normal for mediastinal lymph nodes should generally be considered to be 1.0 cm, as measured in its short axis, except in the subcarinal region. Ninety-five percent or more of lymph nodes in normal subjects measure 1.0 cm or less in the lower paratracheal (4R), right paratracheal (10R), and aortopulmonary window (5) regions. In the subcarinal region, an upper limit of 1.5 cm is usually used. Internal mammary nodes, paracardiac nodes, and paravertebral nodes are not commonly seen on CT in normals.

Significant abnormalities (e.g., micrometastases) can be present in the absence of lymph node enlargement. Also, the significance given to the presence of a minimally enlarged lymph node must be tempered by a knowledge of the patient's clinical history. For example, if the patient is known to have lung cancer, an enlarged lymph node has a significant likelihood of being involved by tumor. However, the same node in a patient without lung cancer is much less likely to be of clinical significance. In the absence of a known disease, a mildly enlarged node must be regarded as likely to be hyperplastic or postinflammatory.

Very large lymph nodes, having a short axis of 2 cm or more, often reflect the presence of neoplasm, such as metastatic tumor or lymphoma, granulomatous disease, or infection, and should be regarded as potentially significant. Although mediastinal lymph nodes can become enlarged in a variety of noninfectious and nongranulomatous inflammatory diseases, they are often smaller than 2 cm.

With progression of disease, a pathologic process involving several contiguous nodes may also involve surrounding mediastinal fat, and several adjacent nodes may fuse to form a single larger mass. Poor definition of node margins or poor definition of the margins of the coalescent node mass can indicate extension of the disease process through the node capsule, or an associated fibrotic or inflammatory reaction. This appearance is most typical of infection, granulomatous disease, and neoplasm. Diffuse infiltration of mediastinal fat may also occur, with individual nodes or node groups becoming unrecognizable (Fig. 8-37). Typically, mediastinal fat appears to be replaced by soft-tissue density. This pattern suggests lymphoma, undifferentiated carcinoma, generalized infection, or granulomatous mediastinitis.

Lymph Node Calcification

Lymph node calcification may be recognized on chest radiographs or CT. CT, of course, is more sensitive. Typically, calcified lymph nodes indicate prior granulomatous disease, including tuberculosis, histoplasmosis and other fungal infections, and sarcoidosis, although a variety of diseases may be associated with this finding.

TABLE 8-13. LYMPH NODE SIZE MEASURED USING CT IN NORMAL SUBJECTS, BY ATS LYMPH NODE STATION

ATS station	Patients with nodes	Number of nodes (± SD)	Maximum number of nodes	Short axis diameter (mm) (± SD)	Upper limits of normal (mm) (mean + 2 SD)
2R	95%	2.1 ± 1.3	6	3.5 ± 1.3	6.1
2L	75%	1.9 ± 1.6	6	3.3 ± 1.6	6.5
4R	100%	3.2 ± 2.0	10	5.0 ± 2.0	9.0
4L	84%	2.1 ± 1.6	7	4.7 ± 1.9	8.5
5	59%	1.2 ± 1.1	3	4.7 ± 2.1	8.9
6	86%	4.8 ± 3.5	12	4.1 ± 1.7	7.5
7	95%	1.7 ± 1.1	6	6.2 ± 2.2	10.6
8R	57%	1.0 ± 1.1	4	4.4 ± 2.6	9.6
8L	45%	0.8 ± 1.2	6	3.8 ± 1.7	7.2
10R	100%	2.8 ± 1.3	7	5.9 ± 2.1	10.1
10L	70%	1.0 ± 0.8	3	4.0 ± 1.2	6.4

(Modified from Glazer GM, Gross BH, Quint LE, et al. Normal mediastinal lymph nodes: number and size according to American Thoracic Society mapping. AJR Am J Roentgenol 1985; 144:261–265.)

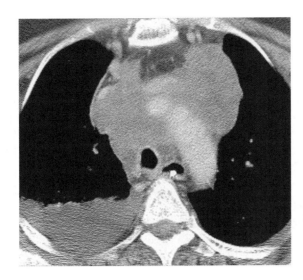

FIG. 8-37. Confluent lymph node mass in a patient with metastatic squamous cell carcinoma involving the pretracheal and prevascular spaces. Individual lymph nodes are not visible.

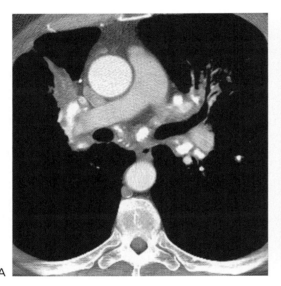

A

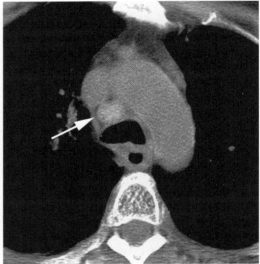

C

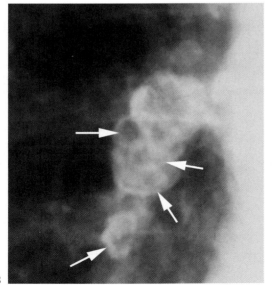

B

FIG. 8-38. Lymph node calcification. **A.** Dense lymph node calcification in sarcoidosis. **B.** Hilar eggshell calcification in silicosis. A number of nodes show ringlike calcification in their periphery *(arrow)*. **C.** Stippled and faint calcification *(arrows)* in metastatic thyroid carcinoma.

Calcification can be dense, involving the node in a homogeneous fashion, stippled, "eggshell" in appearance, or faint and hazy. The abnormal nodes are often enlarged but can also be of normal size. Multiple calcified lymph nodes are often visible, usually in contiguity, and hilar lymph node calcifications are often associated. Dense calcification involving all or most of an abnormal node is typical of previous granulomatous infection or sarcoidosis (Fig. 8-38A).

Eggshell calcification is defined by the presence of calcium in the node periphery, which is often ringlike. Eggshell calcification is most often seen in patients with silicosis (see Fig. 8-38B) or coal workers' pneumoconiosis, sarcoidosis, and tuberculosis, but it also occurs in patients with HD, usually following radiation, and occasionally occurs in patients with other causes of node calcification.

Rarely, lymph node calcification is seen in untreated lymphoma or as a result of metastatic carcinoma, typically mucinous adenocarcinoma or thyroid carcinoma (see Fig. 8-38C). Usually calcification of adenocarcinomas is stippled or faint and difficult to see on plain radiographs. Lymph node calcification may also be seen in patients with metastatic osteogenic sarcoma. Calcified hilar and mediastinal lymph nodes have been observed in AIDS patients with *Pneumocystis jiroveci* (formerly *P. carinii*) infection.

Although calcified lymph nodes generally indicate the presence of old disease, densely calcified nodes can remain functional and can become involved by other processes such as metastatic neoplasm (Table 8-14).

Calcified lymph nodes in the mediastinum or hila may erode into adjacent bronchi, resulting in *broncholithiasis*. This is most common in histoplasmosis and tuberculosis. The calcified node, or broncholith, may be expectorated or result in atelectasis, postobstructive pneumonia, or hemoptysis.

Low-Attenuation or Necrotic Lymph Nodes

After administration of intravenous contrast agent, enlarged lymph nodes may appear to be low in attenuation, often

---

TABLE 8-14. CALCIFIED LYMPH NODES

Common
Infectious granulomatous diseases
  Tuberculosis
  Fungal infections (histoplasmosis)
Sarcoidosis
Silicosis
Hodgkin's disease (usually following treatment)
Rare
Pneumocystis jiroveci (P. carinii) pneumonia
Metastases (mucinous adenocarcinoma)
Amyloidosis
Scleroderma
Castleman's disease

TABLE 8-15. LOW-DENSITY/NECROTIC LYMPH NODES

Common
Infectious granulomatous diseases
  Tuberculosis
  Fungal infections (histoplasmosis)
Metastases
  Lung cancer
  Extrathoracic malignancy
Lymphoma
Rare
Sarcoidosis

---

with an enhancing rim (Fig. 8-39). Typically, low-attenuation nodes reflect the presence of necrosis. They are commonly seen in patients with tuberculosis, fungal infections, and neoplasms such as metastatic carcinoma and lymphoma.

Necrotic lymph nodes are common in patients with active tuberculosis. After injection of intravenous contrast agent, nodes larger than 2 cm in diameter almost always show central areas of low attenuation with peripheral enhancement and an irregular wall. Smaller lymph nodes may also show this finding.

Low-density nodes also occur in patients with metastatic lung cancer (often when the primary tumor also appears necrotic), metastatic seminoma, and metastatic ovarian, thyroid, and gastric neoplasia (Table 8-15). Low-attenuation or necrotic lymph nodes are seen in 10% to 20% of patients with lymphoma, either before or after treatment. They have also been described in patients with a variety of other entities, including sarcoidosis.

Lymph Node Enhancement

Normal lymph nodes may show some increase in attenuation following intravenous contrast infusion. Pathologic lymph nodes with an increased vascular supply may increase significantly in attenuation. The differential diagnosis of densely enhancing mediastinal nodes is limited and includes Castleman's disease (Fig. 8-40A), angioimmunoblastic lymphadenopathy, vascular metastases (e.g., renal cell carcinoma, papillary thyroid carcinoma, lung carcinoma, sarcoma, and melanoma; see Fig. 8-40B), tuberculosis, and sometimes sarcoidosis (Table 8-16).

Differentiation between enhancing lymph nodes and enhancing mediastinal mass should be attempted. Enhancing masses include substernal thyroid and parathyroid lesions, carcinoid tumor, lymphangioma, hemangioma, and paraganglioma.

MR Evaluation of Mediastinal Lymph Nodes

MR is comparable to CT in identifying mediastinal and hilar lymph nodes, even though its spatial resolution is infe-

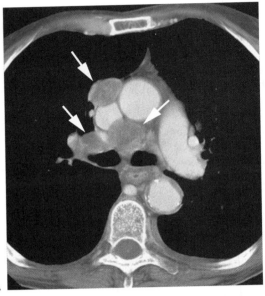

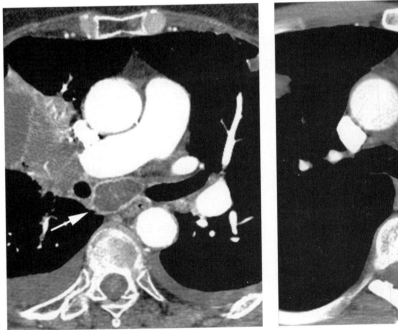

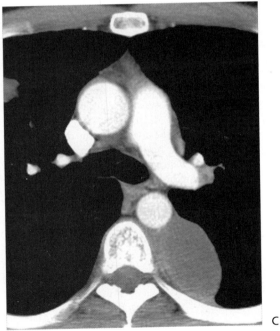

FIG. 8-39. Low-attenuation mediastinal lymph nodes. **A.** Metastatic carcinoma with enlarged low-attenuation lymph nodes *(arrows)*. **B.** Low-attenuation mediastinal lymph node with a densely enhancing rim *(arrow)* in metastatic breast carcinoma. Right lung consolidation and bilateral pleural effusions are also seen. **C.** Low-attenuation paravertebral lymph node metastasis from testicular carcinoma.

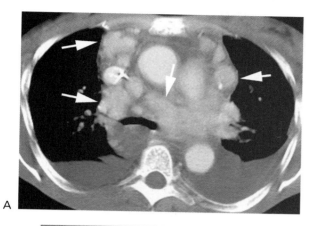

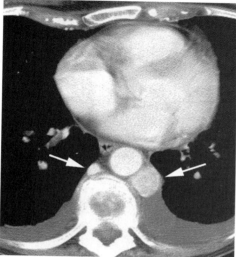

FIG. 8-40. Enhancing lymph nodes. **A.** Multiple enlarged lymph nodes *(arrows)* in multicentric plasma cell type Castleman's disease show dense enhancement. **B.** Enhancing paravertebral (para-aortic) lymph node metastases *(arrows)* from a paraganglioma.

rior. Although there are some differences in the MR characteristics of benign and malignant lymph nodes, their differentiation in individual cases is not possible. Furthermore, MR is unable to detect calcification, rendering identification of granulomatous nodes difficult. Low signal intensity

TABLE 8-16. ENHANCING LYMPH NODES

Common
Metastases (vascular tumors)
Tuberculosis
Rare
Castleman's disease
Sarcoidosis
Angioimmunoblastic lymphadenopathy

has been noted in calcified nodes on T2-weighted images in patients with fibrosing mediastinitis; however, this appearance is nonspecific.

LYMPHOMA

Lymphomas are primary neoplasms of the lymphoreticular system and are classified in two main types: HD and NHL. HD is the less common of the two types, representing about 25% to 30% of cases, but it is more common as a cause of mediastinal involvement. Lymphomas are discussed in detail in Chapter 5.

Hodgkin's Disease

HD has a predilection for thoracic involvement, and up to 85% of patients with HD present with mediastinal adenopathy. HD most often involves the superior mediastinal (prevascular, paratracheal, aortopulmonary) lymph nodes (Figs. 8-41 and 42; see also Figs. 5-1 to 5-7 in Chapter 5); if these nodes appear normal on CT, intrathoracic adenopathy is unlikely to represent HD.

Multiple node groups are commonly involved in patients with HD (see Fig. 8-42). In addition to superior mediastinal node groups, sites of lymph node enlargement, in order of decreasing frequency, include hilar nodes, subcarinal nodes, cardiophrenic angle (paracardiac) lymph nodes, internal mammary nodes, and posterior mediastinal nodes. Enlargement of lymph nodes in a single node group can be seen in some patients with HD, most commonly in the anterior (prevascular) mediastinum. This often indicates the presence of nodular sclerosing HD, which accounts for 50% to 80% of adult HD cases.

In patients with HD, enlarged lymph nodes are variable in appearance. Nodes are usually of homogeneous soft-tissue attenuation, but low attenuation or necrosis may be seen with contrast enhancement. Rarely nodes show fine flecks of calcification in untreated patients. Multiple enlarged lymph nodes are often seen, and they can be well defined and discrete, matted, or associated with diffuse mediastinal infiltration. HD also has a predilection for involvement of the thymus in association with mediastinal lymph node enlargement.

Non-Hodgkin's Lymphoma

The term *non-Hodgkin's lymphoma* refers to a diverse group of diseases, varying in radiologic findings, clinical presentation, course, and prognosis. In comparison to HD, these tumors are less common as causes of thoracic disease.

Thoracic involvement is about half as common with NHL (40% to 50%) as with HD (85%). As with HD, the most common thoracic abnormality in patients with NHL is mediastinal lymph node involvement, although the pat-

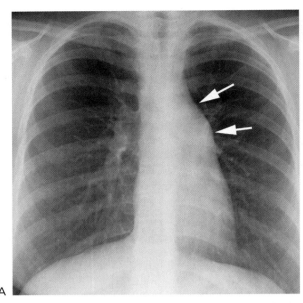
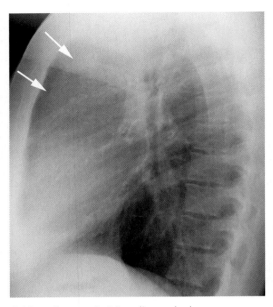

FIG. 8-41. Superior mediastinal lymph nodes in Hodgkin's disease. **A.** PA radiograph shows a mass *(arrows)* in the region of the aortopulmonary window. **B.** An anterior mediastinal mass *(arrows)* is visible on lateral chest radiograph.

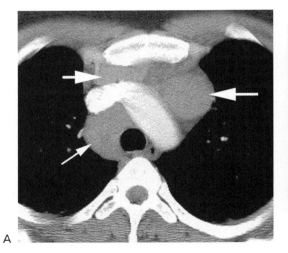
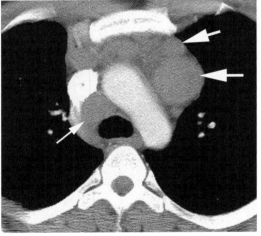

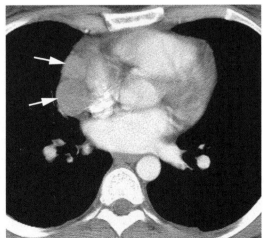

FIG. 8-42. Involvement of multiple lymph node groups in Hodgkin's disease. **A** and **B.** Involvement of pretracheal *(small arrows)* and prevascular *(large arrows)* nodes is common in Hodgkin's disease. **C.** At a lower level, paracardiac lymph node enlargement is also seen *(arrows)*.

tern of lymph node disease is different (see Figs. 5-15 to 5-19 in Chapter 5).

Involvement of one node group is much more common in patients with NHL: 40% of patients with NHL and thoracic involvement have involvement of only one node group. Enlargement of anterior mediastinal, internal mammary, paratracheal, and hilar nodes is much less common with NHL than with HD. Nonetheless, superior mediastinal node involvement is the most common abnormality seen: 35% of patients have superior mediastinal (prevascular and pretracheal) node involvement. Subcarinal lymph nodes, hilar nodes, and cardiophrenic nodes are less often abnormal. Involvement of posterior mediastinal nodal groups is much more common with NHL (10% of cases) than with HD. Rarely, calcification of nodes masses is seen.

LEUKEMIA

Mediastinal lymph nodes can be involved in patients with leukemia, particularly lymphocytic leukemia. On chest radiographs, enlarged mediastinal lymph nodes are visible in less than 20% of cases. Mediastinal lymph node enlargement is more common than hilar node enlargement.

In patients with acute or chronic myelogenous leukemia, masses of malignant myeloid precursor cells may be found in an extramedullary location; these masses are termed granulocytic sarcoma or chloroma. They most commonly are present at the time of first diagnosis of leukemia. In about 50% of cases, masses involve the mediastinum, either as a focal mass or generalized widening (see Figs. 5-34 and 5-35 in Chapter 5). Lymph node enlargement or mediastinal infiltration can be seen. Any portion of the mediastinum can be affected.

CASTLEMAN'S DISEASE

Castleman's disease (also referred to by a number of other terms, including angiofollicular mediastinal lymph node hyperplasia, angiomatous lymphoid hamartoma, and giant mediastinal lymph node hyperplasia) is a disease of unknown etiology. Histologically, two forms of the disease have been described: the hyaline-vascular type and the plasma cell type (Table 8-17). From a clinical standpoint, Castleman's disease (CD) is also classified as localized or multicentric.

The hyaline-vascular type of CD occurs in up to 90% of cases and is characterized histologically by lymph nodes having hypervascular hyaline germinal centers marked by extensive capillary proliferation. Patients with the hyaline-vascular type are usually children or young adults and are usually asymptomatic; their disease behaves in a benign fashion with cure following complete surgical resection. Up to 70% of patients have an asymptomatic, localized mediastinal mass (Fig. 8-43A).

TABLE 8-17. CASTLEMAN'S DISEASE

Angiofollicular lymph node hyperplasia
Hyaline-vascular and plasma cell types
Localized or multicentric
Dense enhancement on CT is typical
Hyaline-vascular type
  90% of cases
  Children or young adults
  Often asymptomatic
  Localized mediastinal or hilar mass
  Behaves in a benign fashion
Plasma cell type
  10% of cases
  Patients 40–50 years old
  Usually multicentric, multiple node groups
    involved
  Systemic illness
  Progressive

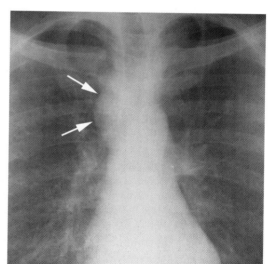

A

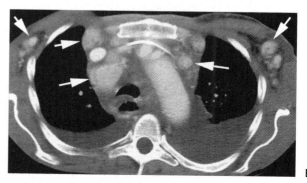

B

FIG. 8-43. Castleman's disease. **A.** Hyaline-vascular type Castleman's disease is manifested as a localized mediastinal mass *(arrows)* in an asymptomatic patient. **B.** Multiple densely enhancing lymph nodes *(arrows)* in a patient with multicentric plasma cell type Castleman's disease.

Unlike the hyaline-vascular type of CD, the plasma cell variety often presents as a multicentric process, associated with generalized lymphadenopathy and hepatosplenomegaly (see Figs. 8-40A and 8-43B). Most cases of multicentric CD are of the plasma cell variant, with some cases having mixed histology. Clinically, multicentric disease occurs in an older population than localized CD, with most patients being in their fifth or sixth decade. It often results in a systemic illness, associated with fever, anemia, infections, and malignancies such as lymphoma or Kaposi's sarcoma. When associated with localized node involvement, such systemic findings usually disappear following total resection; however, the multicentric form of disease is difficult to treat and usually progressive, even with the use of steroids and chemotherapeutic agents.

A plain radiograph may show a well-defined focal mass (localized CD), involving any part of the mediastinum (see Fig. 8-43A), or findings of lymph node enlargement (multicentric CD) (see Figs. 8-40A and 8-43B).

On contrast-enhanced CT, localized CD typically shows dense contrast enhancement; any mediastinal compartment can be involved. Central, dense, or flocculent lymph node calcifications are occasionally seen. Patients with multicentric CD evaluated using contrast-enhanced CT have shown early, dense, uniform enhancement of enlarged mediastinal lymph nodes. Axillary, abdominal, and other lymph node groups may also be involved.

OTHER LYMPHOPROLIFERATIVE DISORDERS

In addition to those diseases listed above, a variety of uncommon lymphoproliferative diseases affecting the lung can be associated with hilar or mediastinal lymph node enlargement. These include posttransplantation lymphoproliferative disorders, angioimmunoblastic lymphadenopathy, lymphoid interstitial pneumonitis, and lymphomatoid granulomatosis. Among these, lymph node enlargement is most common with angioimmunoblastic lymphadenopathy, a disease most common in patients over 50 years of age, characterized by enlarged, hypervascular lymph nodes, constitutional symptoms, and infections.

METASTATIC TUMOR

Metastases to mediastinal or hilar lymph nodes from extrathoracic malignancies are uncommon, occurring in less than 3% of cases. The extrathoracic tumors most likely to metastasize to the mediastinum are carcinomas of the head and neck, genitourinary tract, breast, and malignant melanoma. Metastases are discussed in detail in Chapter 4.

Most metastatic tumors cause lymph node enlargement without distinguishing characteristics. However, enhancing nodes may be seen secondary to metastatic renal cell carcinoma, papillary thyroid carcinoma, lung cancer, sarcomas, and melanoma. Lymph node metastases can also appear cystic or necrotic or calcified. Calcified lymph node metastases are most typical of thyroid carcinoma or mucinous adenocarcinoma.

The location of enlarged nodes is sometimes suggestive of the primary tumor site. Lymph node enlargement involving posterior mediastinal and paravertebral lymph nodes suggests an abdominal location for the primary tumor, and superior mediastinal lymph node involvement suggests a head and neck tumor. Internal mammary lymph node metastases are most like due to breast carcinoma. Paracardiac lymph node enlargement can occur as a result of metastasis from abdominal or thoracic tumors in approximately equal numbers. In studies reviewing the causes of paracardiac lymph node enlargement, although a variety of metastatic tumors were responsible, the most common were colon carcinoma, lung carcinoma, ovarian carcinoma, and breast carcinoma.

SARCOIDOSIS

Mediastinal lymph node enlargement is very common with sarcoidosis, occurring in 60% to 90% of patients at some stage in their disease. About half of these will also show findings of lung disease on plain radiographs. A greater percentage of patients with lymph node enlargement due to sarcoidosis show evidence of lung disease on CT.

Typically, node enlargement involves the hilar as well as mediastinal node groups, and lymph node masses appear bilateral and symmetrical on chest radiographs (Fig. 8-44A); the combination of bilateral hilar and paratracheal node enlargement usually allows the differentiation of sarcoidosis from lymphoma. The combination of (1) right paratracheal, (2) right hilar, and (3) left hilar node enlargement is termed the 1-2-3 pattern and is typical of sarcoidosis. In patients also having aortopulmonary node enlargement, a 1-2-3-4 pattern is said to be present (see Figs. 8-44A and 8-45A). The presence of hilar lymph node enlargement is so typical of sarcoidosis that the absence of this finding in a patient with mediastinal lymphadenopathy should lead one to question the diagnosis.

On chest radiographs, lymph node enlargement is seen, in order of decreasing frequency, in the hilar (85% to 95% of those with lymph node enlargement), right paratracheal (75%), aortopulmonary (50% to 75%), subcarinal (20%), and anterior mediastinal (10% to 15%) regions; internal mammary, paravertebral, and retrocrural lymph node enlargement can also be seen, but these locations are much less common (Table 8-18; see Figs. 8-44 and 8-45). Unilateral hilar lymph node enlargement shown on plain radiographs is seen in less than 5% of cases. Lymph node calcifi-

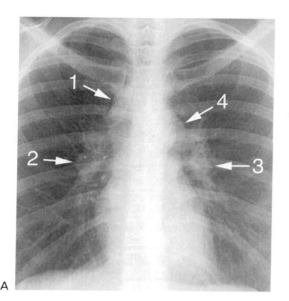

A

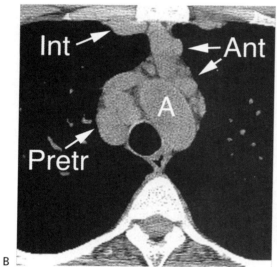

B

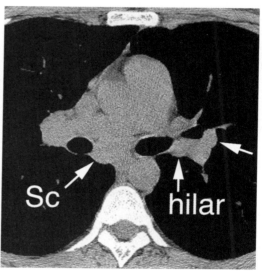

C

FIG. 8-44. Lymph node enlargement in sarcoidosis. **A.** PA chest radiograph shows the 1-2-3-4 pattern of symmetrical hilar and mediastinal lymph node enlargement. *1*, right paratracheal nodes; *2*, right hilar nodes; *3*, left hilar nodes; *4*, aortopulmonary window nodes. **B** and **C.** Enlarged lymph nodes involve the anterior mediastinum *(Ant)*, internal mammary nodes *(Int)*, pretracheal nodes *(Pretr)*, subcarinal space *(Sc)*, and hilar groups *(hilar)*. *A*, aorta.

TABLE 8-18. SARCOIDOSIS: FREQUENCY OF ENLARGED NODES SEEN ON CHEST RADIOGRAPH AND CT BY LYMPH NODE GROUP

Node group	Radiograph	CT
Hilar	85%–95%	90%
Right paratracheal	75%	100%
Aortopulmonary window	50%–75%	90%
Subcarinal	20%	65%
Anterior mediastinal	10%–15%	50%
Posterior mediastinal	<5%	15%

cation may be seen on chest films, appearing dense, stippled, or eggshell in appearance.

On CT, lymph node enlargement is visible in more than 80% to 95% of cases of sarcoidosis, with the great majority showing both hilar and mediastinal lymph node enlargement. A greater frequency of node enlargement is seen on CT than on chest radiographs, and symmetrical adenopathy is more often visible than on chest films.

In patients with sarcoidosis, lymph nodes can be several centimeters in diameter, but sarcoid is not generally associated with large localized masses as is lymphoma. Lymph node calcification is visible on CT in 25% to 50% of cases (see Fig. 8-45). As on chest radiographs, it may appear hazy or dense or have a stippled or eggshell appearance. Rarely nodes appear necrotic or low in attenuation or enhancing on contrast-enhanced scans.

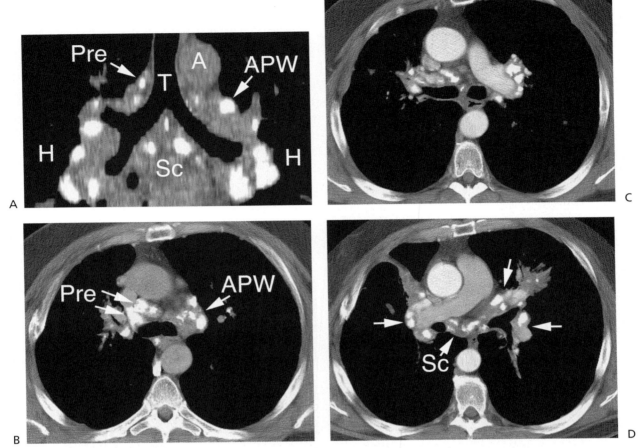

FIG. 8-45. Lymph node enlargement and calcification in sarcoidosis. **A.** Coronal reconstruction shows symmetric mediastinal and hilar involvement with sarcoidosis (i.e., the 1-2-3-4 pattern). The lymph nodes are densely calcified. *Pre,* pretracheal; *APW,* aortopulmonary window; *H,* hilar; *Sc,* subcarinal; *A,* aorta; *T,* trachea. **B.** Calcified pretracheal *(Pre)* and aortopulmonary window *(APW)* nodes in the same patient. **C.** Calcified precarinal and hilar nodes. **D.** Calcified subcarinal *(Sc)* and hilar nodes *(arrows).* Areas of consolidation represent atelectasis due to bronchial narrowing by nodes.

A variety of patterns of pulmonary involvement, from small nodules to large ill-defined masses or pulmonary fibrosis, can also be seen in patients with sarcoidosis (see Chapter 15). However, not all patients with active sarcoidosis show lymph node enlargement on CT. It is common to see typical features of sarcoid lung involvement on high-resolution CT without lymph node enlargement being visible.

INFECTIONS

A variety of infectious agents can cause mediastinal lymph node enlargement during the acute phase of disease. These include tuberculosis, a number of fungal infections including histoplasmosis and coccidioidomycosis, bacterial infections, and viral infections. Typically, there are symptoms and signs of acute infection and chest radiographs show evidence of lung disease, although this is not always the case. In patients with prior granulomatous infection, lymph node calcification is common, with such nodes appearing normal in size or enlarged.

Tuberculosis

Hilar and mediastinal lymph node enlargement is commonly seen on plain radiographs and CT in patients with active tuberculosis (Table 8-19), although it is more frequently seen in children than adults.

Lymph node enlargement is usually present on the side of lung disease (Fig. 8-46A), but involvement of contralateral nodes is sometimes present. Although the presence of lymphadenopathy on chest radiographs in the absence of visible

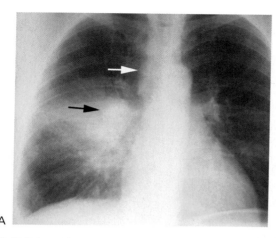

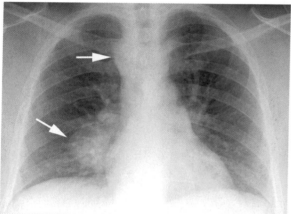

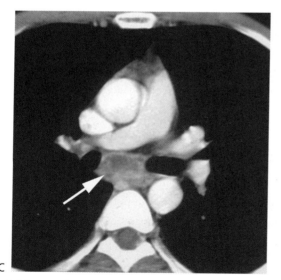

FIG. 8-46. Lymph node enlargement in tuberculosis. **A.** Primary tuberculosis with right lung consolidation, right hilar lymph node enlargement *(black arrow),* and right paratracheal lymph node enlargement manifested by widening of the right paratracheal stripe *(white arrow).* **B.** Tuberculosis in AIDS with right hilar and right paratracheal lymph node enlargement *(arrows).* **C.** Tuberculosis with a low-attenuation, rim-enhancing subcarinal lymph node mass *(arrow).*

TABLE 8-19. LYMPH NODE ENLARGEMENT IN PATIENTS WITH ACTIVE TUBERCULOSIS SHOWN ON CT

Site	ATS designation	% Abnormal
Right paratracheal	2R	80
Left paratracheal	2L	5
Right paratracheal	4R	85
Left paratracheal	4L	10
Right tracheobronchial	10R	65
Subcarinal	7	50
Aortopulmonary	5	35
Right hilar	11R	30
Left hilar	11L	10

lung disease is unusual in tuberculosis, this is not always the case (see Fig. 8-46B).

Right-sided adenopathy usually predominates, and specifically right paratracheal lymph node enlargement is most common (see Figs. 8-46A and B). Bilateral hilar lymph node enlargement is much less common than in sarcoidosis.

In patients with active tuberculosis, nodes larger than 2 cm in diameter commonly show central areas of low attenuation on contrast-enhanced CT, with peripheral rim enhancement (see Fig. 8-46C). The areas of relative low attenuation are not of water density, but range from about 40 to 60 HU; they are usually visible only on contrast-enhanced scans. Areas of low attenuation involving the mediastinum with obliteration of mediastinal fat represent tuberculous mediastinitis or a cold abscess. Rim-enhancing lymph nodes have also been reported in nearly 85% of AIDS patients with tuberculosis.

Three patterns of lymph node enlargement have been reported on MR in patients with tuberculosis, correlating with clinical symptoms and pathologic findings and paralleling the expected CT findings in such patients. In patients with necrosis and active TB, nodes are inhomogeneous with marked peripheral enhancement after injection of contrast material. Nodes with granulomatous inflammation, but without necrosis, appear relatively homogeneous and hyperintense to muscle on both T1- and T2-weighted images and enhance homogeneously after contrast infusion. Inactive fibrocalcific nodes are homogeneous and hypointense on both T1- and T2-weighted images, without enhancement after contrast infusion.

Histoplasmosis

Infection with *Histoplasma capsulatum* is a well-recognized cause of hilar and mediastinal lymph node enlargement. In patients with acute or subacute histoplasmosis, radiographs and CT may show paratracheal, subcarinal, and hilar lymph node enlargement. On CT, irregular enhancement, rim enhancement, and low-attenuation necrosis may be seen, as in patients with tuberculosis. Masses range up to several centimeters in diameter.

FIBROSING MEDIASTINITIS

In some patients with granulomatous disease involving mediastinal lymph nodes, extension of the disease process to involve surrounding mediastinal tissues results in extensive fibrosis (Table 8-20). This is termed fibrosing or granulomatous mediastinitis. Symptomatic encasement and/or compression of a number of mediastinal structures, particularly vessels, and the trachea or esophagus can result. The most common causes are histoplasmosis, tuberculosis, and sarcoidosis, but fibrosing mediastinitis can also be related to autoimmune disease, drugs, or retroperitoneal fibrosis, or it may be idiopathic.

Typically, enlarged lymph nodes seen on CT in patients with granulomatous disease such as histoplasmosis, tuberculosis, and sarcoidosis are sharply defined. Fibrosing mediastinitis is manifested on CT by replacement of low-density mediastinal fat by higher-density fibrous tissue, often associated with calcification. In the presence of fibrosing mediastinitis, discrete enlarged lymph nodes cannot be identified.

Manifestations on CT include hilar and mediastinal mass, stippled or diffuse calcification, and compression and/or encasement of the trachea, main bronchi, or mediastinal vessels (Fig. 8-47). Those structures most often involved are those that have the thinnest walls (e.g., superior vena cava) or the longest mediastinal course (e.g., trachea and left main bronchus and right pulmonary artery). In patients with fibrosing mediastinitis, the most common complications are narrowing or obstruction of the superior vena cava (40%), bronchi (35%), pulmonary artery (20%), and esophagus (10%). Rarely, these findings primarily affect the posterior mediastinum, with esophageal encasement and dysphagia predominating.

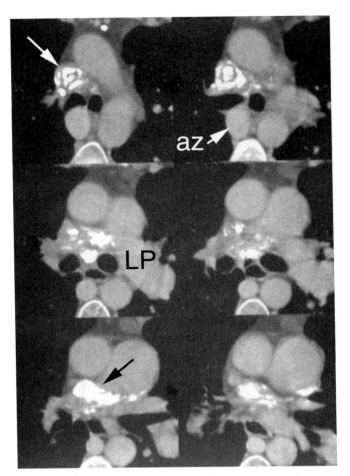

FIG. 8-47. Granulomatous mediastinitis due to histoplasmosis. CT at six levels shows extensive calcifications in the region of the superior vena cava *(white arrow at top left)* resulting in superior vena cava obstruction. The azygos vein *(az)*, serving as a collateral pathway, is enlarged. Calcifications at a lower level result in obstruction of the right pulmonary artery *(black arrow)*, and the left pulmonary artery *(LP)* is enlarged.

FATTY LESIONS

Fat is specifically recognized on CT by its low CT numbers, which vary from −40 to −130 HU. Fat is normally present in the mediastinum, and its amount often increases with age.

Normal fat is unencapsulated and equally distributed throughout the connective tissue matrix of the mediastinum. The contours of the mediastinum are not generally affected by normal amounts of fat. However, accumulations of fat in the anterior cardiophrenic angles, or epicardiac fat pads, can be asymmetric and can suggest the presence of a mass on chest radiographs.

Abnormalities of fat distribution can be diffuse (i.e., mediastinal lipomatosis) or focal (e.g., lipoma or fat-containing diaphragmatic hernias; Table 8-21). In the large majority

TABLE 8-20. FIBROSING MEDIASTINITIS

Causes
  Histoplasmosis
  Tuberculosis
  Sarcoidosis
  Autoimmune diseases
  Drugs
  Retroperitoneal fibrosis
  Idiopathic
Calcification common
Narrows superior vena cava, trachea, left main
  bronchus, right pulmonary artery

TABLE 8-21. MASSES CONTAINING FAT

Lipomatosis and fat pads
Lipoma or liposarcoma
Thymolipoma
Teratoma
Lymphangioma and hemangioma
Hernias containing fat
Extramedullary hematopoiesis

of cases, discovery of the fatty nature of a mass indicates its benign nature.

Mediastinal Lipomatosis

Lipomatosis is a benign condition in which excessive amounts of histologically normal, unencapsulated fat accumulate in the mediastinum. Lipomatosis may be associated with Cushing's syndrome, steroid treatment, or obesity, but these factors are absent in up to half of cases. It is unassociated with symptoms. Lipomatosis is relatively common and is often detected incidentally in patients having chest radiographs or CT.

The excess fat deposition is most prominent in the upper mediastinum, resulting in smooth symmetrical mediastinal widening as shown on chest radiographs (Fig. 8-48A) and convex or bulging mediastinal pleural surfaces on CT. The appearance of smooth mediastinal widening on a plain radiograph is characteristic of mediastinal lipomatosis and in patients with a suitable clinical history usually requires no further evaluation. Tracheal compression or displacement is absent. Less commonly, fat also accumulates in the cardiophrenic angles and paraspinal areas. In patients with lipomatosis, the fat should appear homogeneously low in attenuation, sharply outlining mediastinal vessels and lymph nodes (see Fig. 8-48B). If the fat appears inhomogeneous or the margins of mediastinal structures are ill defined, su-

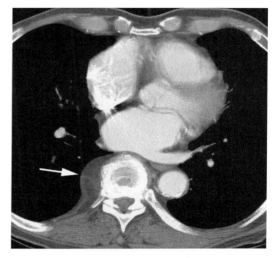

FIG. 8-49. Lipoma. A well-circumscribed fatty lesion is visible in the posterior mediastinum *(arrow)*.

perimposed processes such as mediastinitis, hemorrhage, tumor infiltration, or fibrosis may be present.

Lipoma and Liposarcoma

Mediastinal lipoma is uncommon, constituting approximately 2% of all mediastinal tumors. As with other mesenchymal tumors, lipomas can occur in any part of the mediastinum but are most common in the prevascular space. Lipomas are soft and pliable and do not result in symptomatic compression of adjacent structures unless they are very large. They may or may not be encapsulated. Lipomas appear homogeneously low in attenuation (Fig. 8-49). Their boundaries are typically smooth and sharply defined, and adjacent mediastinal structures appear well defined and sharply marginated.

Mediastinal liposarcoma and lipoblastoma are rare malignant tumors composed largely of fat. Histologic differentia-

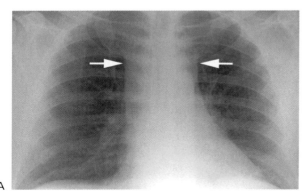

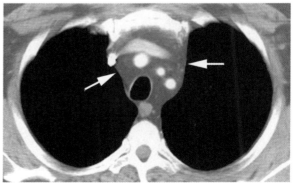

FIG. 8-48. Lipomatosis. **A.** Chest radiograph shows smooth symmetrical widening of the upper mediastinum. **B.** CT shows homogenous fat filling the mediastinum *(arrows)*.

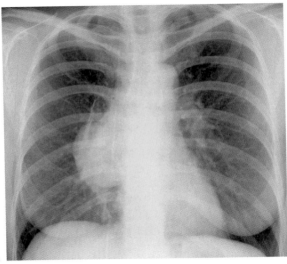

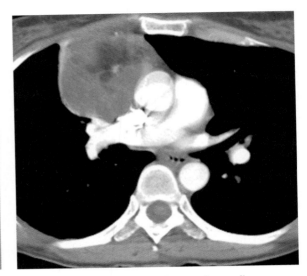

A   B

FIG. 8-50. Liposarcoma. **A.** Chest radiograph shows a right mediastinal mass. **B.** An anterior mediastinal mass contains both fat and soft tissue.

tion between a lipoma and well-differentiated liposarcoma depends on the presence of mitotic activity, cellular atypia, fibrosis, neovascularization, and tumor infiltration. CT findings suggesting liposarcoma or lipoblastoma include (1) inhomogeneous attenuation with evidence of significant amounts of soft tissue within the fatty mass (Fig. 8-50), (2) poor definition of adjacent mediastinal structures, or (3) evidence of infiltration or invasion of mediastinal structures. The diagnosis of a liposarcoma is often difficult using CT.

Hernias Containing Fat

There are several direct connections between the abdomen and mediastinum that permit passage of intraabdominal fat into the thorax.

Omental fat is freely mobile and can herniate through the foramen of Morgagni to create the appearance of a cardiophrenic angle mass, almost always on the right side (Fig. 8-51A). The transverse colon may accompany the omentum in patients with a Morgagni hernia. Fine linear densities are sometimes seen within herniated omental fat and probably represent omental vessels. When seen within a fatty mass, these linear densities should suggest fat herniation rather than a lipoma.

Fat herniation through the foramen of Bochdalek occurs most often on the left side since the presence of the liver limits its occurrence on the right. Although said to be most often located in the posterolateral diaphragm, they can occur anywhere along the posterior costodiaphragmatic

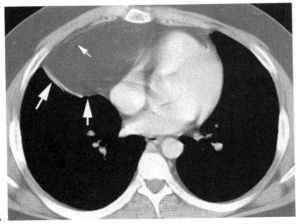

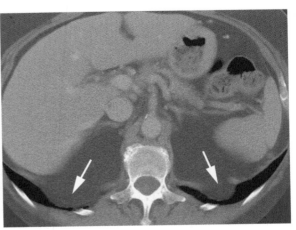

A   B

FIG. 8-51. Fatty hernias. **A.** Morgagni hernia *(large arrows)* projecting into the right cardiophrenic angle. The hernia consists of omentum. Omental vessels *(small arrow)* are visible within the fatty mass. **B.** Bochdalek hernias *(arrows)* containing fat.

margin and are often seen medially (see Fig. 8-51B). Bochdalek hernias in adults usually contain retroperitoneal fat, although kidney is occasionally present. CT has shown that small Bochdalek hernias occur in as many as 5% of normal individuals. Characteristically, a thinning or defect in the diaphragm is visible on CT, marginating the collection of fat. Lateral chest radiographs usually show a rounded mass in the posterior costophrenic angle.

Herniation of perigastric fat through the phrenicoesophageal membrane surrounding and fixating the esophagus to the diaphragm is the first step in the pathogenesis of hiatus hernias. The herniated fat can extend along the aorta and widen the paraspinal line, or it can appear as a retrocardiac mass.

On MRI, fat has high signal intensity on both T1- and T2-weighted sequences, appearing identical to subcutaneous fat.

Other Fatty Masses

Other rare, fatty lesions have been reported to involve the mediastinum. Thymolipoma usually appears on CT as a large fatty mass in the anterior mediastinum, containing wisps or strands of fibrous tissue. Fat is also commonly identifiable as a component of mediastinal germ cell tumors. In the posterior mediastinum, spinal lipomas rarely present as primary mediastinal masses. Fatty transformation of thoracic extramedullary hematopoiesis may be seen in the posterior mediastinum.

MEDIASTINAL CYSTS

Most mediastinal cysts are of congenital origin. Bronchogenic cyst, esophageal duplication cyst, and neurenteric cyst result from abnormalities in foregut development and are termed foregut duplication cysts. Pericardial cysts are mesothelial in origin. Thymic cyst, described above, may be congenital or acquired. Cysts account for about 10% of primary mediastinal masses in both adults and children.

Bronchogenic Cysts

Bronchogenic cysts are most common, representing about 60% of foregut duplication cysts (Table 8-22). They proba-

TABLE 8-22. BRONCHOGENIC CYST

60% of foregut duplication cysts
Wall contains respiratory epithelium, smooth muscle, mucous glands, or cartilage
50% subcarinal; 20% paratracheal; 10% retrocardiac
Round, smooth, sharply defined
Wall thin or invisible on CT; wall may calcify
Fluid contents variable in attenuation on CT (0–40 HU)

bly result from defective growth of the lung bud during fetal development. Bronchogenic cysts are lined by pseudostratified ciliated columnar epithelium, typical of the respiratory system, and frequently are associated with smooth muscle, mucous glands, or cartilage in the cyst wall. Bronchogenic cysts contain fluid, which ranges in color from clear to milky white to brown; the fluid can contain variable amounts of protein and can be serous, hemorrhagic, or highly viscous and gelatinous. Cyst fluid rarely contains milk of calcium.

Bronchogenic cysts can be present in any part of the mediastinum but are most commonly located in the middle or posterior mediastinum, near the carina (50%), in the paratracheal region (20%), adjacent to the esophagus (15%), or in a retrocardiac location (10%). Most occur in contact with the tracheobronchial tree and within 5 cm of the carina. A subcarinal location is most frequently seen. They rarely occur in the anterior mediastinum or the inferior aspect of the posterior mediastinum.

On plain radiographs, bronchogenic cysts appear as smooth, sharply marginated, round or elliptical masses (Fig. 8-52A). They may be large and displace the trachea or bronchi. Subcarinal cysts may result in convexity in the superior aspect of the azygoesophageal recess.

On CT, bronchogenic cysts usually appear rounded or elliptical, smooth in contour; as on chest radiographs, they are sharply marginated (see Figs. 8-52B and 8-53A and B). The wall of a bronchogenic cyst appears thin or is imperceptible (see Fig. 8-52B). Rarely, calcification of the cyst wall is present. Because of the variable composition of the fluid contained within bronchogenic cysts, their attenuation on CT is highly variable. Half of bronchogenic cysts are of water attenuation; in the other half, the CT density ranges from being higher than water to higher than muscle. When dense, bronchogenic cysts may be difficult to distinguish from solid lesions. An important clue to the diagnosis can be their lack of enhancement on scans obtained following intravenous contrast infusion. Mediastinal bronchogenic cysts rarely contain air or become infected, although this is common in patients with pulmonary bronchogenic cysts.

MR is valuable in assessing cysts that do not appear fluid-filled on CT. High signal intensity is characteristically seen within cysts on T2-weighted sequences regardless of the nature of the cyst contents, but a variable pattern of signal intensity may be seen on T1-weighted sequences, presumably because of variable cyst contents and the presence of protein or mucoid material and/or hemorrhage (see Figs. 8-53C and D). A high intensity on T1-weighted images reflects high protein content and is common with bronchogenic cysts.

Large bronchogenic cysts may be associated with symptoms because of compression of adjacent structures such as the trachea and carina, mediastinal vessels, and left atrium. Small, asymptomatic cysts can be followed. However, enlargement over years is typical, and rapid enlargement asso-

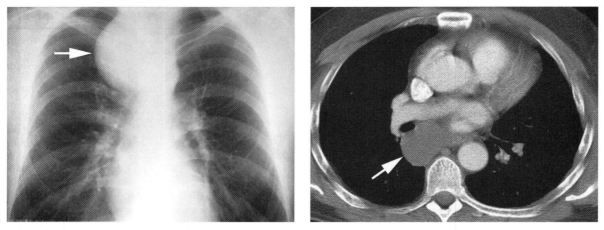

FIG. 8-52. Bronchogenic cysts. **A.** A large smooth round right mediastinal mass *(arrow)* is visible on chest radiograph. **B.** In another patient, a low-attenuation subcarinal bronchogenic cyst *(arrow)* is visible. The cyst wall is invisible.

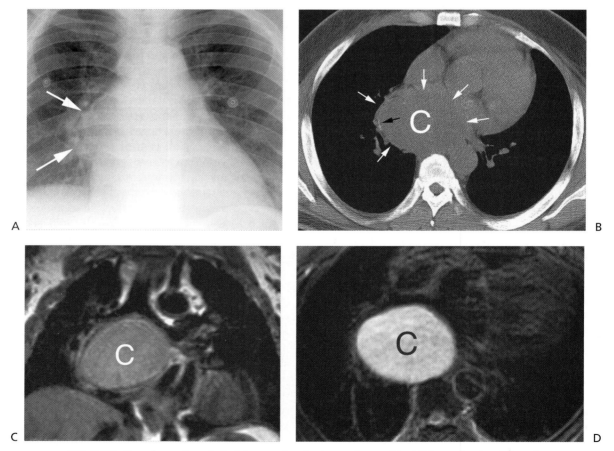

FIG. 8-53. Bronchogenic cyst. **A.** A large subcarinal mass *(arrows)* is visible on chest radiograph. **B.** Unenhanced CT shows a large subcarinal bronchogenic cyst *(C, white arrows)*, appearing slightly less dense than soft tissue. Focal calcification of the cyst wall is visible *(black arrow)* **C.** Coronal T1-weighted MRI shows a large subcarinal cyst. Signal from the cyst *(C)* is due to its protein content. **D.** Transaxial T2-weighted, fat-saturated image shows high signal intensity. This is typical. C, cyst.

ciated with pain can indicate hemorrhage or infection. Because of their tendency to enlarge, surgical management has been traditional. Recently, percutaneous and transbronchial needle aspiration has also been used for the diagnosis and treatment of bronchogenic and esophageal duplication cysts.

Esophageal Duplication Cysts

Esophageal duplication cysts are lined by gastrointestinal tract mucosa and are often connected to the esophagus; unlike bronchogenic cysts, they do not contain cartilage. Sixty percent are found in the lower posterior mediastinum, adjacent to the esophagus, and are sometimes found within its wall. Their appearance on plain radiographs and CT and MRI is indistinguishable from that of bronchogenic cysts, except for their paraesophageal location (Fig. 8-54). Rarely, the cyst wall calcifies.

Neurenteric Cysts

This rare cyst is connected to the meninges through a midline defect in one or more vertebral bodies. They are composed of both neural and gastrointestinal elements, including gastric, salivary gland, adrenal, pancreatic, and intestinal tissues. A connection with the esophagus is often present. The appearance of neurenteric cyst on CT is the same as that of other duplication cysts, but the presence of a vertebral abnormality can point to the diagnosis (Fig. 8-55); vertebral anomalies (e.g., hemivertebrae or butterfly vertebrae) or scoliosis are present in about half of cases. The cysts rarely contain air, because of communication with the esophagus.

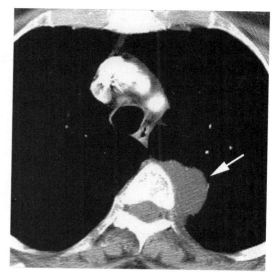

FIG. 8-55. Neurenteric cyst. A low-attenuation paravertebral cystic lesion *(arrow)* is associated with scoliosis.

They frequently cause pain and are generally diagnosed at a young age.

Pericardial Cysts

Pericardial cyst represents a defect in the embryogenesis of the coelomic cavity. The wall of a pericardial cyst is composed of connective tissue and a single layer of mesothelial cells. Most patients are asymptomatic.

On plain radiographs, pericardial cysts are smooth and sharply marginated (Fig. 8-56A). Approximately 90% of

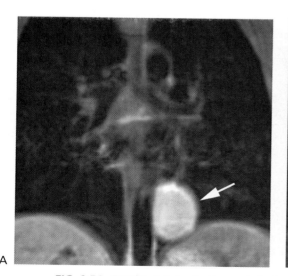
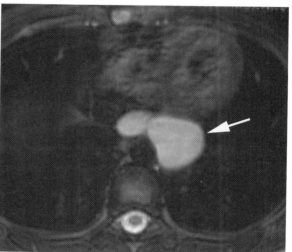

FIG. 8-54. Esophageal duplication cyst. **A.** Coronal MR shows a paraesophageal cyst *(arrow)*. **B.** Transaxial T2-weighted, fat-saturated image shows high signal intensity typical of cyst *(arrow)*. The cyst is paraesophageal in location.

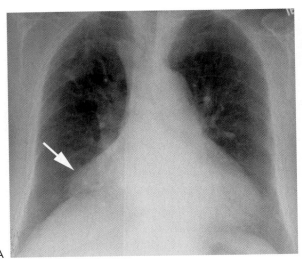
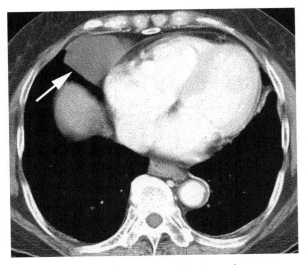

FIG. 8-56. Pericardial cyst. **A.** Chest radiograph shows a mass in the right cardiophrenic angle *(arrow)*. **B.** CT shows a low-attenuation cyst *(arrow)* contacting the pericardium.

pericardial cysts contact the diaphragm, with 65% occurring the right cardiophrenic angle and 25% in the left cardiophrenic angle. In this location, they sometimes are seen to extend into the major fissure, having a lenticular shape on lateral chest films. Ten percent of pericardial cysts do not touch the diaphragm and are seen at higher levels, contiguous with the proximal aorta or pulmonary arteries.

On CT, they appear sharply marginated and have low CT numbers (see Fig. 8-56B); however, pericardial cysts with high CT numbers are occasionally seen. When occurring within the upper mediastinum, they may be seen to have a relationship to the superior pericardial recesses. Pericardial cysts are not always round; they may assume different shapes when studied at different times. On MRI, pericardial cysts containing serous fluid appear less intense than muscle on T1-weighted images.

Mediastinal Pseudocysts

Pancreatic pseudocyst represents an encapsulated collection of pancreatic secretions, blood, and necrotic material. Mediastinal extension of a pancreatic pseudocyst is rare but can occur via the aortic hiatus or esophageal hiatus or through a defect in the diaphragm. Symptoms are generally those of pancreatitis.

Plain radiographs may show a retrocardiac mediastinal mass. CT shows a cystic and low-attenuation mass in the posterior mediastinum or adjacent thoracic cavity, associated with compression or displacement of the esophagus or splaying of the diaphragmatic crura. Mediastinal pseudocysts are commonly located under and posterior to the heart, anterior to the aorta and esophagus, and medial to the inferior vena cava. The fluid can be of water density or higher, depending on the presence of blood or infection.

An abdominal fluid collection is common but not invariably present.

Other Cystic Lesions

Cystic or fluid-filled mediastinal lesion may represent congenital cysts or cystic masses (Table 8-23). Differentiation of an uncomplicated congenital cyst from other cystic encapsulated lesions, such as abscess, chronic hematoma, cystic lymphangioma or hemangioma, cystic teratoma, or other cystic tumor relies on the clinical presentation, findings on correlative radiographic studies, and the location and CT appearance of the cyst. Abscess, hematoma, and cystic tumors commonly demonstrate thick or irregular walls, septations, and mixed-density fluids. Cystic masses of the anterior mediastinum rarely represent a congenital cyst but are

TABLE 8-23. CYSTIC, LOW-ATTENUATION, OR FLUID-FILLED MASSES

Congenital or acquired cysts (bronchogenic, esophageal, neurenteric, pericardial, and thymic)
Necrotic or cystic neoplasms (germ cell tumors, cystic thymoma, lymphoma)
Necrotic lymph nodes
Cystic lymphangioma (hygroma)
Thoracic meningocele
Mediastinal abscess
Mediastinal hematoma
Mediastinal pseudocyst
Cystic goiter
Dilated, fluid-filled esophagus
Pericardial fluid collections

more likely related to the presence of a cystic tumor or a thymic cyst. Anterior or lateral meningocele may closely resemble a congenital cyst, but careful examination of adjacent sections should demonstrate the intraspinal connection of the mass through the neural foramen.

VASCULAR TUMORS

Lymphangiomas and Cystic Hygromas

Lymphangiomas are rare benign lesions of lymphatic origin and represent 1% to 5% of mediastinal tumors; most are present at birth and are detected in the first 2 years of life (Table 8-24). Patients may be asymptomatic, but compression of mediastinal structures can result in chest pain, cough, or dyspnea. Because of a tendency for local growth, surgery is recommended. Lymphangioma can be seen in adults, with or without a history of incomplete resection as a child.

Lymphangiomas are most common in the neck (75%) and axilla (20%). Although 10% of cervical lymphangiomas extend into the mediastinum, less than 5% of lymphangiomas are limited to the mediastinum. In adults, it is common for lymphangioma to be localized to the mediastinum.

Lymphangiomas are classified as capillary, cavernous, or cystic (hygroma), depending on the size of the lymph channels they contain. Cystic lymphangioma is most common, accounting for more than 60% cases of lymphangioma in adults (Fig. 8-57). Cystic lymphangioma may be either unilocular or multilocular and can contain either serous or chylous fluid; thin septations within the mass are sometimes seen. In adults, lymphangiomas are most common in the anterior (25% to 35%) or superior (15% to 35%) mediastinum but are also seen in the middle (20% to 25%) and posterior (15% to 30%) mediastinum. They can be quite large, ranging up to 30 cm in diameter.

On plain radiographs, a focal mass in the upper mediastinum may be visible or diffuse mediastinal widening may be seen (Fig. 8-58). An increase in cervical soft tissues may be associated.

On CT, the attenuation of lymphangioma is usually ho-

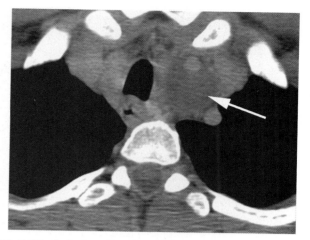

FIG. 8-57. Cystic lymphangioma (hygroma). A low-attenuation lesion *(arrow)* is visible in the superior mediastinum.

mogeneous and near to that of water (see Fig. 8-57), but they can be of higher attenuation or variably composed of a combination of fluid, solid tissue, and fat (see Fig. 8-58); calcification is rare. Although they are usually well circumscribed and localized, they may appear to envelop mediastinal structures. Lymphangioma may be associated with vascular malformations that are easily identifiable following the administration of intravenous contrast. Simple lymphangiomas and hemangiomas composed of capillary-sized, thin-walled channels may appear as solid masses. On MR, heterogeneous signal is typical, with increased signal on T2-weighted images reflecting their fluid content (see Fig. 8-58).

Hemangiomas

Hemangiomas are rare benign vascular tumors, accounting for less than 0.5% of mediastinal masses. They are composed of large interconnecting vascular channels with regions of thrombosis and varying amounts of interposed stroma, such as fat and fibrous tissue. Tumors are categorized according to the size and nature of their vascular spaces as capillary, cavernous, or venous; cavernous hemangiomas make up about 75% of cases. They are well defined and rarely are invasive.

Mediastinal hemangiomas are most common in young patients: about 75% present before the age of 35. One third to one half of cases are asymptomatic, but some patients present with symptoms of compression of mediastinal structures. Occasional cases are associated with peripheral hemangiomas or Osler-Weber-Rendu syndrome.

Hemangiomas most commonly arise in the anterior mediastinum (45% to 70% of cases) and posterior mediastinum (20% to 35% of cases). Extension into the neck may occur (7%). Masses may appear well marginated on CT (70%), inseparable from adjacent mediastinal structures

TABLE 8-24. LYMPHANGIOMA

1%–5% of mediastinal tumors
Usually present in childhood
Compression of mediastinal structures
Most common in neck (75%) and axilla (20%)
10% of cervical masses extend into mediastinum
5% limited to mediastinum
Classified as capillary, cavernous, or cystic (hygroma)
Unilocular or multilocular cystic masses
Contain serous or chylous fluid
May contain fat and enhancing vessels

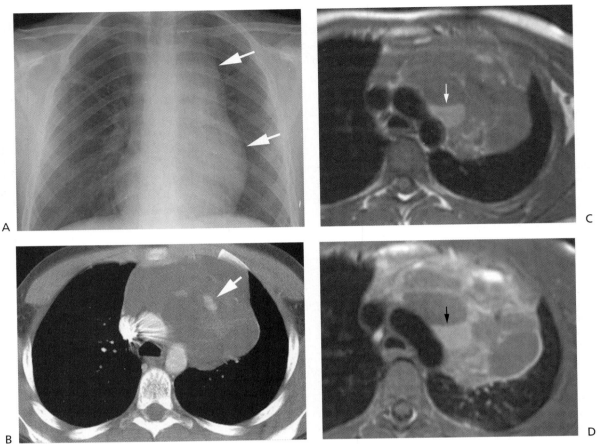

FIG. 8-58. Lymphangioma in a young boy. **A.** Chest radiograph shows a mass *(arrows)* involving the left superior mediastinum, obscuring the left heart border. **B.** Contrast-enhanced CT shows a multicystic mass containing enhancing vessels *(arrow)*. **C.** Transaxial T1-weighted image shows a large cystic mass with a fluid-fluid level *(arrow)*. **D.** Transaxial T2-weighted image shows a complex cystic mass. The fluid-fluid level is visible *(arrow)*.

(21%), or diffusely infiltrative (7%). Apparent infiltration may or may not predict unresectability.

On CT, tumors are often heterogeneous in attenuation on unenhanced scans, and fat is occasionally seen within them. Heterogeneous enhancement is typical following contrast infusion but is not always present. Enhancement may be dense, multifocal, or diffuse, and central or peripheral. Opacified vascular channels can be seen within the mass, with rapid enhancement similar to that of normal mediastinal vessels. Phleboliths, thought to be pathognomonic, are visible in up to 10% of cases on plain radiographs. On CT, punctate calcifications or phleboliths are visible in 10% to 20%.

Other Vascular Lesions

Other mediastinal lesions may be associated with significant enhancement following contrast infusion (Table 8-25).

ESOPHAGUS

At successive levels in the mediastinum, the esophagus is in intimate contact anteriorly with the posterior or posterolateral trachea, the left mainstem bronchus, and the left atrium. The esophagus lies between the aorta on the left and the azygos vein on the right. Intraluminal air or a small amount of fluid is common and a normal finding with CT. Evalua-

TABLE 8-25. ENHANCING MASSES

Mediastinal thyroid glands or masses
Ectopic parathyroid glands or masses
Carcinoid tumors
Lymphangioma
Hemangioma
Paraganglioma
Castleman's disease

tion of esophageal disease is limited if the esophagus is incompletely distended.

CT has several distinct indications in patients with suspected esophageal disease. It is indicated (1) to evaluate and stage patients with esophageal carcinoma and to provide a means for assessing response to therapy and resultant complications, (2) to evaluate and characterize esophageal contour abnormalities detected at esophagography, and their relationship to intrinsic or extrinsic masses, and (3) to evaluate patients with suspected esophageal perforation and to assess the extent of pleural and mediastinal fluid collections.

Esophageal Carcinoma

Esophageal carcinoma represents approximately 10% of all cancers of the gastrointestinal tract. Excluding adenocarcinomas of gastric origin with secondary esophageal involvement, 90% to 95% of esophageal tumors are squamous cell carcinomas. These tumors usually present in an advanced stage, with 5-year survival rates varying between 3% and 20%. This poor prognosis results from rapid submucosal extension of the tumor and early transmural invasion. This leads to early spread to regional and distal lymphatics as well as the liver, adrenals, and lung. Esophageal carcinoma often presents with symptoms of obstruction, and incidental detection with plain radiographs or CT is unusual.

Plain radiographs show some abnormality in about half of patients with esophageal carcinoma, including an abnormal convexity of the azygoesophageal recess (25%), mediastinal widening (20%), a retrotracheal mass (15%) or thickening of the posterior tracheal band (10%), and tracheal displacement (10%).

The CT manifestations of esophageal carcinoma include (1) narrowing of the esophageal lumen or dilatation due to obstruction; (2) thickening of the esophageal wall, either symmetrical or asymmetrical; (3) loss of periesophageal fat planes, with or without evidence of invasion of surrounding organs; and (4) periesophageal adenopathy. Wall thickening must be distinguished from idiopathic muscular hypertrophy of the esophagus.

Mesenchymal Tumors

Benign tumors of the esophagus, arising from components of the esophageal wall, include leiomyoma, fibroma, and lipoma. Unlike esophageal carcinoma, these tumors may be detected incidentally as a mediastinal mass in asymptomatic patients. Leiomyoma is most common and predominates in the middle and lower esophagus. An abnormality in the subcarinal space or involving the azygoesophageal recess may be seen (Fig. 8-59). On lateral radiographs, an abnormality of the posterior tracheal band may be seen.

Esophageal Dilatation

Esophageal dilatation may result from obstructing tumors, stricture, or achalasia. Achalasia or strictures secondary to

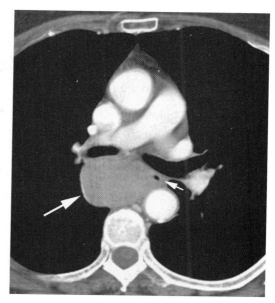

FIG. 8-59. Esophageal leiomyoma. An enhancing mass *(large arrow)* is present in the subcarinal space, contiguous with the esophagus *(small arrow)*.

scleroderma are usually associated with the greatest degree of esophageal dilatation. An increase in air or fluid in the esophageal lumen and retained ingested material are common findings.

With marked esophageal dilatation, or megaesophagus, the esophagus usually projects to the right of the mediastinum, with a marked abnormality of the azygoesophageal recess seen on the chest radiograph (Fig. 8-60A). The left wall of the dilated distal esophagus is often visible in a left retrocardiac location. The trachea may be displaced forward if the upper esophagus is dilated, and there may be thickening of the posterior tracheal band or filling in of the retrotracheal triangle. An air-fluid level may be seen (see Figs. 8-60A and B); this is most common with achalasia. CT shows dilatation of the esophageal lumen with air, air and fluid, and sometimes air-fluid or fat-fluid levels (see Figs. 8-60C and D).

Esophageal Varices

Esophageal or paraesophageal varices occur because of portal hypertension or, less often, systemic venous obstruction. They occasionally result in a chest film abnormality. Findings include convexity of the inferior aspect of the azygoesophageal interface, paravertebral widening (Fig. 8-61A), and dilatation of the azygos arch. Typically, plain film findings are nonspecific, necessitating differentiation from enlarged periesophageal lymph nodes or other posterior mediastinal masses.

CT is able to detect both esophageal and paraesophageal

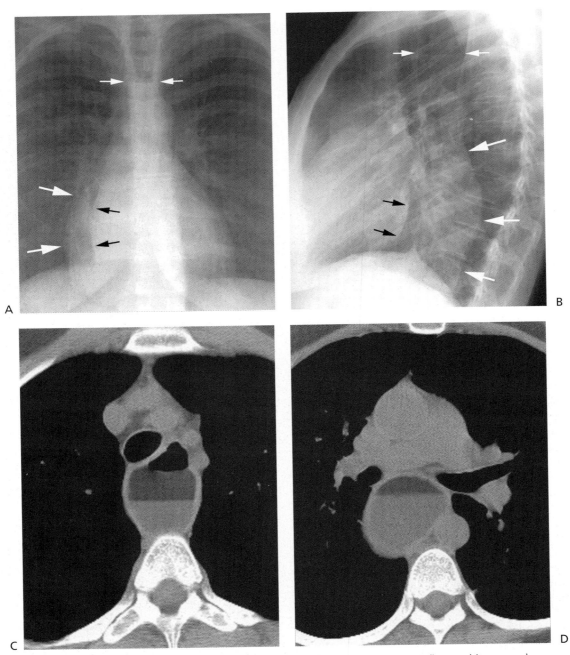

FIG. 8-60. Achalasia. **A.** PA chest radiograph shows the dilated esophagus *(large white arrows)* projecting to the right of the right heart border *(black arrows).* An air-fluid level is visible in the esophagus *(small white arrows).* **B.** Lateral chest radiograph shows the dilated esophagus *(large white arrows)* projecting posterior to the heart border *(black arrows).* The air-fluid level is also visible *(small white arrows)* on the lateral view. **C** and **D.** The dilated esophagus shows air-fluid and fluid-fluid levels.

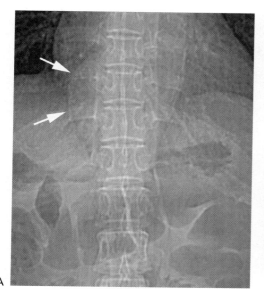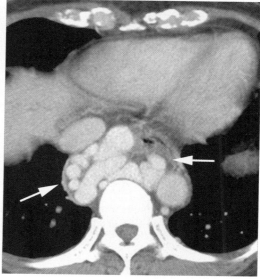

FIG. 8-61. Paraesophageal varices appearing as a mediastinal mass in a patient with hepatitis B and portal hypertension. **A.** Scout view shows a convex right posterior mediastinal mass *(arrows)*. **B.** CT shows very large paraesophageal varices *(arrows)*. The air-filled esophagus is also visible.

varices. Serpiginous soft-tissue opacities may be seen on unenhanced scans, sometimes indenting the wall of the air-filled esophagus (see Fig. 8-61B). Using CT with intravenous contrast, esophageal and paraesophageal varices are easily diagnosed.

Hiatal Hernia

Hiatal hernia represents a protrusion of a portion of the stomach through the esophageal hiatus. The esophageal hiatus is an elliptical opening just to the left of the midline, corresponding superiorly to the level of the tenth thoracic vertebral body. It is margined on each side by the diaphragmatic crura. Variation in the normal appearance of the crura is common.

In patients with hiatal hernia, chest radiographs show characteristic findings of convexity of the lower aspect of the azygoesophageal interface, sometimes with a similar convexity of the preaortic recess in a retrocardiac location. Air or air and fluid may be seen in association with this convexity. On the lateral view, a retrocardiac opacity may be seen but is usually less conspicuous.

In a patient with sliding hiatal hernia, the most common CT abnormality identified is dehiscence of the diaphragmatic crura, visible as widening of the esophageal hiatus on cross section, with projection of a portion of the stomach into the mediastinum. The width of the esophageal hiatus, defined as the distance between the medial margins of the crura, has a maximum normal value of 15 mm. Sliding hiatal hernias are frequently associated with an increase in the amount of fat surrounding the distal esophagus, secondary to herniation of omentum.

MEDIASTINITIS AND MEDIASTINAL ABSCESS

Acute mediastinal infections are uncommon and usually related to surgery, esophageal perforation, or spread of infection from adjacent regions. Infections may be classified as diffuse mediastinitis or mediastinal abscess, depending on their extent. Diffuse mediastinitis has a relatively poor prognosis.

Plain radiographs generally show diffuse mediastinal widening, most commonly involving the upper mediastinum (Fig. 8-62A). Pneumomediastinum and subcutaneous emphysema may be seen in the neck (see Fig. 8-62A); pneumothorax and pleural effusion may also be associated, depending of the cause of the infection. These are common with esophageal perforation, either spontaneous (Boerhaave's syndrome), posttraumatic, or iatrogenic, complicating endoscopy, esophageal dilatation, attempted intubation, or surgery. Distal esophageal perforation usually results in left-sided pleural abnormalities, while upper or midesophageal perforation usually results in right-sided abnormalities.

CT findings in mediastinitis include diffuse or streaky edema and increased attenuation of mediastinal fat; mediastinal widening; localized fluid collections, sometimes with a thick or enhancing wall; pleural or pericardial effusion; lymph node enlargement; and compression of mediastinal

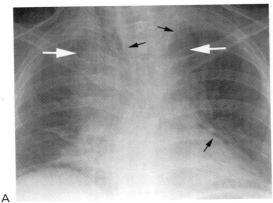
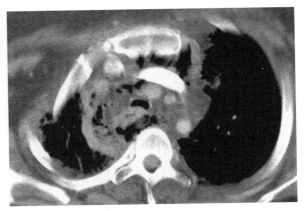

FIG. 8-62. Mediastinitis secondary to esophageal perforation. **A.** The mediastinum is widened *(white arrows)* and streaky pneumomediastinum is visible *(black arrows)*. Air extends into the neck. **B.** CT shows mediastinal widening, increased attenuation of mediastinal fat, and pneumomediastinum.

structures (see Fig. 8-62B). Gas bubbles in the mediastinum, with or without associated fluid collections, are seen in up to half of cases and are an important finding in diagnosis. In patients with an abscess, a localized fluid-filled space is visible, often containing air.

Many cases of mediastinitis occur after median sternotomy. In subjects having CT after an uncomplicated sternotomy, findings can closely mimic the appearance of mediastinitis, and abnormal findings can persist for up to 3 weeks. More than 75% of patients having median sternotomy show retrosternal fluid collections, air, hematoma, or a combination of these in the early postoperative period. However, after 2 weeks, these abnormalities should largely resolve.

PARASPINAL ABNORMALITIES

A wide variety of pathologic processes may involve the paraspinal regions. Most frequently, paraspinal masses are neural in origin, including neurogenic tumors, neurenteric cyst, and anterior or lateral thoracic meningocele, or are related to the spine. Infections involving the spine may lead to the development of paraspinal abscess. In addition, lymphoma and other causes of lymph node enlargement may result in abnormalities in this region; paraspinal lymph nodes freely communicate with lymph nodes in the upper abdomen, and contiguous involvement is common. Since the mediastinum communicates with the retroperitoneal space via the esophageal hiatus, aortic hiatus, and other defects in the diaphragm, diseases can spread between the abdomen and thorax by direct extension; inflammatory masses such as pancreatic pseudocysts can involve the paraspinal mediastinal regions. Rare entities such as extramedullary hematopoiesis, primary myelolipomas of the mediastinum, be-

nign hemangioendotheliomas, aggressive fibromatosis, and fibrosing mediastinitis have been reported in the paravertebral regions.

Neurogenic Tumors

Neurogenic tumors account for about 10% to 20% of primary mediastinal masses in adults and 30% to 35% of mediastinal tumors in children. Seventy-five percent of posterior mediastinal masses are neurogenic tumors. Tumors may arise from peripheral nerves and nerve sheath (neurofibroma, schwannoma, malignant peripheral nerve-sheath tumors) or sympathetic ganglia (ganglioneuroma, ganglioneuroblastoma, neuroblastoma). The most common cell types are schwannoma (35%), ganglioneuroma (25%), neuroblastoma (15% to 20%), ganglioneuroblastomas (7% to 15%), and neurofibroma (5% to 10%), but the incidence varies with the patient's age. Eighty percent are benign.

Nearly 85% of tumors in children are of ganglionic origin, while in adults more than 75% are nerve sheath tumors. Specifically, schwannoma and neurofibroma are more common in adults, while ganglioneuroblastoma and neuroblastoma are more common in children. The mean age at diagnosis is about 5 years for neuroblastoma, 10 years for ganglioneuroblastoma, 20 years for ganglioneuroma, 30 years for neurofibroma, and 40 years for schwannoma.

Neurogenic tumors occurring in the superior mediastinum commonly show a finding termed the "cervicothoracic" sign on plain radiographs. The sign is said to be present if a mediastinal mass shows a sharply marginated border outlined by lung above the level of the clavicles. Only posterior mediastinal masses show this finding. Above the level of the clavicles, anterior and middle mediastinal masses enter the neck and are no longer outlined by lung (i.e., they no longer have a sharply marginated border).

TABLE 8-26. PERIPHERAL NERVE SHEATH TUMORS

Neurilemmoma (schwannoma), neurofibroma, and neurogenic sarcoma
Most common in adults
Round, elliptical, or lobulated paravertebral mass
Often one or two interspaces in length
Rib or vertebral abnormalities in 50%
Lower attenuation than muscle in 70%
One third of patients with neurofibromas have neurofibromatosis
Plexiform neurofibroma: extensive fusiform or infiltrating mass

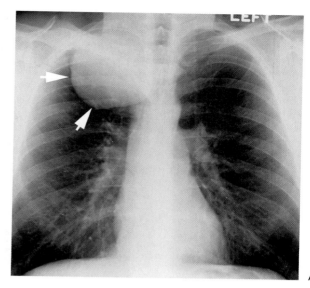

A

Peripheral Nerve Sheath Tumors

Nerve sheath tumors include neurilemmoma (schwannoma), neurofibroma, and neurogenic sarcoma (Table 8-26). Schwannomas are composed of spindle cells densely packed together (Antoni A pattern) or organized more loosely in association with a myxoid stroma (Antoni B pattern); areas of infarction are common. Neurofibromas are also variable in appearance, consisting of spindle cells, a loose myxoid matrix, neurofibrils, and collagen.

On plain radiographs, nerve sheath tumors typically appear as sharply marginated round, elliptical, or lobulated paravertebral masses, although they may be well seen only on the frontal radiograph (Figs. 8-63, 8-64A and B, and 8-65). They tend to be limited to one or two interspaces in

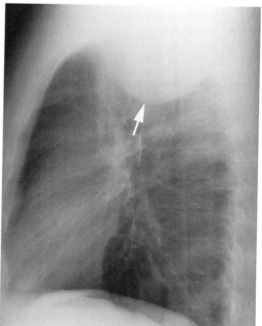

B

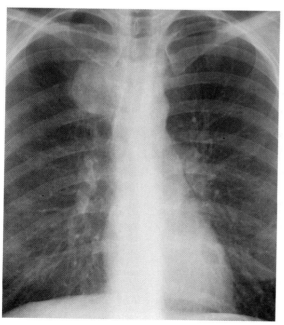

FIG. 8-63. Schwannoma. PA chest radiograph shows a well-defined right mediastinal mass associated with deformity of right-sided ribs.

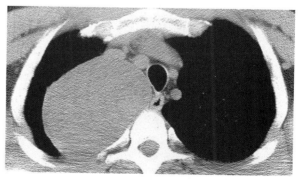

C

FIG. 8-64. Schwannoma. **A.** PA chest radiograph shows a well-defined mass in the superior mediastinum *(arrows)*. **B.** On the lateral view, the mass is relatively posterior in location *(arrow)*. **C.** A well-defined homogeneous mass is visible on CT.

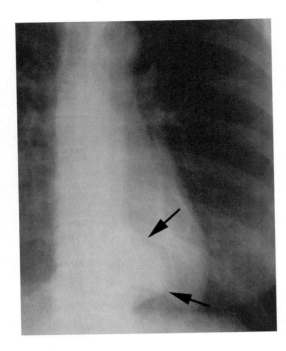

FIG. 8-65. Neurofibroma. A well-defined mass is visible in the left posterior mediastinum *(arrows)*.

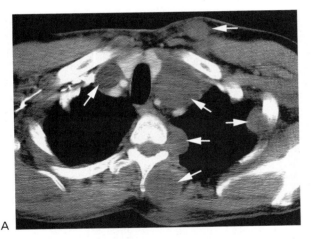

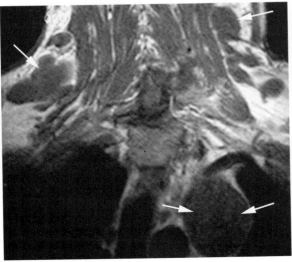

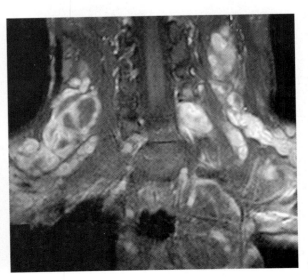

FIG. 8-66. Extensive (plexiform) neurofibromas in neurofibromatosis. **A.** CT shows multiple neurofibromas *(arrows)* in the subcutaneous tissues, along the courses of mediastinal and intercostal nerves, and in a paravertebral location. The masses appear low in attenuation on CT, measuring 15 HU. Enlargement of the left neural foramen is visible, contiguous with a left paravertebral neurofibroma. **B.** T1-weighted MRI of the lower neck and upper mediastinum shows numerous neurofibromas along the courses of cervical and mediastinal *(arrows)* nerves. **C.** Contrast-enhanced MRI shows irregular enhancement. The centers of some lesions appear low in intensity.

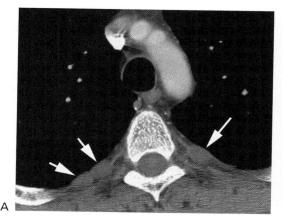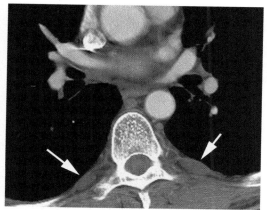

FIG. 8-67. Neurofibromatosis with paravertebral and intercostal neurofibromas. Multiple paravertebral and intercostal neurofibromas are visible *(arrows)*. They appear slightly lower in attenuation than muscle.

length but in some patients can be large. Associated rib or vertebral deformity or enlargement of a neural foramen is visible in about 50% of cases (see Fig. 8-63). Nerve sheath tumors may also be seen in the middle or anterior mediastinum, occurring in relation to the vagus, phrenic, or recurrent laryngeal nerves, or along the courses of intercostal nerves (Figs. 8-66 to 8-68).

On CT, nerve sheath tumors typically appear as well-marginated, smooth, rounded or elliptical masses (see Fig. 8-64C). Enlargement of neural foramina may be better

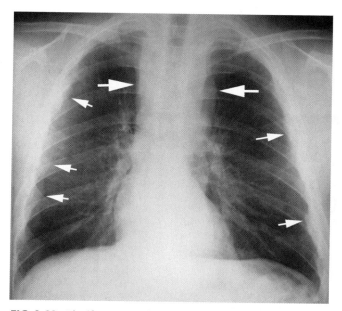

FIG. 8-68. Plexiform neurofibromas in neurofibromatosis. Mediastinal widening *(large arrows)* reflects the presence of multiple, infiltrative neurofibromas along the courses of mediastinal nerves. Extensive intercostal neurofibromas *(small arrows)* mimic the appearance of pleural thickening.

shown on CT than on plain films (see Fig. 8-66A). In over 70% of cases, peripheral nerve or nerve sheath tumors appear to be lower in attenuation than chest wall muscle (see Fig. 8-66A); in the remainder, they are of soft-tissue attenuation. Low-density areas within nerve sheath tumors can be due to the presence of (1) lipid-rich Schwann cells; (2) adipocytes; (3) perineural adipose tissue entrapped by plexiform neurofibromas; or (4) cystic spaces in the tumor. Variable enhancement of the tumor may be seen following contrast infusion; peripheral enhancement is common. Small areas of calcification are seen in 5% to 10% of cases. Extension into the spinal canal is present in 10% and is best demonstrated with MRI.

Neurofibromas may be associated with von Recklinghausen's disease, which can result in vertebral abnormalities including kyphoscoliosis, scalloped vertebrae, and lateral meningocele. More than one third of patients with neurofibromas have neurofibromatosis.

On MRI, neurogenic tumors typically have slightly greater signal intensity than muscle on T1-weighted images and markedly increased signal intensity on T2-weighted or contrast-enhanced images, although often in an inhomogeneous fashion. On T2-weighted or contrast-enhanced images, the center of the lesion may have a higher or lower intensity than its periphery (see Fig. 8-66C).

Plexiform neurofibroma represents an extensive fusiform or infiltrating mass along the course of the sympathetic chains or mediastinal or intercostal nerves (see Figs. 8-66 and 8-68). It is considered pathognomonic of von Recklinghausen's disease. As with localized nerve sheath tumors, plexiform neurofibromas often appear low in attenuation compared to muscle, with CT numbers ranging from 15 to 20 HU on unenhanced scans. They are often multiple and lobulated, have ill-defined margins, and tend to surround mediastinal vessels with loss of normally visible fat planes. They can closely mimic the appearance of extensive

**TABLE 8-27. TUMORS DERIVED FROM
SYMPATHETIC GANGLIA**

Ganglioneuroma, ganglioneuroblastoma, and neuroblastoma
20% of posterior masses in children
Oblong or sausage-shaped paravertebral mass
Calcification in 20%

mediastinal lymph node enlargement. Calcification and contrast enhancement can be seen.

Malignant nerve sheath tumors, termed malignant schwannoma, neurogenic sarcoma, or neurofibrosarcoma, are relatively uncommon but represent up to 15% of nerve sheath tumors. Malignant nerve sheath tumors tend to be large, infiltrating, irregular in contour, and inhomogeneous in attenuation, although these findings are not sufficiently reliable for diagnosis. Both benign and malignant lesions may be symptomatic, rendering clinical differentiation of limited utility. Calcification and some degree of contrast opacification may be present with either benign or malignant tumors.

Tumors Originating From Sympathetic Ganglia

In children, 80% of posterior mediastinal masses are derived from sympathetic ganglia. Included in this group are ganglioneuroma, ganglioneuroblastoma, and neuroblastoma (Table 8-27).

Ganglioneuroma, a benign tumor made up of Schwann cells, collagen, and ganglion cells, is a common neoplasm in teenagers and young adults. On plain radiographs, this tumor often appear as an oblong or sausage-shaped mass in a paravertebral location; they tend to be longer than nerve sheath tumors occurring in a similar location. Ganglioneuroma cannot be distinguished from schwannoma or neurofibroma on the basis of its CT appearance. Calcification is seen in about 20% of cases, and vertebral abnormalities may be seen. On MRI, ganglioneuroma may appear homogenous in intensity on T1- and T2-weighted images or may show a unique whorled appearance of layers of varying intensity.

Approximately 15% of *neuroblastomas* arise in the mediastinum, and almost all are located posteriorly (Fig. 8-69). Mediastinal neuroblastoma is seen almost exclusively in young children under the age of 5 years. It is malignant and may present with a wide variety of signs and symptoms including chest pain, fever, malaise, anemia, Horner's syndrome, and extremity weakness. On CT, neuroblastomas appear as soft-tissue attenuation masses, but up to 40% contain speckled or curvilinear calcifications (see Fig. 8-69C). They are most common in the paravertebral regions and may extend superiorly and inferiorly for several centimeters. Neuroblastoma often shows inhomogeneous enhancement following contrast injection. CT and MR may be used to help determine the presence and extent of mediastinal or vertebral column invasion (see Fig. 8-69D). Invasion of the extradural spinal canal is common, even in the absence of neurologic signs and symptoms. On T2-weighted images, neuroblastoma appears intense (see Fig. 8-69D). MR has the advantage of allowing tumor and surrounding soft tissues to be distinguished more readily than on CT and is more accurate in the recognition of bone marrow involvement. Neuroblastoma may extend from a primary site in the abdomen into the thorax. Most commonly, this occurs by direct invasion through the retrocrural space and into the lower paravertebral regions, often on both sides. In the rare instance of adult neuroblastoma, differentiation from lymphoma may be difficult.

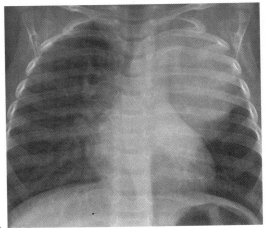
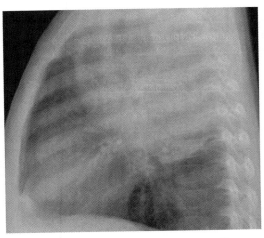

A   B

FIG. 8-69. Mediastinal neuroblastoma in a 16-month-old child. PA **(A)** and lateral **(B)** chest radiographs show a large superior, posterior mediastinal mass. *(Figure continues.)*

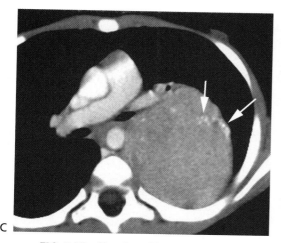
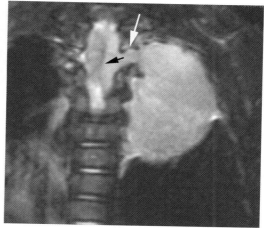

C

D

FIG. 8-69. *(Continued.)* **C.** CT shows a large paravertebral, posterior mediastinal mass containing small areas of calcification *(arrows).* **D.** T2-weighted MRI shows a large mass in the posterior mediastinum. The tumor extends into the spinal canal through a neural foramen *(white arrow),* displacing the spinal cord to the right *(black arrow).*

Ganglioneuroblastoma is found in somewhat older children than neuroblastoma and is less common. Ganglioneuroblastomas are regarded by some as partially matured malignant neuroblastomas and are somewhat intermediate in histology between neuroblastoma and ganglioneuroma. Their imaging characteristics are indistinguishable from neuroblastoma. They can present as either a large, smooth spherical mass or a small, elongated sausage-shaped mass.

Paraganglioma

Paraganglioma (chemodectoma) is a rare tumor originating from neuroectodermal cells located in relation to the autonomic nervous system, especially in the region of the aortopulmonary window (Fig. 8-70) and the posterior mediastinum; it has also been identified within the atria. It accounts for less than 5% of thoracic neurogenic tumors.

Radiographs usually show a well-defined, round or elliptical mass indistinguishable from other neurogenic tumors. It has a predilection for the midthoracic region. On unenhanced CT, paraglionoma has no characteristic features. However, scanning with contrast infusion shows dense enhancement (see Fig. 8-40B).

Patients may be asymptomatic, with the tumor being detected incidentally. About half of patients with paravertebral paraganglioma have symptoms of catecholamine secretion by the tumor or associated tumors in other locations, but catecholamine secretion is rare in patients with aortopulmonary tumors. Compression of mediastinal structures may also result in symptoms.

Identification of hormonally active lesions has been greatly aided recently by use of 131-I metaiodobenzylguanidine (131-I-MIBG) scintigraphy, which localizes cate-

cholamine-producing tumors, including neuroblastoma and carcinoid tumor. Octreotide scintigraphy is also useful in localization of these lesions.

Approximately 10% of paragangliomas are malignant or invasive. Paravertebral paragangliomas are more easily resectable than aortopulmonary tumors and have a better prognosis. Local recurrence is common following surgery in patients with aortopulmonary paraganglioma.

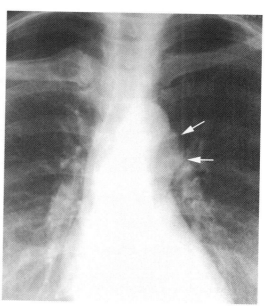

FIG. 8-70. Paraganglioma (chemodectoma). Chest radiograph shows a mass *(arrows)* in the aortopulmonary window.

Anterior or Lateral Thoracic Meningocele

This entity represents anomalous herniation of the spinal meninges through an intervertebral foramen or a defect in the vertebral body. In many patients, this abnormality is associated with neurofibromatosis; most are detected in adults. Meningoceles are described as lateral or anterior, depending on their relationship to the spine. They are slightly more common on the right side.

On chest radiographs, meningocele commonly results in a sharply marginated paravertebral soft-tissue mass associated with scoliosis or rib and vertebral anomalies at the same level (Fig. 8-71A). When scoliosis is present, the meningocele typically occurs at the apex of a convex curve. On CT they appear low in attenuation, as they contain cerebro-spinal fluid (see Fig. 8-71B). MRI is diagnostic (see Figs. 8-71C to E), as is filling of the meningocele with contrast on CT myelography.

Extramedullary Hematopoiesis

Extramedullary hematopoiesis can result in paravertebral masses in patients with severe anemia caused by inadequate production or excessive destruction of blood cells. It can be seen in the presence of thalassemia, hereditary spherocytosis, and sickle cell anemia. These masses are of unknown origin but may arise from herniations of vertebral or rib marrow through small cortical defects, or may arise from lymph nodes or elements of the reticuloendothelial system.

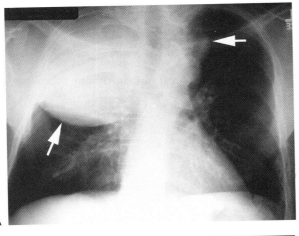

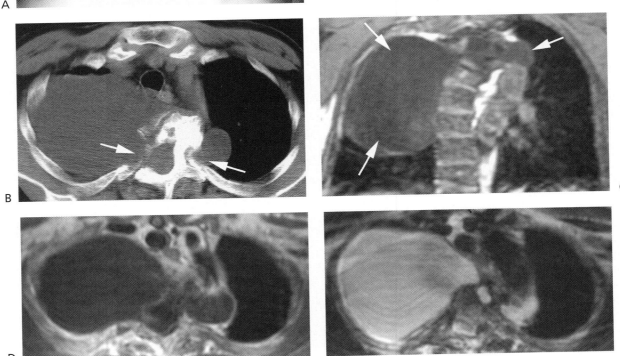

FIG. 8-71. Lateral thoracic meningocele in neurofibromatosis. **A.** PA chest radiograph shows large right and small left mediastinal masses *(arrows)*. Scoliosis and rib deformities are present. **B.** CT shows the large right and small left mediastinal masses. They are low in attenuation. The vertebral body is abnormal in appearance and the neural foramina *(arrows)* are enlarged. **C.** Coronal MRI shows the right and left meningoceles *(arrows)* and associated scoliosis. **D.** T1-weighted MRI shows low intensity typical of fluid. **E.** T2-weighted MRI shows high intensity.

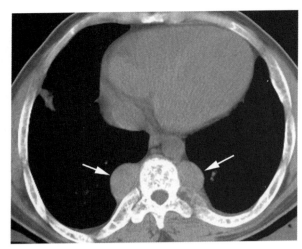

FIG. 8-72. Extrathoracic hematopoiesis. CT in a patient with thalassemia major. Paravertebral masses *(arrows)* reflect hematopoietic tissue. Ribs and vertebral bodies are expanded and show an abnormal trabecular pattern, typical of severe anemia.

Lobulated paravertebral masses, usually multiple and bilateral and caudad to the sixth thoracic vertebra, are typically seen (Fig. 8-72). They appear well marginated. On CT, the paravertebral masses are of homogeneous soft-tissue attenuation (30 to 65 HU) or may show areas of fat attenuation (−50 HU), which may increase in extent after treatment.

The diagnosis can be suggested by the presence of paravertebral masses in a patient with chronic anemia and skeletal abnormalities visible on radiographs or CT findings suggesting a bone marrow abnormality. Coarsening of the trabecular pattern, rib expansion, and periosteal new bone may be seen. Although not always present, splenomegaly may also be visible.

Abnormalities of the Thoracic Spine

Tumors either primary or malignant, infectious spondylitis, or vertebral fracture with associated hemorrhage can produce a paravertebral mass. Frequently, the abnormality is bilateral and fusiform, allowing it to be distinguished from solitary masses such as a neurogenic tumor. Associated abnormalities of the vertebral bodies or discs assist in diagnosis and should be sought.

SELECTED READING

Ahn JM, Lee KS, Goo JM, et al. Predicting the histology of anterior mediastinal masses: comparison of chest radiography and CT. J Thorac Imaging 1996; 11:265–271.

Armstrong EA, Harwood-Nash DCF, Ritz CR, et al. CT of neuroblastomas and ganglioneuromas in children. AJR Am J Roentgenol 1982; 139:571–576.

Balthazar EJ, Naidich DP, Megibow AJ, et al. CT evaluation of esophageal varices. AJR Am J Roentgenol 1987; 148:131–135.

Bashist B, Ellis K, Gold RP. Computed tomography of intrathoracic goiters. AJR Am J Roentgenol 1983; 140:455–460.

Bourgouin PM, Shepard JO, Moore EH, et al. Plexiform neurofibromatosis of the mediastinum: CT appearance. AJR Am J Roentgenol 1988; 151:461–463.

Bragg DG, Chor PJ, Murray KA, et al. Lymphoproliferative disorders of the lung: histopathology, clinical manifestations, and imaging features. AJR Am J Roentgenol 1994; 163:273–281.

Brown LR, Aughenbaugh GL. Masses of the anterior mediastinum: CT and MR imaging. AJR Am J Roentgenol 1991; 157:1171–1180.

Castellino RA, Blank N, Hoppe RT, et al. Hodgkin disease: contributions of chest CT in the initial staging evaluation. Radiology 1986; 160:603–605.

Castellino RA, Hilton S, O'Brien JP, et al. Non-Hodgkin lymphoma: contribution of chest CT in the intitial staging evaluation. Radiology 1996; 199:129–132.

Cohen LA, Schwartz AM, Rockoff SD. Benign schwannomas: pathologic basis for CT inhomogeneities. AJR Am J Roentgenol 1986; 147:141–143.

de Geer G, Webb WR, Gamsu G. Normal thymus: assessment with MR and CT. Radiology 1986; 158:313–317.

Do YS, Im JG, Lee BH, et al. CT findings in malignant tumors of thymic epithelium. J Comput Assist Tomogr 1995; 19:192–197.

Drucker EA, McLoud TC, Dedrick CG, et al. Mediastinal paraganglioma: radiologic evaluation of an unusual vascular tumor. AJR Am J Roentgenol 1987; 148:521–522.

Filly R, Blank N, Castellino R. Radiographic distribution of intrathoracic disease in previously untreated patients with Hodgkin's disease and non-Hodgkin's lymphoma. Radiology 1976; 120:277.

Fitch SJ, Tonkin ILD, Tonkin AK. Imaging of foregut duplication cysts. Radiographics 1986; 6:189–201.

Freundlich IM, McGavran MH. Abnormalities of the thymus. J Thorac Imaging 1996; 58–65

Glazer GM, Gross BH, Quint LE, et al. Normal mediastinal lymph nodes: number and size according to American Thoracic Society mapping. AJR Am J Roentgenol 1985; 144:261–265.

Glazer HS, Molina PL, Siege MJ, Sagel SS. Pictorial essay. Low-attenuation mediastinal masses on CT. AJR Am J Roentgenol 1989; 152:1173–1177.

Glazer HS, Siege MJ, Sagel SS. Pictorial essay. High-attenuation mediastinal masses on unenhanced CT. AJR Am J Roentgenol 1991; 156:45–50.

Glazer HS, Wick MR, Anderson DJ, et al. CT of fatty thoracic masses. AJR Am J Roentgenol 1992; 159:1181–1187.

Hoffman OA, Gillespie DJ, Aughenbaugh GL, et al. Primary mediastinal neoplasms (other than thymoma). Mayo Clin Proc 1993; 68:880–891.

Jolles H, Henry DA, Roberson JP, et al. Mediastinitis following median sternotomy: CT findings. Radiology 1996; 201:463–466.

Kang YS, Rosen K, Clark OH, et al. Localization of abnormal parathyroid glands of the mediastinum with MR imaging. Radiology 1993; 189:137–141.

Kawashima A, Fishman EK, Kuhlman JE, et al. CT of posterior mediastinal masses. Radiographics 1991; 11:1045–1067.

Kirchner SG, Heller RM, Smith CW. Pancreatic pseudocyst of the mediastinum. Radiology 1977; 123:37–42.

Kirks DR, McCormick VD, Greenspan RH. Pulmonary sarcoidosis: roentgenographic analysis of 150 patients. AJR Am J Roentgenol 1973; 117:777–786.

Kirsch CFE, Webb EM, Webb WR. Multicentric Castleman's disease and POEMS syndrome: CT findings. J Thorac Imaging 1997; 12:75–77.

Kiyono K, Sone S, Sakai F, et al. The number and size of normal mediastinal lymph nodes: a postmortem study. AJR Am J Roentgenol 1988; 150:771–776.

Kushihashi T, Munechika H, Motoya H, et al. CT and MR findings in tuberculous mediastinitis. J Comput Assist Tomogr 1995; 19: 379–382.

Lee KS, Im JG, Han CH, et al. Malignant primary germ cell tumors of the mediastinum: CT features. AJR Am J Roentgenol 1989; 153:947–951.

Long JA, Doppman JL, Nienhuis AW. Computed tomographic studies of thoracic extramedullary hematopoiesis. J Comput Assist Tomogr 1980; 4:67–70.

McAdams HP, Rosado de Christenson ML, Moran CA. Mediastinal hemangioma: radiographic and CT features in 4 patients. Radiology 1994; 193:399–402.

McLoud TC, Kalisher L, Stark P, et al. Intrathoracic lymph node metastases from extrathoracic neoplasms. AJR Am J Roentgenol 1978; 131:403–407.

Miyake H, Shiga M, Takaki H, et al. Mediastinal lymphangiomas in adults: CT findings. J Thorac Imaging 1996; 11:83–85.

Moon WK, Im JG, In KY, et al. Mediastinal tuberculous lymphadenitis: MR imaging appearance with clinicopathologic correlation. AJR Am J Roentgenol 1996; 166:21–25.

Moon WK, Im JG, Kim JS, et al. Mediastinal Castleman's disease: CT findings. J Comput Assist Tomogr 1994; 18:43–46.

Mountain CF, Dresler CM. Regional lymph node classification for lung cancer staging. Chest 1997; 111:1718–1723.

Müller NL, Webb WR, Gamsu G. Paratracheal lymphadenopathy: radiographic findings and correlation with CT. Radiology 1985; 156:761–765.

Müller NL, Webb WR, Gamsu G. Subcarinal lymph node enlargement: Radiographic findings and CT correlation. AJR Am J Roentgenol 1985; 145:15–19.

Nicolaou S, Müller NL, Li DKB, et al. Thymus in myasthenia gravis: comparison of CT and pathologic findings and clinical outcome after thymectomy. Radiology 1996; 20:471–474.

Patil SN, Levin DL. Distribution of thoracic lymphadenopathy in sarcoidosis using computed tomography. J Thorac Imaging 1999; 14:114–117.

Reed JC, Hallet KK, Feigin DS. Neural tumors of the thorax: subject review from the AFIP. Radiology 1978; 126:9–17.

Reed JC, Sobonya RE. Morphologic analysis of foregut cysts in the thorax. AJR Am J Roentgenol 1974; 120:851–860.

Rosado de Christenson ML, Pugatch RD, Moran CA, et al. Thymolipoma: analysis of 27 cases. Radiology 1994; 193:121–126.

Rosado de Christenson ML, Templeton PA, Moran CA. Mediastinal germ-cell tumors: radiologic and pathologic correlation. Radiographics 1992; 12:1013–1030.

Sakai F, Sone S, Kiyono K, et al. Intrathoracic neurogenic tumors: MR–pathologic correlation. AJR Am J Roentgenol 1992; 159: 279–283.

Sherrick AD, Brown LR, Harms GF, et al. Radiographic findings of fibrosing mediastinitis. Chest 1994; 106:484–489.

9

SOLITARY AND MULTIPLE NODULES, MASSES, CAVITIES, AND CYSTS

W. RICHARD WEBB

The radiographic assessment of patients with solitary or multiple lung nodules, masses, or cavities is a common clinical problem. Primary or metastatic tumor usually is the main consideration in patients with these findings. However, many other diseases or abnormalities may present with focal lung abnormalities. Some have specific appearances that may suggest the correct diagnosis or limit the differential diagnosis.

THE SOLITARY PULMONARY NODULE

A solitary pulmonary nodule (SPN) usually is defined as a focal opacity, visible on chest radiographs or CT, which fits the following criteria:

1. It is relatively well-defined.
2. It is surrounded, at least partially, by lung.
3. It is roughly spherical in shape.
4. It is 3 cm or less in diameter (Fig. 9-1).

Lesions larger than 3 cm in diameter usually are referred to using the term "mass." This cutoff also is used to distinguish a T1 carcinoma (3 cm or less in diameter) from a T2 carcinoma (more than 3 cm).

Clinical Evaluation

Clinical and historical information is helpful in the differential diagnosis of a solitary lung nodule. Important considerations that increase the likelihood of cancer include a history of smoking, age over 40, occupational exposures (e.g., asbestos), lung fibrosis, coexisting chronic obstructive pulmonary disease (COPD) and emphysema, and a family history of lung cancer. Risk factors for a cancer are reviewed in Chapter 3.

Recent travel history, a positive skin test for tuberculosis (TB) or fungus, or the presence of other diseases (e.g., rheumatoid arthritis) increases the likelihood of a benign SPN. In a patient younger than 30 years of age, cancer is very uncommon as a cause of SPN.

An SPN found in a patient with a history of extrathoracic malignancy may be a metastasis, a primary lung carcinoma, or an insignificant benign lesion. Certain tumors have a propensity to metastasize as SPNs. Among patients with an SPN, those with a history of melanoma, sarcoma, or testicular carcinoma are more than twice as likely to have a solitary metastasis than a bronchogenic carcinoma. On the other hand, patients with an SPN who have a history of carcinoma of the head and neck, bladder, breast, cervix, bile ducts, esophagus, ovary, prostate, or stomach are more than three times as likely to have primary bronchogenic carcinoma than lung metastasis. In patients with other types of tumors, the relative likelihood of metastasis and lung cancer is about equal.

Radiographic Evaluation

The differential diagnosis of a solitary pulmonary nodule is extensive (Table 9-1). In patients with an SPN, plain films and computed tomography (CT) are used to determine the nodule's (1) morphologic characteristics; (2) density (i.e., calcium, fat, or contrast-enhancement); and (3) growth rate.

Morphologic Characteristics

Using plain radiographs or CT, an SPN sometimes may be diagnosed as a specific lesion based on its appearance. Some such lesions include mucous plug, arteriovenous fistula, rounded atelectasis, mycetoma, and focal pleural lesions. These are described later in this chapter.

Much more often, radiographic studies are used to assess less specific morphologic characteristics that suggest that an SPN is likely malignant or likely benign.

Size

The likelihood of malignancy in a nodule or mass is directly related to its size (Table 9-2). The likelihood of cancer is about 35% for a nodule ranging from 0.5 to 1.0 cm in diameter, 50% for an SPN 1.0 to 2.0 cm in diameter, and

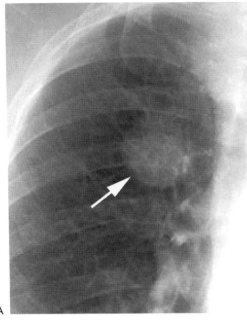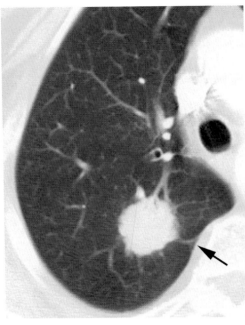

FIG. 9-1. Right upper lobe nodule representing an adenocarcinoma. **A.** Chest radiograph shows a right upper lobe nodule *(arrow)*. This lesion is classified as a nodule because it is relatively well defined, at least partially surrounded by lung, roughly spherical in shape, and 3 cm or less in diameter. Because the nodule exceeds 2 cm in diameter, it is very likely malignant. **B.** CT shows the edge of the nodule to be ill-defined and lobulated, and a pleural tail *(arrow)* extends to the pleural surface.

TABLE 9-1. Differential diagnosis of a solitary pulmonary nodule or mass

Congenital lesions and normal variants
Arteriovenous fistula
Bronchogenic cyst
Congenital cystic adenomatoid malformation
Intrapulmonary lymph node
Mucoid impaction (bronchial atresia)
Pulmonary vein varix
Sequestration
Malignant neoplasms
Carcinoma
Lymphoma
Lymphoproliferative disease
Metastatic neoplasm
Sarcoma (e.g., chondrosarcoma, liposarcoma, fibrosarcoma)
Benign neoplasms and neoplasm-like conditions
Endometrioma
Hamartoma
Lymphoproliferative disease
Miscellaneous benign tumors
  Mesenchymal tumors (e.g., chondroma, lipoma, fibroma)
  Epithelial tumors (e.g., atypical adenomatous hyperplasia,
    mucous gland adenoma)
  Vascular tumors
Infection and parasites
Aspergillosis, angioinvasive
Dirofilaria immitus (dog heartworm)
Echinococcus
Focal (round) pneumonia
Granulomatous infection or granuloma
  Tuberculosis
  Nontuberculous mycobacteria (e.g., *Mycobacterium avium-
    intracellulare* complex)
  Coccidioidomycosis

Histoplasmosis
Cryptococcus
Lung abscess
Mycetoma (aspergilloma)
Pulmonary gangrene
Septic embolism
Inflammatory (noninfectious)
Churg-Strauss syndrome
Focal organizing pneumonia
Rheumatoid nodule
Sarcoidosis
Wegener's granulomatosis
Airways and inhalational disease
Mucoid impaction (mucous plug)
  Asthma
  Allergic bronchopulmonary aspergillosis
  Bronchial atresia
  Bronchiectasis
  Cystic fibrosis
Conglomerate mass or progressive massive fibrosis (e.g., silicosis)
Lipoid pneumonia
Vascular lesions
Arteriovenous fistula
Hematoma
Infarction
Pulmonary artery aneurysm
Pulmonary vein varix
Septic embolism
Idiopathic and miscellaneous
Amyloidosis
Fluid-filled bulla
Round atelectasis

TABLE 9-2. LIKELIHOOD OF MALIGNANCY RELATED TO NODULE DIAMETER

Diameter	Malignancy rate
<1 cm	35%
1–2 cm	50%
2–3 cm	80%
>3 cm	97%

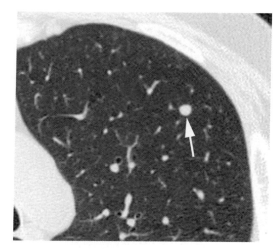

FIG. 9-3. Smooth, sharply marginated, rounded nodule representing a granuloma. Its appearance *(arrow)* is typical of a benign lesion. Its small size also makes malignancy less likely.

more than 85% for an SPN more than 2.0 cm in diameter (see Fig. 9-1). It should be kept in mind, however, that even a very small lesion can represent a carcinoma.

One or more small lung nodules are exceedingly common as an incidental finding on CT scans, and the large majority represent benign lesions such as granuloma or intrapulmonary lymph node. Follow-up CT is the only practical method of evaluating their significance.

Location

About two thirds of lung cancers occur in the upper lobes, and the right upper lobe is most commonly involved (see Fig. 9-1). Sixty percent of cancers presenting as an SPN on chest radiographs are seen in the lung periphery; only 10% are visible in the medial third of the lung.

Metastatic tumor presenting as an SPN tends to be located in the subpleural or outer third of the lung. Two thirds of metastatic lesions occur in the lower lobes.

Edge Appearance

Although plain radiographs do not allow the edge of a lung nodule or mass to be assessed with the precision of CT, cancers can appear to be ill-defined, irregular in contour, spiculated, or lobulated on plain films (see Fig. 9-1).

On CT, malignant nodules are much more likely to have an ill-defined, irregular, lobulated, or spiculated margin (see Figs. 9-1B and 9-2). Benign lesions tend to have a smooth, sharply defined edge (Figs. 9-3 and 9-4; Table 9-3). Nearly 90% of nodules with an irregular or spiculated edge are malignant; only 20% of nodules with a smooth, sharp margin are malignant. Malignancies that tend to have a sharp and smooth edge include metastases (Fig. 9-5) and carcinoid tumor (see Fig. 3-44 in Chapter 3).

The terms *corona radiate* and *corona maligna* have been used to describe the appearance of spiculation associated with a nodule or mass (see Figs. 9-2 and 9-6). Particularly in patients with adenocarcinoma and bronchioloalveolar carcinoma, this appearance reflects the presence of fibrosis surrounding the tumor, although tumor invasion of adja-

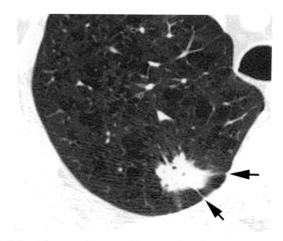

FIG. 9-2. Adenocarcinoma with a spiculated margin seen on CT. Two pleural tails *(arrows)* extend to the pleural surface. This appearance has been termed *corona radiata* or *corona maligna*. The surface of the nodule is lobulated and shows notches, both of which are findings indicating malignancy. Several lucencies within the nodule represent air bronchograms of areas of pseudocavitation, typical findings in adenocarcinoma and bronchioloalveolar carcinoma.

TABLE 9-3. EDGE APPEARANCES AND COMMON DIAGNOSES

Sharply marginated
Granuloma
Hamartoma or benign tumor
Carcinoid tumor
Metastasis
Spiculated (corona radiata) or pleural tail
Bronchioloalveolar carcinoma
Carcinoma
Granuloma or focal scarring

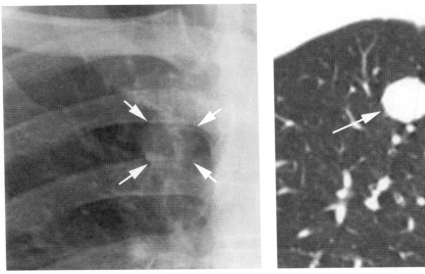
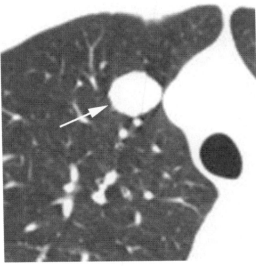

FIG. 9-4. Hamartoma presenting as a sharply defined, round nodule. **A.** Chest radiograph shows a round nodule *(arrows)* in the right upper lobe. **B.** CT shows the nodule *(arrow)* to be rounded in shape and sharply marginated. Slight lobulation may be seen with hamartomas.

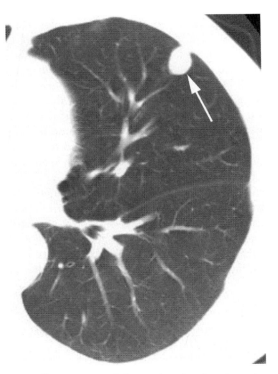

FIG. 9-5. Solitary metastasis from a head and neck carcinoma. A left upper lobe nodule *(arrow)* is smooth and sharply defined on CT. This appearance is common with metastases.

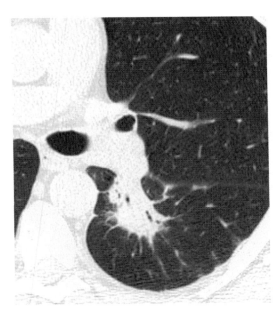

FIG. 9-6. Adenocarcinoma. HRCT shows an irregular, spiculated nodule with multiple pleural tails. Air bronchograms are visible within the nodule.

cent lung also may be present. The fibrosis usually reflects a desmoplastic reaction rather than preexisting lung fibrosis. Spiculation is less common with large cell carcinoma than other cell types that present as a solitary nodule or mass.

In addition, carcinomas can show the presence of a "pleural tail" sign or "pleural tag," in which a thin linear opacity is seen extending from the edge of a lung nodule to the pleural surface (see Figs. 9-1B, 9-2, and 9-6). This tail, which can be from a few millimeters to a few centimeters in length, often is seen in association with spiculation. As with spiculation, it reflects the presence of fibrosis, and often is associated with a dimpling of the visceral pleura. In patients with lung cancer, a pleural tail sign most often is associated with adenocarcinoma or bronchioloalveolar carcinoma; it uncommonly indicates the presence of a large cell carcinoma. The pleural tail sign also can be seen in association with benign lung nodules, which are associated with fibrosis, including various granulomatous diseases. The presence of a spiculated contour is more suggestive of malignancy than a pleural tail.

The "halo" sign, a halo of ground-glass opacity surrounding a nodule, may be seen in some patients with an SPN. It is commonly present in leukemic patients with invasive aspergillosis (Fig. 9-7), but also can be seen in patients with other infections (see Fig. 9-35C) and in some tumors, particularly adenocarcinoma or bronchioloalveolar carcinoma (Fig. 9-8; Tables 9-4 and 9-5). The histologic nature of the halo varies with the disease. In patients with invasive aspergillosis, the halo sign represents hemorrhage; in patients with carcinoma, it reflects the presence of lepidic spread of tumor.

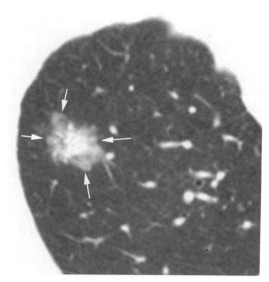

FIG. 9-8. Halo sign in bronchioloalveolar carcinoma. HRCT shows a dense central nodule surrounded by a halo *(arrows)*. In bronchioloalveolar carcinoma, the halo represents the presence of lepidic tumor growth.

TABLE 9-4. CAUSES OF THE HALO SIGN

Fungi: invasive aspergillosis, candidiasis, coccidioidomycosis
Bacteria: tuberculosis, *Nocardia*, *Legionella*
Viruses: cytomegalovirus, herpes
Pneumocystis jiroveci (P. carinii)
Bronchiolitis obliterans with organizing pneumonia
Wegener's granulomatosis
Infarct
Metastatic tumor
Kaposi's sarcoma
Bronchioloalveolar carcinoma
Adenocarcinoma

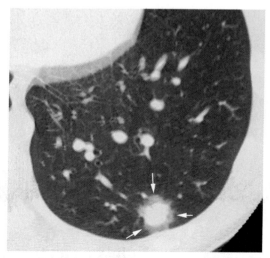

FIG. 9-7. Halo sign in invasive aspergillosis. HRCT in a young patient with leukemia and granulocytopenia shows a dense left lower lobe nodule surrounded by a halo *(arrows)* of ground-glass opacity. In patients with invasive aspergillosis, the halo represent hemorrhage surrounding a septic infarction.

TABLE 9-5. CAUSES OF AIR BRONCHOGRAMS IN SOLITARY PULMONARY NODULES

Adenocarcinoma
Bronchioloalveolar carcinoma
Conglomerate mass
Focal pneumonia
Infarction
Rounded atelectasis
Bronchiolitis obliterans with organizing pneumonia
Lymphoma
Lymphoproliferative diseases
Mycetoma (may mimic a bronchogram)

Shape

Lung carcinomas tend to be irregular in shape, lobulated, or notched (see Figs. 9-1, 9-2, and 9-6). Granulomas often are round (see Fig. 9-3). Hamartomas and metastases may be round, oval, or lobulated (see Figs. 9-4 and 9-5). Scars or areas of atelectasis or scarring may appear linear or angular. A number of other benign lesions (e.g., AVM, mucous plugs) may be identified by their characteristic shapes.

Air Bronchograms and Pseudocavitation

On HRCT, air bronchograms commonly are seen in cancers presenting as an SPN (25% to 65% of cases; see Figs. 9-2 and 9-6). This finding is most typical of adenocarcinoma or bronchioloalveolar carcinoma. Air bronchograms are much less common in benign lesions, but have a variety of causes. An appearance similar to this may be seen with developing mycetoma, representing spaces between fronds of fungus. Small bronchi seen in relation to lung cancers often appear abnormal, being narrowed, obstructed, or irregular in contour.

In addition to air bronchograms, small bubbly lucencies may be seen in cancers (see Fig. 9-2). These may represent air bronchograms, small air-filled cystic areas in the tumor (so-called pseudocavitation), or small cavities. They have the same significance as air bronchograms.

Cavitation

By general agreement, a cyst is an air-filled lesion that has a smooth and uniform wall 3 mm or less in thickness. The term *cavity* usually is used to describe a lesion with a thicker or more irregular wall or a lesion that has *cavitated* (i.e., evolved by developing an air-filled space, regardless of how thick the wall is). Thus, a thin-walled lesion may be either a cyst or a cavity, whereas a thick-walled or irregular lesion is a cavity. An exception to this rule is an infected cyst: surrounding lung inflammation may result in a thick "wall."

Cavitation occurs in about 10% of cancers, most commonly in patients with squamous cell carcinoma (Fig. 9-9A and B; see also Figs. 3-4 and 3-26 in Chapter 3). Approximately 80% of cavitary lung cancers are squamous cell. Cavitation of large cell carcinoma and adenocarcinoma also occurs (see Fig. 9-9C); small cell carcinoma rarely cavitates.

Although a long list of abnormalities may be associated with cysts or cavities, described in Table 9-6 and in detail

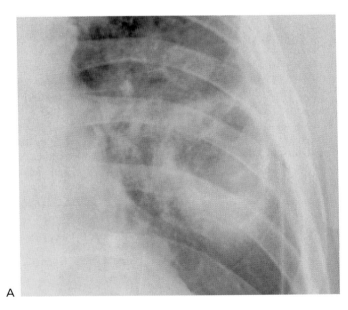

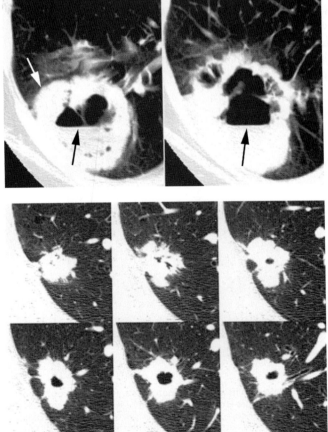

FIG. 9-9. Cavitary carcinoma. **A.** Plain radiograph showing a cavitary left lung mass that represents a squamous cell carcinoma. **B.** Cavitary squamous cell carcinoma shown at two levels. The wall of the cavity is irregular, with several thick nodular regions *(white arrow)*. The cavity contains an air-fluid level *(black arrows)*. This is uncommon in malignancy and may represent hemorrhage or infection. **C.** Cavitary adenocarcinoma shown on HRCT in six contiguous scans. The nodule contains an irregular cavity; is irregular and lobulated in shape, notched, and spiculated; and is associated with pleural tails. It also contains several air bronchograms.

TABLE 9-6. CAUSES OF A CYST OR CAVITY (SOLITARY OR MULTIPLE)

Amyloidosis—solitary or multiple
Aspergillosis, angioinvasive—usually multiple
Aspergillosis, semi-invasive—usually solitary
Bronchogenic cyst—usually single
Bulla—solitary or multiple
Carcinoma
Congenital cystic adenomatoid malformation—solitary, but often multiloculated
Conglomerate mass or progressive massive fibrosis—often bilateral
Cystic bronchiectasis—usually multiple
Cystic lung disease (e.g., histiocytosis, lymphangiomyomatosis)—multiple
Echinococcus—solitary or multiple
Endometrioma
Granulomatous infection
  Tuberculosis
  Nontuberculous mycobacteria (e.g., *Mycobacterium avium-intracellulare* complex)
  Coccidioidomycosis
  Histoplasmosis
  Cryptococcus
Hematoma—solitary or multiple
Intralobar sequestration—may be lucent, cystic, or multicystic
Lung abscess—solitary or multiple
Lymphoma—solitary or multiple
Metastatic neoplasm—usually multiple
Mycetoma—aspergilloma
Papillomatosis—usually multiple
Paragonimiasis—usually multiple
Pneumatocele—solitary or multiple
Pulmonary gangrene—usually solitary
Pulmonary laceration—traumatic
Rheumatoid nodule—usually multiple
Sarcoidosis—usually multiple
Sarcoma—solitary
Septic embolism—usually multiple
Wegener's granulomatosis—usually multiple

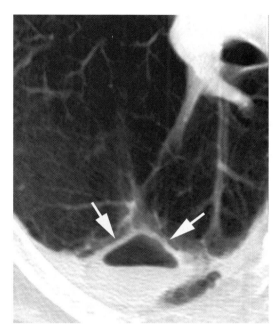

FIG. 9-10. CT scan of a lung abscess. The wall is thin and smooth, measuring less than 5 mm in thickness. An air-fluid level is visible.

below, for practical purposes, radiographic evaluation is directed a determining the likelihood of malignancy. Cavitary malignant lesions tend to have a thick, nodular wall (see Fig. 9-9B and C; see also Figs. and 3-4 and 3-26 in Chapter 3); benign lesions often have a thin, smooth wall (Fig. 9-10). The thickness of the wall of a cavity serves as an indicator of its likelihood of being malignant. Nearly 85% of cavities with a wall measuring more than 15 mm in its thickest portion are malignant (see Fig. 9-9B). If the thickest part of the wall is less than 5 mm, 95% are benign (see Fig. 9-10). Seventy-five percent of cavities with a wall 5 to 15 mm in thickness are benign. If the thickest part of the cavity wall measures 1 mm or less, malignancy is rare. However, thin-walled cystic lesions may rarely be seen with bronchioloalveolar carcinoma or metastases.

Lung cancer resulting in bronchial obstruction also can be associated with an abscess in the distal lung, mimicking a cavitary carcinoma. In addition, lung cancer sometimes can arise in a bulla or cyst, or be associated with a preexisting cavity. In such a case, focal thickening of the cyst or cavity wall or fluid within the cyst may be the only findings suggesting this diagnosis.

Air-crescent Sign

In some patients with a cavitary nodule or lung cyst, a mass or nodule may be present within the cavity. Air outlining or capping the superior aspect of the mass results in a crescent-shaped collection of air, termed the "air-crescent" sign. The most likely cause of this appearance is aspergilloma (mycetoma), but the differential diagnosis includes other entities as well (Table 9-7). Gravitational shift of the intracavitary mass strongly suggests mycetoma and excludes carcinoma.

TABLE 9-7. CAUSES OF THE AIR-CRESCENT SIGN

Aspergilloma (mycetoma)
Angioinvasive aspergillosis with septic infarction
Carcinoma arising in a cyst
Cavitary carcinoma
Clot in a cyst or cavity
Echinococcus
Mucous plug in cystic bronchiectasis
Papillomatosis
Pulmonary gangrene
Rasmussen aneurysm (mycotic pulmonary artery aneurysm in a tubercular cavity)

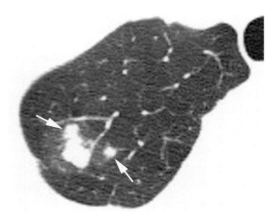

FIG. 9-11. Tuberculosis. A right upper lobe nodule is associated with satellites *(arrows)*. This appearance is most typical of a benign process but sometimes is seen with carcinoma.

TABLE 9-9. CAUSES OF CALCIFICATION OR HIGH ATTENUATION IN A SOLITARY PULMONARY NODULE

Amyloidosis—dense or stippled
Carcinoid tumor—punctate, eccentric
Carcinoma—punctate, eccentric
Conglomerate mass—multiple foci
Dirofilaria immitis
Granuloma—diffuse, central, concentric
Hamartoma or chondroma—popcorn, central
Mucoid impaction in allergic bronchopulmonary aspergillosis or bronchial atresia
Metastases—diffuse, punctate
Talcosis—secondary to talc not calcium
Amiodarone toxicity—due to iodine content

Air-fluid Level

The presence of an air-fluid level in a patient with a cavitary SPN tends to indicate a benign lesion, particularly lung abscess (see Fig. 9-10). Any infected cystic or cavitary lesion may be associated with an air-fluid level. An air-fluid level is uncommon in a cavitary carcinoma, but may be seen in the presence of intracavity hemorrhage or superinfection (see Fig. 9-9B).

Satellite Nodules

Satellite nodules are small nodules seen adjacent to a larger nodule or mass. They tend to predict a benign lesion (Fig. 9-11). Satellites are most common with granulomatous diseases and infections such as TB (Table 9-8). Only a small percentage of carcinomas are associated with satellite nodules. In patients with sarcoidosis, the presence of satellite nodules has been termed the "galaxy" sign.

Feeding Vessel Sign

The "feeding vessel" sign is present if a small pulmonary artery is seen leading directly to a nodule (Fig. 9-12). This appearance is most common with metastasis, infarct, and arteriovenous fistula. It is less common with primary lung carcinoma or benign lesions such as granuloma.

TABLE 9-8. CAUSES OF SATELLITE NODULES

Tuberculosis
Nontuberculous mycobacterial infection
Bacterial infections with endobronchial spread
Fungal infections
Sarcoid
Conglomerate masses (silicosis, coal worker's pneumonoconiosis, talcosis)
Bronchioloalveolar carcinoma
Adenocarcinoma

Density

A lung nodule usually is examined using volumetric HRCT to determine its density before contrast injection. Because of volume averaging, unless an SPN is grossly calcified, CT with thick collimation (5 to 10 mm) usually cannot be used to determine its density accurately. Most cancers appear to be of soft tissue attenuation.

Ground-glass Opacity

With thin collimation, some nodules appear to be of ground-glass opacity. Many focal opacities of ground-glass opacity are inflammatory and resolve on follow-up. However, bronchioloalveolar carcinoma may present as a nodule

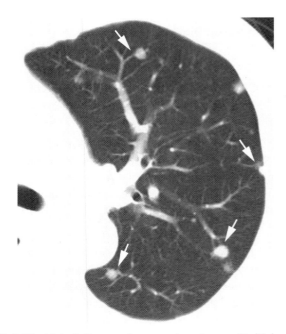

FIG. 9-12. Metastatic nasopharyngeal carcinoma. Multiple nodules *(arrows)* are associated with a feeding vessel.

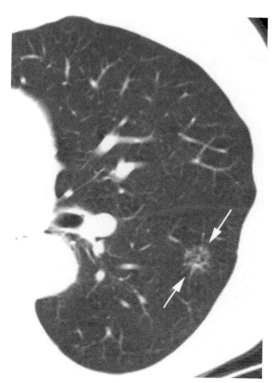

FIG. 9-13. Bronchioloalveolar carcinoma. A spiculated nodule *(arrows)* is visible on CT with 3-mm slice thickness. The nodule is of ground-glass opacity. This appearance may be seen with bronchioloalveolar carcinoma.

entirely of ground-glass opacity, and a high degree of suspicion should be maintained (Fig. 9-13). Follow-up of such a lesion is appropriate.

Calcification or High Attenuation

The presence of calcium in an SPN increases its chances of being benign (Table 9-9). Diagnosing a small nodule as calcified on chest radiographs is somewhat subjective and subject to error. However, if a nodule a few millimeters in diameter is easily seen on radiographs, it probably is calcified.

CT is more sensitive and accurate in diagnosing calcification. Volumetric HRCT images usually should be obtained through a lung nodule to look for calcium. HRCT demonstrates calcification in about 25% of patients with a benign SPN that does not appear calcified on plain radiographs.

The pattern of calcification is important in determining its diagnostic significance. Generally the following four patterns of calcification can be used to predict the presence of a benign lesion with sufficient accuracy to allow appropriate management (Fig. 9-14):

1. Homogeneous calcification (Fig. 9-15)
2. Dense central ("bull's-eye") calcification (Fig. 9-16)
3. Concentric rings of calcium ("target" calcification; Fig. 9-17)
4. Conglomerate foci of calcification involving a large part of the nodule ("popcorn" calcification; Fig. 9-18).

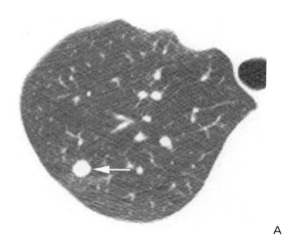

A

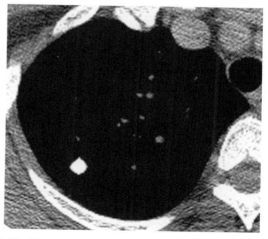

B

FIG. 9-15. Homogeneous calcification. Dense and uniform calcification of a small right upper lobe nodule *(arrow)* is typical of a benign lesion, usually a tuberculoma.

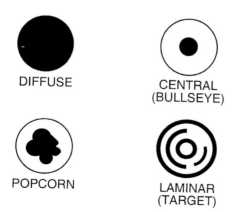

FIG. 9-14. Benign patterns of calcification. With rare exceptions, these indicate the presence of a benign lesion.

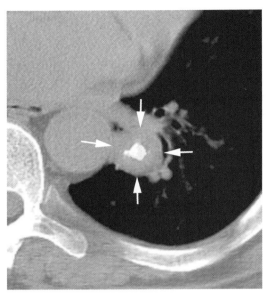

FIG. 9-16. Dense central or "bull's-eye" calcification in a hamartoma. A round lung nodule *(arrows)* adjacent to the descending aorta shows dense central calcification. This is typical of histoplasmoma or hamartoma.

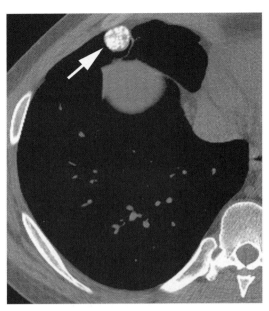

FIG. 9-18. Multiple confluent nodular foci of calcification ("popcorn" calcification; *arrow*) in a hamartoma. This appearance is typical of hamartoma and corresponds to calcification of cartilage nodules.

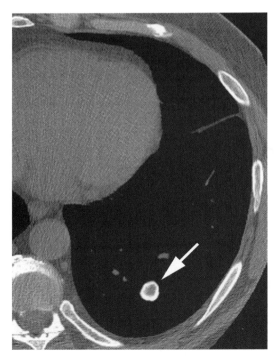

FIG. 9-17. Concentric or "target" calcification *(arrow).* One or more rings of calcium may be seen. This pattern is typical of a histoplasmoma.

The first three of these patterns are most typical of granulomas; the last is more typical of hamartoma. Calcified lesions thought to be benign should be followed radiographically in most cases unless the calcification is diffuse.

Stippled calcification or eccentric foci of calcification (Figs. 9-19 and 9-20) may be seen in benign SPN but are visible in as many as 10% to 15% of cancers; these patterns must be considered indeterminate (see Fig. 9-19).

Calcium in a tumor may reflect dystrophic calcification (occurring in areas of tumor necrosis), engulfing of a preexisting granuloma, or calcification of the tumor itself (as in mucinous adenocarcinoma, carcinoid tumor, or osteogenic sarcoma). A "benign" pattern of calcification occasionally is seen in patients with neoplasm. Carcinoid tumor and mucinous adenocarcinoma can show dense central calcification. Metastases from osteogenic sarcoma or chondrosarcoma can show homogenous calcification, but history of the primary tumor allows a correct diagnosis.

Because of the high likelihood of cancer in patients with

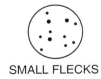

SMALL FLECKS

ECCENTRIC

FIG. 9-19. Indeterminate patterns of calcification. These may be seen in benign or malignant lesions.

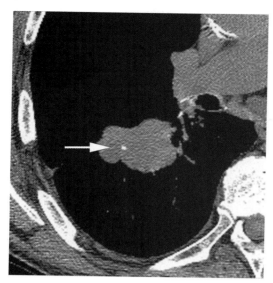

FIG. 9-20. Eccentric calcification in an adenocarcinoma. A lobulated mass shows a small focus of eccentric calcification *(arrow)*.

spiculated nodules or nodules exceeding 2 cm in diameter, it is inadvisable to call such a nodule benign on the basis of visible calcification, unless the calcification is diffuse and dense. A small central calcification is insufficient for determining whether such a nodule is benign.

Usually, a visible inspection of HRCT scans is sufficient for diagnosing calcification. However, measurement of CT numbers can allow the detection of calcification, which is not clearly seen on the scans. This technique is termed *CT nodule densitometry.* Pixels denser than 100 HU indicate the presence of calcification.

High attenuation of a nodule or mass sometimes is seen using CT in patients who do not have calcification. This may be seen in patients with amiodarone toxicity resulting in focal organizing pneumonia: the drug contains iodine, which appears dense. Patients with conglomerate masses from talcosis may show high attenuation due to the talc.

Fat

The presence of fat in an SPN may be diagnosed accurately only on HRCT. On HRCT, fat can be accurately diagnosed if low CT numbers are seen (-40 to -120 HU). This most likely indicates the presence of hamartoma (see Figs. 3-49 and 3-51 in Chapter 3), lipoma, or lipoid pneumonia (see Figs. 21-1 and 21-2 in Chapter 21). On occasion, histoplasmoma may show fat deposition with growth.

In most cases, fat indicates the presence of a hamartoma, although other lesions may be associated with some fat (Table 9-10). Nearly 65% of hamartomas show fat on HRCT, sometimes in association with dense popcorn calcification or flecks of calcium. The presence of fat within a lung nodule is sufficient for calling it benign, although follow-up is appropriate.

TABLE 9-10. CAUSES OF SOLITARY PULMONARY NODULES CONTAINING FAT

Hamartoma
Lipoma
Liposarcoma (primary or metastatic)
Lipoid pneumonia
Histoplasmoma
Teratoma

Water Density

Benign cystic lesions, such as pulmonary bronchogenic cyst, sequestration, congenital cystic adenomatoid malformation (CCAM), or a fluid-filled cyst or bulla (Table 9-11), occasionally may be diagnosed on CT by their water attenuation (0 HU) and very thin or invisible walls (see Fig. 1-6 in Chapter 1). Mucoid impaction also may appear to be of low attenuation. On the other hand, bronchogenic cysts or other cystic lesions may have a higher attenuation because of their protein content. Hematoma may have the attenuation of blood (50 HU) or may be of fluid attenuation, depending on its age.

A necrotic neoplasm, conglomerate mass, or lung abscess or infarction may have a low attenuation center on CT, but these lesions have a thick and perceptible wall.

Contrast Enhancement

Cancers have a greater tendency to opacify following contrast infusion than do some types of benign nodules. Specific contrast enhancement techniques have been suggested to help diagnosis malignancy. When using these techniques, sequential thin-collimation scans must be obtained through the center of a lung nodule for several minutes following contrast injection. Most SPNs show peak enhancement at either 3 or 4 minutes.

One currently recommended protocol uses scans at 1

TABLE 9-11. CAUSES OF FLUID DENSITY SOLITARY PULMONARY NODULES

Bronchogenic cyst
Carcinoma (necrotic or infected)
Congenital cystic adenomatoid malformation
Conglomerate mass (necrotic)
Fluid-filled or infected cyst, cavity, or bulla
Hematoma
Lung abscess (bacterial and fungal)
Lymphoma (necrotic)
Metastatic neoplasm (necrotic)
Mucoid impaction
Sequestration

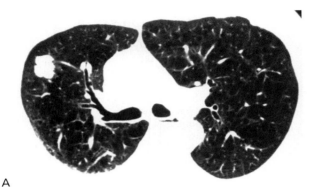

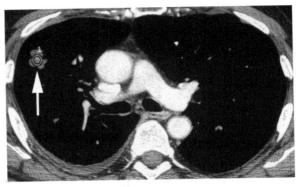

A   B

FIG. 9-21. Enhancement of a carcinoma. **A.** A lobulated right upper lobe nodule shown on HRCT represents a carcinoma. **B.** After contrast enhancement, the region of interest in the center of the nodule *(arrow)* showed an increase in attenuation of 40 HU (change from 8 to 48 HU). This is typical of malignant lesions.

minute intervals for 4 minutes following the start of the injection of 420 mg iodine/kg (usually 75 to 125 mL) at a rate of 2 mL/sec. A region of interest encompassing about 60% of the nodule diameter is used to measure enhancement.

Using this protocol, carcinomas enhance by 14 to 165 HU (median, 38 HU; Fig. 9-21) and benign lesions exhibit a change in CT number of −20 to 96 HU (median, 10 H). Using an enhancement of 15 HU or more to suggest malignancy, this test has a sensitivity of 98%, specificity of 58%, and accuracy of 77%. Specific benign lesions that show significant enhancement include active granulomas, inflammatory lesions, focal pneumonias, and some benign tumors such as hamartoma (Fig. 9-22; Table 9-12). Round atelectasis tends to enhance densely, as does any area of atelectasis.

Although the role of nodule enhancement has not yet been determined, it would seem most appropriate to use this technique when a nodule does not show typical findings of malignancy (e.g., spiculation, nodularity, cavitation, or growth) or typical features of a specific benign lesion. In such patients, this technique may help select which patients require surgery (i.e., if enhancement is present) or which can just be followed carefully (i.e., if enhancement is absent).

Contrast Opacification

Some solitary (or multiple) lesions opacify following contrast injection, thus representing vascular structures (Table 9-13). These have a limited differential diagnosis and specific morphology, described in the following sections.

Growth

Carcinomas grow (Fig. 9-23). The growth rate of an SPN has been used to determine its likelihood of being malignant. *Doubling time*, the time required for a lesion to double in volume, is used to measure growth rate. For easy reference, a 26% increase in nodule diameter is one doubling, and a doubling of diameter means that three volume doublings have occurred. However, not all carcinomas grow in

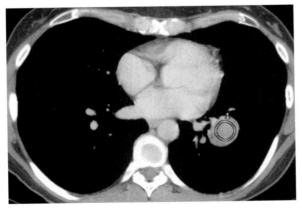

FIG. 9-22. Enhancement of a hamartoma. HRCT through a left lung nodule during contrast enhancement showed an increase in attenuation of 22 HU (increase in attenuation from 20 to 42 HU) following contrast enhancement for the region of interest shown.

TABLE 9-12. CAUSES OF A SOLITARY PULMONARY NODULE WITH CONTRAST ENHANCEMENT

Carcinoma
Carcinoid tumor
Granuloma (active)
Hamartoma or other benign tumor
Hemangioma
Focal pneumonia
Round atelectasis
Vascular metastases

TABLE 9-13. SOLITARY PULMONARY NODULES ASSOCIATED WITH CONTRAST OPACIFICATION

Arteriovenous malformation
Pulmonary vein varix
Pulmonary artery aneurysm

a concentric fashion, and estimating their volume may be difficult (see Fig. 9-23).

The range of doubling times associated with carcinoma has been reported to be 1 week to 16 months, although reported values vary. Doubling times ranging from 1 month to 200 days encompass most cancers, but doubling times of more than 1000 days have been reported for some slow-growing cancers. Average doubling times for different cell types have been estimated as 30 days for small cell carci-noma, 100 days for squamous cell and large cell carcinoma, and 180 days for adenocarcinoma. The doubling time of the slowest growing bronchioloalveolar carcinomas may be more than 3 years. Nearly all carcinomas will show growth over a follow-up period of 2 years.

It has been suggested that a typical lung cancer has dou-bled approximately 30 times by the time it reaches a diame-ter of 1 cm and becomes visible radiographically. Metastasis before the tumor is recognized radiographically probably account for the poor prognosis of many lung cancer pa-tients.

A pulmonary nodule that doubles in volume in less than 1 month or more than 200 days is very likely benign. Slower-growing lesions often are benign tumors or granu-lomas. More rapidly growing lesions usually are inflamma-tory.

However, the overlapping growth rates of benign and

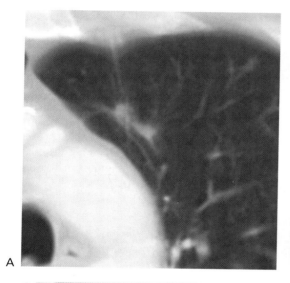
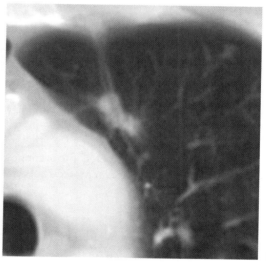
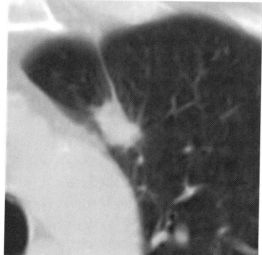

FIG. 9-23. Adenocarcinoma with growth. **A.** Base-line CT shows an irregular and spiculated nodule in the anterior lung. **B.** Follow-up CT 6 months later shows growth, although the lesion's long axis has not changed. **C.** A second follow-up CT scan obtained 1 year after that shown in **A** shows further increase in size.

malignant lesions, particularly among rapidly growing nodules, make it difficult to use doubling time as an absolute indicator that the lesion is benign. Nonetheless, it is generally agreed that a solitary pulmonary nodule that does not grow over a 2-year period most likely is benign and does not require resection. Only rare exceptions to this rule have been reported. Nonetheless, if only 2 years of stability can be demonstrated, further follow-up to ensure stability is a good idea.

If no old examinations are available, or if prior examinations are not old enough to demonstrate lack of growth for 2 years, the diagnostic approach may be based on the patient's age and the plain radiographic appearance of a lesion. If the patient is younger than 30 years of age and the pulmonary nodule appears benign (e.g., it is less than 2 cm, round, and sharply defined), follow-up should be sufficient; lung cancers are rare in patients under the age of 30. However, if the patient is older than 30, has a history of an extrathoracic tumor (which raises the possibility of a solitary metastasis), or if the lesion does not appear benign (i.e., it is large, irregular, ill-defined, or spiculated), further diagnostic procedures must be performed. In most cases CT would be appropriate.

Occasionally a patient with an acute process, such as pulmonary embolism, focal pneumonia, or other inflammatory process, can present with an SPN on chest radiographs. Short-term follow up may be indicated, particularly in patients with acute symptoms. A decrease in size of a nodule suggests it is benign, although lung cancers sometimes show a transient decrease in size because of necrosis.

For a small SPN, CT usually is required for accurate follow-up. When carcinoma is suspected, repeated scans at 3 months, 6 months, 1 year, and 2 years often are recommended.

For very small lung nodules (3 mm or smaller), follow-up at 1 year usually is sufficient. These nodules often are benign. Also, because of their small size, it is difficult to determine growth accurately when they are followed at short intervals, even on HRCT.

PET and SPECT Imaging

Positron emission tomography (PET) obtained following injection of 2-(fluorine-18)-fluoro-2-deoxy-D-glucose (FDG) may be used to characterize pulmonary nodules. FDG is a D-glucose analog labeled with a positron emitter (^{18}F) that is transported through the cell membrane and phosphorylated using normal glycolytic pathways. Increased uptake and accumulation of FDG have been shown to occur in tumor cells, although the effect is nonspecific and may be seen with inflammation.

The degree of FDG accumulation is measured using the standardized uptake ratio (SUR); the SUR of lung cancers usually is more than 2.5. FDG-PET has a sensitivity of about 95% in detecting malignant SPNs 1 cm or more in diameter, with a specificity of about 80% (Fig. 9-24). False-positive studies occur with inflammatory lesions. False-negative scans may occur with carcinoid tumor, bronchioloalveolar carcinoma, and lesions smaller than 1 cm.

Radionuclide single-photon emission computed tomography (SPECT) employing depreotide (a somatostatin analogue), thallium, or FDG also may be used to diagnose malignancy in a large lung nodule but is less sensitive than PET for nodules smaller than 2 cm.

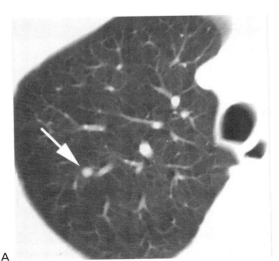
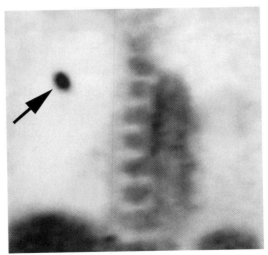

FIG. 9-24. FDG-PET in a patient with adenocarcinoma. **A.** HRCT shows a small right upper lobe nodule *(arrow).* **B.** PET (coronal plane) shows the nodule to have a very high activity *(arrow).* The size of the nodule on PET exceeds its real size. PET is poor at showing the specific location of abnormalities.

Biopsy

Methods for biopsy of an SPN include fiberoptic bronchoscopy (FOB), transthoracic needle biopsy (TNB), and surgery, including video-assisted thoracoscopic surgery (VATS).

Fiberoptic Bronchoscopy

Fiberoptic bronchoscopy with transbronchial biopsy and bronchial washing has a limited role in evaluating SPN. Although transbronchial biopsy is accurate for assessing endobronchial lesions, the yield of FOB for peripheral nodules is less than 60%, and is only 25% to 30% for an SPN smaller than 2 cm. The sensitivity of FOB is best when a bronchus leads directly to or is seen within the SPN (the "positive bronchus" sign; Fig. 9-25).

Transthoracic Needle Biopsy

Transthoracic needle biopsy is often used for assessing an SPN. The sensitivity of TNB in diagnosing cancer is over 90%. Unfortunately, the accuracy of TNB for diagnosing benign disease other than active infections is limited. Malignancy cannot be ruled out if a biopsy is "negative" but no specific benign diagnosis is made; 30% of such cases later prove to represent cancer. Biopsy of nodules smaller than 1 cm in diameter is associated with an increased false-negative rate. Complications include pneumothorax, hemorrhage, and air embolism.

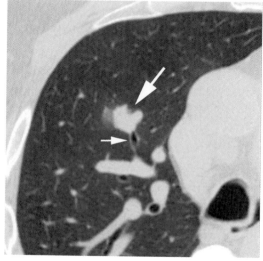

FIG. 9-25. The positive bronchus sign. A small right upper lobe nodule *(large arrow)* with a bronchus *(small arrow)* leading to it. This sign predicts a higher likelihood of a diagnosis being made at bronchoscopy.

Video-assisted Thoracic Surgery

Video-assisted thoracoscopic surgery also is used to assess indeterminate pulmonary nodules. Wedge resections and, less commonly, lobar resections may be performed using either an endoscopic stapler or a laser. CT nodule localization before surgery may be accomplished using methylene blue or a hooked wire.

A Strategy for Nodule Evaluation

If a nodule is definitely benign, based on lack of growth on sequential examinations or CT findings (i.e., it has specific morphologic characteristics of a benign lesion, contains fat, or benign calcification), further evaluation should be limited to plain film or CT follow-up.

If an SPN has benign characteristics on CT (e.g., it is small, smooth, round, and sharply defined) but is not definitely benign, and risk factors for cancer (e.g., history of malignancy, smoking history) are absent, follow-up using radiographs or CT is appropriate. Depending on the clinician's or patient's wishes, needle biopsy or PET may be performed.

If a nodule has malignant characteristics on CT (e.g., it is uncalcified, irregular in shape, or spiculated, or contains air bronchograms), in most cases a surgeon should be consulted. The surgeon may request a needle biopsy or PET scanning.

If a nodule cannot be diagnosed as benign or likely benign, and is not strongly suspicious of malignancy based on CT (i.e., if a decision to resect the nodule or leave it alone cannot be made based on history, radiographs, and CT), further radiologic assessment usually is appropriate. Methods of assessment include nodule enhancement, PET, and needle biopsy, all of which have high sensitivity for carcinoma. If the lesion is too small to biopsy or study using PET, close follow-up may be used to determine its significance.

MULTIPLE NODULES AND MASSES

This section of the chapter reviews the differential diagnosis of multiple large nodules (i.e., 1 cm or larger) and masses (Table 9-14). A nodular pattern of diffuse lung disease (i.e., innumerable nodules 1 cm or less in diameter) is discussed in Chapter 10. Obviously, there is some overlap in differential diagnosis.

Metastases should be considered most likely when multiple nodules or masses are visible (see Chapter 4). The initial evaluation of these abnormalities usually is based on history, clinical studies, and assessment of radiographic findings. Bronchoscopy or percutaneous biopsy may be needed for eventual diagnosis. An organized radiographic approach to the evaluation of multiple nodules and masses is more diffi-

TABLE 9-14. MULTIPLE PULMONARY NODULES OR MASSES

Congenital lesions and normal variants
Arteriovenous fistulas
Intrapulmonary lymph nodes
Malignant neoplasm
Bronchioloalveolar carcinoma
Carcinoma
Lymphoma
Lymphoproliferative disease
Metastatic neoplasm
Benign neoplasms and neoplasm-like conditions
Endometriomas
Lymphoproliferative disease
Multiple chondromas (Carney's triad)
Papillomas (papillomatosis)
Infection and parasites
Aspergillosis, angioinvasive
Bronchopneumonia
Echinococcus
Granulomatous infection or granulomas
   Tuberculosis
   Nontuberculous mycobacteria (e.g., *Mycobacterium avium-intracellulare* complex)
   Coccidioidomycosis
   Histoplasmosis
   Cryptococcus
Lung abscesses
Mycetomas (aspergillomas)
Paragonimiasis
Septic embolism
Inflammatory (noninfectious)
Churg-Strauss syndrome
Focal organizing pneumonia
Rheumatoid nodules
Sarcoidosis
Wegener's granulomatosis
Airways and inhalational disease
Mucoid impaction (mucous plug)
   Asthma
   Alergic bronchopulmonary aspergillosis
   Bronchiectasis
   Cystic fibrosis
Conglomerate masses or progressive massive fibrosis (e.g., silicosis)
Lipoid pneumonia
Vascular lesions
Arteriovenous fistulas
Hematomas
Infarctions
Pulmonary artery aneurysms
Septic embolism
Idiopathic and miscellaneous
Amyloidosis
Fluid-filled bullae
Round atelectasis

cult to devise than for the SPN, but it is based on many of the same principles.

Size

Benign and malignant lesions may be either small or large. A clear-cut relation of size to malignancy does not exist as it does with SPN. There is a tendency for multiple nodular metastases to vary in size (see Fig. 4-8 in Chapter 4), whereas benign processes result in nodules of similar size.

Number

Multinodular metastases may be few in number or innumerable, but a large number of nodules suggests this diagnosis (see Figs. 4-8 to 4-11 in Chapter 4). Most infectious and inflammatory diseases result in less than a dozen nodules.

Location

Metastases, infarction, and septic emboli have a predilection for the lung periphery and the lung bases. Abscesses related to aspiration often are posterior or basal in distribution.

Edge Appearance

Metastases usually are sharply marginated (see Figs. 4-8 to 4-11 in Chapter 4), as are nodules in amyloidosis, rheumatoid nodules, AVMs, hematomas, and Caplan's syndrome. Infectious lesions, diffuse bronchioloalveolar carcinoma (see Figs. 3-8, 3-9, and 3-22 in Chapter 3), lymphoma (see Figs. 5-10 to 5-12 in Chapter 5), conglomerate masses and progressive massive fibrosis, and Wegener's granulomatosis are often ill-defined.

An increase in sharpness of the edge of a lesion with time suggests resolution of a benign inflammatory process. For example, septic emboli, lung abscesses, infections, and Wegener's granulomatosis result in masses that are ill-defined early in their course and become sharply defined as they heal.

The halo sign may be seen in patients with multiple nodules; its differential diagnosis is described in Table 9-4.

Cavitation

As with SPNs, thick-walled cavities are consistent with malignancy, but thick walls may be seen with inflammatory, nonmalignant lesions as well. Very thin-walled cavities usually are benign, although metastatic tumors, particularly squamous cell carcinoma of the head and neck or sarcomas and tracheobronchial papillomatosis, may be associated with thin-walled lesions. As with SPN, an air-fluid level tends to predict benign disease. The differential diagnosis of multiple cystic or cavitary lesions is reviewed in Table 9-6.

Growth

Rapid growth with increase in size over a period of a few days suggests infection (e.g., bacterial infection or fungus or TB in an immunosuppressed patient). Progression over a period of a few weeks is typical of indolent infections (e.g., TB or fungus in an immunocompetent patient), noninfectious inflammatory disease, or rapidly progressing malignancy (Fig. 9-26). Nodules that appear stable over a period of weeks or show slow growth during a few months are likely to be either malignant or due to indolent inflammatory conditions (e.g., rheumatoid nodules). Masses that show little change over a period of months are typical of amyloidosis, AVMs, benign tumors, and conglomerate masses. Some metastatic tumors (e.g., thyroid carcinoma or benign metastasizing leiomyoma) may show very slow growth.

Resolution of lesions with or without treatment suggests benign disease. Slow resolution is typical of hematoma and infarction. Rapid resolution is typical of treated infections.

DIFFERENTIAL DIAGNOSIS OF LUNG NODULES, MASSES, AND CAVITIES

The large number of diseases and abnormalities associated with solitary or multiple nodules, masses, or cysts are reviewed in the following sections in alphabetical order. These are discussed in more detail elsewhere in this book.

Amyloidosis

Patients with localized nodular amyloidosis usually are asymptomatic. Nodular amyloidosis may manifest as single or multiple lung nodules or masses, usually well-defined and round (see Fig. 21-5 in Chapter 21). Bilateral lung nodules are most typical, and they tend to be peripheral or subpleural in location. Nodules range from 0.5 to 5 cm in diameter in most cases, but may be as large as 10 cm. Calcification is visible radiographically in 30% to 50% of cases, and may be stippled or dense. Cavitation may be seen in approximately 5%. Nodules may grow slowly or remain stable over a number of years. Needle biopsy may be diagnostic. Amyloidosis is discussed in detail in Chapter 21.

Arteriovenous Malformation

Congenital arteriovenous malformation, also known as arteriovenous fistula, is associated with Osler-Weber-Rendu syndrome in 35% to 67% of cases. *Simple AVM* represents a single, dilated vascular sac connecting one artery and one vein (see Figs. 1-10 to 1-15 in Chapter 1). It is the most common type and accounts for almost all cases of AVM. Radiographically, a simple fistula appears as a peripheral, well-defined, round, oval, lobulated, or serpentine density. Large vessels (feeders) extending centrally toward the hilum are easily seen on CT. AVM typically are subpleural in location, and more than two thirds are found in the lower lobes. Fistulas are multiple in 35% of patients and bilateral in 10%. Multiple AVM are most common in patients with Osler-Weber-Rendu syndrome. Enlargement of fistulas over a period of months or years is common, and rapid increase in size can occur. Opacification occurs following contrast enhancement. AVM are discussed in detail in Chapter 1.

Aspergillosis

Angioinvasive Aspergillosis

Angioinvasive aspergillosis is characterized by involvement of normal lung tissue by aspergillus organisms, usually resulting in significant tissue damage and necrosis. It almost always occurs in immunosuppressed patients, and is particu-

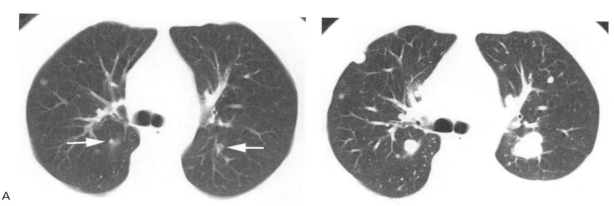

FIG. 9-26. Metastases from a spindle cell sarcoma with rapid growth. **A.** CT scan shows multiple small nodules *(arrows)*. **B.** Follow-up scan 6 weeks later shows marked increase in size. Such rapid growth suggests an infectious or inflammatory process, but may be seen with very rapidly growing neoplasms.

larly common in association with (1) neutropenia in patients with acute leukemia; (2) treatment using corticosteroids or other immunosuppressive agents; (3) organ transplantation; and (4) malignancy. Pathologic examination shows infiltration of lung tissue by fungus, with invasion of small arteries, vascular occlusion, and, often, infarction of involved lung.

Early in the course of disease, ill-defined nodules up to several centimeters in diameter or focal areas of consolidation typically are seen on chest radiographs. At this stage, CT typically shows the halo sign (see Figs. 9-7 and 9-27). The halo and central nodule reflect, respectively, a rim of hemorrhage surrounding a central fungal nodule or infarct. In an immunosuppressed patient, the CT appearance of early invasive aspergillosis with a visible halo sign is sufficiently characteristic to justify a presumptive diagnosis and treatment. However, as described above, the halo sign can be associated with a variety of infectious and noninfectious processes.

If patients with invasive aspergillosis survive their acute infection, nodules often cavitate, showing the air-crescent sign (see Fig. 9-27). The presence of an air crescent in angioinvasive aspergillosis reflects lung necrosis with the presence of a sequestrum or ball of devitalized and necrotic lung occupying part of the cavity. Although this appearance mimics that of a mycetoma, the two conditions are unrelated.

Cavitation, when present, generally occurs about 2 weeks after the appearance of nodular opacities and is associated with a white blood cell count of more than 1000. Thus, the presence of cavitation is generally considered to be a good prognostic sign.

Semi-invasive (Chronic Necrotizing) Aspergillosis

Semi-invasive (chronic necrotizing) aspergillosis typically is associated with slowly progressive upper lobe abnormalities. Most patients have an underlying chronic lung disease such as tuberculosis, chronic obstructive pulmonary disease, fibrosis, or pneumoconiosis. Patients may be mildly immunocompromised (e.g., chronic disease, advanced age, diabetes, poor nutrition, alcoholism, low-dose corticosteroid treatment), but lack the severe immune deficiencies typical of patients with invasive aspergillosis. Pathology reveals a combination of granulomatous inflammation, necrosis, and fibrosis similar to that seen in tuberculosis. Symptoms are nonspecific, consisting of cough, sputum production, weight loss, fever, and hemoptysis.

Radiographs and CT typically show upper lobe consolidation, with progressive cavitation over a period of weeks to months, indistinguishable from TB. It is common to see irregular thickening of the wall of a cavity or frondlike intracavity opacities representing growing fungus. Frank aspergillomas may develop in patients with semi-invasive aspergillosis. These may have a typical (i.e., air-crescent sign) or atypical appearance. With progressive disease, pleural and chest wall involvement may be present.

Bronchiectasis

Bronchiectasis may result in the presence of multiple cystic lung lesions (i.e., cystic bronchiectasis). These often have thin but easily recognizable walls, and may be focal or diffuse in distribution. Air-fluid levels are common, representing secretions and pus, and help to distinguish cystic bronchiectasis from cystic lung diseases such as lymphangiomyomatosis, histiocytosis, and lymphoid (lymphocytic) interstitial pneumonitis. Because the cystic areas communicate with each other (via the bronchial tree), the amount of fluid in each "cyst" is similar or more fluid is seen in cysts located at the lung bases (Fig. 9-28).

Bronchogenic Cyst

Pulmonary bronchogenic cysts are most common in the medial lung and the lower lobes. Uninfected cysts are

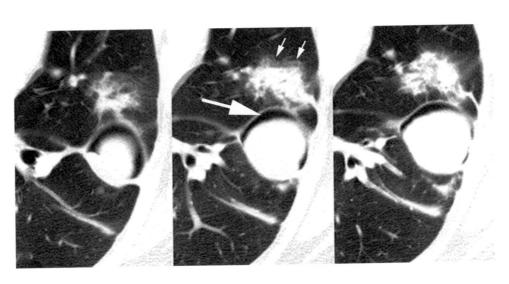

FIG. 9-27. Angioinvasive aspergillosis with halo sign and air-crescent sign. CT scans at three adjacent levels in a patient with leukemia show an air-crescent sign *(large arrow)* outlining a "lung ball" within a cavity. Anterior to it is an ill-defined nodule with a halo sign *(small arrows)*.

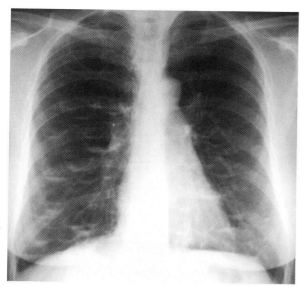

FIG. 9-28. Cystic bronchiectasis. Multiple thin-walled cysts represent cystic bronchiectasis. Air-fluid levels are visible, with the largest amount of fluid being in cysts at the lung bases. This implies communication between the cysts and is diagnostic of bronchiectasis.

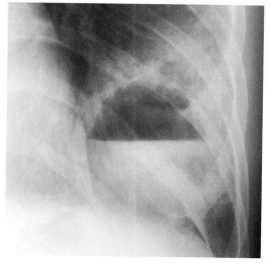

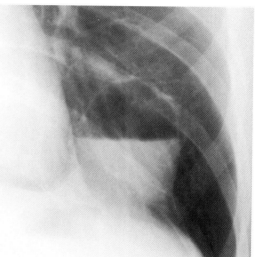

FIG. 9-29. Bronchogenic cyst. **A.** When it is acutely infected, the air- and fluid-filled cyst is very ill-defined, resembling a lung abscess. **B.** After treatment, a thin-walled cystic lesion is visible in the left lung. This was found to represent a bronchogenic cyst. The presence of an air-fluid level indicates prior infection.

sharply circumscribed and round or oval in shape; their wall is invisible on CT or appears very thin. Fluid-filled bronchogenic cysts may appear to contain fluid on CT (0 to 20 HU; see Fig. 1-6 in Chapter 1) or may have high CT numbers (40 to 80 HU). Rarely, the cyst wall may calcify or the cyst may contain milk of calcium and appear dense. Infection eventually occurs in 75% of cases. In the presence of acute infection, a rapid increase in size of the cyst may be seen. In addition, the outer cyst wall may become less well-defined because of surrounding lung inflammation (Fig. 9-29A). A previously infected cyst may contain air, showing a thin and well-defined wall, and may contain an air-fluid level (see Fig. 9-29B and Fig. 1-7 in Chapter 1).

Bronchioloalveolar Carcinoma

Bronchioloalveolar carcinoma (BAC) most often presents as a solitary nodule, often appearing spiculated, containing air bronchograms, and associated with the halo sign or appearing to be entirely ground-glass opacity. However, 40% of patients show radiographic findings of diffuse lung involvement (see Figs. 3-8, 3-9, and 3-22 in Chapter 3). Thirty percent of these demonstrate multiple ill-defined nodules, which may be centrilobular in distribution on HRCT. The nodules are usually 5 mm to 1 cm in diameter and may be patchy in distribution or diffuse. Most (60%) of the remaining patients with diffuse BAC show patchy, lobar, or diffuse consolidation, with air bronchograms. Nodules and consolidation may be seen in combination.

Bullae

By definition, a bulla is a sharply demarcated area of emphysema, measuring 1 cm or more in diameter, and possessing a wall less than 1 mm thick. Bullae usually are a manifestation of paraseptal emphysema but also may be seen in patients with centrilobular emphysema. Bullae usually are subpleural in location, largest at the lung apices, and very thinwalled (Fig. 9-30A); these findings usually allow their accurate diagnosis on chest radiographs or CT. On HRCT, other areas of emphysema usually are visible.

A bulla may contain fluid, showing an air-fluid level or appearing as a focal mass. This may result from infection, hemorrhage, tumor arising in a bulla, or bland fluid accu-

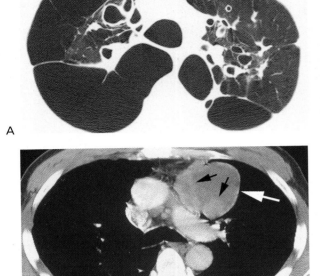

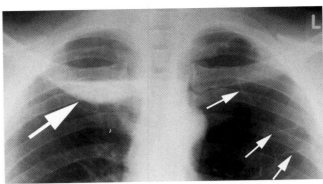

FIG. 9-30. Bullae. **A.** Bullous emphysema with large subpleural bullae. These appear very thin-walled. Bronchiectasis also is visible, resulting in thicker-walled cystic structures in the central lung. **B.** Bullous emphysema with infection. Multiple thin-walled bullae are visible in the left upper lobe *(small arrows)*. An air-fluid level in a right upper lobe bulla *(large arrow)* suggests infection. **C.** Carcinoma arising in a bulla. A patient with bullous emphysema shows a fluid-filled bulla *(white arrow)* in the left upper lobe. Masses *(black arrows)* within the bulla represent carcinoma.

mulation (see Fig. 9-30B and C). The identification of other bullae may be helpful in diagnosis. CT may show the fluid nature of the opacity or associated wall thickening in patients with tumor.

Carcinoma

Approximately one third of lung cancers present radiographically as a solitary pulmonary nodule or lung mass. The most common cell types presenting as a nodule or mass are adenocarcinoma (40%), squamous cell carcinoma (20%), large cell carcinoma (15%), and bronchioloalveolar carcinoma (10%). Nearly two thirds of lung cancers presenting as a lung nodule occur in the upper lobes. Because they usually are not associated with symptoms, they often are relatively large when first detected; nearly 60% are larger than 2 cm, and 25% are larger than 3 cm. The appearances of lung carcinoma are described earlier in this chapter and in Chapter 3.

Multiple lung nodules may occur in patients with lung cancer in the presence of multiple synchronous primary tumors, satellite nodules associated with the primary tumor due to local spread, or hematogenous metastases to lung from the primary lung cancer, or in patients with diffuse bronchioloalveolar carcinoma (see Figs. 3-8, 3-9, and 3-22 in Chapter 3). In patients with metastatic carcinoma, the primary lesions usually is visible as a dominant mass (Fig. 9-31).

Carcinoid Tumor

Carcinoid tumors account for 1% to 2% of tracheobronchial neoplasms. Approximately 20% of carcinoid tumors present as a peripheral nodule or mass. They often are well-defined, round or oval, and slightly lobulated in contour (see Fig. 3-44 in Chapter 3). Calcification is uncommonly seen on radiographs, but is visible on CT in nearly 40%. Approximately 10% to 25% of carcinoid tumors can be classified as *atypical carcinoid tumor* because of histologic features suggesting a more aggressive behavior. Atypical carcinoid tumors tend to present as a lung nodule or mass somewhat larger than seen with carcinoid tumor. Cavitation is rare. Dense enhancement may be seen following contrast infusion. Carcinoid tumor is discussed in Chapter 3.

Churg-Strauss Syndrome

Churg-Strauss syndrome is characterized by a combination of necrotizing vasculitis, extravascular granulomas, and tissue infiltration by eosinophils. Patients with this syndrome usually are middle-aged (average onset, 40 to 50 years), and often have a history of allergic diseases including asthma, nasal polyps, or sinusitis. One or more ill-defined pulmonary nodules, up to 3.5 cm, are seen in 20% of cases. Cavitation is uncommon, a finding that is helpful in distinguishing Churg-Strauss syndrome from Wegener's granulomatosis, which may have a similar presentation. Other common radiographic abnormalities, which may be seen in combina-

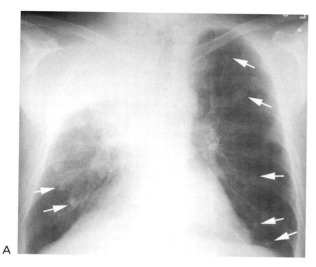

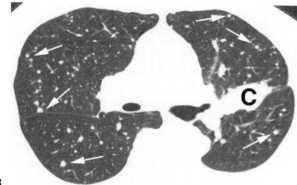

FIG. 9-31. Lung cancer with multiple nodules representing metastases. **A.** A patient with right upper lobe collapse due to right hilar carcinoma shows multiple small nodules *(arrows)* representing metastases. **B.** CT in a patient with left-sided carcinoma *(C)* who shows diffuse nodular metastases *(arrows)*.

tion, consist of transient multifocal areas of consolidation indistinguishable from simple pulmonary eosinophilia or chronic eosinophilic pneumonia. Pulmonary hemorrhage may be associated. Churg-Strauss syndrome is described in detail in Chapter 16.

Congenital Cystic Adenomatoid Malformation

Congenital cystic adenomatoid malformation (CCAM) consists of a multicystic, intralobar mass of disorganized lung tissue. About 70% of cases present during the first week of life, but 10% are diagnosed after the first year. Lower lobes are involved most often, but any lobe can be affected. CCAM often is classified into three types that have different histology, gross pathologic findings, and radiographic appearances.

Type I CCAM (55% of cases) contains one or more cysts, which are larger than 2 cm in diameter (see Fig. 1-8 in Chapter 1). Type I CCAM usually presents as a large, air-filled, multicystic lesion, sometimes with air-fluid levels, which may occupy the entire hemithorax.

Type II CCAM (40% of cases) contains multiple cysts less than 2 cm in diameter. It presents as an air-filled multicystic mass or a solid mass or area of consolidation (see Fig. 1-9 in Chapter 1).

Type III CCAM (5% of cases) contains microscopic (less than 3 to 5 mm) cysts, and presents radiographically as a solid mass.

Types I and II CCAM may become air-filled over a period of days to weeks after birth. They often are associated with progressive air trapping and mediastinal shift to the opposite side. In adults, CCAM usually presents as an air-filled or air- and fluid-filled cystic or multicystic mass.

Conglomerate Masses

Large conglomerate masses may develop in patients with sarcoidosis (see Figs. 15-9 and 15-12 in Chapter 15), long-standing silicosis or coal-worker's pneumoconiosis (see Figs. 18-10 and 18-11 in Chapter 18), and talcosis (see Fig. 18-13 in Chapter 18), and in association with some granulomatous infections. Their appearances are similar. In silicosis, conglomerate masses reflect the presence of progressive massive fibrosis.

These masses represent a conglomeration of small interstitial nodules in combination with a variable degree of fibrosis. A background pattern of multiple small lung nodules often is visible (satellite nodules). Conglomerate masses are typically, but not always, seen in the upper lobes or mid-lung, are usually oval or lenticular in shape, are distinct from the hila, and are separated from peripheral pleural surface (Fig. 9-32). Nearly all have irregular borders. They often are bilateral and symmetrical.

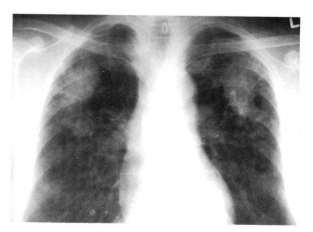

FIG. 9-32. Conglomerate masses (progressive massive fibrosis) in silicosis. Conglomerate masses typically—but not always—are seen in the upper lobes or mid-lung, and usually are oval or lenticular in shape. They often are bilateral and symmetrical.

Distortion of lung architecture usually is evident due to fibrosis and volume loss. Traction bronchiectasis with air bronchograms may be seen within the masses, and surrounding bullae may be present. Calcification in association with conglomerate masses is common. Talcosis, secondary to intravenous injection of talc, is seen almost exclusively in drug users who inject medications intended for oral use; the masses may appear high in attenuation on CT because of the talc they contain. Central necrosis or cavitation may be present, and may indicate superinfection by TB or bacteria. Cavities usually are thick-walled.

Cysts and Cystic Lung Disease

Cyst is a nonspecific term describing the presence of a thin-walled (usually less than 3 mm), well-defined and circumscribed, air- or fluid-containing lesion, 1 cm or more in diameter, and having an epithelial or fibrous wall. The term usually is used to describe the presence of a thin-walled lesion when a more specific diagnosis cannot be made. Cysts may be congenital (e.g., bronchogenic cyst) or acquired (e.g., honeycombing, bullae, pneumatocele). It is not uncommon to see one or more (i.e., up to a few) lung cysts in an asymptomatic patient without known disease. These are usually undiagnosed and are rarely of significance.

Multiple lung cysts as a manifestation of diffuse lung disease are seen in patients with Langerhans' histiocytosis, lymphangiomyomatosis, sarcoidosis, and lymphoid (lymphocytic) interstitial pneumonitis (see Chapter 25).

Lung cysts may contain fluid as a result of accumulated secretions or in the presence of infection, hemorrhage, or tumor. Thickening of the wall of a cyst suggests infection or tumor. Fluid filling cysts is uncommon in patients with cystic lung diseases such as lymphangiomyomatosis, histiocytosis, and lymphoid (lymphocytic) interstitial pneumonitis.

Dirofilaria immitis

Dirofilaria immitis is the dog heartworm. Humans may become infected by a mosquito bite. Larvae travel to right-sided cardiac chambers, but cannot live in humans, and eventually embolize to the pulmonary vascular bed, where they result in an infarct and granulomatous response. A small lung nodule may result, usually less than 2 cm in diameter, rounded, sharply marginated, and subpleural in location (Fig. 9-33). Calcification may be visible on CT. Eosinophilia usually is absent. It is most common in eastern and southern states.

Echinococcus Species

Echinococcus granulosus and *Echinococcus multilocularis* are intestinal tapeworms of canine carnivores such as the dog and wolf. Ova are dispersed in feces and ingested by an intermediate host. Larvae develop in the intestine of the intermediate host and migrate via the circulation to organs such as the liver and lungs, where they develop and encyst. When the larva is consumed by the carnivore (at the same time the intermediate host is consumed), the adult tapeworm develops in the carnivore.

The development of parasites in the intermediate host results in one or more hydatid cysts, usually in the liver or lungs, an occurrence termed *hydatid disease*. Hydatid disease occurs in two forms. In the pastoral form, a dog is the primary host and sheep are the intermediate host; it occurs in sheep-raising countries and is most common in the Mediterranean regions of Europe and North Africa, in South America, and in Australia. In the *sylvatic* or sylvian form, the wolf is the primary host, and wild animals such as deer, moose, or caribou are intermediate hosts; it is endemic in Arctic regions such as Alaska or Siberia. Humans may serve as an intermediate host of either form.

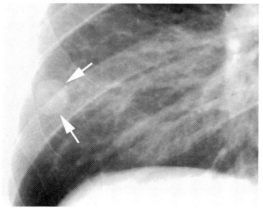
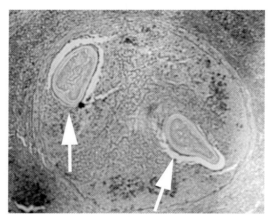

FIG. 9-33. Lung nodule secondary to *Dirofilaria immitis* infection. **A.** A sharply marginated rounded nodule *(arrows)* is visible in the peripheral right lung. **B.** The histologic specimen following resection shows an intravascular worm *(arrows)* within the nodule.

Pulmonary lesions have three components, a knowledge of which is important in understanding the radiographic appearance of pulmonary hydatid cysts. The outermost part is termed the *pericyst*. It consists of compressed lung tissue and fibrosis adjacent to the parasite. The parasite itself is composed of two layers, an outer layer or *ectocyst* and an inner layer or *endocyst*, from which daughter cysts bud.

Uncomplicated pulmonary hydatid cysts are fluid-filled, rounded, and may be quite large (over 10 cm; Fig. 9-34). Pulmonary cysts are solitary in more than half of cases. They occur most commonly in the lower lobes. Rapid growth may be seen. CT may show a wall ranging up to 1 cm in thickness, largely depending on the thickness of the pericyst. Cyst contents are of fluid attenuation on CT, but septations may be visible, representing the walls of daughter cysts. Although common in the liver, calcification of the walls of cysts is rare in the lung. Liver cysts may or may not be present in a patient with lung cysts.

Rupture of the pericyst leads to dissection of air between the pericyst and the ectocyst, forming an air-crescent sign. Rupture of the extocyst, with expulsion of some fluid contents, results in an air-fluid level, and allows the endocyst to collapse. The presence of the endocyst floating on the fluid may be visible as the "water lily" (*camalote*) sign. Rupture of the cyst into the pleural space may result in effusion or seeding of the pleural space with cysts. Rupture of the cyst into a bronchus may be associated with allergic reaction or infection. Mediastinal cysts may be seen. Diagnosis usually is based on serologic tests. Biopsy should be avoided because of risk of rupture.

Endometrioma

Nodules of the endometrium may rarely involve the lung parenchyma. They typically occur in women who have pre-

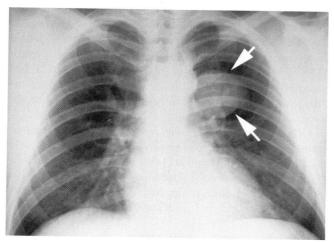

FIG. 9-34. Pulmonary hydatid cyst *(arrows)* resulting from the sylvatic form of disease. A fisherman from Alaska shows a focal rounded opacity.

viously given birth or have had uterine surgery and probably reflect embolism and implantation of endometrial tissue. Pelvic endometriosis need not be present. Pulmonary endometrioma may result in catamenial hemoptysis or pulmonary hemorrhage, symptoms that strongly suggest the diagnosis. Pneumothorax may result if the implants involve the pleural surface. Pulmonary endometrioma usually is solitary, appearing in most cases as a well-defined rounded nodule up to a few centimeters in diameter. Cavitation may occur, with the cavity often appearing thin-walled. Treatment is hormonal or by excision.

Focal Organizing Pneumonia

Organizing pneumonia (OP), also known as bronchiolitis obliterans organizing pneumonia (BOOP), is characterized pathologically by the presence of granulation tissue polyps within bronchioles and alveolar ducts and patchy areas of inflammation in the surrounding lung (organizing pneumonia). Most cases are idiopathic, but OP also may be seen in patients with pulmonary infection, drug reactions, collagen-vascular diseases, Wegener's granulomatosis, and after inhalation of toxic fumes.

Most often, OP presents with patchy, unilateral or bilateral areas of air-space consolidation, which may be peripheral or peribronchial. Small or large nodules are seen, with or without associated consolidation, in up to 50% (see Figs. 13-18 and 13-19 in Chapter 13, and Fig. 17-3 in Chapter 17). Large nodules or masses usually are multiple and may appear very irregular in shape, mimicking carcinoma. A finding termed the "atoll" sign, in which ring-shaped or crescentic opacities are seen, often with ground-glass opacity in the center of the ring (resembling a coral atoll), may be seen with OP. This finding strongly suggests the diagnosis. High-attenuation nodules or masses may be seen in patients with OP related to amiodarone toxicity due to its iodine content. Cavitation and calcification do not occur.

Focal (Round) Pneumonia

Pneumonias may be focal, mimicking the appearance of carcinoma. This configuration has been termed "round pneumonia." Findings suggestive of focal pneumonia include satellite nodules, tree-in-bud, centrilobular nodules (Fig. 9-35A), or a lobular or multilobular pattern, but these do not need to be seen to establish the diagnosis. Focal infections are common with bacterial bronchopneumonia (see Fig. 9-34A), TB, nontuberculous mycobacteria, and fungal infection (see Fig. 9-34B), and occasionally are seen with viral infection or infection with *Pneumocystis jiroveci* (formerly *P. carinii*; see Fig. 9-34C). Focal opacities associated with infection may be solitary or multiple. The halo sign is common with angioinvasive aspergillosis (see Figs. 9-7 and 9-27), but may be seen with focal infection of various causes (see Fig. 9-34C).

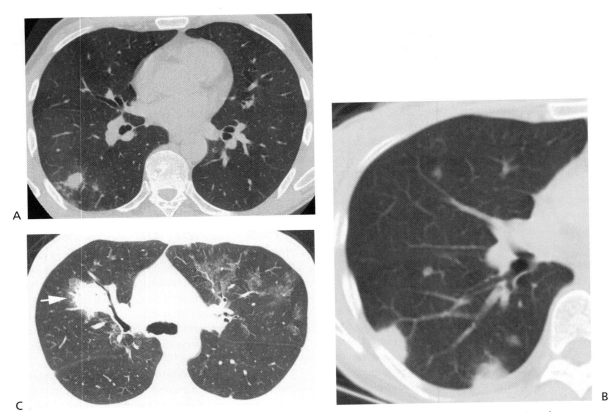

FIG. 9-35. Focal (round) pneumonia. **A.** An irregular nodule is visible in the right lung, associated with satellite nodules in a patient with bacterial infection. This appearance may be seen in patients with infection from a variety of organisms. **B.** Cryptococcal pneumonia with multiple focal areas of consolidation. **C.** *Pneumocystis jiroveci* (*P. carinii*) infection in a patient with AIDS. Patchy ground-glass opacity is visible bilaterally, typical of this infection. A focal mass with a halo sign within the right lung *(arrow)* also represented *Pneumocystis* infection.

Granuloma

Granulomas may be the result of tuberculosis, nontuberculous mycobacteria, and fungal infections, most commonly coccidioidomycosis and histoplasmosis. They usually are well-defined and rounded (see Fig. 9-3). Granulomas associated with surrounding lung fibrosis (common in tuberculosis) may appear very irregular and spiculated in contour, mimicking carcinoma. Granulomas also may be associated with irregular cavities. Calcification is common, but may have a variety of appearances—dense and homogeneous, central, lamellar, eccentric, or stippled.

Granulomas usually are smaller than 2 cm in diameter, and often are solitary or few in number. Numerous small granulomas, a few millimeters in diameter, also may be seen.

Hamartoma

Hamartoma is the most common mesenchymal lung tumor and accounts for more than 75% of benign lung tumors. More than 85% appear radiographically as a solitary pulmo-

nary nodule. Peripheral hamartomas usually are 1 to 4 cm in diameter, well-defined, sharply circumscribed, and often lobulated (see Fig. 9-4 and Figs. 3-50 to 3-52 in Chapter 3). Calcification is visible on plain radiographs in approximately 30% of hamartomas and is seen more commonly on CT. The calcification of hamartomas can be stippled or conglomerate, referred to as "popcorn" calcification. Nearly 65% of hamartomas may be diagnosed using HRCT because of visible fat (-40 to -120 HU), either focal or diffuse or a combination of fat and calcification. Cavitation is rare.

Other benign tumors may arise from mesenchymal or epithelial tissues. They usually are well-defined and rounded. Benign tumors usually are solitary. Multiple chondromas may be associated with Carney's triad (i.e., multiple pulmonary chondromas, gastric epithelioid leiomyosarcoma, and extra-adrenal paraganglioma).

Hematoma and Laceration

Hematomas are often the result of trauma (blunt or penetrating), representing focal lung contusion or pulmonary

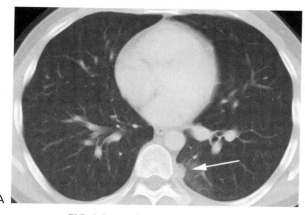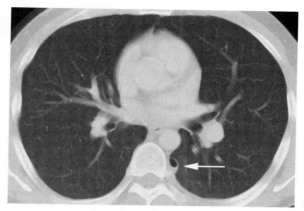

FIG. 9-36. Pulmonary laceration with hematoma in a hockey player with hemoptysis after a "bad body check." **A.** A focal lung opacity *(arrow)* represents a focal hematoma. Some surrounding ground-glass opacity is due to hemorrhage. **B.** At a different level, an air-fluid level *(arrow)* is visible within a focal cystic lesion.

laceration containing blood. Contusion represents focal bleeding without disruption of lung architecture. Traumatic laceration is associated with tearing of lung; a laceration contains blood or air (or both), with air-fluid levels sometimes visible (Figs. 9-36 and 9-37). These lesions usually are thin-walled. They may be solitary or multiple. High-attenuation clot may be detectable using CT. Focal hematoma also may result from other causes of bleeding.

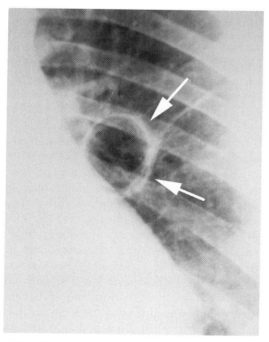

FIG. 9-37. Pulmonary laceration. A cystic air-filled lesion in the left lung *(arrows)* represents a laceration from a stab wound.

Infarction

Focal consolidation distal to a pulmonary embolus may be due to ischemia with focal pulmonary hemorrhage or frank infarction. Because the lung is supplied by both pulmonary and bronchial arteries, pulmonary infarction occurs in the minority (10% to 15%) of patients with pulmonary embolism, and often is associated with underlying cardiovascular disease, the presence of peripheral emboli, or multiple emboli.

Hemorrhage or infarction in the peripheral lung may result in a wedge-shaped or rounded, pleural-based opacity, the classic "Hampton hump." Subpleural opacities are seen more often in the lower lobes, where most emboli occur. On plain films, these opacities usually are not associated with air-bronchograms; the absence of air bronchograms is likely due to blood filling the bronchi. Pulmonary opacities due to hemorrhage usually resolve within a week, but pulmonary infarctions may require months to heal. They typically resolve by maintaining the same shape while decreasing in size, an occurrence called the "melting" sign because of its resemblance to a melting ice cube. Infarctions often leave linear scars.

On CT (Fig. 9-38), a pulmonary infarction may be characterized by the following features:

1. A wedge-shaped opacity (sometimes with a truncated apex)
2. Contact with the pleural surface
3. Convex borders
4. A linear opacity directed from the apex of the density toward the hilum (i.e., its feeding vessel)
5. Scattered areas of low attenuation (necrosis) within the lesion
6. A halo sign due to adjacent hemorrhage

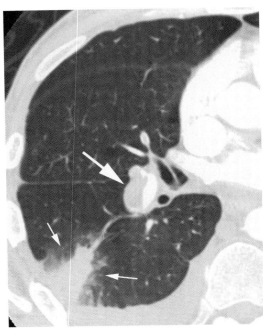

FIG. 9-38. Pulmonary infarction in a patient with pulmonary embolism. CT shows a pulmonary embolus in the right interlobar pulmonary artery *(large arrow)*. A wedge-shaped opacity *(small arrows)* is visible in the peripheral lung, contacting the pleural surface, and associated with surrounding ground-glass opacity (halo sign). A vessel is noted at the apex of the opacity. A pleural effusion is associated.

Some or all of these findings are seen on CT in about half of patients with pulmonary embolism.

Following the administration of a bolus of intravenous contrast medium, the perimeter of an infarct characteristically enhances, possibly because of collateral blood flow from adjacent bronchial arteries, while the center of the lesion remains lucent. Cavitation of an infarction suggests septic embolism or infection of a bland infarct.

Intrapulmonary Lymph Nodes

Intrapulmonary lymph nodes may be visible as small peripheral lung nodules, usually well-defined, smooth, and rounded in contour. They may be located immediately beneath the visceral pleural surface or within 2 cm of the pleura, and are most common at the lung bases. They usually measure a few millimeters in diameter, but may be as large as 1 cm. They are almost always solitary.

Lipoid Pneumonia

Lipoid pneumonia (lung consolidation containing lipid) may be endogenous or exogenous.

Endogenous lipoid pneumonia may occur due to bronchial obstruction with the distal accumulation of lipid-rich cellular debris distal to the obstructing lesion.

Exogenous lipoid pneumonia results from the chronic aspiration of animal, vegetable, or petroleum-based oils or fats. Consolidation, ill-defined masses, or (sometimes) findings of fibrosis are seen on chest radiographs. A posterior or lower lobe distribution is typical. Opacities may be bilateral or unilateral. If a large amount of lipid has been aspirated, CT can show rounded or irregular areas of low-attenuation consolidation (-35 to -75 HU); this appearance is most common in patients with chronic mineral oil aspiration (see Figs. 20-1 and 20-2 in Chapter 20). Because inflammation or fibrosis may accompany the presence of the lipid material, the CT attenuation of the consolidation need not be low, but in many cases small areas of low-attenuation oil are visible within larger masses. In some patients, necrosis and cavitation may be present.

Lung Abscess

Lung abscess is an infected, necrotic, pus-filled cavity. If communication with a bronchus occurs, partial drainage of the abscess contents may occur. With a chronic abscess, the wall of the cavity may be surrounded by granulation tissue or fibrosis.

Lung abscess may result from pyogenic bacteria, mycobacteria, fungal organisms, parasites, and, rarely, viral infections. Many cases are caused by anaerobic organisms in association with poor oral hygiene and periodontal disease, conditions predisposing to aspiration, and old age. Lung abscess may also be associated with infection by *Klebsiella pneumoniae*, *Staphylococcus aureus*, *Pseudomonas aeruginosa*, *Nocardia* spp., *Actinomyces* spp., and TB. They may occur as complications of infarction, cavitary neoplasm, and cavitary conglomerate mass.

In patients with an anaerobic abscess, symptoms include low-grade fever, cough, and sputum production, often of several weeks' duration. In patients with other causes of bacterial abscess, symptoms usually are acute and resemble those of pneumonia.

On plain radiographs, acute lung abscesses usually appear as irregular masses. The outer aspect of an abscess may be very ill-defined because of surrounding inflammation and lung consolidation. An air-fluid level may be seen if communication with a bronchus and partial drainage have occurred.

On CT, when contrast medium is infused, lung abscesses typically show a densely enhancing wall that is variable in thickness and irregular in contour (Fig. 9-39A). The internal wall of the abscess cavity often is shaggy (Fig. 9-40). The outer wall may be sharply marginated and smooth, irregular, or obscured by surrounding consolidation. The contents of a lung abscess appear low in attenuation (i.e., fluid attenuation) compared to the density of the enhancing wall or surrounding consolidated lung. An air-fluid level may be seen (see Fig. 9-10). Bronchi may be seen entering the abscess, an appearance that helps to distinguish lung abscess from empyema.

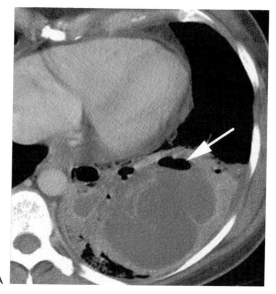 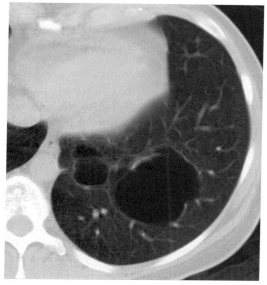

FIG. 9-39. Lung abscess. **A.** Acutely, an irregular, fluid-filled abscess is visible in the left lung on contrast-enhanced CT. Its wall enhances. A small amount of air *(arrow)* is visible within the fluid-filled cavity. **B.** After healing, a thin-walled cystic lesion is visible in the left lower lobe.

With healing, the wall of an abscess becomes thinner and more sharply defined (see Fig. 9-39B). The abscess tends to decrease in size, and the amount of fluid in the abscess decreases. Complete resolution or focal scarring is typical.

In patients with clinical symptoms of infection, the diagnosis of lung abscess usually is not difficult. However, the appearance of a peripheral abscess may overlap that of empyema. This distinction is important to make because empyema is often treated by tube drainage, whereas abscess is not. Several findings usually assist in distinguishing between these two entities.

Lung abscesses typically are round or oval in shape and form acute angles where they touch the pleural surface. Abscesses tend to have an irregularly thick wall in their acute

stage. Because an abscess represents necrotic lung, pulmonary vessels or bronchi may be seen entering an abscess wall or may be seen within its center.

Empyemas typically are oval, lenticular, or crescentic in shape and usually show obtuse angles at the pleural surface. The walls of an empyema cavity tend to be smooth and regular in thickness, although the wall may be partially obscured by adjacent atelectasis. Pulmonary vessels and bronchi are displaced by an empyema.

Lymphoma

Lymphomas may be associated with single or multiple lung nodules, masses, or focal mass-like areas of consolidation. Cavitation may occur. The presence of associated lymph node enlargement is variable. The lymphomas are discussed in detail in Chapter 5.

Hodgkin's disease (HD) involves lung in 10% of patients at the time of presentation. It is uncommon in untreated patients in the absence of radiographically visible mediastinal or ipsilateral hilar adenopathy. However, lung recurrence can be seen without node enlargement in patients with prior mediastinal radiation. Discrete, single or multiple, well-defined or ill-defined, large or small nodules or mass-like lesions, or localized areas of air-space consolidation associated with air bronchograms, may all be seen (see Figs. 5-10 to 5-12 in Chapter 5). These can cavitate, with either thick or thin walls. Peripheral, subpleural masses are common.

Non-Hodgkin's lymphoma (NHL) usually is a disseminated disease, and the lung is involved in 10% to 15% of

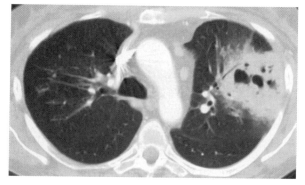

FIG. 9-40. Lung abscess. Both the internal and external walls of the cavitary lesion appear irregular or shaggy. An air bronchogram is seen within the abscess.

cases. Lung involvement may appear as discrete nodules or masses, air-space consolidation, or infiltration contiguous with enlarged lymph nodes (see Figs. 5-21 and 5-29 in Chapter 5). Specific types of NHL include primary pulmonary lymphoma, AIDS-related lymphoma, mycosis fungoides, and plasmacytoma.

NHL is considered primary to the lung if there is no evidence of extrathoracic disease for at least 3 months after the initial diagnosis of lung lymphoma. *Primary pulmonary lymphoma* generally is classified as a low-grade B-cell lymphoma or high-grade lymphoma. Both may present as a solitary nodule or mass, multiple nodules or masses, or multifocal areas of consolidation, with or without associated lymph node enlargement.

AIDS-related lymphoma originates primarily in extranodal locations and commonly involves multiple sites, including the lung. Multiple pulmonary nodules and masses, ranging in size from 1 to 5 cm, are seen most commonly on radiographs or CT. The nodules usually are well-defined. Cavitation may be present but is not common.

Mycosis fungoides is a T-cell lymphoma that primarily affects the skin. Radiographic findings in patients with disseminated disease are similar to those of other lymphomas and include lung nodules, areas of lung consolidation, and hilar or mediastinal lymph node enlargement.

Plasmacytoma usually originates in bone; much less common is extramedullary plasmacytoma. Pulmonary nodules or mass lesions may be seen.

Lymphoproliferative Disease

In addition to Hodgkin's disease and the non-Hodgkin's lymphomas, pulmonary lymphoproliferative diseases represent a spectrum of focal and diffuse lung abnormalities associated with either a benign or malignant course. As with the lymphomas, these may be associated with single or multiple lung nodules, masses, or focal mass-like areas of consolidation, and cavitation may occur.

Focal lymphoid hyperplasia is an uncommon benign condition characterized histologically by localized proliferation of benign mononuclear cells including polyclonal lymphocytes, plasma cells, and histiocytes. Its most common radiologic manifestation is that of a solitary nodule or a focal area of consolidation, often containing air bronchograms (see Fig. 5-31 in Chapter 5). There is no associated lymphadenopathy.

Lymphomatoid granulomatosis encompasses a group of angiocentric, angiodestructive abnormalities characterized by a lymphoid infiltrate and a variable degree of cellular atypia. Progression to lymphoma may occur. The lung is the primary site of disease. Radiographic and CT findings consist of bilateral, poorly defined nodular lesions, ranging from 0.5 cm to 8 cm in diameter, with a basal predominance. Lesions may progress rapidly and cavitate, mimicking Wegener's granulomatosis.

Posttransplantation lymphoproliferative disorder. Several histologic patterns of disease, ranging from a benign proliferation of lymphocytes to overtly malignant lymphoma, can occur after bone marrow or solid organ transplantation. These are known collectively as posttransplantation lymphoproliferative disorder (PTLD). PTLD can manifest as localized or disseminated disease and has a predilection for extranodal involvement. Lung involvement may occur as part of multiorgan disease or in isolation. In 85% of cases, radiographs and CT show single or multiple pulmonary nodules, which may be small or large (0.3 to 5 cm), well-defined or ill-defined (see Fig. 5-33 in Chapter 5). Other findings include patchy or focal consolidation. Hilar or mediastinal lymphadenopathy is common.

Metastatic Neoplasm

Lung nodules are the most common thoracic manifestation of metastatic tumor, usually due to hematogenous spread. See Chapter 4.

Nodules of metastatic tumor tend to be sharply marginated. Poorly marginated nodules may be seen in the presence of surrounding hemorrhage, local invasion of adjacent lung, or lepidic growth. They tend to predominate in the lung bases because of relatively greater blood flow. Individual metastases may arise from the tips of small arteries, suggesting their hematogenous origin (i.e., the feeding vessel sign). Nodules may be of any size.

Cavitation of metastases is not as common as with primary lung carcinoma, but it does occur in 5% of cases. The likelihood of cavitation varies with histology. Cavitation is most common with squamous cell tumors, but it also may be seen in adenocarcinomas and in some sarcomas.

Calcification of metastases occurs most commonly with osteogenic sarcoma, chondrosarcoma, synovial sarcoma, thyroid carcinoma, and mucinous adenocarcinoma.

A subpleural predominance of nodules is common unless the nodules are very numerous. On HRCT, numerous nodules tend to involve the lung in a diffuse fashion without regard for specific anatomic structures, a distribution termed "random."

Multiple nodules are most common, and often the nodules vary in size. Benign nodular disease most often results in nodules of similar size. The size and number of nodules varies greatly. Nodules may be small (i.e., miliary) and very numerous; this appearance often is seen with very vascular tumors. Fewer, larger metastases also may be seen; when these are well-defined, they are referred to as *cannonball metastases.*

Most patients (80% to 90%) with multiple metastases have a history of neoplasm. In some patients, however, history of a primary tumor is lacking at the time of diagnosis; in others, the primary tumor may never be found.

A metastatic tumor occasionally presents as a solitary nodule. About 5% to 10% of solitary nodules represent a solitary metastasis. Solitary metastases are most common with carcinoma of the colon, sarcomas, melanoma, and carcinomas of the kidney and testicle. Solitary metastases more often have a smooth margin than do the lesions of primary lung carcinoma.

Solitary metastases are least common in patients with carcinomas of the head and neck, bladder, breast, cervix, bile ducts, esophagus, ovary, prostate, and stomach; in patients with these tumors, a solitary nodule more likely represents a primary carcinoma.

Multiple pulmonary "leiomyomas" associated with smooth muscle tumors of the uterus in women (*benign metastasizing leiomyoma*) represent pulmonary metastases from a low-grade uterine leiomyosarcoma. Single or multiple lung masses usually are seen. They may be quite large, may calcify, and grow very slowly over a period of years.

Mucoid Impaction (Mucous Plug)

Mucous plugs mimicking the appearance of a lung nodule or nodules may be seen in a variety of conditions, including bronchial atresia (see Figs. 1–4 and 1–5 in Chapter 1), bronchial obstruction by a stricture or tumor, asthma, allergic bronchopulmonary aspergillosis, cystic fibrosis, and other causes of bronchiectasis (Fig. 9-41; see also Figs. 23-10 and 23-11 in Chapter 23). In many cases, the characteristic branching appearance of the mucoid impaction allows it to be distinguished from other causes of a lung nodule. Air trapping or atelectasis may be associated. Mucous plugs often appear low in attenuation on CT, being less dense than the bronchial wall. High-attenuation mucous plugs may be seen on CT in patients with allergic bronchopulmonary aspergillosis and bronchial atresia, most likely due to

calcification. Resolution of the mucous plug, revealing a dilated bronchus, may mimic cavitation of a solid lesion.

Mycetoma (Aspergilloma)

In patients with a preexisting cyst or cavity, a mycetoma or fungus ball can form as a result of saprophytic infection, usually by aspergillus; other fungi occasionally are involved. Patients may be asymptomatic. However, hemoptysis or hemorrhage are common presenting complaints because of inflammation in the wall of the cyst.

Chest radiographs often show a cyst or cavity containing a mass within its dependent portion (Fig. 9-42). Cysts are commonly upper lobe, and often result from prior TB or sarcoidosis (see Figs. 15-17 and 15-18 in Chapter 15). However, early in the development of the mycetoma, thickening of the wall of the preexisting cyst or adjacent pleural thickening may be the only recognizable finding and should sug-

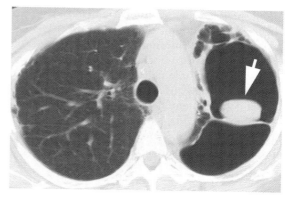

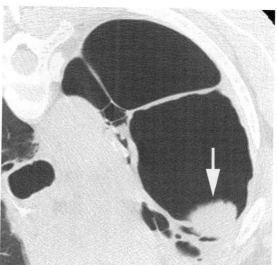

FIG. 9-42. Mycetoma (aspergilloma) seen on chest radiograph. **A.** Cystic lung disease in the left upper lobe is associated with an intracavity mass *(arrow)*. **B.** On the prone image, the mass moves anteriorly *(arrow)*.

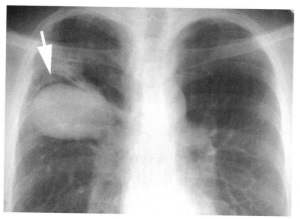

FIG. 9-41. Mucoid impaction in bronchial atresia. A large oval mass in the right upper lobe represents a mucous plug distal to the atretic bronchial segment. Air in the dilated bronchial lumen *(arrow)* outlines the bronchial wall and mucous plug, resulting in an air-crescent sign.

gest the diagnosis. Gravitational shift of the intracavitary mass may be seen with change in the patient's position. A rim of air outlining the top of the mycetoma and the inner wall of the cavity is characteristic, and is termed the "air-crescent" sign.

Although the air-crescent sign is typical of mycetoma, the differential diagnosis of this sign includes the following possibilities: (1) tumor arising in a cyst; (2) clot in a cyst or cavity; (3) necrotizing pneumonia (e.g., invasive aspergillosis) with lung infarction; and (4) *Echinococcus* infection (see Table 9-7).

On CT, a round or oval mass (the fungus ball) can be seen within the cavity, usually in a dependent location. Gravitational shift of the fungus ball may be demonstrated. An air-crescent sign may be seen. The wall of the associated cyst or cavity usually is thick. In patients with a developing mycetoma, the fungus ball can contain multiple bubbles of air.

Papillomatosis

In 2% to 5% of patients with a history of laryngeal papillomas, distal spread occurs, with involvement of the tracheobronchial tree, a condition referred to as *tracheobronchial papillomatosis*. The extension of papillomas to the bronchi, bronchioles, and lung parenchyma is rare but may occur. Papillomas may be visible radiographically as nodular mass lesions within the lung, usually multiple, which often cavitate. Eventually, cavitary lesions may progress to large, thick- or thin-walled cysts. Nodules representing papillomas may be seen within cysts (Fig. 9-43; see also Figs. 3-55 and 3-56 in Chapter 3). Squamous cell carcinoma may develop.

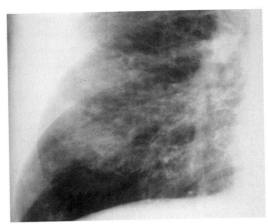

FIG. 9-44. Paragonimiasis in a world traveler with hemoptysis. Radiograph coned to the right lung base shows multiple small nodules. Some cystic or cavitary lesions also are visible.

Paragonimiasis

Paragonimiasis results from infection by the lung fluke *Paragonimus westermani*. It is common in Southeast Asia and thus may be seen in recent immigrants to the United States. It is acquired by eating freshwater crustaceans. Flukes migrate through the bowel wall, peritoneum, diaphragm, and pleura to reach the lungs, where they develop. They may result in the presence of ill-defined nodules or linear opacities, often multiple, with a predominance at the lung bases (Fig. 9-44). Cysts or cavities may also be seen; irregular wall thickening may reflect the presence of the adult worm within a lung cyst.

Pneumatocele

Pneumatoceles are thin-walled, air-filled spaces that typically occur in association with infection. They may increase in size after they develop due to air trapping. These spaces commonly are seen in patients with *P. jiroveci* (*P. carinii*) pneumonia in association with AIDS, but also may be seen in association with *Staphylococcus aureus* or other bacterial infections. In distinction to lung abscess or pulmonary gangrene, the wall of an air-filled pneumatocele tends to be thin-walled and of uniform thickness (Fig. 9-45).

Pulmonary Artery Aneurysm

Pulmonary artery aneurysms are rare. When they occur in relation to lobar, segmental, or smaller arteries, they may present as a lung nodule (Fig. 9-46). CT with contrast medium infusion is diagnostic, resulting in dense opacification. Pulmonary artery aneurysms may be (1) mycotic (see Fig. 9-46); (2) the result of catheter-related complications; or (3) associated with pulmonary hypertension (see Fig. 6-29

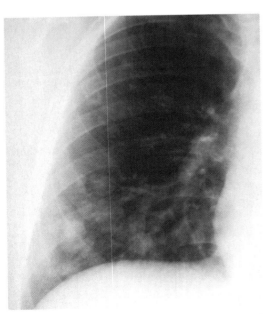

FIG. 9-43. Papillomatosis with multiple nodules. Multiple well-defined nodules are visible, some of which appear to be cavitary.

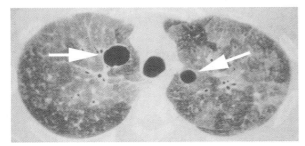

FIG. 9-45. Pneumatoceles in *Pneumocystis jiroveci* (*P. carinii*) pneumonia. High-resolution CT in a patient with AIDS shows ground-glass opacity consistent with *P. jiroveci* pneumonia. Thin-walled pneumatoceles are visible bilaterally.

in Chapter 6) or diseases such as Takayasu's arteritis, Williams syndrome, Behçet's syndrome, and prenatal varicella.

Rasmussen aneurysm is a mycotic aneurysm occurring in relation to an infectious cavity and is most typical of TB.

Pulmonary Vein Varix

Pulmonary vein varix represents a segmental dilatation of a pulmonary vein at or near its junction with the left atrium. Although varix is said to result often from a congenital defect of the vein wall, many varices are associated with elevated pulmonary venous pressure and mitral valve disease. They are radiographically visible as round or oval densities in the medial third of either lung, typically adjacent to the left atrial shadow (Fig. 9-47). On the lateral view, they are noted in the typical location of pulmonary veins. They rarely cause symptoms but can enlarge in response to increasing left atrial pressure, and may rupture with hemorrhage. CT is diagnostic.

Pulmonary Gangrene

Rarely, patients with lung infection develop a sequestrum of necrotic lung within an abscess cavity, identical to that

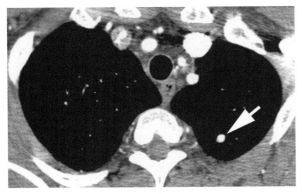

FIG. 9-46. Pulmonary artery aneurysm following septic embolism. A small, densely opacified aneurysm *(arrow)* is visible at the left lung apex.

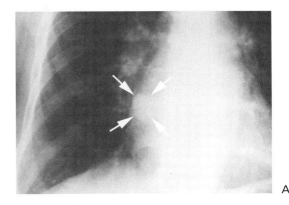

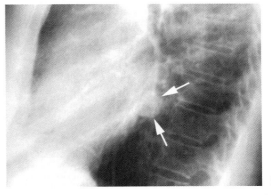

FIG. 9-47. Pulmonary vein varix in mitral stenosis. **A.** On the PA radiograph, a well-defined oval opacity *(arrows)* overlies the shadow of the left atrium. **B.** On the lateral view, the opacity is localized to the junction of the pulmonary veins with the left atrium *(arrows)*.

seen with angioinvasive aspergillosis. This occurrence is termed *pulmonary gangrene*. Lung necrosis may be the result of direct action by bacterial toxins or ischemia resulting from thrombosis of small pulmonary arteries. It may occur in patients infected with *Klebsiella, Streptococcus pneumonia, Haemophilus influenzae, Staphylococcus aureus*, or anaerobic bacteria. The presence of a mass in a cavity or an air-crescent sign is typical on radiographs or CT (Fig. 9-48).

Rheumatoid Nodules and Caplan's Syndrome

Rheumatoid (necrobiotic) nodules are an uncommon manifestation of rheumatoid arthritis. They often are asymptomatic, but tend to appear and disappear in conjunction with subcutaneous nodules. They range in size from a few millimeters to 5 cm or more, and may be solitary or multiple and numerous (Fig. 9-49). Rheumatoid nodules predominate in the lung periphery and typically are well defined. They may cavitate, having thick walls that become thin with healing. Pleural effusion may be associated and cavitary nodules in the periphery may lead to pneumothorax.

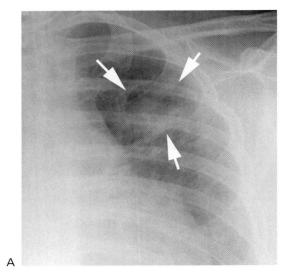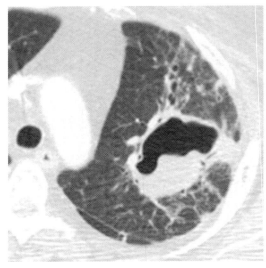

FIG. 9-48. Pulmonary gangrene in *Staphylococcus aureus* infection. **A.** Chest radiograph shows a thin-walled cavity *(arrows)* in the left upper lobe. The cavity contains an ill-defined opacity, representing a sequestrum of necrotic lung. **B.** HRCT shows the thin-walled cavity, a sequestrum of necrotic lung, and an air-crescent sign. This appearance is very similar to that seen with angio-invasive aspergillosis.

Caplan's syndrome is a rare manifestation of rheumatoid arthritis that occurs in coal miners or patients with silicosis. It is characterized by single or multiple lung nodules ranging from a few millimeters to 5 cm in diameter, similar to those seen with rheumatoid nodules. Nodules may have an upper lobe predominance, resembling the appearance of silicosis, but nodules in Caplan's syndrome appear rapidly and in "crops," in contrast to the slow progression of pneumoconiosis.

Round Atelectasis

Round atelectasis represents focal rounded lung collapse, usually associated with pleural thickening or effusion. It typically appears as a focal mass lesion, and is described in detail in Chapter 2.

Round atelectasis often shows characteristic findings on chest radiographs or CT. It usually is (1) round or oval in shape; (2) peripheral in location and abutting the pleural surface; (3) associated with curving of pulmonary vessels or bronchi into the edge of the lesion (the "comet-tail" sign); and (4) associated with an ipsilateral pleural abnormality, either effusion or pleural thickening, with the lesion contacting the abnormal pleural surface. If these criteria for rounded atelectasis are met, a confident diagnosis usually can be made, and radiographic follow-up should be sufficient. Rounded atelectasis is most common in the posterior lower lobes, and sometimes is bilateral or symmetrical (see Figs. 2-42 to 2-46 in Chapter 2).

Sarcoidosis

Large masses or areas of consolidation, measuring 4 cm in diameter or larger, are seen in 15% to 25% of patients with active sarcoidosis (see Figs. 15-8 and 15-9 in Chapter 15).

FIG. 9-49. Rheumatoid nodule. A well-defined nodule *(arrow)* is visible in the peripheral right upper lobe. A central lucency represents cavitation. Focal pleural thickening is visible adjacent to the nodule.

Because they may contain air bronchograms, they sometimes are termed *alveolar sarcoid*. These masses are due to the confluence of large numbers of small interstitial granulomas. They may be parahilar or peripheral in location, and rarely cavitate. On CT, small nodules (satellite nodules) often are visible at the periphery of these masses.

Pulmonary masses also may be seen in patients with end-stage sarcoidosis (see Fig. 15-12 in Chapter 15). Progressive fibrosis may lead to abnormal central conglomeration of parahilar bronchi and vessels, associated with masses of fibrous tissue, typically most marked in the upper lobes. This finding often is associated with bronchial dilation, a finding referred to as *traction bronchiectasis*. It is similar in appearance to that of progressive massive fibrosis in silicosis.

Septic Embolism with Infarction

Septic pulmonary emboli, with or without infarction, generally result in multiple parenchymal abnormalities; rarely does septic embolism present as a solitary lesion. The correct radiographic diagnosis usually is suggested by the finding of relatively well-defined, bilateral peripheral nodules with or without cavitation, especially in the setting of known intravenous drug abuse, or some other known source of sepsis.

In patients with septic embolism, peripheral nodules in varying stages of cavitation often are present, presumably due to intermittent seeding of the lungs by infected material (Fig. 9-50). The feeding vessel sign is visible in 65% of cases (see Fig. 9-50C). CT is helpful in showing the peripheral and subpleural location of the nodules (see Fig. 9-50B and C).

Sequestration

Sequestration represents an area of disorganized pulmonary parenchyma without normal pulmonary arterial or bronchial communications. Sequestration usually receives its blood supply from branches of the thoracic or abdominal aorta. There are two forms of sequestration, intralobar and extralobar.

Intralobar sequestration is more common. Two thirds of intralobar sequestrations are found adjacent to the diaphragm in relation to the posterior basal segment of the left lower lobe. Intralobar sequestration usually presents in adults or older children. Uncomplicated intralobar sequestration can have a variety of appearances. It may appear as (1) a homogeneous and well-defined mass lesion; (2) a cystic or multicystic air and fluid-filled lesion; (3) a hyperlucent and hypovascular region of lung; or (4) a combination of

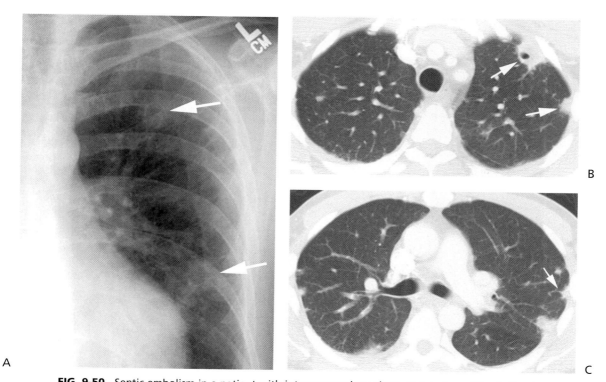

FIG. 9-50. Septic embolism in a patient with intravenous drug abuse and endocarditis. **A.** Chest radiograph shows lung nodules, which appear cavitary *(arrows)*. **B.** CT shows the peripheral nature of the nodules *(arrows)*, relatively well-defined margins, and a variable degree of cavitation. **C.** Several examples of the feeding vessel sign are visible *(arrow)*. The nodules are peripheral in location.

these. Bilateral intralobar sequestrations may occur (see Figs. 1-26 to 1-28 in Chapter 1).

Extralobar sequestration represents an anomaly in which the sequestered tissue is enclosed within its only pleural envelope; it is less common than intralobar sequestration and often is diagnosed in neonates. Approximately 90% of cases are visible at the left lung base, contiguous with the left hemidiaphragm (see Figs. 1-30 and 1-31 in Chapter 1). Extralobar sequestration appears as a sharply marginated mass lesion, which does not contain air (unlike intralobar sequestration). It usually is homogeneous in appearance, but may contain cystic areas. Its supplying artery may be seen on CT.

Wegener's Granulomatosis

Wegener's granulomatosis is a multisystem disease of unknown cause associated with involvement of the upper respiratory tract (nasal, oral, or sinus inflammation), lower respiratory tract (airway or lung), and kidney (see Chapter 19). The presence of antineutrophilic cytoplasmic antibody (C-ANCA) is characteristic, and is seen in 90% of cases.

Patients usually are between the ages of 30 and 60. At presentation, chest radiographic abnormalities are visible in 75% of patients with Wegener's granulomatosis. The most common radiographic abnormality is multiple lung nodules or masses; these are visible in more than half of patients

at presentation. Typically, fewer than a dozen nodules are visible, but they may be more numerous. In most cases, the nodules are bilateral and widely distributed without predominance in any lung region. A solitary nodule or mass may be seen, but this appearance is less common.

Masses usually range from 2 to 4 cm, but may be up to 10 cm in diameter (Fig. 9-51; see also Figs. 19-8 and 19-9 in Chapter 19). Masses are round or oval in shape and may well or poorly defined. Cavitation occurs in approximately 50% of cases. Cavities usually are thick-walled with an irregular inner margin. Air-fluid levels may be present. Calcification of the masses does not occur.

With progression of disease, nodules and masses tend to increase in size and number. With treatment, nodules usually resolve over a period of months. Typically, cavitary nodules and masses become thin-walled and decrease in size with treatment. Complete resolution may occur.

SELECTED READING

Au V, Leung AN. Radiologic manifestations of lymphoma in the thorax. AJR Am J Roentgenol 1997; 168:93–98.

Balakrishnan J, Meziane MA, Siegelman SS, Fishman EK. Pulmonary infarction: CT appearance with pathologic correlation. J Comput Assist Tomogr 1989; 13:941–945.

Bankoff MS, McEniff NJ, Bhadelia RA, et al. Prevalence of pathologically proven intrapulmonary lymph nodes and their appearance on CT. AJR 1996; 167:629–630.

Bernard A, Azorin J, Bellenot F, et al. Resection of pulmonary nodules using video-assisted thoracic surgery. Ann Thorac Surg 1996; 61:202–204.

Calhoun P, Feldman PS, Armstrong P, et al. The clinical outcome of needle aspirations of the lung when cancer is not diagnosed. Ann Thorac Surg 1986; 41:592–596.

Davis SD. CT evaluation for pulmonary metastases in patients with extrathoracic malignancy. Radiology 1991; 180:1–12.

Dewan NA, Shehan CJ, Reeb SD, et al. Likelihood of malignancy in a solitary pulmonary nodule: comparison of Bayesian analysis and results of FDG-PET scan. Chest 1997; 112:416–422.

Gaeta M, Pandolfo I, Volta S, et al. Bronchus sign on CT in peripheral carcinoma of the lung: value in predicting results of transbronchial biopsy. AJR 1991; 157:1181–1185.

Gupta NC, Maloof J, Gunel E. Probability of malignancy in solitary pulmonary nodules using fluorine-18-FDG and PET. J Nucl Med 1996; 37:943–948.

Gurney JW. Determining the likelihood of malignancy in solitary pulmonary nodules with Bayesian analysis. Part 1: theory. Radiology 1993; 186:405–413.

Gurney JW, Lyddon DM, McKay JA. Determining the likelihood of malignancy in solitary pulmonary nodules with Bayesian analysis. Part II: application. Radiology 1993; 186:415–422.

Hasegawa M, Sone S, Takashima S, et al. Growth rate of small lung cancers detected on mass CT screening. Br J Radiol 2000; 73:1252–1259.

Hirakata K, Nakata H, Haratake J. Appearance of pulmonary metastases on high-resolution CT scans: comparison with histopathologic findings from autopsy specimens. AJR Am J Roentgenol 1993; 161:37–43.

Huang RM, Naidich DP, Lubat E, et al. Septic pulmonary emboli: CT-radiographic correlation. AJR Am J Roentgenol 1989; 153:41–45.

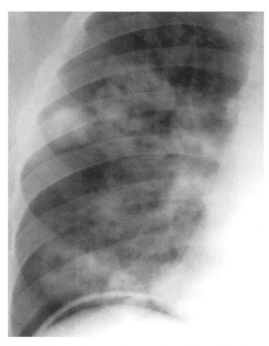

FIG. 9-51. Wegener's granulomatosis with multiple nodules. Multiple poorly marginated nodules are visible in the right lung. Some appear cavitary. Free intraperitoneal air is the result of peritoneal dialysis for associated renal failure.

Jang HJ, Lee KS, Kwon OJ, et al. Bronchioloalveolar carcinoma: focal area of ground-glass attenuation at thin-section CT as an early sign. Radiology 1996; 199:485–488.

Kuhlman JE, Fishman EK, Siegelman SS. Invasive pulmonary aspergillosis in acute leukemia: characteristic findings on CT, the CT halo sign, and the role of CT in early diagnosis. Radiology 1985; 157:611–614.

Kui M, Templeton PA, White CS, et al. Evaluation of the air bronchogram sign on CT in solitary pulmonary lesions. J Comput Assist Tomogr 1996; 20:983–986.

Kushihashi T, Munechika H, Ri K, et al. Bronchoalveolar adenoma of the lung: CT-pathologic correlation. Radiology 1994; 193: 789–793.

Li HQ, Boiselle PM, Shepard JAO, et al. Diagnostic accuracy and safety of CT-guided percutaneous needle aspiration biopsy of the lung: comparison of small and large pulmonary nodules. Am J Roentgenol 1996; 167:105–109.

Libby DM, Henschke CI, Yankelevitz DF. The solitary pulmonary nodule: update 1995. Am J Med 1995; 99:491–496.

Mahoney MC, Shipley RT, Cocoran HL, Dickson BA. CT demonstration of calcification in carcinoma of the lung. AJR 1990; 154: 255–258.

Munden RF, Pugatch RD, Liptay MJ, et al. Small pulmonary lesions detected at CT: clinical importance. Radiology 1997; 202: 105–110.

Nathan MH, Collins VP, Adams RA. Differentiation of benign and malignant pulmonary nodules by growth rate. Radiology 1962; 79:221–231.

Patz EF, Lowe VJ, Hoffman JM. Focal pulmonary abnormalities: evaluation with F-18 fluorodeoxyglucose PET scanning. Radiology 1993; 188:487–490.

Primack SL, Hartman TE, Lee KS, Müller NL. Pulmonary nodules and the CT halo sign. Radiology 1994; 190:513–515.

Quint LE, Park CH, Iannettoni MD. Solitary pulmonary nodules in patients with extrapulmonary neoplasms. Radiology 2000; 217: 257–261.

Remy J, Remy-Jardin M, Giraud F, Wattinne L. Angioarchitecture of pulmonary arteriovenous malformations: clinical utility of three-dimensional helical CT. Radiology 1994; 191:657–664.

Siegelman SS, Khouri NF, Leo FP, et al. Solitary pulmonary nodules: CT assessment. Radiology 1986; 160:307–312.

Siegelman SS, Khouri NF, Scott WW, et al. Pulmonary hamartoma: CT findings. Radiology 1986; 160:313–317.

Theros EG. Varying manifestations of peripheral pulmonary neoplasms: a radiologic-pathologic correlative study. AJR Am J Roentgenol 1977; 128:893–914.

Webb WR. Radiologic evaluation of the solitary pulmonary nodule. AJR Am J Roentgenol 1990; 154:701–708.

Webb WR. The pleural tail sign. Radiology 1978; 127:309–313.

Weisbrod GL, Towers MJ, Chamberlain DW, et al. Thin-walled cystic lesions in bronchioalveolar carcinoma. Radiology 1992; 185: 401–405.

Zwiebel BR, Austin JHM, Grines MM. Bronchial carcinoid tumors: assessment with CT of location and intratumoral calcification in 31 patients. Radiology 1991; 179:483–486.

Zwirewich CV, Vedal S, Miller RR, Müller NL. Solitary pulmonary nodule: high-resolution CT and radiologic-pathologic correlation. Radiology 1991; 179:469–476.

10

PLAIN FILM AND HIGH-RESOLUTION COMPUTED TOMOGRAPHIC ASSESSMENT OF DIFFUSE INFILTRATIVE LUNG DISEASE

W. RICHARD WEBB

Diffuse infiltrative lung diseases (DILD) may be acute or chronic, involving the interstitium, alveolar spaces, or both. Specific DILD are discussed in other chapters in this book. This chapter reviews the radiographic and high-resolution CT (HRCT) diagnosis of DILD, including important findings to look for and the differential diagnosis of various patterns of disease. Airway disease and emphysema, although diffuse lung diseases, are not considered DILDs and are discussed in Chapters 23 and 24.

PLAIN RADIOGRAPHIC ASSESSMENT OF DIFFUSE INFILTRATIVE LUNG DISEASE

On plain radiographs, infiltrative diseases usually are classified according to the pattern of abnormality they produce. There are six basic patterns:

1. Air-space or alveolar consolidation
2. Linear or septal
3. Reticular
4. Nodular
5. Reticulonodular
6. Ground-glass opacity.

Air-space or Alveolar Consolidation

The terms *air-space consolidation* and *alveolar consolidation* refer to diseases associated with pathologic filling of alveoli (i.e., replacement of alveolar air) as a predominant abnormality. As discussed in detail in Chapter 2, radiographic abnormalities indicating the presence of air-space or alveolar disease include (1) confluent or homogeneous opacities obscuring vessels; (2) air bronchograms; (3) ill-defined or fluffy opacities; (4) air alveolograms; (5) "acinar" or air-space nod-

ules; (6) preserved lung volume; and (7) a tendency for opacities to extend to pleural surfaces.

The differential diagnosis of diffuse air-space consolidation is reviewed in detail in Chapter 2 and Table 2-1. It includes the following features:

1. Water (e.g., pulmonary edema)
2. Blood (e.g., pulmonary hemorrhage)
3. Pus (e.g., pneumonia)
4. Cells (e.g., bronchioloalveolar carcinoma, lymphoma, eosinophilic pneumonia, BOOP, hypersensitivity pneumonitis, interstitial pneumonia)
5. Other substances (e.g., lipoprotein in alveolar proteinosis, lipid in lipoid pneumonia).

Linear or Septal Pattern

A linear pattern is defined by the presence of Kerley's A or B lines. Kerley's A and B lines result from thickening of interlobular septa; this pattern also may be referred to as *septal* (Table 10-1).

Kerley B lines are the most common (Fig. 10-1). They are horizontal lines, 1 to 2 cm in length. They are seen in contact with the pleural surface, and are best seen laterally at the costophrenic angles.

TABLE 10-1. LINEAR OR SEPTAL PATTERN: DIFFERENTIAL DIAGNOSIS

Pulmonary edema (hydrostatic most common), typically symmetric
Lymphangitic spread of neoplasm, often asymmetric
Chronic or recurrent pulmonary hemorrhage and hemosiderosis
Pulmonary fibrosis (sarcoidosis most common)

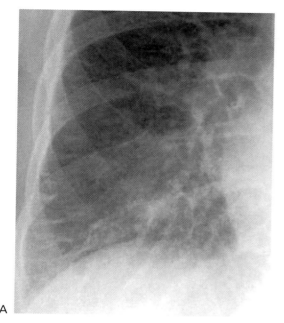

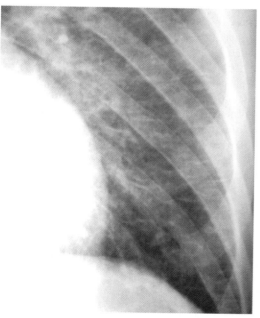

FIG. 10-1. Kerley B lines. Coned-down views of the right and left lateral costophrenic angles in two different patients with cardiogenic interstitial pulmonary edema. Thin horizontal lines in the lung periphery represent Kerley B lines. These represent thickened interlobular septa.

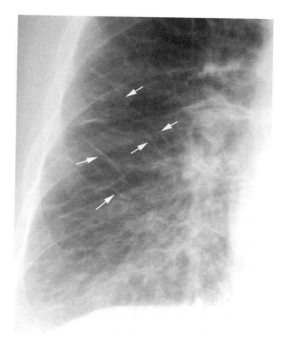

FIG. 10-2. Kerley A lines. A patient with pulmonary edema associated with fluid overload shows multiple Kerley A lines. Thin oblique lines in the parahilar lung *(arrows)* represent A lines. Thickening of the minor fissure also is seen.

The characteristic appearance of Kerley B lines results from the consistent size and regular organization of pulmonary lobules at the lung bases.

Kerley A lines are seen less often. They are oblique in orientation, several cm in length, and are located within the central or parahilar lung.

Kerley A lines (Fig. 10-2) also represent thickened septa,

but their appearance is different from that of B lines because of the different arrangement of pulmonary lobules in the parahilar lungs.

Kerley C lines are seen at the lung bases and represent interlobular septa en face rather than in profile. They result in a nonspecific, reticular pattern and are unimportant in diagnosis, because B lines invariably are visible as well.

Peribronchial cuffing results from thickening of the peribronchovascular interstitium, and also contributes to a linear pattern. This abnormality is seen as thickening of bronchi seen end-on or as lines radiating outward from the hila. To some extent, peribronchial cuffing contributes to the appearance of Kerley A lines on chest radiographs.

Well-defined and easily recognized Kerley's lines are indicative of interstitial lung disease and have a limited differential diagnosis. They are typical of interstitial pulmonary edema and lymphangitic spread of carcinoma. Edema usually is symmetrical. Lymphangitic spread often is asymmetrical; asymmetrical Kerley's lines strongly suggest lymphangitic spread of carcinoma.

Although consolidation may be seen with any type of pulmonary edema (e.g., hydrostatic, increased permeability with or without diffuse alveolar damage, or mixed), a septal pattern more often represents hydrostatic edema or increased permeability edema occurring in the absence of diffuse alveolar damage (see Chapter 11).

A septal pattern also can result from chronic or recurrent pulmonary hemorrhage and hemosiderosis.

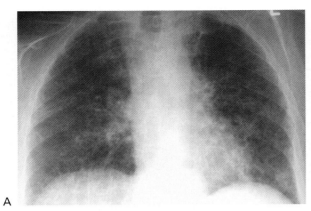
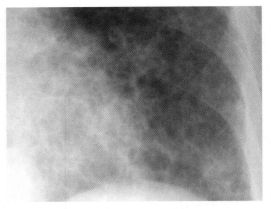

FIG. 10-3. Reticular pattern in rheumatoid lung disease. **A.** Chest radiograph shows decreased lung volumes and irregular reticular opacities at the lung bases. Kerley B lines are inconspicuous. The lines appear to outline spaces 1 cm or less in diameter, representing a medium reticular pattern. **B.** Coned-down view of the left lower lobe in the same patient shows the irregular reticular pattern.

Pulmonary fibrosis sometimes can result in well-defined Kerley's lines, but a reticular pattern is more typical. Kerley's lines in patients with fibrosis are seen most commonly in those patients with sarcoidosis.

Reticular Pattern

"Reticular" means "net-like," which is an excellent description of the appearance of this pattern. A reticular pattern is characterized by multiple intersecting lines, often irregular in appearance, outlining round or irregular spaces (Fig. 10-3). Although a few Kerley lines may be visible, they do not predominate (if they did, the pattern would be a linear one). A reticular pattern indicates the presence of interstitial lung disease (Table 10-2).

The reticular pattern has been subdivided into three subpatterns, based on the size of the "spaces" surrounded by lines: a fine pattern (spaces smaller than 3 mm; Fig. 10-4); a medium pattern (spaces 3 mm to 10 mm; Fig. 10-5); and coarse pattern (spaces larger than 10 mm; Fig. 10-6). It

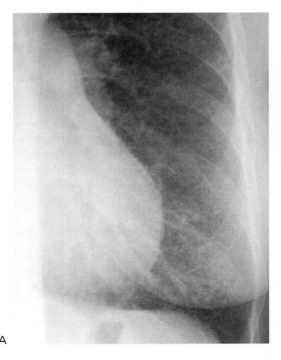
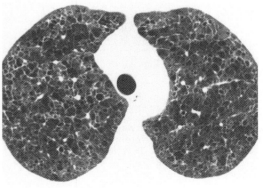

FIG. 10-4. Fine reticular pattern in Langerhans' cell histiocytosis. **A.** Coned-down view of the left lower lobe shows fine reticular opacities. Outlined spaces appear very small. **B.** HRCT shows diffuse cystic disease. Note that the cysts are larger than the "spaces" visible on the chest radiograph, due to their superimposition.

TABLE 10-2. RETICULAR PATTERN: DIFFERENTIAL DIAGNOSIS

Usual interstitial pneumonia
   Idiopathic pulmonary fibrosis
   Collagen vascular disease
   Drug-related fibrosis
   Asbestosis
   End-stage hypersensitivity pneumonitis
   End-stage sarcoidosis
Nonspecific interstitial pneumonia
Radiation
End-stage adult respiratory distress syndrome
Cystic lung disease
   Langerhans histiocytosis
   Lymphangiomyomatosis
   Tuberous sclerosis
   Sjögren's syndrome
   Lymphocytic interstitial pneumonia
   Cystic bronchiectasis
   Pneumonia with pneumatoceles (e.g., pneumocystis)
   Papillomatosis

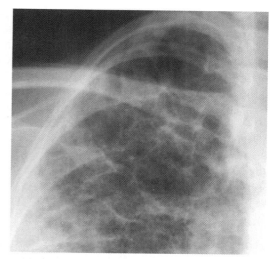

FIG. 10-6. Coarse reticular pattern in cystic lung disease. Coned-down view of the right apex shows reticular opacities outlining spaces exceeding 1 cm.

should be kept in mind, however, that the size of the spaces visible on chest radiograph do not necessary reflect the presence or size of the spaces present pathologically. Superimposition of the reticular opacities often confuses the picture; in the presence of extensive reticulation, the outlined spaces usually appear smaller than they really are (see Fig. 10-4). Medium or coarse patterns are the most common and the most easily seen on chest radiographs.

A medium pattern is typical of patients with pulmonary fibrosis and "honeycombing"; the reticulation often appears to have a peripheral, posterior, and lower lobe predominance (see Figs. 10-3 and 10-5). The abnormality often is best seen on the lateral view, just above the diaphragm, in the posterior costophrenic angle. Because of lung fibrosis, lung volumes usually appear reduced.

Honeycombing with medium reticulation usually indicates the presence of *usual interstitial pneumonia* (UIP). UIP can be seen in a variety of conditions; however, over 90% of cases of honeycombing result from a small group of diseases, including idiopathic pulmonary fibrosis, collagen-vascular disease, drug-related fibrosis, asbestosis, end-stage hypersensitivity pneumonitis, or end-stage sarcoidosis. *Nonspecific interstitial pneumonia* (NSIP) less commonly results in honeycombing; it often is associated with collagen-vascular disease. Honeycombing also may result from radiation lung fibrosis, as an end-stage of acute respiratory distress syndrome, and other entities. Lung volumes are characteristically reduced in the presence of honeycombing.

Some cystic lung diseases (e.g., Langerhan histiocytosis, lymphangiomyomatosis) result in a reticular pattern (i.e.,

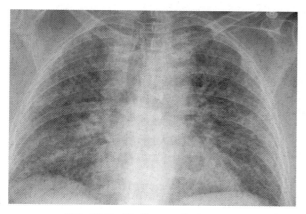 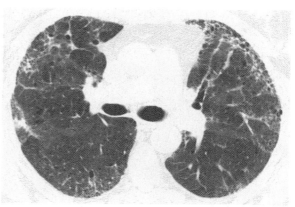

FIG. 10-5. Medium reticular pattern in rheumatoid lung disease. **A.** Chest radiograph shows irregular reticular opacities, best classified as a medium pattern. **B.** HRCT shows reticular opacities associated with honeycombing in the anterior lung.

intersecting lines) because of superimposition of the walls of cysts ranging in size from several millimeters to several centimeters in diameter (see Fig. 10-6). Depending on the size of the cysts, the pattern may be fine, medium, or coarse. This appearance can mimic honeycombing, but significant lung fibrosis is absent, and lung volumes are not reduced. In many such patients, lung volumes appear increased. An upper lobe predominance may be seen rather than predominance at the lung bases, depending on the responsible disease.

A fine reticular pattern may indicate fine lung fibrosis or lung infiltration by a variety of processes (see Fig. 10-4). This pattern is less common, more difficult to see, and less specific.

Nodular Pattern

Innumerable small nodules, ranging from a few millimeters to 1 cm in diameter, may indicate interstitial or air-space disease. The differential diagnosis of multiple larger nodules and masses is reviewed in Chapter 9.

Interstitial nodules usually are sharply marginated, despite being very small (Fig. 10-7). Air-space disease also may result in nodules (air-space or acinar nodules), typically 5 to 10 mm in diameter and poorly marginated. The term *miliary pattern* describes the presence of diffuse or widespread, well-defined nodules, 2 mm or less in diameter (see Fig. 10-7). Miliary nodules usually are interstitial.

Nearly all patients with nodules that are 5 mm or less in size, either well-defined or ill-defined, have a predominant interstitial abnormality; many will have metastases (Fig. 10-8) or a granulomatous disease (see Figs. 10-7 and 10-9; Table 10-3). Granulomatous diseases that may produce this appearance include infections (e.g., miliary tuberculosis and fungus); noninfectious granulomatous diseases (e.g., sarcoid, histiocytosis, hypersensitivity pneumonitis); and some pneumoconioses (primarily silicosis and coal-worker's

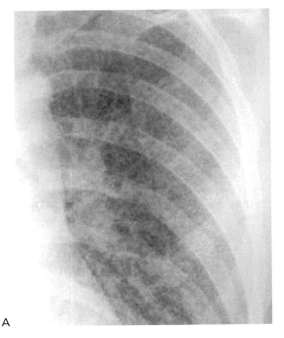

A

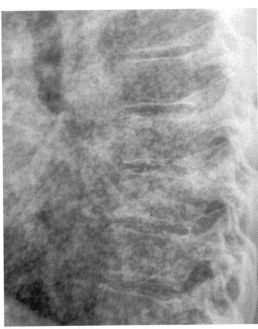

B

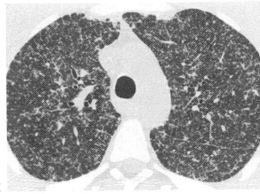

C

FIG. 10-7. Miliary nodules in hematogenous spread of coccidioidomycosis. Coned-down views from PA **(A)** and lateral **(B)** radiographs show innumerable nodules a few millimeters in diameter. **C.** HRCT shows innumerable, very small lung nodules.

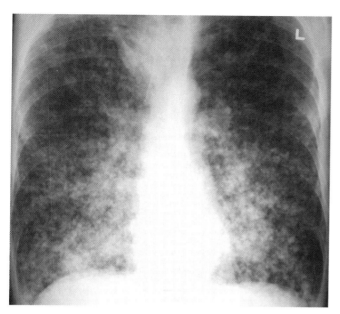

FIG. 10-8. Small nodules in metastatic melanoma. Numerous small nodules are visible, with a basal predominance.

TABLE 10-3. NODULAR PATTERN: DIFFERENTIAL DIAGNOSIS

Metastases: diffuse or basal, well-defined
Diffuse bronchioloalveolar carcinoma (diffuse or patchy, ill-defined)
Miliary tuberculosis (diffuse, well-defined, may be upper lobe)
Miliary fungus (diffuse, well-defined)
Sarcoidosis (upper lobe, may be asymmetric, adenopathy)
Silicosis and coal-worker's pneumoconiosis (posterior, upper lobe predominance, symmetric, adenopathy with eggshell calcification)
Histiocytosis (upper lobe predominance, cysts)
Hypersensitivity pneumonitis (ill-defined)
Endobronchial infection (diffuse or patchy, ill-defined)

pneumoconiosis). Metastases tend to have a basal predominance because of greater blood flow to the bases (see Fig. 10-8); the granulomatous diseases and pneumoconioses, for a variety of reasons, often have an upper lobe predominance.

Nodules measuring 5 to 10 mm in diameter may be seen in these same diseases, but are more typical of infection, particularly endobronchial spread of infection or bronchopneumonia. Common causes include tuberculosis (Fig. 10-10) and other mycobacterial, bacterial, viral infections such as cytomegalovirus or varicella, and *Pneumocystis* infection in patients with AIDS. Other causes of air-space consolidation also may result in ill-defined nodules. Diffuse bronchioloalveolar carcinoma often results in this appearance.

Reticulonodular Pattern

The term *reticulonodular*, indicating a perceived combination of lines and dots, is used commonly by radiologists, but is of limited value in diagnosis. Reticulonodular opacities observed on plain radiographs often are artifactual, resulting from the superimposition of mostly lines or mostly nodules. Thus, it is generally a good idea, if a reticulonodular pattern is detected on plain radiographs, to decide whether a reticular or nodular pattern predominates and use that finding for differential diagnosis. Cases actually characterized histologically by a combination of reticular and nodular opacities are relatively uncommon, but include sarcoidosis, lymphangitic spread of tumor, and diffuse amyloidosis.

Ground-Glass Opacity

Ground-glass opacity represents an increase in lung density without the presence of frank consolidation (Fig. 10-11A).

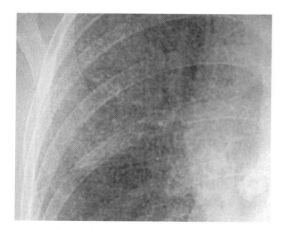

FIG. 10-9. Miliary tuberculosis. Coned-down view of the right upper lobe shows innumerable discrete, very small nodules.

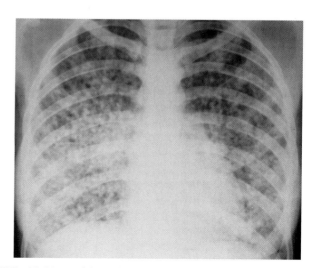

FIG. 10-10. Endobronchial spread of tuberculosis. Ill-defined nodules ranging from 5 to 10 mm in diameter are visible.

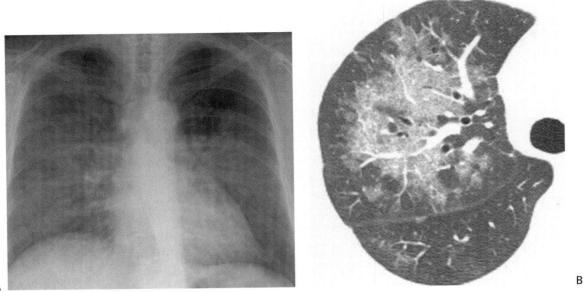

FIG. 10-11. Ground-glass opacity in exogenous lipoid pneumonia. **A.** Chest radiograph shows a subtle increase in lung opacity in the parahilar regions. Parahilar vessels are poorly defined. **B.** HRCT coned down to the right lung shows patchy ground-glass opacity.

A slight fuzziness of pulmonary vessels usually is visible, but this abnormality can be quite subtle and difficult to diagnose with certainty. It is a nonspecific pattern (see the following section on HRCT), and can be seen in the presence of either air-space disease or interstitial disease. Because it is nonspecific, its differential diagnosis is very long. It may be seen with edema, hemorrhage, infections, and a wide variety of different DILDs. When visible on a chest film, it is best evaluated by assessment of the history and clinical presentation in patients with acute symptoms, or by further imaging

(e.g., HRCT) in patients with chronic symptoms (see Fig. 10-11B).

HRCT ASSESSMENT OF DIFFUSE INFILTRATIVE LUNG DISEASES

High-resolution CT (HRCT) techniques optimize the radiographic demonstration of lung architecture and are invaluable in the assessment of patients with suspected DILD.

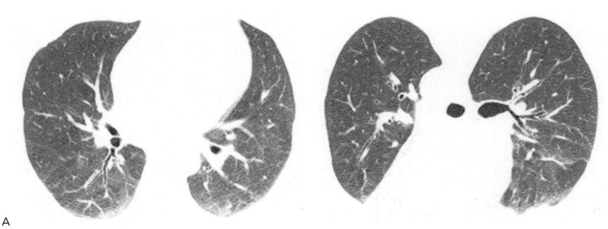

FIG. 10-12. Normal dependent lung collapse and the use of prone scans. **A.** Supine HRCT in a normal subject shows increased opacity in the posterior (dependent) lung. This appearance cannot be distinguished from lung disease. **B.** Prone scan shows that the posterior lung is normal.

The use of thin collimation (1 to 1.5 mm) and a high-resolution algorithm for image reconstruction is essential.

HRCT usually samples lung anatomy (and abnormalities) by obtaining images at spaced levels. Usually, no attempt is made to scan the entire lung.

Scanning at 1-cm intervals in the supine position is commonly employed, and obtaining prone scans also is advisable. Some dependent (posterior) lung collapse often is seen on supine scans (Fig. 10-12A). Prone scans are valuable in distinguishing true posterior lung disease from dependent collapse; posterior lung collapse clears in the prone position (Fig. 10-12B). In patients suspected of having DILD, scanning at 2-cm intervals in both the supine and prone positions is recommended. Patients with normal or minimal chest film abnormalities benefit most from prone scans.

In patients with suspected obstructive disease or emphysema, scans performed at 1-cm intervals with the patient in the supine position usually are adequate. Postexpiratory scans at selected levels can demonstrate air-trapping and may be valuable in diagnosing airway disease in patients with normal inspiratory scans. Appropriate lung windows for HRCT are mean −700 and width 1000 HU or −600/1500 HU.

Normal Anatomy: The Secondary Pulmonary Lobule and Acinus

Secondary pulmonary lobules (also simply known as the pulmonary lobules) range from 1 to 2.5 cm in size and are marginated by connective tissue interlobular septa, which contain pulmonary veins and lymphatics (Figs. 10-13 and 10-14). Within the peripheral lung, interlobular septa are at the lower limit of HRCT resolution. On clinical HRCT in normal patients, a few interlobular septa often can be seen, but they tend to be inconspicuous.

The central portion of the secondary lobule, referred to as the *centrilobular region*, contains the pulmonary artery and bronchiolar branches that supply the lobule. The pulmonary artery supplying a secondary lobule measures somewhat less than 1 mm in diameter and can be seen in normal lungs as a dot or branching structure 5 to 10 mm from the pleural surface; the centrilobular bronchiole normally is invisible.

An *acinus* is the largest unit of lung structure in which all airways participate in gas exchange. Anatomically, it is located distal to a terminal bronchiole and is supplied by a first-order respiratory bronchiole (see Fig. 10-13). Acini average 7 to 8 mm in diameter. A pulmonary lobule usually consists of a dozen or fewer acini, although large lobules may contain twice that number. Acini are not visible on HRCT.

HRCT FINDINGS IN DIFFUSE INFILTRATIVE LUNG DISEASES

Chest films are normal in 10% to 15% of patients with interstitial lung disease. HRCT is more sensitive, specific, and accurate. HRCT characterizes the morphologic abnormalities present much more precisely and allows a more accurate diagnosis than do chest radiographs.

An approach to the HRCT diagnosis of DILD is based

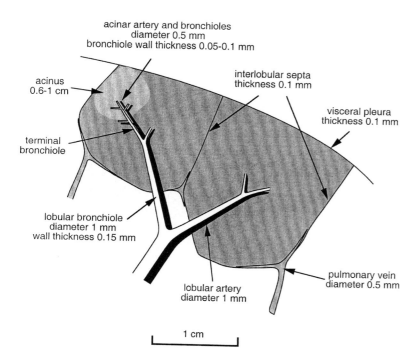

FIG. 10-13. Normal anatomy of the pulmonary lobule. Two lobules are shown.

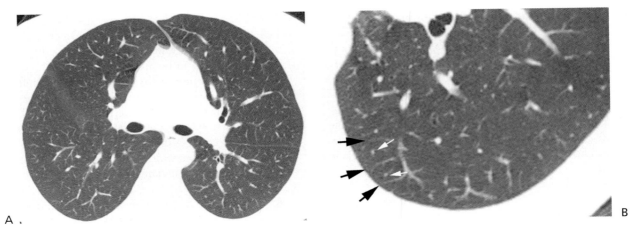

FIG. 10-14. Normal HRCT. **A.** The lung appears homogeneous in attenuation, with posterior lung appearing slightly denser than anterior lung. Fissures are smooth and uniform in thickness. Vessels are smooth in contour and sharply marginated. The most peripheral vessels visible are 5 to 10 mm from the pleural surface and represent centrilobular arteries or, sometimes, veins in interlobular septa. Centrilobular bronchioles and interlobular septa are not visible. **B.** Coned-down HRCT of the left lower lobe. Two pulmonary lobules are outlined by pulmonary veins within interlobular septae *(black arrows)*. Centrilobular arteries are visible as dots *(white arrows)*.

fundamentally on the recognition of specific abnormalities in lung anatomy, together with an assessment of their distribution. Generally speaking, HRCT findings of lung disease can be considered in four groups or categories, which reflect the histologic abnormalities present. These abnormalities include reticular opacities, nodular opacities, increased lung opacity, and decreased lung opacity or cystic lesions.

Within each of these four categories, a relatively short list of findings may be recognized. Although some HRCT findings (e.g., "tree-in-bud" pattern, emphysema, mosaic perfusion, and air-trapping) are features of airways and obstructive lung disease rather than DILD, they are discussed briefly in this chapter to describe an overall approach to HRCT.

Reticular Opacities

Thickening of the interstitial fiber network of the lung by fluid or fibrous tissue, or because of cellular infiltration, results in an increase in reticular lung opacities.

Interlobular Septal Thickening

Thickened interlobular septa can be characterized accurately because they form the margins of pulmonary lobules having a characteristic size and shape. In the peripheral lung, thickened septa measure 1 to 2 cm in length and often are seen extending to the pleural surface; in the central lung, the thickened septa can outline lobules that are 1 to 2.5 cm in diameter and appear polygonal in shape (Figs. 10-15 and

10-16). Visible lobules commonly contain a central dot-like or branching centrilobular artery.

Associated findings, regardless of the cause of septal thickening, often include peribronchial interstitial thickening recognized as peribronchial cuffing, thickening of fissures, and abnormal prominence of the centrilobular arteries (see Fig. 10-16).

Septal thickening can be smooth, nodular, or irregular in contour in different pathologic processes. Smooth septal thickening is most typical of pulmonary edema (see Fig. 10-15), lymphangitic spread of tumor (see Fig. 10-16), or, rarely, amyloidosis (Table 10-4). Nodular septal thickening reflects a perilymphatic distribution of nodules and is typical of lymphangitic spread of tumor and sarcoidosis. Septal thickening is not common in patients with interstitial fibro-

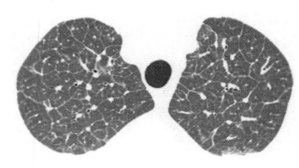

FIG. 10-15. Interlobular septal thickening in interstitial pulmonary edema. Smooth thickening of numerous septa is visible. The thickened septa outline lobules of characteristic size and shape. Pulmonary veins within septa are visible as rounded opacities.

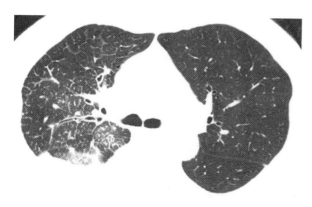

FIG. 10-16. Interlobular septal thickening in lymphangitic spread of lung cancer. Smooth thickening of septa is visible within the right lung. The left lung appears normal. Peribronchial interstitial thickening recognized as peribronchial cuffing on the right. The right bronchi appear thicker-walled than those on the left. A right pleural effusion also is present.

sis, except for those with sarcoidosis; when visible, septal thickening due to fibrosis often is irregular in appearance and associated with lung distortion.

Honeycombing

Honeycombing reflects extensive lung fibrosis with alveolar destruction, and results in a characteristic reticular appear-

TABLE 10-4. SMOOTH INTERLOBULAR SEPTAL THICKENING: DIFFERENTIAL DIAGNOSIS

Lymphangitic spread of tumor (asymmetrical or symmetrical)
Pulmonary edema (symmetrical)
Amyloidosis (rare)

ance. On HRCT, honeycombing may be diagnosed accurately by the presence of thick-walled, air-filled cysts, usually measuring from 3 mm to 1 cm in diameter. Typically, the cysts share walls and occur in several layers at the pleural surface (Fig. 10-17). Early honeycombing usually occurs in a subpleural location, and scattered individual cysts rather than layers of clusters of cysts may be seen (Fig. 10-17C and D).

When honeycombing is present, normal lung architecture is distorted, and secondary lobules are difficult or impossible to recognize. Associated findings of fibrosis, including reticular opacities, traction bronchiectasis, and traction bronchiolectasis, are usually present.

The presence of honeycombing strongly predicts the presence of usual interstitial pneumonia (UIP). The differential diagnosis is that of UIP, and includes idiopathic pulmonary fibrosis (IPF), which accounts for 60% to 70% of cases of honeycombing; collagen-vascular diseases (most

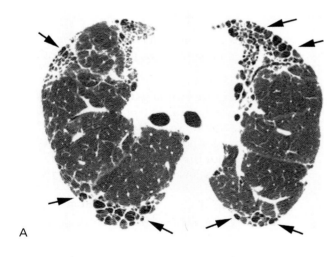

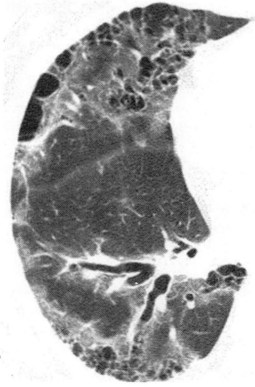

FIG. 10-17. Honeycombing. **A.** Patchy areas of subpleural honeycombing *(arrows)* are visible in a patient with rheumatoid arthritis and lung fibrosis. The cysts share walls and occur in multiple layers in the subpleural lung. **B.** Honeycombing in a patient with scleroderma. Cysts tend to be clustered. Several cysts are larger than 1 cm. *(Figure continues.)*

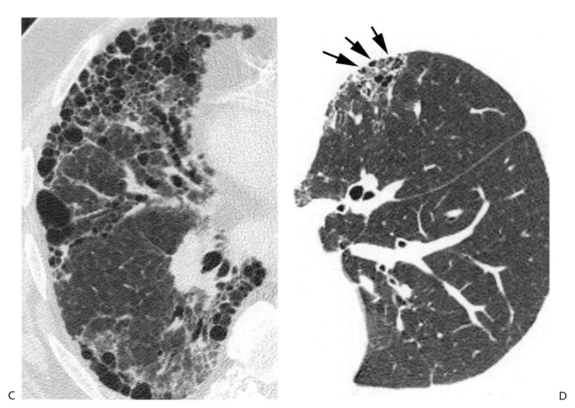

FIG. 10-17. *(Continued.)* **C.** Honeycombing in a patient with idiopathic pulmonary fibrosis. In the posterior lung, cysts are seen in a single layer. **D.** Early honeycombing in a patient with lupus. Focal fibrosis is visible posteriorly on a prone scan. Scattered subpleural honeycomb cysts are visible *(arrows)*.

often rheumatoid arthritis and scleroderma); fibrotic drug reactions; asbestosis, chronic or end-stage hypersensitivity pneumonitis; and, occasionally, sarcoidosis (Table 10-5). This appearance also may be seen with nonspecific interstitial pneumonia (NSIP). It usually is easy to distinguish honeycombing from cystic disease on HRCT (as opposed to plain radiographs), and diseases such as histiocytosis and LAM usually are not considered in the differential diagnosis.

The identification of honeycombing on HRCT is of great clinical importance for the following reasons:

1. It indicates end-stage disease in most patients, although progression can be seen in patients with honeycombing.
2. It indicates that a lung biopsy probably will not prove diagnostic (other than showing UIP).
3. It points to a poor prognosis (20% 5-year survival in patients with IPF).
4. It indicates a low likelihood (5%) that treatment will help.
5. Open lung biopsy rarely is performed when honeycombing is visible on HRCT.

TABLE 10-5. HONEYCOMBING: DIFFERENTIAL DIAGNOSIS

Usual interstitial pneumonia
  Idiopathic pulmonary fibrosis
  Collagen vascular disease (often rheumatoid arthritis or scleroderma)
  Drug-related fibrosis
  Asbestosis
  End-stage hypersensitivity pneumonitis
  End-stage sarcoidosis
Nonspecific interstitial pneumonia
Radiation
End-stage acute respiratory distress syndrome

Nonspecific Reticular Patterns

Reticular patterns other than interlobular septal thickening and honeycombing are somewhat nonspecific, and may indicate lung fibrosis or lung infiltration without fibrosis. The reticular opacities may be very fine and difficult to see or may be coarse and irregular. They often reflect the presence of intralobular interstitial thickening, or thickening of the lung interstitium at a sublobular level (Fig. 10-18).

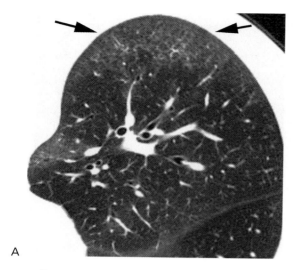

A

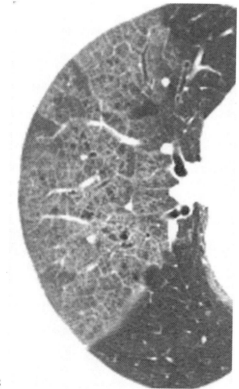

B

FIG. 10-18. Fine reticular opacities (intralobular interstitial thickening). **A.** Prone HRCT in a patient with scleroderma shows fine reticular opacities in the posterior left lung *(arrows)*. This represents mild lung fibrosis. **B.** HRCT in a patient with alveolar proteinosis shows a fine reticular pattern in the right lung associated with ground-glass opacity. Some septal thickening is also visible. This appearance represents interstitial infiltration rather than fibrosis.

A reticular pattern not associated with traction bronchiectasis may represent mild fibrosis (see Fig. 10-18A) or may be seen in association with ground-glass opacity, nodules, or other findings in patients with lung disease (see Fig. 10-18B). When this is the case, it is most appropriate to ignore the reticulation and base the differential diagnosis on the other findings present. When reticular opacities are visible, the presence of "traction bronchiectasis" is important in determining that fibrosis is present.

Traction Bronchiectasis

The term *traction bronchiectasis* refers to bronchial dilatation occurring as a result of lung fibrosis. It typically is associated with a reticular pattern, lung distortion, or honeycombing. Bronchi tend to be quite irregular or corkscrewed in appearance (Fig. 10-19). In comparison to garden variety infectious bronchiectasis, mucous plugging or fluid within the bronchi is absent. The appearance of traction bronchiectasis in the peripheral lung may overlap with that of honeycombing.

Dilatation of small peripheral bronchioles also may be seen in the presence of lung fibrosis, and is termed *traction bronchiolectasis*. Normally, bronchi are not visible in the peripheral 1 to 2 cm of lung; if they are visible, bronchiolectasis is present. If this finding is seen in combination with a reticular pattern, fibrosis is the likely cause.

Traction bronchiectasis and traction bronchiolectasis are very helpful in making the diagnosis of fibrosis when honeycombing is not present (Fig. 10-19B and C). Although the differential diagnosis includes UIP and the diseases that cause honeycombing, some other diseases are more likely when this pattern of fibrosis is present, including sarcoidosis, hypersensitivity pneumonitis, and NSIP (Table 10-6). Because of this possibility and the greater likelihood that treatment may be effective when this pattern is present, lung biopsy may be performed.

Nodules

Nodules as small as 1 to 2 mm in diameter can be detected on HRCT in patients with DILD. Nodules can be classified by (1) their appearance as well-defined (and thus most likely interstitial) or ill-defined (and most likely "air-space"); (2)

TABLE 10-6. TRACTION BRONCHIECTASIS: DIFFERENTIAL DIAGNOSIS

Nonspecific interstitial pneumonia
Usual interstitial pneumonia and its causes (see above)
Sarcoidosis
Hypersensitivity pneumonitis
Radiation
End-stage acute respiratory distress syndrome

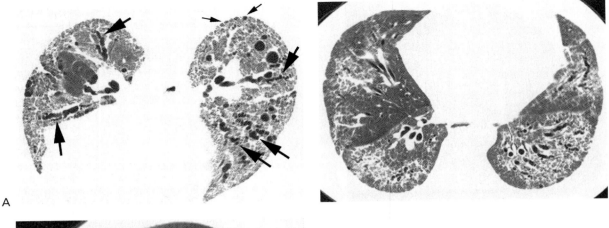

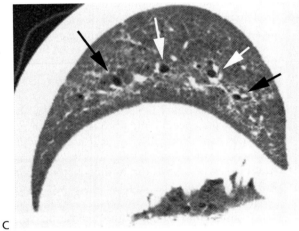

FIG. 10-19. Reticular opacities with traction bronchiectasis. **A.** Prone HRCT in a patient with lung fibrosis shows an extensive reticular pattern associated with multiple irregularly dilated (corkscrewed) bronchi *(large arrows)*. This is termed *traction bronchiectasis*. A few scattered subpleural honeycomb cysts also are visible in the posterior subpleural lung *(small arrows)*. **B.** A patient with rheumatoid arthritis shows reticular opacities with irregular dilatation of multiple bronchi. This finding indicates the presence of lung fibrosis. There is no evidence of honeycombing. **C.** Prone HRCT in a patient with mixed connective tissue disease shows a fine reticular pattern. This appearance is nonspecific, but the presence of multiple dilated bronchi *(arrows)* indicates that lung fibrosis is present. There is no evidence of honeycombing. This appearance probably is due to NSIP.

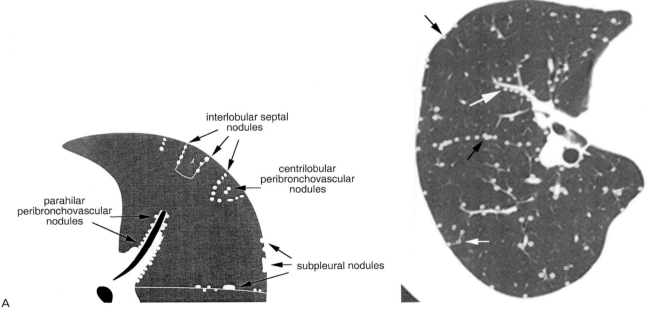

FIG. 10-20. Locations of "perilymphatic" nodules. **A.** Nodules are visible in the subpleural regions and adjacent to fissures, the parahilar region adjacent to vessels and bronchi, the interlobular septa, and the peribronchovascular interstitium in a centrilobular location. **B.** Simulated perilymphatic nodules. Nodules are visible in the subpleural regions *(black arrow)*, peribronchovascular regions *(large white arrow)*, and in relation to interlobular septae *(small white arrow)*.

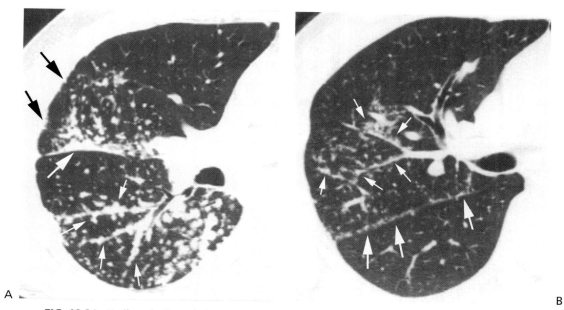

FIG. 10-21. Perilymphatic nodules on HRCT in two patients with sarcoidosis. Nodules involve the subpleural interstitium *(large arrows)* in the lung periphery and adjacent to the fissure. Parahilar peribronchovascular nodules *(small arrows)* also are visible. Septal nodules and centrilobular nodules are visible but less numerous.

their overall distribution; or (3) their specific anatomic distribution relative to lung structures. Although taking account of each of these features is important, recognition of the specific anatomic distribution of nodules is fundamental to their accurate diagnosis.

Nodules can be classified as "perilymphatic," random, or centrilobular in distribution on HRCT.

Perilymphatic Nodules

Perilymphatic nodules occur in relation to lung lymphatics. They usually are well defined. They involve specific lung regions: (1) the subpleural interstitium at the pleural surfaces and fissures; (2) the peribronchovascular interstitium in the parahilar lung; (3) the interlobular septa; and (4) the peribronchovascular interstitium in a centrilobular location (Fig. 10-20).

In clinical practice, perilymphatic nodules usually are the result of sarcoidosis (see Chapter 15), which tends to have a peribronchovascular and subpleural predominance of nodules (Fig. 10-21), or lymphangitic spread of tumor (see Chapter 4), which typically predominates in relation to interlobular septa and the peribronchovascular interstitium (Fig. 10-22 and Table 10-7). Sarcoidosis usually shows more extensive abnormalities in the upper lobes and may be symmetrical or asymmetrical. Lymphangitic spread of carcinoma usually is most severe at the lung bases and often is asymmetrical.

Silicosis and coal-worker's pneumoconiosis (CWP) also may result in this pattern, predominating in the subpleural and centrilobular peribronchovascular regions (see Chapter 18). However, silicosis and CWP are best recognized by a

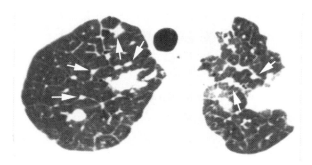

FIG. 10-22. Lymphangitic spread of breast carcinoma. Multiple nodules *(arrows)* are visible in relation to interlobular septa.

TABLE 10-7. PERILYMPHATIC NODULES: DIFFERENTIAL DIAGNOSIS
Sarcoidosis
Lymphangitic spread of tumor
Silicosis and coal-worker's pneumoconiosis
Amyloidosis (rare)
Lymphoid interstitial pneumonitis (rare)

symmetrical, posterior, upper lobe predominance of nodules. Also, an exposure history usually is available. Rarely, amyloidosis (see Chapter 21) or lymphoid interstitial pneumonitis (LIP; see Chapter 13) results in this pattern.

Random Nodules

Random nodules are randomly distributed relative to structures of the secondary lobule and lung, and appear diffuse and uniform in distribution (Figs. 10-23 and 10-7C). Subpleural nodules often are seen. Nodules usually are well-defined.

The random nodule pattern is most typical of miliary

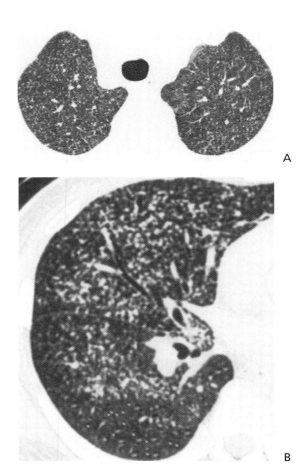

FIG. 10-24. Random nodules in two patients with miliary tuberculosis. **A.** The nodules are small, sharply defined, and diffuse and uniform in distribution. **B.** Nodules involve the pleural surfaces and are diffuse.

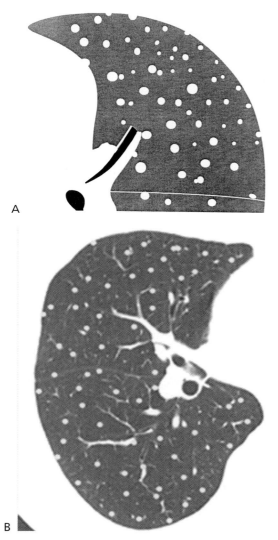

FIG. 10-23. Random nodules. **A.** Nodules may involve the pleural surfaces, peribronchovascular interstitium, and interlobular septa, but do not show a predominance in relation to these structures as is present with a perilymphatic pattern. The overall distribution appears diffuse and uniform. **B.** Simulated random nodules. Compare with Figure 10-20B.

tuberculosis (Fig. 10-24) or fungal infection (see Fig. 10-7C) and hematogenous metastases (Fig. 10-25), but sarcoidosis, when diffuse, also can show this pattern (Table 10-8).

Centrilobular Nodules

Centrilobular nodules often reflect bronchiolar or peribronchiolar abnormalities in a centrilobular location, although abnormalities occurring in relation to small vessels also may result in this finding. The most peripheral nodules often

TABLE 10-8. RANDOM NODULES: DIFFERENTIAL DIAGNOSIS
Miliary infections
Hematogenous metastases
Sarcoidosis

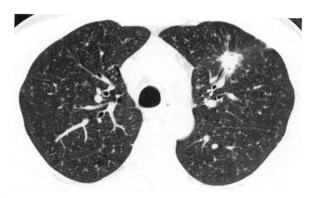

FIG. 10-25. Random nodules of metastatic lung carcinoma. The primary carcinoma is visible in the left upper lobe. The nodules are diffuse and uniform in distribution.

are centered 5 to 10 mm from the pleural surface and do not touch the pleura unless they are large (unlike the other two patterns) (Fig. 10-26). Because the lobules are all of similar size, they tend to be evenly spaced. Nodules may be well- or ill-defined, or a centrilobular rosette of small nodules may be seen (Fig. 10-27). Nodules may involve the lung diffusely or be patchy.

Centrilobular nodules can be seen in endobronchial spread of tuberculosis or other causes of bronchopneumonia (see Fig. 10-27A); endobronchial spread of tumor (e.g.,

bronchioloalveolar carcinoma [BAC]; see Fig. 3-8 in Chapter 3); hypersensitivity pneumonitis (see Fig. 10-27B and C); bronchiolitis obliterans organizing pneumonia (BOOP); silicosis and coal-worker's pneumoconiosis; histiocytosis; or vascular diseases such as vasculitis and pulmonary edema (Table 10-9).

When centrilobular nodules are the predominant finding, diseases involving the small airways are most likely. Consider infection, hypersensitivity and pneumonitis (which may be diagnosed by history), and remember BAC.

Centrilobular Tree-in-bud Pattern

When a centrilobular distribution of nodules is present, the "tree-in-bud" pattern should be sought (see Fig. 10-26A). This finding nearly always represents the presence of dilated and fluid-filled (with mucus or pus) centrilobular bronchioles (Fig. 10-28). Nodular branching opacities are visible in the lung periphery, and these are considerably larger than normal branching vessels. Trees-in-bud, which are centrilobular, tend to be centered 5 to 10 mm from the pleural surface when they are seen in the peripheral lung. Centrilobular nodules or clusters of nodules (rosettes) also may be seen.

The presence of the tree-in-bud pattern is of great value in the differential diagnosis. Because this finding represents dilatation and impaction of small centrilobular bronchioles,

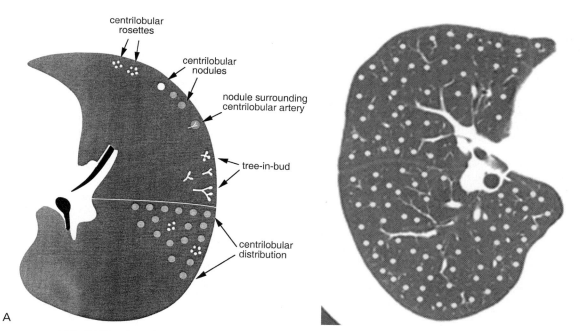

FIG. 10-26. Centrilobular nodules. **A.** Nodules spare the pleural surfaces unless they are large, and tend to be centered 5 to 10 mm from the pleural surface or fissures. Because lobules are of similar size, nodules tend to appear evenly spaced. Nodules may be well- or ill-defined, or may appear as a rosette of smaller nodules. The finding of the tree-in-bud pattern, which almost always represents dilatation and impaction of bronchioles, also is centrilobular in location. **B.** Simulated centrilobar nodules. Compare with Figure 10-20B.

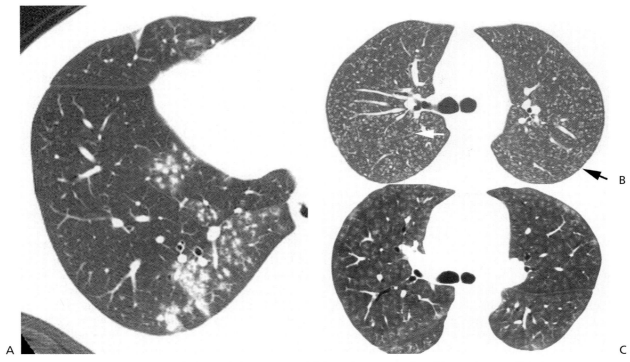

FIG. 10-27. Centrilobular nodules. **A.** Bacterial bronchopneumonia with patchy centrilobular nodules in the lower lobe. The most peripheral nodules are centered 5 to 10 mm from the pleural surface and spare the pleura. Small rosettes also are visible. **B.** Centrilobular nodules in hypersensitivity pneumonitis. Note that the nodules spare the fissure *(arrows)* and pleural surface. The nodules are diffuse and appear evenly spaced. **C.** Hypersensitivity pneumonitis with centrilobular nodules of ground-glass opacity.

it confirms the presence of airway disease. Furthermore, the tree-in-bud appearance almost always indicates the presence of infection (e.g., tuberculosis, *Mycobacterium avium* complex, bacteria, fungus) or infected airway disease (e.g., bronchiectasis, cystic fibrosis; Fig. 10-28). Rarely, it may be due to asthma with mucous plugging, allergic bronchopulmonary aspergillosis, or endobronchial spread of tumor (Table 10-10).

This finding means the diagnosis should be made by examination or culture of sputum. If not, bronchoalveolar lavage is likely to be diagnostic.

Distribution of Nodules: A Diagnostic Algorithm

It is possible to distinguishing these three specific distributions—perilymphatic, random, or centrilobular nodules (or tree-in-bud)—on HRCT by using a simple algorithm (Fig. 10-29).

The first step is to look for subpleural nodules and nodules seen in relation to the fissures. If they are absent, the nodules are centrilobular. Once it has been confirmed that the nodules are centrilobular, the presence of tree-in-bud should be sought.

If pleural or fissural nodules are present, then the pattern

TABLE 10-9. CENTRILOBULAR NODULES: DIFFERENTIAL DIAGNOSIS

Endobronchial spread of infection (bacteria, virus, tuberculosis, mycobacteria, fungus)
Endobronchial spread of tumor (bronchioloalveolar carcinoma)
Hypersensitivity pneumonitis
Bronchiolitis obliterans organizing pneumonia
Silicosis and coal-worker's pneumoconiosis
Histiocytosis
Pulmonary edema
Vasculitis

TABLE 10-10. TREE-IN-BUD: DIFFERENTIAL DIAGNOSIS

Endobronchial spread of infection (bacteria, tubercu-losis, mycobacteria, fungus)
Airways diseases with infection (e.g., cystic fibrosis, bronchiectasis)
Mucous plugging (asthma, allergic bron-chopulmonary aspergillosis)
Bronchioloalveolar carcinoma (rare)

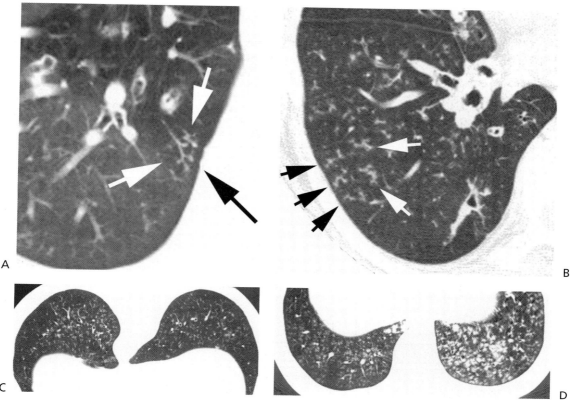

FIG. 10-28. Tree-in-bud. **A.** The tree-in-bud *(arrows)* in the right lower lobe in a patient with cystic fibrosis. A branching opacity in the peripheral lung (i.e., the tree) represents a dilated centrilobular bronchiole impacted with mucus and pus. Small, rounded opacities at the tips of the branches (i.e., the buds) represent peribronchiolar inflammation. Bronchial wall thickening and mosaic perfusion also are visible. **B.** Several examples of the tree-in-bud *(arrows)* in another patient with airway infection. These appear larger than normal branching vessels in the peripheral lung, visible posteriorly. **C.** Bilateral tree-in-bud in a patient with *Pseudomonas bronchopneumonia.* **D.** Centrilobular nodules and tree-in-bud in a patient with *Haemophilus influenzae* bronchopneumonia.

is either perilymphatic or random. These two patterns are then distinguished by looking at the distribution of other nodules. If they are patchy in distribution, particularly if a distinct peribronchovascular or septal distribution is present, then the nodules are perilymphatic; if the nodules are diffuse and uniform, the pattern is random. Using this approach, 94% of cases can be classified accurately.

Increased Lung Opacity

Increased lung opacity may be classified as consolidation or ground-glass opacity.

Air-space Consolidation

Air-space consolidation is said to be present when alveolar air is replaced by fluid, cells, or other substances. On HRCT, consolidation results in an increase in lung opacity

associated with obscuration of underlying vessels. Air bronchograms may be present.

If another pattern also is present (e.g., small nodules), the consolidation probably represents confluent disease and should be ignored for the purposes of differential diagnosis.

The differential diagnosis of consolidation is based primarily on the duration of symptoms. In patients with acute symptoms, pneumonia, pulmonary edema, pulmonary hemorrhage, and acute respiratory distress syndrome are most likely (see Table 10-10). Among patients with chronic symptoms, the most common causes of this finding include chronic eosinophilic pneumonia (Fig. 10-30A), bronchiolitis obliterans organizing pneumonia (BOOP; Fig. 10-30B), and interstitial pneumonia such as UIP or NSIP (Table 10-11). BAC also may result in this pattern.

Ground-glass Opacity

Ground-glass opacity is a nonspecific term referring to a hazy increase in lung opacity that is not associated with

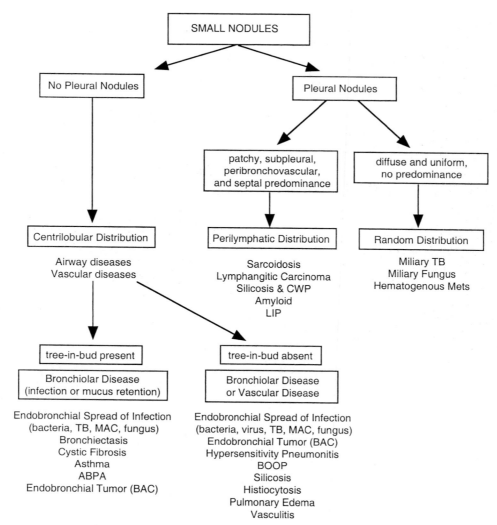

FIG. 10-29. Algorithm for classification and diagnosis of multiple small nodules.

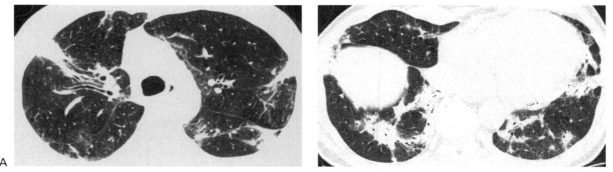

FIG. 10-30. Consolidation. **A.** Homogeneous areas of consolidation are visible in the peripheral lung. This represents chronic eosinophilic pneumonia. **B.** Patchy areas of consolidation with air bronchogram in a patient with bronchiolitis obliterans organizing pneumonia.

TABLE 10-11. AIR-SPACE CONSOLIDATION: DIFFERENTIAL DIAGNOSIS

Acute symptoms
  Pneumonia
  Pulmonary edema
  Pulmonary hemorrhage
  Acute respiratory distress syndrome
Chronic symptoms
  Chronic eosinophilic pneumonia or other eosinophilic disease
  Bronchiolitis obliterans organizing pneumonia
  Interstitial pneumonias
  Lipoid pneumonia
  Bronchioloalveolar carcinoma

TABLE 10-12. GROUND-GLASS OPACITY: DIFFERENTIAL DIAGNOSIS

Acute symptoms
  Pulmonary edema
  Hemorrhage
  Pneumonia (e.g., *Pneumocystis jiroveci* (*P. carinii*) or viral pneumonias)
  Diffuse alveolar damage
  Acute interstitial pneumonia
  Hypersensitivity pneumonitis (acute)
Chronic symptoms
  Nonspecific interstitial pneumonia
  Usual interstitial pneumonia (rare)
  Desquamative interstitial pneumonitis
  Hypersensitivity pneumonitis
  Alveolar proteinosis
  Sarcoidosis
  Lipoid pneumonia
  Bronchioloalveolar carcinoma

obscuration of underlying vessels (see Figs. 10-11B, 10-18B, and 10-31), although they may appear fuzzy. This finding can reflect the presence of a number of diseases, and can be seen in patients with either minimal interstitial thickening or minimal air-space disease. Although ground-glass opacity is a nonspecific finding, its presence is very significant. As with consolidation, the differential diagnosis is based primarily on the duration of symptoms.

In patients with acute symptoms, the presence of ground-glass opacity reflects active disease such as pulmonary edema (Fig. 10-31A) or hemorrhage, pneumonia (e.g., *Pneumocystis carinii* or viral pneumonias (Fig. 10-31B and C), diffuse alveolar damage, acute interstitial pneumonia, and hypersensitivity pneumonitis (Table 10-12).

In patients with subacute or chronic symptoms, ground-glass opacity usually (60% to 80% of cases) indicates an acute, active, and potentially treatable process, such as

NSIP, desquamative interstitial pneumonitis, hypersensitivity pneumonitis (Fig. 10-31D), alveolar proteinosis (see Figs. 10-18B and 10-32), sarcoidosis, lipoid pneumonia (see Fig. 10-11B), and BAC (see Table 10-11). Because of its association with active lung disease, the clinical diagnosis should be pursued. The presence of this finding often leads to lung biopsy, depending on the clinical status of the patient.

The combination of ground-glass opacity and interlobular septal thickening is termed "crazy paving" (see Fig. 10-32). This appearance is nonspecific and may be seen with a variety of acute lung diseases such as *Pneumocystis* or viral

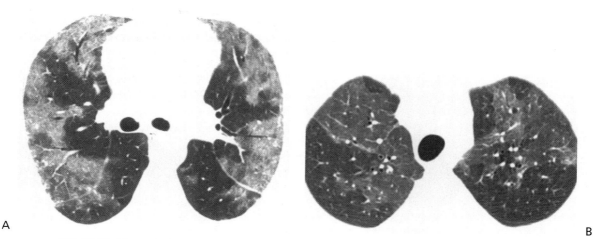

FIG. 10-31. Ground-glass opacity. **A.** A peripheral increase in lung attenuation represents ground-glass opacity. Vessels remain visible in the dense lung regions. This patient had acute dyspnea due to pulmonary edema. **B.** Patchy ground-glass opacity is visible in the upper lobes. This immunosuppressed patient had symptoms of acute fever and cough. Bronchoscopy revealed cytomegalovirus pneumonia. *(Figure continues.)*

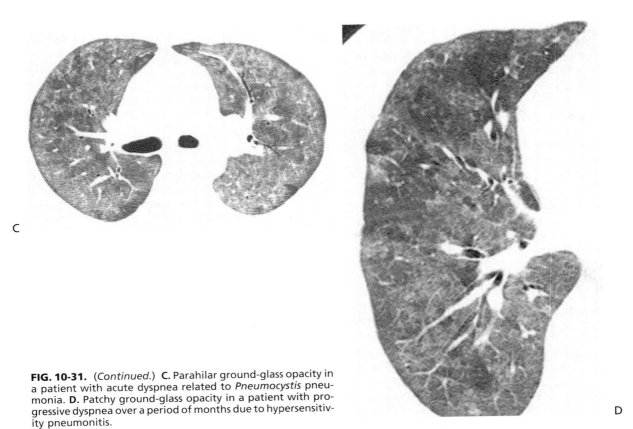

C

D

FIG. 10-31. (*Continued.*) **C.** Parahilar ground-glass opacity in a patient with acute dyspnea related to *Pneumocystis* pneumonia. **D.** Patchy ground-glass opacity in a patient with progressive dyspnea over a period of months due to hypersensitivity pneumonitis.

pneumonia, edema, hemorrhage, and ARDS. Among patients with chronic lung disease, it often is the result of alveolar proteinosis.

When ground-glass opacity is associated with reticulation and findings of fibrosis such as traction bronchiectasis (Fig. 10-33), and particularly when they are seen in the same

lung regions, the ground-glass opacity is likely to be due to fibrosis rather than active disease. In this situation, it is necessary to hedge in the interpretation; in most cases the differential diagnosis for traction bronchiectasis listed in Table 10-6 should be used rather than that listed in Table 10-12. Biopsy may be warranted, and can be directed to areas showing the least evidence of fibrosis.

Decreased Lung Opacity and Cystic Lesions

Geographic areas of decreased lung attenuation may represent emphysema, mosaic perfusion, or air-trapping (on expi-

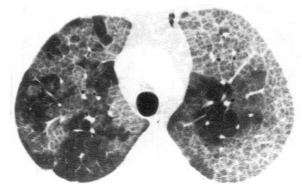

FIG. 10-32. Ground-glass opacity with "crazy paving." Patchy ground-glass opacity is associated with interlobular septal thickening in the abnormal regions. This represents alveolar proteinosis.

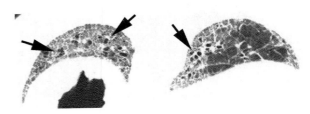

FIG. 10-33. Ground-glass opacity associated with traction bronchiectasis. Fibrosis in the posterior lung bases is associated with ground-glass opacity and reticulation. The presence of traction bronchiectasis (*arrows*) indicates that the ground-glass opacity is likely due to fibrosis.

ratory scans). Circumscribed areas of decreased lung attenuation may represent emphysema or lung cysts.

Emphysema

Emphysema results in areas of very low attenuation, usually less than -950 HU. The appearance of emphysema is characteristic and depends on the type of emphysema present (Fig. 10-34). Typical appearances are as follows:

Centrilobular emphysema: focal areas of lucency without visible walls, usually with an upper lobe predominance (see Fig. 24-6 in Chapter 24)

Panlobular emphysema: large areas of low attenuation, usually diffuse and associated with decreased vessel size (see Fig. 24-9 in Chapter 24)

Paraseptal emphysema: subpleural lucencies marginated by interlobular septae or subpleural bullae, usually with an upper lobe predominance (see Fig. 24-11 in Chapter 24).

Lung Cysts

Lung cyst is a nonspecific term, used to describe a thin-walled (usually less than 3 mm), well-defined and circumscribed, air-containing lesion, 1 cm or more in diameter. Cysts may be seen in cystic lung disease, or may represent bullae in association with emphysema, honeycombing in patients with fibrosis, pneumatoceles in association with pneumonia, or cystic bronchiectasis (see Table 10-12). Bullae, honeycombing, pneumatoceles, and cystic bronchiectasis usually can be distinguished from cystic lung disease by

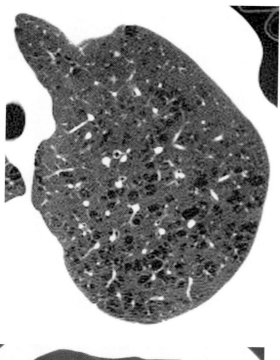

A

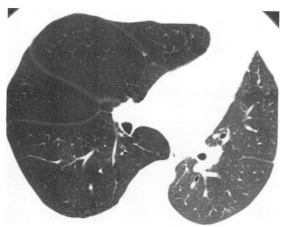

B

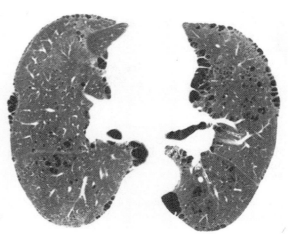

C

FIG. 10-34. Appearances of emphysema. **A.** Centrilobular emphysema. Focal areas of lucency without visible walls are visible in the left upper lobe. **B.** Panlobular emphysema in a patient with a left lung transplant. The right lung is hyperlucent, and vessels are reduced in size and number. **C.** Paraseptal emphysema. Subpleural lucencies marginated by interlobular septae and subpleural bullae are visible.

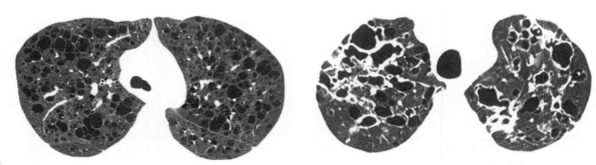

FIG. 10-35. Lung cysts. **A.** HRCT in a young woman with lymphangiomyomatosis. Multiple lung cysts are visible, having thin but easily discernible walls. In this disease, the cysts usually are interspersed within areas of normal-appearing lung and appear rounded. **B.** Lung cysts in histiocytosis. The cysts are more irregular in shape than those in patients with lymphangiomyomatosis, and have an upper lobe predominance. In this patient, the cysts appear thick-walled.

associated findings. Scattered lung cysts may be seen in some patients with hypersensitivity pneumonitis.

Cystic lung diseases (i.e., lung disease characterized by numerous cysts) are rare. Lymphangiomyomatosis (LAM) and Langerhans' histiocytosis often are associated with multiple lung cysts as a primary manifestation. The cysts have a thin but easily discernible wall, ranging up to a few millimeters in thickness (Fig. 10-35). In these diseases, the cysts usually are interspersed with areas of normal-appearing lung. LAM occurs only in women of childbearing age, and typically the cysts are uniformly distributed, round, and similar in size and shape (see Fig. 10-35A). In patients with histiocytosis, the cysts can be irregularly or bizarrely shaped (see Fig. 10-35B), have an upper lobe predominance, and tend to spare the costophrenic angles. Multiple cysts also may be seen in lymphoid interstitial pneumonia (LIP), particularly in patients with Sjögren's syndrome (Table 10-13).

Mosaic Perfusion

Patchy areas of decreased lung attenuation sometimes can be recognized on HRCT in patients with abnormal lung perfusion and reduced regional pulmonary blood volume (Fig. 10-36). The term *mosaic perfusion* is used to describe this appearance. Mosaic perfusion most often results from airway disease such as cystic fibrosis or bronchiolitis obliterans; in this setting, abnormal regional lung ventilation leads to vasoconstriction and decreased perfusion. Mosaic perfusion also can be seen with vascular obstruction (e.g., chronic pulmonary embolism; Table 10-14).

Key to diagnosing mosaic perfusion as the cause of inhomogeneous lung attenuation on HRCT is recognizing the presence of reduced vessel size in relatively lucent lung regions (see Figs. 10-36A and 10-38A). If abnormal bronchi are visible in lucent lung regions (see Fig. 10-36A), and bronchi appear normal in relatively dense regions, airway disease very likely is the cause.

Air-trapping on Expiratory Computed Tomography

In patients with mosaic perfusion resulting from airway disease, air-trapping often is visible on expiratory scans in lucent lung regions. Although mosaic perfusion and air-trapping look the same, and often are related, they are distinct findings. Mosaic perfusion is an inspiratory scan finding, and air-trapping is an expiratory scan finding. Also, in some

---

TABLE 10-13. LUNG CYSTS: DIFFERENTIAL DIAGNOSIS

Common causes of cysts
  Bullae
  Honeycombing
  Pneumatoceles in association with pneumonia
  Cystic bronchiectasis
  Cysts in hypersensitivity pneumonitis
Cystic lung disease (uncommon)
  Lymphangiomyomatosis
  Langerhans histiocytosis
  Tuberous sclerosis
  Sjögren's syndrome
  Lymphoid interstitial pneumonia
  Papillomatosis

TABLE 10-14. MOSAIC PERFUSION: DIFFERENTIAL DIAGNOSIS

Airway diseases
  Large airway diseases (e.g., cystic fibrosis, bronchiectasis)
  Small airway diseases (e.g., bronchiolitis obliterans, small airway infection, or mucous plugging)
Vascular diseases
  Chronic pulmonary embolism
  Other causes of vascular obstruction

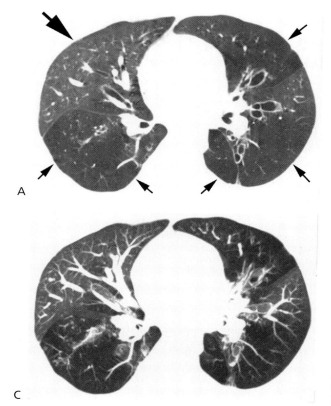

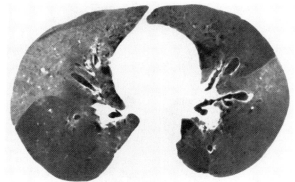

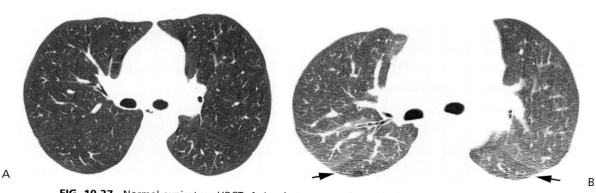

FIG. 10-36. Mosaic perfusion due to bronchiolitis obliterans. **A.** HRCT shows decreased lung attenuation in the lower lobes and left upper lobe *(small arrows)*. Note that vessels appear smaller in these regions than in the relatively dense right upper lobe *(large arrow)*. This is typical of mosaic perfusion. Abnormal bronchi are also seen in the lucent lung regions, suggesting an airway disease as the cause. **B.** Minimum-intensity projection from a stack of HRCT images at the same level shows the density differences between lung regions resulting from differences in lung perfusion. **C.** Maximum intensity projection at the same level shows the difference in vascular size between lucent and dense lung regions.

patients with airway disease, air-trapping may be visible on expiratory scans even though inspiratory scans are normal.

A variety of techniques can be used to obtain expiratory scans. Postexpiratory scans may be obtained following exhalation (i.e., the patient breathes out and suspends respiration). Dynamic expiratory scans are more sensitive. These are obtained with a spiral scanner by continuing to rotate the gantry as the patient exhales, obtaining a series of five

or six scans at a single level. This may be done with reduced milliamperage settings so that the entire dynamic series equals the radiation dose of a single HRCT slice.

Normally, lung attenuation increases homogeneously in attenuation on expiratory scans (usually by more than 100 HU), although dependent lung increases more than nondependent lung (Fig. 10-37). In the presence of air-trapping, lung remains lucent on expiration, with little increase in

FIG. 10-37. Normal expiratory HRCT. **A.** Inspiratory scan shows the lung to be homogeneous in attenuation. **B.** Following expiration, the lung increases in attenuation. Posterior, dependent lung usually increases in density more than nondependent lung. Mild air-trapping posterior to the major fissures in the superior segments of the lower lobes *(arrows)* is common in healthy individuals.

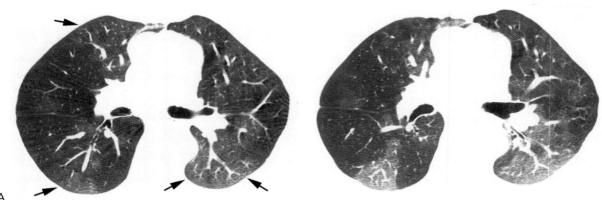

FIG. 10-38. Mosaic perfusion and air-trapping in a patient with bronchiolitis obliterans secondary to lung transplant rejection. **A.** Inspiratory scan shows inhomogeneous lung attenuation due to mosaic perfusion. Several lung regions *(arrows)* appear relatively dense and contain larger vessels. Other lung regions appear relatively lucent and contain small vessels. **B.** Expiratory scan shows a normal increase in attenuation of the dense regions shown in **A.** The relatively lucent regions in **A** show little change in attenuation on the expiratory scan due to air-trapping.

measured attenuation, and shows little change in volume (see Fig. 10-38). Patchy air-trapping is characteristic of small airway diseases. Larger areas of air-trapping (e.g., an entire lobe) suggest a large airway abnormality. Air-trapping on HRCT is associated principally with airway disease and bronchiolitis; its appearance is discussed in detail in Chapter 23.

SELECTED READING

Aquino SL, Gamsu G, Webb WR, Kee SL. Tree-in-bud pattern: frequency and significance on thin section CT. J Comput Assist Tomogr 1996; 20:594–599.

Arakawa H, Webb WR. Expiratory high-resolution CT scan. Radiol Clin North Am 1998; 36:189–209.

Austin JH, Müller NL, Friedman PJ, et al. Glossary of terms for CT of the lungs: recommendations of the Nomenclature Committee of the Fleischner Society. Radiology 1996; 200:327–331.

Colby TV, Swensen SJ. Anatomic distribution and histopathologic patterns in diffuse lung disease: correlation with HRCT. J Thorac Imag 1996; 11:1–26.

Felson B. A new look at pattern recognition of diffuse pulmonary disease. AJR Am J Roentgenol 1979; 133:183–189.

Godwin JD, Müller NL, Takasugi JE. Pulmonary alveolar proteinosis: CT findings. Radiology 1988; 169:609–613.

Gruden JF, Webb WR, Naidich DP, McGuinness G. Multinodular disease: anatomic localization at thin-section CT—multireader evaluation of a simple algorithm. Radiology 1999; 210:711–20.

Gruden JF, Webb WR, Warnock M. Centrilobular opacities in the lung on high-resolution CT: diagnostic considerations and pathologic correlation. AJR Am J Roentgenol 1994; 162:569–574.

Johkoh T, Müller NL, Cartier Y, et al. Idiopathic interstitial pneumonias: diagnostic accuracy of thin-section CT in 129 patients. Radiology 1999; 211:555–560.

Lee KS, Kim TS, Han J, et al. Diffuse micronodular lung disease: HRCT and pathologic findings. J Comput Assist Tomogr 1999; 23:99–106.

Leung AN, Miller RR, Müller NL. Parenchymal opacification in chronic infiltrative lung diseases: CT-pathologic correlation. Radiology 1993; 188:209–214.

Mayo JR. High resolution computed tomography: technical aspects. Radiol Clin North Am 1991; 29:1043–1049.

Müller NL, Miller RR. Diseases of the bronchioles: CT and histopathologic findings. Radiology 1995; 196:3–12.

Müller NL, Miller RR. Computed tomography of chronic diffuse infiltrative lung disease: part 1. Am Rev Respir Dis 1990; 142: 1206–1215.

Müller NL, Miller RR. Computed tomography of chronic diffuse infiltrative lung disease: part 2. Am Rev Respir Dis 1990; 142: 1440–1448.

Primack SL, Hartman TE, Hansell DM, Müller NL. End-stage lung disease: CT findings in 61 patients. Radiology 1993; 189: 681–686.

Webb WR. High resolution lung computed tomography: normal anatomic and pathologic findings. Radiol Clin North Am 1991; 29:1051–1063.

11

PULMONARY EDEMA, THE ACUTE RESPIRATORY DISTRESS SYNDROME, AND RADIOLOGY IN THE INTENSIVE CARE UNIT

W. RICHARD WEBB

Chest radiographs often are obtained daily in critically ill patients in the intensive care unit. Radiographs are used to detect significant changes in cardiopulmonary status; to search for pleural abnormalities; to evaluate the position of the numerous tubes, lines, and catheters used in monitoring and treatment; and to detect complications arising from the use of monitoring and support devices.

Radiographs obtained routinely or following placement of a tube or catheter show significant abnormalities not suspected clinically in 35% to 65% of patients in the ICU, and these findings often result in an intervention or change in treatment. The American College of Radiology (www.acr.org) recommends daily portable radiographs in patients requiring mechanical ventilation and those with acute cardiac or pulmonary disease. Radiographs are also recommended following placement of support and monitoring devices such as endotracheal tubes, tracheostomy tubes, central venous catheters, nasogastric tubes, chest tubes, pacemakers, and intraaortic balloon pump.

RADIOGRAPHIC TECHNIQUE

Adequate radiographs are difficult to obtain in the ICU. Portable chest radiographs usually are done using relatively low kilovoltage, long exposure times, no grids, and short source (tube)-to-detector (film or digital medium) distance. These result in high-contrast films, often with portions of the mediastinum or pulmonary parenchyma poorly seen (note: digital techniques help solve this problem), motion-related blur, and increased scatter radiation. The American College of Radiology has recommended technical standards for the performance of bedside portable radiographs (Table 11-1).

Even if the technique is optimized, it often is not possible to obtain the desired radiographs because of the patient's inability to cooperate. Patients in the ICU often are too ill to be positioned for radiographic examinations. Portable radiographs are performed in the anteroposterior (AP) projection, usually supine or semierect rather than upright. Position must be taken into account in interpreting radiographs for the presence of cardiomegaly, pulmonary vascular congestion, and pleural effusion. Furthermore, variation in patient position from day to day also must be considered.

PULMONARY DISEASE IN THE CRITICALLY ILL PATIENT

Common pulmonary complications that occur in patients in the ICU and other critically ill patients include pulmonary edema (hydrostatic; increased capillary permeability), the acute respiratory distress syndrome (ARDS), atelectasis, pneumonia, aspiration, pulmonary embolism, and pulmo-

TABLE 11-1. AMERICAN COLLEGE OF RADIOLOGY TECHNICAL STANDARDS FOR BEDSIDE PORTABLE RADIOGRAPHS

1. 72-inch source to image distance and upright position when possible (although this is uncommonly possible in ICU patients), or
2. 40-inch or more source to image distance for supine or semierect radiographs in uncooperative patients
3. kVp of 70–100 should be used in radiographs obtained without a grid
4. kVp of more than 100 may be used for radiographs obtained with a grid
5. Exposure times as short as possible
6. Technical parameters such as mAs, kVp, distance, and patient position should be recorded (to allow consistency in performance)

nary hemorrhage. To some extent, the radiographic distribution of pulmonary disease, the time course of radiographic abnormalities, and associated radiographic findings may help in reaching a useful differential diagnosis. However, the radiographic findings in a patient in the ICU with acute pulmonary disease may be nonspecific, and knowledge of the clinical history or physical findings often is essential in suggesting the appropriate diagnosis.

PULMONARY EDEMA AND THE ACUTE RESPIRATORY DISTRESS SYNDROME

Pulmonary edema often is classified as either hydrostatic (cardiogenic) or due to increased capillary permeability (noncardiogenic). It should be recognized, however, that it is not always possible—or entirely appropriate—to make a simple distinction between hydrostatic and permeability edema. A classification as (1) hydrostatic edema, (2) increased permeability edema associated with diffuse alveolar damage (DAD), (3) increased permeability edema without associated DAD, and (4) mixed edema agrees better with pathology, physiology, and radiology. Although these types of edema cannot always be distinguished on the basis of plain film or CT findings, their appearances do tend to differ.

HYDROSTATIC PULMONARY EDEMA

Hydrostatic pulmonary edema results from alterations in the normal relation between intra- and extravascular hydrostatic and oncotic pressures. In most cases, an increased intravascular pressure due to pulmonary venous hypertension is the predominant cause, resulting in loss of fluid into the interstitium. This may result from left heart failure, left atrial or pulmonary venous obstruction, volume overload in renal failure, or overhydration. Low intravascular oncotic pressure resulting from hypoalbuminemia, liver failure, or renal failure also can also result in increased interstitial transudation of fluid.

Radiographic abnormalities associated with hydrostatic or cardiogenic pulmonary edema may be difficult to evaluate on portable radiographs. Heart size is difficult to determine accurately on portable AP radiographs, particularly when lung volume is reduced. Pulmonary vascular congestion also may be difficult to identify with certainty because of patient position. Upper lobe vessels appear larger than normal when patients are supine or semierect. Similarly, dilatation of the azygos vein, useful as a sign of increased right atrial pressure, occurs normally in the supine position. The apparent width of the mediastinum (vascular pedicle) is increased by supine position, AP projection, and decreased inspiratory level.

Plain radiographs and high-resolution CT (HRCT) may show findings of interstitial or air-space edema or both.

Associated pleural effusion is common, but may be difficult to see on supine radiographs.

Interstitial Edema

Interstitial edema is manifested on chest radiograph or CT by interlobular septal thickening (Kerley's A or B lines), subpleural edema with thickening of the fissures, peribronchial cuffing, poor definition of pulmonary vessels, "perihilar haze," and ground-glass opacity.

Interlobular Septal Thickening (Kerley's Lines)

Kerley's B lines result from thickening of interlobular septa (Fig. 11-1; see also Fig. 10-1 in Chapter 10). They are horizontal, are 1 to 2 cm in length, touch the pleural surface, and are best seen laterally at the costophrenic angles. Their characteristic appearance results from the regular organization of pulmonary lobules at the lung bases.

Kerley's A lines (see Fig. 11-1; see also Fig. 10-2 in Chapter 10) are less commonly seen. They are oblique, several centimeters in length, and are seen within the central or perihilar lung. They also represent thickened septa, but their appearance is different from that of B lines because of the different organization of lobules in this location.

In patients with Kerley's lines, HRCT shows interlobular septal thickening (Fig. 11-2; see also Fig. 10-15 in Chapter 10).

Subpleural Edema

The subpleural interstitial space is contiguous with peripheral interlobular septa. If interlobular septal thickening and Kerley's lines are present, subpleural interstitial thickening often is visible as well. It is recognized as thickening of the fissures (see Figs. 11-1B and 11-2). This finding also may be due to pleural effusion thickening the fissure.

Peribronchial Cuffing

Thickening of the peribronchovascular interstitium often occurs in patients with interstitial edema, resulting in apparent bronchial wall thickening, or *peribronchial cuffing* (see Fig. 11-2). On chest radiographs, peribronchial cuffing is easiest to recognize in the perihilar regions where bronchi are seen end-on; sometimes lines radiating outward from the hila reflect the thickened peribronchial interstitium. Thickening of the peribronchovascular interstitium is seen on CT as bronchial wall thickening.

Poor Definition of Perihilar Vessels and Perihilar Haze

Edema fluid surrounding pulmonary vessels blurs their margins, making them difficult to see or poorly defined on chest

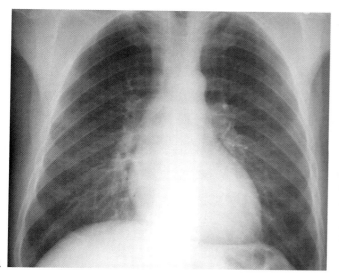
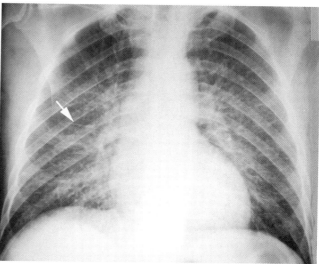

FIG. 11-1. Acute hydrostatic pulmonary edema with Kerley's lines in a patient with aortic stenosis and fluid overload. **A.** Baseline chest radiograph is normal. **B.** One hour later, after rapid infusion of fluid, Kerley's A and B lines are visible, with a perihilar predominance. Thickening of the right minor fissure also is visible *(arrow)* as a result of subpleural edema. The patient was acutely short of breath.

radiographs. This finding is easiest to recognize when comparison films are available. Poor definition of lower lobe vessels usually is the first abnormality noted in pulmonary edema and may be seen when Kerley's lines are unrecognizable.

Poor definition of hilar or perihilar vessels is a common finding in patients with mild pulmonary edema (Fig. 11-3). This finding, sometimes referred to as *perihilar haze*, often is often useful in diagnosing pulmonary edema in

bedridden patients with lower lobe atelectasis or pneumonia in whom the lower lobe vessels cannot be assessed. This appearance may progress to a frank "batwing" pattern of pulmonary edema.

Ground-glass Opacity

An overall increase in lung water or interstitial thickening often is recognizable as a poorly defined, generalized in-

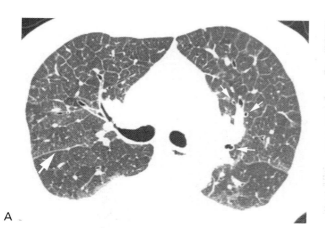
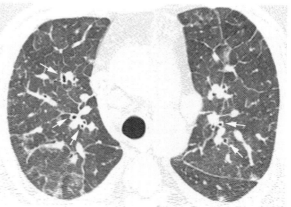

FIG. 11-2. Interlobular septal thickening on HRCT in acute hydrostatic pulmonary edema in two different patients. **A.** There is extensive thickening of interlobular septa. Subpleural edema results in thickening of the fissures *(large arrow)*. Apparent parahilar bronchial wall thickening ("peribronchial cuffing") results from edema fluid thickening the peribronchovascular interstitium *(small arrows)*. Bilateral pleural effusions also are present. **B.** Interlobular septal thickening and thickening of the left major fissure are visible. Peribronchial cuffing *(arrows)* is well seen in this case. Patchy areas of increased lung attenuation represent ground-glass opacity, which may be seen with or without septal thickening in patients with interstitial edema.

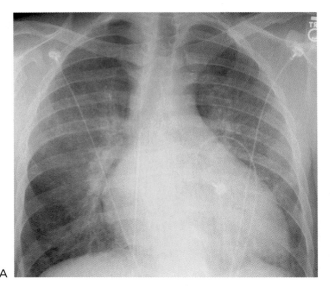
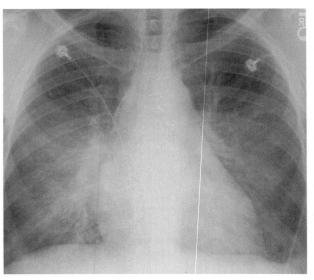

FIG. 11-3. Poor definition of perihilar and lower lobe vessels ("perihilar haze") in two patients with hydrostatic edema. **A.** Chest radiograph in a patient with congestive heart failure and cardiomegaly shows poor definition of perihilar and lower lobe vessels as the first sign of pulmonary edema. **B.** In another patient with cardiomegaly and pulmonary edema, hazy opacity obscures perihilar and lower lobe vessels.

crease in lung density, or ground-glass opacity. It may be difficult to recognize on chest radiographs in the absence of comparison films, but is easily seen on HRCT (Fig. 11-4). In patients with perihilar haze visible on chest radiographs, ground-glass opacity often is seen on HRCT.

On HRCT, ground-glass opacity due to edema may be perihilar and perivascular (see Fig. 11-4B), peripheral and subpleural (see Fig. 10-31A in Chapter 10), patchy and lobular in distribution, or centrilobular (Fig. 11-5). It may

be seen in combination with septal thickening (see Fig. 11-2B) or in isolation.

Air-space Edema

With an increase in interstitial pressure and a worsening of edema, fluid overflows the interstitium and fills the alveoli. Findings of air-space edema are the same as those of air-space consolidation. They include ill-defined or confluent

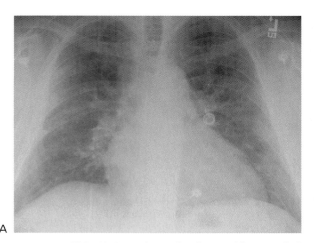
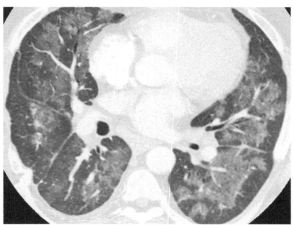

FIG. 11-4. Hydrostatic edema with ground-glass opacity. **A.** Chest radiograph in a patient with edema shows poor definition of perihilar vessels and a subtle increase in lung density. **B.** HRCT shows patchy perihilar ground-glass opacity. Thickening of the fissures and small pleural effusions are present, but septal thickening is absent in this patient.

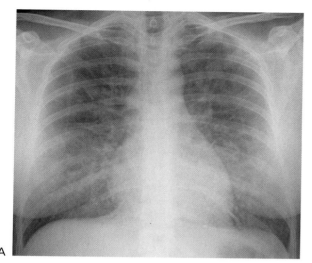

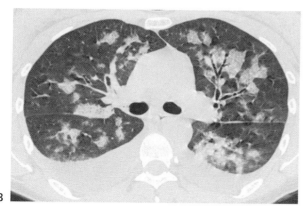

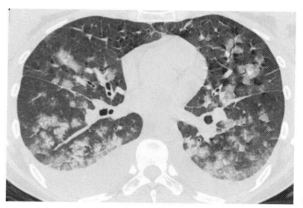

FIG. 11-5. Acute hydrostatic edema due to fluid overload, with ground-glass opacity. **A.** Chest radiograph shows poor definition of perihilar and lower lobe vessels, an increase in lung density, and thickening of the minor fissure. Linear opacities in the perihilar regions represent peribronchial cuffing and Kerley's A lines. **B.** HRCT obtained several hours later shows patchy perihilar and perivascular areas of ground-glass opacity, some appearing lobular. Thickening of the fissures, septal thickening, and peribronchial cuffing also are present. Bilateral pleural effusions are visible. **C.** At a lower level, thickening of fissures, septal thickening, and patchy lobular and centrilobular ground-glass opacity is visible.

opacities with obscuration of underlying vessels and "acinar" or air-space nodules. Air bronchograms may be seen in some patients, but are not always visible. HRCT may show frank consolidation or dense ground-glass opacity in patients with the appearance of consolidation on plain radiographs. Homogeneous dense consolidation is unusual on HRCT in patients with edema unless atelectasis is associated.

Air-space edema may be patchy, multifocal, or diffuse, but usually it is bilateral and symmetric. In upright patients, a basal distribution often is visible. A perihilar "batwing" or "butterfly" distribution occurs occasionally, often related to rapid accumulation of edema fluid (Fig. 11-6). This pattern also has been attributed to better clearance of edema fluid in the lung periphery because of a richer lymphatic network in this region, but why it is seen in some patients and not in others is unclear.

Unilateral or Asymmetric Edema

Hydrostatic edema usually is bilateral and symmetric. In patients with edema, variations in the distribution of the edema fluid may result from variations in blood flow or hydrostatic pressure (or other mechanisms). Unilateral or asymmetric edema may be seen due to ipsilateral or contralateral abnormalities in blood flow or hydrostatic pressure (Table 11-2).

The most common cause of ipsilateral edema is the decubitus position (Fig. 11-7). Right upper lobe edema may be seen in patients with papillary muscle rupture and mitral regurgitation; this is caused by a jet or regurgitant blood directed into the right superior pulmonary vein (Fig. 11-8).

Patients with decreased blood flow to one lung (e.g., pulmonary artery occlusion) tend to develop edema on the opposite side. This also may be seen in patient with unilateral lung abnormalities resulting in decreased blood flow, such as Swyer-James syndrome (Fig. 11-9).

Course and Clearing of Hydrostatic Edema

Hydrostatic edema may appear rapidly in association with acute heart failure or fluid overload (see Fig. 11-1). Often

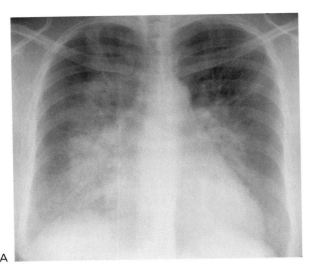

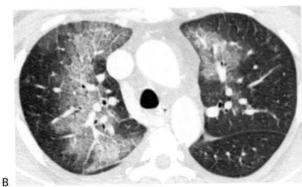

FIG. 11-6. Hydrostatic pulmonary edema with a perihilar or "batwing" appearance of consolidation. **A.** Chest radiograph shows perihilar consolidation. Air bronchograms are visible. **B** and **C.** HRCTs at two levels show dense ground-glass opacity in a perihilar distribution.

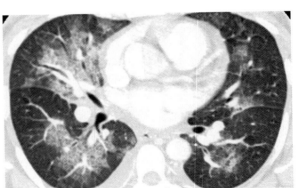

TABLE 11-2. UNILATERAL PULMONARY EDEMA

Unilateral edema associated with ipsilateral abnormalities
Decubitus position
Reexpansion edema
Pulmonary vein occlusion
Congenital or acquired systemic to pulmonary artery shunt
   (e.g., Blalock-Taussig)
Papillary muscle rupture and mitral regurgitation with a jet
   effect

Unilateral edema associated with contralateral abnormalities
Pulmonary artery occlusion (e.g., pulmonary embolism, tumor)
Hypoplastic pulmonary artery or interruption of the pulmonary
   artery
Swyer-James syndrome
Unilateral emphysema or bullae
Transient atelectasis

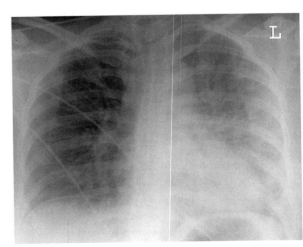

FIG. 11-7. Unilateral left-sided pulmonary edema. Postoperative radiograph in a patient who had a right nephrectomy in the left lateral decubitus position. Note free air under the right hemidiaphragm secondary to surgery.

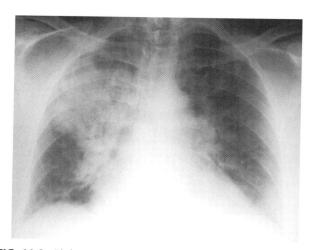

FIG. 11-8. Right upper lobe edema due to acute myocardial infarction with papillary muscle rupture, prolapse of the posterior leaflet of the mitral valve, and acute mitral regurgitation. Note cardiomegaly.

the radiograph becomes abnormal at the same time that symptoms appear. However, it is important to recognize that hydrostatic edema may be visible on chest radiographs before the symptoms develop (clinical lag) or after pulmonary venous pressure has returned to normal (radiographic lag).

Because hydrostatic edema is relatively low in protein, it may show rapid clearing with improvement in patient status. Similarly, a gravitational shift in the distribution of edema fluid may occur within minutes to hours of a change in patient position. Air-space edema reacts more slowly than interstitial edema to changes in patient status.

Although a progression of edema from an interstitial to an air-space pattern may be seen with worsening, this is not always the case. Many patients show air-space edema as the initial finding. Similarly, in patients with air-space edema, the edema does not typically assume an interstitial appearance as it clears.

INCREASED PERMEABILITY EDEMA WITH DIFFUSE ALVEOLAR DAMAGE: ACUTE RESPIRATORY DISTRESS SYNDROME

Permeability edema is a manifestation of capillary endothelial injury with resultant loss of fluid and protein into the lung interstitium. It results in a high-protein edema and, therefore, is slow to clear. It often is associated with respiratory epithelial injury and DAD. This combination results in ARDS.

ARDS is characterized by diffuse lung injury with progressive dyspnea and hypoxemia over a period of hours to days. Specific criteria for the diagnosis of ARDS include the following:

1. Acute onset
2. Hypoxemia despite high inspired oxygen concentration: (PaO_2/FIO_2 200 mmHg or less)
3. Characteristic bilateral radiographic abnormalities
4. Normal pulmonary artery wedge pressure
5. Absence of elevated left atrial pressure

ARDS can be related to a variety of pathologic processes, including the following:

1. Infection (e.g., pneumonia and sepsis)
2. Inhalation or aspiration of toxic or irritating substances
3. Trauma with lung or extrathoracic injury

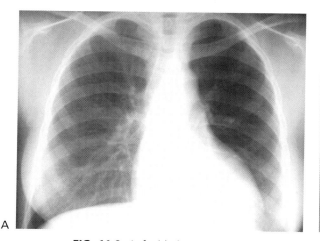
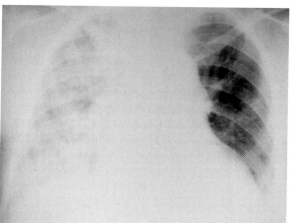

A

B

FIG. 11-9. Left-sided Swyer-James syndrome with predominant right-sided pulmonary edema. **A.** Baseline chest radiograph shows a hyperlucent and hypovascular left upper lobe. This appearance is typical of Swyer-James syndrome. **B.** Subsequently, congestive heart failure with cardiomegaly is associated with pulmonary edema. The edema spares the left upper lobe.

4. Hemodynamic abnormalities (e.g., shock, high altitude, anaphylaxis)
5. Hematologic disorders (e.g., disseminated intravascular coagulation, transfusion reaction)
6. Embolic disease (e.g., fat embolism, amniotic fluid embolism)
7. Drugs, either therapeutic or nontherapeutic
8. Metabolic disorders (e.g., pancreatitis, ketoacidosis)
9. Neurologic disease (e.g., head injury, stroke).

An idiopathic form of ARDS is termed acute interstitial pneumonia (AIP). AIP is discussed in Chapter 13. Most simply, the mechanism of lung injury in ARDS may be considered to be *direct,* in which the lungs themselves are injured (e.g., pneumonia, aspiration, and inhalational injury) or *indirect,* in which extrapulmonary abnormalities (e.g., sepsis, shock, pancreatitis) lead to lung injury (Table 11-3).

The Stages of Acute Respiratory Distress Syndrome

ARDS is considered to occur in stages, within the time frame of hours, days, weeks, and months (Table 11-4), which have close pathologic and radiographic correlates.

Pathologic Abnormalities

Pathologic abnormalities in ARDS are similar regardless of its cause. The histologic abnormalities occurring in ARDS are usually referred to as diffuse alveolar damage.

Hours. Within hours of the precipitating insult, endothelial cell edema, widening of intracellular junctions, congestion of capillaries, and limited interstitial pulmonary edema and hemorrhage are present. These manifestations represent the early exudative (injury) stage of ARDS.

Days. The period from a day to a week after the initial insult is characterized by progressive capillary endothelial injury, necrosis of alveolar lining cells (type I pneumocytes), proteinaceous interstitial and alveolar edema, and hemorrhage. Hyaline membranes form within the alveoli. This represents the late exudative (injury) stage.

Weeks. The proliferative (reparative) stage usually occurs from 1 week to 1 month following the onset of ARDS. It is characterized by proliferation of type II pneumocytes, which reline the denuded alveolar walls, organization of the alveolar exudates, fibroblast proliferation within the alveolar walls and interstitium, and deposition of collagen.

TABLE 11-3. DIRECT AND INDIRECT CAUSES OF ACUTE RESPIRATORY DISTRESS SYNDROME

Direct injury
Pneumonia (including virus, bacteria, mycoplasma, fungus, tuberculosis, *Pneumocystis jiroveci* [*P. carinii*] pneumonia, rickettsia)
Miliary tuberculosis or other disseminated infections
Inhalation (smoke, toxic gases, oxygen in high concentration)
Aspiration (gastric acid, ingested substances, drowning, chemicals, blood)
Thoracic trauma with contusion or crush injury
Thoracic radiation
Cardiopulmonary bypass
Fat embolism
Air embolism
Amniotic fluid embolism
Reexpansion or reperfusion edema
Sickle cell crisis
Acute interstitial pneumonia
Usual interstitial pneumonia with acute exacerbation

Indirect injury
Sepsis (particularly gram negative organisms)
Shock
Toxic shock syndrome
Disseminated intravascular coagulation
Extrathoracic trauma
Burns
Neurogenic edema
Drugs
Anaphylaxis
Transfusion reactions
Leukoagglutinin reactions
Diabetic ketoacidosis
Pancreatitis
Uremia
High altitude

Months. In many patients, these abnormalities resolve, and little respiratory disability results. In patients with more severe lung injury, interstitial fibrosis develops. This is termed the *fibrotic stage* of ARDS.

Radiographic Abnormalities

Hours. Radiographs typically are normal for the first 12 to 24 hours after the acute injury, despite the presence of dyspnea (Fig. 11-10A). This latent period is suggestive of ARDS (Table 11-4).

Days. Radiographs typically become abnormal within 24 hours of the inciting insult and the development of symptoms. Radiographs show bilateral patchy areas of air-space consolidation; these tend to have a more peripheral distribution than those seen in patients with hydrostatic edema (see Fig. 11-10B and C). They increase over time and eventually become confluent (see Fig. 11-10D and E). Dependent atelectasis often develops. Air bronchograms are more common

TABLE 11-4. THE STAGES OF ACUTE RESPIRATORY DISTRESS SYNDROME

Time Frame	Stage	Pathologic Findings	Radiologic Findings
Hours	Early exudative (injury)	Endothelial edema, early edema	Normal
Days	Late exudative (injury)	Progressive endothelial injury, necrosis of alveolar lining cells, progressive alveolar edema and hemorrhage	Patchy consolidation, often peripheral, progressive confluence, dependent atelectasis
Weeks	Proliferative (reparative)	Proliferation of alveolar lining cells, organization of alveolar exudates, fibroblast proliferation in alveolar walls	Slow resolution of consolidation, development of reticular opacities
Months	Fibrosis	Depending on the degree of injury, resolution or fibrosis	Persistence of reticular opacities and honeycombing, often anterior

than with hydrostatic edema. Interstitial abnormalities may be present, but Kerley's lines are distinctly uncommon. Pleural effusion is much less common and smaller than in patients with hydrostatic edema.

Because of the more severe lung injury occurring with ARDS and the presence of proteinaceous edema fluid, hyaline membranes, and hemorrhage, radiographic abnormalities clear much more slowly with ARDS than with hydrostatic edema. Radiographic improvement, with increased lung volumes and decrease in lung opacity, may occur within the first week, but this often reflects positive pressure ventilation rather than improvement in lung abnormalities.

Mechanical ventilation (see Fig. 11-10D) usually is required to maintain oxygenation. High ventilator pressures often are necessary for ventilation in patients with ARDS,

and barotrauma with pneumothorax and pneumomediastinum often occurs during this stage.

On HRCT, pulmonary edema occurring secondary to ARDS generally is associated with ground-glass opacity or consolidation, with predominance in dependent lung regions (see Fig. 11-10C). Opacities can be diffuse or patchy. Interlobular septal thickening is less commonly seen than in hydrostatic edema. Depending on the etiology of the edema, opacities may predominate in the peripheral and subpleural regions, or can spare the lung periphery. Unilateral or bilateral pleural effusions may be seen, but they typically are small.

Differences may be seen in the CT appearances of patients with ARDS due to pulmonary disease (e.g., pneumonia) and those with ARDS resulting from extrapulmonary

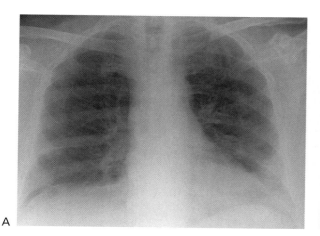
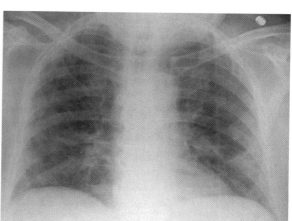

FIG. 11-10. Acute respiratory distress syndrome (ARDS) associated with sepsis. **A.** The initial radiograph is normal despite the presence of dyspnea. **B.** The next day, patchy opacities are visible peripherally, with a predominance at the lung bases. *(Figure continues.)*

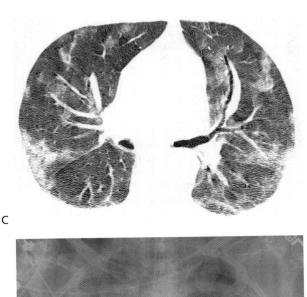

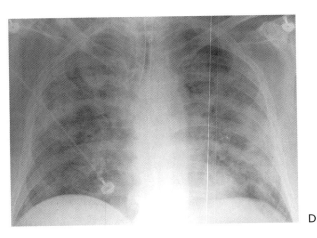

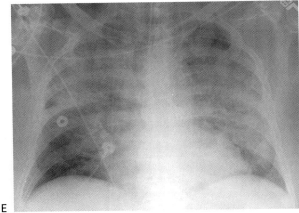

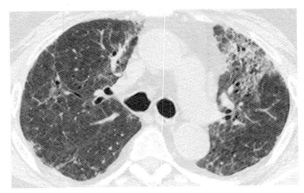

FIG. 11-10. *(Continued.)* **C.** HRCT obtained at the same time as the image shown in **B** shows patchy peripheral areas of consolidation and ground-glass opacity. These are nonspecific but typical of early ARDS. **D.** Twelve hours after the image shown in **B** was obtained, there has been progressive consolidation, with a peripheral predominance. An endotracheal tube has been placed for mechanical ventilation. **E.** Three days after the image shown in **D** was obtained, there has been progressive confluent consolidation, and air bronchograms are visible.

causes (e.g., sepsis). In patients with ARDS due to pulmonary disease, consolidation and ground-glass opacity are equally prevalent, and lung abnormalities often are asymmetric, reflecting the presence of the predisposing lung disease. In patients with an extrathoracic cause of ARDS, ground-glass opacity is predominant, and symmetric lung involvement is more typical (see Fig. 11-10C).

The CT findings in patients with pulmonary fat embolism syndrome, a cause of ARDS, include diffuse ground-glass opacity, focal areas of consolidation or ground-glass opacity, or nodules. Focal abnormalities predominate in the upper lobes. Gravity-dependent opacities predominate in the lower lobes.

Weeks. After 1 week, consolidation may begin to resolve slowly, being replaced by reticular opacities, or may assume a more patchy appearance. Progression of consolidation after 1 week may indicate superimposed pneumonia. Over time, consolidation clears in patients with ARDS, but ground-glass opacity and findings of lung fibrosis may persist.

Months. In patients with pulmonary fibrosis resulting from ARDS, chest films show a persisting reticular pattern or findings of honeycombing. Reticulation and honeycombing may be seen on HRCT, and tend to have a striking anterior distribution (Fig. 11-11). This unusual distribution probably reflects the fact that patients with ARDS typically develop posterior lung atelectasis and consolidation during the

FIG. 11-11. Anterior lung fibrosis in a patient recovering from ARDS. There is asymmetric reticulation with traction bronchiectasis and mild honeycombing. The posterior lung also is abnormal, but to a lesser degree.

exudative stage of disease; it is thought that this consolidation protects the posterior lung regions from the adverse effects of mechanical ventilation, including high ventilatory pressures and high oxygen tension.

PERMEABILITY EDEMA WITHOUT DIFFUSE ALVEOLAR DAMAGE

Permeability pulmonary edema may occur without accompanying DAD in patients with drug reactions, interleukin-2 treatment, transfusion reaction, or Hantavirus pulmonary syndrome, or as a result of a mild insult of a type usually resulting in ARDS, such as air embolism or toxic shock syndrome. It has been suggested that the absence of a pulmonary epithelial injury in such patients reduces the extent of alveolar edema.

In patients with permeability pulmonary edema occur-

ring in the absence of DAD, radiographic abnormalities typically resemble hydrostatic edema, with interlobular septal thickening being a predominant feature in many cases (Fig. 11-12). Edema may clear rapidly, because of the absence of epithelial injury.

MIXED EDEMA

Mixed permeability and hydrostatic edema may be seen in diseases resulting in increased intravascular pressure and capillary endothelial injury. A mixed etiology is thought to exist in patients with neurogenic pulmonary edema, reexpansion edema, high-altitude pulmonary edema, reexpansion or reperfusion edema, edema associated with tocolytic therapy, posttransplantation edema, postpneumonectomy or post–volume reduction edema, and edema related to air embolism; in some drug reactions (Fig. 11-13); and in patients with ARDS who are overhydrated or develop renal

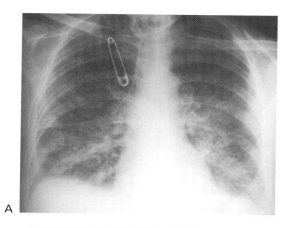

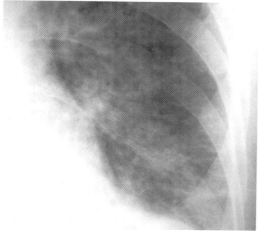

FIG. 11-12. Acute drug reaction (to bleomycin) showing permeability pulmonary edema. **A.** Chest radiograph shows increased reticular opacities at the lung bases with Kerley's lines. Although this appearance resembles hydrostatic edema, the heart size is normal. **B.** Coned-down view of the left base shows Kerley's B lines.

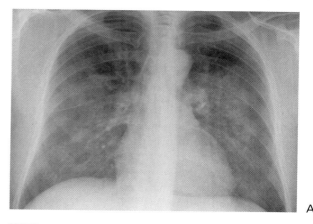

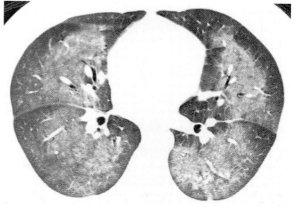

FIG. 11-13. Mixed permeability and hydrostatic pulmonary edema in a patient with cocaine abuse. Transient hypertension and capillary leak are thought to be responsible. **A.** Chest radiograph shows a perihilar "batwing" appearance of pulmonary edema. **B.** HRCT shows perihilar ground-glass opacity, with sparing of the lung periphery. This cleared over a period of a few days.

or heart failure. As would be expected, the radiographic appearances of these different types of edema are variable.

DISTINGUISHING THE TYPES OF EDEMA

Although it is sometimes impossible to distinguish among these types of edema, attention to specific findings allows more than two thirds of cases to be classified correctly.

In hydrostatic edema, findings of cardiomegaly and vascular congestion often are valuable in making the diagnosis. Radiographic findings of edema often appear soon after the inciting incident and may change rapidly. The presence of interstitial edema with Kerley's lines suggests hydrostatic edema, although they may be seen in patients with permeability edema without DAD and in mixed edema. Pleural effusion is common with hydrostatic edema and may be large.

In patients with ARDS, radiographic abnormalities often are delayed 24 hours after the onset of symptoms, and radiographic abnormalities change slowly. Air bronchograms are more typical of ARDS and Kerley's lines are unusual. Pleural effusions are uncommon and usually small.

SPECIFIC CAUSES OF PULMONARY EDEMA

Neurogenic Pulmonary Edema

Pulmonary edema developing in patients with head trauma, intracranial hemorrhage, increased intracranial pressure, seizures, or other acute neurologic conditions most likely occurs because of both hydrostatic mechanisms and increased permeability (i.e., mixed edema). Sympathetic discharge resulting from central nervous system injury results in systemic vasoconstriction, increased systemic blood pressure, and acute left heart failure. The edema fluid may be high in protein, indicating increased permeability. Edema may appear very rapidly, within minutes of the responsible episode (i.e., flash pulmonary edema). The appearance is usually that of air-space edema (Fig. 11-14). Clearing occurs within 1 or 2 days.

Reexpansion Pulmonary Edema

Rapid reexpansion of lung after being collapsed for more than 2 or 3 days may result in focal edema of the reexpanded lung. It typically occurs within 2 to 4 hours of reexpansion, but may progress for 1 or 2 days. It typically appears as air-space edema.

Two mechanisms probably are responsible. First, following collapse, lung perfusion decreases, lung becomes hypoxemic, surfactant production decreases, and lung become less compliant. Because of this, a more negative intrapleural pressure is required (during thoracentesis or chest tube

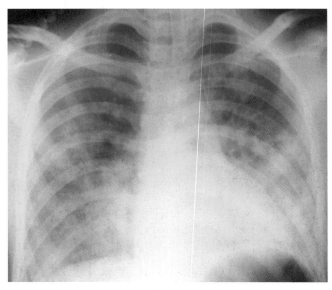

FIG. 11-14. Neurogenic pulmonary edema following head trauma. Bilateral consolidation is visible.

drainage) to achieve lung reexpansion. This may contribute to development of edema by hydrostatic mechanisms. Secondly, prolonged hypoxemia with release of free radicals may result in capillary endothelial injury, with increased permeability edema developing with reperfusion. A transient decrease in pulmonary lymphatic or venous return has also been suggested as a contributing mechanism. Edema usually resolves in less than 1 week.

Although the edema usually is localized to the part of lung that was previously collapsed, it sometimes may be seen in other lobes or in the opposite lung. This occurrence may be due to the release of free radicals and vasoactive substances into the blood stream following reperfusion of hypoxemic lung. Reexpansion pulmonary edema usually appears as consolidation or ground-glass opacity (Figs. 11-15 and 11-16).

Reexpansion edema usually is not problematic, but in some cases, it may result in a worsening of the patient's symptoms even though lung compression due to the pleural air or fluid collection has been alleviated. In patients with large pleural collections, slow removal over a period of days may be appropriate, reducing the chance that reexpansion edema will occur.

High-altitude Pulmonary Edema

Pulmonary edema may develop after rapid ascent to high altitude, usually in excess of 10,000 feet. Edema usually develops between 12 hours and 3 days after ascent; most cases occur in the first day. Less commonly, it develops in people with prolonged residence at high altitude.

Reduction in the partial pressure of oxygen in inspired air

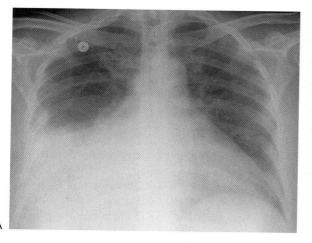

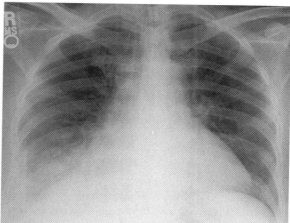

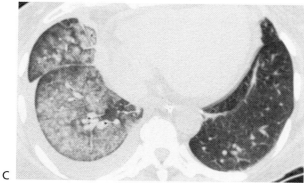

FIG. 11-15. Reexpansion pulmonary edema following thoracentesis. **A.** A patient with cardiomegaly shows a right-sided pleural effusion. **B.** Radiograph following thoracentesis shows a small residual effusion and increased opacity in the right lower lobe due to reexpansion edema. **C.** HRCT shows a small residual right sided effusion and ground-glass opacity involving right middle and lower lobes. The opacities show a centrilobular predominance.

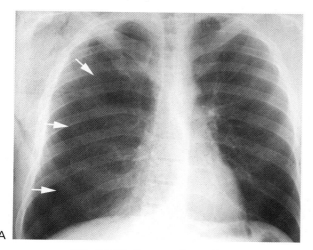

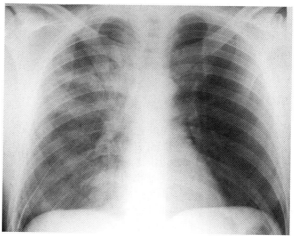

FIG. 11-16. Reexpansion pulmonary edema following evacuation of pneumothorax. **A.** Chest radiograph following trauma shows a large right pneumothorax *(arrows)* and subcutaneous emphysema. **B.** Following rapid lung reexpansion using a chest tube, patchy consolidation is visible in the right lung.

is responsible for this type of edema. In susceptible people, it results in patchy spasm of some small pulmonary arteries, resulting in high pressure in those arterial branches that remain patent. This high pressure not only results in hydrostatic edema, but also injures the capillary endothelium, leading to increased permeability. Patchy air-space edema typically is seen. Administration of oxygen or a return to sea level results in resolution within 1 or 2 days.

ATELECTASIS

Atelectasis often develops in patients in the ICU because of depressed sensorium, pain, endotracheal intubation, mechanical ventilation, and the supine position. Particularly in postsurgical patients, areas of basal atelectasis are common and typically appear in the first 24 to 48 hours. Obstruction of small peripheral airways by retained secretions is the usual cause.

A localized area of consolidation is the most common radiographic finding with atelectasis, and its radiographic appearance is impossible to distinguish from pneumonia or aspiration unless associated findings of volume loss are visible. On AP portable radiographs, signs of lower lobe volume loss include depression of the hilum, a vertical orientation of the main bronchus, crowding of segmental lower lobe bronchi, and a visible and vertically oriented major fissure. Left lower lobe atelectasis is almost universal in patients having open heart surgery with cold cardioplegia.

Because the mucous plugging resulting in atelectasis in these patients usually is peripheral and involves small bronchi, air bronchograms often are visible within collapsed lung. Small pleural effusions can be present.

Areas of consolidation resulting from atelectasis may change rapidly in appearance, a finding that helps to distinguish them from pneumonia. Acute opacification of a hemithorax may represent atelectasis and drowned lung; little volume loss may be seen in this situation.

PNEUMONIA

Pneumonias occur in 10% to 20% of patients in the ICU. They are associated with high mortality because these patients often are debilitated; hospital-acquired infections are notoriously antibiotic-resistant and difficult to treat; and normal mechanisms of mucociliary clearance are suppressed or made ineffective by oxygen therapy and mechanical ventilation. Gram-negative organisms such as *Pseudomonas* and *Klebsiella* species often are responsible.

Although the diagnosis of pneumonia usually is based on the association of fever, culture of pathogenic organisms from the sputum, and an abnormal chest radiograph, a patient in the ICU may have each of these findings without having pneumonia. Endotracheal intubation often results

in tracheal colonization by pathogenic bacteria without producing pneumonia. Many such patients will also have some sort of pulmonary abnormality on chest radiographs, usually representing atelectasis, aspiration, or pulmonary edema. A misdiagnosis of pneumonia is common, and bacteriologic confirmation of pneumonia may not be obtained.

Radiographically, pneumonias may appear as localized or diffuse areas of air-space consolidation, often patchy and inhomogeneous. Depending on the organism responsible and the patient's immunocompetence, pneumonias generally appear and progress over a few days. Uncommonly, pneumonia shows a dramatic worsening in consolidation over a matter of hours; this occurrence is more typical of atelectasis, pulmonary edema, aspiration, or hemorrhage. Within 1 or 2 days of appropriate antibiotic treatment, a pneumonic consolidation should stabilize and begin to clear. Further, progression suggests superinfection with a

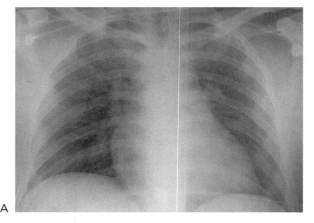

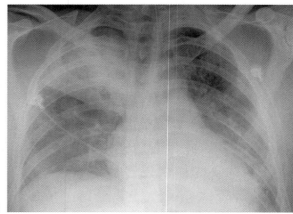

FIG. 11-17. Acute aspiration. **A.** Baseline radiograph appears normal. **B.** Several hours later, following an acute aspiration, there has been rapid appearance of right upper lobe and left lower lobe consolidation, with lesser consolidation at the right base. The distribution of consolidation varies with the patient position at the time of aspiration.

second organism, a mixed infection, or a superimposed second process such as pulmonary edema.

ASPIRATION

Aspiration of bland substances such as water, blood, or neutralized gastric contents elicits little inflammatory response and does not result in severe lung disease unless the volume of aspirated fluid is large. Radiographs may show areas of consolidation in dependent portions of lung resulting from the aspirated substance, but these areas rapidly clear with ventilatory therapy or coughing.

Aspiration of irritating substances, particularly acid gastric contents with a pH less than 2.5, causes marked inflammation of pulmonary parenchyma and results in pulmonary edema. Patients in the ICU are predisposed to aspiration of gastric contents because of nasogastric or endotracheal intubation, diminished level of consciousness, and a supine position. Inflation of the cuff of the endotracheal tube does not entirely prevent aspiration.

In general, within several hours of aspiration of acid material, the patient experiences fever, dyspnea, and hypoxemia. Radiographs usually show rapidly appearing and progressing consolidation, homogeneous or patchy, favoring dependent areas of lung (Fig. 11-17). HRCT may show ground-glass opacity (often acute) or consolidation (Fig. 11-18). Within the next few days, clinical improvement and at least some clearing of consolidation should occur. If the patient worsens and the radiograph fails to show clearing or worsens, superimposed infection or ARDS must be suspected. Pleural effusion is not generally associated with aspiration unless pneumonia supervenes (see Fig. 11-18B).

PULMONARY EMBOLISM

Pulmonary embolism may be considered in the differential diagnosis of early ARDS. Both conditions are characterized by progressive respiratory insufficiency in the face of a normal or slightly abnormal radiograph. However, the diffuse consolidation typically occurring with ARDS rarely is seen in patients with pulmonary embolism. Rather, pulmonary embolism usually produces more localized areas of consolidation, and pleural effusion is common. The diagnosis of pulmonary embolism in ICU patients primarily rests with spiral CT.

PULMONARY HEMORRHAGE

Pulmonary parenchymal hemorrhage can occur in anticoagulated patients, patients with a bleeding diathesis, patients with pulmonary vasculitis, and patients with Goodpasture's syndrome, among others. Typically, areas of consolidation appear rapidly, are bilateral, and are associated with a drop in hematocrit. Resolution may be slow. Aspiration of blood from the trachea resulting from traumatic intubation can produce a similar appearance. Hemoptysis need not be present in patients with significant pulmonary hemorrhage. Pulmonary hemorrhage syndromes are discussed in Chapter 19.

PLEURAL EFFUSION

Pleural effusion may be extremely difficult—if not impossible—to distinguish from basal areas of consolidation on portable supine or semierect radiographs. Costophrenic

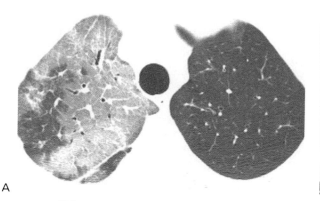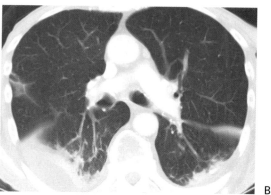

A   B

FIG. 11-18. Aspiration. **A.** HRCT in a patient with acute aspiration shows ground-glass opacity in the right upper lobe. **B.** Aspiration pneumonias in a different patient. Consolidation involves dependent lung regions. Small pleural effusions thickening the fissures suggest superimposed infection.

angle blunting and a meniscus often are absent, and poor definition of the ipsilateral hemidiaphragm or homogeneous opacity in the inferior hemithorax may be the only findings visible. The presence of air bronchograms indicates that at least some consolidation is present but does not rule out the presence of fluid; in fact, the lung consolidation and air bronchograms may reflect atelectasis secondary to effusion.

Unless diagnostic thoracentesis is being considered, small pleural fluid collections rarely are significant in patients in the ICU, and the differentiation of fluid and consolidation may not be necessary. If a definite diagnosis of effusion is desired in a bedridden patient, decubitus films can be taken by rolling the patient onto a hard surface (e.g., a resuscitation board). If decubitus films are unobtainable, taking two films, one supine and one erect, may allow a diagnosis of effusion to be made.

In patients in the ICU, the presence or absence of pleural effusion usually does not help in diagnosing the cause of coexisting lung disease. Although pleural effusion is uncommonly associated with ARDS, aspiration, and hemorrhage, patients with these diseases may have pleural effusion resulting from another process, such as congestive heart failure, recent surgery, or abdominal disease.

Large pleural effusions, significantly reducing ventilation and pulmonary function usually are treated by thoracentesis or pleural drainage tubes.

MECHANICAL VENTILATION AND PULMONARY BAROTRAUMA

Mechanical ventilators commonly are used in the ICU to treat ventilatory or respiratory failure. High peak ventilator pressure and continuous positive airway pressure usually are employed in the treatment of hypoxemia resulting from ARDS, edema, and other respiratory diseases.

Ventilator therapy may alter the appearance of lung disease. Increasing ventilator pressures result in increased lung volume and produce an apparent clearing of lung consolidation, whereas decreasing pressure produces a decrease in lung volume and an apparent worsening of disease. Thus, knowledge of changes in ventilator settings is helpful in allowing the correct interpretation of radiographs.

Barotrauma

The use of mechanical ventilators and high ventilatory pressures can result in barotrauma with alveolar rupture and subsequent development of pneumomediastinum, subcutaneous emphysema, pneumothorax, and air within the retroperitoneum or free within the abdominal cavity. Prompt recognition of extra-alveolar air is important, because pneumothorax may be life-threatening in patients with this complication.

In a small minority of patients, extra-alveolar air first

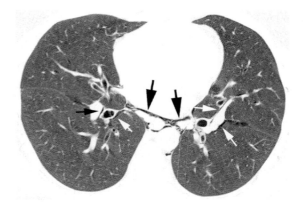

FIG. 11-19. Interstitial emphysema and pneumomediastinum. In a postoperative patient, streaks of air *(small arrows)* are seen surrounding the central bronchi and vessels. This appearance represents interstitial emphysema. Although this is thought to be the first manifestation of barotrauma, it is not commonly seen in adults. Interstitial emphysema leads directly to pneumomediastinum. In this patient mediastinal air is seen surrounding the esophagus and aorta *(large arrows)*.

may be recognized in the pulmonary interstitial space as collections of perivascular air *(interstitial emphysema;* Fig. 11-19) or as irregular bubbles within areas of consolidation. Subpleural blebs may develop and threaten impending pneumothorax due to their rupture. Interstitial emphysema visible on plain radiographs is very uncommon in adults.

From the interstitial space, air dissects centrally to produce pneumomediastinum (Fig. 11-20; see also Fig. 11-19).

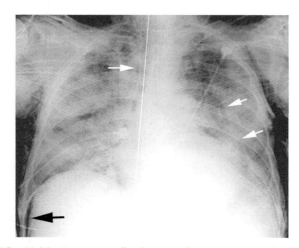

FIG. 11-20. Pneumomediastinum, subcutaneous emphysema, and retroperitoneal air. In a patient with barotrauma, pneumomediastinum *(white arrows)* is visible outlining the tracheal wall and displacing the mediastinal pleura laterally. The presence of subcutaneous emphysema, seen outlining the pectoralis major muscles, is presumptive evidence of pneumomediastinum in the absence of penetrating trauma or chest tube placement. A crescent of air lateral to the liver *(black arrow)* is retroperitoneal. Free air in the abdomen is seen above the liver rather than lateral to it.

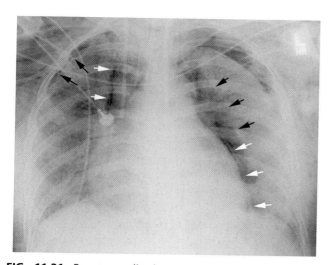

FIG. 11-21. Pneumomediastinum, subcutaneous emphysema, and pneumothorax. In a patient with barotrauma, pneumomediastinum *(white arrows)* is visible, outlining and displacing the mediastinal pleura laterally. Bilateral pneumothorax is present *(black arrows)*. Little lung collapse had occurred despite the presence of pneumothorax (likely under tension because of mechanical ventilation). This is due to underlying lung consolidation. Subcutaneous emphysema is present.

This may be visible a lucency adjacent to the mediastinal structures or outlining specific mediastinal structures, such as the aorta or trachea. Air outlining the tracheal wall is common with pneumomediastinum.

Pneumopericardium may occur because of interstitial air dissecting along pulmonary vessels. This finding is relatively common in infants but is uncommon in adults, except following cardiac surgery or pericardial intervention.

In the absence of penetrating trauma or chest tube placement, the presence of subcutaneous emphysema is evidence that pneumomediastinum is present, even if it is not visible (see Fig. 11-20).

Pneumothorax may result from rupture of mediastinal air into the pleural space, but the opposite is not true—pneumothorax does not lead to pneumomediastinum under normal circumstances. In mechanically ventilated patients, pneumothorax should be considered to be under tension; this is commonly the case. With tension pneumothorax, the diaphragm often is depressed, and the mediastinum may be displaced to the opposite side. However, because of underlying lung disease (i.e., consolidation), significant lung collapse on the side of the pneumothorax may not occur even in the presence of tension (Fig. 11-21). In supine patients, pneumothorax may be seen in atypical

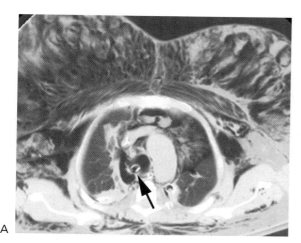

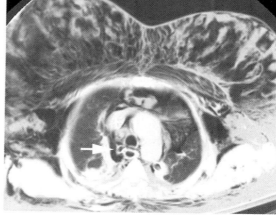

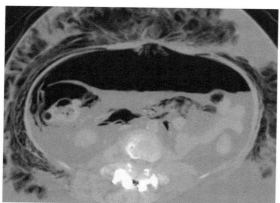

FIG. 11-22. Endotracheal tube penetrating the trachea, resulting in pneumomediastinum, pneumothorax, extensive subcutaneous emphysema, and pneumoperitoneum. **A** and **B.** The endotracheal tube *(arrows)* penetrates the trachea, with its tip free within the mediastinum *(arrow in* **B***).* Extensive extra-alveolar air is present. **C.** Both retroperitoneal and intraperitoneal air are present.

locations, either medial to the lungs or at the lung base (see Chapter 26). Care must be taken to distinguish skin folds from pneumothorax.

Air dissecting inferiorly from the mediastinum can reach the retroperitoneum (Fig. 11-22; see also Fig. 11-20) and may rupture into the peritoneal space, producing free abdominal air (see Fig. 11-22C). Retroperitoneal air is seen lateral to the liver; free air is seen above it. Almost all patients with ventilator-related abdominal air will also have a visible pneumomediastinum.

TUBES AND LINES AND THEIR COMPLICATIONS

The first step in interpreting a radiograph of a patient in the ICU is an evaluation of indwelling catheters and tubes. Misplaced catheters can result in serious complications. Tube or catheter misplacement occurs in about 10% of cases.

Endotracheal Tubes

Mechanical ventilators require the use of an endotracheal tube. The tube's tip should be positioned several centimeters above the tracheal carina. The tracheal carina often is visible; if it is not visible, it can be located by looking for the main bronchi. If it still is not visible, it may be assumed to be near the level of the undersurface of the aortic arch (Fig. 11-23) or near the level of the T4-5 vertebral bodies.

The ideal position for an endotracheal tube depends on the degree of extension or flexion of the patient's neck. An endotracheal tube's tip may descend as much as 3 cm when the neck is flexed from a neutral position and may ascend as much as 5 cm with neck extension. With the patient's neck in a neutral position, the tube's tip should lie approximately 4 to 7 cm above the carina. If the neck is extended, the tip should be higher (7 to 9 cm above the carina) to allow for possible downward migration. If the neck is flexed, the reverse is true, and the tip should be lower (2 to 4 cm above the carina).

Flexion and extension of the neck can be judged by the position of the patient's mandible on the chest radiograph. In a neutral position, the mandible overlies the lower cervical spine. If the mandible is higher, the neck is extended; if it is lower, the neck is flexed. It is simplest to remember that the tube tip moves in the same direction as the chin on flexion or extension of the neck.

Placing an endotracheal tube too low usually results in its entering the right main bronchus (Fig. 11-24A). This position can produce right lung overinflation, alveolar rupture and pneumothorax, or right upper lobe or left lung collapse because of lack of ventilation of these areas. Intubation of the left main bronchus is less common because of its more horizontal orientation (see Fig. 11-24B).

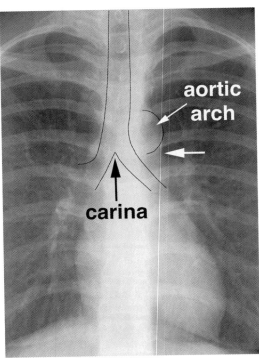

FIG. 11-23. Relation of the carina to the aortic arch. If the carina is not clearly visible, it is located near the level of the undersurface of the rounded opacity of the aortic arch (*white arrow*).

A tube placed too high may lodge in the hypopharynx or larynx (Fig. 11-25), resulting in poor ventilation or gastric distention. If the tube tip or cuff lies at the level of the vocal cords, ulceration and scarring may result, leading to stricture.

Esophageal intubation may be recognized by an unusual tube course, with the tube not overlying the tracheal air column or because of gastric distention (Fig. 11-26). A lateral view is very helpful in diagnosis; although the trachea and esophagus overlap on the frontal projection, they can be easily distinguished on the lateral view.

Overinflation of the tube cuff or balloon (see Fig. 11-25) results in ulceration of the tracheal wall, with perforation or scarring and stricture as complications. Overinflation may be recognized if there is a bulge in the tracheal air column at the site of the balloon, several centimeters above the tube tip. Tracheal stenosis or tracheal malacia may occur as a late complication of endotracheal intubation. These complications have been minimized by the use of low-pressure balloons, but they still occur.

Rarely, tracheal perforation occurs with intubation (see Fig. 11-22). The endotracheal tube may have an abnormal course, or pneumomediastinum may be present.

Tracheostomy Tubes

A tracheostomy tube is placed if a patient requires chronic mechanical ventilation or for upper airway obstruction. The

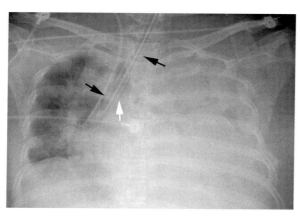

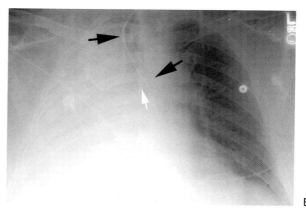

FIG. 11-24. Intubation of a main bronchus. **A.** Right main bronchus intubation. The endotracheal tube *(black arrows)* enters the right main bronchus. The tracheal carina is indicated by the white arrow. Left lung collapse has resulted. **B.** Left main bronchus intubation. The endotracheal tube *(black arrows)* extends into the proximal left main bronchus. This is less common than intubation of the right main bronchus. Right lung collapse has resulted. The *white arrow* indicates the location of the carina.

tube tip position relative to the carina is not critical, because this is determined by the location of the tracheostomy stoma. Tracheostomy tubes that are angled relative to the tracheal lumen may cause erosion of the tracheal wall, with perforation or subsequent tracheal stenosis, or may occasionally fall out. Tracheostomy balloons may be overinflated.

Central Venous Catheters

Central venous catheters used for measuring central venous pressure or for intravenous infusion of fluids often are placed by means of percutaneous puncture of the internal jugular or subclavian veins. Complications of subclavian puncture include laceration of the subclavian or carotid artery (Fig. 11-27); mediastinal hemorrhage (Fig. 11-28); or

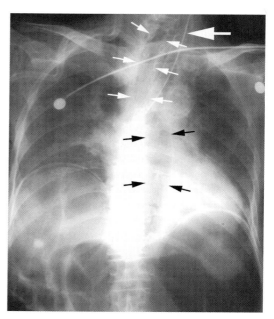

FIG. 11-25. Endotracheal tube located too high. The tube tip is just below the vocal cords *(large arrows)* at the level of C6. The tube balloon *(small arrows)* is overinflated and at the level of the piriform sinuses.

FIG. 11-26. Esophageal intubation. The endotracheal tube *(large white arrow)* does not overlie the shadow of the tracheal *(small white arrows)*. Below the level of the tube tip, the esophagus *(black arrows)* is dilated and air-filled. The stomach and bowel are dilated by air.

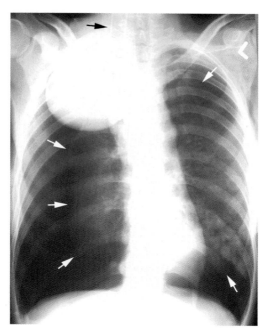

FIG. 11-27. Chest radiograph following attempted bilateral sub-clavian and internal jugular vein catheter placement. A catheter *(black arrow)* overlies the right neck. A large mass at the right apex represents an extrapleural hematoma due to laceration of the right carotid artery. Bilateral pneumothoraces *(white arrows)* also are present, with mediastinal shift to the left. The heart appears small, suggesting tension with decreased venous return. This patient subsequently died.

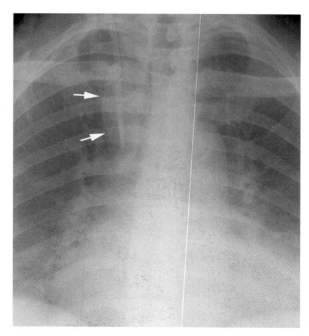

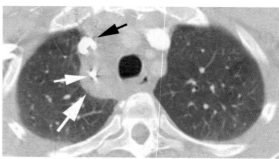

FIG. 11-28. Mediastinal hemorrhage following catheter placement. **A.** Chest radiograph shows a catheter overlying the superior vena cava. The mediastinum is widened *(arrows)*. Blood return from the catheter was poor. **B.** CT shows the catheter *(small white arrow)* to be extravascular and associated with mediastinal hematoma *(large white arrow)*. The catheter should be within the right brachiocephalic vein *(black arrow)*.

infusion of intravenous fluids into the mediastinum or pleural space (Fig. 11-29); pneumomediastinum; and pneu-mothorax (see Fig. 11-27). Pneumothorax is most common, occurring in more than 5% of patients (see Fig. 11-27). Because of these possible complications, a portable chest radiograph should be obtained after every attempted or suc-cessful subclavian or jugular puncture.

A catheter placed properly should be in the superior vena cava. Because many catheters have two or three lumens, each with a different orifice, the catheter tip should be as near to the azygos arch as possible. This position allows each orifice, which may be as much as 5 cm proximal to the tip, to be distal to the last venous valve (this valve is located at the junction of the internal jugular and subclavian veins, at the level of the inner aspect of the first rib).

It usually is not desirable to place a catheter in the right atrium; this may result in dysrhythmia or injection of undi-luted toxic drugs into the heart. If the chest radiograph shows the catheter tip to be at the level of the lower aspect of the bronchus intermedius, it generally is considered to be at the junction of the SVC and RA. A catheter below this level is in the RA. It should be kept in mind that the relative positions of the catheter and RA change with inspi-ratory level. A catheter in the SVC may appear to be in the RA on an expiratory radiograph. Catheters directed laterally

against the wall of the SVC are at risk for perforation. This occurs most often with catheters placed via the left subcla-vian vein or left internal jugular vein.

Catheters may inadvertently extend into smaller veins, increasing the risk of inaccurate pressure measurements, thrombosis, or perforation (Fig. 11-30). Such catheters show unusual courses or angulation. A catheter placed in a persistent left superior vena cava (Fig. 11-31) may mimic placement in a small vein.

Occasionally, a catheter may be placed in the subclavian artery rather than in the vein (Fig. 11-32). Its course usually appears abnormal. Because the artery is superior to the vein, it may be seen above the clavicle or overlying the aortic arch.

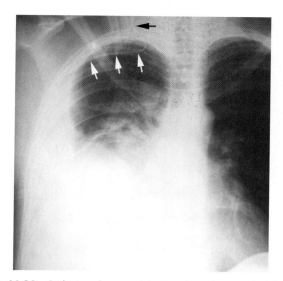

FIG. 11-29. Catheter placement in the pleural space. A right internal jugular catheter *(black arrow)* follows an unusual course and is directed laterally *(white arrows)* at a level above the clavicle (and the subclavian vein). This catheter is within the right pleural space. A large right pleural effusion is due to intravenous fluid infusion.

A catheter taking an unusual course may be free within the mediastinum or pleural space rather than within a vein, and fluids should be administered with care. A good return of blood through the catheter does not ensure proper positioning.

Improperly placed catheters sometimes can be sheared off at the needle tip and embolize to the heart or pulmonary arteries (Fig. 11-33). Perforation, infection, and thrombosis can result.

Improper technique may lead to air embolism, with air visible in the pulmonary artery.

Pulmonary Artery (Swan-Ganz) Catheters

Swan-Ganz catheters are double-lumen, balloon-tipped catheters allowing measurement of pulmonary arterial and wedge pressures when the balloon is inflated. Normally the tube tip should lie within a large central pulmonary artery; with inflation of the balloon, the tube tip migrates distally to a wedged position. If the catheter lies in a small (lobar or segmental) artery, it may remain wedged with the balloon uninflated, and thrombosis and pulmonary infarction or pulmonary artery aneurysm can result (Fig. 11-34). Care also must be taken that the balloon does not remain inflated between measurements; continued inflation also may result

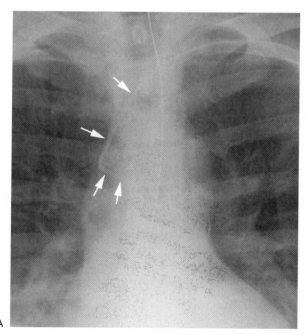
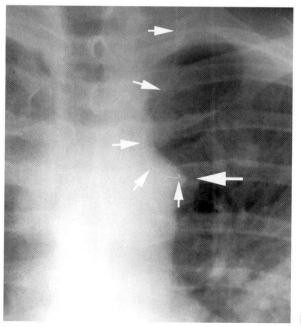

A

B

FIG. 11-30. Atypical catheter placements. **A.** Catheter extending into the azygos vein. A left venous catheter *(arrows)* shows sharp angulation at the level of the azygos arch. **B.** Catheter extending into the left superior intercostal vein. A left internal jugular venous catheter *(small arrows)* descends along the left mediastinum and is directed laterally at the level of the aortic arch. The close relation of the catheter to an "aortic nipple" *(large arrow)* indicates its position in the superior intercostal vein.

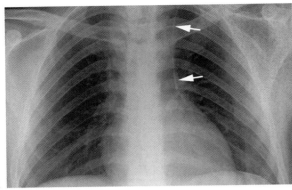
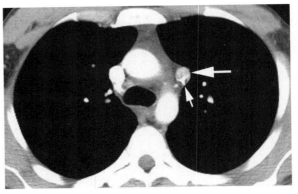

FIG. 11-31. Catheter placement in a persistent left superior vena cava. **A.** A left internal jugular venous catheter *(white arrows)* descends along the left mediastinum. This course is typical of a persistent left superior vena cava. However, this catheter position also may be extravascular or in a small mediastinal vein (e.g., internal mammary or left pericardiophrenic vein). **B.** CT shows the catheter *(small arrow)* to be within a persistent left superior vena cava *(large arrow)*.

in infarction. Coiling of the catheter within the heart should be avoided. Coiling can result in knotting or sudden peripheral migration of the catheter with wedging.

Transvenous Pacemakers

Transvenous pacemaker leads normally are positioned with the tip in the apex of the right ventricle, pointing to the left, anteriorly, and inferiorly. Placement of the tip into the coronary sinus usually results in a superior and posterior deviation of the pacemaker lead.

A bipolar pacemaker has a second lead, which normally is positioned in the right atrium, often with its tip directed laterally against the right atrial wall. In some circumstances, this lead is placed in other locations. The lead may be intentionally positioned in the coronary sinus.

Rarely, pacemaker leads perforate the coronary sinus or myocardium, resulting in pericardial tamponade or diaphragmatic pacing (with hiccoughs). If this occurs, the lead tip may be seen very close to the edge of the heart shadow or may project beyond it.

Pacemaker failure may result from poor lead position, fracture of the pacemaker lead usually near the pacemaker (this often is difficult to see), or failure of the pacemaker itself. Some patients play with their pacemaker device (so-called "twiddler's syndrome"), which may result in coiling

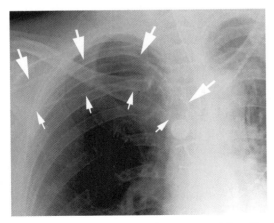

FIG. 11-32. Subclavian artery catheter. A peripherally placed right venous catheter *(small arrows)* is visible in the typical location of the subclavian vein, beneath and overlying the clavicle. A second catheter, placed using a subclavian approach *(large arrows)* is too high to be within the subclavian vein, and its tip is medially located, overlying the aortic arch rather than the superior vena cava.

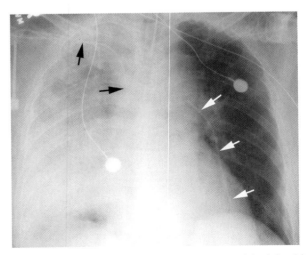

FIG. 11-33. Catheter embolization. A patient with right-sided pneumonia shows a right subclavian catheter *(white arrows)* in a normal position. A previously placed catheter *(black arrows)* was sheared off and has embolized to the left pulmonary artery.

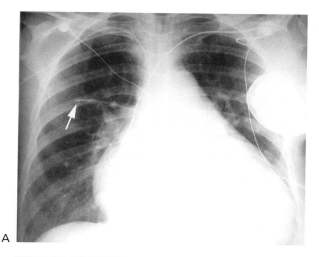

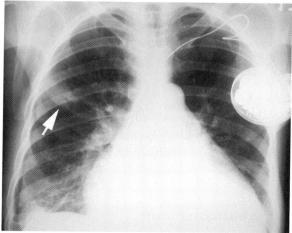

FIG. 11-34. Peripheral location of a Swan-Ganz catheter with infarction. **A.** A patient with cardiomegaly shows a peripherally located (segmental or subsegmental) Swan-Ganz catheter *(arrow)*. The catheter should overlie the large hilar vessels. **B.** Following withdrawal of the catheter 1 day later, a focal opacity representing a lung infarction is visible in the right lung *(arrow)*.

of the pacemaker wire around the pacemaker and retraction of the lead tip into the right atrium or vena cava.

Pleural Drainage Tubes

Pleural drainage tubes commonly are used to evacuate pneumothorax or pleural effusion. Ideally, tubes placed for pneumothorax should occupy the least dependent portion of the pleural space (anterosuperior in a bedridden patient). For treatment of pleural fluid, tubes should be placed within the dependent portion of the pleural space (posteroinferior).

If a tube functions poorly, it may be occluded or kinked, it may be positioned in the chest wall or with its side hole (marked by a discontinuity in the radiopaque tube marker) outside the thoracic cavity, or may be positioned in the

major fissure with the two adjacent lobes occluding the tube. A tube located within the major fissure is most easily recognized by comparing its position on the frontal and lateral radiographs, and localizing this to the plane of the fissure.

Rarely, the lung may be perforated during tube placement with the tube tip lying within lung parenchyma. Obviously, such tubes function poorly and lead to pneumothorax. CT may be needed to confirm this location.

Nasogastric Tubes

Nasogastric tubes or feeding tubes occasionally may be placed in the tracheobronchial tree (Figs. 11-35 and 11-36). This placement may result in perforation of the visceral pleural surface and pneumothorax (see Fig. 11-36),

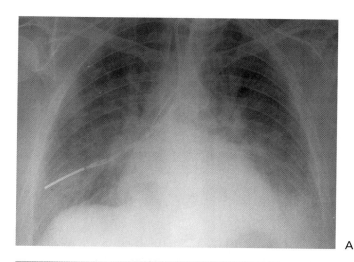

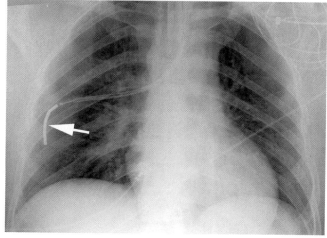

FIG. 11-35. Feeding tubes placed in the tracheobronchial tree. **A.** A tube is placed in the right lower lobe, and is oriented along the course of bronchi. **B.** In another patient, the tube follows the course of bronchi in the central lung, but curves in a manner inconsistent with an endobronchial location in the periphery *(arrow)*. This suggests perforation of the pleural surface and a location within the pleural space.

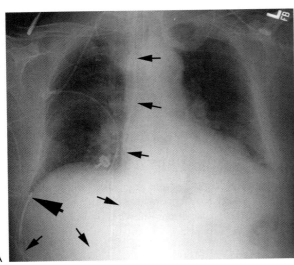

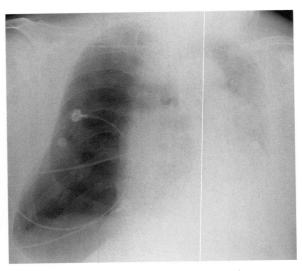

FIG. 11-36. Pleural feeding tube placement with pneumothorax. **A.** A feeding tube *(arrows)* overlies the tracheobronchial tree in a central location, but is positioned with its tip *(large arrow)* in the lateral costophrenic angle. **B.** Following removal of the tube, a tension pneumothorax is present. The mediastinum is displaced to the left, and the left lung is collapsed.

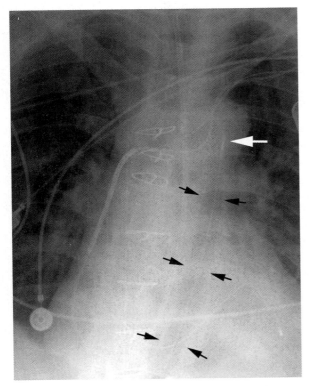

FIG. 11-37. Aortic balloon pulp. The balloon tip *(white arrow)* is radiopaque, and is properly positioned slightly below the superior aspect of the aortic arch. In this patient, the balloon *(black arrows)* was inflated at the time the radiograph was performed, and is visible as a long lucency overlying the descending aorta.

bronchial obstruction and atelectasis, or delivery of a tube feeding into the lung, which may result in severe pneumonia. Coiling of a nasogastric tube in the hypopharynx can contribute to aspiration. If the tube is coiled in the esophagus, gastric distention and aspiration may result.

Aortic Balloon Pump

A catheter-based, gas-filled intraaortic balloon pump may be used to improve peripheral blood flow in patients with left ventricular failure and low cardiac output. The long (nearly 30 cm), sausage-shaped balloon may be visible when inflated as a relative lucency within the descending aorta (Fig. 11-37). The catheter itself is difficult to see, although a small radiopaque line usually marks its tip. Ideally, the catheter tip is positioned just below the origin of the left subclavian artery, and therefore should overlie the aortic knob on the radiograph (see Fig. 11-37). If advanced too far, the catheter may occlude the left vertebral artery; if located too low, it is less effective, and its lower portion may partially obstruct the renal arteries.

SELECTED READING

Bartsch P. High altitude pulmonary edema. Respiration 1997; 64: 435–443.

Bernard GR, Artigas A, Brigham KL, et al. The American-European Consensus Conference on ARDS. Definitions, mechanisms, relevant outcomes, and clinical trial coordination. Am J Respir Crit Care Med 1994; 149:818–824.

Desai SR, Wells AU, Rubens MB, et al. Acute respiratory distress syndrome: CT abnormalities at long-term follow-up. Radiology 1999; 210:29–35.

Gluecker T, Capasso P, Schnyder P, et al. Clinical and radiologic features of pulmonary edema. Radiographics 1999; 19:1507–1531.

Goodman LR, Fumagalli R, Tagliabue P, et al. Adult respiratory distress syndrome due to pulmonary and extrapulmonary causes: CT, clinical, and functional correlations. Radiology 1999; 213: 545–552.

Hommeyer SH, Godwin JD, Takasugi JE. Computed tomography of air-space disease. Radiol Clin North Am 1991; 29: 1065–1084.

Ketai LH, Godwin JD. A new view of pulmonary edema and acute respiratory distress syndrome. J Thorac Imaging 1998; 13: 147–171.

Müller-Leisse C, Klosterhalfen B, Hauptmann S, et al. Computed tomography and histologic results in the early stages of endotoxin-injured pig lungs as a model for adult respiratory distress syndrome. Invest Radiol 1993; 28:39–45.

Murata K, Herman PG, Khan A, et al. Intralobular distribution of oleic acid–induced pulmonary edema in the pig: evaluation by high-resolution CT. Invest Radiol 1989; 24:647–653.

Owens CM, Evans TW, Keogh BF, Hansell DM. Computed tomography in established adult respiratory distress syndrome. Correlation with lung injury score. Chest 1994; 106:1815–1821.

Storto ML, Kee ST, Golden JA, Webb WR. Hydrostatic pulmonary edema: high-resolution CT findings. AJR Am J Roentgenol 1995; 165:817–820.

12

PULMONARY INFECTIONS

MICHAEL B. GOTWAY, WILLIAM G. BERGER, AND JESSICA W.T. LEUNG

Pulmonary infections are among the most common causes of morbidity and mortality worldwide and contribute substantially to annual medical expenditures in the United States. The various causes of pulmonary infection are numerous, and the clinical presentations of pulmonary infection are frequently nonspecific.

MECHANISMS

Microorganisms gain access to the respiratory system and cause infection in a variety of ways. The most common route of entry is inoculation via the tracheobronchial tree, usually by the inhalation of aerosolized respiratory droplets, less commonly by the aspiration of oropharyngeal secretions, and rarely by the direct extension of organisms into the respiratory system from adjacent sources, such as infected mediastinal or hilar lymph nodes. Pulmonary infection may also occur through inoculation via the pulmonary vasculature, usually in the presence of a definable extrapulmonary infectious source, such as endocarditis. Finally, pulmonary infection may occur as a result of extension of an infectious process from an adjacent organ, such as transdiaphragmatic spread from a liver abscess or esophageal rupture with esophagopulmonary fistula formation.

Whether or not overt pulmonary infection takes place depends on a variety of factors, including the number of inoculating organisms, the integrity of the host's immune system, and the virulence of the infecting organisms. Many organisms exhibit characteristics that enhance the likelihood of pulmonary infection and promote tissue destruction.

PATTERNS

Pathologically, pulmonary infections may be divided into infections involving the central airways (tracheobronchitis), the small airways (bronchiolitis), and the pulmonary parenchyma (pneumonia).

Pneumonia is subdivided into several categories: lobar pneumonia, bronchopneumonia, and interstitial pneumo-

nia. Lung abscess is an additional pattern of pulmonary infection that may be seen with lobar pneumonia or bronchopneumonia.

Imaging manifestations often are sufficiently different to allow recognition of these patterns of infection. Although it is usually not possible to suggest a specific microbiological diagnosis in individual cases, specific patterns tend to be associated with specific organisms.

Tracheobronchitis

Infection of the central airways may predominantly affect the trachea, the central bronchi, or both. Tracheobronchitis is usually the result of viral infection.

Viral tracheobronchitis, also known as croup, is a common infection in children, particularly those under the age of 3 years. Narrowing of the subglottic trachea may be seen on chest radiographs.

In adults, viral tracheobronchitis is usually of little clinical consequence, and patients rarely undergo imaging. Occasionally viral infections impair host immunity sufficiently to predispose to bacterial superinfection, in which case the radiographic pattern will primarily be that of a bacterial pneumonia.

Bacterial tracheitis is rare. It most often affects children, although adults may be affected as well. It often occurs after an upper respiratory viral infection. The most common etiologic agents are *Staphylococcus aureus* and *Haemophilus influenzae*; anaerobes and *Corynebacterium diphtheriae* are rare causes. Bacterial tracheitis produces inflammatory exudates that may lead to obstruction of the tracheal lumen.

Bacterial bronchial infections in adults are most common in patients with chronic obstructive pulmonary disease (COPD) or cystic fibrosis. Bacterial bronchitis is usually diagnosed clinically and treated conservatively. Imaging is not necessary in most cases, although airway wall thickening may be visible on chest radiographs. Often chest radiographs are performed to exclude associated pneumonia. CT, particularly high-resolution CT (HRCT), may show airway wall thickening, and air-trapping may be evident on postexpiratory imaging.

Airway inflammation and stenoses may result from tuberculosis. Smooth, tapered narrowings affecting the lobar bronchi and associated with bronchial wall thickening are most typical. The distal trachea may be involved, usually in concert with mainstem bronchial involvement.

Acute tracheobronchitis may be seen with *Aspergillus fumigatus* infection. It is an uncommon form of invasive aspergillosis occurring in immunosuppressed patients. Radiographs and CT are often normal in this form of disease. Focal airway wall thickening or plaques are seen on CT in some cases (Fig. 12-1).

Bronchiolitis

The term *bronchiolitis* refers to inflammation of small airways, particularly membranous and respiratory bronchioles.

Acute bronchiolitis consists of predominantly peribronchiolar neutrophilic and lymphocytic inflammation associated with necrosis of the respiratory epithelium. The organisms most commonly associated with acute bronchiolitis are viruses, especially respiratory syncytial virus (RSV), but also parainfluenza virus, adenovirus types 3, 7, and 21, and rhinoviruses. *Mycoplasma pneumoniae* and *Chlamydia* spp. may also cause acute bronchiolitis. Bacterial and fungal organisms involving the large airways may also result in infectious bronchiolitis.

Most clinically significant viral bronchiolar infections are encountered in small children. RSV is the most common offending agent and usually afflicts children between the ages of 2 months and 2 years. Infants below the age of 6 weeks may be relatively protected by maternal IgG.

Chest radiographic findings of acute bronchiolitis may show a combination of peribronchiolar thickening, perihilar linear opacity, and peribronchiolar consolidation, often bilateral (Fig. 12-2A). Air-trapping, manifested as areas of increased lucency, is also common in patients with acute bronchiolitis. Air-trapping may be effectively demonstrated with postexpiratory imaging. In very young patients who are unable to cooperate with the instructions required for postexpiratory imaging, lateral decubitus imaging may be used to demonstrate air-trapping.

CT and HRCT manifestations of acute bronchiolitis include patchy areas of atelectasis, frequently combined with bronchial wall thickening and mosaic perfusion (see Fig. 12-2B), the latter due to air-trapping.

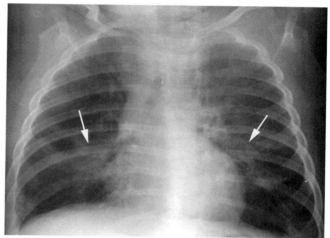

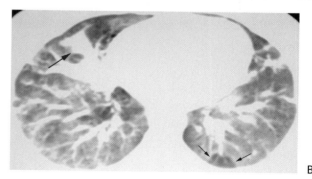

FIG. 12-2. Viral bronchiolitis in a 3-year-old boy. **A.** Frontal chest radiograph shows bilateral perihilar linear opacities *(arrows)* consistent with bronchial wall thickening and atelectasis. **B.** Axial CT image shows patchy atelectasis *(large arrow)* and lobular air-trapping *(small arrows)*.

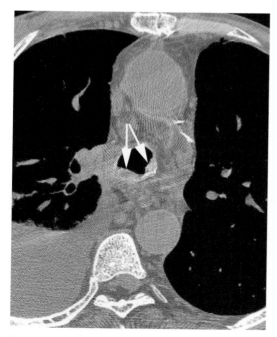

FIG. 12-1. *Aspergillus* tracheobronchitis. Axial CT image in an immunosuppressed heart transplant recipient shows irregular, mildly high-attenuation plaques *(arrows)* along the posterior and left lateral tracheal wall, consistent with *Aspergillus* tracheobronchitis.

Acute bronchiolitis, particularly related to adenovirus infection acquired during early childhood, may result in the Swyer-James syndrome (constrictive bronchiolitis or bronchiolitis obliterans). Histopathology in the Swyer-James syndrome shows constrictive bronchiolitis, chronic bronchiolitis, bronchiectasis, and some destruction of the lung parenchyma.

The Swyer-James syndrome is usually encountered incidentally in a patient undergoing radiography for unrelated reasons. Patients occasionally complain of dyspnea on exertion. Many patients provide a history of childhood infection.

Inspiratory chest radiographs in patients with Swyer-James syndrome show increased lucency involving all or part of one lung. The inspiratory volume of the affected lung or lobe is usually normal or perhaps slightly diminished. The area of lucency shows attenuated peripheral vasculature. The hilum on the affected side is usually small (Fig. 12-3A). Postexpiratory imaging shows air-trapping in the affected lung or lobe, with shift of the mediastinum away from the affected side. CT and HRCT easily demonstrate the findings of Swyer-James syndrome. CT shows increased lucency with diminished vascular size in the affected area in most patients (see Fig. 23-23 in Chapter 23). Bronchiectasis is often seen as well (see Fig. 12-3B). Air-trapping, manifesting as failure of the expected increase in lung attenuation (and decrease in volume) following exhalation, or a paradoxical decrease in attenuation following exhalation, is always present.

Lobar Pneumonia

Lobar pneumonia is typically caused by organisms such as *Streptococcus pneumoniae* (*Pneumococcus*) and *Klebsiella*

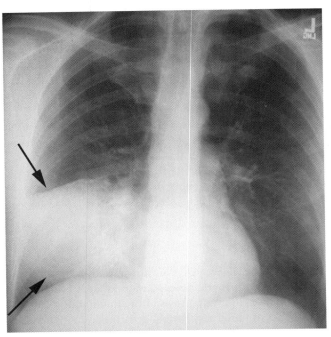

FIG. 12-4. Lobar pneumonia. Frontal chest radiograph shows homogeneous right middle lobe consolidation *(arrows)*, representing pneumococcal pneumonia.

pneumoniae. This pattern is characterized by the initial development of peripheral opacity that rapidly evolves into confluent, homogeneous consolidation (see Fig. 12-4 and Fig. 2-12 in Chapter 2), often conforming to anatomic boundaries such as the interlobar fissures. Lobar pneumonia

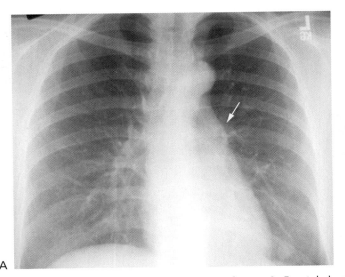

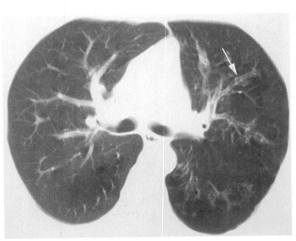

FIG. 12-3. Swyer-James syndrome. **A.** Frontal chest radiograph shows a diminutive left hilum *(arrow)* and relatively decreased attenuation throughout the left upper lobe. Note leftward shift of the trachea, indicating diminished left upper lobe volume. **B.** Axial CT image shows relatively decreased attenuation of the left upper lobe associated with irregular bronchial wall thickening and dilation *(arrow)*.

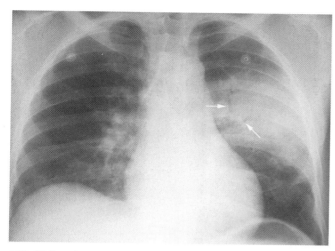

FIG. 12-5. Air-space pneumonia: air bronchograms. Frontal chest radiograph in a patient with pneumococcal pneumonia shows homogenous consolidation associated with tubular lucencies *(arrows)*, representing air bronchograms.

uncommonly affects the entire lobe, and the term *air-space pneumonia* is often used instead. Air bronchograms are common with lobar or air-space pneumonia (Fig. 12-5). Usually, lobar or air-space pneumonia is nonsegmental, meaning that it easily crosses pulmonary segments (bronchopneumonia is usually segmental and patchy). Lobar or air-space pneumonia may produce expansion of a lobe, the "bulging fissure" sign (see Fig. 12-6 and Fig. 2-12 in Chap-

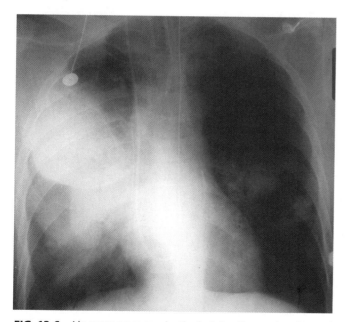

FIG. 12-6. Air-space pneumonia: the bulging fissure sign. Frontal chest radiograph shows homogenous right upper lobe consolidation associated with inferior displacement of the major fissure. *Klebsiella pneumoniae* was recovered in both blood and sputum.

ter 2); this sign has been associated with *K. pneumoniae* infection but probably is more commonly the result of pneumococcal pneumonia owing to its greater prevalence. If the patient survives the infection, air-space pneumonia usually heals without sequelae.

Bronchopneumonia

Bronchopneumonia begins with infection of the airway mucosa and subsequently extends into the adjacent alveoli. The bronchopneumonia pattern consists of patchy areas of consolidation that may be initially limited to one or more pulmonary segments (Fig. 12-7), but it then progresses to multifocal, often bilateral, consolidation (see Fig. 2-4 in Chapter 2). Air-space nodules (also known as acinar nodules) are commonly encountered with the bronchopneumonia pattern. These nodules are ill defined and usually range from 5 to 10 mm in size; they represent infection of the terminal and respiratory bronchioles with peribronchiolar consolidation. Because of the prominent airway involvement with bronchopneumonia, some volume loss is common. The bronchopneumonia pattern is often associated with virulent organisms such as *S. aureus* or gram-negative organisms. Because these organisms are commonly aggressive, tissue destruction is common and complications such as abscess may occur. Healing of bronchopneumonia often results in scarring.

Interstitial Pneumonia

Infectious interstitial pneumonias are commonly caused by viruses, *M. pneumoniae,* and *Pneumocystis carinii* pneumonia. The latter has been renamed *Pneumocystis jiroveci.* Pathologically, inflammation in interstitial pneumonia is primarily limited to the pulmonary interstitium, although not exclusively so. The classic chest radiographic appearance of interstitial pneumonia is bilateral, symmetrical linear or reticular opacities (Fig. 12-8). Interstitial pneumonias, particularly *P. jiroveci* pneumonia, may produce a fine granular or ground-glass pattern on chest radiography that subsequently evolves to consolidation if not treated. Ground-glass opacity or consolidation is usually associated with alveolar filling superimposed on the interstitial abnormality. Treated infectious interstitial pneumonias typically resolve without sequelae, if the patient survives.

Lung Abscess

A lung abscess represents a localized infection that undergoes tissue destruction and necrosis. When a communication with the tracheobronchial tree is present, cavitation and an air-fluid level may be evident (see Fig. 12-9 and Figs. 9-10, 9-39, and 9-40 in Chapter 9). The inner wall of an abscess varies from smooth to shaggy and irregular, and maximum wall thickness usually ranges from 5 to 15

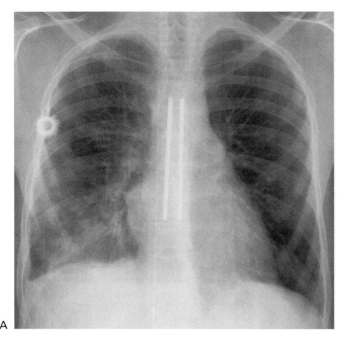

A

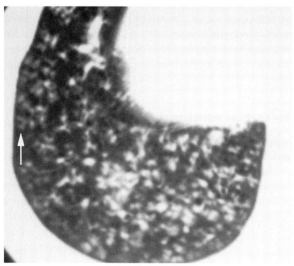

B

FIG. 12-7. Bronchopneumonia. **A.** Frontal chest radiograph shows patchy right lower lobe consolidation, consistent with bronchopneumonia. **B.** Axial CT image shows numerous small nodules throughout the right lower lobe, some with a branching appearance *(arrow)* typical of tree-in-bud. This represents endobronchial spread of infection.

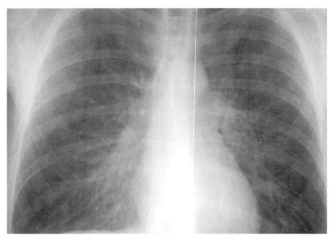

FIG. 12-8. Infectious interstitial pneumonia. Frontal chest radiograph shows diffuse, bilateral interstitial prominence. *Pneumocystis jiroveci* (*P. carinii*) was recovered with sputum induction.

A

B

FIG. 12-9. Pulmonary abscess. **A.** Frontal chest radiograph shows a focal lucency within the right upper lobe associated with an air-fluid level *(arrows)*, representing a pulmonary abscess. **B.** Axial CT image shows that the right upper lobe abscess is composed of several distinct cavities. Note presence of air-fluid levels *(arrows)*.

mm. Pulmonary abscesses are most commonly caused by mixed anaerobic infections, followed in frequency by *S. aureus* and *Pseudomonas aeruginosa*. Such infections are often the result of aspiration. Consequently, lung abscess is often encountered in patients at risk for aspiration, such as patients with poor dental hygiene, impaired consciousness, esophageal motility disorders, and neurologic diseases. Multiple abscesses may result from septic embolism.

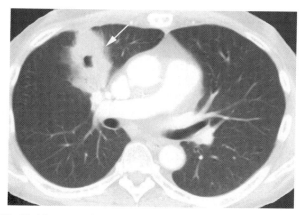

FIG. 12-10. *Nocardia asteroides* infection in a heart transplant recipient. Axial CT image shows nodular right lung consolidation with central cavitation *(arrow)*. *N. asteroides* was recovered following biopsy of this lesion.

APPROACH TO IMAGING OF THE IMMUNOCOMPROMISED PATIENT

Imaging of immunocompromised patients, including those with HIV infection or organ transplantation and patients with bone marrow transplantation or suppression, requires special consideration. An organized approach to the imaging evaluation of such patients is critical to ensure accurate and timely diagnosis.

It is critical to understand the pathogenesis of the various causes of immunosuppression for such patients and to recognize that the use of any prophylactic medications may alter the interpretation of imaging studies. For example, the pathogenesis of immunosuppression for patients with HIV infection is related to progressive depletion of T-cell immunity (specifically depletion of CD4 cells). Because opportunistic infections occur with greater frequency as the CD4 cell count falls, awareness of the CD4 cell count is critical for accurate interpretation of imaging studies. Furthermore, because the use of highly active antiretroviral therapy (HAART) has dramatically changed the course of HIV infection, every effort should be made to determine whether a patient is receiving HAART before providing a differential diagnosis for abnormal thoracic imaging findings.

For patients with bone marrow suppression from chemotherapy or bone marrow transplantation and for patients with organ transplantation, certain infectious and noninfectious complications are more likely to occur at different times following the institution of chemotherapy or transplantation. Awareness of these time courses is important for accurate diagnosis.

Imaging of immunosuppressed patients usually begins with chest radiography. While chest radiographic findings in immunosuppressed patients are often nonspecific, recognizing certain basic radiographic patterns is important. The discussion below details a basic imaging approach to the immunosuppressed patient.

Focal Air-space Opacities

Infected immunosuppressed patients with focal air-space opacities are most likely to have bacterial infection, particularly if such opacities are unilateral, if they show air bronchograms and/or pleural effusions, or if either a segmental or lobar distribution is evident. This is true for patients with HIV infection, regardless of CD4 count, and is generally the case for patients with immunosuppression unrelated to HIV infection. With advancing severity of immunosuppression, infection with *Mycobacterium tuberculosis* (MTB) must be considered as a cause of focal air-space consolidation. Although uncommon in patients with HIV infection, *Nocardia asteroides* infection may present with focal, often masslike, air-space opacity, particularly in organ transplant recipients (Fig. 12-10). This pattern may reflect lobar pneumonia or bronchopneumonia.

Multifocal Air-space Opacities

When bilateral opacities are present, the differential diagnosis must be expanded, and it becomes very important to integrate information regarding the degree of immunosuppression in the imaging assessment of such patients. Bilateral opacities may represent bacterial pneumonia, but for severely immunosuppressed patients (HIV infection with CD4 cell counts below 200 cells/µl, and non–HIV-immunosuppressed patients with neutropenic fever), opportunistic infections, such as *P. jiroveci* (*P. carinii*) pneumonia (PCP), fungal infections (most commonly *Cryptococcus neoformans* and *A. fumigatus*), and, less commonly, viruses and infection with unusual bacterial organisms, such as mycobacteria and *N. asteroides*, must be considered. Fungal, mycobacteria, or *N. asteroides* infections are more likely if the radiographic abnormalities are nodular in appearance, whereas PCP or viral infections are more likely when opacities are interstitial-appearing (see Fig. 12-8) or have a ground-glass appearance and are unaccompanied by either pleural effusion or lymphadenopathy.

Linear (Interstitial-appearing) Opacities

Linear, or interstitial-appearing, radiographic abnormalities in immunosuppressed patients may reflect atypical pneumonia, such as viral infections or PCP. These infections usually occur in HIV-infected patients with CD4 cell counts below 200 cells/µl and in bone marrow transplant patients between 1 and 6 months after transplantation, although viral infections may occur in lung transplant recipients any time after lung transplantation. PCP is, however, very uncommon in patients receiving appropriate prophylactic therapy.

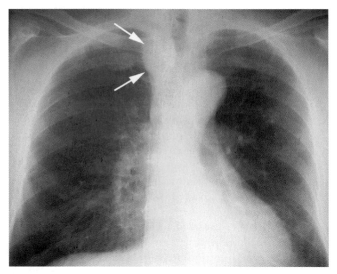

FIG. 12-11. *Mycobacterium tuberculosis* infection in an AIDS patient with a low CD4 cell count. Frontal chest radiograph shows right paratracheal lymph node enlargement *(arrows)*.

Cavitation

Cavitation within either focal or diffuse lung parenchymal opacities in immunosuppressed patients is usually caused by bacterial infection, including *N. asteroides* (see Fig. 12-10) and mycobacterial infections, and fungal infection. In patients with severe bone marrow suppression, such as chemotherapy patients or patients several weeks after bone marrow transplantation, bilateral, multifocal, nodular opacities that quickly undergo cavitation are very suggestive of invasive aspergillosis.

Cavitation of upper lobe parenchymal opacities may occur in relatively immunocompetent patients with mycobacterial infections. Cavitation in mycobacterial infections in HIV-infected patients with CD4 cell counts below 200 cells/μl is uncommon, however, and the presence of cavitation within focal or diffuse opacities in such patients favors either necrotizing pyogenic pneumonia or fungal infection.

Pleural Effusions

Pleural effusions are commonly present in immunosuppressed patients with pyogenic bacterial infections of any etiology. They may be present in patients with fungal infections, although they are extremely uncommon in patients with PCP.

Lymphadenopathy

Lymphadenopathy is commonly encountered in immunosuppressed patients with pyogenic bacterial infections, although enlarged nodes are usually seen only with CT and not on chest radiographs. Visibly enlarged nodes on chest radiographs in HIV-infected patients with CD4 cell counts below 200 cells/μl should specifically suggest the diagnosis of MTB (Fig. 12-11). The development of lymphadenopathy in patients who have recently been started on HAART therapy has been associated with mycobacterial infection. It has been postulated that HAART allows the reconstituted immune system to react to latent pulmonary infection. It is therefore important to know whether an HIV-infected patient is taking HAART, and when HAART was started, if lymphadenopathy is encountered on chest radiographs in patients with AIDS.

SPECIFIC INFECTIONS

The epidemiology, pathogenesis, clinical presentation, and imaging findings of specific infections (Table 12-1) are reviewed in this section.

Bacteria

Gram-positive Cocci

Streptococcus pneumoniae

S. pneumoniae is overwhelmingly the most common cause of pneumonia associated with gram-positive cocci (Table 12-2). Numerous antigenic types have been identified. Pneumococcus may colonize nearly 20% of the population, and this figure is higher in COPD patients.

The development of pneumococcal pneumonia has been associated with several risk factors, including advanced age, immunosuppression, chronic heart, lung, and renal disease, sickle cell disease, cirrhosis, prior splenectomy, and hematologic malignancies. *S. pneumoniae* is the most commonly isolated pathogen in hospitals, and pneumococcal pneumonia is the most common cause of pneumonia requiring hospitalization or resulting in death. In recent years, the emergence of resistant strains of *S. pneumoniae* has caused great concern in the medical community.

Pulmonary infection with *S. pneumoniae* is typically preceded by colonization of the nasopharynx. Once the organism reaches the lower respiratory tract, infection is facilitated by several virulence factors, including the antiphagocytic properties of the organism's capsule as well as the organism's ability to elaborate various proteins that augment the infection.

Pneumococcal pneumonia classically presents with the abrupt onset of high fever, cough that may be productive of rusty brown sputum, shaking chills, and pleuritic chest pain. Manifestations of pneumococcal pneumonia in the elderly may be somewhat atypical and are occasionally overshadowed by other chronic illnesses. Physical examination may reveal crackles, dullness to percussion, decreased breath sounds, and bronchial breathing.

TABLE 12-1. CLASSIFICATION OF IMPORTANT PULMONARY INFECTIONS BY ORGANISM

Bacteria
Gram-positive cocci
  Streptococcus pneumoniae
  Staphylococcus aureus
  Streptococcus pyogenes
Gram-positive bacilli
  Bacillus anthracis
  Rhodococcus equi
Gram-negative cocci
  Moraxella catarrhalis (*Branhamella catarrhalis*)
  Neisseria meningitides
Gram-negative rods
  Escherichia coli
  Klebsiella pneumoniae
  Pseudomonas aeruginosa
  Yersinia pestis
  Serratia and *Enterobacter* spp.
Gram-negative coccobacilli
  Haemophilus influenzae
  Legionella pneumophila
  Bordetella species
  Bartonella henselae and *quintana*
  Francisella tularensis
Anaerobic bacteria

Mycobacteria
Mycobacterium tuberculosis
Mycobacterium bovis
Nontuberculous mycobacteria
  M. avium complex
  M. kansasii
  M. abscessus

Actinomyces
Nocardiosis
Actinomycosis

Fungi
Histoplasmosis
Coccidioidomycosis
North American blastomycosis
South American blastomycosis (paracoccidioidomycosis)
Cryptococcosis

Aspergillosis
  Invasive aspergillosis
  Semiinvasive aspergillosis
  Aspergilloma
Zygomycosis
Pneumocystis jiroveci (*P. carinii*) pneumonia

Mycoplasma, Chlamydia, and Rickettsiae pneumonias
Mycoplasma pneumoniae
Chlamydia
  C. trachomatis
  C. psittaci
  C. pneumoniae
Rickettsiae

RNA viruses
Influenza virus
Parainfluenza virus
Respiratory syncytial virus
Coronaviruses
Hantaviruses
Togaviruses (rubella)

DNA viruses
Herpesviruses
  Herpes simplex
  Varicella-zoster
Cytomegalovirus
Epstein-Barr virus
Adenoviruses

Parasites: protozoans, roundworms (nematodes), and flatworms
Amebiasis
Toxoplasmosis
Ascariasis
Strongyloidiasis
Dirofilariasis
Tropical eosinophilia
Toxocariasis (visceral larval migrans)
Paragonimiasis
Schistosomiasis
Echinococcosis (hydatid disease)
Cysticercosis

Complications of pneumococcal pneumonia include empyema, meningitis, disseminated intravascular coagulation, hepatocellular damage, renal damage, and the acute respiratory distress syndrome (ARDS). Pneumococcal pneumonia may leave the patient vulnerable to superinfection by other bacterial organisms.

TABLE 12-2. *STREPTOCOCCUS PNEUMONIAE*

Most common pneumonia associated with gram-positive cocci
Most common pneumonia requiring hospitalization or resulting in death
Air-space (lobar) pneumonia often with air bronchograms
Multifocal consolidation consistent with a bronchopneumonia less common
Pleural effusion in <50%

Imaging Findings. Pneumococcal pneumonia appears on the chest radiograph as classical air-space pneumonia: consolidation extending to pleural surfaces, often with air bronchograms (Fig. 12-12). Volume loss is minimal. Pneumococcal pneumonia may also present with patchy, multifocal consolidation consistent with bronchopneumonia or, rarely, as an interstitial-appearing process associated with some air-space consolidation. Occasionally, pneumococcal pneumonia appears as a focal nodule or mass (Fig. 12-13), often referred to as "round pneumonia." Cavitation and abscess formation are uncommon. Pleural disease, either pleural effusion or empyema, is found in 50% or fewer patients.

With appropriate treatment, pneumococcal pneumonia may completely resolve within 14 days, although complete resolution may take longer in elderly or very ill patients.

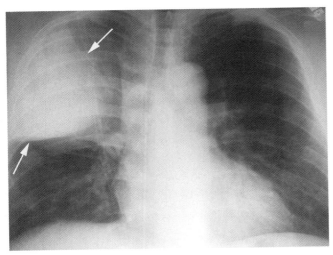

FIG. 12-12. Pneumococcal pneumonia. Frontal chest radiograph shows homogenous right upper lobe consolidation *(arrows)* associated with air bronchograms.

Staphylococcus aureus

S. aureus is an uncommon cause of community-acquired pneumonia but an important cause of nosocomial pneumonia (Table 12-3). It possesses several virulence factors that allow the organism to infect susceptible hosts. While *S. aureus* infection usually occurs via the tracheobronchial tree, hematogenous spread of organisms to the lungs from staphylococcal endocarditis or cellulitis is another common mode of pulmonary infection.

S. aureus pneumonia uncommonly occurs in otherwise healthy outpatients, although it has a well-recognized propensity for occurring following influenza infection. When pneumonia occurs in these settings, abrupt onset of chest

TABLE 12-3. *STAPHYLOCOCCUS AUREUS*

Common cause of nosocomial pneumonia
Associated with influenza and hematogenous pulmonary dissemination from endocarditis
Usually bronchopneumonia with patchy lower lobe consolidation
Cavitation frequent
Pneumatoceles may be seen.
Septic emboli
Pleural effusion in nearly 50%; empyema may result.

pain, fever, cough, and purulent sputum, occasionally with hemoptysis, is typical. Factors that place patients at risk for pneumonia include COPD and other chronic illnesses, advanced age, immunosuppression, and cystic fibrosis. Most commonly, *S. aureus* pneumonia is encountered in hospitalized patients and presents with fever and cough productive of purulent, occasionally blood-streaked, sputum. The mortality rate associated with *S. aureus* pneumonia in hospitalized patients is often substantial.

Imaging Findings. *S. aureus* usually causes a bronchopneumonia, with homogeneous or patchy, often multifocal, consolidation (Fig. 12-14), often predominating in the lower lobes. Volume loss is common, but air bronchograms are not. Abscess formation with cavitation is frequent (see Fig. 9-48 in Chapter 9). Occasionally pneumatoceles are seen, especially in children. Pneumatoceles, unlike abscesses, appear as thin-walled cystic structures that may contain air-fluid levels. The inner wall of a pneumatocele is usually thin

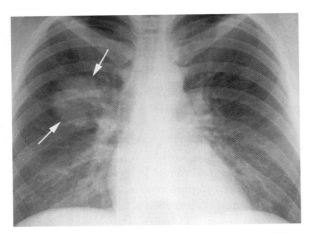

FIG. 12-13. Round pneumonia caused by pneumococci. Frontal chest radiograph shows a round, masslike opacity within the right upper lobe *(arrows)*. Pneumococci were recovered in the patient's sputum, and the opacity resolved following antibiotic therapy.

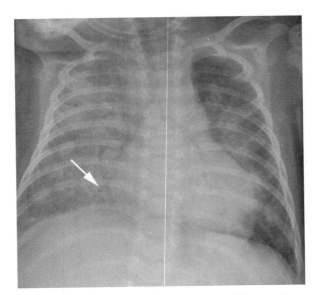

FIG. 12-14. Staphylococcal pneumonia. Frontal chest radiograph shows bilateral consolidation, associated with air bronchograms *(arrow)*. Staphylococcal pneumonia was proven by blood and sputum culture.

and regular, unlike that of a pulmonary abscess. Pneumatoceles tend to resolve spontaneously in weeks or a few months following infection.

On CT or HRCT, pneumonia usually appears as segmental consolidation often associated with centrilobular nodules or tree-in-bud.

Pleural effusions occur in nearly 50% of patients with *S. aureus* pneumonia; empyema may complicate such effusions. The latter may be suggested when loculation is present, particularly when extensive pleural thickening (the "split-pleura" sign) is seen on CT.

Hematogenous dissemination ("septic embolization") of *S. aureus* to the lungs, as may be encountered with intravenous drug abuse and bacterial tricuspid valve endocarditis, typically presents as multiple poorly defined nodules that cavitate over a period of several days (Fig. 12-15A). These nodules are usually peripherally located and predominate in the lower lobes. CT may show the presence of cavitation (see Fig. 12-15B) to better advantage than radiography and may also reveal that the nodules are closely associated with pulmonary vessels; this association, termed the "feeding vessel sign," is typical of processes that are hematogenously disseminated to the lung. Wedge-shaped areas of peripheral consolidation, representing septic pulmonary infarction, are commonly seen in patients with septic embolization. Diffuse alveolar damage rarely follows septic embolization. The imaging manifestations of septic embolization are not specific to *S. aureus* and may be encountered with other bacterial pathogens, such as *Staphylococcus epidermidis*.

Streptococcus pyogenes

Streptococcus pyogenes, a gram-positive organism that is usually arranged in chains on smear, predominantly causes pneumonia in the very young and the elderly.

Pathologically, a bronchopneumonia pattern is usually observed with *S. pyogenes*. Much like *S. aureus*, *S. pyogenes* pneumonia frequently follows other respiratory infections, especially measles and whooping cough (*Bordetella pertussis*), although the frequency of these two infections has declined and *S. pyogenes* pneumonia is rarely seen.

S. pyogenes pneumonia usually presents with high fever, cough productive of purulent sputum, pleuritic chest pain, and shaking chills. The sputum may be blood-streaked. Rarely, *S. pyogenes* pneumonia is accompanied by other *S. pyogenes* infections, such as scarlet fever and toxic shock syndrome.

S. pyogenes pulmonary infection typically causes patchy, segmental, multifocal consolidation that is often accompanied by pleural effusion. Unlike *S. aureus* pneumonia, pneumatocele formation is uncommon with *S. pyogenes* pneumonia, although lung abscesses may occur.

Other Gram-positive Cocci

Other gram-positive cocci that rarely produce pulmonary infection include *Streptococcus viridans, Streptococcus fecalis* (*Enterococcus*), and *Streptococcus agalactiae*. These organisms usually produce a bronchopneumonia pattern that is radiographically indistinguishable from *S. pyogenes* pneumonia or *S. aureus* pneumonia.

Gram-positive Bacilli

Bacillus anthracis

Bacillus anthracis is an encapsulated gram-positive rod that forms spores (Table 12-4). The organism is most commonly found in agricultural areas, especially in Central and South America, Eastern and Southern Europe, Asia, the Middle East, and Africa. The spores are found in soil. Once they germinate, they are ingested by an animal, usually wild or domestic herbivores such as sheep, cattle, camels, and goats.

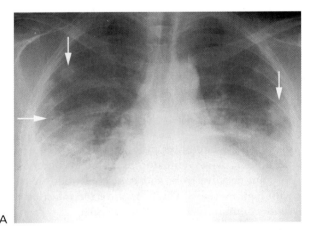

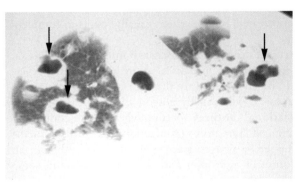

A

B

FIG. 12-15. Infective endocarditis with septic embolization. **A.** Frontal chest radiograph shows multiple, bilateral, peripheral nodules and cavities *(arrows)* representing septic emboli in a patient with *Staphylococcus aureus* infection of the tricuspid valve. **B.** Axial CT shows multiple bilateral cavities *(arrows)* representing septic embolization.

TABLE 12-4. *BACILLUS ANTHRACIS*

Most common in agricultural areas (Central and South America, Eastern and Southern Europe, Asia, the Middle East, and Africa)
Contact with animals or their tissues
Three forms: cutaneous, gastrointestinal, and inhalational
Inhalational anthrax occurs when spore-containing dust is inhaled
Mediastinal widening, due to lymphadenopathy
Progressive pleural effusions

Individuals who come in contact with these animals or their tissues may be exposed and become infected. Therefore, the highest-risk occupations include farmers, individuals who work with animal hides, and butchers.

Anthrax was largely unknown in the United States until October 2001, shortly following the terrorist attacks on the World Trade Center and Pentagon on Sept. 11, 2001. From Oct. 4 to Nov. 20, 2001, 22 cases of anthrax (11 inhalational, 11 cutaneous) occurred following exposure to mail contaminated with anthrax spores. Five of the 11 patients with inhalational anthrax died.

Anthrax infection occurs in three forms: cutaneous, gastrointestinal, and inhalational. Humans usually become infected when they inhale spores after being exposed to infected animals or animal tissue. Rarely, infection is acquired through ingestion of undercooked meat from infected animals.

Inhaled anthrax spores are ingested by macrophages and are transported to the pulmonary lymphatics and eventually into the mediastinal and hilar lymph nodes. There the organisms may germinate and produce endotoxin, which results in hemorrhage and edema within the affected nodes. The organisms may then reach the bloodstream and cause sepsis.

Cutaneous anthrax occurs when the organism enters a host through an abrasion or laceration on the skin while an individual is handling infected animal tissue. This may be fatal if not treated, but treatment usually results in complete recovery.

Gastrointestinal anthrax occurs if infected animal tissue is ingested; it results in nausea, anorexia, vomiting, fever, and abdominal pain. Severe diarrhea is often present, and hematemesis is occasionally noted.

Inhalational anthrax occurs when spore-containing dust is inhaled. Symptoms of infection may initially resemble an upper respiratory tract viral infection, although an abrupt onset of high fever and chest pain occurs in some individuals. Inhalational anthrax often progresses to respiratory failure and shock. Inhalational anthrax is often fatal, although early antibiotic treatment may be curative for some patients.

Imaging Findings. Chest radiographic manifestations of anthrax include mediastinal widening, due to bulky lymphadenopathy, and progressively enlarging pleural effusions. Hilar lymphadenopathy may also be present. Lung opacity is usually minimal in comparison to the lymph node enlargement and pleural effusions. CT often shows high-attenuation lymphadenopathy and may also show peribronchiolar thickening resulting from lymphatic stasis.

Rhodococcus equi

Rhodococcus equi is a weakly acid-fast coccobacillus that has been primarily associated with pulmonary infection in immunocompromised individuals, particularly AIDS patients. The organism lives in soil, and human infection occurs via inhalation. Once a susceptible host inhales the organisms, they enter and replicate within alveolar macrophages. The presence of the organism induces an inflammatory response within the pulmonary parenchyma. Infection with *R. equi* is usually subacute in nature. Patients present with fever, productive cough, and chest pain. Infection with *R. equi* carries a high mortality. Imaging findings of *R. equi* pulmonary infection include rounded areas of consolidation, often with cavitation.

Gram-negative Cocci

Moraxella catarrhalis (Branhamella catarrhalis)

Infection with *Moraxella catarrhalis* usually occurs in patients with chronic illnesses such as COPD or patients on corticosteroid therapy. Other forms of immunocompromise may also place patients at risk for infection. *M. catarrhalis* is frequently found in the oral cavity. Upper and lower respiratory tract infection may occur in susceptible hosts. Patients present with fever and cough, usually mild. Infection with *M. catarrhalis* is usually mild, manifesting as a bronchopneumonia or bronchitis, and radiographic findings are nonspecific. Complications such as pleural effusion and empyema are uncommon.

Neisseria meningitides

Pulmonary infection with *N. meningitides* is uncommon and may occur with or without associated meningitis. Either lobar pneumonia or bronchopneumonia patterns may occur, occasionally with pleural effusion.

Gram-negative Rods

Gram-negative rods are an important cause of nosocomial pneumonia. Most ventilator-associated pneumonias are due to gram-negative rods, and these infections are associated with high mortality. Gram-negative rod infection may also cause community-acquired pneumonia.

Escherichia coli

Escherichia coli is a normal inhabitant of the small and large bowel and may also be found within the oropharynx and nasopharynx following antibiotic treatment. Pulmonary infection occurs when the organism is aspirated into the lower respiratory tract. Gram-negative rods, including *E. coli*, typically cause a bronchopneumonia pattern.

Patients with *E. coli* pulmonary infection are usually either hospitalized or have chronic illnesses; they usually present with fever, cough productive of yellow sputum, shortness of breath, and pleuritic chest pain. When infection occurs in the outpatient setting, abrupt onset of fever, productive cough, pleuritic chest pain, and shortness of breath are the major presenting features.

The typical radiographic pattern of *E. coli* pulmonary infection is lower lobe bronchopneumonia. Pleural effusion is common.

Klebsiella pneumoniae

Although several *Klebsiella* species are known, *K. pneumoniae* is the most important organism from the point of view of human infection. *K. pneumoniae* classically affects older patients, particularly chronic alcoholics (Table 12-5). Other chronic illnesses, such as diabetes mellitus and COPD, are associated with a higher prevalence of *K. pneumoniae* infection.

K. pneumoniae is occasionally a normal commensal in the human gastrointestinal tract. The organism may also colonize the upper airway in some patients, particularly those who are hospitalized. Lower respiratory tract infection may occur when oral secretions are aspirated. Bronchopneumonia and air-space pneumonia patterns may be observed, and tissue necrosis and abscess formation are common.

K. pneumoniae usually presents with rapid onset of fever, painful respiration, and shortness of breath. Cough productive of purulent green sputum is suggestive of *K. pneumoniae* infection, although occasionally the sputum is red and gelatinous ("currant jelly" sputum). Patients are usually quite ill and may even be hypotensive.

Imaging Manifestations. When *K. pneumoniae* presents with an air-space pattern, nonsegmental homogeneous consolidation resembling pneumococcal pneumonia is present. Air bronchograms are commonly seen. *K. pneumoniae* is known for its peculiar tendency to produce a large volume of consolidation, which causes expansion of a lobe, resulting in the bulging fissure sign (see Fig. 12-6). Pulmonary abscess formation is common, as is pleural effusion and empyema. A bronchopneumonia pattern may be seen with *K. pneumoniae* pulmonary infection, especially when the infection is hospital-acquired.

Pseudomonas aeruginosa

P. aeruginosa is typically found in soil and water, but also in small numbers in the gastrointestinal tract of humans. *P. aeruginosa* is a common cause of nosocomial pneumonia, particularly in patients in the intensive care unit (Table 12-6). The organism typically lives within moist areas, such as showers, sinks, nebulizers, respiratory therapy equipment, and so forth. Infection with *P. aeruginosa* pneumonia is associated with numerous risk factors, including COPD, immunosuppression, mechanical ventilation, and prolonged antibiotic use.

Aspiration of organisms colonizing the upper respiratory tract is the usual cause of respiratory infection with *P. aeruginosa*. The organism elaborates a number of toxins and virulence factors that contribute to the ability to cause infection. The pattern of infection is bronchopneumonia, with peribronchiolar microabscess formation, hemorrhage, and associated inflammation being common.

Patients usually present with fever, shaking chills, cough productive of purulent sputum (occasionally blood-streaked), and shortness of breath. Mortality in ventilator patients or patients in the intensive care unit is high.

Imaging Findings. Chest radiographs show a pattern typical of bronchopneumonia, including segmental, often multifocal, patchy consolidation that favors the lower lobes. Pleural effusions may occur, as may empyema. Cavitation may also be seen (see Fig. 12-9). Tree-in-bud or centrilobular nodules may be seen on HRCT (see Fig. 10-28C in Chapter 10). The pattern of *P. aeruginosa* infection is insufficiently specific to distinguish it from other causes of bronchopneumonia.

Yersinia pestis

Yersinia pestis is the gram-negative rod that causes plague. Historically, it has caused great epidemics, one of the largest of which occurred throughout Europe from 1347 to 1367, killing over one quarter of the population. While public health measures have largely controlled this disease, *Y. pestis* is still endemic in several areas of the world, including South

---

TABLE 12-5. *KLEBSIELLA PNEUMONIAE*

Risk factors: old age, chronic alcoholism, chronic illness, chronic obstructive pulmonary disease
Occurs with aspiration
Green sputum
Lobar pneumonia, sometimes bulging fissure sign
Abscesses common
Bronchopneumonia may be seen

TABLE 12-6. *PSEUDOMONAS AERUGINOSA*

Nosocomial pneumonia, particularly in intensive care patients
Risk factors: chronic obstructive pulmonary disease, immunosuppression, mechanical ventilation, antibiotic use
Bronchopneumonia pattern, lower lobe involvement
Cavitation

America, China, parts of eastern and southern Africa, and the western United States. The disease usually occurs in the late spring through early fall. It affects men more commonly than women.

Y. pestis usually infects wild rodents (squirrels are the most important disease reservoir in the United States), although dogs and cats may become infected as well. In urban areas, rats are an important disease reservoir. The disease is transferred from animal to animal or animal to person by the bite of a tick or flea. Rare cases of plague occur following the inhalation of the organism from other infected patients.

Following a bite from an infected flea or tick, a local skin reaction occurs, after which regional lymphadenopathy develops. Infected lymph nodes are usually very enlarged and tender, and the skin overlying these lymph nodes is often discolored, giving rise to the "buboes" of **bubonic plague**. A septicemic phase may then occur, which affects the lungs and produces pneumonic plague. Person-to-person disease transmission may occur during this phase.

Y. pestis has several virulence factors that promote infection. The organism has a capsule that resists phagocytosis, and several surface antigens allow the organism to resist destruction and multiply within monocytes even if phagocytosed.

Pathologically, *Y. pestis* produces a severe bronchitis and bronchiolitis that rapidly evolves into severe bronchopneumonia. The air spaces may become filled with hemorrhage, edema, organisms, macrophages, and neutrophils, and alveolar necrosis is common.

Patients with pneumonic plague present with high fever, cough productive of bloody fluid, pleuritic chest pain, dyspnea, and cyanosis. Tender peripheral lymphadenopathy is often present. Prior to antibiotics, plague was uniformly fatal within 1 week of presentation. If antibiotic therapy is instituted in a timely fashion, recovery is the rule.

Pneumonic plague presents as severe, bilateral bronchopneumonia without cavitation, simulating ARDS. Pleural effusions may be present. Occasionally, regional lymph node enlargement is present, and this may be a clue to the diagnosis in endemic areas. Rarely, lymphadenopathy occurs without visible lung parenchymal abnormalities.

Serratia and *Enterobacter* Species
Both *Serratia* (*Serratia marcescens*) and *Enterobacter* spp. can cause pneumonia in debilitated, chronically ill patients, particularly those in the hospital. Bronchopneumonia patterns are typical. Pleural effusions are common with both organisms.

Gram-negative Coccobacilli

Haemophilus influenzae
H. influenzae is by far the most important human pathogen within the *Haemophilus* genus. This infection is particularly

---

TABLE 12-7. HAEMOPHILUS INFLUENZAE

Risk factors: chronic obstructive pulmonary disease, chronic illness, alcoholism, immunodeficiency
Bronchitis and bronchopneumonia pattern
Lobar pneumonia less common

---

common in COPD patients (Table 12-7). Other risk factors include chronic illnesses such as diabetes, alcoholism, and immunodeficiency. *H. influenzae* also commonly afflicts young children and the elderly.

H. influenzae typically causes bronchitis in adults. In patients with viral respiratory infections, *H. influenzae* may cause a bronchopneumonia pattern; the air-space pneumonia pattern is less commonly observed. *H. influenzae* is a major cause of epiglottitis in both children and adults.

The clinical presentation of *H. influenzae* pneumonia consists of fever, cough productive of purulent sputum, and shortness of breath, usually superimposed on a background of chronic illness.

Imaging Findings. Chest radiography usually shows multifocal, bilateral patchy consolidation that favors the lower lobes. An air-space pneumonia pattern is occasionally encountered. Centrilobular nodules or tree-in-bud may be seen on HRCT (see Fig. 10-28D in Chapter 10). Pleural effusions occur in about half of affected patients. Cavitation is uncommon.

Legionella pneumophila
Identified as the etiologic agent causing the pneumonia affecting the attendees of the National Convention of the American Legion in Philadelphia in 1976, *Legionella pneumophila* is recognized as the pathogen that causes the vast majority of cases of legionellosis. *Legionella* pneumonia is a fairly common cause of lower respiratory tract infection and is a frequent cause of nosocomial infection (Table 12-8). The organism is not part of the normal human flora; rather, *Legionella* resides in natural water sources. The organism is indigenous to freshwater lakes and streams, and human infection may occur when *Legionella* contaminates water systems, such as air conditioners and condensers. The organism may also contaminate showerheads and the like. Despite

---

TABLE 12-8. LEGIONELLA PNEUMOPHILA

Resides in natural water sources, contamination of water systems
Risk factors: old age, chronic obstructive pulmonary disease, steroid use, chronic illness, immunodeficiency
Bronchopneumonia or lobar pneumonia
Cavitation in immunosuppressed patients
Pleural effusion in 30%–60%

the frequency of *Legionella* nosocomial infection and the propensity of the organism to reside within sources of moisture, *Legionella* pneumonia is an uncommon cause of pulmonary infection in ventilator patients.

Legionella pneumonia usually affects older men, usually those with underlying chronic illnesses. Risk factors for infection include COPD, corticosteroid use, immunosuppression (including both AIDS and following organ transplantation), and malignancy.

Pathologically, *Legionella* causes a bronchopneumonia pattern of infection more commonly than an air-space pattern.

Legionella pneumonia may present with a wide range of severity, ranging from nearly asymptomatic to fulminant respiratory failure. On the mild end of the spectrum is the flulike illness known as Pontiac fever; and on the severe end is respiratory failure with diffuse alveolar damage. The typical presentation is a middle-aged to elderly man with underlying chronic illness such as COPD, presenting with nonproductive cough, fever, headache, myalgia, mental status changes, and gastrointestinal symptoms, particularly diarrhea. As the disease progresses, shortness of breath and chest pain may occur and the cough may become productive.

Central nervous system symptoms, gastrointestinal symptoms, and renal insufficiency are more commonly encountered in patients with *Legionella* pneumonia than other bacterial pneumonias. Electrolyte disturbances, such as hyponatremia, are also common.

Imaging Findings. *Legionella* pneumonia often causes peripheral focal consolidation that rapidly progresses to involve an entire lobe or perhaps several lobes on the side of initial presentation (see Fig. 2-13 in Chapter 2). Soon after, the consolidation becomes bilateral in the majority of patients, and this progression tends to occur even with proper antibiotic therapy. Cavitation is uncommon in immunocompetent patients but occurs frequently in immunocompromised patients. Pleural effusion is encountered in 30% to 60% of patients. Radiographic clearing of *Legionella* pneumonia is slow compared to other bacterial pneumonias.

Bordetella Species

B. pertussis is by far the most important organism in the *Bordetella* genus to cause human disease. *B. pertussis* is the pathogen that causes the majority of cases of whooping cough. *B. pertussis* infection results in extensive mucous production, bronchitis, and bronchiolitis in infected patients. Infection can range from mild to quite serious, and bronchiectasis can result from severe infections.

Whooping cough classically presents in patients under the age of 2. The characteristic component of the infection is paroxysmal coughing that ends with a "whoop." Posttussive emesis may also occur. Adult infection is more common than previously recognized. Infection in adults may not fol- low the same pattern as in children, although the infection can be severe in some individuals.

Imaging Findings. The radiographic manifestations of *B. pertussis* infection include multifocal atelectasis and consolidation, occasionally accompanied by hilar lymphadenopathy. Radiographic abnormalities are most commonly found in the lower lobes, and central opacities obscuring the cardiac borders are common.

Bartonella henselae and *quintana*

Bartonella henselae and *quintana* are the causative agents of cat-scratch disease and bacillary angiomatosis in patients with AIDS.

B. henselae and *quintana* pulmonary infections occur almost exclusively in patients with AIDS. Cat-scratch disease is an infection that primarily affects children and causes local lymphadenopathy. The mode of transmission of thoracic bacillary angiomatosis is unknown, but because cat-scratch disease is transmitted by animal–human contact, a similar mechanism may apply for thoracic bacillary angiomatosis.

B. henselae and *quintana* infection produces extensive vascular proliferation, commonly involving the skin, mucous membranes, and internal organs, including the lungs.

Patients infected with *B. henselae* and *quintana* may present with fever, chest pain, weight loss, and night sweats. Hemoptysis has also been reported. Palpable lymphadenopathy may be evident on physical examination. The infection usually responds rapidly to antibiotic therapy.

Imaging Findings. Bacillary angiomatosis most commonly causes lung nodules. If large enough, the nodules may show intense enhancement. Large pleural effusions are often evident, and mediastinal lymphadenopathy is common. Enlarged lymph nodes often show extensive enhancement.

Francisella tularensis

Francisella tularensis is the cause of tularemia. This disease usually occurs in small animals, but human infection may occur when individuals come in contact with infected animals or insect vectors.

Infection is usually acquired by contact with infected animals, often through an open cut or skin abrasion while handling animal hides. Infection may also occur by ingesting contaminated meat or being bitten by infected insect vectors, such as ticks or deer flies. Infection is most frequently encountered in rural areas.

Several patterns of *F. tularensis* infection have been described. The most common patterns of pulmonary infection are the **typhoidal** and **ulceroglandular** forms of the disease. The typhoidal form of tularemia results from the ingestion of meat or water contaminated with organisms, whereas the ulceroglandular form of the disease results from direct patient skin inoculation through the handling of contaminated skins or hides. A rare pulmonary form of tularemia acquired by inhalation has been reported in laboratory employees working with *F. tularensis.*

The ulceroglandular form of tularemia causes ulcerated skin lesions and regional lymphadenopathy. The typhoidal form of the disease causes bacteremia. Clinical pneumonia develops in one third and three quarters of patients with the ulceroglandular and typhoidal forms of the disease, respectively. Patients present with high fever, weakness, and headaches, often with variable pharyngeal symptoms ranging from mild inflammation to ulcerative tonsillitis.

A nonspecific air-space pattern of pneumonia is most often encountered in patients with tularemia. Pleural effusion and hilar or mediastinal lymphadenopathy are also seen in nearly 50% of affected patients.

Anaerobic Bacteria

The major anaerobic bacteria implicated in human disease include organisms of the genus *Bacteroides, Fusobacterium, Porphyromonas,* and *Prevotella* (all gram-negative bacilli), *Clostridium, Actinomyces,* and *Eubacterium* (gram-positive bacilli), *Peptostreptococcus* and *Peptococcus* (gram-positive cocci), and *Veillonella* (gram-negative coccus).

These organisms are normally found in the oral cavity, and they may result in disease when aspirated (Table 12-9). Therefore, conditions that favor the occurrence of aspiration, such as impaired consciousness, seizure, stroke, drug ingestion, and alcoholism, or conditions that impair the ability to clear aspirated secretions, such as obstructing endobronchial lesions or bronchostenoses, favor the development of anaerobic pulmonary infections. Additionally, factors that favor overgrowth of these organisms in the oral cavity, particularly poor dental hygiene or gingivitis, also predispose to the development of pulmonary anaerobic infections. Tonsillitis or chronic sinus infections are also associated with pulmonary anaerobic infections.

Pulmonary or pleural anaerobic infection begins with aspiration of infectious material from the oral cavity. Anaerobic bacterial infection produces a bronchopneumonia pattern, often associated with tissue necrosis; the latter produces radiographic evidence of cavitation.

TABLE 12-9. ANAEROBIC BACTERIA

Organisms are normally found in the oral cavity
Risk factors: poor dental hygiene or gingivitis
Pneumonia occurs with aspiration.
Few symptoms; foul-smelling sputum, fever, nonproductive cough
Involves gravitationally dependent regions
  Superior segments of lower lobes and posterior segments of upper lobes
  Right lower lobe more common than left lower lobe
Bronchopneumonia or lung abscess most common
Empyema may be associated.

Patients may initially present with fever and nonproductive cough, and then develop a foul-smelling sputum production once abscess formation occurs. Chest pain and hemoptysis may also occur. Quite often, anaerobic infection presents with few symptoms, making the infection difficult to diagnose.

Imaging Findings

Because anaerobic pulmonary infection is strongly related to aspiration, anaerobic bronchopneumonia most commonly involves the gravitationally dependent regions of lung: the superior segments of the lower lobes and the posterior segments of the upper lobes in the recumbent patient, and the basal segments of the lower lobes in upright patients (Fig. 12-16). As a result of the relatively vertical orientation of the right mainstem bronchus, the right lung is more commonly involved by aspiration events than is the left lung.

Bronchopneumonia in a basilar and dependent distribution is the most common radiographic abnormality in patients with aspiration-induced anaerobic infection. Pleural effusion commonly accompanies the lung parenchymal abnormalities. Occasionally, pleural effusion or empyema, without significant lung parenchymal abnormality, is the primary manifestation of anaerobic infection. Parenchymal cavitation is common and may evolve into a discrete lung abscess. Necrotizing pneumonia, manifesting as areas of consolidation with multiple areas of cavitation, is common. Lymphadenopathy may be present, and the radiographic appearance occasionally resembles pulmonary carcinoma. With treatment, cavities may slowly close, but residual scarring and bronchiectasis may occur.

Mycobacteria

Mycobacteria are aerobic, non–spore-forming rods with unusually long doubling times. Numerous species of mycobacteria exist in nature, but the mycobacteria that cause human disease may be divided into two broad groups: the **tuberculosis complex** and the **nontuberculous,** or **atypical,** mycobacteria.

Another classification scheme for mycobacteria groups the organisms according to their rate of growth on solid medium: rapid growers usually show visible colonies within 7 days, and slow growers require longer than 7 days to form visible colonies. Organisms classified as rapid growers that cause human pulmonary disease include *Mycobacterium abscessus, Mycobacterium fortuitum,* and *Mycobacterium chelonae.* Organisms in the slow-growing group that cause pulmonary infection in humans include MTB, *Mycobacterium avium* complex, and *Mycobacterium kansasii.* This classification scheme is useful from a clinical standpoint because rapid-growing mycobacteria are usually resistant to first-line antituberculosis drugs. Grouping mycobacteria into the tuberculosis complex and nontuberculous mycobacteria is more useful from an imaging standpoint.

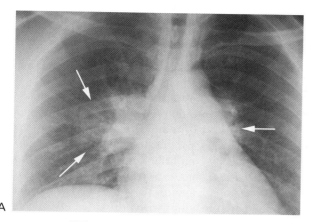
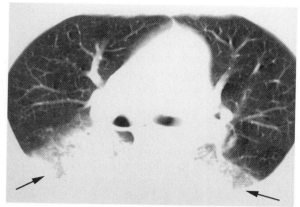

FIG. 12-16. Aspiration pneumonia. **A.** Frontal chest radiograph shows bilateral poorly defined opacities in the superior segments of both lower lobes *(arrows).* **B.** Axial CT image shows air-space opacity within the superior segments of the lower lobes *(arrows),* associated with volume loss. The right lung is more abnormal than the left. The relatively vertical orientation of the right mainstem bronchus predisposes the right lower lobe to aspiration pneumonia.

The major organisms that cause human disease in the tuberculosis complex include MTB, *Mycobacterium bovis, Mycobacterium africanum,* and *Mycobacterium microti.*

Mycobacterium tuberculosis

Tuberculosis has been an infection of importance throughout history. Although MTB infection rates had been steadily declining in the United States, worldwide MTB infection rates remain quite high. It has been estimated that at least 3 million people are infected with MTB throughout the world.

Numerous factors influence the likelihood of contracting tuberculosis. These include socioeconomic status, immune system integrity, age, general state of health, gender, and ethnicity. Patients with low socioeconomic status are at relatively higher risk for acquiring tuberculosis infection. Such patients often include those living in crowded housing conditions, individuals living in inner-city areas, homeless individuals, and drug abusers. Immunosuppressed patients, especially AIDS patients, are clearly at higher risk than the general population for the development of tuberculosis. Patients treated with corticosteroids or those who have undergone organ transplantation are also at increased risk for the development of MTB infection. Chronic illnesses, including diabetes mellitus, silicosis, and alveolar proteinosis, also place patients at increased risk for the development of tuberculosis. Very young and elderly patients are also at relatively increased risk for MTB infection, and men are more commonly affected than women. Finally, African-American and Native American patients are at relatively higher risk for tuberculosis compared with other ethnic groups. In North America, immigrants from areas of the world that have a high prevalence of tuberculosis are at high risk for the development of infection.

MTB infection occurs with the inhalation of airborne respiratory droplets containing the organisms. Many factors influence the likelihood of contagion, including the presence of cavitation on imaging examinations, the burden of organisms, and the severity of cough. Person-to-person transmission is also more likely if exposure occurs in a poorly ventilated area or if contact with the infectious person is prolonged, such as occurs in relatively confined situations such as prisons, schools, and nursing homes.

Several different patterns of tuberculous infection have been described, differing in pathologic, clinical, and radiologic manifestations. These include primary MTB, progressive primary MTB, and postprimary MTB.

Primary Tuberculosis. Primary tuberculosis is said to occur when clinical infection occurs following the first exposure to the organism. Ultimately, the ability of MTB to cause human infection is related to the organism's ability to survive dormant within host macrophages for long periods of time and to incite a T-cell–mediated, delayed hypersensitivity response by the infected host. The host organism, under normal circumstances, will sequester the MTB organism by forming granulomas. Usually, these granulomas show **caseous necrosis**, a pattern characteristically, but not exclusively, associated with tuberculous infection. This initial infection has been termed the **Ghon focus** and usually heals by the development of a fibrous capsule around the focus of infection, which often calcifies. Shortly after the infection occurs, organisms may spread through the lymphatics to hilar and mediastinal lymph nodes, where a similar histopathologic reaction may occur. The combination of the lung parenchymal and lymph node MTB infection has been termed the **Ranke complex**. Organisms within the Ghon focus often gain access to the bloodstream and may disseminate to extrathoracic organs, but usually host defenses are sufficient to prevent overt infection from developing in extrathoracic sites. Although the pulmonary, lymphatic, and extrathoracic foci of infection are usually inactive at this point, organisms remain viable and may serve as the nidus for reactivation of disease when the circumstances are favorable.

Primary MTB infection in children is usually asymptomatic and may be detected only with the conversion of skin tests. When symptoms occur, cough and fever are most common. In contrast, adults with primary MTB infection are usually symptomatic and may present with weight loss, failure to thrive, fever, cough, and hemoptysis. Night sweats may also occur.

Imaging Findings. Patients with primary MTB most often show no radiologic abnormalities. If overt infection occurs, the pattern is usually one of air-space consolidation (Fig. 12-17), often involving an entire lobe. The right lung is more commonly affected than the left, although no definite zonal predominance is seen. Cavitation in primary MTB is unusual, and miliary dissemination is similarly uncommon.

Atelectasis is often encountered in children with primary MTB and may be related to airway compression by enlarged lymph nodes. Less commonly, rupture of an infected lymph node into an adjacent bronchus may cause endobronchial dissemination of infection associated with atelectasis. Adults with primary MTB uncommonly present with pulmonary atelectasis.

Radiographic abnormalities in primary MTB infections are often slow to resolve, even with prompt treatment. Air-space opacities may take more than 6 months to clear, and lymphadenopathy may take even longer to resolve. The pulmonary lesion in primary MTB often heals with calcification, leaving a residual nodule; infected lymph nodes may heal in a similar fashion.

Lymphadenopathy commonly occurs in children with primary MTB infection. Usually hilar lymph nodes are involved (Fig. 12-18), and mediastinal lymph nodes, particularly in the right paratracheal region, may be enlarged as well. Unilateral lymphadenopathy is more often seen than bilateral disease, and occasionally lymph node enlargement is the only radiographic finding present. Lymphadenopathy is uncommon in adults with primary MTB unless they are immunocompromised (see below; see Fig. 12-11). Lymph nodes actively infected with MTB quite commonly show central low attenuation, representing necrosis, on contrast-enhanced CT (Fig. 12-19).

Pleural effusion may occur in patients with primary MTB infection (see Fig. 12-17). Often when tuberculosis is discovered as the cause of pleural effusion, no parenchymal focus of disease is radiographically evident; this pattern is considered characteristic of primary MTB pleural infection. Usually such effusions are small and unilateral (Table 12-10).

Progressive Primary Tuberculosis. Rarely, a parenchymal focus of primary MTB infection becomes rapidly progressive. Extensive consolidation and cavitation develop, either at the site of the initial pulmonary parenchymal focus of infection or in the apical and posterior segments of the

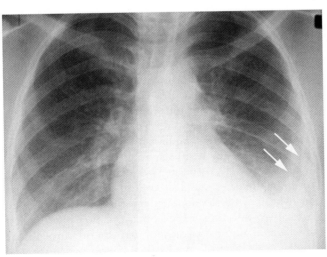

FIG. 12-17. Primary *Mycobacterium tuberculosis* infection. Frontal chest radiograph shows left lower lobe consolidation associated with a small left effusion *(arrows)*. MTB was recovered in the sputum, and the radiographic abnormalities resolved with antituberculous therapy.

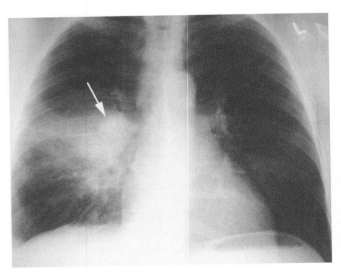

FIG. 12-18. Lymphadenopathy associated with primary *Mycobacterium tuberculosis* infection. Frontal chest radiograph in a young patient shows enlargement of right hilar lymph nodes *(arrow)* associated with parenchymal consolidation. Mild right paratracheal lymph node enlargement is also present.

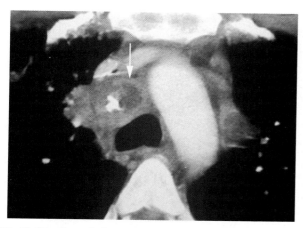

FIG. 12-19. Necrotic lymphadenopathy due to *Mycobacterium tuberculosis* infection. Axial contrast-enhanced CT in a patient with AIDS shows low attenuation and calcification within right paratracheal lymph nodes *(arrow)*.

TABLE 12-11. POSTPRIMARY *MYCOBACTERIUM TUBERCULOSIS*

Reactivation of latent infection
Most often involves apical and posterior segments of upper
  lobes and superior segments of lower lobes
Often associated with progressive disease
Cavitation common; endobronchial spread may occur
Fatigue, night sweats, weight loss, low-grade fever, hemoptysis
Radiographic findings:
  Poorly defined areas of consolidation
  Cavitation visible in 20%–45%
  Tree-in-bud or centrilobular nodules on HRCT
  Lymphadenopathy and effusions uncommon
  Miliary spread
  Airway stenosis
  Tuberculoma

upper lobes. Thus, progressive primary MTB infection may closely resemble postprimary MTB infection.

Postprimary (Reactivation) Tuberculosis. Usually postprimary MTB occurs as a result of previously latent infection (Table 12-11). During the initial infection, organisms may be transported by the bloodstream to the apical and posterior segments of the upper lobes and to the superior segments of the lower lobes. Later reactivation of infection in these regions may be favored by the relatively high oxygen tension in these lung segments, and tends to occur when host defenses become impaired. The latent organisms then become active, inflammation with necrosis occurs, and overt infection develops. Unlike the healing that commonly occurs with primary MTB infection, postprimary MTB infection is often associated with progressive disease. As the inflammation mounts, tissue destruction occurs and caseous material liquefies and may acquire communication with the tracheobronchial tree, producing the characteristic patho-

logic and radiologic finding of postprimary MTB: cavitation. The presence of cavitation tends to promote worsening infection by allowing more oxygen to reach the inflammatory focus, and also creates the opportunity for endobronchial spread of infection and communication of infection to others.

If host defenses triumph, cavities in postprimary MTB usually heal by scar formation. Bronchiectasis, volume loss, and areas of emphysema are common sequelae. Chronic cavities, often very thin-walled, may persist.

Typical clinical manifestations of postprimary MTB include failure to thrive, fatigue, night sweats, weight loss, and low-grade fever. Hemoptysis may occur and is commonly due to bronchiectasis, although the presence of this symptom has been associated with active disease. The presence of chest pain may indicate spontaneous pneumothorax, and shortness of breath may herald the presence of extensive tuberculous bronchopneumonia or developing ARDS.

Imaging Findings. The most typical finding of postprimary MTB is that of poorly defined areas of consolidation favoring the apical and posterior segments of the upper lobes (Fig. 12-20) and to a lesser extent the superior segments of the lower lobes. Opacities may also be found in other segments. Often small poorly defined opacities, or satellite nodules, are seen on the periphery of the dominant foci of consolidation (see Fig. 9-11 in Chapter 9). On HRCT, such nodules characteristically show centrilobular branching linear patterns, or so-called tree-in-bud opacities (Fig. 12-21). These opacities represent impaction of small airways with pus. Areas of cavitation are seen in 20% to 45% of patients with active postprimary MTB on chest radiographs, but small cavities are more easily appreciated with CT and HRCT. Cavities may be thick- or thin-walled; air-fluid levels are relatively uncommon.

Lymphadenopathy is uncommon in postprimary MTB, as are pleural effusions. When effusions occur, they are often

TABLE 12-10. *PRIMARY MYCOBACTERIUM TUBERCULOSIS*

Clinical infection following first exposure
Ghon focus: local infection
Ranke complex: local infection with lymph node spread
Often asymptomatic in children
Adults: weight loss, fever, cough, hemoptysis
Radiographs may be normal.
Air-space consolidation, may be lobar; often slow to clear
Atelectasis in children
Cavitation and miliary spread uncommon
Lymphadenopathy common in children, uncommon in adults
Pleural effusion may be seen without lung disease.

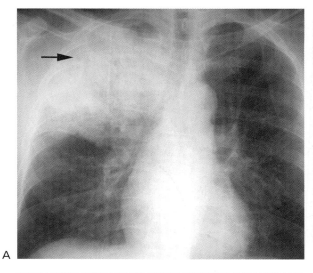

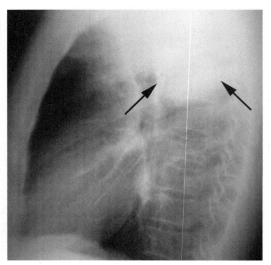

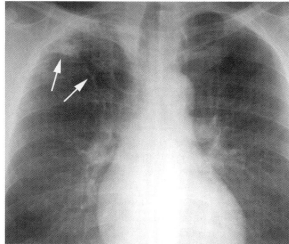

FIG. 12-20. Postprimary *Mycobacterium tuberculosis* infection. **A.** Frontal chest radiograph at presentation shows right upper lobe consolidation with cavitation *(arrow)*. Sputum smears were positive for acid-fast bacilli. **B.** Lateral chest radiograph at presentation shows that the majority of the consolidation is located in the apical and posterior segments of the right upper lobe *(arrows)*, characteristic of postprimary *M. tuberculosis* infection. **C.** Frontal chest radiograph performed 18 months after presentation shows right upper lobe volume loss and scarring *(arrows)*, consistent with prior *M. tuberculosis* infection. Note tracheal deviation toward right upper lobe.

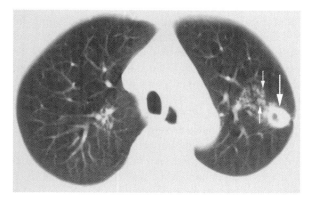

FIG. 12-21. Postprimary *Mycobacterium tuberculosis* infection. Axial CT image shows a cavity in the apical-posterior segment of the left upper lobe *(large arrow)*, with small surrounding centrilobular nodules *(small arrows)*, representing endobronchial dissemination of infected material.

discovered in elderly patients, and a parenchymal focus of infection is frequently evident.

Occasionally, poorly defined nodules ranging in size from 2 to 10 mm are seen in a patchy distribution, spatially separated from areas of cavitation. These nodules often represent endobronchial spread of MTB infection (Fig. 12-22). Endobronchial spread of infection usually occurs as a result of spillage of caseous material from cavities, although rarely it occurs following rupture of an infected lymph node into a bronchus; the latter mechanism may allow an endobronchial spread pattern of infection to occur in primary MTB infection.

MTB infection may result in a miliary pattern. This pattern manifests as numerous, well-defined nodules that measure 1 to 2 mm in size, diffusely distributed throughout the lungs (Fig. 12-23). On HRCT, these small nodules show a random distribution (Fig. 12-24). The miliary pattern represents hematogenous dissemination of infection from a pulmonary nidus and may be seen in both primary and

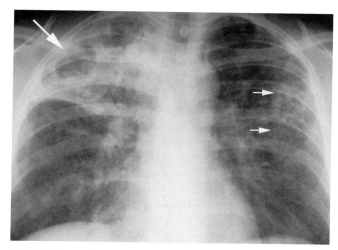

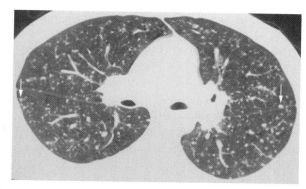

FIG. 12-24. Miliary spread of *Mycobacterium tuberculosis* infection. Axial HRCT image shows numerous, bilateral, randomly distributed small nodules *(arrows)* representing miliary spread of MTB infection.

FIG. 12-22. Endobronchial spread of *Mycobacterium tuberculosis* infection. Frontal chest radiograph shows right upper lobe cavitation *(large arrow)* associated with numerous small nodules in the left upper lobe *(small arrows)*, representing airway spread of infectious material.

postprimary disease. Radiographs occasionally appear normal in patients with miliary tuberculosis.

MTB may affect the main or lobar bronchi, and the pattern is usually one of bronchial obstruction associated with airway wall thickening and inflammation. Airway strictures most commonly involve the left mainstem bronchus. Tracheal disease is less common and is usually accompanied

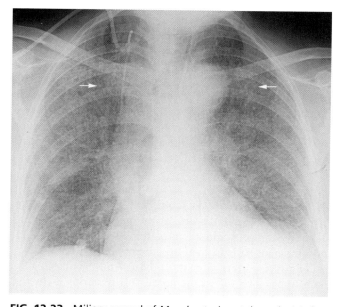

FIG. 12-23. Miliary spread of *Mycobacterium tuberculosis* infection. Frontal chest radiograph shows innumerable, bilateral, diffusely distributed small nodules representing miliary (hematogenous) spread of MTB infection.

by bronchial disease; MTB preferentially affects the distal portion of the trachea. Airway lesions usually result from local extension of infection from affected lymph nodes or lung parenchyma. They are less commonly related to endobronchial or hematogenous dissemination of MTB. Active infection appears as irregular or smooth circumferential airway thickening and narrowing, often accompanied by lymphadenopathy and strandlike densities within the mediastinum. Chronic airway stenoses from MTB are due to fibrosis and are not generally accompanied by other signs of active infection. Chronic stenoses are associated with less wall thickening than with acute infection.

Occasionally, MTB infection manifests as a solitary pulmonary nodule, or tuberculoma. Tuberculomas may result from either primary or postprimary MTB infection. Tuberculomas appear as rounded nodules, often circumscribed (see Fig. 12-21), but occasionally with a spiculated margin, and are usually located in the upper lobes. Small satellite nodules are often present as well. These lesions often do not show enhancement following CT performed with intravenous contrast administration, although peripheral enhancement may occur. Calcification may develop over time.

Active versus Inactive Tuberculosis. Radiologists are often asked to determine whether a particular radiographic pattern suggests the presence of active tuberculous infection, or more frequently whether active tuberculous infection can be confidently excluded by radiography. In general, one must have prior radiographs for comparison to determine disease activity, and the radiographic pattern should be stable for 6 months or more before suggesting that disease is not active. An exception to this rule is that one may confidently assume that calcified lung nodules represent inactive disease.

Radiographic patterns that usually suggest active disease include consolidation, endobronchial spread patterns (see Fig. 12-22), the miliary pattern (see Figs. 12-23 and 12-24), and cavities (see Fig. 12-22). On HRCT, centrilobular nodules, particularly when tree-in-bud opacities are present (see Fig. 12-21), usually suggest active disease. Such nodules often resolve with treatment. Findings more often associated with inactive disease include bronchiectasis, linear opacities, and calcified nodules.

AIDS and Tuberculosis. AIDS is a major risk factor for the development of tuberculosis. This phenomenon is at least in part related to the fact that HIV adversely affects macrophage function and also destroys CD4 lymphocytes, both of which are part of the normal host defense mechanisms involved in combating MTB.

The radiographic manifestations of MTB in patients with AIDS depend on the CD4 count. Patients with relatively preserved immunity (CD4 counts above 200 cells/μL) usually present with the typical postprimary pattern of MTB infection seen in immunocompetent patients. These findings include upper lobe consolidation, cavitation, and nodules, usually without pleural effusion or lymphadenopathy. Patients who are comparatively immunosuppressed, usually with CD4 counts less than 200 cells/μL, present with a pattern of disease resembling primary MTB infection. Such findings include consolidation associated with lymphadenopathy. Often the lymphadenopathy is the dominant or only finding, and on CT, affected lymph nodes may show low central attenuation with peripheral enhancement following contrast administration (Fig. 12-25). HRCT commonly shows centrilobular nodules, often with tree-in-bud patterns. Pleural effusions may also occur. Normal radiographs are occasionally encountered in patients with AIDS and MTB, and extrapulmonary dissemination is also more frequent in this setting than in immunocompetent patients.

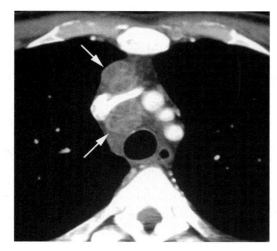

FIG. 12-25. Low-attenuation lymph nodes due to *Mycobacterium tuberculosis* infection in AIDS. Axial CT image shows low-attenuation lymphadenopathy anterior and posterior to the left brachiocephalic vein and superior vena cava *(arrows)*.

Mycobacterium bovis

The BCG (bacille Calmette-Guérin) vaccine, composed of an avirulent strain of *Mycobacterium bovis*, is used to generate immunity against MTB in certain high-risk patients. BCG has also been used as an immune stimulant in the treatment of certain conditions, particularly carcinoma of the bladder. Although the organism used for this vaccine is not usually pathogenic in humans, in certain populations, particularly immunosuppressed patients, disseminated disease may develop, often manifesting as a miliary pattern on chest radiographs and HRCT.

Nontuberculous Mycobacteria

Nontuberculous mycobacteria (NTMB) include at least 20 organisms that potentially cause human disease, although only a fraction of these organisms are important as a cause of thoracic infection. The NTMB have been subclassified according to Runyon criteria, based on their rate of growth and the presence or absence of pigment production: photochromogens (*M. kansasii*), scotochromogens (*Mycobacterium szulgai* and *Mycobacterium gordonae*), the nonphotochromogens (*M. avium* complex), and the rapid growers (*M. fortuitum*, *M. abscessus*). Most NTMB are inhabitants of natural water sources, such as lakes, rivers, and ponds, and some species may be found in soil or on animals. Infection may occur by various routes, including inhalation, ingestion, direct inoculation, or iatrogenic infection.

Many patients who develop NTMB infections are chronically ill. Risk factors include COPD, bronchiectasis, silicosis, cystic fibrosis, and AIDS. Other conditions associated with NTMB infection include diabetes mellitus, alcoholism, malignancy, and achalasia.

The pathologic patterns of most NTMB infections are similar to that of MTB infection. Pathologic features of NTMB infection include tissue destruction, necrosis, and cavitation, and occasionally endobronchial spread of infection or miliary disease. Often these disease patterns are superimposed on underlying chronic pulmonary abnormalities, complicating the pathologic appearance of NTMB infection.

For many patients, the symptoms of NTMB infection are indistinguishable from those of MTB pulmonary infection. One of the most common presenting symptoms is chronic cough.

***M. avium-intracellulare* Complex.** *M. avium-intracellulare* complex (MAC) is one of the most common human NTMB pathogens, and several patterns of infection in immunocompetent patients have been described (Table 12-12).

The first pattern resembles that of postprimary MTB, with upper lobe (often the apical and posterior segments) consolidation, cavities, scar formation, and small nodules suggesting endobronchial spread of infection. Pleural effusions and lymphadenopathy are relatively infrequent. This pattern of MAC infection is most often encountered in

TABLE 12-12. *MYCOBACTERIUM AVIUM COMPLEX (MAC): PATTERNS OF DISEASE*

MAC resembling postprimary *Mycobacterium tuberculosis*
 Most often in older men with mild immunocompromise or chronic obstructive pulmonary disease
MAC infection associated with bronchiectasis and nodules
 Usually women >60 years of age
 Often involves right middle lobe and lingula
 Patchy consolidation, bronchiectasis, nodules, and tree-in-bud
MAC with hypersensitivity pneumonitis
 Patchy ground-glass opacity or small nodules
 "Hot-tub lung"

older men with some degree of mild underlying immunocompromise, such as COPD.

The second pattern of MAC infection consists of bronchiectasis and centrilobular nodules. The bronchiectasis and nodules may be found in all lobes, but they predominate in the right middle lobe and lingula (Fig. 12-26). Large nodules (more than 1 cm) are seen in some patients (see Fig. 12-26C). Patchy consolidations, representing foci of organizing pneumonia, are also seen. This pattern of infection most often affects older (more than 60 years of age) women.

A third pattern of MAC infection resembles hypersensitivity pneumonitis, with patchy ground-glass opacities and poorly defined ground-glass centrilobular nodules, and air-trapping. MAC in this context is usually acquired via exposure to contaminated hot tubs, and the term "hot-tub lung" has been applied to this exposure (see Fig. 16-6 in Chapter 16).

M. kansasii. The radiographic pattern of *M. kansasii* infection closely resembles that of postprimary MTB (Fig. 12-27). Several studies examining the differences in the radiographic abnormalities between these two infections have found no consistent feature that can distinguish the two infections, except that pleural effusions are very uncommon with *M. kansasii* infection.

M. abscessus. *M. abscessus* pulmonary infection may be more common than previously thought. *M. abscessus* tends to cause bronchiectasis and centrilobular nodules, often with tree-in-bud morphology, predominating in the right middle lobe and lingula.

Nontuberculous Mycobacteria in AIDS. NTMB infection, especially MAC, is very common in patients with AIDS, and the incidence of infection rises as the CD4 cell count falls. Most patients with clinically overt MAC infection have CD4 cell counts below 50 cells/μL. Although MAC is often found in the sputum of patients with advanced AIDS, true pulmonary disease due to MAC is rela-

tively uncommon. Clinically overt MAC infection in patients with AIDS often presents with small nodules, usually centrilobular in distribution, combined with air-space consolidation. Mediastinal lymph node enlargement may occur. Enlarged lymph nodes may show low attenuation, although this finding is more predictive of MTB than MAC infection. Occasionally patients present with solitary pulmonary nodules resembling pulmonary carcinoma (Fig. 12-28). Hepatosplenomegaly is common.

M. kansasii infection may also occur in patients with AIDS and may present with upper lobe consolidation and thin-walled cavities. Other concurrent infections are common.

Actinomyces

The actinomyces resemble fungi morphologically and are often classified with fungi, but they respond to antibiotics and are more appropriately considered bacteria. Disease is usually caused by *Nocardia* and *Actinomyces*.

Nocardiosis

The most important disease-causing *Nocardia* sp. is *N. asteroides*. Nocardia are aerobic, gram-positive, weakly acid-fast organisms that live in soil. Human disease is acquired via inhalation of the organism, although person-to-person transmission can occur (Table 12-13). *Nocardia* infection may occur in otherwise healthy patients but is most common in patients with underlying immunodeficiency, such as transplant recipients on immunosuppressive therapy, patients with connective tissue disease on corticosteroid therapy, patients with malignancy on cytotoxic therapy, or patients with AIDS. *N. asteroides* has a propensity for infecting patients with alveolar proteinosis.

N. asteroides infection usually appears as either bronchopneumonia or multiple nodules, often accompanied by a neutrophilic exudate. Cough, chest pain, and fever are the most common presenting symptoms, and the course of the illness is often protracted. However, the disease course may be quite rapid in severely immunocompromised patients. In such patients, dissemination may occur, often affecting the brain.

Imaging Findings

Chest radiography or CT may show one or more areas of consolidation (i.e., bronchopneumonia) or a solitary pulmonary nodule or mass, which may be cavitary (see Figs. 12-10 and 12-29). Multiple nodules, either large or small, may be seen, particularly in immunosuppressed patients (Fig. 12-30). Nodules are often sharply defined. Cavitation may occur. Areas of decreased attenuation may be seen on CT within nodules or areas of consolidation, due to necrosis. Pleural effusion or empyema occurs in nearly 50% of patients. Chest wall invasion is uncommon but may occur.

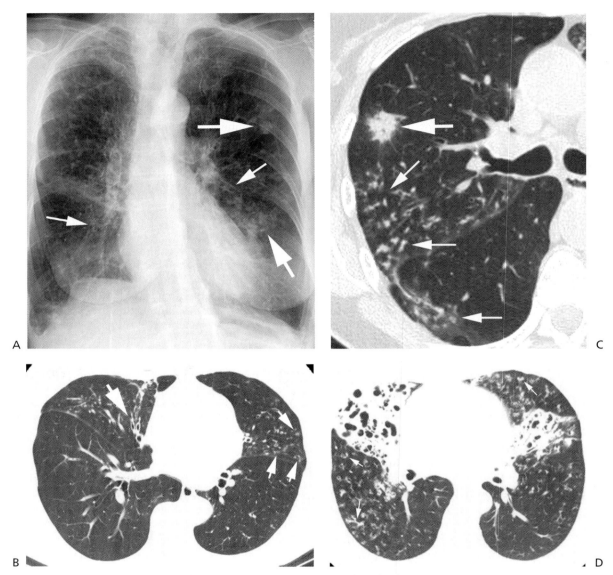

FIG. 12-26. Spectrum of *Mycobacterium avium* complex (MAC) infection. **A.** Chest radiograph in a 72-year-old woman with MAC infection. Ill-defined nodular opacities *(large arrows)* are associated with bronchial wall thickening *(small arrows)* in the middle lobe and lingula. **B.** HRCT in a 70-year-old woman with MAC. Right middle lobe bronchiectasis *(large arrow)* is associated with centrilobular nodules (and tree-in-bud) *(small arrows)*. **C.** HRCT of the right lung in an elderly woman with MAC. Small nodules and tree-in-bud are visible *(small arrows)*. Large nodules *(large arrow)* are also due to MAC. **D.** Axial HRCT image in a 67-year-old woman shows extensive right middle lobe and lingular bronchiectasis with centrilobular nodules and "tree-in-bud" opacities *(arrows)*.

Actinomycosis

Among the various species within the genus *Actinomyces*, *Actinomyces israelii* is the most important cause of human infection. *A. israelii* is an anaerobic or microaerophilic organism that occasionally stains in a weakly gram-positive fashion. The organisms uncommonly show minimal acid-fast staining characteristics if a weak decolorizing solution is used. *A. israelii* forms mycelia that, in tissue, may cluster to form sulfur granules. These granules are so named because of their yellow color, although they contain relatively little actual sulfur.

A. israelii is a normal inhabitant of the oropharynx. The organism causes disease when it is aspirated into the lungs or swallowed into the gastrointestinal tract. The organism is ubiquitous and no specific factors predisposing to infec-

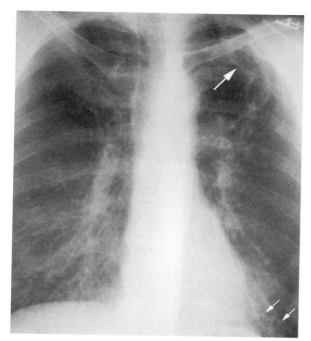

FIG. 12-27. *Mycobacterium kansasii* infection. Frontal chest radiograph shows a left upper lobe cavity *(large arrow)* and numerous small nodules in the lower lobes *(small arrows)*, representing endobronchial spread of infection.

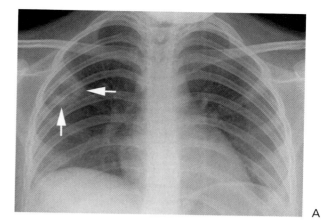

A

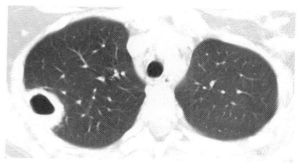

B

FIG. 12-29. *Nocardia* infection. **A.** Chest radiograph in an immunosuppressed patient shows a cavitary mass in the right upper lobe *(arrows)*. **B.** CT shows a cavity containing an air-fluid level.

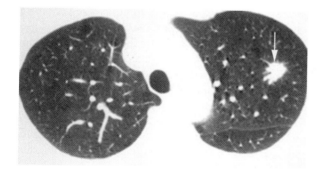

FIG. 12-28. *Mycobacterium avium* complex infection in AIDS. Axial CT image shows a spiculated nodule *(arrow)* in the left upper lobe mimicking the appearance of carcinoma. Resection revealed that the nodule was caused by *M. avium* complex infection.

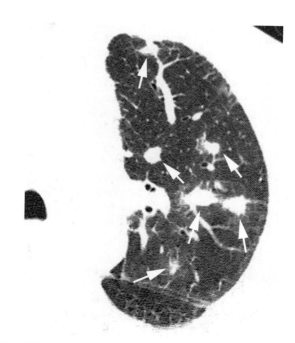

FIG. 12-30. *Nocardia* infection in a patient with a heart transplant. CT shows multiple left lung nodules *(arrows)*.

TABLE 12-13. NOCARDIOSIS

Organisms live in soil.
Acquired via inhalation of the organism; human-to-human spread less common
Immunodeficiency usually present
Bronchopneumonia pattern or multiple nodules
Cavitation may occur.
Pleural effusion in 50%
Chest wall involvement may occur

tion are found in many patients, although alcoholics may be relatively predisposed to *A. israelii* infection due to their increased risk of aspiration and poor oral hygiene. The organism usually causes mandibular osteomyelitis following dental extraction, with gastrointestinal and thoracic disease occurring less commonly.

When the organism reaches the lungs, it has a propensity for causing abscesses and sinus tracts. Acute and chronic inflammation, often with some degree of fibrosis, is present surrounding the sulfur granules.

A. israelii infection may start as a nonproductive cough that may become purulent over time, occasionally accompanied by hemoptysis. Fever may also be present. Pleuritic chest pain may occur if the infection involves the pleural space. If the infection remains untreated, patients may develop stigmata of chronic pulmonary disease, such as weight loss, and digital clubbing. As infection extends into the pleural space and then into the chest wall, bronchopleural-cutaneous fistulas and sinus tracts may develop. *A. israelii* infection may also invade the diaphragm and extend into the abdomen, into the mediastinum, or through the lung apex into the neck. Extrathoracic dissemination may occur.

Imaging Findings

A. israelii typically causes lower lobe peripheral air-space consolidation that may progress to abscess formation if proper therapy is not instituted in a timely fashion. On CT, foci of air-space consolidation may show areas of low attenuation, representing microabscess formation. If a frank abscess occurs, pleural effusion and empyema commonly develop, and chest wall invasion may also occur. The latter usually appears as a chest wall mass, often with periosteal reaction involving the ribs or frank rib destruction. A pattern particularly suggestive of *A. israelii* chest wall infection is wavy periosteal reaction affecting several contiguous ribs; this pattern may be seen in the absence of associated empyema. Although chest wall invasion has classically been associated with *A. israelii* infection, it is becoming very uncommon due to effective early antibiotic treatment.

A. israelii may present on chest radiography as a mass, often with cavitation, simulating lung carcinoma. Rare reported manifestations of thoracic *A. israelii* infection include endobronchial lesions, isolated pleural effusions, a miliary pattern, and biapical consolidation resembling pulmonary tuberculosis. For patients who develop chronic *A. israelii* pulmonary infection, extensive lung fibrosis and architectural distortion may occur.

Fungal Infections

Certain fungi—including *Histoplasma capsulatum*, *Coccidioides immitis*, North American blastomycosis, *Paracoccidioides brasiliensis*, and *Blastomyces dermatitidis*—are endemic to particular geographic areas and in these regions tend to affect otherwise healthy persons; these fungi are known as

endemic fungi. These organisms typically live in soil as saprophytes and infect humans when their spores are inhaled.

Histoplasmosis

H. capsulatum is by far the most important *Histoplasma* species from a human disease perspective. Infection with *H. capsulatum* is usually asymptomatic, but clinically overt infection may result from overwhelming innoculation or infection in immunocompromised patients.

H. capsulatum normally lives in soil. The organism thrives in nitrogen-rich environments and is thus often found in soil contaminated with guano from bats or birds. Particularly high-risk environments include caves, pigeon roosts, chicken houses, or other environments where guano becomes concentrated.

H. capsulatum infection occurs most commonly in individuals living in the Ohio and Mississippi River valleys in the United States, and less commonly in South America, Africa, Southeast Asia, and Europe. In these areas, infection is endemic, with 70% or more of the population showing positive histoplasmin skin tests.

H. capsulatum exists in a mycelial form in soil and may produce microconidia that may be inhaled by humans. The initial polymorphonuclear leukocytic response to the inhaled microconidia is ineffective in killing the organisms, and soon lymphocytes and macrophages are recruited. These cells are capable of killing the microconidia and the budding yeast into which microconidia transform. The recruitment of lymphocytes is part of the cell-mediated immunity that is important in the pathogenesis of *H. capsulatum* infection, and granulomatous inflammation very similar to tuberculosis is common. Early in the course of infection, spread to lymph nodes is ubiquitous, and extrathoracic dissemination, often to the liver, spleen, bone marrow, and lymph nodes, is also frequent. Healing with the formation of a fibrous capsule around the inflammatory focus usually occurs, often with calcification.

The vast majority of *H. capsulatum* infections are not associated with symptoms. When symptoms are associated with clinical evidence of infection, the term "acute histoplasmosis" is often used. Patients often present with fever, headache, chest pain, and cough, usually mild. Uncommonly, overwhelming exposures may produce severe infection, with hemoptysis, pericarditis, and even ARDS.

Imaging Findings

In the majority of patients with *H. capsulatum* infection, the chest radiograph appears normal. When findings are present, nonspecific multifocal areas of consolidation are often found. If infection is severe, the pattern may resemble bacterial air-space pneumonia. Lymphadenopathy is common, but pleural effusions are not.

In patients with large exposures, diffusely distributed,

variably sized but usually small (occasionally small enough to resemble a miliary pattern) nodules may be seen, usually associated with lymphadenopathy. Such nodules may eventually undergo calcification when healing occurs (Fig. 12-31).

The development of a solitary pulmonary nodule from *H. capsulatum* infection, or **histoplasmoma**, is a well-recognized pattern of disease. Such nodules are often circumscribed, measuring up to 3 cm and occasionally more (Fig. 12-32), and often contain central "bull's-eye" or "target" calcification (see Fig. 9-16 in Chapter 9). Adjacent satellite nodules may be present, and calcified lymph nodes are also common. Occasionally histoplasmomas are multiple but usually not more than five in number.

Uncommonly, lymphadenopathy is the only abnormality seen on chest radiography. Enlarged lymph nodes may compress adjacent bronchi, causing atelectasis.

Chronic pulmonary histoplasmosis may appear as upper lobe fibrocavitary consolidation that closely resembles postprimary MTB. Often these findings are superimposed on COPD, and air-fluid levels within bullae and increasing wall thickness of bullae may be seen. Over time, linear opacities develop, indicating the presence of fibrosis.

H. capsulatum infection of mediastinal lymph nodes may result in extensive necrosis and fibrosis of the affected lymph nodes (see Fig. 8-47 in Chapter 8). This pattern of infection may result in granulomatous or fibrosing mediastinitis, with venous obstruction, bronchial stenoses, and narrowing of the pulmonary arteries visible on CT scanning; the former is recognized by the formation of extensive mediastinal venous collateral vessels. Soft-tissue masses in the distribution of

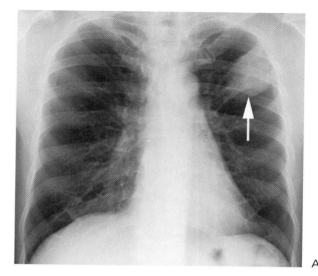
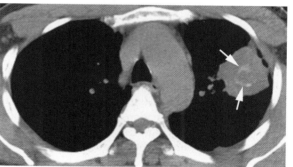

FIG. 12-32. Histoplasmoma. **A.** Chest radiograph shows a left upper lobe mass *(arrow)*. **B.** CT shows ringlike calcification *(arrows)*.

lymph node stations are present, and *H. capsulatum* may be assumed to be the cause when extensive calcifications of lymph nodes are seen. Esophageal obstruction and esophageal diverticula may occur.

Acute disseminated histoplasmosis usually occurs in very young children or in severely immunocompromised individuals, such as AIDS patients or transplant recipients. The typical radiographic appearance is a miliary pattern, and the liver, spleen, lymph nodes, adrenal glands, and bone marrow are often affected. The disease course may be fulminant (Table 12-14).

Coccidioidomycosis

Coccidioides immitis is a dimorphic fungus that exists in soil in a mycelial form. The mycelia produce arthrospores that may cause human infection when inhaled (Table 12-15). Once in tissue, the organisms exist as spherules and may undergo reproduction while in this form.

C. immitis infection is endemic in the Southwestern United States, Northern Mexico, and areas of Central and

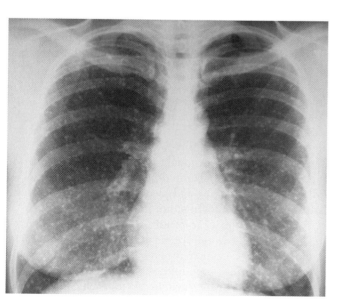

FIG. 12-31. Healed histoplasmosis with multiple calcified nodules. This appearance reflects healing of diffuse nodular histoplasmosis.

TABLE 12-14. HISTOPLASMOSIS

Organisms live in soil.
Thrives in nitrogen-rich environments (soil contaminated with guano); high-risk environments: caves, pigeon roosts, and chicken houses
Ohio and Mississippi River valleys
Infection usually asymptomatic; if not, fever, headache, chest pain, cough
Radiographs may be normal.
Radiographic findings:
    Patchy pneumonia
    Lymphadenopathy common
    Effusion uncommon
    Diffuse small nodules due to large exposure, may calcify
    Histoplasmoma, central "bull's-eye" or "target" calcification
    Chronic disease may mimic postprimary *Mycobacterium tuberculosis.*
    Fibrosing mediastinitis
    Miliary spread, usually in children or immunocompromised patients

South America. Strong winds may carry infection beyond these areas, and travel through endemic areas may account for other cases that are noted outside endemic areas of the country. Within endemic regions, infection rates (often measured by conversion of skin tests) are high. Risk factors associated with *C. immitis* infection include living in endemic areas and immunosuppression. It has been suggested that Filipinos, Native Americans, and African-Americans are at relatively higher risk for infection than whites. Miniepidemics have occurred in situations when soil has been disturbed in endemic areas, such as construction projects and earthquakes.

C. immitis infection has traditionally been divided into

TABLE 12-15. COCCIDIOIDOMYCOSIS

Organisms live in soil.
Southwestern United States, Northern Mexico, Central and South America
Infection often asymptomatic
Primary infection pattern: usually occurs at initial exposure
    Resembles bronchopneumonia
    Unilateral consolidation
    Hilar lymphadenopathy may be present.
    Resolves in most patients
Persistent primary infection: infection lasting >6 weeks
    Progressive pneumonia
    Development of nodular lesions, often with cavitation
    Cavities may be thin-walled.
    Calcification uncommon
Disseminated infection
    Male Filipino, Native American, African-American, and immunocompromised patients
    Miliary pattern often with lymph node enlargement

primary infection, persistent primary infection, and disseminated infection patterns. The primary infection pattern usually occurs at initial exposure. When inhaled, *C. immitis* arthrospores develop into sporangia, which induce pulmonary inflammation. Initially the pattern of inflammation resembles bronchopneumonia, but later granulomatous inflammation develops. In most patients, the inflammatory focus resolves without sequelae.

In a few individuals, the initial site of inflammation progresses and necrosis develops. Such progressive disease may occupy an entire lobe or even a whole lung, and hilar and mediastinal lymph node involvement is common in this setting.

Persistent primary infection with *C. immitis* is said to be present when primary infection lasts longer than 6 weeks. This pattern of infection may result in progressive pneumonia or the formation of nodular lesions, often with central necrosis, residing within a fibrous capsule.

Disseminated infection tends to occur in male Filipino, African-American, and immunocompromised patients. Using the lungs as an entry portal, *C. immitis* infection may disseminate to the brain and meninges, bones, skin, joints, and kidneys. Radiographic evidence of coincident pulmonary infection is usually present but occasionally is lacking. Miliary disease with *C. immitis* infection may occur and is usually accompanied by evidence of extrathoracic infection.

For most patients, primary *C. immitis* infection is asymptomatic. In some cases, flulike symptoms are present, including fever, cough, headache, and chest pain. An erythematous rash may also be encountered. A syndrome known as "valley fever" has been noted with *C. immitis* infection; it consists of a flulike constellation of symptoms in addition to erythema nodosum or erythema multiforme and arthralgias. Peripheral blood eosinophilia may be present in patients with valley fever.

Patients with persistent primary *C. immitis* pneumonia are often symptomatic, whereas those with nodular lesions are not.

Imaging Findings

When chest radiographic findings are present, primary *C. immitis* pulmonary infection usually manifests as unilateral air-space consolidation, often in the lower lobe (Fig. 12-33). The consolidation occasionally shows the tendency to resolve in one area and recur in other ("phantom infiltrates"). Hilar lymphadenopathy and pleural effusions, usually ipsilateral to the consolidation, are present in a few cases.

Progressive primary infection is associated with increasing multifocal pneumonia or the development of pulmonary nodules, either of which may cavitate. Occasionally, consolidation resolves into a peripheral nodule, which may then undergo progressive cavitation into a thin-walled ("grapeskin") cyst, which then spontaneously resolves (Fig. 12-34). Such nodules are more commonly single than multiple, and they calcify very few patients.

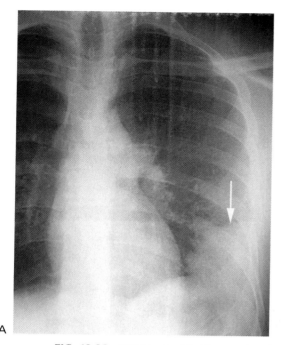
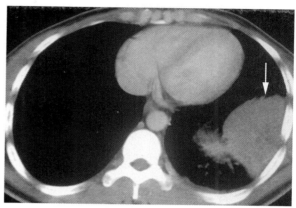

FIG. 12-33. Primary coccidioidomycosis pulmonary infection proven by serology and bronchoscopy. **A.** Frontal chest radiograph shows homogenous left lower lobe consolidation *(arrow)*. Left hilar enlargement reflects lymphadenopathy. **B.** Axial CT image shows homogenous left lower lobe masslike opacity *(arrow)* without air bronchograms.

Similar to MTB and histoplasmosis, a progressive form of *C. immitis* infection has been described, variously referred to as chronic progressive coccidioidomycosis or progressive coccidioidal pneumonia. Radiographically, chronic progressive coccidioidomycosis appears as upper lobe consolidation associated with linear opacities and cavitation (Fig. 12-35) and therefore may closely resemble either postprimary MTB or chronic histoplasmosis.

Disseminated coccidioidomycosis occurs most frequently in immunocompromised patients, African-Americans, or Filipinos. A miliary pattern is often present on chest radiographs or CT (Fig. 12-36), usually accompanied by hilar or mediastinal lymphadenopathy. Extrathoracic dissemination occurs frequently, often affecting the bones, brain and meninges, and spleen.

North American Blastomycosis

North American blastomycosis is caused by *Blastomyces dermatitidis*. This organism resides in soil but may assume a yeast form at body temperature.

B. dermatitidis is endemic in the central and southeastern United States and Canada (especially the Ohio and Mississippi River valleys, particularly Wisconsin) but may also be found in Central and South America and parts of Africa. Infection occurs by the inhalation of aerosolized fungal spores, often in previously healthy individuals, and has been associated with people living and working in wooded areas. Certain risk factors for *B. dermatitidis* have been identified, including immunosuppression and corticosteroid therapy. Similar to the other endemic fungi, disseminated disease is more likely in immunosuppressed patients.

Following inhalation of the organisms, bronchopneumonia occurs. The initial neutrophilic reaction is subsequently replaced with lymphocytes and macrophages and granulomatous inflammation, although caseous necrosis is uncommon.

B. dermatitidis infection may be asymptomatic, much like the other endemic fungi, but the frequency of asymptomatic primary infection may be less than the other endemic fungi. Symptomatic infection presents either as a flu-like illness or as an acute bronchopneumonia, with fever, chills, sputum production, and chest pain. Musculoskeletal symptoms and skin findings may be present.

Imaging Findings

Infection with *B. dermatitidis* may present as consolidation resembling other causes of bronchopneumonia. Occasionally disease is rapidly progressive, with the development of multifocal bilateral air-space opacities or even ARDS. Miliary disease has been reported. Extrathoracic dissemination may occur, especially in immunocompromised patients, usually affecting the skin, musculoskeletal structures, and characteristically the genitourinary tract.

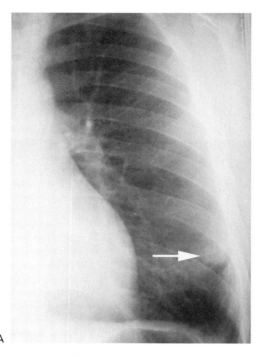

A

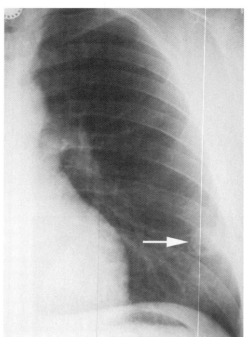

B

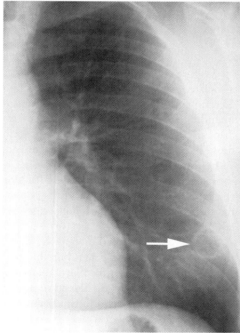

C

FIG. 12-34. Progressive primary coccidioidomycosis pulmonary infection proven by percutaneous transthoracic biopsy. **A.** Frontal chest radiograph at presentation shows a subpleural left lower lobe nodule *(arrow)*. **B.** Frontal chest radiograph several months after presentation shows cavitation *(arrow)*. **C.** Frontal chest radiograph 1 year after presentation shows that the left lower lobe nodule has evolved into a thin-walled cavity *(arrow)*, assuming the "grapeskin" morphology characteristic of chronic pulmonary coccidioidomycosis infection.

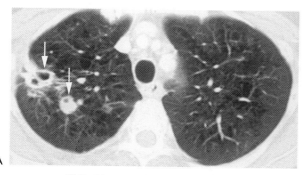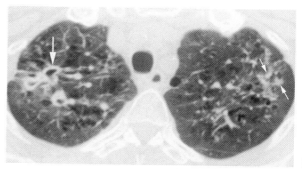

FIG. 12-35. Chronic progressive primary coccidioidomycosis pulmonary infection. **A.** Axial CT image shows thin-walled cavities *(arrows)* in the right upper lobe. **B.** Axial CT image obtained several months later, and after the initiation of antifungal therapy, shows persistence of the right upper lobe cavities *(large arrow)* and development of nodular opacities in the left upper lobe *(small arrows)*. Sputum examination was persistently positive for *Coccidioides immitis.*

South American Blastomycosis (Paracoccidioidomycosis)

The causative agent of South American blastomycosis is *Paracoccidioides brasiliensis.* Much like *B. dermatitidis, P. brasiliensis* exists in soil as a mycelial form but converts to a yeast form at body temperature.

P. brasiliensis is endemic in Central and South America. Patients outside these regions with *P. brasiliensis* infection usually have a history of travel to an endemic area. Asymptomatic infection may show no gender predilection, but clinically apparent infection is far more common in men than women. Infection occurs following inhalation of the organisms, and dissemination may then occur. Patients at greatest risk for the development of infection are those who come in contact with soil in endemic regions, such as farmers and manual laborers.

Much like the other endemic fungi, cell-mediated immunity is important in the host response to *P. brasiliensis* infection. Patterns of infection include bronchopneumonia, nodules with or without cavitation, and miliary disease. A combination of granulomatous inflammation and a neutrophilic infiltrate may be seen pathologically.

Patients may be asymptomatic or present with a flulike illness. Immunocompromised patients are at higher risk for developing disseminated disease and may present with hepatosplenomegaly, lymphadenopathy, and possibly central nervous system or gastrointestinal findings.

Imaging Findings

The imaging manifestations of *P. brasiliensis* pulmonary infection are similar to the other endemic fungi and include air-space consolidation and single or multiple nodules (Fig. 12-37) that may cavitate. Lymphadenopathy may occur, either alone or together with pulmonary parenchymal disease.

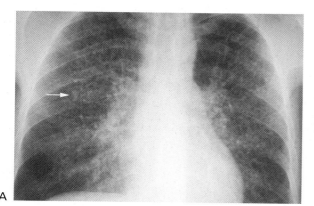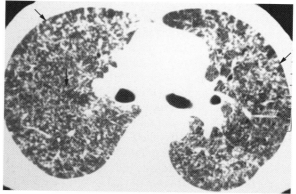

FIG. 12-36. Hematogenous dissemination of coccidioidomycosis pulmonary infection in AIDS. **A.** Frontal chest radiograph shows numerous bilateral small nodules, some of which are larger *(arrow)* than is typical for miliary *Mycobacterium tuberculosis* infection. **B.** Axial chest CT shows numerous, variably sized, randomly distributed nodules *(arrows)*, consistent with hematogenous dissemination.

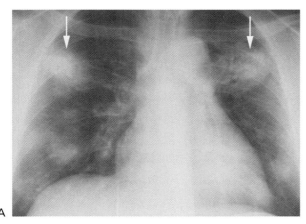
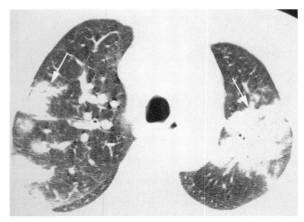

FIG. 12-37. Paracoccidioidomycosis proven by transthoracic needle biopsy. **A.** Frontal chest radiograph shows bilateral, poorly defined masses *(arrows).* **B.** Axial CT image shows poorly defined areas of nodular consolidation *(arrows).* Note presence of air bronchograms within left upper lobe opacity.

Cryptococcus

C. neoformans is the most common etiologic agent resulting in cryptococcosis. Unlike the endemic fungi, *C. neoformans* exists only in a yeast form in both nature and when it infects humans. The organism often has a characteristic capsule that becomes visible with India ink preparations. Two variants of *C. neoformans* cause human disease: *C. neoformans* variant *neoformans* and *C. neoformans* variant *gattii.*

C. neoformans is typically found in pigeon droppings, although it is unclear if contact with pigeons actually results in a demonstrably increased risk of developing cryptococcosis. *C. neoformans* variant *gattii* is found mostly in tropical regions and may infect otherwise healthy adults, whereas *C. neoformans* variant *neoformans* is found worldwide and primarily causes disease in immunocompromised patients.

Inhalation of the yeast provides the route for infection. It is likely that the capsule of the organism contributes to its ability to cause disease because organisms without a capsule are usually easily destroyed by neutrophils. Infection by *C. neoformans* may take the form of single or multiple nodules, bronchopneumonia, or miliary nodules. The pattern of inflammation is variable, occasionally with elements of a granulomatous response in some and a suppurative response in others. In patients with AIDS, there may be little inflammation associated with the organisms.

C. neoformans infection in otherwise healthy patients is often asymptomatic. When symptoms occur, a flulike illness is common. Patients with AIDS and *C. neoformans* infection may present with a variety of respiratory complaints as well as headache. The latter may indicate the presence of meningitis and may occur in the absence of radiographic evidence of pulmonary disease.

Imaging Findings

In healthy patients, cryptococcal infection usually manifests as one or more peripheral, circumscribed nodules, usually without cavitation. Less commonly, air-space consolidation is seen.

In patients with AIDS, a diffuse interstitial pattern, variously described as reticular or nodular, resembling *P. jiroveci* pneumonia (Fig. 12-38), may be seen. A miliary pattern may occur (Fig. 12-39), as may single (Fig. 12-40) or multiple nodules (see Fig. 9-35B in Chapter 9), occasionally with cavitation (Fig. 12-41). Lymph node enlargement is uncommon, as is pleural effusion. Dissemination to extrathoracic structures is common in patients with AIDS, particularly to the brain and meninges.

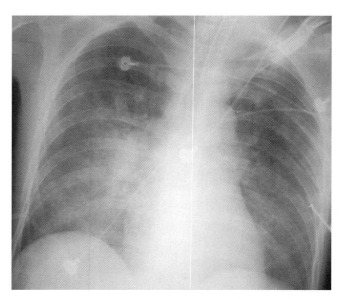

FIG. 12-38. Cryptococcosis in AIDS. Frontal chest radiograph shows bilateral linear and ground-glass opacity that resembles *Pneumocystis jiroveci* pneumonia. Bronchoscopy proved cryptococcal pneumonia.

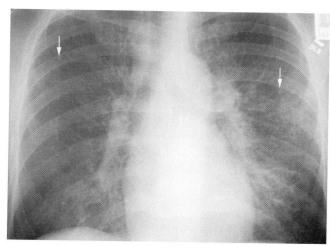

FIG. 12-39. Cryptococcosis in AIDS. Frontal chest radiograph shows innumerable, bilateral, very small, and well-defined pulmonary nodules *(arrows)*, consistent with a miliary pattern, proven to represent pulmonary cryptococcosis. Note right paratracheal and bilateral hilar lymphadenopathy.

Candida

Several species of *Candida* are capable of causing human disease, but *Candida albicans* is the most common and most important. *C. albicans* is found in the gastrointestinal tract and on the skin of normal individuals, but clinically overt pulmonary infection almost always occurs in the setting of immunosuppression. Such conditions include cytotoxic therapy for malignancy, AIDS, chronic antibiotic use, organ transplant recipients, chronic granulomatous disease of childhood, and patients with severe burns. As with other fungi, cell-mediated immunity is important for the prevention of *C. albicans* infection.

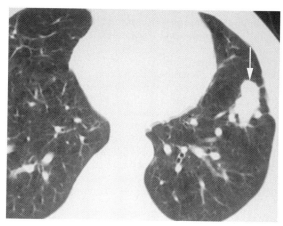

FIG. 12-40. Cryptococcosis in AIDS. Axial CT image shows an irregular left lower lobe nodule *(arrow)* with associated pleural reaction. Percutaneous biopsy recovered *Cryptococcus neoformans*.

C. albicans pulmonary infection usually occurs in the setting of multiorgan involvement in patients with disseminated disease. In this circumstance, the lungs show numerous small nodules with associated inflammation. Very rarely, *C. albicans* infection occurs as a result of aspiration of organisms from the oral cavity into the lungs. Symptoms of infection are nonspecific and include purulent cough and fever. Findings suggesting extrathoracic dissemination are often present.

The most common chest radiographic appearance of *C. albicans* pulmonary infection is focal or multilobar consolidation (Fig. 12-42), occasionally with linear abnormalities suggesting an interstitial component. Cavitation and lymphadenopathy are not features of *C. albicans* pulmonary infection. A miliary pattern may occur. HRCT may show multiple nodules with areas of ground-glass opacity and consolidation; the nodules may be poorly defined or circumscribed.

Aspergillus

Aspergillus species are ubiquitous fungi found throughout nature that may result in disease in susceptible hosts when inhaled. The most important *Aspergillus* species from a human infectious disease point of view is *A. fumigatus*. The organism exists in a mycelial form with hyphae that characteristically branch at 45-degree angles, and may be found throughout nature.

Infections caused by *A. fumigatus* have traditionally been classified into four different forms: invasive aspergillosis, semi-invasive aspergillosis (also known as chronic necrotizing aspergillosis), allergic aspergillosis (including allergic bronchopulmonary aspergillosis [ABPA] and hypersensitivity pneumonitis; see Chapters 16 and 23), and aspergilloma. An uncommon manifestation of *A. fumigatus* infection that primarily affects AIDS patients, known as obstructing bronchial aspergillosis, also has been described.

Aspergillus infection may occur when a susceptible host inhales the organism. Various risk factors for the development of *A. fumigatus* infection exist, and each is related to a particular pattern of infection.

Invasive Aspergillosis

In normal hosts, inhaled *Aspergillus* organisms are rapidly destroyed by macrophages, with neutrophils providing additional immunity. The presence of granulocytopenia or neutropenia allows *Aspergillus* spores to germinate and develop into hyphae; the latter may invade tissues.

Aspergillus hyphae may invade the pulmonary vasculature, causing thrombosis, pulmonary hemorrhage, and infarction. This occurrence, termed **angioinvasive aspergillosis**, accounts for about 80% of cases of invasive aspergillosis (Table 12-16). *Aspergillus* within airways may invade the airway wall and peribronchial or peribronchiolar lung, a condition known as **airway invasive aspergillosis**

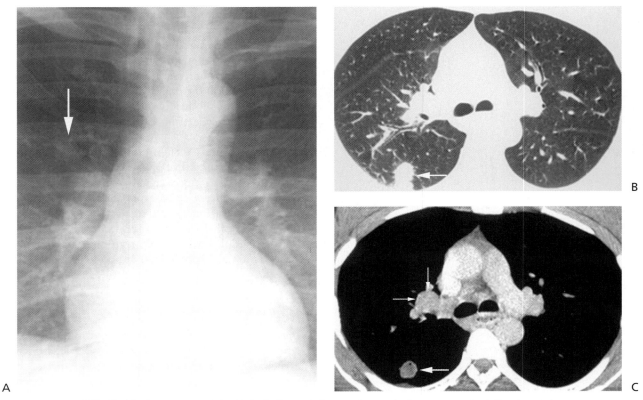

A

B

C

FIG. 12-41. Cryptococcosis in AIDS. **A.** Frontal chest radiograph shows a poorly defined nodule in the right lung *(arrow)* associated with right hilar lymphadenopathy. **B.** Axial CT image photographed in lung windows shows a spiculated nodule *(arrow)* within the superior segment of the right lower lobe. **C.** Axial CT image photographed in soft tissue windows shows that the nodule *(larger arrow)* is low in attenuation (necrotic) and contains a small amount of air due to cavitation. Right hilar lymphadenopathy *(smaller arrows)* is also present.

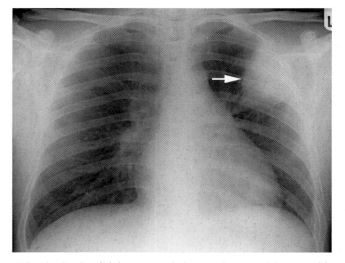

FIG. 12-42. Candidal pneumonia in a patient receiving steroids for collagen-vascular disease. Chest radiograph shows a focal left upper lobe pneumonia *(arrow)*.

TABLE 12-16. INVASIVE ASPERGILLOSIS

Associated with granulocytopenia and neutropenia
Severely immunocompromised patients; transplant recipients; patients with hematologic malignancy; AIDS
Occurs in three forms:
   Angioinvasive aspergillosis
      80% of cases of invasive aspergillosis
      Results in thrombosis, pulmonary hemorrhage, infarction
      Patchy consolidations or multiple, ill-defined nodules
      Halo sign on CT in early disease
      Air crescent sign after 2 weeks
   Airway invasive aspergillosis (*Aspergillus* bronchopneumonia)
      15% of cases of invasive aspergillosis
      Results in thrombosis, pulmonary hemorrhage, infarction
      Patchy air-space opacity
      Centrilobular nodules, centered on airways
      Tree-in-bud on HRCT
Acute tracheobronchitis
      5% of cases of invasive aspergillosis
      Invasion of the walls of trachea or bronchi
      Radiographs often normal; CT may show plaques in airways

or *Aspergillus* bronchopneumonia. This manifestation accounts for about 15% of cases of invasive aspergillosis. A third form of invasive aspergillosis, termed **acute tracheobronchitis**, results in more limited invasion of the trachea or bronchi; it accounts for about 5% of cases of invasive aspergillosis. Pathologically, ulcerated mucosa, fungal hyphae, mucus, and sloughed epithelial cells, combined with extensive submucosal inflammation, are present.

Invasive aspergillosis is primarily an infection of severely immunocompromised patients, such as bone marrow transplant recipients, patients with hematologic malignancy, patients treated with high doses of corticosteroids, and patients with AIDS. Invasive aspergillosis is characterized by tissue invasion and destruction caused by *Aspergillus* organisms. Less commonly, invasive aspergillosis is seen in patients with milder forms of immunocompromise, such as obstructive lung disease and interstitial fibrosis. Rarely, invasive aspergillosis develops in patients with normal immune systems following massive inhalation of spores, a condition known as **primary invasive aspergillosis**.

Usually the immune defect predisposing to invasive aspergillosis is known. Nonproductive cough, shortness of breath, and chest pain are some of the more common symptoms encountered. Fever may also occur, but often the febrile response is blunted in patients with severe immunodeficiency, especially those receiving high-dose corticosteroid therapy. The time course of angioinvasive aspergillosis following bone marrow transplantation is frequently predictable. Infection is typically encountered at the point of most profound immunosuppression, generally about 15 to 25 days after induction chemotherapy or bone marrow transplantation. Risk is maximal while the white blood cell count remains below 500 cells/mm^3.

Imaging Findings. The imaging manifestations of invasive aspergillosis depend on the type of invasion present.

Angioinvasive Aspergillosis. Chest radiographs are often abnormal but nonspecific, revealing patchy segmental or lobar consolidations or multiple, ill-defined nodular opacities. Nodular opacities may show the "halo" sign on CT (Fig. 12-43; see also Fig. 9-7 in Chapter 9), a halo of ground-glass opacity surrounding a denser central nodule; this finding correlates with the presence of hemorrhage (the halo) surrounding a region of septic infarction (the central nodule). As the patient's immune system recovers, about 2 weeks after the onset of infection, chest radiography or CT may demonstrate the "air-crescent" sign (see Fig. 9-27 in Chapter 9). The air-crescent sign consists of a nodular opacity that represents retracted, infarcted lung associated with crescentic or circumferential cavitation. Although this finding is not specific for angioinvasive aspergillosis, it is highly characteristic in the proper clinical setting. It is seen in nearly 50% of patients with invasive aspergillosis, particu-

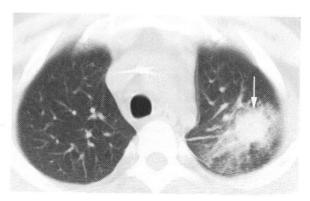

FIG. 12-43. Invasive aspergillosis in a bone marrow transplant patient. Axial CT image shows a left upper lobe nodule *(arrow)* with surrounding ground-glass opacity. This combination represents the halo sign.

larly those in whom the initial lesion was consolidation or a mass.

Airway Invasive Aspergillosis (Aspergillus Bronchopneumonia). Radiographs usually show as patchy air-space opacity, often accompanied by small nodules. The radiographic appearance is nonspecific and the differential diagnosis is extensive and includes pyogenic bronchopneumonia, pulmonary hemorrhage, noncardiogenic pulmonary edema, and other acute lung injury patterns. CT shows multifocal areas of air-space consolidation or nodules that may be peribronchiolar in distribution (Fig. 12-44). Small centrilobular nodules, indicative of bronchiolitis, may also be seen.

Acute Tracheobronchitis. Chest radiography is unrevealing, but CT may reveal multifocal irregular plaques within the trachea, which are occasionally high in attenuation due to the ability of *Aspergillus* to fix calcium (see Fig. 12-1). Bronchoscopy is the procedure of choice for diagnosis and will reveal raised, white fungal plaques coating the airways.

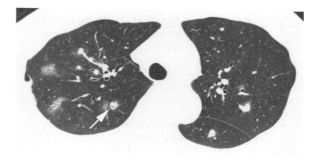

FIG. 12-44. Airway invasive aspergillosis in an immunosuppressed patient. Ill-defined nodules are visible bilaterally. A nodule on the right *(arrow)* surrounds a small bronchus.

Semi-invasive Aspergillosis

Semi-invasive aspergillosis, also known as chronic necrotizing aspergillosis, commonly occurs in patients with low-grade forms of immunocompromise, such as COPD, low-dose corticosteroid use, alcoholism, tuberculosis, diabetes mellitus, and collagen vascular diseases (Table 12-17). Risk is compounded in those with preexisting structural lung disease, such as pneumoconioses or prior radiation treatment. Tissue invasion occurs following the inhalation of spores, but the time course of semi-invasive aspergillosis is different from that of angioinvasive aspergillosis. Tissue invasion and infarction occurs over months with the former and over days or weeks with the latter.

Patients with semi-invasive aspergillosis present with low-grade fever and productive cough, often over a period of months. Hemoptysis may also occur. These symptoms may be superimposed on a background of chronic illness.

Imaging Findings. Semi-invasive aspergillosis mimics the appearance of active TB. It often presents with irregular upper lobe consolidation and pleural thickening that slowly progresses to cavitation over weeks or months. The upper lobe disease commonly contacts thickened pleura. The cavity may contain an internal opacity resembling an aspergilloma, largely consisting of fungus. Irregular strands may be seen extending from the intracavitary mass to the cavity wall (Fig. 12-45). Occasionally, regions of high attenuation are visible within the cavity on CT. This probably represents calcification occurring in relation to the fungus.

Aspergilloma

Aspergilloma, or mycetoma, is a saprophytic infection that occurs in patients with underlying structural lung disease. Patients with mycetoma generally have normal immunity, although coexistent chronic diseases are often present. Pathologically, aspergilloma consists of a combination of fungal hyphae, cellular debris, and mucus within a cavity. The cavity wall commonly consists of fibrous tissue, inflammatory cells, and granulation tissue, the latter derived from the bronchial circulation. The most common cause of underlying structural lung disease in patients with aspergilloma is cavitary disease from prior TB. Structural lung disease due to sarcoidosis is the second most common condition predisposing to aspergilloma formation. Bullae, abscesses, and bronchiectasis are less common predisposing factors. The preexisting lung disease presumably impairs normal clearance of the organisms, allowing infection to occur. Characteristically, the fungus does not usually produce tissue invasion.

Often patients with aspergilloma are asymptomatic. When symptoms are present, cough, weight loss, and hemoptysis are common. Hemoptysis may range from minor blood streaking to massive, life-threatening hemorrhage. The latter is commonly temporized with bronchial embolization, although pulmonary resection may be required. Although the overall prognosis of patients with aspergilloma is good, death from massive hemoptysis may occur and rare cases of severe local parenchymal destruction and even dissemination have occurred.

Imaging Findings. Aspergilloma usually appears as a round or oval mass partially filling a cavity and creating the characteristic finding of the air-crescent sign (Fig. 12-46A). If the fungus ball completely fills the pulmonary cavity, the air-crescent sign may not be discernible. Aspergillomas often show mobility with decubitus imaging.

Aspergillomas are usually located in the upper lobes, adjacent to the pleura, which may be thickened. Aspergillomas rarely calcify, and they may diminish or remain unchanged in size over time. An air-fluid level is usually not present within the cavity. The cavity itself is usually thin-walled, although thickening of cavity walls before a discrete internal opacity is seen may indicate early infection.

CT shows a mobile, intracavitary mass (see Fig. 12-46B and C; see also Fig. 9-42 in Chapter 9) and may also reveal small fungal strands bridging the fungus ball and the cavity wall in cases when the air-crescent sign is not visible on chest

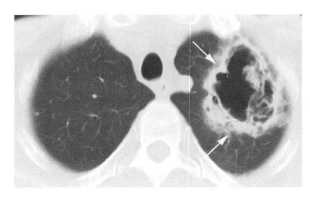

FIG. 12-45. Semi-invasive aspergillosis in a patient with diabetes mellitus. Axial CT image through the lung apices shows an irregular left upper lobe cavity *(arrows)*. Internal opacities reflect the presence of fungus.

TABLE 12-17. SEMI-INVASIVE ASPERGILLOSIS

Also known as chronic necrotizing aspergillosis
Associated with mild immunocompromise (chronic obstructive pulmonary disease, low-dose corticosteroid use, alcoholism, tuberculosis, diabetes, collagen-vascular diseases)
Low-grade fever, productive cough, often over a period of months
Mimics active *Mycobacterium tuberculosis* radiographically
Progressive upper lobe consolidation
Cavitation
Pleural thickening
Mass within the cavity due to fungus

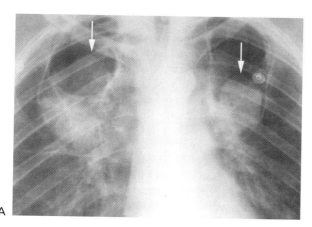

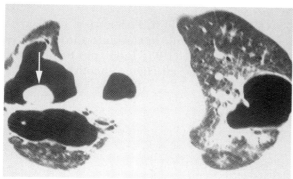

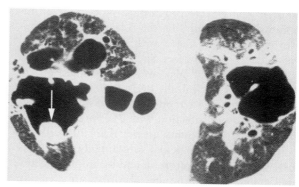

FIG. 12-46. Aspergilloma. **A.** Frontal chest radiograph shows biapical aspergillomas *(arrows)* in a patient with sarcoidosis. **B.** Axial HRCT supine image shows a dependent opacity *(arrow)* within the right upper lobe opacity. **C.** Axial prone HRCT image shows that the intracavitary opacity *(arrow)* is mobile.

radiographs. CT may also demonstrate foci of increased attenuation within the fungal ball, presumably reflecting calcium. As with chest radiography, CT may reveal thickening of the wall of a preexisting cavity before the fungus ball is evident.

Zygomycosis

Zygomycosis includes fungal infections caused by a variety of organisms, the most important of which include *Rhizopus*, *Rhizomucor*, and *Mucor*. Mucormycosis is probably the most common of these infections affecting the thorax.

The fungi that cause zygomycoses are found worldwide, usually in decaying matter. These organisms produce spores that may result in disease when inhaled. Disease almost always occurs in patients with impaired immunity, including patients with diabetes mellitus (especially in the context of ketoacidosis), corticosteroid therapy, AIDS (often when corticosteroid therapy is employed concomitantly), hematologic malignancy, lymphoma, and chronic renal failure. In particular, neutropenic patients are at risk for zygomycoses.

The pattern of infection caused by the zygomycotic fungi is variable, depending on the degree of underlying immunity. An extensive neutrophilic infiltrate may be present, but granulomatous inflammation is rare. Vascular invasion by the fungal organisms is common.

Patients with zygomycotic infections, especially mucormycosis, present with chest pain, fever, and hemoptysis; the latter can be massive. The organisms can be very destructive, and invasion of the mediastinum, pleura, chest wall, and spine may occur. Bronchopleural-cutaneous fistulas may also result from mucormycosis. Vascular catastrophes, such as pulmonary artery aneurysms, pulmonary vein thrombosis with subsequent pulmonary infarction, and superior vena cava thrombosis, may also occur.

Imaging Findings
Chest radiography in patients with mucormycosis may show multifocal, occasionally bilateral, air-space consolidation, a single nodule or mass, or multiple ill-defined nodules or masses. CT scanning may show a ground-glass halo surrounding nodular abnormalities; this finding represents hemorrhage resulting from pulmonary vascular thrombosis. An air-crescent sign may also occur, especially as the patient's immune system recovers following chemotherapy. Pleural effusions and lymphadenopathy may also occur.

Pneumocystis jiroveci (Pneumocytis carinii)

P. jiroveci, previously known as *P. carinii*, was initially classified as a protozoan but is now thought to be a fungus. The organism exists as a cyst containing trophozoites, which may then be liberated to develop into cysts themselves.

P. jiroveci pneumonia occurs almost exclusively in patients with underlying disease. Patients with AIDS are most vulnerable, with transplant recipients on immunosuppression and patients on low-dose corticosteroid therapy for vasculitis or connective tissue disorders also at risk. Patients with malignancies undergoing cytotoxic therapy are also at relatively increased risk for infection with *P. jiroveci*. *P. jiroveci* infection in the general population, as evidenced by the presence of IgG antibodies against the organism's surface antigens, is common and is usually asymptomatic in immunocompetent individuals.

Infection with *P. jiroveci* probably occurs as a result of reactivation of a latent infection, occurring because of immunosuppression. Furthermore, the risk of developing infection with *P. jiroveci* increases with worsening immunosuppression. Exogenous sources, such as animal reservoirs or other patients, may still play some role in infection.

The development of clinically overt *P. jiroveci* infection is strongly related to CD4 lymphocyte function. In patients with AIDS, the risk of infection with *P. jiroveci* is low in patients with CD4 cell counts greater than 200 cells/μl, but the risk of infection increases substantially with CD4 counts below this level. Neutrophil and macrophage activity, as well as humoral immunity, also play some role in the pathogenesis of *P. jiroveci* infection.

P. jiroveci infection causes alveolar inflammation with an eosinophilic exudate containing cysts and trophozoites as well as other material. Lymphocytes and plasma cells may also be present. The organisms are identifiable within the exudate when a sputum sample is obtained, either by sputum induction or with bronchial lavage. Hyaline membrane formation, interstitial edema, and type II pneumocyte hyperplasia are often present to a variable degree. *P. jiroveci* infection less commonly is associated with granulomatous inflammation, cyst formation, calcification, and interstitial fibrosis.

Infection usually presents with a variable duration of dyspnea on exertion, shortness of breath, a dry, nonproductive cough, and high fever. Patients with AIDS who are infected with *P. jiroveci* are usually severely immunocompromised (CD4 cell count less than 200 cells/μl) and are usually not on trimethoprim-sulfamethoxazole prophylaxis. Hypoxia is common, and serum levels of lactate dehydrogenase are often elevated.

Diagnosis is usually established with the demonstration of organisms on sputum induction. In patients at risk for infection with *P. jiroveci* but with negative sputum induction results, bronchoscopy with bronchial lavage usually establishes the diagnosis.

Imaging Findings

The earliest chest radiographic manifestation of *P. jiroveci* infection is bilateral perihilar ground-glass opacity or interstitial thickening (see Fig. 12-8) or poor definition of pulmonary vessels (Figs. 12-47A and 12-48A). Later, multifocal air-space consolidation may be present, particularly if the patient has been ill for some time. Pleural effusions are characteristically absent.

Some patients with AIDS and *P. jiroveci* infection develop cystic areas, termed pneumatoceles. Such pneumatoceles are characteristically thin-walled and are usually found in the upper lobes. The presence of these lesions may predispose to the development of pneumothorax.

Atypical chest radiographic manifestations of *P. jiroveci* infection include an upper lobe distribution, focal consolidation, single or multiple nodules, cavitation of a nodule, lymphadenopathy, and pleural effusions. A normal chest radiograph occurs uncommonly in patients with AIDS and *P. jiroveci* infection.

CT, in particular HRCT, shows multifocal ground-glass opacity predominantly in a perihilar distribution (see Figs. 12-47 and 12-48); HRCT shows this finding in all AIDS patients with this infection. Smooth interlobular septal

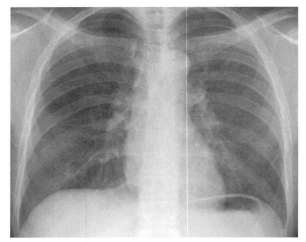

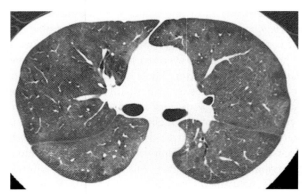

FIG. 12-47. *Pneumocystis jiroveci* pneumonia in a patient being treated with steroids for collagen-vascular disease. **A.** Chest radiograph shows subtle perihilar ground-glass opacity with poor definition of pulmonary vessels. **B.** HRCT shows diffuse, patchy ground-glass opacity typical of *Pneumocystis* pneumonia. The lung periphery is spared.

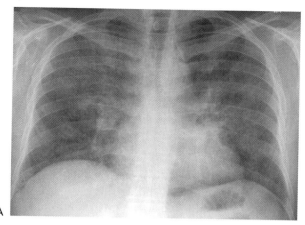
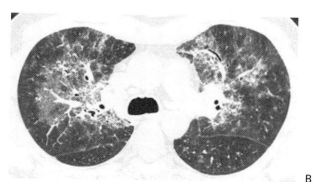

FIG. 12-48. *Pneumocystis jiroveci* pneumonia in an AIDS patient. **A.** Chest radiograph shows perihilar ground-glass opacity, interstitial opacities, and poor definition of pulmonary vessels. **B.** HRCT shows perihilar ground-glass opacity and reticular opacities. The lung periphery is spared. Ground-glass opacity is always seen on HRCT in AIDS patients with *Pneumocystis* pneumonia.

thickening may be present, and foci of consolidation are often encountered. Pneumatoceles and pneumothorax may also be evident (Fig. 12-49). Patients with a granulomatous response to *P. jiroveci* infection may show small nodules in addition to ground-glass opacities. Rarely, evidence of fibrosis may be seen in patients who have recovered from *P. jiroveci* infection. Larger nodules or masses are occasionally seen (Table 12-18; see Fig. 9-35C in Chapter 9).

Mycoplasma, Chlamydia, and Rickettsiae Pneumonias

Mycoplasma pneumoniae

Mycoplasmas are the smallest free-living culturable organisms. They share some similarities with bacteria, but their

lack of a cell wall and certain genetic features make them distinctly different than most bacteria. There are several distinct *Mycoplasma* spp., but *Mycoplasma pneumoniae* is the most important from the human infectious disease standpoint.

M. pneumoniae is a common cause of community-acquired pneumonia. *M. pneumoniae* pulmonary infection occurs mostly in younger patients, and infection is particularly common among military recruits. Infection is transmitted by person-to-person contact and respiratory droplets; infection rates peak in the fall and winter.

M. pneumoniae causes infection by both direct cytotoxicity and damage incurred from the host inflammatory response. A peribronchiolar mononuclear cell infiltrate is one of the more common pathologic findings, although neutrophilic infiltration, chronic inflammatory cell infiltration, fibrosis, diffuse alveolar damage, organizing pneumonia, and

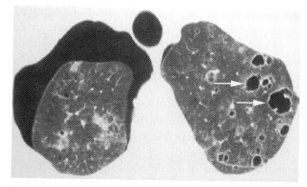

FIG. 12-49. *Pneumocystis jiroveci* pneumonia with pneumatoceles and pneumothorax in an AIDS patient with a low CD4 cell count. Axial HRCT image shows numerous thin-walled cysts *(arrows)*, representing pneumatoceles, surrounded by ground-glass opacity. Pneumothorax is present on the right side, likely due to rupture of a pneumatocele.

TABLE 12-18. PNEUMOCYSTIS JIROVECI (PNEUMOCYSTIS CARINII)

Associated with AIDS, with transplant recipients on immunosuppression, low-dose corticosteroid therapy, cytotoxic therapy for malignancy
Associated with low CD4 count (<200)
Shortness of breath, dry, nonproductive cough, and high fever
Hypoxia, elevated lactate dehydrogenase level
Radiographs and HRCT
  Perihilar ground-glass opacity
  Air-space consolidation may be present.
  Effusion rare
  Pneumatoceles may develop.
  May present with pneumothorax
HRCT is highly sensitive in AIDS patients.
  Ground-glass opacity visible in all patients

pulmonary hemorrhage are additional reported pathologic features.

Upper respiratory tract infectious symptoms may precede overt *M. pneumoniae* infection. Patients develop nonproductive cough, headache, malaise, and fever, somewhat resembling a viral infection, although unlike viral infections, arthralgias and myalgias are usually absent. Rarely, infection is severe, resulting in hypoxemic respiratory failure, particularly in patients with sickle cell disease. Superimposed bacterial infection occurs rarely.

Patients with *M. pneumoniae* may develop extrathoracic disease manifestations, including aseptic meningitis, encephalitis, and transverse myelitis (among other neurologic syndromes), hemolysis, venous thrombosis, pericarditis, and myocarditis, and skin rashes.

Imaging Findings

The earliest chest radiographic findings are commonly interstitial in appearance, consisting of fine linear opacities followed by segmental air-space consolidation. Occasionally these patterns are seen separately rather than sequentially. Pleural effusion occurs in fewer than 20% of patients, and lymphadenopathy is uncommon.

CT scanning typically shows patchy, segmental and lobular consolidation or ground-glass opacity (Fig. 12-50), sometimes associated with thickening of the perihilar interstitium. Mosaic perfusion may be seen due to small airway obstruction. Air-trapping may be present on expiratory scans.

Chlamydia

Chlamydia spp. are obligate intracellular organisms that possess their own cell walls and share some other characteristics with other bacteria. They exist in an extracellular form known as elementary bodies and then change to reticular bodies once they enter a cell. Three *Chlamydia* spp. are important in the pathogenesis of human disease: *Chlamydia trachomatis*, *Chlamydia psittaci*, and *Chlamydia pneumoniae*.

Chlamydia trachomatis

C. trachomatis infection usually causes a sexually transmitted disease, but an infant born through the birth canal of an infected patient may acquire pulmonary infection. Pathologically, *C. trachomatis* causes peribronchiolar inflammation, but few data regarding the pathologic appearance of *C. trachomatis* infection are available. Infants born to mothers infected with *C. trachomatis* may acquire pneumonia; such patients manifest disease shortly after birth, usually between 2 days and 2 weeks, and always by 6 months of age. Cough and tachypnea, often in the absence of significant fever, are common. Radiographs of infants infected with *C. trachomatis* often show multifocal air-space consolidation combined with interstitial opacities and areas of air-trapping. Patchy areas of atelectasis are often seen.

Chlamydia psittaci

C. psittaci primarily infects birds. Humans usually acquire the disease from pigeons, parakeets, or poultry following inhalation of dried bird excrement containing the organisms. Peribronchiolar mononuclear inflammatory cell infiltration that eventually extends into the alveoli is one of the more common pathologic findings of *C. psittaci* pneumonia. Hyaline membrane formation may occur. Patients with *C. psittaci* pneumonia usually present with fever, nonproductive cough, headache, fever, and chills. The illness is usually mild, with cases of overwhelming infection with hypoxemic respiratory failure occurring rarely.

Chest radiographs in patients with *C. psittaci* pneumonia may show perihilar linear opacities, air-space consolidation, and multifocal or diffuse ground-glass opacities. Hilar lymph node enlargement has been reported as a common finding on the radiographs of patients infected with *C. psittaci*.

Chlamydia pneumoniae

C. pneumoniae is a fairy common cause of community-acquired pneumonia. The disease is rarely severe or fatal. Patients with *C. pneumoniae* pulmonary infection usually present with pharyngitis, fever, and nonproductive cough. The disease is usually self-limited.

The imaging appearances of *C. pneumoniae* pulmonary infection are nonspecific and include air-space consolidation, linear opacities simulating interstitial disease, or a combination of these findings. Pleural effusions occur in about one fifth of patients and may be moderate in size. The radiographic pattern of *C. pneumoniae* infection tends to progress to multilobar opacities over time.

Rickettsiae

Rickettsiae are small obligate intracellular organisms that cause disease when humans are bitten by the arthropods,

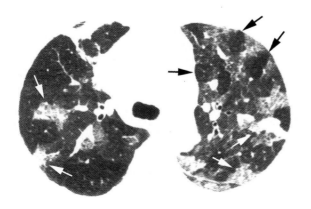

FIG. 12-50. Mycoplasmal pneumonia. HRCT shows patchy, lobular areas of ground-glass opacity and consolidation *(white arrows)*. Lobular lucencies *(black arrows)* reflect mosaic perfusion due to small airway abnormalities.

often ticks, in which the organisms live. The Rickettsia that most commonly causes human pulmonary disease is *Cox-iella burnetii*.

C. burnetii causes Q fever. The organism usually lives in a variety of wild and domestic animals and insects, most notably ticks. Humans may acquire disease when bitten by the arthropod vector, although disease can be transmitted to humans by inhalation when humans come into contact with animals infected by the bacteria.

Few data regarding the pathologic appearance of Q fever are available. Interstitial and alveolar inflammation associated with hemorrhage, edema, and necrosis may occur.

Patients with Q fever present with fever, myalgia, malaise, headache, chills, nonproductive cough, and occasionally shortness of breath and chest pain. Extrathoracic disease manifestations, such as meningoencephalitis, myocarditis, venous thrombosis, and hepatitis, often occur.

Chest radiographs in patients with Q fever often show multifocal, bilateral, basilar predominant areas of consolidation that may be somewhat rounded. Segmental or lobar consolidation may also occur. Pleural effusions are uncommon. Areas of linear atelectasis may also be seen.

Viruses

The viruses that cause thoracic infection are usually transmitted from person to person by hand-to-hand contact, contact with infected surfaces, or aerosol transmission. Viral organisms may be deposited in the nasopharynx and cause upper respiratory infection only, although smaller organisms may be carried into the lungs, causing lower respiratory tract infections such as bronchitis, bronchiolitis, and pneumonia.

Viruses infect cells by interaction with various receptors on cell membranes. Once the virus enters the cell, the virus undergoes replication. This replication may kill the host cell, releasing more viruses to infect other cells. Alternatively, the viral replication may not kill the cell, but the virus continues to replicate within the cell and releases virions. In this situation, the infected cells may express viral antigens that may provoke a reaction from the host immune system. Last, viral infection may result in the virus incorporating itself into the DNA of the host cell, only to cause disease later upon reactivation of this latent infection.

Viral infections may be classified into the RNA virus group and the DNA virus group. RNA viruses include myxoviruses (including influenza virus, parainfluenza virus, respiratory syncytial virus, and measles), coronaviruses, hantaviruses, togaviruses, reoviruses, picornaviruses, arenaviruses, and retroviruses. The DNA virus group includes herpesviruses, adenoviruses, papovaviruses, and poxviruses.

RNA Viruses

Influenza Virus
Influenza is responsible for up to 16 million excess respiratory illnesses per year in the United States among patients below the age of 20 years, and up to 4 million excess respiratory illnesses among those 20 years and older. Each year, approximately 150,000 hospitalizations result from influenza, and as many as 35,000 deaths occur from influenza-related complications. Influenza occurs sporadically, in epidemics, and in worldwide pandemics. Transmission of influenza virus occurs by respiratory droplets, although direct transmission from animals to humans may occur.

Influenza outbreaks tend to occur in the winter. Patients at greatest risk for contracting disease include those with diabetes mellitus, COPD, chronic renal disease, cystic fibrosis, or heart disease, the elderly, immunocompromised patients, and cigarette smokers.

Influenza viruses are divided into types A, B, and C. Type A is most often responsible for serious illnesses, and both epidemics and pandemics are almost exclusively caused by influenza A. Type B influenza tends to cause upper respiratory tract infections, and type C influenza causes sporadic, mild, lower respiratory tract infections. Influenza pulmonary infection causes hemorrhagic and edematous consolidation with diffuse alveolar damage and an associated mononuclear cell inflammatory infiltrate. Infection with influenza renders the host more susceptible to superinfection, usually with bacteria such as pneumococci and staphylococci. Such superinfection may prove fatal.

Influenza infection presents with dry cough, headache, myalgia, low-grade fever, and conjunctivitis. Young children may present with croup or otitis media. When overt pulmonary infection occurs, symptoms of bronchitis occur, followed shortly by signs of severe illness, including cyanosis, hypoxemia, shortness of breath, and chest pain. Bacterial superinfection may be heralded by the onset of purulent cough and worsening fever and chest pain, often in a patient who was improving.

Chest radiography often shows multifocal patchy consolidation that may be unilateral or bilateral. When unilateral, the pulmonary opacities may rapidly progress to bilateral disease. Pleural effusion is relatively uncommon. CT and HRCT may show multifocal patchy air-space consolidation and ground-glass opacities. Imaging findings are usually nonspecific and resemble noncardiogenic pulmonary edema.

Parainfluenza Virus
Parainfluenza viruses are classified into types 1 through 4. Types 1, 2, and 3 are responsible for the majority of human disease. Parainfluenza virus types 1 and 2 usually cause outbreaks of croup or acute bronchiolitis in young children, usually in the fall and winter. Parainfluenza type 3 may cause pneumonia and acute bronchiolitis in children, often in the spring. Parainfluenza viral infections are usually self-limited.

Because parainfluenza viral infection is usually self-limited, little information regarding the pathologic characteristics of infection is available. Infection with parainfluenza virus does render the host more susceptible to bacterial superinfection.

In children, parainfluenza viral infection usually results in croup or, less commonly, acute bronchiolitis. Symptoms of parainfluenza viral acute bronchiolitis include coughing, dyspnea, and wheezing; physical examination may disclose crackles. Parainfluenza viral infection in adults usually causes tonsillitis and pharyngitis. Lower respiratory tract infection by a parainfluenza viral infection is rare in adults.

Radiographs in children with croup may show smooth subglottic tracheal narrowing, the so-called "steeple" sign. Acute bronchiolitis may manifest as a combination of multifocal atelectasis and areas of air-trapping. HRCT may more effectively demonstrate these findings but is rarely indicated unless the patient is immunocompromised and the diagnosis is not straightforward. When parainfluenza virus pneumonia occurs, radiographs are often normal or may show only vague ground-glass opacity or interstitial prominence. HRCT reveals multifocal ground-glass opacity in many patients.

Respiratory Syncytial Virus

Respiratory syncytial virus (RSV) is an important cause of both upper and lower respiratory tract disease in infants and young children. Sporadic infection may occur, but outbreaks often occur in schools or nurseries. Infection is transmitted by respiratory droplets or hand-to-hand contact, often in the winter. Infants with congenital heart disease or pulmonary bronchodysplasia are at particularly high risk.

RSV may cause direct bronchiolar and pulmonary parenchymal damage, although hypersensitivity may also contribute to the pathogenesis of infection. The size of the viral inoculum may also play a role in the pathogenesis of RSV bronchiolar and pulmonary parenchymal infection. In children, RSV typically causes upper respiratory tract symptoms such as pharyngitis, rhinitis, and otitis media. Lower respiratory tract infection produces coughing, dyspnea, wheezing, and intercostal retractions. Physical examination may reveal crackles.

In adults, RSV usually causes symptoms of the common cold, and lower respiratory tract infection is rare. When the latter occurs, it usually affects chronically ill, debilitated, elderly, or immunocompromised patients and produces symptoms suggestive of pneumonia. Respiratory failure resulting from ARDS may occur.

Chest radiographs in patients with RSV infection commonly show perihilar linear opacities, bronchial wall thickening, patchy areas of consolidation, and areas of air-trapping (see Fig. 12-2). Often the radiographic findings seem unimpressive in comparison to the patient's clinical presentation. Hilar lymphadenopathy may occur in a few patients. HRCT may show patchy areas of ground-glass opacity and interstitial thickening (Fig. 12-51).

Measles (Rubeola) Virus

The incidence of measles infection has been dramatically reduced in recent years due to the introduction of immuni-

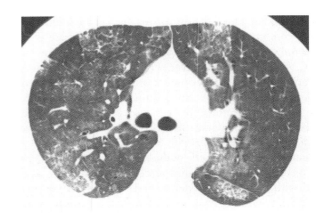

FIG. 12-51. Respiratory syncytial virus pneumonia in an adult. HRCT shows patchy ground-glass opacity associated with interstitial thickening. Interlobular septal thickening is visible.

zation programs. Epidemics, particularly in underdeveloped countries, are still a problem. Adults may rarely contract the disease, possibly from lack of exposure to the infection during childhood.

Measles classically produces giant cell pneumonia, manifest as multinucleated giant cells containing viral inclusions, infiltrating the alveoli and bronchial epithelium. Giant cell pneumonia is characteristic of measles but may also be seen with parainfluenza and RSV infection.

Patients with measles viral infection initially usually present with fever, myalgia, headache, conjunctivitis, cough, and rhinorrhea, followed by the characteristic skin rash. Measles pneumonia develops either before or at the onset of the skin rash and presents with worsening cough and dyspnea. Bacterial superinfection may occur with measles infection, usually after the patient has begun to improve clinically, and presents with worsening purulent cough, fever, and chest pain.

Measles pneumonia usually manifests on chest radiography as bilateral patchy air-space consolidation associated with perihilar linear opacities, bronchial wall thickening, and small nodules. Radiographs in children may show lymph node enlargement, but radiographs in adults usually do not. CT of measles pneumonia may show multifocal ground-glass opacity and consolidation, often with small nodular opacities.

Coronaviruses

Until 2002, coronaviruses were considered relatively unimportant respiratory pathogens, causing only coryza and pharyngitis and other upper respiratory tract ailments. However, in the fall of 2002, a new respiratory illness, known as severe acute respiratory syndrome (SARS), began in southern China. The disease rapidly spread throughout Asia, Europe, and North America (especially Canada) over the ensuing months. By spring 2003, over 4,400 worldwide cases of SARS had been reported, with 263 deaths (as of April 23, 2003) related to the infection (mortality approximately 4%).

The World Health Organization defined SARS cases as either suspect or probable. A suspect case was defined as a patient presenting after November 1, 2002, with fever greater than 38°C; cough or dyspnea; close contact with a SARS patient; history of travel to an affected area or residence within the affected area, all within 10 days prior to the onset of symptoms. A probable case was defined as a suspect case with radiographic evidence of opacities consistent with pneumonia or respiratory distress syndrome, or autopsy results consistent with respiratory distress syndrome without an identifiable cause.

Patients presenting with SARS range from the second through seventh decades of life, and no definite gender predilection has been noted. Affected patients may either have underlying chronic illnesses or be previously healthy.

Viral isolation methods, histology, electron microscopy, and other sophisticated methods have shown that the causative agent of SARS is a coronavirus. The infection is transmitted by respiratory droplets or direct contact. The predominant pattern of the lungs found at autopsy is diffuse alveolar damage with hyaline membrane formation. Some of the tissue damage induced by SARS may be related to a cell-mediated host response.

The most common presenting symptoms of SARS include fever, dyspnea, nonproductive cough, malaise, chills or rigors, and myalgias. The disease course may be mild, or hypoxemic respiratory failure may occur. Factors associated with increased risk of death include advanced age, underlying chronic illness, elevated lactate dehydrogenase levels, and high absolute neutrophil count at presentation.

Imaging Findings. Radiographic abnormalities begin to appear about 12 days after viral exposure (range, 4 to 26 days), or about 5 days after the onset of fever. Patients may present with a normal chest radiograph, but abnormalities usually develop within a matter of a few days following an initially normal radiograph. Radiographic abnormalities in patients with SARS consist of poorly marginated consolidation that may start focally and remain unilateral until resolution, that may start focally and progress to bilateral multifocal opacities, or thay may first be detected as multifocal bilateral opacities. When progression of radiographic abnormalities occurs, it often does so rapidly, usually over a period of a few days. Radiographic abnormalities tend toward a lower lobe predominant location and peripheral distribution. Lymphadenopathy does not occur and pleural effusions are quite rare in patients with SARS. Radiographic clearing may be delayed relative to clinical improvement. Volume loss and scarring have been reported in a few patients.

The HRCT findings of SARS include lower lobe predominant ground-glass opacity associated with thickening of the interlobular septa, occasionally with consolidation. In some patients, a peripheral distribution of the opacities is seen. Nearly half of patients who have undergone HRCT for SARS show some findings of fibrosis, including architectural distortion, traction bronchiectasis, and coarse linear opacities. Such changes may be more likely to occur in older men, patients admitted to the intensive care unit, patients with relatively higher peak levels of lactate dehydrogenase, and patients with more extensive radiographic abnormalities.

Hantaviruses

There are several antigenically different hantaviruses known to cause human disease, such as hemorrhagic fever with renal syndrome and the hantavirus pulmonary syndrome. The natural reservoir of hantaviruses is rodents, in particular the deer mouse. Hantavirus pulmonary syndrome is most commonly encountered in rural areas, especially in the Southwestern United States. Human disease is acquired by the inhalation of dried rodent excrement containing the virus.

Hantavirus infection causes both interstitial and air-space edema accompanied by lymphocytic infiltration, but with little evidence of vascular thrombosis or hyaline membrane formation.

Patients with hantavirus pulmonary syndrome present with fever, myalgia, and headache that progresses to worsening cough, shortness of breath, and then hypotension. Hypoxemia respiratory failure may occur. The death rate approaches 50%.

Chest radiographic findings of hantavirus pulmonary syndrome include peribronchiolar thickening, perihilar indistinctness, and interlobular septal thickening. Air-space consolidation may also be encountered. For patients who do not present with air-space consolidation on the initial chest radiograph, subsequent films may show developing consolidation. Pleural effusions occur in more than half of patients and may be large.

Togaviruses (Rubella)

Rubella is the only significant togavirus from a human respiratory infection viewpoint. Infants born to mothers infected with rubella during the first trimester may develop congenital anomalies. The teratogenic effects of congenital rubella infection include pulmonary abnormalities such as pulmonary artery stenoses and interstitial pneumonitis.

Infants born with pulmonary arterial stenoses from congenital rubella infection may be largely asymptomatic, or they may develop pulmonary arterial hypotension and right heart failure. Interstitial pneumonitis related to congenital rubella infection may be mild or may produce fulminant respiratory failure.

DNA Viruses

Herpesviruses

Numerous antigenically different types of herpesviruses are known to exist, but herpesvirus types 1, 2, 6, 8, varicella-zoster virus, cytomegalovirus, and Epstein-Barr virus are the most important from the standpoint of human disease.

Herpesviruses infect patients and incorporate themselves into the cell of the host, and there may remain latent for the lifetime of the individual. On occasion, particularly when the host becomes immunocompromised, the herpes infection reactivates and causes clinically overt disease. While reactivation episodes are usually minor, they may become quite significant in immunocompromised patients.

Herpes Simplex. Herpes simplex virus type 1 (HSV-1) and herpes simplex virus type 2 (HSV-2) infections usually cause mucosal ulcerations following reactivation of latent infection.

HSV-1 infection is often acquired during childhood and usually affects the oral cavity. Following reactivation of latent disease, lower respiratory tract infection may occur if the organisms are transported into the trachea and bronchi, as could occur with aspiration or endotracheal intubation. However, overt oral cavity infection is not always present, implying that other mechanisms are operative. Patients with HSV-1 infection of the trachea and bronchi are often severely immunocompromised. Tracheobronchial involvement is suggested by the presence of fever and productive cough, occasionally in the presence of the oral ulcerative lesions. Symptoms of HSV-1 pneumonia are nonspecific. Chest radiographs may show multifocal consolidation due to bronchopneumonia. CT and HRCT also show patchy, multifocal ground-glass opacity and consolidation, often associated with small nodules.

HSV-2 pulmonary infection is acquired during birth as the fetus passes through the infected maternal birth canal. The newborn may present with fever, jaundice, seizure, and signs of pneumonia. Radiographs may show patchy air-space consolidation, usually without effusions.

HSV-6 causes roseola (a childhood skin infection). Pulmonary disease is exceedingly rare, usually occurring in immunocompromised patients.

HSV-8 (also called Kaposi's sarcoma–associated herpesvirus) has been implicated in the pathogenesis of both Kaposi's sarcoma and primary effusion lymphoma (previously known as body cavity–based lymphoma). Primary effusion lymphoma presents with fluid accumulation in body cavities, especially the pleural space and peritoneal cavity. Body cavity–based lymphoma tends to present in patients with AIDS and a low CD4 cell count; shortness of breath is commonly present, and the pleural effusions may be quite large. Kaposi's sarcoma is discussed in Chapter 4.

Varicella-zoster Virus. Hematogenous dissemination of the varicella virus develops soon after the organism is in-haled, and the organism subsequently invades the respiratory epithelium. Viral replication eventually results in a second viremic episode, which causes the skin eruption. If pneumonia occurs, the virus will induce diffuse alveolar damage and produce giant cell pneumonia.

Varicella represents the initial varicella-zoster infection in previously uninfected patients, also called chickenpox. Varicella is a very contagious skin infection that usually affects children. About one in six patients with skin infection caused by varicella develop coincident pulmonary infection; this figure is higher for patients ill enough to be admitted to the hospital or for immunocompromised patients. Zoster, also known as shingles, represents reactivation of a latent herpes varicella-zoster infection. Pulmonary infection may occur with either form of herpes varicella-zoster, although it is more commonly seen with varicella. Varicella pneumonia presents as high fever that is usually rapidly followed by a painful skin rash. Chest pain, nonproductive cough, and shortness of breath are common. Radiographic abnormalities often persist after clinical improvement.

Varicella pneumonia appears on chest radiography as diffuse small nodules in the range of 5 to 10 mm that progress to air-space consolidation rather rapidly. Hilar lymphadenopathy is common, but pleural effusion is rare. Radiographic clearing of pulmonary opacities may take weeks or months. Some patients develop multiple bilateral small calcified pulmonary nodules measuring 2 to 3 mm without hilar lymph node calcification.

Cytomegalovirus

Congenital cytomegalovirus (CMV) infection may occur by transplacental spread of the organism, or neonatal infection may occur when the fetus passes through an infected birth canal. Acquired infection with CMV is very common; infection is usually asymptomatic. Pulmonary infection with CMV is usually significant only in patients with impaired immunity. Cell-mediated immunity is particularly important in defense against CMV infection. Clinically overt CMV infection usually occurs as a result of reactivation of latent disease, although reinfection from an endogenous source can occur.

CMV infection may cause direct cellular damage, although the host reaction to infection also contributes to the infectious process. Nevertheless, it is clear that in most patients from whom CMV is isolated, the organism is not a primary pulmonary pathogen. When CMV infects cells, it often produces a characteristic pattern of intranuclear inclusions that fill most of the nucleus and are separated from the remaining nuclear membrane by a characteristic halo, resulting in the so-called owl-eye appearance.

Congenital CMV infection presents with hepatosplenomegaly, jaundice, chorioretinitis, microcephaly, seizures, and thrombocytopenic purpura; mental retardation often results. Neonatal CMV infection, acquired through maternal transmission from an infected birth canal, is often asymptomatic.

CMV infection acquired in childhood or adulthood is often asymptomatic or presents with low-grade fever, lymphadenopathy, and organomegaly.

In immunocompromised patients, CMV infection presents with nonproductive cough, fever, and shortness of breath. Diagnosis rests on demonstrating the presence of the organism and viral inclusions, usually with associated tissue damage, to prove that CMV is the culprit organism.

Imaging Findings. CMV infection usually occurs in the setting of impaired immunity. Chest radiographic findings associated with CMV infection include bilateral reticulation or interstitial opacities, diffuse ground-glass opacities, or multifocal consolidation; chest radiographs may be normal (Fig. 12-52). Diffuse, small nodules are a less common pattern of infection with CMV, and lobar consolidation in CMV infection is uncommon. Bilateral opacities are more commonly encountered than unilateral disease.

CT may reveal multifocal, bilateral areas of ground-glass opacity and foci of air-space consolidation, occasionally accompanied by small centrilobular nodules (see Fig. 12-52; see also Fig. 10-31B in Chapter 10). Small pleural effusions are encountered in less than half of patients, and lymphadenopathy is infrequent.

Epstein-Barr Virus

Epstein-Barr virus (EBV) infects B lymphocytes and cells lining the pharynx. Direct person-to-person transmission is most common, although spread via blood transfusions may also occur.

EBV causes infectious mononucleosis, which presents as hepatosplenomegaly, lymphadenopathy, pharyngitis, and fever. When intrathoracic involvement occurs, lymphade-nopathy is the most common manifestation; interstitial pneumonia may occur but is rare.

Patients with infectious mononucleosis present with fever, malaise, weakness, a minimally productive cough, and pharyngitis. One of the most compelling physical examination findings of infectious mononucleosis is splenomegaly.

EBV is an important pathogen in the pathogenesis of lymphoproliferative disorders, especially Burkitt's lymphoma, lymphomas in patients with AIDS, and posttransplant lymphoproliferative disease.

Adenoviruses

Sporadic adenoviral infection is not an uncommon cause of respiratory infection in childhood. Epidemic outbreaks of adenoviral infection have been reported in military recruits and other situations in which the living quarters are close.

Adenoviral infection causes bronchitis and bronchiolitis that in severe cases progresses to hemorrhagic bronchopneumonia with edema and hyaline membranes.

Adenoviral infection usually presents with pharyngitis, fever, myalgia, malaise, and cough. Disease is usually mild, but rare cases of hypoxemic respiratory failure occur. As discussed previously, adenoviral infection may result in bronchiectasis and bronchiolitis obliterans, including Swyer-James syndrome.

Adenoviral pneumonia may present on chest radiography with multifocal bilateral bronchopneumonia associated with air-trapping. In one of the largest series detailing the chest radiographic appearance of adenoviral infection, lobar collapse was a common event; the right upper lobe was particularly commonly involved. Resolution of infection may be complete but occasionally results in pulmonary scarring, especially when infection occurs in patients under the age of 2 years.

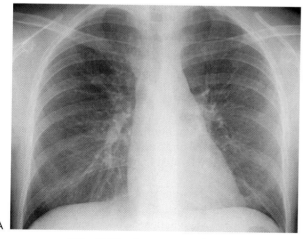
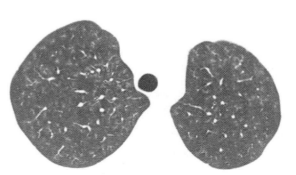

FIG. 12-52. Cytomegalovirus infection in an immunosuppressed patient. **A.** Chest radiograph is normal. **B.** Axial CT image shows multiple small centrilobular areas of ground-glass opacity.

Parasites: Protozoans, Roundworms (Nematodes), and Flatworms

Amebiasis

Amebiasis is caused by the protozoan *Entamoeba histolytica*. The organism usually causes amebic dysentery, with pulmonary disease occurring as a complication of colon or liver disease.

Amebic dysentery is most prevalent in underdeveloped countries, where transmission of the organism from person to person occurs by the fecal–oral route. In the United States, many cases of amebic dysentery occur in immigrants who have been in the United States for only a short time. Pulmonary amebiasis is far more common in men and usually occurs in young to middle-aged adults.

The life cycle of *E. histolytica* begins with the host ingesting cysts in contaminated food or water. The cyst form of the organism is acid-resistant, so it is capable of passing through the stomach and into small intestine unharmed. Once in the small intestine, *E. histolytica* excysts and forms trophozoites, which then migrate to the colon. From there, organisms may be passed in feces to complete the life cycle of the organism.

The organisms may be transported to the liver, where an amebic abscess may form; such abscesses are almost always located in the cranial portion of the liver, usually in the right lobe. From there, direct transdiaphragmatic spread of infection may cause pleural effusion or lung abscess formation. Very rarely, pulmonary or pleural infection forms in the absence of a liver abscess by extension of the organisms through the hemorrhoidal veins, the transdiaphragmatic lymphatics or the thoracic duct, or the hepatic veins.

Patients with pulmonary or pleural amebic abscesses usually present with right upper quadrant pain, fever, and cough. Chest pain may also be present. Patients may also expectorate the characteristic "anchovy paste" or "chocolate sauce" material that usually represents amebic abscesses. Rarely, biloptysis occurs. Gastrointestinal symptoms are often, but not invariably, present.

Amebic pulmonary infection usually presents as lower lobe air-space consolidation, usually on the right, often accompanied by a pleural effusion (Fig. 12-53). The latter may be quite large. Cavitation within the consolidation may occur. Amebic abscesses in the liver, uncomplicated by pulmonary abscesses, often cause elevation of the right diaphragm with basilar atelectasis; a small pleural effusion may be present.

Toxoplasmosis

Toxoplasmosis is caused by the protozoan *Toxoplasma gondii*. *T. gondii* is an intracellular protozoan that commonly causes human infection, although such infections are often not clinically apparent. *T. gondii* is distributed worldwide.

Human infection is extremely common but usually asymptomatic.

The organism's definitive host is the cat, and mice or rats may serve as an intermediate host. Humans acquire disease when they ingest the oocyte form of the parasite in contaminated water or food or in undercooked meat. Once ingested, the oocyte excysts and forms trophozoites, which may cross the intestine and disseminate through the bloodstream. The trophozoites usually travel to the heart, skeletal muscle, and brain most commonly, where they may remain viable and cause infection when the host becomes immunocompromised. *T. gondii* can also be transmitted from women to their fetuses by the transplacental route.

Most infections caused by *T. gondii* are asymptomatic. When symptoms are present, they most often include low-grade fever and lymphadenopathy; the presentation somewhat resembles mononucleosis. Immunocompromised patients may develop disseminated disease; when *T. gondii* pneumonia occurs in this setting, fever, dry cough, and shortness of breath may be encountered. Neurologic symptoms, due to *T. gondii* brain infection, may occur.

Overt pulmonary infection in patients without impaired immunity is uncommon. Chest radiographs may show bilateral linear opacities suggesting an interstitial process, perhaps accompanied by hilar lymphadenopathy. HRCT will reveal patchy areas of ground-glass opacity, possibly with some foci of consolidation.

Ascariasis

Ascaris lumbricoides is a nematode (roundworm) that causes the majority of cases of the infection known as ascariasis. *Ascaris suum* may also cause this infection.

A. lumbricoides infection is acquired by the ingestion of food or water contaminated by worm's ova. The larval forms of the worm develop within the ovum inside the small intestine of the host. Once the larval forms hatch, they may burrow through the wall of the small intestine to reach the portal venous circulation. The larvae may then migrate to the pulmonary capillary circulation, and then into the alveoli. From there, the larva may migrate into the proximal airways and into the larynx, where they are swallowed. Eventually they reach the small intestine and develop into adult worms, where they may produce eggs that are passed in the feces to complete the worm's life cycle. *A. lumbricoides* infection is most commonly encountered in Southeast Asia, Africa, and Central and South America. However, infection does occur in the United States, especially in the southeastern region.

Although the worms can be comparatively large (often over 30 cm in length), *A. lumbricoides* infection is usually asymptomatic. Most patients who experience symptoms develop gastrointestinal complaints. As the worms migrate through the lungs, they can cause bronchopneumonia, pro-

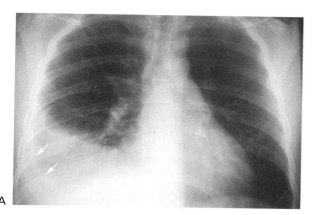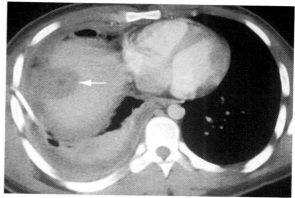

FIG. 12-53. Amebic pneumonia and liver abscess. **A.** Frontal chest radiograph shows right lower lobe pneumonia and right pleural effusion *(arrows)*, initially interpreted as community-acquired pneumonia and parapneumonic effusion. The patient's symptoms and the radiographic abnormalities failed to resolve with therapy directed toward community-acquired pneumonia. **B.** Axial CT image through the cranial aspect of the liver shows right lower lobe consolidation and a low-attenuation lesion within the liver *(arrow)*.

ducing symptoms of chest pain, shortness of breath, cough, and hemoptysis.

When pulmonary infection is present, air-space consolidation is usually encountered. Pneumonia may be caused by the migration of the larvae or by vomiting with aspiration. Often the air-space opacities are transient.

Strongyloidiasis

Strongyloides stercoralis is the nematode (roundworm) that causes most cases of strongyloidiasis. *S. stercoralis* infection is endemic in tropical areas, although infection does occur in the United States. Immunocompromised patients, particularly those with AIDS, are at increased risk.

Human infection with *S. stercoralis* begins with larvae penetrating the skin of the human host, after which they travel to the lungs via the bloodstream. Once the larvae reach the lungs, they migrate through the airways into the larynx, then into the esophagus, and finally into the small intestine. There, the larvae develop into adult worms and lay eggs. The eggs may be passed in feces to perpetuate the life cycle, although eggs also have the ability to develop into larval forms while still in the intestine. Once larvae form in the intestine, they may directly penetrate the intestinal wall and migrate to the lungs and back to the gut. This ability is termed autoinfection and allows the organism to perpetuate infection within the host.

Most patients with *S. stercoralis* infection are asymptomatic. When symptoms occur, cough, shortness of breath, and hemoptysis may be seen.

Chest radiography in patients with *S. stercoralis* infection may show patchy areas of air-space consolidation. Other patterns, such as nodular consolidation, small nodules, or reticulation, have been reported. Pleural effusions occur in a few patients.

Dirofilariasis

Dirofilaria are nematodes. Several species of *Dirofilaria* may cause dirofilariasis, but the most common species is *Dirofilaria immitis*.

D. immitis infection is primarily encountered in the eastern United States, although the infection has been seen in Europe, Canada, and South America. Adults are far more commonly affected than children. Dogs are the most common definitive hosts for *D. immitis*; the organism is the cause of dog heartworm. The infection is transmitted by mosquito bites, and humans become intermediate hosts when they are bitten by an infected mosquito. Because the filaria cannot complete their life cycles in humans, the organisms die and are transported to the pulmonary arterial circulation, where they may incite an inflammatory reaction.

Patients with *D. immitis* infection are usually asymptomatic. Cough, hemoptysis, and chest pain may occur. The diagnosis is usually discovered upon biopsy of a pulmonary nodule. Serum eosinophilia may occur but is not marked.

The typical chest radiographic appearance of *D. immitis* infection is a peripheral, circumscribed solitary pulmonary nodule (see Fig. 9-33 in Chapter 9). Less commonly, multiple nodules or air-space consolidation is seen.

Tropical Eosinophilia

Tropical eosinophilia refers to an asthma-like condition caused primarily by two nematodes: *Wuchereria bancrofti* and *Brugia malayi*. As the name implies, the disease is seen most commonly in the tropics. Tropical eosinophilia is most commonly seen in Southeast Asia, Africa, India, and the West Indies.

Tropical eosinophilia is acquired when an infected mosquito bites a person and injects the larvae into the lymphatics. Larvae mature into adult worms in the lymphatics and produce microfilariae; the latter reach the bloodstream and are ingested by an uninfected mosquito, thus completing the life cycle. As the microfilariae travel the bloodstream, they may become trapped within pulmonary capillaries and induce a hypersensitivity reaction.

Patients often present with a mildly productive cough, occasionally with hemoptysis. Low-grade fever, weight loss, and other constitutional symptoms may occur. Blood eosinophilia is common.

Chest radiographs in patients with tropical eosinophilia usually show a basilar predominant, symmetric, small nodular or reticular and nodular pattern. Lymphadenopathy may occur. Pleural effusions are uncommon.

Toxocariasis (Visceral Larval Migrans)

Toxocara canis and *Toxocara catis* are the two organisms that cause the roundworm infection toxocariasis. The former organism generally infects dogs and the latter cats. Toxocariasis occurs in tropical and temperate regions alike, with symptomatic human disease occurring more commonly in the former.

Dogs and cats normally serve as the definitive hosts for *Toxocara* sp. The parasite eggs reach the soil when the definitive hosts pass them, through feces, into soil. Toxocariasis may occur when humans, often children, ingest soil containing the eggs of the organism. Once ingested, the eggs develop into larvae in the intestine of the human host and are then carried in the bloodstream to various organs, including the brain, liver, eyes, lungs, and heart. The larvae cannot develop properly in these organs and instead migrate into the surrounding tissues, where they often eventually die, evoking a host granulomatous inflammatory reaction.

Patients are often asymptomatic. When clinically overt pulmonary infection occurs, cough, shortness of breath, and symptoms referable to other involved organs (such as the brain) may be present.

Patchy, poorly defined areas of air-space consolidation may be encountered on chest radiographs during the course of pulmonary infection.

Paragonimiasis

Paragonimiasis is caused by worms of the flatworm genus *Paragonimus*. Most human disease is caused by infestation by *Paragonimus westermani*. Paragonimiasis occurs most frequently in Southeast Asia and less commonly in South and Central America and Africa. The infection is particularly common in the Philippines. North American disease occurs in immigrants from these regions or from comparatively rare infections by a related organism found in North America, *Paragonimus kellicotti*.

Humans acquire paragonimiasis by ingesting the organism when they eat infected shellfish. The ingested organisms, called *metacercariae*, develop in the small intestine of the human host and then migrate through the intestinal wall into the peritoneum. From there, the organisms burrow through the diaphragm into the lungs, where they develop into adult worms. In the lungs, adult worms lay eggs that are either coughed up or swallowed and excreted in feces, where they reach the soil. In the soil, the eggs develop into miracidia, which can then infect freshwater snails. Within the snails, the miracidia develop further and form cercariae, which then infect shellfish (crab and crayfish) to complete the life cycle.

The typical symptoms of fever, cough, and chest pain occur when the organisms are migrating through the lung parenchyma. Hemoptysis becomes a common symptom in patients with chronic disease.

Imaging Findings

Chest radiographs in patients infected with *P. westermani* often show basilar predominant small, thin-walled cystic lesions or ring shadows, perhaps accompanied by poorly defined areas of nodular consolidation (see Fig. 9-44 in Chapter 9). The cystic areas are usually small, often less than 1 cm, but may be as large as 5 cm. Patchy areas of nonsegmental consolidation may also be seen, and the ring shadows, nodules, and consolidation may be seen together or separate from one another. On CT, there may be crescentic thickening of a portion of the cystic lesions, perhaps representing the worm itself.

Pleural effusions occur in more than half of patients. The pulmonary parenchymal lesions may calcify in chronic cases.

In patients immigrating to the United States from endemic regions, a pattern resembling postprimary TB has been described.

Schistosomiasis

Schistosomiasis is caused by flatworms of the genus Schistosoma; the species *Schistosoma mansoni*, *Schistosoma japonicum*, *Schistosoma mekongi*, and *Schistosoma haematobium* are the most important etiologic agents of this infection.

Schistosomiasis is a very important parasitic infection worldwide. *S. mansoni* and *S. haematobium* are endemic in the Middle East and Africa, whereas *S. japonicum* is endemic in Japan, China, and the Philippines. *S. mekongi* infection occurs in Southeast Asia. *S. mansoni* may also be found in South America and the West Indies. Schistosomiasis infection in North America is most often encountered in individuals emigrating from endemic regions.

Cercariae living in water in endemic regions may infect humans when they drink infected water, or the organisms may burrow into skin when humans work in infected waters. Once the cercariae penetrate human integument, they change into a form known as a schistosomula and migrate into the pulmonary venous circulation. From here, the organisms migrate to the hepatic portal circulation and develop further. The worms then migrate to the mesenteric venous circulation (*S. mansoni, S. japonicum, S. mekongi*) or the perivesicular veins (*S. haematobium*), and then adult worms reproduce in these venules. Laden with eggs, the adult female worm burrows into the submucosa of either the bowel or bladder and lays eggs, which then may be passed into water via feces or urine. In the water, the eggs develop into miracidia, which then infect snails. Within the snail, cercariae develop, eventually to leave the snail to infect humans and complete the organism's life cycle.

The release of eggs into human tissue by the adult female worm precipitates a host inflammatory response and is usually the cause of clinically overt disease. These eggs may produce inflammation within the wall of the organ in question (either bladder or bowel), or they may be released into the associated venous circulation and embolize downstream organs. In the cases of *S. japonicum*, *S. mansoni*, and *S. mekongi*, the eggs may travel the mesenteric venous system to the liver; eggs released by *S. haematobium* may reach the inferior vena cava and travel to the lungs. If cirrhosis develops, eggs from the organisms that typically inhabit the mesenteric vasculature may also reach the lungs through collateral circulation. Once these eggs reach the lungs, they may extend through the capillaries into the surrounding tissue and induce a fibrotic reaction that obliterates small vessels, inducing pulmonary hypertension.

A transitory febrile reaction, associated with gastrointestinal symptoms, cough, and constitutional findings, may occur with initial infection. As eggs embolize to the lungs, patients may develop cough, shortness of breath, and hypoxemia. Chronically, pulmonary hypertension, which develops in a minority of patients and usually after repeated infection, presents with right heart failure. *S. haematobium* may cause hematuria.

Imaging Findings

Transient opacities (a Löeffler-like syndrome) may occur on chest radiography as the schistosomes enter the pulmonary circulation shortly after infection. The migration of the eggs from the pulmonary vessels into the surrounding tissues, and the host inflammatory reaction that results, may produce radiographically evident abnormalities, commonly focal or multifocal consolidation. Pulmonary hypertension caused by schistosomiasis has the same appearance as other causes of pulmonary hypertension: dilation of the main and central pulmonary arteries with peripheral tapering. Cirrhosis may be caused by the organisms that inhabit the mesenteric venous circulation.

Echinococcosis (Hydatid Disease)

Echinococcosis is primarily caused by the tapeworms (Cestodes) *Echinococcus granulosus* and *Echinococcus multilocularis*. *E. granulosus* is responsible for most cases of hydatid disease.

Epidemiology

E. granulosus causes infection in two basic varieties, the pastoral and sylvatic forms, that differ in terms of their definitive and intermediate hosts and the geographic disease distribution. The clinical and imaging appearances are also slightly different between these two disease forms.

The intermediate hosts for the more common pastoral variety of echinococcosis are domestic farm animals, such as sheep, cows, pigs, and horses; dogs are the usual definitive hosts. This form of the disease is endemic in southeastern Europe, North Africa, the Middle East, and Russia.

The definitive hosts for the sylvatic form of echinococcosis are canines such as foxes, wolves, and coyotes. The intermediate hosts for the sylvatic disease form are moose, deer, and the like. This form of echinococcosis is found primarily in Alaska and Canada.

The definitive hosts for *E. multilocularis* are also canines, including dogs, foxes, and wolves. The intermediate hosts include various rodents. *E. multilocularis* is endemic in southern Europe (especially Switzerland and Germany), Alaska, Russia, and Canada.

The normal life cycle begins with the usual intermediate hosts ingesting the eggs, passed from definitive hosts, in contaminated food, water, or soil. The eggs develop into larvae in the gut of the intermediate host and eventually penetrate through the intestinal wall and migrate into the portal venous system and then to the liver. Many larvae are trapped in the liver, but some escape the liver and come to rest in the pulmonary circulation. Most larvae are killed, but some develop into cysts containing immature worms. The life cycle is completed when the definitive host feeds on the remains of the intermediate host, and the cysts develop into adult worms in the gut of the definitive hosts.

Humans acquire disease by the ingestion of food, water, or soil contaminated by intermediate-host feces containing the organisms (which usually live in the small intestine of the intermediate host). In this fashion, humans become an inadvertent intermediate host.

About 60% to 70% of cases of *E. granulosus* occur in the liver, and 15% to 30% occur in the lung parenchyma. The few remaining cases occur in a variety of other organs, including the brain, heart, and kidneys. Lung abnormalities are more common than liver findings in the sylvatic form of the disease.

The hydatid cysts that occur in intermediate hosts consist of an outer fibrotic capsule called the **pericyst**, an outer **exocyst**, and an inner **endocyst**. The endocyst produces fluid and gives rise to immature forms called **brood cap-**

sules. Larval forms develop within these brood capsules. Daughter cysts may develop directly from the larval forms within the brood capsules or directly from the exocyst, creating the overall appearance of a multilocular cystic lesion on imaging studies.

E. multilocularis has a life cycle similar to *E. granulosus*. However, the structure of the cyst that forms in *E. multilocularis* is different than that of *E. granulosus*. In contrast to *E. granulosus*, the exocyst is rather poorly formed and the pericyst does not form at all.

Hydatid disease causes symptoms by compression of adjacent structures or by rupture of a cyst with an ensuing host inflammatory response, although most patients remain asymptomatic. Cyst rupture may be heralded by sudden onset of cough, hemoptysis, chest pain, fever, and systemic hypersensitivity. Purulent sputum production may occur with bacterial superinfection of hydatid cysts.

Imaging Findings

Chest radiographs in patients with echinococcosis often show a single, lower lobe, circumscribed nodule or mass of variable size, ranging from 1 cm to more than 15 cm (see Fig. 9-34 in Chapter 9). Multiple lesions are seen in 20% to 30% of patients. Pulmonary hydatid cysts grow slowly and, unlike their liver counterparts, usually do not calcify.

Pulmonary hydatid cysts may change shape with respiration and are often irregularly deformed by adjacent anatomy, such as vessels or mediastinal structures.

If the cyst acquires a communication with the tracheobronchial tree, several radiographic patterns may occur. If the pericyst ruptures, allowing air to gain access to the potential space between the pericyst and exocyst, a meniscus or crescent sign may be observed. This sign is not very common overall and is practically seen only with the pastoral form of echinococcosis. If a communication develops between the tracheobronchial tree and the endocyst, an air-fluid level may form within the cyst, accompanied by surrounding pulmonary parenchymal consolidation that represents expelled cyst fluid. Additionally, once tracheobronchial communication with the cyst occurs, the cyst membrane may collapse and float on the resulting air-fluid level, creating a irregular contour to the air-fluid level, representing the characteristic "waterlily (camalote)" sign.

CT often shows that the rounded or oval lesions in patients with pulmonary echinococcosis have fluid attenuation. CT may also effectively show the collapsed cyst membranes as well as the configuration of daughter cysts. CT also effectively shows chest wall invasion or pleural extension by the cysts. In the uncommon patient in whom hydatid pulmonary disease results from extension of an infectious focus from the liver across the diaphragm, CT may show the cystic liver lesion in continuity with pulmonary and pleural disease.

Cysticercosis

The larval form of the tapeworm *Taenia solium* is the cause of cysticercosis. The adult *T. solium* tapeworms usually live asymptomatically in the intestine of the human definitive host. Cysticercosis is endemic in parts of Africa, Europe (especially Spain and Portugal), and Central America.

Humans acquire infection by ingesting undercooked meat containing cysticerci from an intermediate host, usually a pig. The ingested immature forms develop into adult worms within the human gut, shedding eggs in the feces, which are in turn eaten by the intermediate host, completing the organism's life cycle. Humans may also serve as both intermediate and definitive hosts, creating a pattern known as **autoinfection**. This occurs when humans ingest the eggs of the tapeworm directly, or if the eggs are regurgitated back into the stomach. With autoinfection, the ingested eggs hatch into immature forms that migrate through the intestinal wall into the mesenteric veins and are then carried to various organs, such as the brain, eyes, and skeletal muscle, where they develop into cysticerci. Cysticercosis is often asymptomatic. Neurologic involvement may cause seizures, and respiratory muscle involvement may cause chest pain.

Cysticercosis may present as small calcified nodules, which may be oval or cigar shaped, and are often seen in the musculature of the thorax on chest radiographs.

SELECTED READING

Antonio GE, Wong KT, Hui DS, et al. Thin-section CT in patients with severe acute respiratory syndrome following hospital discharge: preliminary experience. Radiology 2003; 228:810–815.

Brecher CW, Aviram G, Boiselle PM. CT and radiography of bacterial respiratory infections in AIDS patients. AJR Am J Roentgenol 2003; 180:1203–1209.

Erasmus JJ, McAdams HP, Farrell MA, Patz EF, Jr. Pulmonary nontuberculous mycobacterial infection: radiologic manifestations. Radiographics 1999; 19:1487–1505.

Franquet T, Müller NL, Gimenez A, et al. Spectrum of pulmonary aspergillosis: histologic, clinical, and radiologic findings. Radiographics 2001; 21:825–837.

Gotway MB, Dawn SK, Caoili EM, et al. The radiologic spectrum of pulmonary *Aspergillus* infections. J Comput Assist Tomogr 2002; 26:159–173.

Grinblat L, Shulman H, Glickman A, et al. Severe acute respiratory syndrome: radiographic review of 40 probable cases in Toronto, Canada. Radiology 2003; 228:802–809.

Gruden JF, Huang L, Turner J, et al. High-resolution CT in the evaluation of clinically suspected *Pneumocystis carinii* pneumonia in AIDS patients with normal, equivocal, or nonspecific radiographic findings. AJR Am J Roentgenol 1997; 169:967–975.

Kim EA, Lee KS, Primack SL, et al. Viral pneumonias in adults: radiologic and pathologic findings. Radiographics 2002; 22: S137–S149.

Leung AN. Pulmonary tuberculosis: the essentials. Radiology 1999; 210:307–322.

Leung AN, Brauner MW, Gamsu G, et al. Pulmonary tuberculosis: comparison of CT findings in HIV-seropositive and HIV-seronegative patients. Radiology 1996; 198:687–691.

Lieberman D, Ben-Yaakov M, Lazarovich Z, et al. *Chlamydia pneumoniae* community-acquired pneumonia: a review of 62 hospitalized adult patients. Infection 1996; 24:109–114.

Lieberman D, Porath A, Schlaeffer F, Boldur I. *Legionella* species community-acquired pneumonia. A review of 56 hospitalized adult patients. Chest 1996; 109:1243–1249.

McAdams HP, Rosado de Christenson ML, Lesar M, Templeton PA, Moran CA. Thoracic mycoses from endemic fungi: radiologic-pathologic correlation. Radiographics 1995; 15:255–270.

McAdams HP, Rosado de Christenson ML, Templeton PA, et al. Thoracic mycoses from opportunistic fungi: radiologic-pathologic correlation. Radiographics 1995; 15:271–286.

Porath A, Schlaeffer F, Pick N, et al. Pneumococcal community-acquired pneumonia in 148 hospitalized adult patients. Eur J Clin Microbiol Infect Dis 1997; 16:863–870.

Reittner P, Muller NL, Heyneman L, et al. *Mycoplasma pneumoniae* pneumonia: radiographic and high-resolution CT features in 28 patients. AJR Am J Roentgenol 2000; 174:37–41.

Saurborn DP, Fishman JE, Boiselle PM. The imaging spectrum of pulmonary tuberculosis in AIDS. J Thorac Imaging 2002; 17:28–33.

Sider L, Gabriel H, Curry DR, Pham MS. Pattern recognition of the pulmonary manifestations of AIDS on CT scans. Radiographics 1993; 13:771–776.

Sullivan KM, Monto AS, Longini IM, Jr. Estimates of the US health impact of influenza. Am J Public Health 1993; 83:1712–1716.

13

THE IDIOPATHIC INTERSTITIAL PNEUMONIAS

W. RICHARD WEBB

The idiopathic interstitial pneumonias (IIPs) are a heterogeneous group of diffuse lung diseases occurring without known cause, and associated with varying degrees of interstitial lung inflammation and fibrosis. The IIPs have been classified by a consensus committee of the American Thoracic Society and the European Respiratory Society into seven types, based on their histologic pattern, clinical features, and radiographic appearances (Table 13-1). Each of the IIPs is referred to using an acronym. Knowing these acronyms is appropriate, as they are in common usage.

In order of decreasing frequency, the IIPs are as follows:

1. Idiopathic pulmonary fibrosis (IPF)
2. Nonspecific interstitial pneumonia (NSIP)
3. Cryptogenic organizing pneumonia (COP)
4. Acute interstitial pneumonia (AIP)
5. Respiratory bronchiolitis–interstitial lung disease (RB-ILD)
6. Desquamative interstitial pneumonia (DIP)
7. Lymphoid interstitial pneumonia (LIP)

In this classification, a distinction is made between the histologic pattern of the IIP and the idiopathic clinical syndrome associated with it. In several cases, these have different names (see Table 13-1).

Although the IIPs are designated as idiopathic, identical histologic patterns, radiographic appearances, and clinical symptoms may occur in association with specific diseases

TABLE 13-1. IDIOPATHIC INTERSTITIAL PNEUMONIAS: CLASSIFICATION AND DIFFERENTIAL DIAGNOSIS

Histologic pattern	Idiopathic clinical syndrome	Differential diagnosis of the histologic pattern
Usual interstitial pneumonia (UIP)	Idiopathic pulmonary fibrosis (IPF)	Collagen-vascular disease, asbestosis, drug toxicity, radiation, chronic hypersensitivity pneumonitis, familial pulmonary fibrosis
Nonspecific interstitial pneumonia (NSIP)	Nonspecific interstitial pneumonia (NSIP)	Collagen-vascular disease, hypersensitivity pneumonitis, drug toxicity, infection, immunodeficiency
Organizing pneumonia (OP); also known as bronchiolitis obliterans organizing pneumonia (BOOP)	Cryptogenic organizing pneumonia (COP)	Infection, bronchial obstruction, aspiration, drug reactions, collagen vascular disease, toxic-fume inhalation, radiation pneumonitis, hypersensitivity pneumonitis
Diffuse alveolar damage (DAD)	Acute interstitial pneumonia (AIP)	Acute respiratory distress syndrome (ARDS) of known cause (e.g., sepsis, shock, infection, drug toxicity, toxic inhalations, trauma)
Respiratory bronchiolitis (RB)	Respiratory bronchiolitis–interstitial lung disease (RB-ILD)	Smoking (usually), inhalations
Desquamative interstitial pneumonia (DIP)	Desquamative interstitial pneumonia (DIP)	Smoking (usually), inhalations
Lymphoid interstitial pneumonia (LIP)	Lymphoid interstitial pneumonia (LIP)	Collagen-vascular diseases (particularly Sjögren's syndrome, rheumatoid arthritis, and lupus), immunologic disorders (e.g., Hashimoto's thyroiditis, autoimmune hemolytic anemia, myasthenia gravis, pernicious anemia, chronic active hepatitis), infection, immunodeficiency (e.g., AIDS), drug toxicity

or exposures, including collagen-vascular disease, drug reactions, smoking, and infection (see Table 13-1). It is helpful to think of the histologic patterns seen in the IIP as having a differential diagnosis, with one of the possible causes being an idiopathic syndrome (see Table 13-1). Since the radiographic appearances of the IIP parallel their histologic patterns, this approach allows the appropriate radiographic or high-resolution CT (HRCT) differential diagnosis to be suggested.

USUAL INTERSTITIAL PNEUMONIA AND IDIOPATHIC PULMONARY FIBROSIS

Idiopathic pulmonary fibrosis (IPF) is the IIP associated with the histologic pattern termed *usual interstitial pneumonia* (UIP).

Histologically, UIP is characterized by a heterogeneous pattern with foci of normal lung, interstitial inflammation, fibroblastic proliferation, interstitial fibrosis, and honeycombing. Histologic abnormalities appear to represent different stages in the temporal evolution of fibrosis, a combination of end-stage and more active lesions. This is termed *temporal heterogeneity*; it is characteristic of UIP and is not seen in other idiopathic interstitial pneumonias. Lung involvement is patchy, although there is a predominance in the subpleural and basal lung regions (Table 13-2).

UIP may be associated with collagen-vascular disease, asbestosis, drug toxicity, radiation, chronic hypersensitivity pneumonitis, or familial pulmonary fibrosis. Idiopathic UIP is termed idiopathic pulmonary fibrosis. IPF accounts for about 70% of cases of UIP.

IPF occurs most frequently in patients older than 50 (see Table 13-2). Symptoms include progressive dyspnea, cough, weight loss, and finger clubbing; symptoms usually precede presentation by 6 months. Pulmonary function tests (PFTs) show restriction with a reduced diffusing capacity. Treatment is largely ineffective. IPF has a poor prognosis, with a mean survival of 3 to 4 years from the onset of symptoms. The 5-year survival rate is 20%. Lung transplantation may be required.

The diagnosis of IPF is limited to patients with histologic findings of UIP; in other words, if it is not UIP, it is not IPF. Histologic diagnosis requires an open lung biopsy; transbronchoscopic biopsy is not sufficient for diagnosis but may be used to exclude other causes of lung disease.

In the absence of lung biopsy, a diagnosis of IPF may be based on a combination of clinical, functional, and HRCT findings. IPF is considered likely if all four major criteria and three of four minor criteria are present (Table 13-3). These criteria outline common features of this disease.

Radiographic Findings

In 80% of patients with UIP/IPF, radiographs show a bilateral reticular pattern predominantly involving the lower lung zones and subpleural lung regions (Figs. 13-1 and 13-

---

TABLE 13-2. USUAL INTERSTITIAL PNEUMONIA (UIP) AND IDIOPATHIC PULMONARY FIBROSIS (IPF): HISTOLOGIC, CLINICAL, AND HRCT FEATURES

UIP: histologic pattern
Characteristics
  Temporal inhomogeneity
  Dense fibrosis, often with honeycombing
  Fibroblastic foci
  Patchy lung involvement
  Subpleural and basal predominance
Differential diagnosis
  Idiopathic (IPF)
  Collagen-vascular disease
  Asbestosis
  Drug toxicity
  Radiation
  Chronic hypersensitivity pneumonitis
  Familial pulmonary fibrosis

IPF: idiopathic clinical syndrome
Age >50 years
Progressive dyspnea; duration of symptoms 3 months or more
Velcro rales
Pulmonary function tests: restriction and impaired gas exchange
Treatment largely ineffective
Mean survival 3–4 years
HRCT findings highly accurate in diagnosis
  Honeycombing
  Reticulation
  Subpleural and basal predominance
  Little ground-glass opacity

---

2). In its earliest stages, a fine reticular pattern may be visible in the posterior costophrenic angles on the lateral radiograph (see Fig. 13-1B), and the lateral radiograph is often more sensitive than the PA view in making this diagnosis. As fibrosis progresses, the reticular pattern becomes coarse;

TABLE 13-3. CRITERIA FOR A CLINICAL DIAGNOSIS OF IDIOPATHIC PULMONARY FIBROSIS

Major criteria
Exclusion of known causes of infiltrative lung disease such as exposures, drugs, and connective tissue disease
Abnormal pulmonary function tests with evidence of restriction and impaired gas exchange
HRCT findings of bibasilar reticulation with minimal ground-glass opacity
Transbronchial lung biopsy or bronchoalveolar lavage showing no evidence of another disease

Minor criteria
Age >50 years
Insidious onset of dyspnea on exertion
Duration of illness of ≥3 months
Bibasilar inspiratory crackles (so-called Velcro rales)

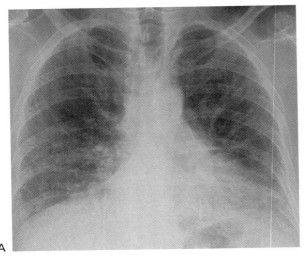

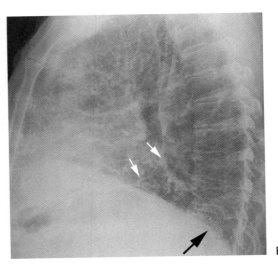

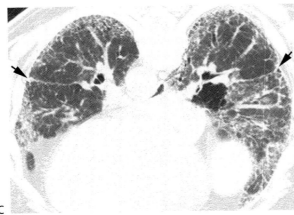

FIG. 13-1. Chest radiograph and HRCT in a patient with histologically proven idiopathic pulmonary fibrosis. **A.** PA radiograph shows reduced lung volumes. There is an increase in reticular opacities in the lung periphery and at the lung bases. This appearance and distribution are typical of idiopathic pulmonary fibrosis. **B.** Lateral view shows increased reticular opacities in the posterior costophrenic angles *(black arrow).* A major fissure *(white arrows)* is bowed posteriorly because of more severe fibrosis in the lower lobe. **C.** Prone HRCT shows extensive subpleural reticular opacities with mild honeycombing. The major fissures *(arrows)* are displaced posteriorly because of lower lobe fibrosis.

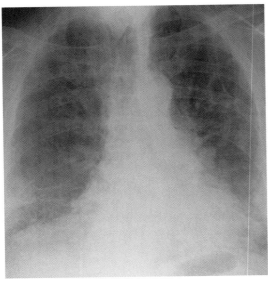

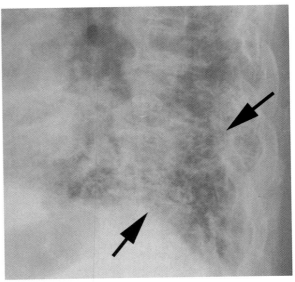

FIG. 13-2. Chest radiograph and HRCT in a patient with idiopathic pulmonary fibrosis. **A.** PA radiograph shows ill-defined reticular opacities at the lung bases. **B.** Coned-down lateral view shows a coarse reticular pattern *(arrows)* in the posterior costophrenic angles. *(Figure continues.)*

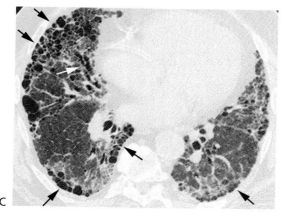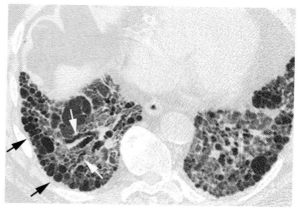

FIG. 13-2. *(Continued.)* **C and D.** HRCT shows extensive subpleural honeycombing *(black arrows)*, reticular opacities, and traction bronchiectasis *(white arrows)*. The honeycomb cysts range from a few millimeters to 2 cm in diameter.

cystic areas of honeycombing are visible in about half of cases (see Fig. 13-2). Pleural thickening or effusion is very uncommon.

Because of lung fibrosis, decreased lung volume is typical (see Fig. 13-1A), and serial chest radiographs are often used to monitor progressive reduction in lung volume with time. Because of greater fibrosis and volume loss in the lower lobes, the major fissures may be seen to bow posteriorly (see Fig. 13-1B).

A combination of clinical and radiographic findings is sufficient to make an accurate diagnosis of IPF in about 70% of cases. In 10% of cases, the radiograph appears normal.

HRCT Findings

On HRCT, UIP/IPF is usually characterized by the presence of honeycombing, irregular reticular opacities, and traction bronchiectasis (see Figs. 13-2 and 13-3 and Table 13-2). In many cases of IPF, findings of honeycombing predominate. Honeycomb cysts usually range from 2 mm to 2 cm in diameter but may be larger. Honeycombing may be asymmetrical (Fig. 13-4).

On HRCT, findings of UIP/IPF typically predominate in the peripheral, subpleural regions and in the lung bases. A subpleural predominance is evident on HRCT in 80% to 95%, and either concentric (Fig. 13-5A) or patchy (Fig. 13-6) subpleural honeycombing is characteristic (see Fig. 13-3). In approximately 70% of patients the fibrosis is most severe in the lower lung zones; in about 20% all zones are involved to a similar degree. If the upper lobes appear abnormal, the extent and severity of abnormalities are typically less than at the lung bases. Subpleural, basal honeycombing associated with irregular reticular opacities in the upper lobes is characteristic of IPF.

Ground-glass opacity may be seen in patients with UIP/

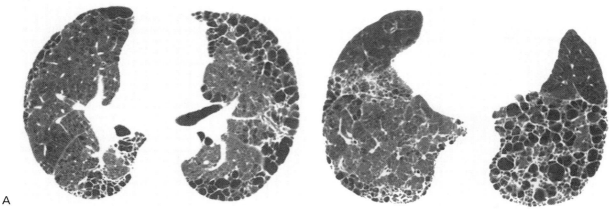

FIG. 13-3. HRCT in idiopathic pulmonary fibrosis with honeycombing. **A.** Concentric subpleural honeycombing is visible. **B.** Near the lung bases, honeycomb cysts are more numerous. Most cysts are less than 2 cm in size.

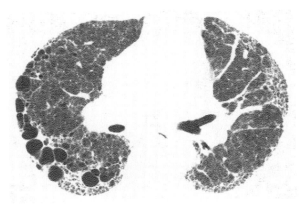

FIG. 13-4. Asymmetrical honeycombing in idiopathic pulmonary fibrosis. Subpleural reticulation and honeycombing are present. The honeycomb cysts are much larger on the right.

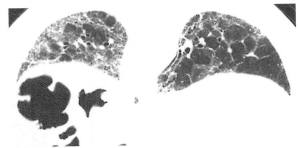

FIG. 13-7. Ground-glass opacity in idiopathic pulmonary fibrosis. Prone HRCT shows patchy ground-glass opacity. These regions also show irregular reticular opacities and traction bronchiectasis and bronchiolectasis, indicating the presence of fibrosis. Ground-glass opacity is rare in idiopathic pulmonary fibrosis as an isolated finding.

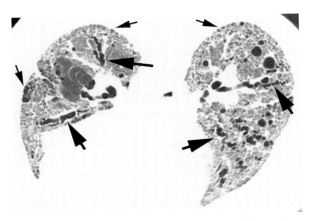

FIG. 13-5. Reticular opacities, traction bronchiectasis, and honeycombing in idiopathic pulmonary fibrosis. Prone HRCT shows a diffuse reticular pattern at the lung bases, with traction bronchiectasis *(large arrows)* and mild subpleural honeycombing *(small arrows)*.

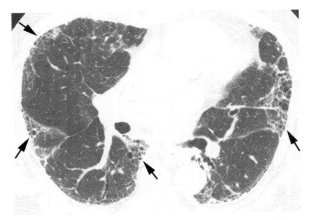

FIG. 13-6. Patchy subpleural reticular opacities and honeycombing in idiopathic pulmonary fibrosis. Areas of honeycombing *(arrows)* involve the peripheral lung in a patchy fashion.

IPF, but this finding typically reflects the presence of fine lung fibrosis and is seen in association with reticulation and traction bronchiectasis in the same lung regions (Fig. 13-7); ground-glass opacity is rare as an isolated finding.

Mediastinal lymph node enlargement is visible on CT in more than 70% of cases. The enlarged nodes typically measure less than 15 mm.

A confident HRCT diagnosis of UIP may be based on the presence of reticular opacities associated with honeycombing and/or traction bronchiectasis, with a predominant basal and subpleural distribution. If these findings are present, the accuracy of HRCT in making the diagnosis of UIP exceeds 90%. In the absence of an associated disease, IPF is very likely the diagnosis. In patients with typical HRCT and clinical findings, lung biopsy is uncommonly performed.

In the vast majority of patients with IPF, serial HRCT scans show an increase in the extent of reticulation and honeycombing. This progression usually occurs gradually over several months or years. Occasionally patients develop fulminant and sometimes fatal acute exacerbations (*accelerated decline*) characterized by consolidation or ground-glass opacity (Fig. 13-8); biopsy typically shows diffuse alveolar damage. When such exacerbations occur, pulmonary function decreases in a series of acute stair-step increments coincident with the exacerbation.

NONSPECIFIC INTERSTITIAL PNEUMONIA

Nonspecific interstitial pneumonia (NSIP) is less common than UIP. The histologic pattern and the IIP are both called NSIP.

According to its most general definition, it is characterized histologically by the presence of varying proportions of interstitial inflammation and fibrosis without any specific features that would allow a diagnosis of UIP, DIP, OP, or AIP. Alternatively, it is thought by some to be a specific

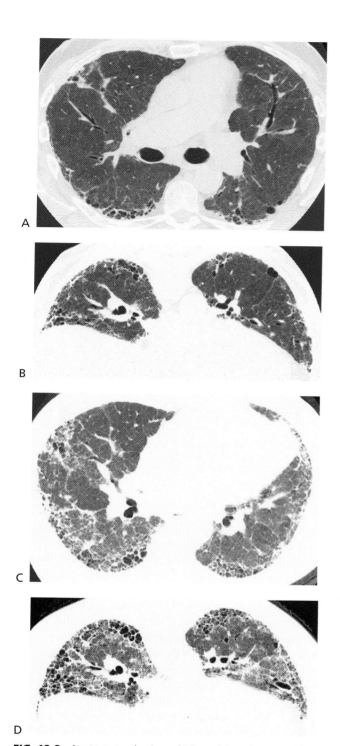

FIG. 13-8. Acute exacerbation of idiopathic pulmonary fibrosis. Supine **(A)** and prone **(B)** HRCTs show subpleural reticulation and honeycombing in the lower lobes, typical of IPF. Supine **(C)** and prone **(D)** HRCTs at the time of an acute exacerbation show progression of honeycombing and an increase in ground-glass opacity. This reflects diffuse alveolar damage.

TABLE 13-4. NONSPECIFIC INTERSTITIAL PNEUMONIA: HISTOLOGIC, CLINICAL, AND HRCT FEATURES

Histologic pattern
Cellular pattern
  Mild to moderate chronic interstitial inflammation
  Type II pneumocyte hyperplasia
  Dense fibrosis absent
Fibrotic pattern
  Mild to moderate chronic interstitial inflammation
  Fibrosis lacking the temporal heterogeneity and/or patchy
    distribution of usual interstitial pneumonia (UIP)
  Fibroblastic foci absent or inconspicuous
Differential diagnosis
  Idiopathic (nonspecific interstitial pneumonia)
  Collagen-vascular disease
  Hypersensitivity pneumonitis
  Drug toxicity
  Infection
  Immunodeficiency

Idiopathic clinical syndrome
Age 40–50 years (younger than UIP)
Progressive dyspnea, for 18 months or more (longer than UIP)
Pulmonary function tests: restriction and impaired gas
  exchange (less severe than UIP)
Treatment (steroids) usually effective
Prognosis good
HRCT findings
  Ground-glass opacity
  Irregular reticulation
  Patchy consolidation
  Honeycombing absent, inconspicuous, or minimal
  Concentric subpleural and basal predominance
  Subpleural sparing may be present

---

pathologic entity, not a "nonspecific" diagnosis. NSIP may demonstrate cellular or fibrotic patterns (Table 13-4). Unlike UIP, histologic lesions in patients with NSIP are temporally homogeneous, appearing to represent the same stage in evolution of disease.

NSIP may be idiopathic or may be associated with collagen-vascular diseases, hypersensitivity pneumonitis, drug toxicity, infection, or immunodeficiency. An association with collagen-vascular diseases is particularly common, and NSIP is the most common histologic abnormality present in patients with collagen disease and a lung abnormality.

Clinically, patients with NSIP present with symptoms similar to idiopathic pulmonary fibrosis, including dyspnea and cough, with an average duration of 18 to 30 months (see Table 13-4). Average age at diagnosis is 40 to 50 years. Patients typically respond to treatment with steroids and the prognosis is good, although this varies with the degree of fibrosis present.

Radiographic Findings

The radiographic findings consist mainly of ill-defined opacity, ground-glass opacity, or consolidation predomi-

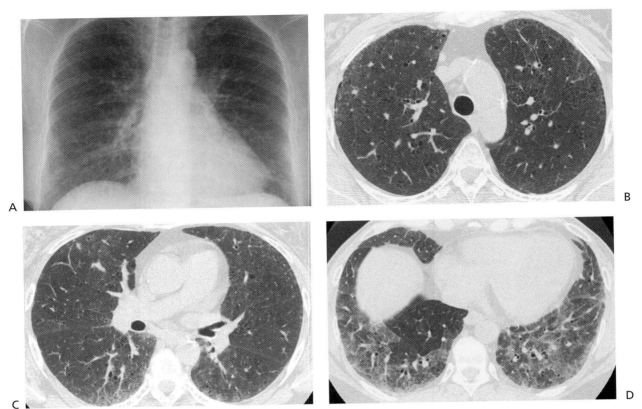

FIG. 13-9. Nonspecific interstitial pneumonia. **A.** Chest radiograph shows a subtle increase in opacity at the lung bases. **B–D.** HRCTs at three levels show an increase in ground-glass opacity and reticular opacities, which is predominant at the lung bases and in the lung periphery.

nantly involving the lower lung zones (Figs. 13-9A and 13-10A). Other manifestations include a reticular pattern or a combination of reticular and air-space patterns. In 10% or more of cases, the chest radiograph is normal.

CT Findings

Because the histology associated with NSIP is variable, HRCT shows a variable combination of ground-glass opacity, irregular reticular opacities, and patchy consolidation, usually with a peripheral and basal predominance.

Although honeycombing may be present in patients with NSIP, it is uncommon and tends to be inconspicuous, particularly in comparison to UIP and IPF. The presence of reticulation and honeycombing correlates with the fibrotic pattern of NSIP. The cellular pattern results in ground-glass opacity.

In most cases, patchy or concentric subpleural ground-glass opacity with a lower lobe predominance is seen on HRCT; superimposed reticulation is common (see Figs. 13-9 to 13-13). Although it predominates in the peripheral lung, NSIP may show sparing of the immediate subpleural region, a finding that helps distinguish it from UIP and

IPF (see Figs. 13-11 to 13-13). Reticular opacities often indicate fibrosis and persist after treatment; ground-glass opacities largely resolve with treatment (Fig. 13-14). Abnormalities may be quite subtle and visible with certainty only on prone scans.

There is considerable overlap between the HRCT findings seen in NSIP and those present in other interstitial pneumonias. Abnormalities seen on HRCT in patients with NSIP can mimic those of DIP (predominantly ground-glass opacities), COP (air-space consolidation), AIP (air-space consolidation), and occasionally UIP (predominantly lower lobe reticulation with or without honeycombing). The diagnosis of NSIP should be strongly considered if HRCT shows an abnormality in subpleural and basal lung, without honeycombing.

CRYPTOGENIC ORGANIZING PNEUMONIA

Organizing pneumonia (OP) is a histologic pattern characterized by the presence of patchy areas of organizing pneumonia, consisting largely of mononuclear cells, foamy macrophages, and organizing fibrosis in peripheral air-

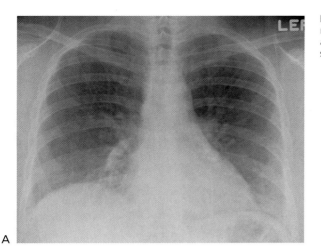

A

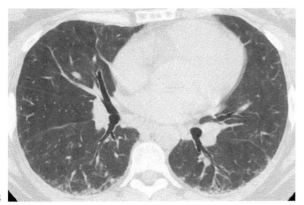

B

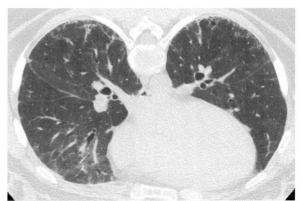

C

FIG. 13-10. Nonspecific interstitial pneumonia. **A.** Chest radiograph shows a subtle increase in ground-glass opacity at the lung bases. Supine (**B**) and prone (**C**) HRCTs show subpleural reticular opacities and ground-glass opacity.

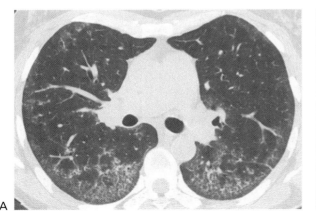

A

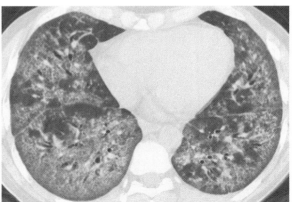

B

FIG. 13-11. Nonspecific interstitial pneumonia with ground-glass opacity. Supine HRCTs show a ground-glass opacity with some superimposed reticulation. There is sparing of the immediate subpleural lung.

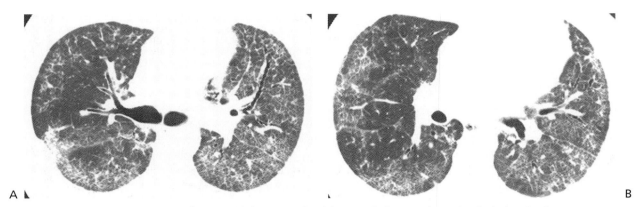

FIG. 13-12. Nonspecific interstitial pneumonia with ground-glass opacity and reticulation. Supine HRCTs show a combination of ground-glass opacity and reticulation. There is sparing of the immediate subpleural lung. This finding helps to distinguish nonspecific interstitial pneumonia from usual interstitial pneumonia.

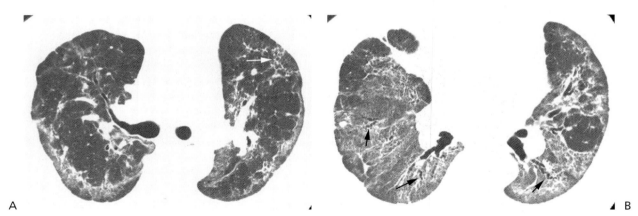

FIG. 13-13. Nonspecific interstitial pneumonia with fibrosis. Supine HRCTs show a reticular opacities and ground-glass opacity. The presence of traction bronchiectasis indicates that fibrosis is present. There is sparing of the immediate subpleural lung. Honeycombing is absent.

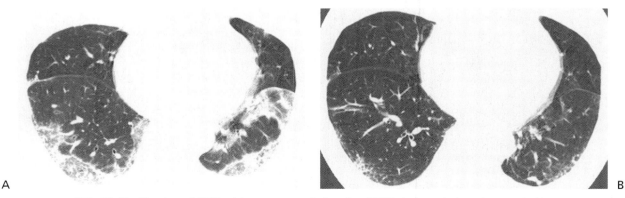

FIG. 13-14. Clearing of NSIP with treatment. **A.** Baseline HRCT shows subpleural ground-glass opacity with superimposed reticulation and focal areas of consolidation. **B.** After treatment with steroids, there has been a significant reduction in ground-glass opacity and consolidation. Some reticulation persists, due to fibrosis.

TABLE 13-5. ORGANIZING PNEUMONIA (OP) AND CRYPTOGENIC ORGANIZING PNEUMONIA (COP): HISTOLOGIC, CLINICAL, AND HRCT FEATURES

OP: histologic pattern
Also known as bronchiolitis obliterans organizing pneumonis
Characteristics
    Organizing fibrosis in distal air spaces
    Lack of interstitial fibrosis
    Patchy distribution
    Mild chronic interstitial inflammation
Differential diagnosis
    Idiopathic (COP)
    Pulmonary infection
    Bronchial obstruction
    Aspiration
    Drug reactions
    Collagen-vascular diseases
    Toxic-fume inhalation
    Radiation pneumonitis
    Hypersensitivity pneumonitis

COP: idiopathic clinical syndrome
Mean age 55 years
Several months of cough, fever, dyspnea
PFT: restriction and impaired gas exchange (less severe than
    usual interstitial pneumonia)
Treatment (steroids) effective
Prognosis very good
HRCT findings
    Patchy consolidation
    Patchy ground-glass opacity
    Subpleural or peribronchial distribution
    Small, ill-defined nodules
    Large nodules or masses
    Focal consolidation
    Atoll sign

spaces, including bronchioles, alveolar ducts, and alveoli (Table 13-5). This histologic pattern is also known as *bronchiolitis obliterans organizing pneumonia* (BOOP), although OP is now the preferred term.

Most examples of OP are idiopathic, termed *cryptogenic organizing pneumonia* (COP). However, OP also may be seen in association with a variety of diseases, including pulmonary infection, bronchial obstruction, aspiration, drug reactions, and collagen-vascular diseases, and after toxic-fume inhalation. It may also accompany radiation pneumonitis, hypersensitivity pneumonitis, UIP, NSIP, and other patterns.

Patients with COP typically present with a several-month history of nonproductive cough, low-grade fever, malaise, and shortness of breath. Mean age is 55. PFTs characteristically show a restrictive pattern. Clinically and functionally, the findings may be similar to IPF, although the duration of symptoms in patients with COP is shorter and systemic symptoms are more common. Patients usually respond well to corticosteroid therapy and have a good prognosis.

Radiographic Findings

The characteristic radiologic features of OP/COP consist of patchy, unilateral or bilateral areas of air-space consolidation. Small nodular opacities or larger nodules may be seen as the only finding or, more commonly, are seen in association with areas of air-space consolidation. In some patients consolidation is peripheral, a pattern similar to that seen in chronic eosinophilic pneumonia.

HRCT Findings

HRCT findings in patients with OP/COP vary and may include the following:

1. Patchy consolidation (80% of cases) or ground-glass opacity (60%), often with a subpleural and/or peribronchial distribution (Figs. 13-15 to 13-18)
2. Small, ill-defined nodules (30% to 50% of cases) which may be peribronchial or peribronchiolar (i.e., centrilobular; Fig. 13-19)
3. Large nodules or masses, which may be irregular in shape (see Figs. 13-16 and 13-19)
4. Focal or lobar consolidation (Fig. 13-20)
5. The "atoll" sign, in which ring-shaped or crescentic opacities are seen, often with ground-glass opacity in the center of the ring (thus resembling a coral atoll; see Figs. 13-18A and 13-21)

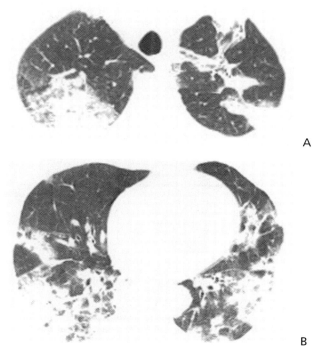

A

B

FIG. 13-15. HRCT in cryptogenic organizing pneumonia/bronchiolitis obliterans organizing pneumonia. The classic appearance of COP/BOOP is patchy subpleural and peribronchial consolidation. In this patient, subpleural consolidation predominates.

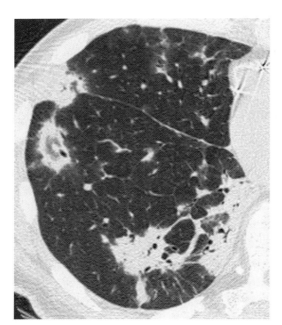

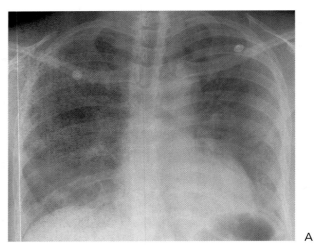

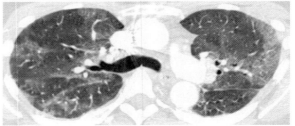

FIG. 13-16. Subpleural and peribronchial consolidation in cryptogenic organizing pneumonia/bronchiolitis obliterans organizing pneumonia. HRCT shows irregular nodular areas of consolidation, many occurring in relation to bronchi. Air bronchograms are visible within the opacities.

FIG. 13-17. Patchy ground-glass opacity in cryptogenic organizing pneumonia/bronchiolitis obliterans organizing pneumonia. **A.** Chest radiograph shows an increase in lung opacity. **B.** HRCT shows patchy areas of ground-glass opacity.

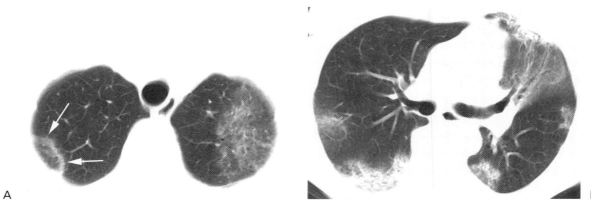

FIG. 13-18. Consolidation and ground-glass opacity in cryptogenic organizing pneumonia/bronchiolitis obliterans organizing pneumonia. **A.** CT through the upper lobes shows ground-glass opacity in the left upper lobe and a ring-shaped opacity surrounding ground-glass opacity *(arrows)*. This represents the "atoll" sign. **B.** CT shows patchy areas of consolidation and ground-glass opacity with a subpleural predominance.

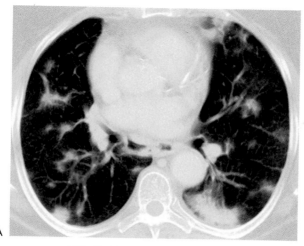

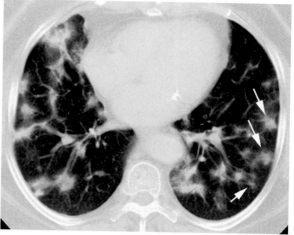

FIG. 13-19. Irregular nodular opacities in cryptogenic organizing pneumonia/bronchiolitis obliterans organizing pneumonia. **A.** CT shows irregular nodular opacities. A subpleural area of consolidation is visible in the posterior left lower lobe. **B.** At a lower level, multiple irregular nodular opacities are visible, many occurring in relation to bronchi. Some of the small nodules *(arrows)* in the left lower lobe appear centrilobular in location.

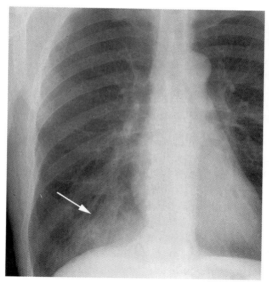

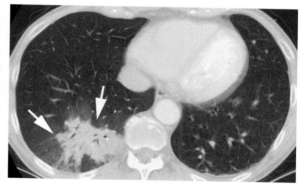

FIG. 13-20. Focal consolidation in cryptogenic organizing pneumonia/bronchiolitis obliterans organizing pneumonia. **A.** Chest radiograph shows focal consolidation in the right lower lobe *(arrow)*. **B.** HRCT shows an irregular peripheral area of consolidation in the right lower lobe *(arrows)*, containing air bronchograms.

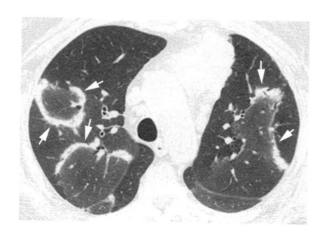

FIG. 13-21. The "atoll" sign in cryptogenic organizing pneumonia/bronchiolitis obliterans organizing pneumonia. Crescentic regions of consolidation *(arrows)* surround or outline areas of ground-glass opacity.

OP/COP often involves the lower lung zones to a greater degree than the upper lung zones. A pattern of patchy peripheral or peribronchial consolidation is common, seen in more than 70% of cases, and should be sufficient to suggest the diagnosis in a patient with a typical history of progressive dyspnea and low-grade fever.

Other findings in patients with OP/COP include small pleural effusions, present in 30% to 35% of cases, irregular linear opacities, mild honeycombing, and "crazy paving," with a superimposition of ground-glass opacity and interlobular septal thickening.

ACUTE INTERSTITIAL PNEUMONIA

Acute interstitial pneumonia (AIP) is a fulminant disease of unknown cause, usually occurring in a previously healthy person. It is associated with the histologic pattern of *diffuse alveolar damage* (DAD) with alveolar hyaline membranes and diffuse, active interstitial fibrosis (Table 13-6). The appearance of DAD in AIP is indistinguishable from DAD in patients with acute respiratory distress syndrome (ARDS) caused by sepsis, shock, infection, drug toxicity, toxic inhalations, trauma, or other insults.

The mean age at presentation is 50. A prodromal illness associated with symptoms of a viral upper respiratory infection is often present, followed by rapidly increasing dyspnea and respiratory failure. Patients with AIP usually require mechanical ventilation within 1 to 2 weeks of the onset of

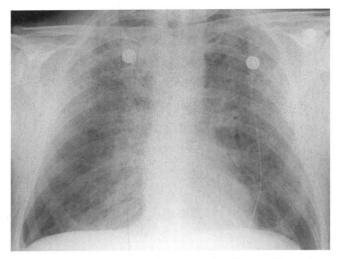

FIG. 13-22. Acute interstitial pneumonia. Chest radiograph at presentation shows diffuse, ill-defined areas of ground-glass opacity and consolidation.

symptoms. Fifty percent or more die within 6 months of presentation.

Because of its acute presentation and a histologic pattern identical to that of ARDS, AIP has been referred to as idiopathic ARDS. It was formerly known as *Hamman-Rich syndrome*.

Radiographic Findings

Chest radiographs show bilateral air-space consolidation or ground-glass opacity that is diffuse (50%) or may predominate in the upper (25%) or lower (25%) lung zones (Figs. 13-22 to 13-24). Honeycombing may be seen late in the disease. Findings are similar to other causes of ARDS.

HRCT Findings

There is little reason to obtain HRCT in a patient with AIP. Findings are similar to those of any patient with ARDS.

In the early stages of AIP, HRCT shows patchy bilateral ground-glass opacity and consolidation, which tend to be diffuse or patchy, indistinguishable from other causes of ARDS. Abnormalities are most severe in the posterior lungs (see Figs. 13-23C and 13-24C). Architectural distortion, traction bronchiectasis, and honeycombing may be seen as the disease progresses.

DESQUAMATIVE INTERSTITIAL PNEUMONIA, RESPIRATORY BRONCHIOLITIS, AND RESPIRATORY BRONCHIOLITIS–INTERSTITIAL LUNG DISEASE

Desquamative interstitial pneumonia (DIP) is a rare condition characterized histologically by the presence of numer-

---

TABLE 13-6. DIFFUSE ALVEOLAR DAMAGE (DAD) AND ACUTE INTERSTITIAL PNEUMONIA (AIP): HISTOLOGIC, CLINICAL, AND HRCT FEATURES

DAD: histologic pattern
Characteristics
  Diffuse distribution
  Uniform temporal appearance
  Hyaline membranes
  Alveolar wall thickening due to organizing fibrosis
  No evidence of infection
Differential diagnosis
  Any cause of ARDS

AIP: idiopathic clinical syndrome
Idiopathic acute respiratory distress syndrome (ARDS) or Hamman-Rich syndrome
Mean age 50 years
Prodromal illness suggesting viral infection
1–2 weeks of progressive dyspnea
Pulmonary function tests: restriction and impaired gas exchange
Severe hypoxemia
Prognosis poor (50% die)
Radiographic features of ARDS
HRCT findings
  Diffuse or patchy consolidation
  Diffuse or patchy ground-glass opacity
  Posterior, lower lobe predominance

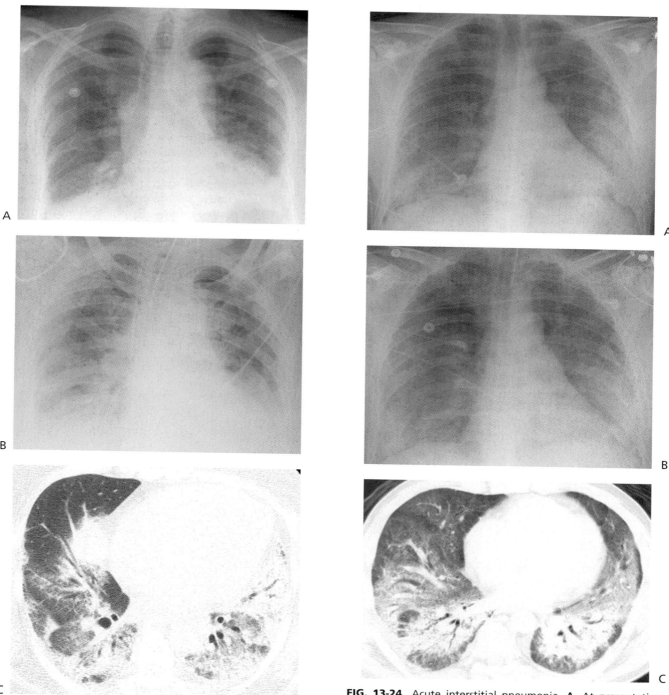

FIG. 13-23. Acute interstitial pneumonia proved at autopsy. **A.** At presentation, chest radiograph shows ill-defined consolidation at the lung bases. **B.** After 1 week, the patient is intubated and consolidation has progressed. The appearance is similar to other causes of acute respiratory distress syndrome. **C.** HRCT shows ground-glass opacity and consolidation.

FIG. 13-24. Acute interstitial pneumonia. **A.** At presentation, chest radiograph shows ill-defined consolidation at the lung bases. **B.** After 1 day, the patient is intubated and consolidation has progressed. **C.** HRCT shows consolidation at the lung bases.

ous macrophages filling alveoli, mild inflammation of alveolar walls, and minimal fibrosis. DIP is typically diffuse in distribution (Table 13-7).

Although DIP is classified as an IIP, more than 90% of patients with DIP are cigarette smokers. In most cases, DIP is considered to be a smoking-related disease. It also can be seen in association with toxic inhalation, drug reactions, Langerhans cell histiocytosis, leukemia, asbestosis, and hard-metal pneumoconiosis.

If the alveolar macrophage infiltrate is localized, having a peribronchiolar predominance, it is usually referred to as *respiratory bronchiolitis* (RB) rather than DIP (see Table 13-7). RB is a common incidental finding in the lungs of asymptomatic smokers. If the histologic finding of RB is associated with pulmonary symptoms, the resulting syndrome is called *respiratory bronchiolitis–interstitial lung disease* (RB-ILD). The association between smoking and RB and RB-ILD is even stronger than with DIP.

Basically DIP, RB, and RB-ILD represent different degrees of lung involvement by the same process, with RB being the mildest and most localized and DIP being most extensive. RB and RB-ILD are more common than DIP (see Table 13-7).

DIP and RB-ILD occur most commonly in patients between 30 and 50 years of age. The clinical symptoms usually consist of slowly progressive dyspnea and dry cough.

The prognosis of patients with DIP and RB-ILD is very good. Smoking cessation leads to an improvement in symptoms. Patients who continue to smoke may improve clinically, but those with persistent complaints may benefit from oral steroid therapy. It has been suggested that RB may be the precursor to chronic airway abnormalities or centrilobular emphysema in susceptible individuals.

Radiographic Findings

The most common abnormality on chest radiographs in patients with DIP is ground-glass opacities seen in the lower lung zones (Fig. 13-25A). However, in up to 25% of patients with DIP, the chest radiographs are normal. Chest radiographs in patients with RB-ILD can be normal or can

TABLE 13-7. DESQUAMATIVE INTERSTITIAL PNEUMONIA (DIP), RESPIRATORY BROCHIOLITIS (RB), AND RESPIRATORY BRONCHIOLITIS–INTERSTITIAL LUNG DISEASE (RB-ILD): HISTOLOGIC, CLINICAL, AND HRCT FEATURES

DIP and RB: histologic patterns
DIP characteristics
  Diffuse distribution
  Intraalveolar macrophages
  Minimal fibrosis
RB characteristics
  Bronchiolocentric (peribronchiolar) distribution
  Intraalveolar macrophages
  Minimal fibrosis
Differential diagnosis
  90% cigarette smokers (DIP), RB higher incidence
  Idiopathic
  Inhalations
  Drug reactions
  Langerhans cell histiocytosis
  Leukemia
  Asbestosis
  Hard-metal pneumoconiosis

DIP and RB-ILD: idiopathic clinical syndromes
Age 30–50
Progressive cough and dyspnea
Pulmonary function tests: restriction and impaired gas exchange
Prognosis very good with smoking cessation or steroids
DIP HRCT findings
  Diffuse or patchy ground-glass opacity
  Posterior, lower lobe predominance in 60%–75%
  Fibrosis rare
  Cystic lucencies or emphysema
  Air trapping on expiratory scans
RB-ILD HRCT findings
  Normal
  Centrilobular or patchy ground-glass opacity
  Upper lobe predominance in 60%–75%
  Bronchial wall thickening

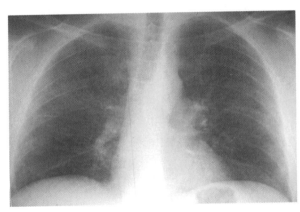

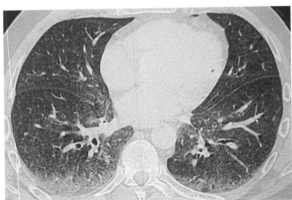

FIG. 13-25. Desquamative interstitial pneumonia. **A.** Chest radiograph shows reduced lung volume and hazy ground-glass opacity in the peripheral lung. **B.** HRCT shows ground-glass opacity in the peripheral lung.

show nonspecific bilateral, ill-defined opacities, usually with a lower zonal predominance.

HRCT Findings

In patients with DIP, the predominant abnormality on HRCT consists of areas of ground-glass opacity (see Figs. 13-25 and 13-26). A subpleural and lower lobe predominance is seen in 60% to 75%; a diffuse distribution may also be seen. Although reticular opacities are commonly associated with the ground-glass opacity, honeycombing or obvious fibrosis is rare.

Because of its association with smoking, centrilobular emphysema may be visible. Small cystic lucencies, not representing emphysema, may also be seen in patients with DIP (see Fig. 13-26A). Patchy air trapping may be seen on expiratory scans, presumably associated with smoking-related small airway disease (see Fig. 13-26B).

Not all patients with RB-ILD show abnormalities on HRCT. When abnormal, HRCT findings include centrilobular ground-glass opacity nodules (40% of cases), patchy ground-glass opacities (50%), and thickening of bronchial walls, probably related to smoking and bronchitis.

Unlike patients with DIP, an upper lobe predominance is typical of RB-ILD. A small percentage of patients (25%) show some reticular opacities due to fibrosis. The fibrosis in RB-ILD is mild and tends to involve mainly the lower lung zones.

LYMPHOID INTERSTITIAL PNEUMONIA

Lymphoid interstitial pneumonia (LIP) is characterized histologically by a dense lymphoid interstitial infiltrate consisting predominantly of lymphocytes, plasma cells, and histiocytes (Table 13-8). Alveolar walls are extensively involved. Lymphoid follicles may be present. If the interstitial infiltrate occurs primarily in relation to small airways, in associa-

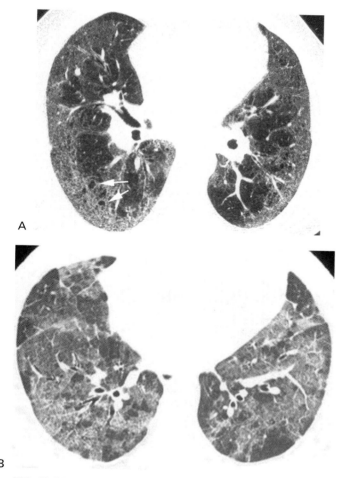

FIG. 13-26. Desquamative interstitial pneumonia in two different patients. **A.** Peripheral ground-glass opacity associated with small cystic lesions *(arrows)*. These may resolve with treatment. **B.** Patchy ground-glass opacity associated with fine reticulation. Areas of lucency likely reflect air trapping.

TABLE 13-8. LYMPHOID INTERSTITIAL PNEUMONIA (LIP): HISTOLOGIC, CLINICAL, AND HRCT FEATURES

Histologic pattern
Characteristics
  Diffuse interstitial and alveolar wall involvement
  Infiltration by lymphocytes, plasma cells, and histiocytes
  Lymphoid hyperplasia
Differential diagnosis
  Idiopathic (rare)
  Collagen-vascular diseases
    Sjögren's syndrome
    Rheumatoid arthritis
    Systemic lupus erythematosus
  Immunologic disorders
    Hashimoto's thyroiditis
    Autoimmune hemolytic anemia
    Myasthenia gravis
    Pernicious anemia
    Chronic active hepatitis
    Primary biliary cirrhosis
  Infection
  Immunodeficiency (e.g., AIDS)
  Drug toxicity

Idiopathic clinical syndromes
Age 40–50
Progressive cough and dyspnea
Dysproteinemia in 75%
Pulmonary function tests: restriction and impaired gas exchange
Steroids helpful in treatment
HRCT findings variable
  Diffuse or patchy areas of ground-glass opacity
  Poorly defined centrilobular nodules
  Small well-defined nodules or septal thickening
  Isolated cystic airspaces (suggestive of LIP)
  Diffuse cystic disease

tion with lymphoid follicles, the abnormality may be termed follicular bronchiolitis.

LIP is considered by some to be a lymphoproliferative disease rather than an IIP, but this question remains unsettled.

LIP is rarely idiopathic and frequently occurs in association with collagen-vascular diseases (particularly Sjögren syndrome, rheumatoid arthritis, and lupus), immunologic disorders (e.g., Hashimoto's thyroiditis, autoimmune hemolytic anemia, myasthenia gravis, pernicious anemia, chronic active hepatitis), infection, immunodeficiency (e.g., AIDS), and drug toxicity. LIP in AIDS patients usually occurs in children; otherwise, most patients with LIP are adults (mean age, 50 years). LIP is more common in women.

The presentation of LIP is often that of the underlying disease (if present). The main clinical symptoms are cough and dyspnea, progressing over a period of a few years. Steroids are helpful in treatment, but about one third of patients progress to lung fibrosis.

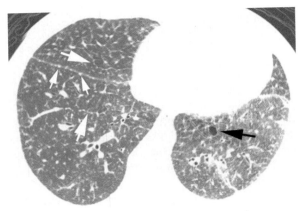

FIG. 13-28. Biopsy-proven lymphoid interstitial pneumonia in a woman with AIDS. Small, sharply defined nodules are visible, particularly along the right major fissure *(small white arrows)*. Interlobular septal thickening and nodules are visible *(large white arrows)*. Ground-glass opacity is also present on the left side, and a single cyst is visible in the left lower lobe *(black arrow)*.

Radiographic and HRCT Findings

Radiographs most often show a reticular pattern predominantly involving the lower lung zones. Less common abnormalities include a nodular pattern or air-space consolidation.

HRCT findings vary and reflect the predominant sites of lymphocytic infiltration. The HRCT findings of LIP include the following:

1. Diffuse or patchy areas of ground-glass opacity (Fig. 13-27A) or consolidation (see Fig. 5-32 in Chapter 5)
2. Poorly defined centrilobular nodules (see Fig. 13-27A)
3. Small, well-defined nodules or septal thickening (Fig. 13-28; see also Fig. 5-32 in Chapter 5) mimicking lymphangitic spread of carcinoma

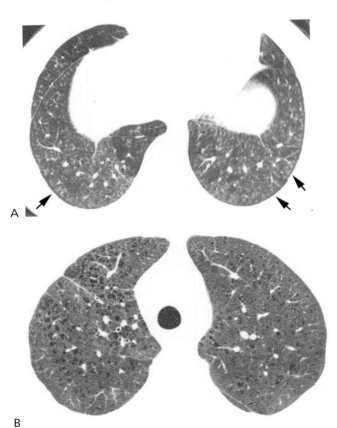

FIG. 13-27. Biopsy-proven lymphoid interstitial pneumonia in a 20-year-old woman with a history of juvenile rheumatoid arthritis. **A.** HRCT shows patchy areas of ground-glass opacity at the lung bases. In some areas *(arrows)* the ground-glass opacities appear predominantly centrilobular. **B.** HRCT through the upper lobes shows thin-walled cysts also typical of lymphoid interstitial pneumonia.

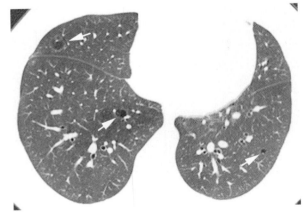

FIG. 13-29. Lung cysts in a patient with Sjögren's syndrome and lymphoid interstitial pneumonia. Several isolated lung cysts are visible *(arrows)*.

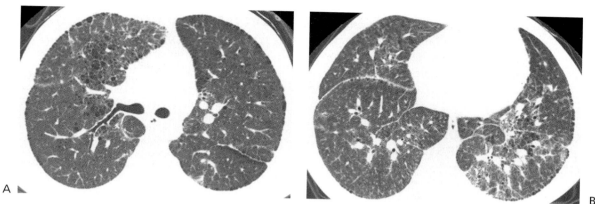

FIG. 13-30. Cystic disease mimicking honeycombing in lymphoid interstitial pneumonia associated with juvenile rheumatoid arthritis. **A.** Scattered and clustered cysts, many subpleural in location, are visible in the upper lobes. **B.** HRCT at the lung bases shows ground-glass opacity, interlobular septal thickening, and subpleural cysts. The predominance of cysts in the upper lobes is unusual in honeycombing.

4. Isolated cystic air spaces, which may appear perivascular and are usually limited in number (see Figs. 13-28 and 13-29)
5. Diffuse cystic appearance resembling honeycombing (see Figs. 13-27B and 13-30)

Alveolar wall infiltration results in ground-glass opacity or consolidation; lymphocytic infiltration predominantly involving bronchioles (follicular bronchiolitis) results in ill-defined centrilobular nodules; interstitial infiltration results in a perilymphatic pattern of nodules or septal thickening.

TABLE 13-9. HRCT FINDINGS IN THE INTERSTITIAL PNEUMONIAS

Histologic pattern	Idiopathic clinical syndrome	HRCT findings	Distribution	Key HRCT findings
UIP	IPF	Reticulation Honeycombing Traction bronchiectasis Ground-glass opacity rare	Peripheral, basal, subpleural, patchy	Subpleural, basal honeycombing
NSIP	NSIP	Ground-glass opacity Reticulation Consolidation Honeycombing uncommon	Peripheral, basal, subpleural, concentric	Concentric subpleural ground-glass opacity without honeycombing
OP (BOOP)	COP (idiopathic BOOP)	Patchy consolidation Centrilobular nodules Large nodules Focal consolidation Atoll sign	Basal, subpleural, peribronchovascular	Patchy subpleural and peribronchial consolidation or nodules
DAD	AIP	Consolidation Ground-glass opacity	Diffuse, lower lobe predominance	Typical findings of ARDS
RB	RB-ILD	Centrilobular nodules Patchy ground-glass opacity	Diffuse, upper lobe predominance	Centrilobular nodules of ground-glass opacity
DIP	DIP	Ground-glass opacity Reticulation Cysts	Peripheral, lower lobe predominance	Diffuse ground-glass opacity
LIP	LIP	Ground-glass opacity Centrilobular nodules Septal thickening or nodules Cysts	Diffuse	Ground-glass opacity or air-filled cysts

UIP, usual interstitial pneumonia; IPF, idiopathic pulmonary fibrosis; NSIP, nonspecific interstitial pneumonia; OP, organizing pneumonia; COP, cryptogenic organizing pneumonia; BOOP, bronchiolitis obliterans organizing pneumonia; DAD, diffuse alveolar damage; AIP, acute interstitial pneumonia; RB, respiratory bronchiolitis; ILD, interstitial lung disease; DIP, desquamative interstitial pneumonia; LIP, lymphoid interstitial pneumonia.

The presence of air-filled lung cysts is most suggestive of LIP and is typical of Sjögren's syndrome (see Chapter 14). The presence of these cysts may reflect the presence of bronchiolar obstruction associated with follicular bronchiolitis.

A RADIOGRAPHIC APPROACH TO THE DIAGNOSIS OF THE INTERSTITIAL PNEUMONIAS

The radiologist is often asked to suggest a diagnosis based on HRCT in a patient with chronic and progressive respiratory symptoms. In these patients, the diagnosis is most often sarcoidosis, hypersensitivity pneumonitis, or an interstitial pneumonia. Fortunately, the HRCT appearances of these entities are sufficiently different to provide guidance.

The HRCT appearances seen in the interstitial pneumonias are usually very helpful in suggesting the diagnosis. HRCT findings and the key findings in diagnosis are listed in Table 13-9. A few important rules should be remembered:

1. Honeycombing with a basal and subpleural predominance is highly suggestive of UIP/IPF. Lung biopsy is rarely performed when HRCT shows these findings.
2. Concentric lower lobe ground-glass opacity without honeycombing suggests NSIP. In a patient with collagen-vascular disease, biopsy is uncommonly performed.
3. Patchy or nodular subpleural or peribronchial consolidation is typical of COP.
4. ARDS with typical plain film or CT findings, without known cause, may be AIP.
5. Diffuse or centrilobular ground-glass opacity in a smoker is typical of DIP or RB-ILD.
6. Cystic air spaces or ground-glass opacity may represent LIP. LIP is usually associated with other diseases.

SELECTED READING

Akira M, Yamamoto S, Sakatani M. Bronchiolitis obliterans organizing pneumonia manifesting as multiple large nodules or masses. AJR Am J Roentgenol 1998; 170:291–295.

American Thoracic Society/European Respiratory Society International Multidisciplinary Consensus Classification of the Idiopathic Interstitial Pneumonias. Am J Respir Crit Care Med 2002; 165:277–304.

Colby TV, Myers JL. The clinical and histologic spectrum of bronchiolitis obliterans including bronchiolitis obliterans organizing pneumonia (BOOP). Semin Respir Dis 1992; 13:119–133.

Hartman TE, Primack SL, Swensen SJ, et al. Desquamative interstitial pneumonia: thin-section CT findings in 22 patients. Radiology 1993; 187:787–790.

Hartman TE, Swensen SJ, Hansell DM, et al. Nonspecific interstitial pneumonia: variable appearance at high-resolution chest CT. Radiology 2000; 217:701–705.

Heyneman LE, Ward S, Lynch DA, et al. Respiratory bronchiolitis, respiratory bronchiolitis-associated interstitial lung disease, and desquamative interstitial pneumonia: different entities or part of the spectrum of the same disease process? AJR Am J Roentgenol 1999; 173:1617–1622.

Johkoh T, Müller NL, Cartier Y, et al. Idiopathic interstitial pneumonias: diagnostic accuracy of thin-section CT in 129 patients. Radiology 1999; 211:555–560.

Johkoh T, Müller NL, Pickford HA, et al. Lymphocytic interstitial pneumonia: thin-section CT findings in 22 patients. Radiology 1999; 212:567–572.

Johkoh T, Müller NL, Taniguchi H, et al. Acute interstitial pneumonia: thin-section CT findings in 36 patients. Radiology 1999; 211:859–863.

Katzenstein AL, Myers JL. Idiopathic pulmonary fibrosis: clinical relevance of pathologic classification. Am J Respir Crit Care Med 1998; 157:1301–1315.

Lee KS, Kullnig P, Hartman TE, Müller NL. Cryptogenic organizing pneumonia: CT findings in 43 patients. AJR Am J Roentgenol 1994; 162:543–546.

Müller NL, Colby TV. Idiopathic interstitial pneumonias: high-resolution CT and histologic findings. Radiographics 1997; 17:1016–1022.

Park JS, Lee KS, Kim JS, et al. Nonspecific interstitial pneumonia with fibrosis: radiographic and CT findings in seven patients. Radiology 1995; 195:645–648.

Primack SL, Hartman TE, Ikezoe J, et al. Acute interstitial pneumonia: radiographic and CT findings in nine patients. Radiology 1993; 188:817–820.

14

COLLAGEN-VASCULAR DISEASES

W. RICHARD WEBB

Collagen-vascular diseases may be associated with focal or diffuse pulmonary abnormalities. The type and frequency of lung abnormalities vary with the specific disease. The two most common conditions associated with diffuse infiltrative lung disease are rheumatoid arthritis and progressive systemic sclerosis (scleroderma).

Most collagen-vascular diseases can cause chronic interstitial pneumonia with clinical, radiographic, high-resolution CT (HRCT), and pathologic features indistinguishable from those of usual interstitial pneumonia (UIP). However, collagen-vascular disease is often associated with pathologic findings other than UIP, including nonspecific interstitial pneumonia (NSIP), bronchiectasis, bronchiolitis obliterans, lymphoid interstitial pneumonia (LIP), and organizing pneumonia (OP), also known as bronchiolitis obliterans organizing pneumonia (BOOP).

As a general rule, HRCT in patients with lung disease resulting from collagen-vascular disease shows a finer reticular pattern and less honeycombing than is typically seen in patients with UIP and idiopathic pulmonary fibrosis (IPF), and ground-glass opacity is more common as a predominant abnormality.

RHEUMATOID ARTHRITIS

Rheumatoid arthritis (RA) is commonly associated with thoracic abnormalities, including interstitial pneumonia and fibrosis, pleural effusion or pleural thickening, necrobiotic nodules, organizing pneumonia (OP), bronchiectasis, and bronchiolitis obliterans (Table 14-1).

Clinical evidence of arthritis precedes the development of pulmonary or pleural disease in about 90% of patients, and 90% have a positive serum rheumatoid factor. Although RA is twice as common in women, extraarticular manifestations of RA, including lung disease, are more common in men. Radiographic findings vary with the manifestation of RA present (see Table 14-1).

Pleural Disease

Pleural disease, either pleural effusion or pleural thickening, is common in patients with RA, being seen in up to 40%

of patients at autopsy. However, radiographic evidence of pleural thickening or pleural effusion is present in only 5% to 20% of patients, and it often is asymptomatic. Pleural effusions are usually small and unilateral, being more common on the right. Generally, effusion is not associated with radiographic evidence of lung disease. On HRCT, pleural effusion is visible more often than on radiographs and is seen in more than 40% of patients with findings of interstitial pneumonia.

Interstitial Pneumonia and Fibrosis

Interstitial pneumonia and fibrosis, the most common pulmonary manifestation of RA, is most common in middle-aged men. Dyspnea is common. Histologically it may appear as either NSIP or UIP.

TABLE 14-1. RHEUMATOID ARTHRITIS

Arthritis precedes lung disease in 90%
Lung disease more common in men
Pleural effusion or pleural thickening in 5%–20%
Interstitial pneumonia 10%–25%
   Histologic pattern may be nonspecific interstitial pneumonia, usual intersitial pneumonia, OP/BOOP
   Ground-glass, reticulation, honeycombing
   Reticulation usually finer than IPF
   Basal and peripheral predominance
   Immediate subpleural sparing may be present (atypical with IPF)
   Anterior upper lobe honeycombing (atypical with IPF)
   Consolidation with OP/BOOP
Rheumatoid nodules
   Peripheral, well-defined
   Caplan's syndrome
Bronchiectasis in 20%
Bronchiolitis obliterans rare
Lymphocytic interstitial pneumonia or follicular bronchiolitis
   Cystic appearance
   Centrilobular nodules
Pulmonary hypertension

IPF, idiopathic pulmonary fibrosis; OP/BOOP, organizing pneumonia/bronchiolitis obliterans organizing pneumonia.

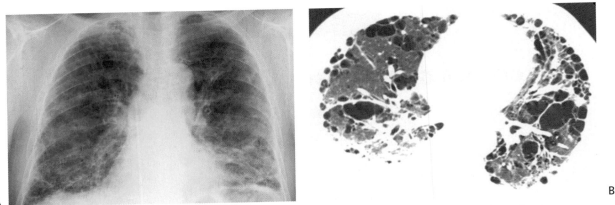

FIG. 14-1. Pulmonary fibrosis with honeycombing in a man with rheumatoid arthritis. **A.** Chest radiograph shows a coarse reticular pattern typical of honeycombing. Lung volume is reduced. **B.** Extensive honeycombing is visible on HRCT. A right pleural effusion is also present.

Although pulmonary function abnormalities are present in up to 40% of patients with RA, only about 5% to 10% of patients with RA have radiologically detectable interstitial disease.

On HRCT, interstitial pneumonia may be associated with a spectrum of abnormalities ranging from ground-glass opacity to fine reticulation and coarse reticulation with honeycombing. Findings of pulmonary fibrosis (irregular reticulation, traction bronchiectasis, honeycombing) are seen on HRCT in about 10% of patients; ground-glass opacity is seen in 15%.

The appearance of RA with interstitial fibrosis may be indistinguishable from that of IPF (Figs. 14-1 and 14-2). However, because some cases are associated with the histologic pattern of NSIP (see Chapter 13), reticular opacities visible in RA tend to be finer than those seen with IPF (Figs. 14-3 and 14-4), and honeycombing is less common and less severe. Also, anterior upper-lobe honeycombing

appears to be more common in the collagen-vascular diseases than in IPF (see Figs. 14-2B and 14-4B).

Predominance in the posterior and subpleural lung and at the lung bases is typical of reticular opacities and ground-glass opacity (Fig. 14-5). Relative sparing of the immediate subpleural lung may be seen, a finding associated with the histologic pattern of NSIP (see Fig. 14-4).

OP/BOOP may also occur in patients with RA, having typical radiographic and CT features of patchy consolidation or nodules (see Chapter 13).

Rheumatoid Nodules

Rheumatoid (necrobiotic) nodules are an uncommon manifestation of RA. Their histology is identical to that of subcutaneous nodules. They are often asymptomatic but tend to appear and disappear in conjunction with subcutaneous nodules. They range in size from a few millimeters to 5 cm

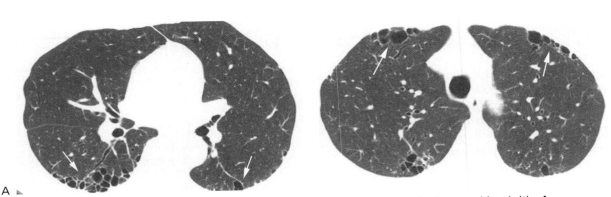

FIG. 14-2. Pulmonary fibrosis with honeycombing in a woman with rheumatoid arthritis. **A.** Patchy subpleural honeycombing *(arrows)* is visible in the posterior lung. **B.** Patchy honeycombing is also present in the upper lobes. Anterior upper-lobe honeycombing *(arrows)* is more common in collagen-vascular diseases than in idiopathic pulmonary fibrosis.

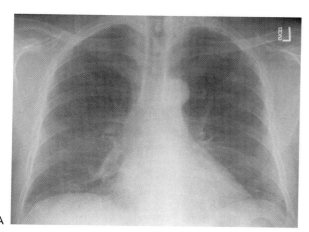

FIG. 14-3. Pulmonary fibrosis in rheumatoid arthritis with reticular opacities. **A.** Chest radiograph shows some reduction in lung volume and a mild nonspecific reticular abnormality at the lung bases. **B.** Fine reticular opacities are visible at the lung bases with evidence of traction bronchiectasis. There is no evidence of honeycombing. **C.** At a higher level, reticular opacities are less severe and predominate on the left. A distinct subpleural and lower-lobe predominance is visible.

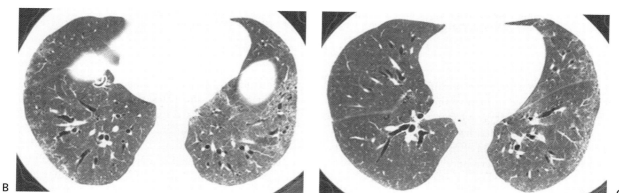

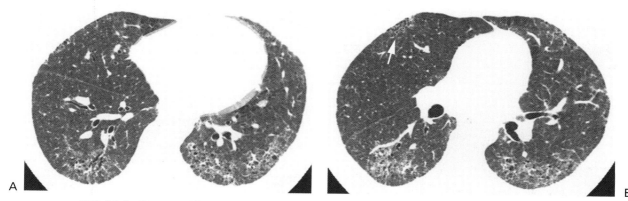

FIG. 14-4. Rheumatoid arthritis with reticular opacities and subpleural sparing. **A.** Fine reticular opacities are visible at the lung bases with evidence of traction bronchiectasis. Although there is a predominance in the subpleural lung, the immediate subpleural lung is less severely involved. This appearance tends to be associated with the histologic pattern of nonspecific interstitial pneumonia. **B.** At a higher level, subpleural sparing is also visible. Despite the absence of lower-lobe honeycombing, patchy honeycombing is visible in the anterior upper lobe *(arrow)*. This finding suggests a collagen-vascular disease.

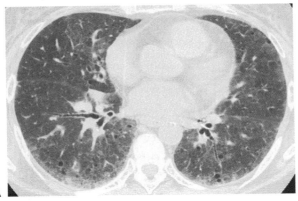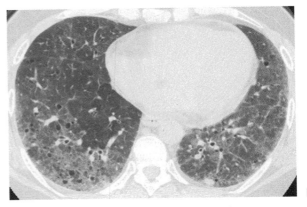

FIG. 14-5. Ground-glass opacity in a woman with rheumatoid arthritis. **A.** HRCT shows patchy ground-glass opacity with a subpleural predominance. **B.** The abnormality is more extensive at the lung bases. Small cystic lucencies are visible within the abnormal lung. These may represent traction bronchiectasis associated with lung fibrosis or cysts associated with LIP.

or more and may be solitary or multiple and numerous. Rheumatoid nodules predominate in the lung periphery and are typically well defined (Fig. 14-6; see also Fig. 9-49 in Chapter 9). They may cavitate, having thick walls that become thin with healing. Pleural effusion may be associated, and cavitary nodules in the periphery may lead to pneumothorax.

Caplan's Syndrome

Caplan's syndrome is a rare manifestation of RA occurring in coal miners or patients with occupational exposures to silicates. Nodules are present that resemble necrobiotic nod-

ules histologically but are characterized by concentric layers of light collagen and black dust-laden cells. Caplan's syndrome is characterized by single or multiple lung nodules ranging from a few millimeters to 5 cm in diameter, similar to rheumatoid nodules. The nodules may cavitate. An upper-lobe predominance may be seen, resembling silicosis or coal-worker's pneumoconiosis, but nodules in Caplan's syndrome appear rapidly in "crops" in contrary to the slow progression of silicosis.

Bronchiectasis

Bronchiectasis is associated with RA, particularly in smokers. It may reflect chronic infection, which has an increased incidence in rheumatoid patients or, associated with infection, it may be a factor in the development of RA. Also, bronchiectasis is commonly present in patients with bronchiolitis obliterans (Fig. 14-7). On CT, it is present in 20% of patients.

Bronchiolitis Obliterans

Bronchiolitis obliterans (see Chapter 23) is a rare manifestation of RA. Although it is often associated with penicillamine treatment, this is not always the case. Radiographs are normal or show increased lung volumes. HRCT may show bronchiectasis, mosaic perfusion, and air trapping (see Fig. 14-7).

Follicular Bronchiolitis and Lymphoid Interstitial Pneumonia

Follicular bronchiolitis is also a rare airway manifestation of RA, characterized by dyspnea. A lymphocytic infiltrate in the walls of small airways is present histologically. Radio-

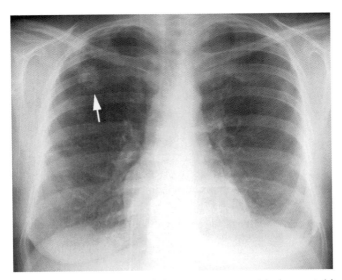

FIG. 14-6. Rheumatoid nodule. A young man with rheumatoid arthritis shows a well-defined nodule in the peripheral right upper lobe. Small pleural effusions are also present (*arrow*).

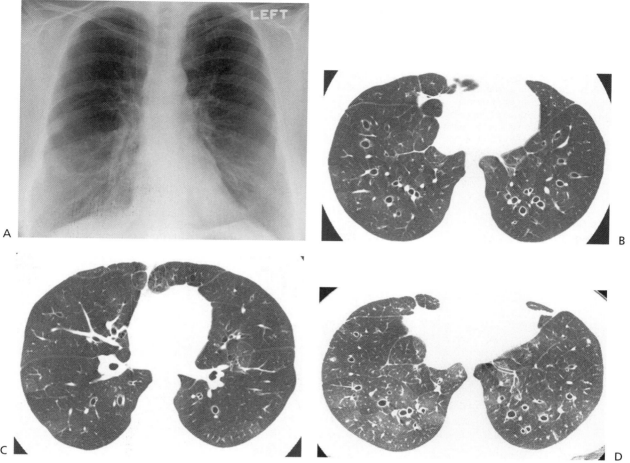

FIG. 14-7. Bronchiectasis and bronchiolitis obliterans in a young woman with rheumatoid arthritis. **A.** Chest radiograph shows large lung volume. **B** and **C.** HRCT scans at two levels show extensive bronchiectasis and regional differences in lung attenuation due to mosaic perfusion. **D.** Postexpiratory HRCT at the same level as **B** shows patchy air trapping typical of bronchiolitis obliterans.

graphs may show a reticular or reticulonodular pattern. HRCT shows small centrilobular nodules or tree-in-bud. More extensive lymphocytic infiltrations may be associated with findings of LIP such as ground-glass opacity or lung cysts (see Fig. 14-5; see also Figs. 13-27 and 13-30 in Chapter 13).

Pulmonary Hypertension

Pulmonary hypertension usually occurs secondary to pulmonary fibrosis. Rarely it develops in the absence of lung disease, perhaps related to vasculitis.

PROGRESSIVE SYSTEMIC SCLEROSIS (SCLERODERMA)

Progressive systemic sclerosis (PSS), also known as scleroderma, is a generalized disease of connective tissue often associated with vasculitis. Women outnumber men by three to one. Only 1% present with pulmonary symptoms, but up to 75% have evidence of pulmonary disease at some point in their disease course.

PSS leads to some degree of interstitial fibrosis in nearly all patients. PSS is commonly associated with NSIP, UIP, pulmonary vasculitis, and pulmonary hypertension (Table 14-2).

Interstitial Pneumonia and Fibrosis

As with RA, chest radiographs may appear normal despite abnormal pulmonary function tests. The incidence of radiographically recognizable interstitial disease is about 25%. Chest radiographs may show a reticular abnormality with lower-lobe predominance indistinguishable from that of IPF. In early cases, ill-defined ground-glass opacity may be seen in the bases (Fig. 14-8A). With progression, the reticu-

TABLE 14-2. SCLERODERMA

Lung disease in 75%
More common in women
Interstitial pneumonia
   Histologic pattern may be interstitial pneumonia, usual
      intersitial pneumonia, organizing pneumonia/bronchiolitis
      obliterans organizing pneumonia
   Ground-glass, reticulation, honeycombing
   HRCT appearances similar to rheumatoid arthritis
Pleural effusion or thickening in 35%
Esophageal dilatation in 40%–80%
Mediastinal lymph node enlargement in 60%

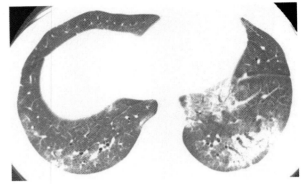

FIG. 14-9. Scleroderma with consolidation. HRCT shows peripheral consolidation and ground-glass opacity in the lower lobes. Subpleural sparing is visible on the left. This may indicate an organizing pneumonia/bronchiolitis obliterans organizing pneumonia or nonspecific interstitial pneumonia.

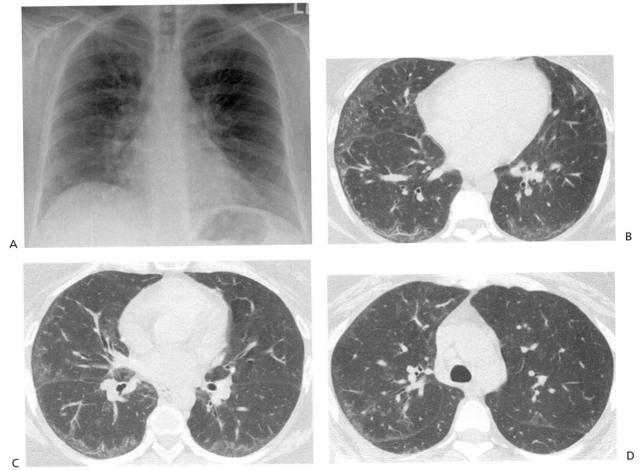

FIG. 14-8. Scleroderma with ground-glass opacity. **A.** Chest radiograph shows a very subtle increase in opacity at the lung bases. **B–D.** HRCT scans at three levels show ground-glass opacity and minimal reticulation with a subpleural and lower-lobe predominance. The immediate subpleural lung is relatively spared. This appearance usually reflects the presence of an nonspecific interstitial pneumonia pattern at biopsy and is typical of early scleroderma.

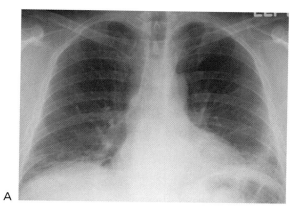
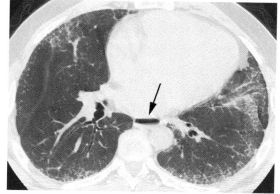

FIG. 14-10. Scleroderma with fine reticular opacities and esophageal dilatation. **A.** Chest radiograph shows reduced lung volume and ill-defined reticular opacities at the lung bases. **B.** HRCT at the lung bases shows a fine reticular pattern without definite honeycombing. The esophagus *(arrow)* is dilated and filled with air and fluid.

lation may progress from fine to coarse, associated with progressive loss of lung volume.

HRCT findings of interstitial fibrosis in PSS are similar to those of IPF, including (1) ground-glass opacity (see Fig. 14-8), (2) consolidation (Fig. 14-9), (3) fine reticular opacities (Fig. 14-10), (4) coarse or irregular reticulation (Fig. 14-11), (5) traction bronchiectasis (see Fig. 14-11), and (6)

honeycombing (Fig 14-12). Abnormalities typically show a subpleural and lower-lobe predominance and often involve the lung periphery in a concentric fashion. As with other collagen diseases, there is a tendency for PSS to show a finer reticular pattern than is typical of IPF, and honeycombing is less frequent. Ground-glass opacity is more common than with IPF.

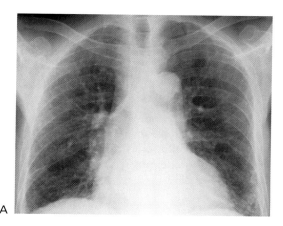

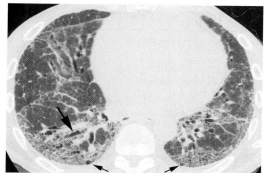
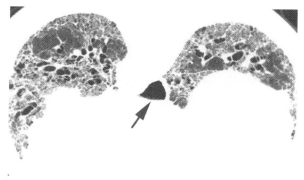

FIG. 14-11. Scleroderma with coarse reticulation and traction bronchiectasis. **A.** Chest radiograph shows reticular opacities laterally at the lung bases. **B.** HRCT at the lung base shows coarse reticulation with traction bronchiectasis *(large arrow)*. Very early honeycombing *(small arrows)* may be present. **C.** Prone HRCT at the lung base shows the reticular pattern and traction bronchiectasis. The esophagus *(arrow)* is dilated and air-filled. Except for the presence of esophageal dilatation, this appearance is indistinguishable from idiopathic pulmonary fibrosis.

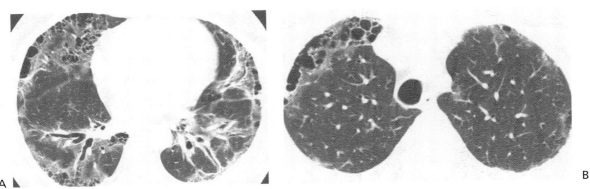

FIG. 14-12. Scleroderma with honeycombing. **A.** HRCT at the base shows extensive honeycombing associated with ground-glass opacity. **B.** HRCT through the upper lobes shows anterior upper-lobe honeycombing.

The HRCT appearance may reflect the histologic pattern present. Ground-glass opacity often is due to NSIP (see Fig. 14-9). Relative subpleural sparing, as sometimes seen in patients with RA, may reflect NSIP (see Figs. 14-9 and 14-10). Consolidation may indicate NSIP or OP/BOOP (see Fig. 14-9). Reticulation, traction bronchiectasis, or honeycombing may indicate fibrotic NSIP or UIP.

Interstitial pneumonia associated with PSS follows a less progressive course and has a better long-term prognosis than IPF. Improvement following treatment is more common in patients with a prominent ground-glass component than in those with predominant reticular abnormalities.

Pleural Disease

Pleural effusion or thickening is less common than with other collagen diseases and is visible on radiographs in 10% to 15%. On CT, diffuse pleural thickening is seen in one third of cases.

Other Findings

Asymptomatic esophageal dilatation is present in 40% to 80% of cases (see Figs. 14-10B and 14-11C). Pulmonary hypertension may occur due to lung disease or vasculitis, but this is more typical of CREST syndrome (see below). Enlarged mediastinal nodes are seen on CT in approximately 60% of cases.

CREST SYNDROME

CREST syndrome (limited systemic sclerosis) is a variant of PSS (Table 14-3). It is defined by the presence of calcification (subcutaneous), Raynaud's phenomenon, esophageal dysmotility, sclerodactyly, and telangiectasia. Pulmonary hypertension is more common than in PSS, occurring in nearly 10% of patients. Otherwise, pleural and pulmonary manifestations of CREST syndrome are similar to those of PSS but tend to be less severe and are associated with a better prognosis.

SYSTEMIC LUPUS ERYTHEMATOSUS

Systemic lupus erythematosus (SLE) is a multisystem autoimmune disease that is associated with increased circulating serum antinuclear antibodies (ANA) in 95% of cases. Clinical diagnosis is based on the presence of at least 4 of the following 10 features: rash, discoid lupus, photosensitivity, oral ulcers, arthritis, serositis, renal disorders, neurologic disorders, hematologic disorders, or immunologic disorders. SLE is much more common in women than in men. Over 50% of patients with SLE develop pleural or pulmonary disease (Table 14-4).

Pleural and Pericardial Disease

Pleural disease is the most common abnormality present. Pleural effusion or pleural thickening occurs in 70% of cases, and pleural effusion is visible on chest radiographs in 35% of patients presenting with SLE. Effusions are usually bilateral and small.

TABLE 14-3. CREST SYNDROME

Variant of scleroderma
Findings
  Calcification (subcutaneous)
  Raynaud's phenomenon
  Esophageal dysmotility
  Sclerodactyly
  Telangiectasia
Pulmonary hypertension in 10%
Pleural and pulmonary disease similar to progressive systemic
  sclerosis but less severe

TABLE 14-4. SYSTEMIC LUPUS ERYTHEMATOSUS

Pleural effusion or pleural thickening in 70%
Pericardial effusion or cardiomegaly in 35%
Lung disease
  Pneumonia most common
  Lupus pneumonitis in 5%
  Pulmonary hemorrhage
  "Shrinking lung syndrome"
  Organizing pneumonia/bronchiolitis obliterans organizing
    pneumonia
  Pulmonary fibrosis in 30%–35% on HRCT
    Findings similar to other collagen-vascular diseases
  Bronchiectasis
  Pulmonary hypertension

Pericardial effusion or cardiomegaly is present in 35% of cases on chest radiographs. Pericardial effusion is seen much more commonly on CT than on chest radiographs. Cardiomegaly may also reflect lupus cardiomyopathy.

Pulmonary Disease

A variety of pulmonary abnormalities may be seen in SLE. These often appear nonspecific on chest radiographs, resulting in focal or patchy opacities predominant at the lung bases.

Pneumonia

Pneumonia, usually bacterial, is the most common cause of pulmonary abnormality in SLE, accounting for two thirds

of cases of lung disease. It may be related to immunosuppression due to SLE or to drug treatment.

Lupus Pneumonitis

Lupus pneumonitis occurs in about 5% of cases and is characterized by fever, dyspnea, cough, and sometimes hemoptysis. It tends to be associated with concurrent multisystem involvement. Chest radiographs and CT show patchy unilateral or bilateral areas of consolidation or ground-glass opacity, with or without pleural effusion. A lower-lobe predominance may be seen. Histology may show diffuse alveolar damage, capillaritis, or hemorrhage often associated with immune complexes visible on immunofluorescent staining. The diagnosis is usually made by exclusion of other manifestations, such as pneumonia.

Diffuse Pulmonary Hemorrhage

Diffuse pulmonary hemorrhage occurs in a few patients with SLE and is likely a manifestation of lupus pneumonitis. It typically presents with worsening anemia and progressive lung consolidation on radiographs (Fig. 14-13). Hemoptysis is variably present. Lupus nephritis is commonly associated, making this a pulmonary-renal syndrome. Radiographic improvement may be rapid, occurring within several days. Consolidation is typically replaced by an interstitial abnormality during resolution.

"Shrinking Lung" Syndrome

Progressive loss of lung volume, so-called shrinking lung syndrome, is a common manifestation of SLE. The etiology is unclear, but it is thought to be due to diaphragmatic

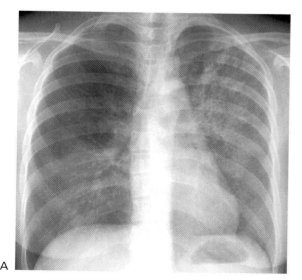
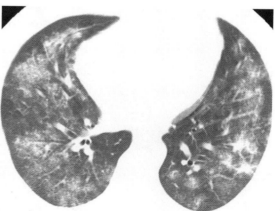

FIG. 14-13. Systemic lupus erythematosus with pulmonary hemorrhage. **A.** Chest radiograph shows areas of consolidation and ground-glass opacity involving the left lung and right lower lobe. Hemoptysis was present. **B.** CT in a different patient shows patchy consolidation and ground-glass opacity with subpleural sparing.

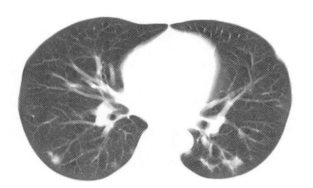

FIG. 14-14. Systemic lupus erythematosus with organizing pneumonia/bronchiolitis obliterans organizing pneumonia (OP/BOOP). CT in a patient with systemic lupus erythematosus and low-grade fever shows ill-defined nodules in the posterior lung. Infection was considered. Lung biopsy showed OP/BOOP.

dysfunction or pleuritic chest pain with restriction of respiration. Patients present with dyspnea. Radiographs show progressive loss of volume in the lower lobes, sometimes associated with linear or focal areas of atelectasis, but obvious parenchymal abnormalities are usually absent. In some patients, this appearance on chest radiographs correlates with mild lung fibrosis.

Organizing Pneumonia (OP/BOOP)

OP/BOOP occurring in SLE shows typical findings of patchy lower-lobe consolidation or ill-defined nodular opacities (Fig. 14-14) with a peripheral or peribronchial distribution. Symptoms include low-grade fever and dyspnea. Its appearance closely mimics pneumonia.

Pulmonary Fibrosis

Pulmonary fibrosis is uncommon in SLE compared with other collagen-vascular diseases. Biopsy may show NSIP or less likely UIP. Pulmonary fibrosis is evident on radiographs in approximately 3% to 5% of patients, showing a basal predominance of reticular opacities. The incidence of HRCT abnormalities consistent with fibrosis is 30% to 35%.

HRCT findings of interstitial pneumonia and fibrosis include ground-glass opacity, fine reticulation, traction bronchiectasis, and honeycombing in advanced cases (Figs. 14-15 and 14-16). Ground-glass opacity is seen in 10% to 15% of patients with SLE, and consolidation is seen in 5% to 10%. These may be associated with pneumonia, lupus

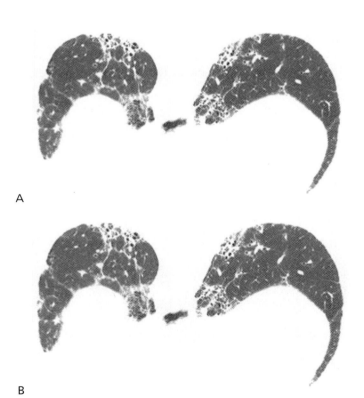

FIG. 14-15. Systemic lupus erythematosus with reticular opacities and traction bronchiectasis. Prone HRCT scans at two levels show patchy reticular opacities with traction bronchiectasis.

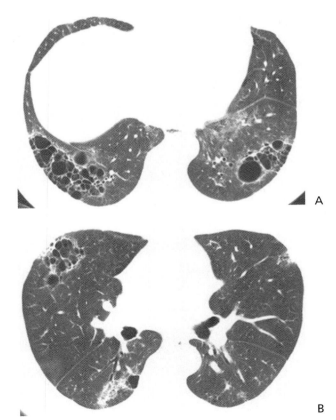

FIG. 14-16. Systemic lupus erythematosus with patchy honeycombing. HRCT scans at the lung base (**A**) and through the mid-lung (**B**) show patchy areas of honeycombing and consolidation. Anterior lung honeycombing is present (**B**).

pneumonitis, pulmonary hemorrhage, interstitial pneumonia, or occasionally BOOP. There is a tendency for fibrosis in patients with SLE to be finer than in patients with IPF, and honeycombing is very uncommon. Lung fibrosis predominates in the periphery and at the lung bases, although anterior upper-lobe involvement is common (see Fig. 14-16). Fibrosis tends to be patchy rather than concentric (see Figs. 14-15 and 14-16).

Airway Disease

Bronchial wall thickening and bronchiectasis are seen on HRCT in about 20% of patients but are uncommonly visible on chest radiographs.

Pulmonary Hypertension

Pulmonary hypertension is rare in SLE. It may be secondary to lung disease or pulmonary emboli or may be similar to primary pulmonary hypertension.

POLYMYOSITIS-DERMATOMYOSITIS

Polymyositis-dermatomyositis (PM-DM) is a group of disorders characterized by weakness in the proximal limb muscles. About 50% of patients show a characteristic rash diagnostic of dermatomyositis. PM-DM is often associated with nuclear and cytoplasmic antibodies. Women are involved twice as often as men. Carcinoma, which may originate from a number of different sites, is associated in 5% to 15% of cases (Table 14-5).

PM-DM is less commonly associated with pulmonary involvement than other connective tissue diseases. The reported incidence of pulmonary function abnormalities is about 30%, and approximately 5% of patients show chest radiographic abnormalities. The pattern of involvement is typically that of NSIP, UIP, or OP/BOOP. Involvement of the diaphragm can lead to diaphragmatic elevation and decreased lung volumes.

HRCT findings of PM-DM include (1) ground-glass

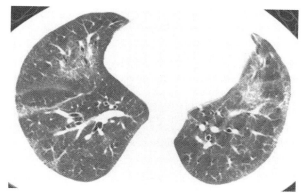

FIG. 14-17. Dermatomyositis with ground-glass opacity. Patchy and subpleural ground-glass opacity is visible on HRCT at the lung bases.

opacity (90% of abnormal cases; Fig. 14-17), (2) fine reticular opacities indicating fibrosis (90%; Fig. 14-18), (3) consolidation (50%), and (4) honeycombing (15%) with a basal and subpleural predominance. The pattern of lung fibrosis is similar to that of other collagen diseases. Consolidation at the lung bases has been associated with OP/BOOP.

After treatment with corticosteroids and immunosuppressants, abnormal findings typically improve (with the exception of fibrosis and honeycombing).

TABLE 14-5. POLYMYOSITIS-DERMATOMYOSITIS

More common in women
Carcinoma in 5%–15%
Lung involvement less common than with other collagen diseases
  Pattern may be interstitial pneumonia, usual interstitial pneumonia, organizing pneumonia/bronchiolitis obliterans organizing pneumonia
  HRCT findings similar to other collagen diseases

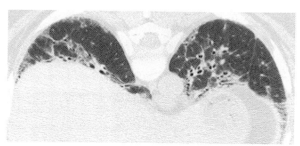

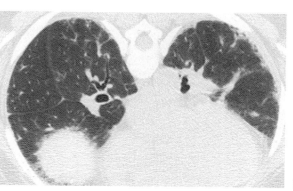

FIG. 14-18. Dermatomyositis with reticular opacities. Prone HRCT scans at two levels show reticulation in the posterior lung bases. Traction bronchiectasis is present (**A**), indicative of fibrosis.

TABLE 14-6. MIXED CONNECTIVE TISSUE DISEASE

Findings of progressive systemic sclerosis, systemic lupus erythematosus, and polymyositis-dermatomyositis
Pleural effusion or thickening in 10%
Lung involvement in 80%
    Pattern may be interstitial pneumonia, usual interstitial pneumonia, organizing pneumonia/bronchiolitis obliterans organizing pneumonia
    HRCT findings similar to other collagen diseases
Pulmonary hemorrhage
Pulmonary hypertension

MIXED CONNECTIVE TISSUE DISEASE

Mixed connective tissue disease (MCTD) is associated with clinical and laboratory findings overlapping those of PSS, SLE, and PM-DM. High titers of circulating antibodies against small nuclear ribonucleoprotein (snRNP) are required for diagnosis (Table 14-6).

MCTD is commonly associated with radiologic and functional evidence of interstitial lung disease or pleural effusion, with a prevalence of up to 80%. Pulmonary vasculitis with pulmonary hypertension and pulmonary hemorrhage are also associated with MCTD.

More than two thirds of patients with MCTD have abnormal pulmonary function tests, but chest radiographic abnormalities are visible in only about 20%. The interstitial lung disease of MCTD appears identical to that of other collagen-vascular diseases on histologic examination, radiographs, and HRCT (Fig. 14-19). Pleural effusion or pleural thickening is present in less than 10% of cases of MCTD.

SJÖGREN'S SYNDROME

Sjögren's syndrome (SS) consists of the clinical triad of keratoconjunctivitis sicca (dryness of the cornea and conjunc-

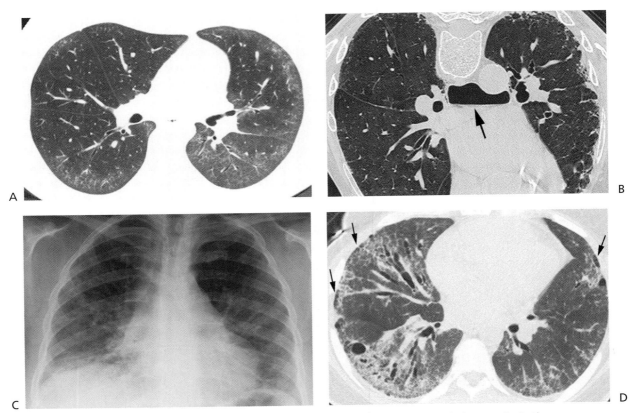

FIG. 14-19. Manifestations of mixed connective tissue disease with ground-glass opacity in three different patients. **A.** Concentric peripheral ground-glass opacity and fine reticulation are visible with sparing of the immediate subpleural lung. This appearance is typical of nonspecific interstitial pneumonia. **B.** Prone HRCT shows reticular opacities in the lung periphery. The esophagus is dilated and filled with air and fluid *(arrow)*. **C.** Chest radiograph shows decreased lung volumes with reticular opacities at the lung bases. **D.** HRCT in the same patient as **C** shows reticular opacities in the lung periphery with traction bronchiectasis and early honeycombing *(arrows)*.

TABLE 14-7. SJÖGREN'S SYNDROME

Primary or secondary (associated collagen disease)
Triad of
    keratoconjunctivitis sicca
    xerostomia
    parotid swelling
More common in women
Lymphocytic interstitial pneumonia and follicular bronchiolitis
    Lung cysts characteristic
Lung disease with pattern of interstitial pneumonia, usual
    intersitial pneumonia, organizing pneumonia/bronchiolitis
    obliterans organizing pneumonia
    HRCT similar to other collagen diseases
Tracheobronchial gland inflammation
Pleuritis with or without effusion
Focal lymphoid hyperplasia and lymphoma
    Lung nodules or masses

TABLE 14-8. ANKYLOSING SPONDYLITIS

Upper lobe fibrosis in 1%
Apical pleural thickening
Cystic lung destruction, bronchiectasis, paraseptal emphysema
Associated aspergilloma

tiva), xerostomia (dryness of the mouth and lips), and recurrent swelling of the parotid gland (Table 14-7). Although SS can occur in isolation (primary SS), most patients have coexistent collagen-vascular disease (secondary SS), most commonly rheumatoid arthritis (less often SLE and PSS). Primary SS is associated with nuclear and cytoplasmic antibodies. SS occurs in patients ranging from 40 to 70 years of age and is much more common in women.

Pleuropulmonary manifestations are relatively common and include LIP, follicular bronchiolitis, NSIP, UIP, OP/BOOP, tracheobronchial gland inflammation, and pleuritis with or without effusion. Focal lymphoid hyperplasia and lymphoma have an increased incidence in SS.

The frequency of reported radiographic abnormalities ranges from 2% to 30%. The most common radiographic finding consists of a reticular or reticulonodular pattern, usually with a basal predominance. This pattern may be caused by LIP, interstitial fibrosis, or occasionally lymphoma.

HRCT findings are largely nonspecific, including ground-glass opacity, fibrosis, and bronchiectasis, typically present in the lower lobes.

A characteristic appearance is that of multiple lung cysts occurring as an isolated abnormality (see Fig. 13-29 in Chapter 13) or in association with ground-glass opacity. These reflect the presence of LIP, which is common in this disease. The HRCT manifestations of LIP in SS are similar to those seen in LIP associated with other conditions (see Chapter 13).

Lymphoma in patients with SS may result in diffuse interstitial infiltration or multiple nodules. Focal lymphoid hyperplasia may present as solitary or multiple lung nodules (see Fig. 5-31 in Chapter 5).

ANKYLOSING SPONDYLITIS

Upper-lobe and apical lung fibrosis is seen in less than 1% of patients with ankylosing spondylitis, usually 10 years or more after the onset of the disease. Histologic abnormalities include nonspecific inflammation, fibrosis, and sometimes bronchiolitis obliterans or lipid pneumonia (Table 14-8).

Radiologically, the process begins as apical pleural thickening; an apical infiltrate characteristically develops and progresses to cystic lung destruction. It may be unilateral or bilateral. The chest radiographic findings may closely mimic those of tuberculosis. Symptoms are usually absent, but the cavities become secondarily infected, most commonly by *Aspergillus fumigatus*. HRCT more commonly shows abnormalities than do chest radiographs. The most common findings are bronchiectasis, paraseptal emphysema, and apical fibrosis.

SELECTED READING

Aquino SL, Webb WR, Golden J. Bronchiolitis obliterans associated with rheumatoid arthritis: findings on HRCT and dynamic expiratory CT. J Comput Assist Tomogr 1994; 18:555–558.

Arroliga AC, Podell DN, Matthay RA. Pulmonary manifestations of scleroderma. J Thorac Imag 1992; 7:30–45.

Bankier AA, Kiener HP, Wiesmayr MN, et al. Discrete lung involvement in systemic lupus erythematosus: CT assessment. Radiology 1995; 196:835–840.

Bhalla M, Silver RM, Shepard JO, McLoud TC. Chest CT in patients with scleroderma: prevalence of asymptomatic esophageal dilatation and mediastinal lymphadenopathy. AJR Am J Roentgenol 1993; 161:269–272.

Fenlon HM, Casserly I, Sant SM, Breatnach E. Plain radiographs and thoracic high-resolution CT in patients with ankylosing spondylitis. AJR Am J Roentgenol 1997; 168:1067–1072.

Fenlon HM, Doran M, Sant SM, Breatnach E. High-resolution chest CT in systemic lupus erythematosus. AJR Am J Roentgenol 1996; 166:301–307.

Franquet T, Giménez A, Monill JM, et al. Primary Sjögren's syndrome and associated lung disease: CT findings in 50 patients. AJR Am J Roentgenol 1997; 169:655–658.

Fujii M, Adachi S, Shimizu T, et al. Interstitial lung disease in rheumatoid arthritis: assessment with high-resolution computed tomography. J Thorac Imag 1993; 8:54–62.

Gamsu G. Radiographic manifestations of thoracic involvement by collagen vascular diseases. J Thorac Imag 1992; 7:1–12.

Kim JS, Lee KS, Koh EM, et al. Thoracic involvement of systemic lupus erythematosus: clinical, pathologic, and radiologic findings. J Comput Assist Tomogr 2000; 24:9–18.

Mino M, Noma S, Taguchi Y, et al. Pulmonary involvement in polymyositis and dermatomyositis: sequential evaluation with CT. AJR Am J Roentgenol 1997; 169:83–87.

Prakash UB. Respiratory complications in mixed connective tissue disease. Clin Chest Med 1998; 19:733–746.

Primack SL, Müller NL. Radiologic manifestations of the systemic autoimmune diseases. Clin Chest Med 1998; 19:573–586.

Remy-Jardin M, Remy J, Cortet B, et al. Lung changes in rheumatoid arthritis: CT findings. Radiology 1994; 193:375–382.

Remy-Jardin M, Remy J, Wallaert B, et al. Pulmonary involvement in progressive systemic sclerosis: sequential evaluation with CT, pulmonary function tests, and bronchoalveolar lavage. Radiology 1993; 188:499–506.

Schurawitzki H, Stiglbauer R, Graninger W, et al. Interstitial lung disease in progressive systemic sclerosis: high-resolution CT versus radiography. Radiology 1990; 176:755–759.

Schwarz MI. Pulmonary and cardiac manifestations of polymyositis-dermatomyositis. J Thorac Imag 1992; 7:46–54.

Tanoue LT. Pulmonary involvement in collage vascular disease: a review of the pulmonary manifestations of the Marfan syndrome, ankylosing spondylitis, Sjögren's syndrome, and relapsing polychondritis. J Thorac Imag 1992; 7:62–77.

Taorimina VJ, Miller WT, Gefter WB, Epstein DM. Progressive systemic sclerosis subgroups: variable pulmonary features. AJR Am J Roentgenol 1981; 137:277–285.

Tazelaar HD, Viggiano RW, Pickersgill J, Colby TV. Interstitial lung disease in polymyositis and dermatomyositis. clinical features and prognosis as correlated with histologic findings. Am Rev Respir Dis 1990; 141:727–733.

Wiedemann HP, Matthay RA. Pulmonary manifestations of sytemic lupus erythematosus. J Thorac Imag 1992; 7:1–18.

15

SARCOIDOSIS

W. RICHARD WEBB

Sarcoidosis is a systemic disorder of unknown cause, characterized by the presence of noncaseating granulomas. It may involve almost any organ, but most morbidity and mortality result from pulmonary disease. Pulmonary manifestations are present in 90% of patients. Approximately 25% of patients have respiratory symptoms at diagnosis, usually dyspnea, weight loss, fatigue, and sometimes fever or night sweats. Erythema nodosum is common.

Pulmonary lesions may resolve spontaneously or progress to fibrosis; 20% to 25% of patients have permanent functional impairment. Hilar and mediastinal lymph node enlargement is a common finding.

Sarcoidosis has been described as occurring in stages based on plain radiographic findings:

Stage 0: No visible abnormalities (10% of cases)
Stage 1: Hilar or mediastinal lymph node enlargement not associated with visible lung disease (50% of cases)
Stage 2: Hilar or mediastinal lymph node enlargement associated with visible lung disease (30% of cases)
Stage 3: Diffuse lung disease without lymph node enlargement (10% of cases)
Stage 4: This designation is sometimes used to refer to end-stage fibrosis.

The utility of this staging system is limited, although there is some correlation between the stage and the course of disease. Radiographic abnormalities resolve in 65% of stage 1 patients, 50% of stage 2 patients, and 20% of stage 3 patients. However, patients in one stage need not progress to the next. This staging system is not used with CT, which is much more sensitive than radiographs in detecting both lymph node enlargement and lung disease.

LYMPH NODE ABNORMALITIES

Mediastinal lymph node enlargement is very common with sarcoidosis, occurring in 60% to 90% of patients at some stage in their disease. No more than half of patients with lymph node enlargement also show findings of lung disease on plain radiographs. A greater percentage of patients with lymph node enlargement show evidence of lung disease on CT.

Typically, node enlargement involves the hilar and mediastinal nodes, and lymph node masses usually appear bilateral and symmetrical on chest radiographs. The combination of (1) right paratracheal, (2) right hilar, and (3) left hilar node enlargement, termed the 1-2-3 pattern, is typical of sarcoidosis (Fig. 15-1; see also Figs. 8-44 and 8-45 in Chapter 8). Aortopulmonary window lymph node enlargement may also be seen, a finding sometimes referred to as the 1-2-3-4 pattern (see Fig. 15-1A).

In patients with enlarged nodes, chest radiographs show abnormalities, in order of decreasing frequency, in the hila (85% to 95%), right paratracheal region (75%), aortopulmonary window (50% to 75%), subcarinal space (20%), and anterior mediastinum (10% to 15%; Fig. 15-2). The presence of hilar lymph node enlargement is so typical of sarcoidosis that the absence of this finding in a patient with mediastinal lymphadenopathy should lead you to question the diagnosis. Enlarged internal mammary, paravertebral, and retrocrural lymph nodes can also be seen but are much less common. Unilateral hilar lymph node enlargement is seen in less than 5% of cases. Lymph nodes may show dense, stippled, or eggshell calcification.

On CT, lymph node enlargement is visible in more than 80% of patients with sarcoidosis, with most showing both hilar and mediastinal lymph node enlargement (see Fig. 15-1B and C; see also Figs. 8-44 and 8-45 in Chapter 8). However, because CT can show lymph nodes not easily evaluated on radiographs, the frequency of involvement of specific regions is somewhat different on CT. Specifically, hilar lymph node enlargement is not invariably seen on CT in patients with mediastinal adenopathy. In patients with enlarged nodes, CT shows abnormalities, in order of decreasing frequency, in the right paratracheal space (100%), aortopulmonary window (95%), hila (90%), subcarinal space (65%), prevascular space (50%), and posterior mediastinum (15%). Symmetry, or bilateral node involvement, is visible more often on CT than on radiographs.

Lymph node masses in sarcoidosis may be quite large. Lymph node calcification is visible on CT in 25% to 50%

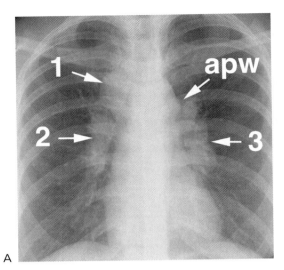

A

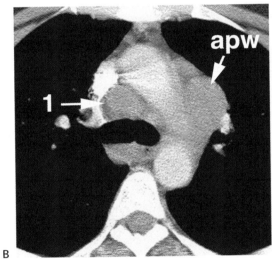

B

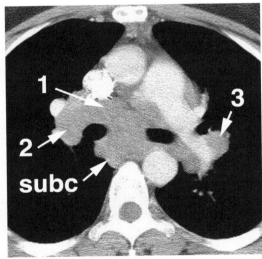

C

FIG. 15-1. The 1-2-3 pattern of lymph node enlargement in sarcoidosis. **A.** On a chest radiograph, lymph node enlargement is visible in the right paratracheal mediastinum *(1)*, right hilum *(2)*, and left hilum *(3)*. The presence of aortopulmonary window lymph node enlargement *(apw)* makes it a 1-2-3-4 pattern. **B** and **C.** On CT, lymph node enlargement is visible in the right paratracheal mediastinum *(1)*, right hilum *(2)*, and left hilum *(3)*. Aortopulmonary window *(apw)* and subcarinal *(subc)* lymph node enlargement is also visible.

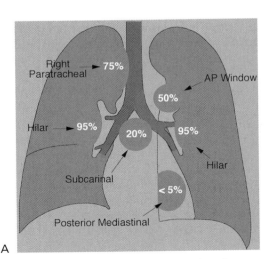

A

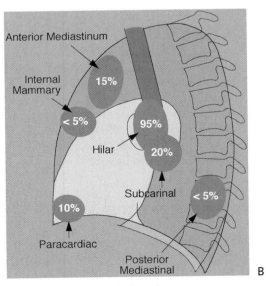

B

FIG. 15-2. Frequency of lymph node enlargement in patients with sarcoidosis as shown on posteroanterior **(A)** and lateral **(B)** radiographs.

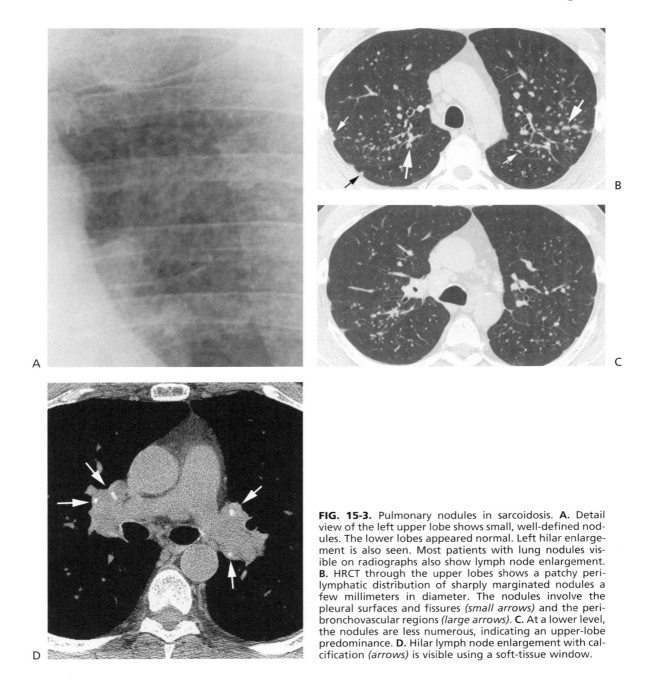

FIG. 15-3. Pulmonary nodules in sarcoidosis. **A.** Detail view of the left upper lobe shows small, well-defined nodules. The lower lobes appeared normal. Left hilar enlargement is also seen. Most patients with lung nodules visible on radiographs also show lymph node enlargement. **B.** HRCT through the upper lobes shows a patchy peri-lymphatic distribution of sharply marginated nodules a few millimeters in diameter. The nodules involve the pleural surfaces and fissures *(small arrows)* and the peribronchovascular regions *(large arrows)*. **C.** At a lower level, the nodules are less numerous, indicating an upper-lobe predominance. **D.** Hilar lymph node enlargement with calcification *(arrows)* is visible using a soft-tissue window.

of cases and may be hazy or dense or show a stippled or eggshell appearance (Fig. 15-3D; see also Figs. 8-38A and 8-45 in Chapter 8). Rarely nodes appear necrotic or low in attenuation or enhance on CT.

LUNG DISEASE

Nodules

In patients with sarcoidosis, pulmonary granulomas are found in relationship to lymphatics in the peribronchovas-

cular interstitial space, subpleural interstitial space, and, to a lesser extent, the interlobular septa. This is termed a **peri-lymphatic** distribution (see Figs. 10-20 and 10-21 in Chapter 10). Although sarcoid granulomas are microscopic in size, they often coalesce to form macroscopic nodules several millimeters or more in diameter.

Plain Radiographs

Lung disease is visible on chest radiographs in about 40% of patients and is usually associated with lymph node en-

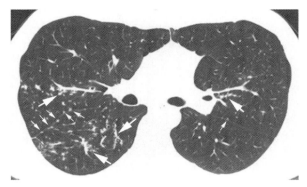

FIG. 15-4. Perilymphatic distribution of nodules on HRCT. Nodules are small, well-defined, and several millimeters in diameter. They are located in relation to the subpleural interstitium in relation to the major fissures *(small arrows)* and the peribronchovascular interstitium adjacent to central vessels *(large arrows)*, giving them a knobby appearance. Their distribution is patchy.

largement (i.e., stage 2). Lung abnormalities are often bilateral and symmetrical as seen on radiographs, with an upper-lobe predominance in up to 80% of cases and a diffuse distribution in most others. A lower-lobe predominance is unusual.

A nodular pattern is most common on chest radiographs, being seen in about half of cases (see Figs. 15-3A and 15-6A). Nodules may appear well-defined or ill-defined and fuzzy and usually range from a few millimeters to 1 cm in diameter; a reticulonodular pattern is seen in an additional 25%.

Radiographs are relatively insensitive in showing lung abnormalities. In patients with radiographic stage 1 disease

(i.e., no visible lung disease), 80% to 90% show lung lesions on high-resolution CT (HRCT) or transbronchial biopsy.

HRCT

HRCT typically shows small nodules. Nodules appear as small as a few millimeters in diameter; they tend to be sharply defined despite their small size.

In most cases, a perilymphatic distribution of nodules is recognizable on HRCT (see Figs. 15-3B and C and 15-4 to 15-6; see also Figs. 10-20 and 10-21 in Chapter 10). Sarcoid granulomas frequently predominate in relation to (1) the parahilar peribronchovascular interstitium (i.e., vessels and bronchi), (2) interlobar fissures, and (3) the peripheral subpleural regions. A distribution of nodules in relation to these three regions is highly suggestive of sarcoidosis. Interlobular septal thickening or nodules occurring in relation to septa may also be seen (see Figs. 15-5 and 15-6B), but this is not usually a predominant feature. Also, peripheral peribronchovascular nodules may appear centrilobular in location (see Fig. 15-6C). In occasional patients with extensive disease, nodules appear diffuse and "random" in distribution (see Fig. 10-23 in Chapter 10).

An upper-lobe predominance of nodules is common but not invariable (see Figs. 15-3, 15-4, and 15-6). Sarcoid often appears patchy in distribution, with some lung regions being very abnormal while others appear normal. In up to 50% of patients, nodules may be few or focal (Fig. 15-7), being localized to small areas in one or both lungs.

Nodules may calcify (Fig. 15-8). These may be associated with calcified hilar or mediastinal lymph nodes.

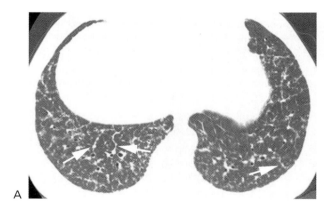

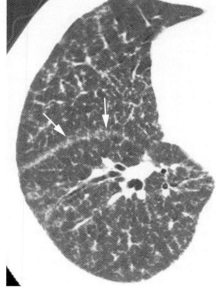

FIG. 15-5. Perilymphatic nodules on HRCT in sarcoidosis predominating in relation to interlobular septa. **A.** A scan at the lung base shows numerous thickening septa containing nodules *(arrows)*. The pleural surfaces are also abnormal. **B.** At a higher level, nodules are visible involving the fissure *(arrows)*.

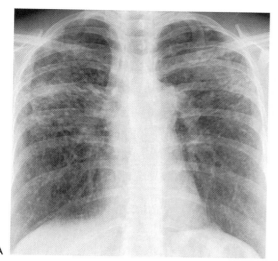

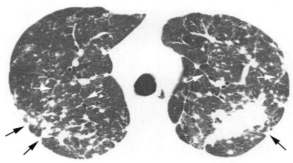

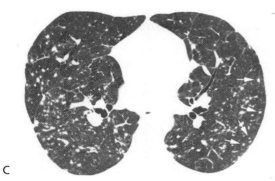

FIG. 15-6. Perilymphatic nodules in sarcoidosis. **A.** Chest radiograph shows many lung nodules, having an upper-lobe predominance. Some confluence is visible in the upper lobes. Elevation of the hila indicates some upper-lobe volume loss, likely due to superimposed lung fibrosis. **B.** HRCT through the upper lobes shows multiple small lung nodules involving the lungs in a patchy fashion. Subpleural nodules *(black arrows)* and septal thickening *(white arrows)* are visible. Confluence of multiple peribronchovascular nodules is noted in the posterior lungs. **C.** HRCT at a lower level shows fewer lung nodules *(arrows)*. The distribution is patchy. Subpleural nodules and peribronchovascular nodules are both seen. Some of the peripheral peribronchovascular nodules appear centrilobular in location.

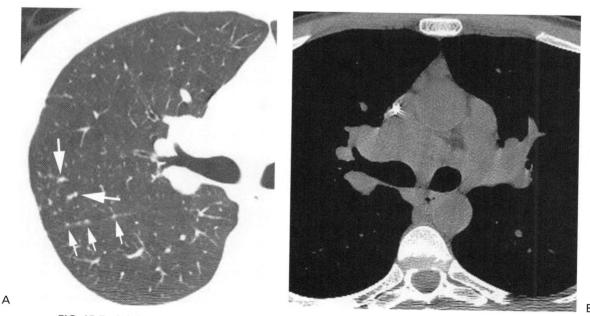

FIG. 15-7. Subtle perilymphatic nodules in sarcoidosis. **A.** HRCT shows a few nodules in relation to the major fissure *(small arrows)*. Peribronchovascular nodules in relation to small peripheral vessels *(large arrows)* are also seen. **B.** Hilar and mediastinal lymph node enlargement is also visible.

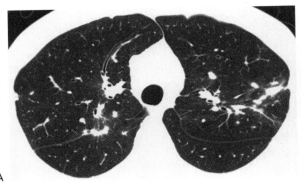

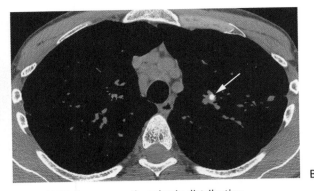

FIG. 15-8. Lung nodule calcification in sarcoidosis. **A.** HRCT shows a perilymphatic distribution of nodules. **B.** Soft-tissue window scan shows mediastinal lymph node enlargement. A left lung nodule is densely calcified *(arrow)*.

Large Nodules and Masses

Large ill-defined opacities with or without air bronchograms, having the appearance of consolidation, can be seen on chest radiographs and CT in patients with sarcoid. These may be peripheral in location or parahilar (see Figs. 15-6A and B, 15-9, and 15-10). Although these opacities have been referred to as alveolar sarcoid, they result from the confluence of large numbers of interstitial granulomas.

Large nodules (1 to 4 cm in diameter) are seen in 15% to 25% of patients on CT (see Figs. 15-6B, 15-9, and 15-10). These rarely cavitate. On CT, small nodules (i.e., satellite nodules) are often visible at the periphery of these masses (see Figs. 15-9 and 15-10). This appearance has been termed the "galaxy" sign. It is often seen in patients with masses related to sarcoid but may be seen in other granulomatous diseases and some patients with neoplasm.

Ground-Glass Opacity

Patients with sarcoidosis sometimes show patchy areas of ground-glass opacity on HRCT, which may be superimposed on a background of interstitial nodules (Fig. 15-11). This finding usually reflects the presence of numerous

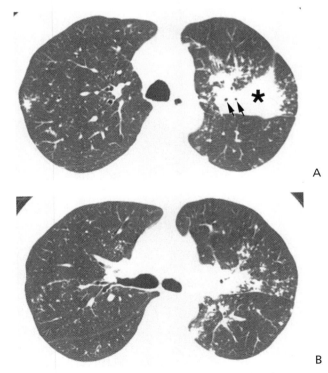

FIG. 15-10. Confluent sarcoid granulomas resulting in a mass. **A.** Confluence of peribronchovascular nodules on the left *(*)* results in a large mass. Discrete satellite nodules are visible on the edge of the mass. Air bronchograms *(arrows)* are visible within the mass. This appearance has been termed alveolar sarcoidosis. **B.** At a lower level, a patchy perilymphatic distribution of nodules is visible.

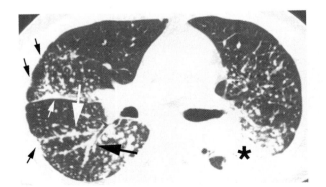

FIG. 15-9. Confluent sarcoid granulomas resulting in a mass. HRCT shows a perilymphatic distribution of nodules involving the pleural surfaces and fissure *(small arrows)* and peribronchovascular interstitium *(large arrows)*. Confluence of peribronchovascular nodules on the left *(*)* results in a mass. Discrete satellite nodules are visible on the edge of the mass, resulting in the galaxy sign.

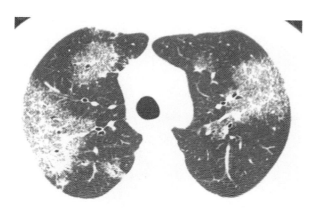

FIG. 15-11. Ground-glass opacity in sarcoidosis. HRCT shows clusters of many very small nodules with superimposed ground-glass opacity.

very small granulomas. It is similar in etiology to alveolar sarcoid.

Reticular Opacities and Fibrosis

In many patients with stage 2 and 3 disease, radiographic abnormalities resolve with time. A persistent reticular pat-

tern is seen on chest radiographs in 15% of cases; it is indicative of fibrosis and may be associated with honeycombing. Because active disease is patchy, areas of fibrosis are usually patchy in distribution.

Reticular opacities usually have an upper-lobe predominance. Parahilar masses, usually in the upper lobes, may be visible due to peribronchial fibrosis. Upper-lobe volume loss with upward retraction of the hila is common (see Figs. 15-6A and 15-12A). Areas of emphysema or air-filled cysts may also be seen in the peripheral lung.

The most common early HRCT finding of fibrosis is posterior displacement of the main and upper-lobe bronchi associated with irregular reticular opacities (see Figs. 15-12 and 15-13). Progressive fibrosis leads to masses of peribronchovascular fibrous tissue with central conglomeration of parahilar bronchi and vessels, typically most marked in the upper lobes (Fig. 15-14). This finding is frequently associated with traction bronchiectasis; the only other diseases that commonly result in this appearance are silicosis and talcosis.

Honeycombing with lung cysts can be present in patients with sarcoidosis but is relatively uncommon. The honeycombing seen in patients with sarcoidosis usually involves the middle- and upper-lung zones, with relative sparing of the lung bases (Fig. 15-15); it may also involve central or

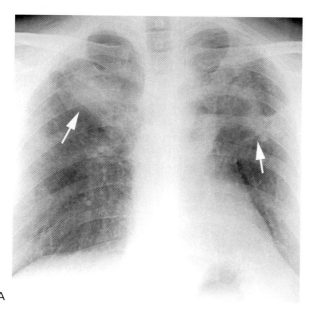

A

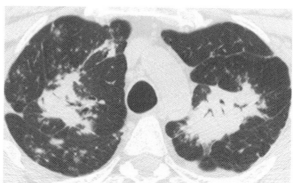

B

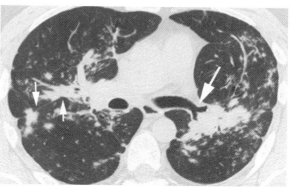

C

FIG. 15-12. Conglomerate masses and early lung fibrosis in sarcoidosis. **A.** Chest radiograph shows upward retraction of the hilar associated with masslike opacities in the upper lobes *(arrows)*. **B.** Masses with air bronchograms are visible in the upper lobes on HRCT. **C.** Posterior displacement of the upper lobe bronchi *(large arrow)* is an early sign of fibrosis. Distortion of lung architecture with displacement of the fissures *(small arrows)* and curving of pulmonary vessels also indicates volume loss and fibrosis.

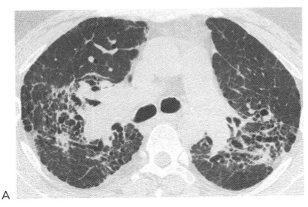

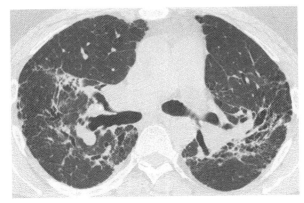

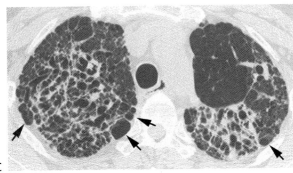

FIG. 15-13. Lung fibrosis in sarcoidosis. **A** and **B.** HRCT scans show posterior displacement of the hila and upper-lobe bronchi, associated with irregular reticular opacities and traction bronchiectasis. **C.** Extensive traction bronchiectasis is visible in the upper lobes, with areas of subpleural emphysema *(arrows).*

peribronchovascular lung, a finding atypical of idiopathic pulmonary fibrosis (IPF). Rarely, the honeycombing may involve mainly the lower-lung zones and mimic the appearance seen in IPF.

CT is helpful in assessing the presence and extent of some complications of sarcoidosis. Even though true cavitary sarcoidosis is rare, cystic lesions representing emphysema, bullae, or traction bronchiectasis are common in pa-

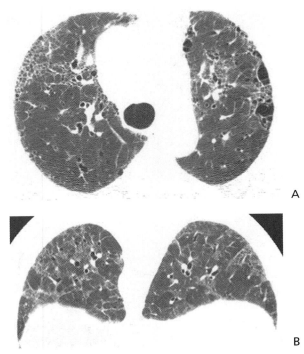

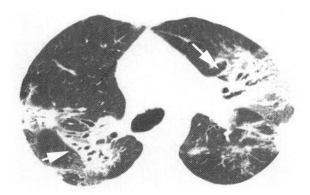

FIG. 15-14. Lung fibrosis in sarcoidosis. HRCT shows peribronchovascular masses of fibrous tissue *(arrows)* with central conglomeration of bronchi and traction bronchiectasis. The right upper-lobe bronchi are displaced posteriorly. Other patchy areas of fibrosis are also visible.

FIG. 15-15. Honeycombing in sarcoidosis. **A.** Honeycombing is visible in the upper lobes. Central or peribronchovascular lung fibrosis is also present. **B.** Prone HRCT at the lung base shows interlobular septal thickening and findings of lung fibrosis, but honeycombing is absent. This distribution would be very unusual with idiopathic pulmonary fibrosis.

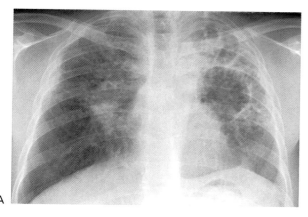

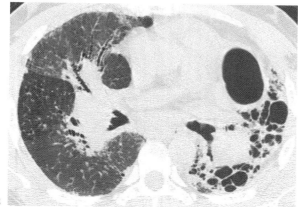

FIG. 15-16. End-stage sarcoidosis with fibrosis and cystic lesions. **A.** Chest radiograph shows reduced lung volume, upward retraction of the hila, and cystic lesion in the left upper lobe. **B.** HRCT shows extensive lung fibrosis with traction bronchiectasis and multiple cystic lesions in the left upper lobe. Enlargement of the hila represents pulmonary hypertension.

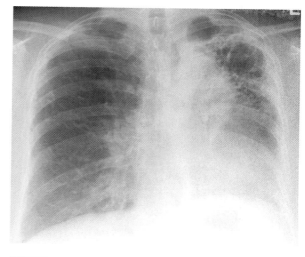

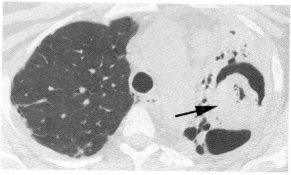

FIG. 15-18. End-stage sarcoidosis with an aspergilloma. **A.** Chest radiograph shows extensive left upper-lobe fibrosis with volume loss and cystic abnormalities. **B.** HRCT shows a fungus ball *(arrow)* within a left upper-lobe cyst.

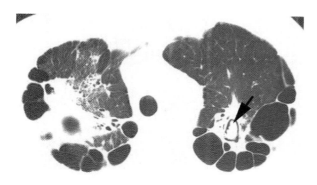

FIG. 15-17. End-stage sarcoidosis with an aspergilloma. HRCT shows upper-lobe fibrosis, traction bronchiectasis, and emphysema. An aspergilloma *(arrow)* is present within a left upper-lobe cyst.

tients with extensive fibrosis (see Figs. 15-13C and 15-16 to 15-18). Superimposed mycetoma (aspergilloma) can be readily detected with CT and is very common, being seen in as many as 10% of patients with end-stage sarcoidosis (see Figs. 15-17 and 15-18).

Bronchial and Bronchiolar Abnormalities

Airway involvement is common in sarcoidosis. Bronchial abnormalities have been reported in as many as 65% of patients, primarily consisting of nodular bronchial wall thickening or small endobronchial lesions (Fig. 15-19). HRCT may show small endobronchial granulomas. Obstruction of lobar or segmental bronchi by endobronchial granulomas or enlarged peribronchial lymph nodes may result in atelectasis; the right middle lobe is commonly involved (Fig. 15-20).

Small airway involvement by granulomas or fibrosis may result in obstruction, manifested on HRCT as mosaic perfusion on inspiratory scans (Fig. 15-21A) and air trapping on expiratory scans (see Fig. 15-21B).

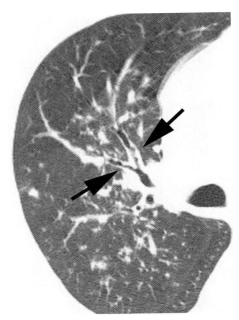

FIG. 15-19. Airway involvement in sarcoidosis. HRCT shows nodular narrowing of the right upper-lobe bronchus *(arrows)*.

Pleural Disease

About 1% of patients with sarcoidosis develop pleural abnormalities, either pleural effusion or pleural thickening. These may reflect pleural involvement by sarcoidosis.

Cardiac Abnormalities

Sarcoidosis commonly involves the heart and may result in cardiomyopathy, arrhythmias, valvular lesions, and heart failure. Cardiomegaly is sometimes seen and may be a clue to the diagnosis. Pulmonary hypertension may occur in patients with lung fibrosis.

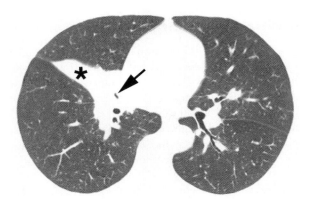

FIG. 15-20. Right middle-lobe collapse due to sarcoidosis. Narrowing of the right middle-lobe bronchus *(arrow)* is associated with middle-lobe atelectasis *(*)*.

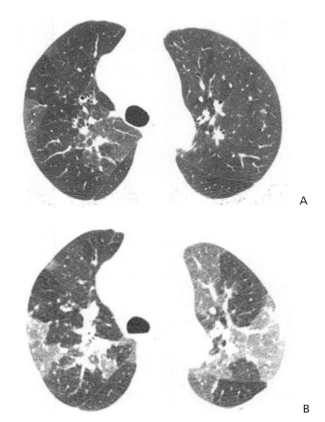

FIG. 15-21. Small airway involvement with sarcoidosis. **A.** Inspiratory scan shows nonhomogenous lung attenuation because of mosaic perfusion. **B.** Expiratory scan shows air trapping.

SELECTED READING

Brauner MW, Grenier P, Mompoint D, et al. Pulmonary sarcoidosis: evaluation with high-resolution CT. Radiology 1989; 172: 467–471.

Brauner MW, Lenoir S, Grenier P, et al. Pulmonary sarcoidosis: CT assessment of lesion reversibility. Radiology 1992; 182:349–354.

Hamper UM, Fishman EK, Khouri NF, et al. Typical and atypical CT manifestations of pulmonary sarcoidosis. J Comput Assist Tomogr 1986; 10:928–936.

Hansell DM, Milne DG, Wilsher ML, Wells AU. Pulmonary sarcoidosis: morphologic associations of airflow obstruction at thin-section CT. Radiology 1998; 209:697–704.

Kirks DR, McCormick VD, Greenspan RH. Pulmonary sarcoidosis: roentgenographic analysis of 150 patients. AJR Am J Roentgenol 1973; 117:777–786.

Lee KS, Kim TS, Han J, et al. Diffuse micronodular lung disease: HRCT and pathologic findings. J Comput Assist Tomogr 1999; 23:99–106.

Lenique F, Brauner MW, Grenier P, et al. CT assessment of bronchi in sarcoidosis: endoscopic and pathologic correlations. Radiology 1995; 194:419–423.

Lynch DA, Webb WR, Gamsu G, et al. Computed tomography in pulmonary sarcoidosis. J Comput Assist Tomogr 1989; 13: 405–410.

McLoud TC, Epler GR, Gaensler EA, et al. A radiographic classification for sarcoidosis: physiologic correlation. Invest Radiol 1982; 17:129–138.

Müller NL, Kullnig P, Miller RR. The CT findings of pulmonary sarcoidosis: analysis of 25 patients. AJR Am J Roentgenol 1989; 152:1179–1182.

Müller NL, Mawson JB, Mathieson JR, et al. Sarcoidosis: correlation of extent of disease at CT with clinical, functional, and radiographic findings. Radiology 1989; 171:613–618.

Nishimura K, Itoh H, Kitaichi M, et al. Pulmonary sarcoidosis: correlation of CT and histopathologic findings. Radiology 1993; 189:105–109.

Padley SP, Padhani AR, Nicholson A, Hansell DM. Pulmonary sarcoidosis mimicking cryptogenic fibrosing alveolitis on CT. Clin Radiol 1996; 51:807–810.

Patil SN, Levin DL. Distribution of thoracic lymphadenopathy in sarcoidosis using computed tomography. J Thorac Imaging 1999; 14:114–117.

Remy-Jardin M, Beuscart R, Sault MC, et al. Subpleural micronodules in diffuse infiltrative lung diseases: evaluation with thin-section CT scans. Radiology 1990; 177:133–139.

Remy-Jardin M, Giraud F, Remy J, et al. Pulmonary sarcoidosis: role of CT in the evaluation of disease activity and functional impairment and in prognosis assessment. Radiology 1994; 191: 675–680.

Traill ZC, Maskell GF, Gleeson FV. High-resolution CT findings of pulmonary sarcoidosis. AJR Am J Roentgenol 1997; 168: 1557–1560.

16

ALLERGIC LUNG DISEASES: HYPERSENSITIVITY PNEUMONITIS AND EOSINOPHILIC LUNG DISEASE

W. RICHARD WEBB

HYPERSENSITIVITY PNEUMONITIS

Hypersensitivity pneumonitis (HP), also known as extrinsic allergic alveolitis, is an allergic lung disease caused by the inhalation of antigens contained in a variety of organic dusts. Farmer's lung, the best-known HP syndrome, results from the inhalation of fungal organisms (thermophilic actinomycetes) growing in moist hay. Many other HP syndromes have been reported, and the list continues to grow. As with farmer's lung, HP syndromes are usually named after the setting in which exposure occurs or the organic substance involved. These include bird fancier's lung (antigen: bird proteins), mushroom worker's lung (antigen: thermophilic actinomycetes), malt worker's lung (*Aspergillus* species), maple-bark disease (*Cryptostroma* species), bagassosis (thermophilic actinomycetes in sugarcane fibers), and building-associated HP and hot-tub lung (mycobacteria). In about 50% of cases, the responsible antigen cannot be found.

Acute exposure of susceptible individuals to an offending antigen produces fever, chills, dry cough, and dyspnea; long-term exposure can produce progressive shortness of breath with few or minimal systemic symptoms. Recurrent acute episodes are common with recurrent exposure.

Although the mechanisms by which HP occurs are unclear, it is associated with circulating antibodies (IgG and IgM). These, however, are not specific to HP, as they are commonly present in exposed individuals who are asymptomatic. There is a reduced incidence of HP in tobacco smokers. The prognosis of HP is good if the patient is removed from the antigenic environment. If not, progressive fibrosis can lead to significant respiratory disability and death.

The radiographic and pathologic abnormalities occurring in patients with HP are similar regardless of the organic antigen responsible. These abnormalities can be classified into acute, subacute, and chronic stages. Often manifestations of more than one stage coexist.

Acute Stage

Exposure to large amounts of antigen in susceptible individuals may result in acute lung injury with dyspnea (Table 16-1). The acute stage of HP is characterized by alveolar filling by a neutrophilic inflammatory exudate and pulmonary edema or hemorrhage due to diffuse alveolar damage.

Radiographs typically show ill-defined air-space consolidation, predominantly in the middle and lower lung zones, but they may be normal even in the face of marked symptoms. Ill-defined air-space nodules can also be seen with acute exposure. High-resolution CT (HRCT) in this stage may show bilateral air-space consolidation and small, ill-defined, centrilobular nodular nodules.

Subacute Stage

After resolution of the acute abnormalities, which may take several days, or between episodes of acute exposure, a poorly defined nodular pattern or an ill-defined increase in lung density with obscuration of vascular margins (i.e., ground-glass opacity) may be visible on radiographs (Fig. 16-1). This appearance correlates with the presence of alveolitis; interstitial infiltrates; small, irregular, poorly defined granulomas; and cellular bronchiolitis. Histologic abnormalities are usually most severe in a peribronchiolar distribution. As in patients with acute disease, radiographs may be normal

TABLE 16-1. ACUTE HYPERSENSITIVITY PNEUMONITIS

Exposure to large amounts of antigen
Acute dyspnea
Acute lung injury with diffuse alveolar damage, edema, or hemorrhage
Air-space consolidation on radiographs and HRCT

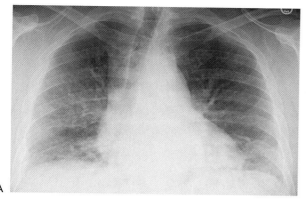

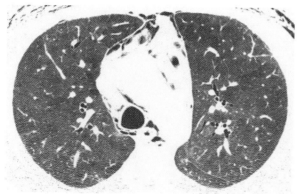

FIG. 16-1. Subacute hypersensitivity pneumonitis. **A.** Chest radiograph shows reduced lung volumes and ill-defined increased lung opacity at the lung bases. **B.** HRCT shows patchy ground-glass opacity typical of subacute hypersensitivity pneumonitis. Pneumomediastinum and subcutaneous emphysema are also present.

Typical HRCT findings include patchy ground-glass opacity (50% to 70%; see Figs. 16-1B, 16-2, and 16-3) or small ill-defined centrilobular nodules of ground-glass opacity, usually 3 to 5 mm in diameter (40% to 70%; see Figs. 16-2 and 16-4 to 16-9). These abnormalities are often seen in conjunction and may be diffuse or most marked in the middle or lower lung zones. The presence of ground-glass opacity nodules or patchy ground-glass opacity in a patient with known antigen exposure and typical symptoms is usually diagnostic in clinical practice.

Another common manifestation of subacute HP is the presence of focal areas of decreased opacity (mosaic perfusion) on inspiratory HRCT (75% to 85%; see Figs. 16-2B, 16-7, 16-8) or air trapping on expiratory HRCT (90%; see

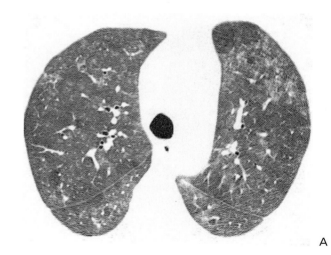

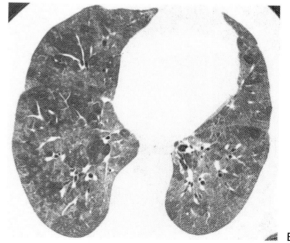

FIG. 16-2. Subacute hypersensitivity pneumonitis in a bird fancier. **A.** HRCT through the upper lobes shows patchy areas of ground-glass opacity and ill-defined nodular opacities with a centrilobular predominance. **B.** HRCT at the lung base shows patchy ground-glass opacities. Focal areas of relatively lucency represent mosaic perfusion. The combination of patchy ground-glass opacity and areas of lucency is termed the headcheese sign and is typical of hypersensitivity pneumonitis.

in the face of symptoms and an abnormal biopsy (Table 16-2).

HRCT is often first performed in the subacute stage of HP, weeks to months following first exposure to the antigen. HRCT is more sensitive than chest radiographs in HP and may show typical features when chest films are normal.

TABLE 16-2. SUBACUTE HYPERSENSITIVITY PNEUMONITIS

Ongoing or recurrent exposure to antigen
Interstitial infiltrates, poorly defined granulomas, cellular bronchiolitis
HRCT
  Patchy ground-glass opacity
  Centrilobular nodules
  Mosaic perfusion
  "Headcheese" sign
  Air trapping
  Lung cysts
May progress to fibrosis

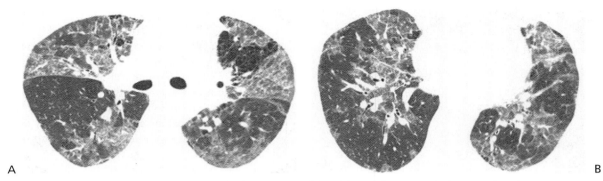

A   B

FIG. 16-3. Subacute hypersensitivity pneumonitis with patchy ground-glass opacity. Scans through the upper and lower lobes show patchy areas of ground-glass opacity.

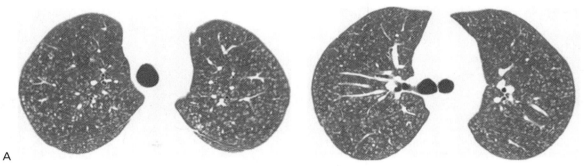

A   B

FIG. 16-4. Subacute hypersensitivity pneumonitis with diffuse centrilobular nodules. Scans through the upper lobes show diffuse centrilobular nodules. The nodules do not involve the fissures or peripheral pleural surface. This appearance correlates with the presence of peribronchiolar infiltrates and ill-defined granulomas.

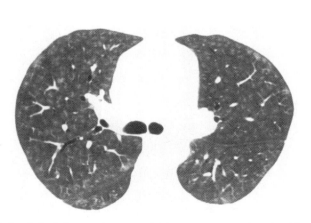

FIG. 16-5. Subacute hypersensitivity pneumonitis in a bird fancier, with ill-defined centrilobular nodules of ground-glass opacity. The nodules surround small vessels and spare the pleural surfaces. The chest radiograph in this patient was normal.

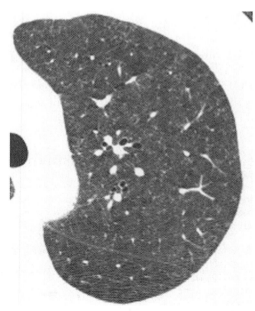

FIG. 16-6. Subacute hypersensitivity pneumonitis with diffuse centrilobular nodules, representing "hot-tub lung." Small, ill-defined nodules are visible.

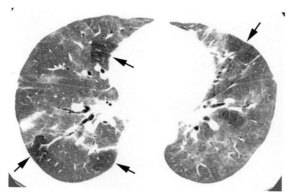

FIG. 16-7. Subacute hypersensitivity pneumonitis with the head-cheese sign. HRCT shows patchy ground-glass opacity and consolidation. Also, areas of lucency *(arrows)* containing small vessels represent mosaic perfusion. The combination of ground-glass opacity and mosaic perfusion constitutes the headcheese sign. It reflects lung infiltration (the ground-glass opacity) and bronchiolar obstruction with air trapping (areas of decreased attenuation).

Figs. 16-8 and 16-9). These areas usually have sharply defined margins and a configuration consistent with involvement of single or multiple adjacent pulmonary lobules. The areas of decreased attenuation and air trapping are due to the bronchiolitis seen in patients with HP with small airway obstruction.

A combination of increased lung attenuation (ground-glass opacity) and decreased lung attenuation (mosaic perfusion) on inspiratory scans is termed the headcheese sign because it resembles the sausage of the same name (see Figs. 16-2B, 16-7, and 16-8). The headcheese sign is common in HP and suggestive of the diagnosis. In some patients with hypersensitivity pneumonitis, evidence of expiratory air trapping is seen in the absence of inspiratory scan abnormalities.

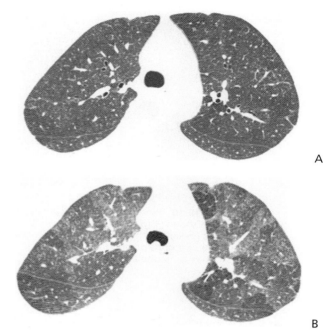

FIG. 16-9. Subacute hypersensitivity pneumonitis with air trapping. **A.** Inspiratory scan shows a fine nodular appearance and subtle mosaic perfusion. **B.** Expiratory scan shows patchy air trapping with geographic areas of lucency. Anterior bowing of the posterior tracheal membrane indicates a good expiration.

In about 10% of patients with HP, thin-walled lung cysts are visible, ranging in size from a few millimeters to more than 2 cm in diameter. In most patients, fewer than five cysts are visible. The cysts are randomly distributed and often associated with ground-glass opacity or mosaic perfusion. They likely result from bronchiolitis and bronchiolar obstruction.

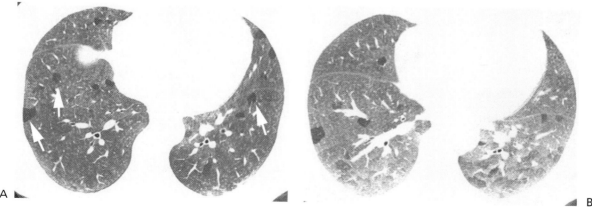

FIG. 16-8. Subacute hypersensitivity pneumonitis with air trapping. **A.** Inspiratory scan shows diffuse ground-glass opacity and centrilobular nodules, with numerous focal, lobular areas of lucency *(arrows)* due to mosaic perfusion. The combination of ground-glass opacity and mosaic perfusion constitutes the headcheese sign. **B.** Expiratory scan at the same level shows air trapping in the lucent lung regions.

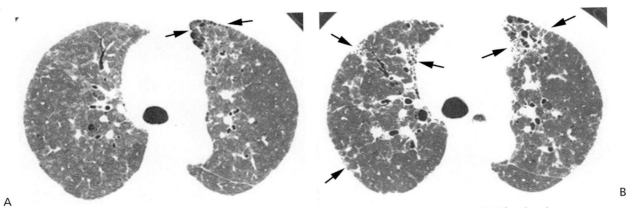

FIG. 16-10. Progression of subacute hypersensitivity pneumonitis to fibrosis in a bird fancier. **A.** HRCT shows diffuse ground-glass opacity and ill-defined ground-glass opacity nodules. Focal fibrosis is present in the left upper lobe *(arrows)* with early honeycombing. **B.** HRCT 15 months later shows progression of honeycombing and reticulation due to fibrosis *(arrows)*. Ground-glass opacity has diminished.

Findings of subacute HP usually resolve within weeks to months if exposure to the antigen is ended or the patient is treated. If exposure is ongoing or repeated exposure occurs, radiographic findings of fibrosis often develop (Fig. 16-10), being superimposed on the nodular opacities typical of subacute disease.

Chronic Stage

The chronic stage of HP is characterized by the presence of fibrosis, which may develop months or years after the initial exposure (Table 16-3).

On chest radiographs, radiographic findings of fibrosis

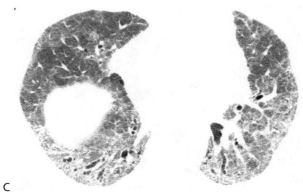

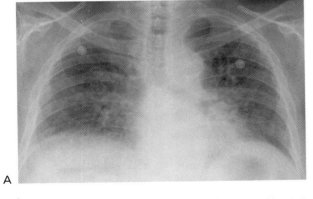

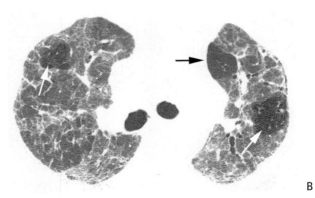

FIG. 16-11. Chronic HP with fibrosis. **A.** Chest radiograph shows marked reduction in lung volume with poorly defined reticular opacities at the lung bases. **B.** HRCT through the upper lobes shows findings of fibrosis with irregular reticular opacities and traction bronchiectasis. Some superimposed ground-glass opacity is also visible. Focal lucencies *(arrows)* reflect mosaic perfusion and the headcheese sign. **C.** HRCT at the lung bases shows similar findings. Traction bronchiectasis is visible in both lower lobes.

TABLE 16-3. CHRONIC HYPERSENSITIVITY PNEUMONITIS

Fibrosis
HRCT
    Irregular reticular opacities
    Traction bronchiectasis
    Honeycombing
    Distribution usually different than idiopathic pulmonary fibrosis
    Often appears patchy and parahilar rather than subpleural
Superimposed findings of subacute hypersensitivity pneumonitis may be present

include irregular reticular opacities that predominate in the middle lung or lower lung zones and may be parahilar, peribronchovascular, or peripheral in distribution (Fig. 16-11A). A patchy distribution is common. In some cases, fibrosis in HP can mimic the appearance of idiopathic pulmonary fibrosis (IPF) with honeycombing.

On HRCT, chronic HP is characterized by fibrosis, although findings of subacute disease are often superimposed (Figs. 16-11 to 16-13). CT scans show irregular reticular

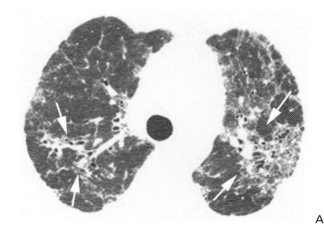

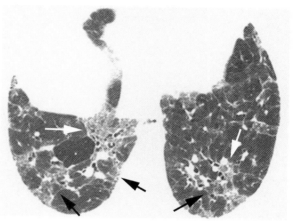

FIG. 16-13. Chronic HP with fibrosis. **A.** HRCT through the upper lobes shows patchy irregular reticular opacities. Traction bronchiectasis is visible bilaterally, with a patchy and parahilar predominance *(arrows)*. **B.** At the lung bases, areas of fibrosis *(arrows)* are patchy and lack the subpleural predominance of IPF. Lobular lucencies are also visible.

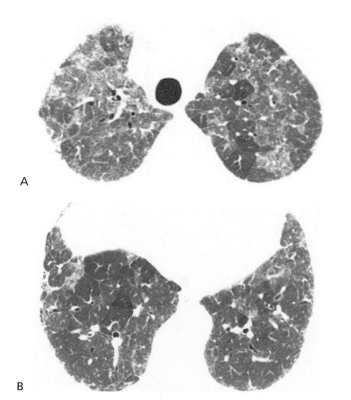

FIG. 16-12. Chronic HP with fibrosis. **A.** HRCT through the upper lobes shows ground-glass opacity, the headcheese sign, and irregular reticular opacities indicating early fibrosis. **B.** At the lung bases, irregular reticular opacities indicative of fibrosis and areas of mosaic perfusion predominate.

opacities that may be associated with patchy bilateral areas of ground-glass opacity (90%), small ill-defined nodules (60%), areas of reduced lung attenuation due to mosaic perfusion, and air trapping on expiratory scans. In HP, fibrosis is often patchy in distribution or parahilar (see Fig. 16-13), lacking the subpleural predominance of IPF; in some cases it is predominantly subpleural. Honeycombing is not common (20% of cases), but unlike IPF, it may be upper lobe in distribution or often appears patchy or peribronchovascular rather than subpleural (Fig. 16-14). Findings of fibrosis in patients with chronic HP most often show a mid-lung or lower lung zone predominance or are evenly distributed throughout the upper, middle, and lower lung zones. Relative sparing of the lung bases, seen in many patients with chronic HP, allows distinction of this entity from IPF, in which the fibrosis usually predominates in the lung bases (Fig. 16-15).

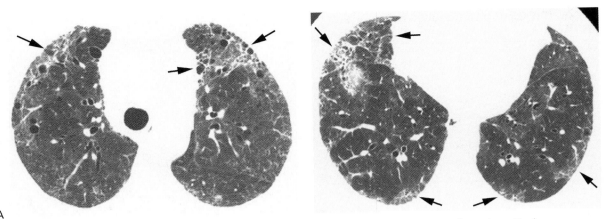

FIG. 16-14. Chronic HP with fibrosis. **A.** HRCT through the upper lobes shows irregular reticular opacities, traction bronchiectasis, and honeycombing *(arrows).* **B.** At the lung bases, patchy areas of fibrosis *(arrows)* are visible.

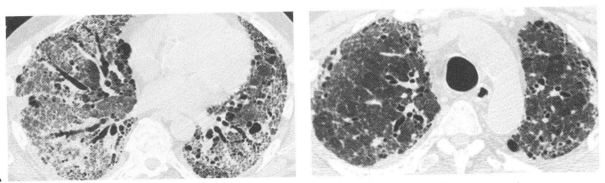

FIG. 16-15. End-stage chronic HP with fibrosis and honeycombing. **A.** HRCT at the lung bases shows extensive lung fibrosis with mild subpleural honeycombing, traction bronchiectasis, and irregular reticulation. **B.** Similar findings are noted in the upper lobes.

EOSINOPHILIC LUNG DISEASE

The term *eosinophilic lung disease* describes a group of entities characterized by an abundant accumulation of eosinophils in the pulmonary interstitium and air spaces. Peripheral blood eosinophilia is commonly present. Diagnostic criteria include (1) radiographic or CT findings of lung disease in association with peripheral eosinophilia, (2) biopsy-confirmed lung tissue eosinophilia, and (3) increased eosinophils at bronchoalveolar lavage.

The disorders can be classified into those of unknown cause and those with a known cause (Table 16-4). Some overlap exists between these categories.

IDIOPATHIC EOSINOPHILIC LUNG DISEASE

Common idiopathic eosinophilic lung diseases include (1) simple pulmonary eosinophilia, (2) chronic eosinophilic

TABLE 16-4. CLASSIFICATION OF EOSINOPHILIC LUNG DISEASE

Idiopathic eosinophilic lung disease
Simple pulmonary eosinophilia
Chronic eosinophilic pneumonia
Acute eosinophilic pneumonia
Hypereosinophilic syndrome
Churg-Strauss syndrome
Bronchocentric granulomatosis

Idiopathic eosinophilic lung disease and angiitis
Wegener's granulomatosis
Polyarteritis
Collagen-vascular diseases

Eosinophilic lung disease with a known cause
Drugs
Parasitic disease and tropical pulmonary eosinophilia
Fungi
Bronchocentric granulomatosis

pneumonia, (3) acute eosinophilic pneumonia, (4) hypereosinophilic syndrome, and (5) Churg-Strauss syndrome. These conditions reflect a spectrum, being associated with symptoms ranging from mild to severe and radiographic abnormalities ranging from focal to diffuse.

Other idiopathic diseases also may be associated with blood or tissue eosinophilia and may be considered in the differential diagnosis of eosinophilic lung disease. Vasculitis is typically present. These diseases include Wegener's granulomatosis (see Chapter 19), polyarteritis, and collagen-vascular diseases such as rheumatoid arthritis, scleroderma, CREST syndrome, polymyositis-dermatomyositis, and Sjögren's syndrome (see Chapter 14). They are sometimes included in a category of eosinophilic lung disease with angiitis.

Simple Pulmonary Eosinophilia (Loeffler's Syndrome)

Simple pulmonary eosinophilia, also known as Loeffler's syndrome, is characterized by blood eosinophilia and radiographic findings of focal areas of consolidation, which are usually transient (Table 16-5). Although similar findings can be seen in association with a number of etiologic agents, particularly parasites and drug reactions, the term *simple pulmonary eosinophilia* should be limited to cases in which the cause is unknown. Approximately one third of patients with this pattern have idiopathic disease. The disease may be self-limited.

Patients typically have cough and mild shortness of breath; often a history of asthma or atopic disease is present. Pathologically, eosinophils and histiocytes accumulate in the alveolar wall and alveoli.

The radiographic manifestations are characteristic and consist of patchy transient (fleeting) and migratory areas of consolidation that usually clear spontaneously within 1 month. These may be single or multiple and usually have ill-defined margins. On radiographs and HRCT, the areas of consolidation often have a predominantly peripheral distribution. On HRCT, areas of ground-glass opacity, focal areas of consolidation, or large nodules may be seen.

TABLE 16-5. SIMPLE PULMONARY EOSINOPHILIA (LOEFFLER'S SYNDROME)

Idiopathic
Blood eosinophilia
Mild dyspnea
History of asthma or atopy often present
Focal consolidation, usually transient or fleeting
May be self-limited

TABLE 16-6. CHRONIC EOSINOPHILIC PNEUMONIA

Idiopathic
Blood eosinophilia
Fever, weight loss, dyspnea, often severe
Patchy peripheral consolidation, often persistent
Patchy ground-glass opacity
Mimics organizing pneumonia/bronchiolitis obliterans organizing pneumonia, but usually shows an upper lobe predominance
Rapid resolution with steroids

Chronic Eosinophilic Pneumonia

Chronic eosinophilic pneumonia is an idiopathic condition characterized by extensive filling of alveoli and interstitial infiltration by a mixed inflammatory infiltrate consisting primarily of eosinophils (Table 16-6). Chronic eosinophilic pneumonia is usually associated with increased eosinophils in the peripheral blood. Clinically, patients present with fever, cough, weight loss, malaise, and shortness of breath. Symptoms are often severe and last 3 months or more. Life-threatening respiratory compromise may occur, but this is unusual.

Radiographically, chronic eosinophilic pneumonia is characterized by the presence of homogeneous peripheral air-space consolidation, "the photographic negative of pulmonary edema" (Figs. 16-16, 16-17; see also Fig. 2-9A in Chapter 2). Consolidation may be patchy. This pattern can remain unchanged for weeks or months unless steroid therapy is given; chronic eosinophilic pneumonia responds

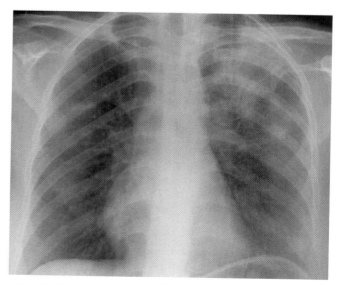

FIG. 16-16. Chronic eosinophilic pneumonia. Chest radiograph shows patchy consolidation with an upper-lobe predominance.

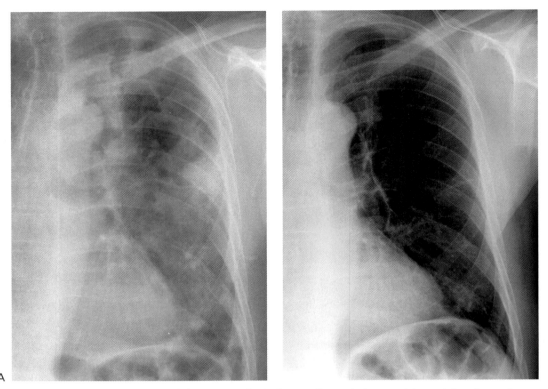

A   B

FIG. 16-17. Chronic eosinophilic pneumonia. **A.** Chest radiograph shows patchy peripheral consolidation. **B.** Following steroid treatment, the abnormalities have resolved.

promptly to the administration of steroids. An upper-lobe predominance is common (see Fig. 16-17).

The combination of blood eosinophilia, peripheral consolidation visible on radiographs, and rapid response to steroid therapy is often sufficiently characteristic to obviate the need for lung biopsy. However, this classic radiologic picture is seen in only about 50% of cases. The diagnosis may

be difficult in patients with minimal blood eosinophilia or those in whom the peripheral distribution of infiltrates is not apparent.

On CT, chronic eosinophilic pneumonia is characterized by (1) consolidation, often peripheral and patchy in distribution (90%; Figs. 16-18 and 16-19), (2) patchy or peripheral ground-glass opacity (80%), sometimes associated with

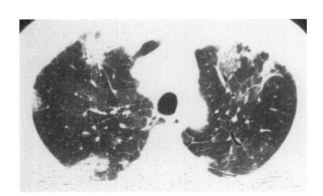

FIG. 16-18. Chronic eosinophilic pneumonia. HRCT shows patchy areas of consolidation involving the peripheral lung.

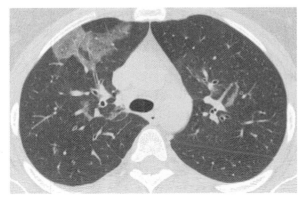

FIG. 16-19. Chronic eosinophilic pneumonia. HRCT shows patchy ground-glass opacity in the peripheral right upper lobe. Similar abnormalities were visible at other levels.

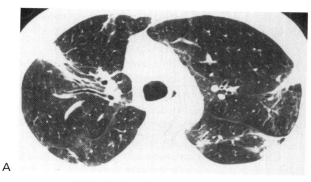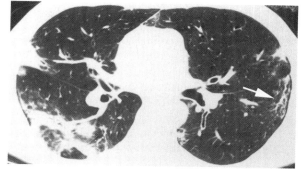

FIG. 16-20. Chronic eosinophilic pneumonia. HRCTs at two levels show patchy consolidation in the peripheral lung. A bandlike opacity is visible (*arrow* in **B**), paralleling the pleural surface. This appearance mimics that of organizing pneumonia/bronchiolitis obliterans organizing pneumonia.

"crazy-paving," (3) linear or bandlike opacities (Fig. 16-20), usually seen during resolution (5%), and (4) an upper-lobe predominance of abnormalities.

An appearance identical to that of chronic eosinophilic pneumonia can be seen in patients with simple pulmonary eosinophilia or Loeffler's syndrome. Simple pulmonary eosinophilia, however, is usually self-limited and associated with pulmonary infiltrates that are transient or fleeting. With simple pulmonary eosinophilia, areas of consolidation can appear and disappear within days; chronic eosinophilic pneumonia has a more protracted course, and areas of consolidation remain unchanged over weeks or months.

The presence of peripheral air-space consolidation can be considered only suggestive of chronic eosinophilic pneumonia in the appropriate clinical setting (i.e., in patients with eosinophilia). An identical appearance of peripheral air-space consolidation can be seen in organizing pneumonia (OP/BOOP) although OP/BOOP often involves the lower-lung zones to a greater degree.

Acute Eosinophilic Pneumonia

Acute eosinophilic pneumonia is an acute febrile illness associated with rapidly increasing shortness of breath and hypoxemic respiratory failure (Table 16-7). The diagnosis is based on clinical findings of acute respiratory failure and the presence of markedly elevated numbers of eosinophils in bronchoalveolar lavage fluid. Response to steroids is

prompt and the prognosis is good, with no residual disability.

The radiographic manifestations are similar to those of pulmonary edema. The earliest radiographic manifestation is reticular opacities, frequently with Kerley B lines. This progresses over a few hours or days to bilateral interstitial opacities and air-space consolidation involving mainly the lower lung zones. Small bilateral pleural effusions are present in most patients.

The HRCT findings of acute eosinophilic pneumonia include bilateral areas of ground-glass opacity, smooth interlobular septal thickening, small pleural effusions, and occasionally areas of consolidation. The combination of ground-glass opacity and septal thickening may result in the appearance of "crazy paving."

Hypereosinophilic Syndrome

Hypereosinophilic syndrome is characterized by blood eosinophilia present persistently for at least 6 months, associated with multiorgan tissue infiltration by mature eosinophils (Table 16-8). An underlying cause may or may not be evident. The main causes of morbidity and mortality are cardiac and central nervous system involvement. Pulmonary and pleural involvement occurs in approximately 40% of

---

TABLE 16-7. ACUTE EOSINOPHILIC PNEUMONIA

Idiopathic
Eosinophilia on bronchoalveolar lavage
Rapidly progressing respiratory failure
Radiographic findings resemble pulmonary edema

TABLE 16-8. HYPEREOSINOPHILIC SYNDROME

Idiopathic
Blood eosinophilia
Multiorgan infiltration by eosinophils
Pulmonary and pleural involvement in 40%
Ground-glass opacity or areas of consolidation
Cardiac involvement: cardiomegaly, pulmonary edema, pleural effusion
Poor prognosis

cases. Pulmonary symptoms include cough, wheezing, and shortness of breath.

The radiographic manifestations are nonspecific and consist of transient hazy ground-glass opacity or areas of consolidation. Cardiac involvement eventually leads to cardiomegaly, pulmonary edema, and pleural effusion. The prognosis is poor.

The predominant HRCT finding is bilateral pulmonary nodules, 1 cm or less in diameter, mainly involving the peripheral lung regions. Nodules may show the halo sign.

Churg-Strauss Syndrome

Churg-Strauss syndrome (also known as Churg-Strauss granulomatosis or allergic granulomatosis and angiitis) is a multisystem disorder characterized by the presence of (1) necrotizing vasculitis, (2) extravascular granuloma formation, and (3) eosinophilic infiltration of various organs, particularly the lungs, skin, heart, nerves, gastrointestinal tract, and kidneys. Not all of these three findings need be present (Table 16-9).

Patients with this syndrome are usually middle-aged (average onset 40 to 50 years) and often have a history of allergic diseases, including asthma, nasal polyps, or sinusitis. Criteria for diagnosis include (1) asthma, (2) blood eosinophilia greater than 10%, (3) a history of allergy, (4) neuropathy, (5) migratory or transient pulmonary opacities visible radiographically, (6) sinus abnormalities, and (7) extravascular eosinophilia on biopsy. The presence of four or more of these criteria is 85% sensitive and nearly 100% specific for Churg-Strauss syndrome. Churg-Strauss syndrome may

be associated with antineutrophil cytoplasmic antibody (ANCA), usually P-ANCA (perinuclear pattern).

Cough and hemoptysis are common, but symptoms may reflect the involvement of various organs, including skin rash, diarrhea, neuropathy, and congestive heart failure.

Patients usually respond well to treatment with steroids, but without treatment they may die within months. With treatment, the 5-year survival rate is good, up to 80%. Associated renal failure is associated with a poor prognosis.

Churg-Strauss syndrome may evolve in three phases:

1. An allergic phase with rhinitis, sinusitis, and asthma as the primary features
2. An eosinophilic phase associated with blood and tissue eosinophilia, usually involving the lung and gastrointestinal tract. Lung abnormalities usually resemble simple pulmonary eosinophilia or chronic eosinophilic pneumonia.
3. A systemic or small-vessel vasculitis phase in which other organs (heart, skin, musculoskeletal system, nervous system, and kidney) are also involved. This may occur years after the development of eosinophilia.

Radiographic abnormalities are common. Pulmonary opacities have been identified in 50% to 70% of patients in the eosinophilic or vasculitic phases of the disease, often consisting of transient multifocal areas of consolidation indistinguishable from simple pulmonary eosinophilia or chronic eosinophilic pneumonia. Pulmonary nodules or masses, hemorrhage, pulmonary edema, and pleural effusions may be present. In 40% of cases, pulmonary radiographic abnormalities precede the development of systemic vasculitis. Involvement of the heart may result in cardiomegaly with findings of congestive heart failure; otherwise, pleural effusion is uncommon.

HRCT findings are variable and nonspecific, reflecting the different pulmonary manifestations of this disease. Findings include (1) consolidation or ground-glass opacity (60%), which may have a peripheral distribution or be patchy and geographic; (2) pulmonary nodules or masses (20%) ranging from 0.5 to 3.5 cm in diameter, which may appear centrilobular or may contain air bronchograms; (3) bronchial wall thickening or bronchiectasis (35%); and (4) interlobular septal thickening due to pulmonary edema (5%). Although cavitation of nodules or masses may occur, it is much less common than with Wegener's granulomatosis, which it may resemble clinically and radiographically. The absence of cavitation is helpful in distinguishing Churg-Strauss syndrome from Wegener's granulomatosis.

EOSINOPHILIC LUNG DISEASE HAVING A SPECIFIC ETIOLOGY

Known causes of eosinophilic lung disease include drugs, parasites, and fungi.

TABLE 16-9. CHURG-STRAUSS SYNDROME

Idiopathic
Multisystem disorder
  Necrotizing vasculitis
  Extravascular granulomas
  Eosinophilic infiltration
History of atopy
Neuropathy
Sinus disorders
Renal involvement
P-ANCA
Three phases
  Allergic phase with rhinitis, sinusitis and asthma
  Eosinophilic phase
    Blood and tissue eosinophilia
    Findings of simple pulmonary eosinophilia or chronic eosinophilic pneumonia
  Systemic or small vessel vasculitis phase
    Heart, kidney, musculoskeletal and nervous systems involved
    Nodules or masses; may cavitate
Responds well to steroids

Drug-related Diseases

Drugs are an important cause of eosinophilic lung disease. Many drugs have been reported to be associated with eosinophilic lung disease; implicated drugs include antibiotics, nonsteroidal anti-inflammatory agents, and cytotoxic drugs. Reactions range from those similar to simple pulmonary eosinophilia to those imitating acute eosinophilic pneumonia.

Parasitic Infestations

Parasites most commonly result in findings similar to simple pulmonary eosinophilia. Most cases are due to roundworms such as *Ascaris lumbricoides, Toxocara, Ancylostoma,* and *Strongyloides stercoralis.*

Tropical pulmonary eosinophilia is caused by the worms *Wuchereria bancrofti* and *Brugia malayi,* with most cases being reported in India, Africa, South America, and Southeast Asia. In the Far East, the lung fluke *Paragonimus westermani* is typically responsible. Symptoms are nonspecific but include fever, weight loss, dyspnea, cough, and hemoptysis. CT findings reported in paragonimiasis include patchy lung consolidation, cystic lesions filled with air or fluid, pneumothorax, and pleural effusion.

Fungal Disease

The primary fungal disease associated with pulmonary eosinophilia is allergic bronchopulmonary aspergillosis, characterized by asthma, peripheral eosinophilia, central bronchiectasis, mucus plugging, and an allergic reaction to *Aspergillus fumigatus.* It is described in detail in Chapter 23. However, other patterns of disease may result from exposure to fungus, including hypersensitivity pneumonitis, eosinophilic pneumonia, and bronchocentric granulomatosis.

Bronchocentric Granulomatosis

The characteristic histologic abnormality seen in patients with bronchocentric granulomatosis is necrotizing granulomatous inflammation centered around bronchioles and small bronchi (Table 16-10). It may be associated with com-

plete destruction of the airway mucosa and filling of the airway lumen with necrotic material. In asthmatic subjects, bronchocentric granulomatosis is most commonly associated with *Aspergillus,* and fungal hyphae are often present within these lesions. Bronchocentric granulomatosis may also be seen in patients with mycobacterial infection or noninfectious inflammatory diseases such as rheumatoid arthritis, and in immunosuppressed patients.

Bronchocentric granulomatosis is generally considered a hypersensitivity reaction. Patients are usually young; one third have a history of asthma; and peripheral eosinophilia is seen in half of cases. Tissue eosinophilia is also present in asthmatic patients. This process may be associated with allergic bronchopulmonary aspergillosis (ABPA) in asthmatic patients, but abnormalities in bronchocentric granulomatosis tend to be more focal than those seen with ABPA. Symptoms are often mild, with fever, cough, chest pain, and hemoptysis.

Chest radiographs may show a nodule or focal area of consolidation. CT findings include a spiculated mass lesion or lobar consolidation with associated mild volume loss. Mucoid impaction may be present. The abnormalities predominantly involve the upper lobes. Masses and consolidation represent necrotic tissue associated with consolidation or eosinophilic pneumonia.

SELECTED READING

Adler BD, Padley SP, Müller NL, et al. Chronic hypersensitivity pneumonitis: high-resolution CT and radiographic features in 16 patients. Radiology 1992; 185:91–95.

Allen JN, Davis WB. Eosinophilic lung diseases. Am J Respir Crit Care Med 1994; 150:1423–1438.

Arakawa H, Webb WR. Air trapping on expiratory high-resolution CT scans in the absence of inspiratory scan abnormalities: correlation with pulmonary function tests and differential diagnosis. AJR Am J Roentgenol 1998; 170:1349–1353.

Bain GA, Flower CD. Pulmonary eosinophilia. Eur J Radiol 1996; 23:3–8.

Buschman DL, Waldron JA, Jr., King TE, Jr. Churg-Strauss pulmonary vasculitis. High-resolution computed tomography scanning and pathologic findings. Am Rev Respir Dis 1990; 142:458–461.

Cheon JE, Lee KS, Jung GS, et al. Acute eosinophilic pneumonia: radiographic and CT findings in six patients. AJR Am J Roentgenol 1996; 167:1195–1199.

Ebara H, Ikezoe J, Johkoh T, et al. Chronic eosinophilic pneumonia: evolution of chest radiograms and CT features. J Comput Assist Tomogr 1994; 18:737–744.

Gaensler EA, Carrington CB. Peripheral opacities in chronic eosinophilic pneumonia: the photographic negative of pulmonary edema. AJR Am J Roentgenol 1977; 128:1–13.

Hansell DM, Moskovic E. High-resolution computed tomography in extrinsic allergic alveolitis. Clin Radiol 1991; 43:8–12.

Hansell DM, Wells AU, Padley SP, Müller NL. Hypersensitivity pneumonitis: correlation of individual CT patterns with functional abnormalities. Radiology 1996; 199:123–128.

Kang EY, Shim JJ, Kim JS, Kim KI. Pulmonary involvement of idiopathic hypereosinophilic syndrome: CT findings in five patients. J Comput Assist Tomogr 1997; 21:612–615.

Kim Y, Lee KS, Choi DC, et al. The spectrum of eosinophilic lung

---

TABLE 16-10. BRONCHOCENTRIC GRANULOMATOSIS

Necrotizing granulomas centered on bronchioles and bronchi
Hypersensitivity reaction
Peripheral eosinophilia
History of asthma in one third
Associated with *Aspergillus*, mycobacteria, inflammatory diseases
Nodules, masses, focal consolidation, mucoid impaction
Upper lobe predominance

disease: radiologic findings. J Comput Assist Tomogr 1997; 21: 920–930.

King MA, Pope-Harman AL, Allen JN, et al. Acute eosinophilic pneumonia: radiologic and clinical features. Radiology 1997; 203: 715–719.

Lynch DA, Newell JD, Logan PM, et al. Can CT distinguish hypersensitivity pneumonitis from idiopathic pulmonary fibrosis? AJR Am J Roentgenol 1995; 165:807–811.

Mindell HJ. Roentgen findings in farmer's lung. Radiology 1970; 97:341–346.

Primack SL, Müller NL. Radiologic manifestations of the systemic autoimmune diseases. Clin Chest Med 1998; 19:573–586.

Remy-Jardin M, Remy J, Wallaert B, Müller NL. Subacute and chronic bird breeder hypersensitivity pneumonitis: sequential evaluation with CT and correlation with lung function tests and bronchoalveolar lavage. Radiology 1993; 198:111–118.

Silver SF, Müller NL, Miller RR, Lefcoe MS. Hypersensitivity pneumonitis: evaluation with CT. Radiology 1989; 173:441–445.

Ward S, Heyneman LE, Flint JD, et al. Bronchocentric granulomatosis: computed tomographic findings in five patients. Clin Radiol 2000; 55:296–300.

Winn RE, Kollef MH, Meyer JI. Pulmonary involvement in the hypereosinophilic syndrome. Chest 1994; 105:656–660.

Worthy SA, Müller NL, Hansell DM, Flower CD. Churg-Strauss syndrome: the spectrum of pulmonary CT findings in 17 patients. AJR Am J Roentgenol 1998; 170:297–300.

17

IATROGENIC LUNG DISEASES: DRUG-INDUCED LUNG DISEASE AND RADIATION PNEUMONITIS

W. RICHARD WEBB

DRUG-INDUCED LUNG DISEASE

Many drugs, both therapeutic and illicit, can be associated with lung disease. However, drug-induced lung disease is manifested in a limited number of ways. Specific pathologic reactions occurring with pulmonary drug toxicity include the following:

1. Hydrostatic and increased permeability pulmonary edema
2. Diffuse alveolar damage and the acute respiratory distress syndrome (ARDS)
3. Pulmonary hemorrhage
4. Organizing pneumonia (OP/BOOP)
5. Eosinophilic pneumonia and hypersensitivity reactions
6. Chronic interstitial pneumonitis with fibrosis
7. Systemic lupus erythematosus (SLE)
8. Pulmonary vasculitis and pulmonary hypertension
9. Bronchiolitis obliterans

Each of these patterns is characteristically associated with a different group of drugs, although many drugs can result in more than one type of lung reaction, and some overlap between these patterns is common. In most cases, the radiographic appearances of a drug-related lung disease are non-specific and the diagnosis must be based on observing a temporal relationship between the administration of a drug and the development of pulmonary abnormalities.

Because of the large number of drugs associated with drug reactions and the variety of patterns possible, a high degree of suspicion must be maintained when evaluating patients with unexplained lung disease, regardless of what it looks like or what drug treatment is being employed. Prompt recognition of drug-induced lung disease is important because early abnormalities may resolve completely if the drug is discontinued or appropriate therapy is instituted.

Radiographic abnormalities associated with drug-related lung injury vary with the pathologic pattern present, and with a few exceptions, the appearance of each pattern tends to appear the same regardless of the drug involved. High-resolution CT (HRCT) is more sensitive than chest radiography in defining the radiographic abnormalities.

Pulmonary Edema

Hydrostatic pulmonary edema may result from drugs affecting the heart or systemic vasculature (Table 17-1). An example would be cocaine. Findings are typical of any cause of hydrostatic edema. Pleural effusion may be present.

Increased-permeability pulmonary edema also may occur. Onset is usually sudden. Increased-permeability pulmonary edema occurring without diffuse alveolar damage results in typical findings of pulmonary edema, including

TABLE 17-1. DRUGS ASSOCIATED WITH PULMONARY EDEMA

Aspirin and salicylates
BCNU
Cocaine
Chlordiazepoxide
Codeine
Cyclophosphamide
Cytosine arabinoside
Heroin
Hydrochlorothiazide
Interleukin-2
Lidocaine
Methadone
Methotrexate
Nitrofurantoin
Nonsteroidal anti-inflammatory drugs
OKT3
Propoxyphene
Tocolytics (ritodrine and terbutaline)
Trimethoprim-sulfamethoxazole
Tricyclic antidepressants

interlobular septal thickening (Kerley's lines; see Fig. 11-12 in Chapter 11), ground-glass opacity (see Fig. 11-13 in Chapter 11), and to a lesser extent, consolidation. This occurrence is typical of interleukin-2, but many other drugs are capable of causing pulmonary edema. These include aspirin, nitrofurantoin, heroin, and cytotoxic agents such as methotrexate, cyclophosphamide, and BCNU. Unlike with hydrostatic edema, pleural effusion is typically absent. Prompt resolution may occur with appropriate treatment.

Diffuse Alveolar Damage

Diffuse alveolar damage (DAD) with ARDS can be caused by a variety of drugs, most typically cytotoxic agents (e.g., bleomycin, busulfan, and cyclophosphamide), nitrofurantoin, and amiodarone (Table 17-2). As with pulmonary edema, onset is usually sudden and occurs within a few days of the onset of chemotherapy.

DAD reflects a more serious injury than with increased-permeability pulmonary edema. The acute or exudative stage of DAD occurs in the first week after injury and is characterized by necrosis of alveolar pneumocytes, edema, hemorrhage, and hyaline membrane formation. Radiographs and CT typically show extensive bilateral parenchymal consolidation, usually most marked in the dependent lung regions; interlobular septal thickening and Kerley's lines are typically absent (Fig. 17-1). Other than a temporal relationship to chemotherapy, there are no clinical or CT findings that allow this appearance to be distinguished from other causes of ARDS. The reparative stage of DAD, characterized by cellular hyperplasia and fibrosis, occurs after 1 to 2 weeks. Depending on the severity of the lung injury, abnormalities may regress, stabilize, or progress to honeycombing.

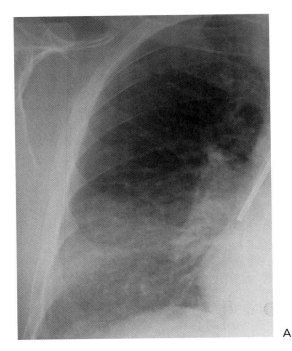

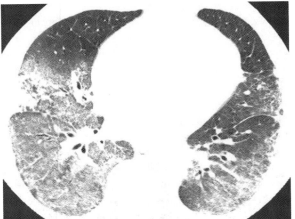

FIG. 17-1. Diffuse alveolar damage resulting from treatment with doxorubicin (Adriamycin). **A.** Chest radiograph coned to the right lung shows basilar consolidation. **B.** HRCT shows ground-glass opacity and consolidation with a basal and dependent predominance.

TABLE 17-2. DRUGS ASSOCIATED WITH DIFFUSE ALVEOLAR DAMAGE

Amiodarone
BCNU
Bleomycin
Busulfan
Chlorambucil
Cyclophosphamide
Cytosine arabinoside
Gold
Methotrexate
Mitomycin
Melphalan
Nitrofurantoin
Oxygen
Penicillamine
Tricyclic antidepressants
Vinblastine and vinca alkaloids

Pulmonary Hemorrhage

Drug-related diffuse pulmonary hemorrhage is uncommon. Typical causes include anticoagulants, cyclophosphamide, and penicillamine. Hemoptysis may or may not be present (Table 17-3). Radiographic and HRCT findings are typical of pulmonary hemorrhage, with bilateral patchy ground-glass opacity or consolidation (see Chapter 19). Pleural effusion is typically absent.

**TABLE 17-3. DRUGS
ASSOCIATED WITH PULMONARY
HEMORRHAGE**

Anticoagulants
Amphotericin B
Crack cocaine
Cyclophosphamide
Cytosine arabinoside
Penicillamine
Quinidine

Organizing Pneumonia/Bronchiolitis Obliterans Organizing Pneumonia

Organizing pneumonia/bronchiolitis organizing pneumonia (OP/BOOP) has been described with methotrexate, gold, penicillamine, nitrofurantoin, amiodarone, bleomycin, and busulfan (Table 17-4). Symptoms include progressive cough, dyspnea, and fever. Like other causes of OP/BOOP (see Chapter 13), this pattern is characterized by consolidation or ground-glass opacity that may have a patchy or nodular distribution and may predominate in a peribronchial or subpleural location (Figs. 17-2 and 17-3). Lung nodules with or without the atoll sign may be present (Figs. 17-2A and 17-3). OP/BOOP tends to predominate in the lower lobes (see Fig. 17-3).

Hypersensitivity Reactions and Eosinophilic Pneumonia

Hypersensitivity reactions can be attributed to a large number of drugs but are most commonly due to methotrexate, nitrofurantoin, bleomycin, procarbazine, BCNU, cyclophosphamide, nonsteroidal anti-inflammatory drugs, and sulfonamides; their presence is unrelated to the cumulative drug dose (Table 17-5).

TABLE 17-4. DRUGS ASSOCIATED WITH ORGANIZING PNEUMONIA/BRONCHIOLITIS OBLITERANS ORGANIZING PNEUMONIA

Amiodarone
Bleomycin
Busulfan
Cyclophosphamide
Gold
Interferon
Methotrexate
Nitrofurantoin
Penicillamine
Sulfasalazine

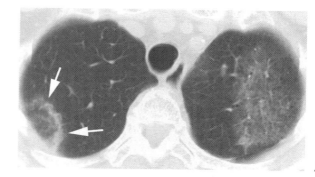

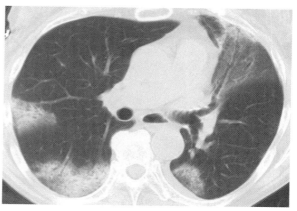

FIG. 17-2. Organizing pneumonia/bronchiolitis organizing pneumonia (OP/BOOP) occurring in association with chemotherapy for breast carcinoma. **A.** CT through the lung apex shows ground-glass opacity in the left upper lobe and a ring of ground-glass opacity in the right upper lobe *(arrows)*, representing the atoll sign of OP/BOOP. **B.** CT shows patchy subpleural areas of consolidation and ground-glass opacity typical of OP/BOOP.

Hypersensitivity reactions may have features of simple eosinophilia (Loeffler's syndrome), chronic eosinophilic pneumonia, or acute eosinophilic pneumonia. Cough and dyspnea, with or without fever, can be acute in onset or progress over a period of several months following institution of treatment. A peripheral eosinophilia is present in up to 40%. These reactions are characterized on chest radiographs and HRCT by patchy areas of consolidation or ground-glass opacity, which may be chronic or relatively acute, transient, and fleeting. A peripheral and subpleural distribution may be seen.

Chronic Interstitial Pneumonitis and Fibrosis

Both usual interstitial pneumonia (UIP) and nonspecific interstitial pneumonia (NSIP) have been associated with drug injury; in some cases the pattern may overlap that of OP/BOOP or DAD. The clinical and radiographic presentations are often identical to those of idiopathic pulmonary fibrosis. A long list of drugs has been implicated in the

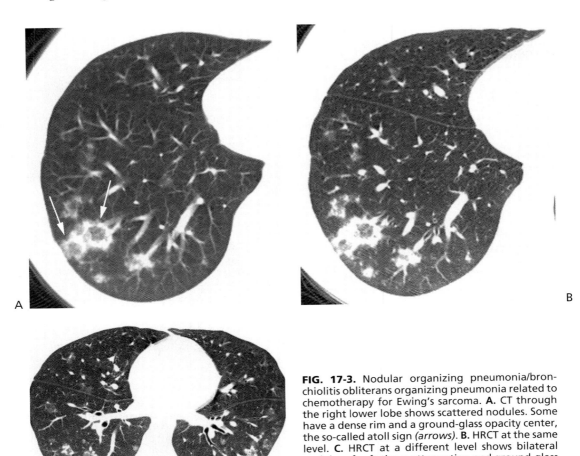

FIG. 17-3. Nodular organizing pneumonia/bronchiolitis obliterans organizing pneumonia related to chemotherapy for Ewing's sarcoma. **A.** CT through the right lower lobe shows scattered nodules. Some have a dense rim and a ground-glass opacity center, the so-called atoll sign *(arrows)*. **B.** HRCT at the same level. **C.** HRCT at a different level shows bilateral nodules of soft-tissue attenuation and ground-glass opacity visible in both lower lobes. Some nodules show the atoll sign.

TABLE 17-5. DRUGS ASSOCIATED WITH EOSINOPHILIC PNEUMONIA AND HYPERSENSITIVITY REACTIONS

BCNU
Bleomycin
Cyclophosphamide
Diphenylhydantoin
Erythromycin
Ethambutol
Fluoxetine
Gold
Imipramine
Isoniazid
Methotrexate
Nitrofurantoin
Nonsteroidal anti-inflammatory drugs
Paraaminosalicylic acid
Penicillamine
Penicillin
Procarbazine
Sulfasalazine
Tetracycline

TABLE 17-6. DRUGS ASSOCIATED WITH CHRONIC PNEUMONITIS AND FIBROSIS

Adriamycin
Amiodarone
BCNU
Bleomycin
Busulfan
Chlorambucil
Cyclophosphamide
Gold
Methotrexate
Mitomycin
Nitrofurantoin
Penicillamine
Sulfasalazine
Tocainide

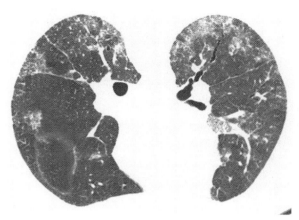

FIG. 17-4. Interstitial pneumonia with fibrosis following chemotherapy. Prone HRCT shows subpleural ground-glass opacity and fine reticular opacities. This appearance is consistent with a nonspecific interstitial pneumonia pattern or early usual interstitial pneumonia pattern.

development of chronic pneumonitis, but this pattern is most commonly the result of cytotoxic chemotherapeutic agents such as bleomycin, busulfan, methotrexate, doxorubicin, and carmustine (BCNU; Table 17-6). Nitrofurantoin, amiodarone, gold, and penicillamine are noncytotoxic drugs that can also result in this type of reaction.

Plain radiographs in patients with chronic pneumonitis and fibrosis typically show a mixture of reticulation and consolidation; abnormalities are usually bilateral and symmetric, with a predominant lower lung zone involvement.

The most common pattern seen on HRCT in patients with chronic pneumonitis and fibrosis includes irregular reticular opacities (Fig. 17-4), honeycombing (Fig. 17-5), architectural distortion, and traction bronchiectasis, with or

without associated consolidation; ground-glass opacity may be seen in early cases (see Figs. 17-4 to 17-8). As on chest radiographs, HRCT abnormalities are usually bilateral and symmetric, with a predominant lower lung zone involvement. A peripheral and subpleural distribution of abnormalities is common, particularly in patients with bleomycin toxicity. Patchy fibrosis may be seen in patients receiving nitrofurantoin. The extent of abnormalities depends on the severity of lung damage. Mild damage is often limited to the posterior subpleural lung regions of the lower lung zones. In patients with more severe abnormalities, there is greater involvement of the remaining lung parenchyma.

Systemic Lupus Erythematosus

Systemic lupus erythematosus (SLE) related to drug treatment is indistinguishable clinically and radiographically from idiopathic SLE (Table 17-7). Pleural effusions and pericardial effusions are the most common manifestations.

Pulmonary Vasculitis and Pulmonary Hypertension

The use of various drugs may result in acute or chronic abnormalities of small vessels within the lung, with histologic abnormalities including pulmonary vasculitis, plexogenic arteriopathy, and pulmonary venoocclusive disease (Table 17-8).

The radiographic appearances of these vary with the specific abnormalities present. Pulmonary vasculitis may result in an appearance similar to that of pulmonary edema or pulmonary hemorrhage, with patchy or diffuse consolidation or ground-glass opacity. Plexogenic arteriopathy shows findings of pulmonary hypertension, with enlargement of

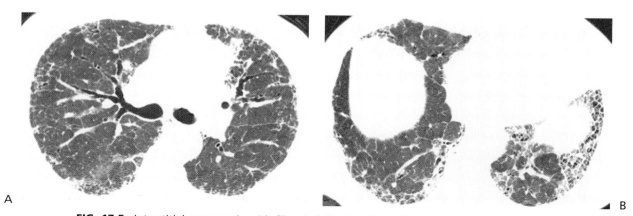

A   B

FIG. 17-5. Interstitial pneumonia with fibrosis following chemotherapy with methotrexate. **A.** HRCT through the upper lobes shows irregular reticular opacities and traction bronchiectasis. **B.** HRCT through the lung bases shows honeycombing with a subpleural predominance. This appearance is that of usual interstitial pneumonia and is indistinguishable from that of idiopathic pulmonary fibrosis.

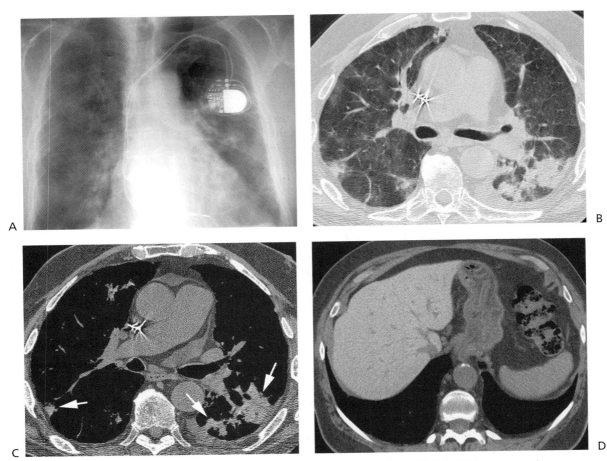

FIG. 17-6. Amiodarone treatment with organizing pneumonia/bronchiolitis obliterans organizing pneumonia (OP/BOOP). **A.** Chest radiograph shows cardiomegaly, a pacemaker, and patchy lung consolidation. **B.** HRCT shows patchy areas of consolidation and ground-glass opacity in the lung periphery. This appearance is typical of OP/BOOP. The presence of a small left pleural effusion is not typical of OP/BOOP but may reflect heart failure. **C.** HRCT with a soft-tissue window shows the areas of lung consolidation to be denser than soft tissue *(arrows)*. This is common in patients with amiodarone toxicity. However, dense lung may be seen in any patient on long-term amiodarone treatment who has lung consolidation; dense lung does not imply toxicity. **D.** CT through the upper abdomen shows the liver to be dense.

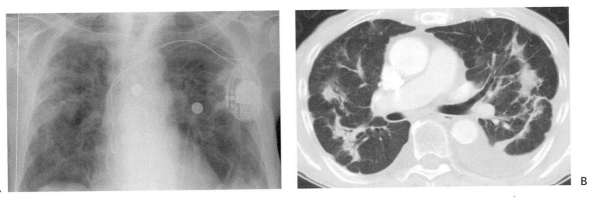

FIG. 17-7. Amiodarone treatment with lung fibrosis. **A.** Chest radiograph shows a pacemaker and streaky areas of fibrosis in the peripheral lungs. **B.** HRCT shows irregular reticular opacities, traction bronchiectasis, and nodular areas of consolidation in the lung periphery. This appearance resembles a combination of organizing pneumonia/bronchiolitis obliterans organizing pneumonia and lung fibrosis. The left pleural effusion is likely related to heart failure.

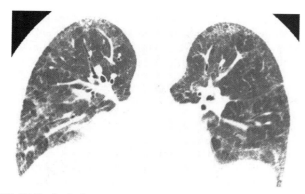

FIG. 17-8. Amiodarone treatment with lung fibrosis. Prone HRCT shows peripheral reticular opacities representing nonspecific interstitial pneumonia or usual interstitial pneumonia.

TABLE 17-7. DRUGS ASSOCIATED WITH SYSTEMIC LUPUS ERYTHEMATOSUS

Anticonvulsants
Beta blockers
Digitalis
Gold
Hydralazine
Isoniazid
Levodopa
Nitrofurantoin
Nonsteroidal anti-inflammatory drugs
Penicillamine
Penicillin
Phenothiazines
Procainamide
Quinidine
Streptomycin
Sulfonamides
Thiouracil

TABLE 17-8. DRUGS ASSOCIATED WITH PULMONARY VASCULITIS AND PULMONARY HYPERTENSION

Amphetamines (pulmonary hypertension)
Anorectic drugs such as fenfluramine and phenformin (pulmonary hypertension)
Anticonvulsants
Cocaine (pulmonary hypertension)
Hydralazine
Busulfan
Penicillin
Phenothiazines
Quinidine
Sulfonamides
Thiouracil

TABLE 17-9. DRUGS ASSOCIATED WITH BRONCHIOLITIS OBLITERANS

Gold
Penicillamine
Sulfasalazine

central pulmonary arteries. Pulmonary venoocclusive disease mimics hydrostatic edema, but with normal heart size.

Bronchiolitis Obliterans

The least common lung reaction to drugs is bronchiolitis obliterans, a finding described primarily in association with penicillamine therapy for rheumatoid arthritis (Table 17-9). However, the role of penicillamine is controversial, as bronchiolitis obliterans can be seen in patients with rheumatoid arthritis who have not been treated with this drug. Bronchiolitis obliterans has also been seen in patients treated with sulfasalazine. Chest radiographs may show large lung volumes. The abnormalities seen on HRCT consist of bronchial wall thickening and a pattern of mosaic perfusion, similar to that seen with other causes of bronchiolitis obliterans (see Figs. 10-36 and 10-38 in Chapter 10 and Figs. 23-21 and 23-22 in Chapter 23); air trapping on expiratory scans is typically present.

REACTIONS TO SPECIFIC DRUGS

Drug reactions may occur during treatment with a wide variety of agents. The highest incidence of adverse effects occurs with cytotoxic agents: up to 10% of patients receiving cytotoxic chemotherapeutic agents develop an adverse reaction. Some of the more common drugs to result in significant pulmonary disease are described below. Commonly used illicit drugs also are responsible for drug reactions, but lung abnormalities resulting from illicit drug use may also reflect injection of particulate matter (i.e., talc) or inhalation of toxic substances.

Amiodarone

Amiodarone is an iodinated drug used in the treatment of refractory cardiac tachyarrhythmias. It accumulates in the liver and lung, where it becomes entrapped in macrophage lysosomes. It results in pulmonary toxicity in 5% of patients.

Pathologic reactions to amiodarone include DAD, OP/BOOP (see Fig. 17-6), and chronic pneumonitis with fibrosis (see Figs. 17-7 and 17-8). The radiographic patterns of pulmonary reaction to amiodarone vary and include focal or diffuse areas of consolidation, reticular opacities, and less commonly ill-defined nodules or masses (see Fig. 17-6).

Regions of consolidated lung in patients with amiodarone-related lung toxicity appear denser than soft tissue on unenhanced CT because of their high iodine content (see Fig. 17-6C). However, dense lung may also be seen in any patient on long-term amiodarone treatment who develops lung consolidation or collapse. Patients with amiodarone pulmonary toxicity almost always show increased liver attenuation on CT (see Fig. 17-6D), although this finding is also present in patients treated with amiodarone who do not have drug toxicity.

Aspirin and Salicylates

As many as 5% of asthmatics are sensitive to aspirin; use causes bronchospasm. This may be related to inhibition of prostaglandin synthesis.

Salicylate-induced increased permeability pulmonary edema can occur when the blood salicylate level exceeds 40 mg/dl, particularly in the elderly or in smokers. This may represent a direct toxic effect on capillary permeability. Treatment may require mechanical ventilation; resolution within a week is typical.

Bleomycin

Bleomycin is a cytotoxic drug used in the treatment of lymphomas and some carcinomas. Bleomycin pulmonary toxicity is the most common pulmonary disease related to chemotherapy, with an incidence of about 4%. Toxicity is related to cumulative doses exceeding 400 mg. Associated risk factors for development of lung disease include recent radiation, oxygen therapy, renal disease, and advanced age.

A wide variety of reactions to bleomycin have been reported, including pulmonary edema (see Fig. 11-12 in Chapter 11), diffuse alveolar damage with respiratory failure, chronic pneumonitis with fibrosis, OP/BOOP, and hypersensitivity reactions. Radiographic and CT appearances vary accordingly.

Pneumonitis with pulmonary fibrosis typically presents 1 to 2 months after the onset of treatment with progressive dyspnea and cough. Chest radiographs show reticulation, ground-glass opacity, and sometimes consolidation with a predominant subpleural and lower-lobe predominance. With severe or progressive disease, more diffuse involvement of the lower, middle, and upper lungs is typically visible. HRCT is more sensitive than radiographs in detecting early disease. Some abnormalities resolve following cessation of treatment in patients with early disease.

A unique manifestation of bleomycin-related lung toxicity is the presence of multiple pulmonary nodules mimicking the appearance of metastases and having histologic characteristics of OP/BOOP.

Busulfan

Busulfan is an alkylating agent used in treating chronic myeloproliferative diseases, and clinically recognized lung toxic-

ity occurs in about 5% of cases. It usually results in findings of chronic pneumonitis and fibrosis, OP/BOOP, or DAD. Radiographic and HRCT findings include patchy or diffuse consolidation or reticulation.

Cocaine and Crack

Use of sympathomimetic agents such as cocaine (or its derivative crack), either by injection or inhalation, may cause hydrostatic pulmonary edema by inducing ischemia-related transient myocardial dysfunction, severe peripheral vasoconstriction with transient left ventricular failure, cardiac arrhythmia, or frank myocardial infarction. Cocaine or crack may also cause acute lung injury with increased permeability pulmonary edema (see Fig. 11-13 in Chapter 11), pulmonary hemorrhage, or pulmonary hypertension. HRCT commonly reveals multifocal ground-glass opacities, occasionally centrilobular in distribution, associated with interlobular septal thickening. Because pulmonary edema, pulmonary hemorrhage, and acute lung injury may be radiographically indistinguishable and may occur in combination, the development of respiratory failure after cocaine or crack use, associated with evidence of bilateral air-space opacities, clearing rapidly following cessation of drug use, has been termed "crack lung."

Cyclophosphamide (Cytoxan)

Cyclophosphamide is an alkylating agent used in the treatment of a variety of malignancies and autoimmune diseases and is commonly used in combination with other therapeutic agents; pulmonary toxicity occurs in less than 1% of cases. Histologic findings associated with lung injury are similar to those seen in patients with bleomycin toxicity and include chronic pneumonitis and fibrosis, OP/BOOP, DAD, pulmonary edema, and hypersensitivity reactions. Radiographic appearances vary accordingly.

Heroin and Narcotics

Use of heroin or other narcotics may result in increased-permeability pulmonary edema. Possible mechanisms include a toxic effect on the alveolar capillary membrane, effects on the central nervous system with neurogenic edema, hypoxemia, and hypersensitivity. Symptoms of dyspnea typically occur from minutes to a few hours after injection. Radiographs show typical findings of increased-permeability edema, with parahilar ground-glass opacity or consolidation, but the appearance may be complicated by associated aspiration. Hemorrhage may also be present. Resolution often occurs within 1 to 2 days.

Interleukin-2

Interleukin-2 is a T-cell growth factor used as an immune system stimulator for treating cancers, particularly melanoma and renal cell carcinoma. It may cause increased-permeability pulmonary edema by a direct toxic effect on the capillary endothelium. Symptoms typically begin within 2 to 8 days of the onset of treatment. Radiographs show typical findings of interstitial or air-space edema. Pleural effusion, an unusual finding with increased-permeability edema, is common. Clearing occurs within days of drug cessation.

Methotrexate

Methotrexate is a folate antagonist used in the treatment of malignancies and inflammatory diseases. Pulmonary toxicity occurs in 5% to 10% of cases and is unrelated to the duration of treatment or the cumulative dose.

In contrast to many other cytotoxic agents, methotrexate often results in reversible abnormalities. Symptoms usually develop within weeks of the onset of treatment and include fever, cough, and dyspnea. In most cases, the histologic appearance resembles hypersensitivity pneumonitis or less often OP/BOOP or DAD; peripheral eosinophilia is present in half of cases. Chest radiographs show ill-defined reticular opacities, ground-glass opacity, or consolidation. A basal predominance is typical. HRCT usually shows ground-glass opacity as the predominant abnormality. Radiographic abnormalities usually regress following discontinuation of the drug. Some residual fibrosis may be seen. However, fibrosis and honeycombing may result (see Fig. 17-5).

Nitrofurantoin

Nitrofurantoin is an antibiotic used for treatment of urinary tract infections. It may result in either acute or chronic reactions; acute reactions are much more common, accounting for 90% of cases of toxicity. SLE related to nitrofurantoin has also been reported.

Acute nitrofurantoin toxicity is a hypersensitivity reaction and usually begins from 1 day to 2 weeks after initiation of therapy. Symptoms include fever, cough, and dyspnea; peripheral eosinophilia is present in most patients. Chest radiographs show an interstitial abnormality with Kerley's lines (i.e., pulmonary edema) or consolidation, which may be symmetric or asymmetric. Pleural effusion, usually small and unilateral, is present in one third of cases. Discontinuation of the drug results in clearing, usually within days.

Chronic nitrofurantoin reaction occurs from 2 months to years after the beginning of continuous treatment. It is unrelated to acute toxicity. Insidious cough and dyspnea are most common; fever is absent and eosinophilia is uncommon. Radiographs show a diffuse reticular abnormality with a basal predominance due to chronic pneumonitis and fibrosis. The appearance closely resembles idiopathic pulmonary fibrosis. Discontinuing the drug should result in some improvement over a period of months. Steroid treatment may also be effective, but mortality is 10%.

Nonsteroidal Anti-inflammatory Drugs

These drugs have been associated with a hypersensitivity reaction with acute onset of dyspnea, cough, low-grade fever, and eosinophilia. They may also be associated with SLE.

OKT3

OKT3 is a monoclonal antibody directed against T cells that is used to treat rejection of solid organ transplants. Pulmonary edema is a common complication in patients who are fluid overloaded prior to the institution of treatment. Consequently, chest radiographs are routinely obtained before treatment begins to exclude preexisting pulmonary edema or heart failure.

Tocolytic Drugs

Tocolytic drugs used to treat premature labor (e.g., ritodrine and terbutaline) result in increased-permeability pulmonary edema in about 1% of cases. Onset is typically 2 to 3 days after treatment. Increased risk is associated with overhydration, twin gestation, and use of steroids. Rapid recovery is typical.

Tricyclic Antidepressants

Overdose of tricyclic antidepressants may be associated with increased-permeability pulmonary edema or DAD with development of ARDS as a direct toxic effect.

RADIATION PNEUMONITIS AND FIBROSIS

Following external-beam thoracic radiotherapy, approximately 40% of patients develop radiographic abnormalities and 7% develop symptomatic radiation pneumonitis.

The development and appearance of radiation lung injury depend on a number of factors, including (1) the volume of lung irradiated, (2) the shape of the radiation fields, (3) the radiation dose, (4) the number of fractions of radiation given, (5) the time period over which the radiation is delivered, (6) prior irradiation, (7) whether chemotherapy is also employed, (8) corticosteroid therapy withdrawal, (9) preexisting lung disease, (10) the type of radiation used, and (11) individual susceptibility.

Generally speaking, radiation is best tolerated by the patient if given in smaller doses, over a long period of time, and to a single lung or a small lung region. For unilateral radiation with fractionated doses, radiographic findings of radiation pneumonitis are seldom detected with doses below 3000 cGy, are variably present with doses between 3000 and 4000 cGy, and are nearly always visible at doses of 4000 cGy. Its likelihood is increased by a second course of radiation, the withdrawal of corticosteroid treatment, and the use of concomitant chemotherapy. Radiographic findings of radiation pneumonitis are usually not associated with symptoms, although low-grade fever, cough, and dyspnea are present in some patients.

Radiation Pneumonitis

Pulmonary abnormalities related to radiation injury have been divided into early and late manifestations. The early stage of radiation lung injury, referred to as radiation pneumonitis, occurs within 1 to 3 months after radiation therapy is completed and is most severe 3 to 4 months following treatment. Radiation pneumonitis is associated with histologic findings of diffuse alveolar damage, intra-alveolar proteinaceous exudates, and hyaline membranes. Depending on the severity of lung injury, these abnormalities may resolve completely, but more often they undergo progressive organization, leading eventually to fibrosis.

Radiation Fibrosis

The late stage of radiation-induced lung injury, termed radiation fibrosis, develops gradually in patients with radiation pneumonitis when complete resolution does not occur. Radiation fibrosis evolves within the previously irradiated field 6 to 12 months following radiation therapy and usually becomes stable within 2 years of treatment. Histologically, dense fibrosis with obliteration of lung architecture and traction bronchiectasis are present. Patients can present with radiation fibrosis without a previous history of acute pneumonitis.

Radiographic and CT Findings

The hallmark of radiation pneumonitis on radiographs or CT is homogeneous or patchy ground-glass opacity or con-

---

TABLE 17-10. RADIATION PNEUMONITIS AND FIBROSIS

Occurrence is multifactorial
Seldom occurs below 3000 cGy
Nearly always visible above 4000 cGy
Radiation pneumonitis
  1–3 months after radiation is completed
  Most severe 3–4 months after radiation
  Diffuse alveolar damage
  Radiographs and HRCT
    Homogeneous or patchy ground-glass opacity
      or consolidation
    Edges correspond to radiation ports
    Abnormalities outside of ports in 20%
Radiation fibrosis
  6–12 months after radiation is completed
  Unchanging after 2 years
  Fibrosis and traction bronchiectasis
  Radiographs and HRCT
    Persisting abnormalities after 9 months
    Dense consolidation
    Edges correspond to radiation ports
    Traction bronchiectasis typical
    May mimic honeycombing
    Ipsilateral volume loss

---

solidation corresponding closely to the location of the radiation ports (Fig. 17-9). Abnormalities are typically nonanatomic and do not tend to respect normal lung boundaries such as lobar fissures or lung segments. Volume loss can be seen; this is due to obstruction of bronchioles by inflammatory exudate, loss of surfactant, or both. Large airways are patent, and air bronchograms are commonly visible. Pleural thickening is sometimes seen adjacent to irradiated areas.

Although findings of radiation pneumonitis are characteristically confined to areas of irradiated lung, relatively

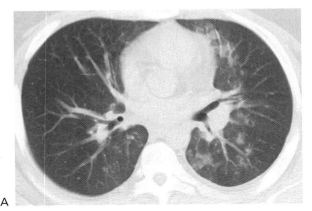 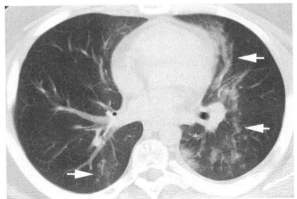

FIG. 17-9. Acute radiation pneumonitis. **A.** Patchy areas of ground-glass opacity are visible in a paramediastinal distribution following mediastinal radiation. **B.** The areas of abnormality are nonanatomic but have straight margins corresponding to the radiation ports *(arrows)*. Little volume loss is present at this stage.

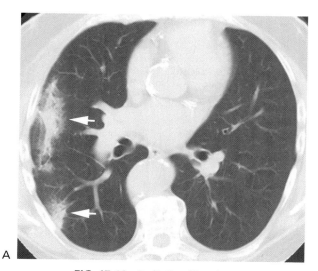
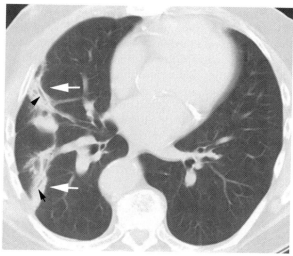

FIG. 17-10. Radiation fibrosis 12 months following axillary radiotherapy. CTs at two levels show consolidation in the peripheral lung. The abnormal areas have a straight edge *(white arrows)* due to the port used. Dense consolidation is typical of fibrosis. Traction bronchiectasis *(black arrows)* indicates that fibrosis is present.

mild abnormalities (ground-glass opacity or consolidation) are detected outside the radiation portal in as many as 20% of cases, perhaps related to a hypersensitivity reaction or OP/BOOP (Table 17-10).

Persistence or progression of radiographic or CT abnormalities more than 9 months after treatment likely indicates fibrosis (Fig. 17-10). The development of radiation fibrosis can be recognized by the appearance of streaky opacities, progressive volume loss, progressive dense consolidation (see Figs. 17-10 and 17-11), traction bronchiectasis (see Figs. 17-10B and 17-11), or pleural thickening within the irradiated lung. Fibrosis and volume loss typically result in a

sharper demarcation between normal and irradiated lung regions than is seen in patients with radiation pneumonitis (see Figs. 17-10 and 17-11). This gives the abnormal lung regions a characteristically straight and sharply defined edge. Occasionally, the appearance mimics honeycombing (Fig. 17-12), although the distribution is related to the radiation ports and is quite different from that of idiopathic pulmonary fibrosis. The adjacent lung may appear hyperinflated and may show bullae. The ipsilateral hemithorax may be reduced in volume (see Fig. 17-11).

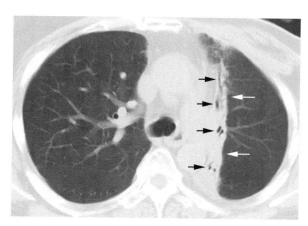

FIG. 17-11. End-stage radiation fibrosis. HRCT shows dense paramediastinal fibrosis with a sharp edge *(white arrows)*. Traction bronchiectasis *(black arrows)* is extensive. The ipsilateral hemithorax is reduced in volume compared with the opposite side.

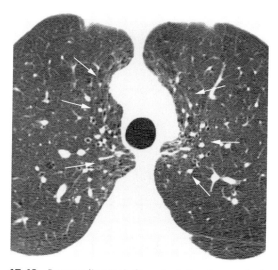

FIG. 17-12. Paramediastinal fibrosis following radiation for Hodgkin's disease. HRCT shows paramediastinal reticulation, traction bronchiectasis, and honeycombing *(arrows)*.

Although pleural thickening is a common manifestation of radiation, pleural effusions are uncommon. Effusion related to radiation typically develops within 6 months of treatment, in conjunction with radiation pneumonitis, and resolves spontaneously. Rapid accumulation of fluid suggests malignancy.

Mediastinal lymph node calcification, particularly after radiation of lymphomas, the development of thymic cysts, pericarditis, and cardiomyopathy may also be seen.

SELECTED READING

Aquino SL, Webb WR, Golden J. Bronchiolitis obliterans associated with rheumatoid arthritis: findings on HRCT and dynamic expiratory CT. J Comput Assist Tomogr 1994; 18:555–558.

Aronchick JM, Gefter WB. Drug-induced pulmonary disorders. Semin Roentgenol 1995; 30:18–34.

Bellamy EA, Husband JE, Blaquiere RM, Law MR. Bleomycin-related lung damage: CT evidence. Radiology 1985; 156: 155–158.

Bush DA, Dunbar RD, Bonnet R, et al. Pulmonary injury from proton and conventional radiotherapy as revealed by CT. AJR Am J Roentgenol 1999; 172:735–739.

Cooper JA Jr. Drug-induced lung disease. Adv Intern Med 1997; 42: 231–268.

Cooper JAD, White DA, Matthay RA. Drug-induced pulmonary disease, part 1: cytotoxic drugs. Am Rev Respir Dis 1986; 133: 321–340.

Cooper JAD, White DA, Matthay RA. Drug induced pulmonary disease, part 2: noncytotoxic drugs. Am Rev Respir Dis 1986; 133:488–503.

Davis SD, Yankelevitz DF, Henschke CI. Radiation effects on the lung: clinical features, pathology, and imaging findings. AJR Am J Roentgenol 1992; 159:1157–1164.

Gotway MB, Marder SR, Hanks DK, et al. Thoracic complications of illicit drug use: an organ system approach. Radiographics 2002; 22:119–135.

Kuhlman JE. The role of chest computed tomography in the diagnosis of drug-related reactions. J Thorac Imaging 1991; 6:52–61.

Kuhlman JE, Teigen C, Ren H, et al. Amiodarone pulmonary toxicity: CT findings in symptomatic patients. Radiology 1990; 177: 121–125.

Libshitz HI. Radiation changes in the lung. Semin Roentgenol 1993; 28:303–320.

Logan PM. Thoracic manifestations of external beam radiotherapy. AJR Am J Roentgenol 1998; 171:569–577.

Movsas B, Raffin TA, Epstein AH, Link CJ Jr. Pulmonary radiation injury. Chest 1997; 111:1061–1076.

Padley SPG, Adler B, Hansell DM, Müller NL. High-resolution computed tomography of drug-induced lung disease. Clin Radiol 1992; 46:232–236.

Pietra GG. Pathologic mechanisms of drug-induced lung disorders. J Thorac Imag 1991; 6:1–7.

Rosenow EC, Myers JL, Swensen SJ, Pisani RJ. Drug-induced pulmonary disease: an update. Chest 1992; 102:239–250.

Rossi SE, Erasmus JJ, McAdams HP, et al. Pulmonary drug toxicity: radiologic and pathologic manifestations. Radiographics 2000; 20: 1245–1259.

Saxon RR, Klein JS, Bar MH, et al. Pathogenesis of pulmonary edema during interleukin-2 therapy: correlation of chest radiographic and clinical findings in 54 patients. AJR Am J Roentgenol 1991; 156: 281–285.

18

PNEUMOCONIOSES

W. RICHARD WEBB

The term *pneumoconiosis* refers to the presence of lung disease related to dust inhalation. Inhaled dusts may be toxic, resulting in fibrosis and disability (e.g., asbestosis and silicosis), or may be relatively inert, associated with radiographic abnormalities but causing little dysfunction (e.g., stannosis and baritosis). Organic dusts result in hypersensitivity pneumonitis (see Chapter 16).

CLASSIFICATION OF PNEUMOCONIOSES

The International Labour Office (ILO) has classified the plain radiographic abnormalities occurring in patients with dust exposure for the purpose of comparative epidemiological studies. This system provides a semiquantitative method for assessing the type and extent of abnormalities present. Classifications using this system are nonspecific, however, and it has little role in diagnosis. Furthermore, this system is complicated and difficult to remember unless used on a regular basis. Limited familiarity with ILO system is appropriate (Table 18-1).

A combination of letters and numbers is used to indicate the type and extent (profusion) of opacities present.

Opacity Type

The type of opacity, either small or large, is indicated by a letter, either small or large.

Small rounded opacities are well circumscribed and nodular. They are indicated as p, q, or r, depending on their diameter. Nodules up to 1.5 mm in diameter are p, opacities 1.5 to 3 mm are q, and those between 3 and 10 mm are r.

Small irregular opacities are linear or reticular in appearance and are indicated as s, t, or u according to their thickness. Opacities up to 1.5 mm are s, those 1.5 to 3 mm are t, and those 3 to 10 mm are u.

Large opacities are larger than 10 mm. These are classified as A if a single lesion or cluster of several opacities is more than 10 mm and 5 cm or less in diameter. B indicates one or more opacities larger or more numerous than those in A, with a combined area not exceeding that of the right upper lung zone. C is used for opacities larger than B.

Profusion

The number of small rounded or irregular opacities is indicated by the term *profusion*. Profusion is graded using four numbers with the following definitions, most easily determined by comparison to a standard reference set of radiographs:

0. Small opacities absent or less profuse than indicated by 1
1: Small opacities definitely present but few in number (normal lung markings are still visible)
2: Numerous small opacities (normal lung markings partially obscured)
3: Very numerous small opacities (normal lung markings usually obscured)

TABLE 18-1. INTERNATIONAL LABOUR OFFICE CLASSIFICATION OF PNEUMOCONIOSES

Opacity type	
Small rounded opacities (diameter)	
p	≤1.5 mm
q	>1.5 to 3 mm
r	>3 to 10 mm
Small irregular opacities (thickness)	
s	≤1.5 mm
t	>1.5 to 3 mm
u	>3 to 10 mm
Large opacities (diameter)	
A	One or a cluster of several opacities >10 mm to 5 cm
B	Larger or more numerous than A, not larger than the right upper lobe
C	Larger than B
Profusion (of small opacities)	
0	Absent or less profuse than 1
1	Definitely present but few in number (normal lung markings are still visible)
2	Numerous small opacities (normal lung markings partially obscured)
3	Very numerous small opacities (normal lung markings usually obscured)

These categories may be further subdivided based on these four numerical categories. If in interpreting a radiograph more than one of these four categories was seriously considered but was determined not to be the profusion present, it is indicated following the final classification and separated from it by a slash. For example, if a patient is determined to have a profusion of 1, but 2 was also considered, this is indicated as 1/2. If no alternative was considered, the number is listed twice (e.g., 1/1). This leads to the following possibilities for profusion:

0/0	1/0	2/1	3/2
0/1	1/1	2/2	3/3
	1/2	2/3	

Also, 0/− may be used to indicate an obvious lack of small opacities, while 3/+ indicates a profusion much higher than 3/3.

Extent

In patients with large opacities, the lung is divided equally into three zones (upper, middle, and lower) using horizontal lines.

Accuracy of the ILO System

The National Institute of Occupational Safety and Heath (NIOSH) has established a course and examination for the purpose of certifying physicians in the use of the ILO classification system. Completion of the course establishes the physician as an "A reader." Passing an examination confers "B reader" status. B readers must be recertified every 4 years. Trained readers show less interobserver variability in interpreting pneumoconiosis radiographs than untrained physicians.

Nonetheless, ILO categories are nonspecific and need not indicate lung disease or the presence of pneumoconiosis. Approximately 5% of subjects without occupational exposure have radiographs interpreted as having a 1/0 profusion of small opacities, usually considered to be abnormal and consistent with pneumoconiosis.

ASBESTOSIS AND ASBESTOS-RELATED DISEASE

Asbestos is a silicate mineral composed of various amounts of magnesium, iron, calcium, and sodium. Asbestos is found in nature in the form of thin fibers and is classified as amphibole or serpentine, depending on its fiber type.

The toxicity of asbestos appears to be related to the fibrous form of the mineral and its durability after inhalation. Amphibole asbestos has fibers that are thin and straight,

allowing them to penetrate deeply into the lung, and is most likely to result in disease. Amphiboles important in industry and often responsible for asbestos-related disease include crocidolite, amosite, and tremolite. Serpentine asbestos fibers are curved. Chrysotile is the only commonly used serpentine asbestos; it is less likely to result in disease than the amphiboles.

Asbestos has a variety of uses, particularly in the construction industry. Asbestos exposure may occur in the mining of asbestos, in the production of asbestos products and their installation during construction, and during repair or removal of asbestos-containing materials.

Asbestos-related abnormalities include asbestosis, asbestos-related rounded atelectasis, and asbestos-related pleural disease. A significantly increased incidence of mesothelioma, lung cancer, and extrathoracic neoplasms (e.g., peritoneal mesothelioma and gastrointestinal, renal, oropharyngeal, and laryngeal carcinomas) is also associated with asbestos exposure. Most patients with asbestos-related abnormalities have no symptoms.

Asbestosis

The lung disease associated with asbestos fiber inhalation is known as asbestosis (Table 18-2). Asbestosis is defined as interstitial pulmonary fibrosis associated with the presence of intrapulmonary asbestos bodies or asbestos fibers.

TABLE 18-2. LUNG DISEASE IN ASBESTOS EXPOSURE

Asbestosis
Interstitial lung fibrosis due to asbestos exposure
Asbestos bodies within the lung
Related to length and intensity of exposure, other factors
Correlation with severity of pleural disease
20–30 years after start of exposure
Radiographs
  ILO s, t, or u
  Shaggy heart sign
  Honeycombing
HRCT
  Findings of usual interstitial pneumonia
  Appearance mimics idiopathic pulmonary fibrosis
  Associated pleural disease visible in most

Rounded atelectasis
Does not necessarily indicate "asbestosis"
Related to visceral or parietal pleural thickening
Seen in 10%
May be preceded by parenchymal bands or crow's foot
Typical CT findings
  Round or oval
  Abutting the pleura
  Comet-tail sign
  Ipsilateral pleural disease
  Volume loss
Atypical findings common

Asbestos bodies are visible on microscopy and consist of translucent asbestos fibers coated with protein and iron. Amphiboles are usually responsible for asbestos bodies. Uncoated asbestos fibers are much more numerous in the lung than asbestos bodies.

Asbestosis results from inflammation associated with inhaled asbestos fibers. The development of asbestosis depends on the duration and intensity of exposure, although host-related factors such as tobacco smoking are also involved. There is a significant correlation between the presence and severity of pleural disease and the presence and severity of asbestosis.

Symptoms of asbestosis include dyspnea and finger clubbing, usually occurring 20 to 30 years after the start of exposure. Symptoms are progressive even without continued exposure. Pulmonary function tests show restrictive abnormalities. Associated findings of airway obstruction may reflect associated smoking-related disease (i.e., emphysema) or asbestos-related bronchiolar fibrosis. Longstanding exposure may result in significant respiratory dysfunction leading to cor pulmonale and death. Risk of death is related to the severity of fibrosis determined clinically, functionally, or radiographically.

After inhalation, asbestos fibers are first deposited in the respiratory bronchioles and alveolar ducts, but deposition becomes diffuse with longer and more extensive exposure. In patients with asbestosis, the earliest changes of fibrosis are peribronchiolar. As fibrosis progresses, it involves alveolar walls throughout the lobule and interlobular septa. Honeycombing can be seen in advanced cases. Visceral pleural thickening often overlies areas of parenchymal fibrosis. In asbestosis, abnormalities are usually most severe in the lower lungs, in the posterior lungs, and in a subpleural location.

The diagnosis of asbestosis usually is based on indirect evidence, including a combination of chest radiographic abnormalities, restrictive abnormalities on pulmonary function tests, appropriate physical findings, and known exposure to asbestos. These findings are limited in accuracy, however, being both nonspecific and insensitive in early disease.

Although many cases of asbestosis resulted from exposure before, during, or in the years after World War II, asbestosis is decreasing in incidence, and new cases with obvious findings are uncommon.

Radiographic Findings

Asbestosis usually results in irregular reticular opacities (ILO classification s, t, or u) on chest radiographs. In its earliest stages, asbestosis appears as a fine reticulation in the lung bases, often best seen posteriorly on the lateral view (Fig. 18-1A and B). As it progresses, reticulation becomes coarser and more obvious, partially obscuring the heart borders (known as the shaggy heart sign). In more advanced stages,

honeycombing may be visible and the abnormalities become more extensive, involving the mid-lungs. Radiographic findings of asbestosis are not usually detected until 10 years after exposure, and the latent period is sometimes as long as 40 years. Also, as many as 10% to 15% of patients with proven asbestosis have normal chest films.

The combination of these findings with typical pleural abnormalities should suggest the diagnosis (see Fig. 18-1). However, plain film findings of pleural disease are absent in about 20% of patients with radiographic evidence of asbestosis.

High-resolution CT Findings

On high-resolution CT (HRCT), asbestosis can result in a variety of findings, depending on the severity of the disease. In general, HRCT findings reflect the presence of interstitial fibrosis and are similar to those seen in patients with usual interstitial pneumonia and idiopathic pulmonary fibrosis. Although none of these findings are specific for asbestosis, the presence of parietal pleural thickening in association with lung fibrosis is highly suggestive (see Fig. 18-1C–E).

Thickening of interlobular septa, fine reticulation (intralobular interstitial thickening), traction bronchiectasis, architectural distortion, subpleural lines, and findings of honeycombing can all be seen, depending on the severity of disease. Honeycombing, common in advanced asbestosis, typically predominates in the peripheral and posterior lung (Figs. 18-1 to 18-3).

Patients with asbestosis usually show a number of HRCT findings indicative of lung fibrosis, and the abnormalities are usually bilateral and often somewhat symmetrical (see Figs. 18-1 to 18-3). The presence of focal or unilateral HRCT abnormalities should not be considered sufficient for making this diagnosis.

Parenchymal bands, linear opacities 2 to 5 cm in length, often extending to the pleural surface, are common in patients with asbestosis and asbestos exposure (Fig. 18-4). These often reflect coarse scars or areas of atelectasis adjacent to pleural plaques or areas of visceral pleural thickening. Several parenchymal bands occurring in the same location may give the appearance of a crow's foot; this abnormality is often related to overlying visceral or parietal pleural thickening and may precede the development of rounded atelectasis. These findings do not necessarily indicate asbestosis.

Rounded Atelectasis and Focal Fibrotic Masses

The term *rounded atelectasis* refers to the presence of focal lung collapse, with or without folding of the lung parenchyma (see Table 18-2). It is typically associated with pleural disease and thus is common in asbestos exposure. Focal masslike lung opacities reflecting the presence of rounded atelectasis or focal subpleural fibrosis are seen in

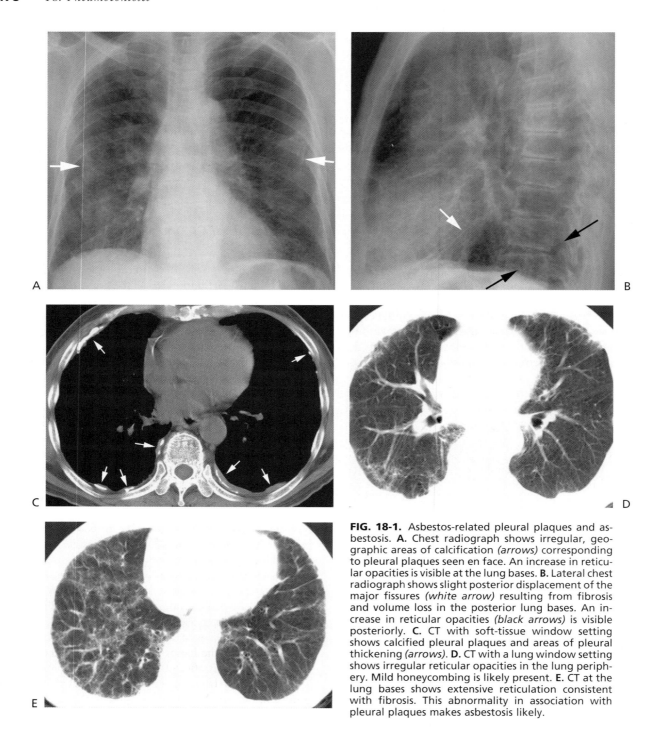

FIG. 18-1. Asbestos-related pleural plaques and asbestosis. **A.** Chest radiograph shows irregular, geographic areas of calcification *(arrows)* corresponding to pleural plaques seen en face. An increase in reticular opacities is visible at the lung bases. **B.** Lateral chest radiograph shows slight posterior displacement of the major fissures *(white arrow)* resulting from fibrosis and volume loss in the posterior lung bases. An increase in reticular opacities *(black arrows)* is visible posteriorly. **C.** CT with soft-tissue window setting shows calcified pleural plaques and areas of pleural thickening *(arrows).* **D.** CT with a lung window setting shows irregular reticular opacities in the lung periphery. Mild honeycombing is likely present. **E.** CT at the lung bases shows extensive reticulation consistent with fibrosis. This abnormality in association with pleural plaques makes asbestosis likely.

10% of patients with significant asbestos exposure; they are usually related to adjacent visceral pleural fibrosis and measure 2 cm to more than 5 cm in diameter. It is important to distinguish these masses from lung cancer, which has an increased incidence in asbestos-exposed individuals.

Plain films show a focal mass in association with pleural thickening, often contacting the pleural surface. It may be associated with curving of pulmonary vessels or bronchi into the edge of the lesion, the so-called comet-tail sign (see Fig. 2-42 in Chapter 2). CT is more accurate in making this diagnosis (see Chapter 2).

Rounded atelectasis is most common in the posterior lower lobes and is sometimes bilateral or symmetrical. It may have acute or obtuse angles where it contacts the pleura.

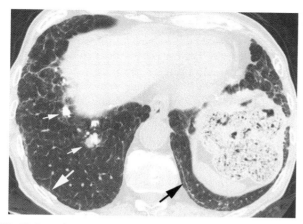

FIG. 18-2. Asbestosis. HRCT shows pleural plaques *(large white arrow)* at the peripheral pleural surface. Irregular nodular opacities *(small arrows)* at the lung base represent pleural plaques on the surface of the diaphragm, projecting into the lung. Irregular reticular opacities, thickening of interlobular septa, and a subpleural line *(black arrow)* are visible at the lung bases. Subpleural lines may reflect underlying pleural disease.

If the criteria for rounded atelectasis listed above are met, a confident diagnosis can usually be made. However, atypical cases are frequently encountered in patients with asbestos exposure, having appearances best described as lenticular, wedge-shaped, or irregular, and often are separated from the thickened pleura by aerated lung (see Figs. 2-45 and 2-46 in Chapter 2). If these lesions can be shown to be unchanged in size over several years, they are likely benign; if not, needle biopsy may be necessary to distinguish them from cancer. FDG-PET scanning may also be of value;

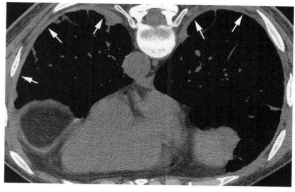

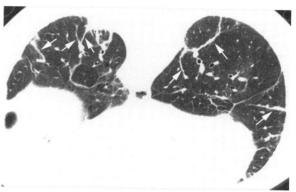

FIG. 18-4. Diffuse pleural thickening in asbestos exposure with parenchymal bands. **A.** HRCT shows diffuse (concentric) pleural thickening *(arrows)*. **B.** Lung window at the same level shows coarse linear opacities *(arrows)* extending to the abnormal pleural surface. These are termed parenchymal bands; when grouped together they resemble a crow's foot. These need not represent asbestosis but usually represent coarse scars or areas of atelectasis. They may precede the development of rounded atelectasis.

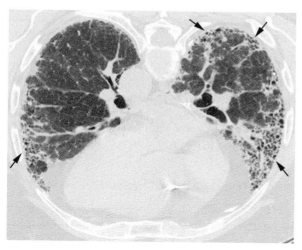

FIG. 18-3. Asbestosis with honeycombing. In a patient with asbestos exposure and pleural thickening, HRCT shows honeycombing *(arrows)* with a peripheral and basal predominance. Except for the presence of pleural thickening, this appearance is identical to that of IPF.

round atelectasis does not show the intense activity typical of cancer.

Asbestos-related Pleural Disease

Pleural disease is the most frequent thoracic manifestation of asbestos exposure (Table 18-3). Manifestations include pleural plaques, asbestos-related pleural effusion, and diffuse pleural thickening. Mesothelioma, a tumor commonly associated with asbestos exposure, is discussed in Chapter 26.

Pleural Plaques and Parietal Pleural Thickening

Pleural plaques are the most common and the most characteristic feature of asbestos exposure. They develop 10 to 20 years after the onset of exposure. They are composed of dense fibrous tissue and contain asbestos fibers, and calcification is common. Plaques nearly always involve the parietal pleural surfaces and are frequently seen overlying ribs in the posterolateral thorax and the domes of the diaphragms.

TABLE 18-3. ASBESTOS-RELATED PLEURAL DISEASE

Pleural plaques
10–20 years after the onset of exposure
Nearly always parietal pleural
Overlie ribs
Most often posterolateral and domes of diaphragms
Spare apices and costophrenic angles
Radiographs
    Calcified in 10%–15% of cases
    Irregular and "geographic"
CT
    Mesa shaped
    Often appear as high attenuation
    Calcified in 15%–20% of cases
    Parietal pleural thickening may be seen without plaques

Visceral pleural thickening
Lateral lower lobes
May be associated with rounded atelectasis

Benign exudative pleural effusion
Early finding
First 10 years after exposure
3% of exposed individuals
Small, unilateral or bilateral

Diffuse pleural thickening
5% of patients
Related to prior benign pleural effusion
Radiographs and CT
    One fourth of the chest wall
    May involve costophrenic angles

They tend to spare the apices and costophrenic angles. Plaques have "square shoulders" and appear mesa-shaped in cross section and 2 to 10 mm thick.

Thin areas of focal parietal pleural thickening without thick plaques may be seen early in the course of disease in patients with asbestos exposure.

Visceral Pleural Thickening

Visceral pleural thickening may occur, usually along the lateral pleural surface of the lower lobes. Overlying rounded atelectasis may be seen.

Benign Exudative Pleural Effusion

Benign exudative pleural effusion can be an early manifestation of asbestos exposure, being the only finding present in the first 10 years after exposure; it occurs in 3% of exposed individuals. Effusions may be associated with pleuritic pain and are often serosanguineous. Asbestos-related pleural effusions can be unilateral or bilateral and may be persistent or recurrent. They are usually less than 500 ml. Diagnosis is by exclusion; malignant mesothelioma must be considered in the differential diagnosis.

Diffuse Pleural Thickening

Diffuse pleural thickening is seen in up to 5% of patients with pleural disease. Diffuse pleural thickening usually represents a synthesis and fusion of thickened visceral and parietal pleural layers, and it is usually related to the presence of prior asbestos-related benign pleural effusion.

Radiographic Findings of Pleural Disease

Although plain radiographs may be diagnostic of asbestos-related plaques in some patients, they are only about 10% to 40% sensitive in detecting pleural plaques.

Pleural plaques are usually visible in the lower half of the thorax and may be seen en face or in profile along the lateral pleural surfaces (see Figs. 18-1 and 18-6; also see Fig. 26-10 in Chapter 26), most numerous between the sixth and tenth ribs, or in relation to the domes of the hemidiaphragms; they spare the costophrenic angles. Because they are often posterolateral in location, bilateral oblique views are often advantageous in demonstrating their presence.

In profile, they are often visible internal to ribs, up to 1 cm in thickness, and sharply contrasted with adjacent normal pleura. They are calcified in 10% to 15% of cases; diaphragmatic plaques are most often calcified. When seen en face, plaques appear round or irregular and "geographic" in shape. En face plaques are difficult to recognize as such unless calcified and may mimic lung nodules. Focal or diffuse thickening of the fissures may also be seen, indicative of visceral pleural disease, but is less common. Plaques are usually bilateral.

Pleural effusion occurring as a result of asbestos exposure has no distinguishing characteristics. It may or may not be associated with plaques.

Diffuse pleural thickening appears as a diffuse or concentric increase in pleural thickness. It is often considered to be present if pleural disease continuously involves at least one quarter of the chest wall. It may affect the costophrenic angles, an uncommon occurrence with plaques.

Collections of extrapleural fat may mimic asbestos-related pleural thickening. These occur in a distribution similar to that of plaques, involving the lower portion of the posterolateral thorax, but are usually longer, have tapering margins, are smooth and symmetrical, and are sometimes seen as lower in attenuation than soft tissue.

CT and HRCT Findings of Pleural Disease

CT and HRCT are considerably more sensitive than chest radiographs in detecting pleural abnormalities. On HRCT, parietal pleural thickening is easiest to see internal to visible rib segments (Fig. 18-5; also see Fig. 26-10 in Chapter 26). Thickened pleura measuring as little as 1 to 2 mm can be readily diagnosed in this location. Pleural thickening is also easy to recognize in the paravertebral regions. In the paraver-

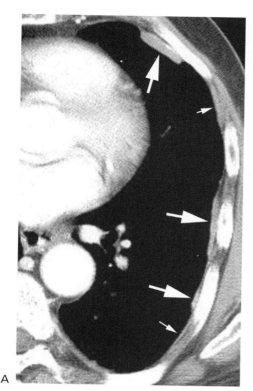

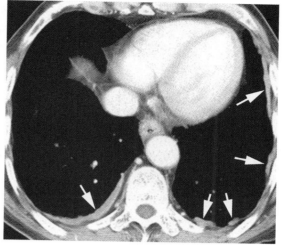

FIG. 18-5. Asbestos-related pleural thickening. **A.** Coned CT of the left hemithorax shows focal areas of pleural thickening and pleural plaques *(large arrows)*. Pleural thickening may be diagnosed most easily internal to ribs. A thin layer of fat may separate the thickening pleura from the rib. A similar linear density seen between the ribs *(small arrows)* is normal and represents innermost intercostals muscle. **B.** CT at a different level shows plaques and concentric areas of pleural thickening *(arrows)*.

tebral regions, the intercostal muscles are anatomically absent, and any distinct stripe of density indicates pleural thickening.

Asbestos-related pleural thickening appears smooth and sharply defined. Early pleural thickening is discontinuous. Plaques are usually bilateral (see Fig. 18-5B), although they appear unilateral in up to one third of cases. The presence of bilateral pleural plaques or focal pleural thickening is strongly suggestive of asbestos exposure, particularly when

calcification is also seen. Pleural calcification is visible on HRCT in about 15% to 20% of patients. Often, even when not grossly calcified, asbestos-related areas of pleural thickening appear denser than adjacent intercostal muscles, likely because of their mineral content.

Since the dome of the diaphragm lies roughly in the plane of the CT scan, the detection of uncalcified pleural plaques on the diaphragmatic surface can be difficult (see Figs. 18-2 and 18-6). In some patients, however, diaphrag-

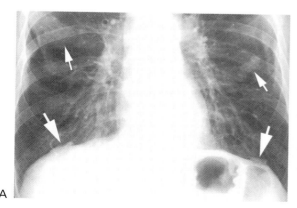

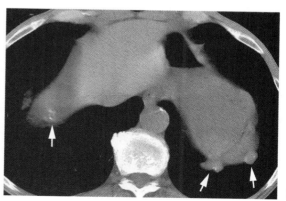

FIG. 18-6. Asbestos-related pleural thickening. **A.** Chest radiograph shows geographic opacities *(small arrows)* overlying the lung bases, representing pleural plaques. Pleural plaques are also visible at the domes of the hemidiaphragms *(large arrows)*. **B.** CT shows plaques *(arrows)* on the surface of the diaphragm.

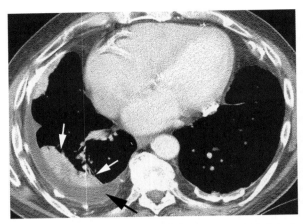

FIG. 18-7. Asbestos-related pleural plaques, rounded atelectasis, and pleural effusion due to mesothelioma. Extensive pleural thickening with calcification is visible. A right pleural effusion *(black arrow)* is also visible. It is unusual to see benign pleural effusion with such marked pleural thickening, and in this case the pleural effusion reflects mesothelioma. Rounded atelectasis is visible in the adjacent lung *(white arrows)*.

matic pleural plaques are visible deep in the posterior costo-phrenic angle, below the lung base; in this location, the pleural disease can be localized with certainty to the parietal pleura because only parietal pleura is present below the lung base. Pleural plaques along the mediastinum have been considered unusual in patients with asbestos-related pleural disease but are visible on CT scans in about 40% of patients. Paravertebral pleural thickening is also common.

On CT, diffuse pleural thickening is defined by the presence of a sheet of thickened pleura 8 cm in a craniocaudal dimension by 5 cm along the cross-sectional surface of the thorax (see Fig. 18-4); extensive calcification is uncommon. Diffuse pleural thickening may be associated with significant impairment of pulmonary function.

Benign pleural effusion is an early finding of asbestos-related pleural disease. Although it may be seen in association with pleural plaques, it is unusual in patients with extensive pleural disease. Pleural effusion may also indicate the presence of mesothelioma (Fig. 18-7).

SILICOSIS AND COAL-WORKER'S PNEUMOCONIOSIS

Silicosis and coal-worker's pneumoconiosis (CWP) result from the inhalation of different inorganic dusts, have different histology, and should be considered distinct diseases. However, their radiographic and HRCT appearances are quite similar, and they cannot be easily or reliably distinguished in individual cases.

Silicosis

Silicosis is caused by inhalation of dust containing silica (silicon dioxide or SiO_2) (Table 18-4). Heavy-metal mining and hard-rock mining are the occupations most frequently associated with chronic silicosis. Pathologically, the primary pulmonary lesion seen in patients with silicosis is a centri-lobular, peribronchiolar nodule consisting of layers of lami-nated connective tissue, termed a *silicotic nodule*. The nodules measure from 1 to 10 mm in diameter, and although diffuse, they are usually most numerous in the upper lobes and parahilar regions. Focal emphysema (also known as focal-dust emphysema) surrounding the nodule is common.

The diagnosis of silicosis requires the combination of an appropriate history of silica exposure and characteristic findings on the chest radiograph. The risk of silicosis is dose-related and usually becomes evident 10 to 20 years after the onset of exposure. Progression of disease both ra-diographically and clinically may occur for years after exposure has ended. Large conglomerate masses of silicotic nodules, so-called progressive massive fibrosis, may result.

A unique manifestation of acute exposure to large amounts of silica is termed *silicoproteinosis;* except for the presence of inhaled silica, it is indistinguishable from idio-pathic pulmonary alveolar proteinosis.

Coal-worker's Pneumoconiosis

CWP results from inhalation of coal dust containing little if any silica; exposure to other carbonaceous materials, such as graphite (pure carbon), may result in a similar disease (Table 18-5). As with silicosis, a history of 10 years or more of exposure is necessary to consider the diagnosis. The characteristic lesion of CWP is the *coal macule,* a 1- to 5-mm focal accumulation of coal dust surrounded by a small amount of fibrous tissue. As in patients with silicosis, these abnormalities tend to surround respiratory bronchioles and are therefore primarily centrilobular in location. With progression, coal macules are surrounded by small areas of focal emphysema.

TABLE 18-4. SILICOSIS

Dust containing silicon dioxide
Heavy-metal mining and hard-rock mining
10–20 years after the onset of exposure
Silicotic nodule
  Peribronchiolar
  Laminated connective tissue
  Upper lobes and parahilar regions
Progression after exposure—progressive massive fibrosis
Silicoproteinosis
  Acute silicosis with alveolar proteinosis

TABLE 18-5. COAL-WORKER'S PNEUMOCONIOSIS

Dust containing coal or carbon
Coal mining
10–20 years after the onset of exposure
Coal macule
   Peribronchiolar
   Coal dust and small amount fibrosis
   Upper lobes and parahilar regions
Progression to conglomerate masses

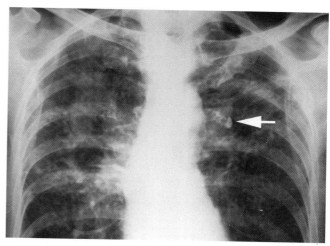

FIG. 18-8. Small lung nodules in silicosis. Small nodules are visible in the upper lobe bilaterally. Hilar enlargement is also visible. Calcification of a lymph node or nodule is visible in the left upper lobe.

Radiographic and HRCT Findings

Small Lung Nodules

The earliest and most characteristic plain radiographic finding in patients with both silicosis and CWP consists of small well-circumscribed nodules, usually measuring 2 to 5 mm in diameter but up to 10 mm in patients with silicosis (Table 18-6). These may be diffuse but mainly involve the upper and posterior lung zones (Fig. 18-8). These nodules indicate

TABLE 18-6. RADIOGRAPHIC AND HRCT FINDINGS IN SILICOSIS AND COAL-WORKER'S PNEUMOCONIOSIS (CWP)

Simple or uncomplicated silicosis and CWP
Well-circumscribed nodules usually measuring 2 to 5 mm
Predominate in the posterior upper lungs
ILO p, q, or r
Centrilobular and subpleural distribution on HRCT
Nodules in silicosis
   May be up to 10 mm
   Better defined
   More likely to calcify (10%–20%)
Complicated silicosis/CWP
Large opacities and conglomerate masses
Worsening symptoms, particularly in silicosis
Silicosis
   Termed progressive massive fibrosis
   Numerous aggregated nodules associated with dense fibrous
     tissue
CWP
   Amorphous black mass of dust surrounded by some fibrous
     tissue
Masses may cavitate (ischemia, tuberculosis, bacterial infection)
ILO A, B, C
Lenticular masses in upper lobes
   Upper lobe nodules decrease in number
   Satellite nodules
   Calcification common
   Adjacent emphysema may be present
Lymph node enlargement
Hilar and mediastinal node enlargement in 30%–40%
Calcification common
Eggshell calcification typical of silicosis

simple or uncomplicated silicosis or CWP. They are indicated as p, q, or r, in the ILO system.

The nodules of silicosis tend to be better defined than those of CWP and are more likely to calcify. Calcification of nodules is eventually visible in 10% to 20% of patients with silicosis and tends to involve the entire nodule. Calcification in CWP may first involve the center of individual nodules.

HRCT is superior to both conventional CT and chest radiography in the detection of small nodules in patients with silicosis and CWP. Simple silicosis or simple CWP is characterized by small nodules that tend to be centrilobular and subpleural. Most typically, nodules show a distinct predominance in the posterior upper lobes and appear symmetrical (Fig. 18-9). Calcification of the nodules is seen in up to 30% of cases. More severe silicosis or CWP is characterized on CT by an increase in the number and size of nodules.

Large Opacities and Conglomerate Masses

The appearance of large opacities (by definition more than 1 cm), also known as conglomerate masses or progressive massive fibrosis, indicates the presence of complicated silicosis or CWP. Large opacities tend to develop with time and progression of the disease. They are indicated as A, B, or C in the ILO system.

In patients with silicosis, these masses represent a conglomeration of numbers of silicotic nodules associated with dense fibrous tissue; in CWP, they consist of an amorphous black mass surrounded by some fibrous tissue. In both silicosis and CWP, these masses can undergo necrosis and cavitation. Cavitation is related to ischemia, tuberculosis (which

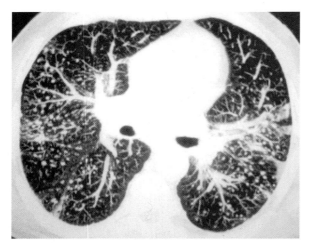

FIG. 18-9. HRCT of silicosis. Multiple small well-defined lung nodules are visible. The nodules are bilateral and symmetrical and show a posterior and upper lobe predominance. This distribution is characteristic. (Courtesy of Luigia Storto.)

has an increased incidence in both silicosis and CWP), or anaerobic bacterial infection.

On plain radiographs these masses are first seen in the midportion or periphery of the upper lung zones and migrate toward the hila with time, leaving emphysematous spaces between them and the pleural surface. On the lateral radiograph, these masses may appear lenticular in shape, often oriented posteriorly, paralleling the major fissure (Fig. 18-10; also see Fig. 9-32 in Chapter 9).

Small nodules may also be visible. However, because these masses develop from conglomeration of small nodules, their appearance is associated with a corresponding decrease in the number of small nodules visible. Although usually bilateral, they may be unilateral or asymmetrical. Progressive massive fibrosis may also occur in the lower lobes, but it is less common in this location.

On CT, conglomerate masses are usually seen to be associated with a background of small nodules (Fig. 18-11). Conglomerate masses are usually oval and often have irregular borders. Apical scarring and adjacent bullae may be seen and are more conspicuous in patients with silicosis than in those with CWP. Calcification in association with conglomerate masses is common (see Fig. 18-11B). Areas of necrosis, visible as low attenuation, with or without cavitation may be present. Increased reticular opacities are not a prominent feature of silicosis or CWP, but honeycombing is occasionally visible.

Although simple silicosis and simple CWP cause few symptoms and little clinical impairment, the development of complicated silicosis or CWP is associated with symptoms and a deterioration of lung function. Patients with silicosis usually have greater respiratory impairment for a given degree of radiographic abnormality than do patients with CWP. Furthermore, the complicated form of silicosis has a poorer prognosis than does simple silicosis, but this is not necessarily the case with CWP. In patients with silicosis, the size of the conglomerate masses is often related to the severity of symptoms.

Caplan's Syndrome

Caplan's syndrome in patients with CWP or silicosis and rheumatoid arthritis may also be seen, with large necrobiotic nodules superimposed on small nodules. Caplan's syndrome (see Chapter 14) is more common with CWP than silicosis.

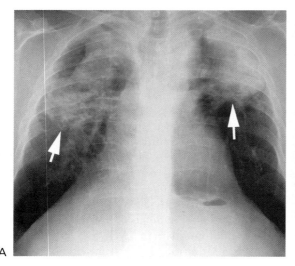

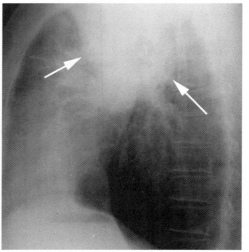

FIG. 18-10. Progressive massive fibrosis in silicosis. Posteroanterior (**A**) and lateral (**B**) radiographs show typical irregular masses *(arrows)* in both upper lobes, associated with volume loss.

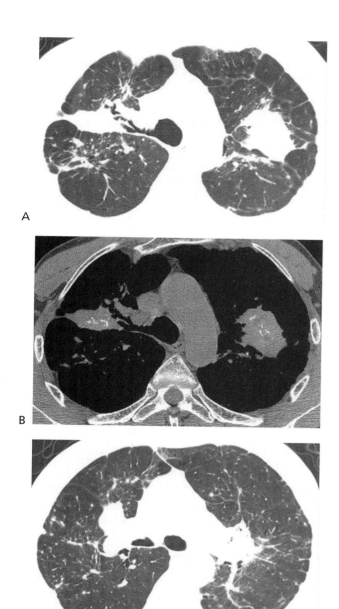

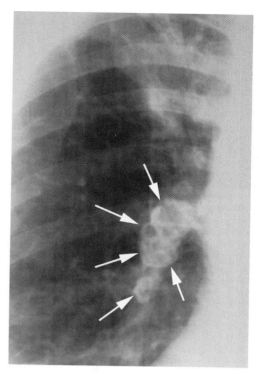

FIG. 18-12. Eggshell calcification in silicosis. Right hilar lymph node enlargement with typical eggshell calcification is visible (*arrows*). An ill-defined upper lobe mass reflects progressive massive fibrosis.

FIG. 18-11. Progressive massive fibrosis in silicosis. **A.** HRCT shows bilateral upper-lobe masses associated with distortion of lung architecture. This appearance is typical of progressive massive fibrosis. Small (satellite) nodules are seen adjacent to the larger mass. **B.** Soft-tissue window shows calcification within the masses, common in silicosis. **C.** Lung window scan at a lower level shows multiple small nodules typical of silicosis. Hilar enlargement is visible.

Lymph Node Enlargement

On plain radiographs, hilar lymphadenopathy is visible in many patients (see Fig. 18-8). The lymph nodes are often calcified. Characteristic peripheral "eggshell" calcification is seen in about 5% of cases of silicosis (Fig. 18-12) and is almost pathognomonic of this entity in a patient with

exposure. Calcification of mediastinal lymph nodes may also be seen. Eggshell calcification is not typical of CWP; when it is seen in a patient with CWP, it reflects the presence of silica in the coal dust. On CT, hilar or mediastinal lymph node enlargement is visible in 30% to 40% of patients with silicosis or CWP.

TALCOSIS

Talc is magnesium silicate occurring in thin sheets. Talcosis, or lung disease related to talc, may result from inhalation or intravenous injection. However, talc is less pathogenetic than asbestos or silica.

Inhalation of talc may result in pneumoconiosis similar to asbestosis, although more mild in degree. Findings include pleural thickening or calcification, sometimes associated with interstitial fibrosis. However, mined talc or commercially available talc is often contaminated with other minerals, such as asbestos or silica. If this is the case, the resulting pneumoconiosis may more closely resemble asbestosis or silicosis (talco-asbestosis and talco-silicosis, respectively).

Talcosis secondary to intravenous injection of talc is seen almost exclusively in drug users who inject medications in-

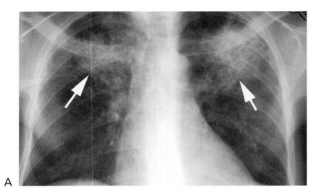

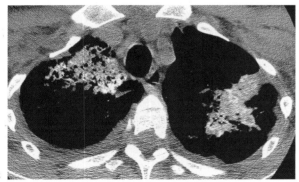

FIG. 18-13. Talcosis with progressive massive fibrosis. **A.** Chest radiograph shows ill-defined upper-lobe masses similar to those seen in silicosis (*arrows*). **B.** On HRCT, the masses contain high-attenuation talc.

tended for oral use, which contain talc as an inert ingredient. When drug users inject a solution of crushed tablets, numerous talc particles become trapped within pulmonary arterioles and capillaries. The particles result in small granulomas composed of multinucleated giant cells surrounded by a small amount of fibrous tissue.

The initial radiologic manifestations of injection talcosis consist of numerous discrete nodules 1 mm or less in diameter. Follow-up chest radiographs show gradual coalescence of the nodules toward the parahilar regions of the upper lobes. Eventually talcosis results in conglomerate masses in the upper lobes, which closely resemble the progressive massive fibrosis seen in silicosis (Fig. 18-13A). On HRCT, the small nodules may appear centrilobular. The confluent para-hilar masses may be seen to contain high-attenuation material representing talc (see Fig. 18-13B).

MISCELLANEOUS SILICA AND SILICATE PNEUMOCONIOSES

Exposure to a variety of other substances containing varying amounts of silica (as in silicosis) and silicates (as in asbestosis) can result in a pneumoconiosis resembling one or both

of these, or a mixture of the two. However, radiographic and clinical abnormalities are usually less profound than in silicosis or asbestosis.

INERT DUST PNEUMOCONIOSIS

Some dusts are not fibrogenic when inhaled. They result in few symptoms because of the absence of fibrosis but may result in significant radiographic abnormalities.

Siderosis results from inhalation of dust containing iron. The most common occupations involved are electric-arc welders and oxyacetylene welders, who may inhale fine particles of iron oxide during their work. Little fibrosis results, but the particles accumulate in macrophages aggregated in relation to peribronchiolar and peribronchial lymphatics. Plain radiographs show small nodules with a parahilar predominance that may appear dense; these may clear with time. HRCT shows small centrilobular nodules, some of which have a fine branching appearance. Focal areas of consolidation may appear very high in attenuation due to the presence of iron.

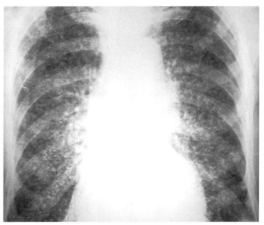

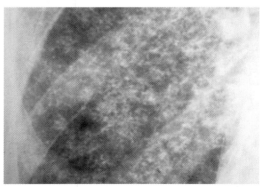

FIG. 18-14. Stannosis in a tin miner. **A.** Chest radiograph shows numerous small very dense nodules predominating in the middle lung zones. **B.** Coned-down view shows the very dense nodules. These represent accumulations of tin but result in little fibrosis.

Stannosis results from inhalation of tin, often by miners or refiners. The tin accumulates in macrophages surrounding small airways. Ill-defined nodules or thin, dense branching opacities may be seen, which may be very dense (Fig. 18-14).

Other such pneumoconioses with a similar appearance include baritosis (barium), argyrosiderosis (silver and iron), antimony, and rare earth exposure.

BERYLLIOSIS

Exposure to beryllium can occur in the ceramics industry, in nuclear weapons production, or in fluorescent lamp manufacture. Acute berylliosis results from massive exposure and has the appearance of acute lung injury with pulmonary edema or acute respiratory distress syndrome. Chronic berylliosis is a systemic granulomatous lung disease resulting from occupational exposure to beryllium over a period of years. A latent period of years between exposure and presentation is typical. Chronic berylliosis is indistinguishable from sarcoidosis histologically and radiographically, although a history of exposure and hypersensitivity to beryllium allow the diagnosis to be made. It may have a poor prognosis.

ALUMINUM

Inhalation of dusts containing metallic or oxidized aluminum has been associated with pulmonary fibrosis, granuloma formation, desquamative interstitial pneumonia, and alveolar proteinosis, but pneumoconiosis related to aluminum dust is rare. HRCT may show subpleural or diffuse honeycombing resembling idiopathic pulmonary fibrosis, centrilobular nodules resembling those seen in silicosis, or irregular reticulation.

HARD-METAL PNEUMOCONIOSIS

Hard metal is an alloy of tungsten carbide and cobalt, sometimes mixed with other metals. Exposure to hard metal re-sults in interstitial inflammation with fibrosis and lung destruction, which may develop within a few years of exposure. Radiographic and CT findings include coarse reticular opacities, consolidation, architectural distortion, and subpleural bullae. On CT, traction bronchiectasis may be seen. The distribution may be patchy or with a lower-lobe predominance.

SELECTED READING

Aberle DR, Balmes JR. Computed tomography of asbestos-related pulmonary parenchymal and pleural diseases. Clin Chest Med 1991; 12:115–131.

Akira M. Uncommon pneumoconioses: CT and pathologic findings. Radiology 1995; 197:403–409.

Akira M, Yamamoto S, Yokoyama K, et al. Asbestosis: high-resolution CT-pathologic correlation. Radiology 1990; 176:389–394.

Akira M, Yokoyama K, Yamamoto S, et al. Early asbestosis: evaluation with high-resolution CT. Radiology 1991; 178:409–416.

Balaan MR, Weber SL, Banks DE. Clinical aspects of coal workers' pneumoconiosis and silicosis. Occup Med 1993; 8:19–34.

Gamsu G, Salmon CJ, Warnock ML, Blanc PD. CT quantification of interstitial fibrosis in patients with asbestosis: a comparison of two methods. AJR Am J Roentgenol 1995; 164:63–68.

Gevenois PA, de Maertelaer V, Madani A, et al. Asbestosis, pleural plaques and diffuse pleural thickening: three distinct benign responses to asbestos exposure. Eur Respir J 1998; 11:1021–1027.

Mossman BT, Churg A. Mechanisms in the pathogenesis of asbestosis and silicosis. Am J Respir Crit Care Med 1998; 157:1666–1680.

Newman LS, Buschman DL, Newell JD, Lynch DL. Beryllium disease: assessment with CT. Radiology 1994; 190:835–840.

Remy-Jardin M, Degreef JM, Beuscart R, et al. Coal worker's pneumoconiosis: CT assessment in exposed workers and correlation with radiographic findings. Radiology 1990; 177:363–371.

Shida H, Chiyotani K, Honma K, et al. Radiologic and pathologic characteristics of mixed dust pneumoconiosis. Radiographics 1996; 16:483–498.

Staples CA. Computed tomography in the evaluation of benign asbestos-related disorders. Radiol Clin North Am 1992; 30:1191–1207.

Ward S, Heyneman LE, Reittner P, et al. Talcosis associated with IV abuse of oral medications: CT findings. AJR Am J Roentgenol 2000; 174:789–793.

19

DIFFUSE PULMONARY HEMORRHAGE AND PULMONARY VASCULITIS

W. RICHARD WEBB

DIFFUSE PULMONARY HEMORRHAGE

Making a specific diagnosis of pulmonary hemorrhage based on radiographic findings is difficult. Lung consolidation visible radiographically in association with hemoptysis and anemia strongly suggests the diagnosis. However chest radiographic and CT findings are often nonspecific (Fig. 19-1), and hemoptysis may be lacking even in patients with sufficient hemorrhage to result in anemia.

For the purposes of differential diagnosis, diffuse pulmonary hemorrhage should be distinguished from focal pulmonary hemorrhage occurring as a result of abnormalities such as bronchiectasis, chronic bronchitis, active infection (e.g., tuberculosis), chronic infection, neoplasm, pulmonary embolism, or other vascular abnormalities such as arteriovenous fistula.

Diffuse pulmonary hemorrhage can result from a variety of diseases. The differential diagnosis of diffuse pulmonary hemorrhage includes (1) anti–glomerular basement membrane disease (Goodpasture's syndrome), (2) idiopathic pulmonary hemosiderosis, (3) small vessel vasculitis associated with antineutrophilic cytoplasmic antibody (ANCA; Wegener's granulomatosis, Churg-Strauss syndrome, microscopic polyangiitis), (4) collagen-vascular diseases (particularly systemic lupus erythematosus [SLE]) and immune complex–related vasculitis, (5) drug reactions, (6) anticoagulation, and (7) thrombocytopenia (see Fig. 19-1).

Goodpasture's syndrome, vasculitis syndromes, and collagen-vascular diseases are often associated with a combination of pulmonary hemorrhage and renal abnormalities and may be termed *pulmonary-renal syndromes.*

Radiographic Findings of Diffuse Pulmonary Hemorrhage

Radiographic findings in diseases causing diffuse pulmonary hemorrhage may be identical. In general, radiographs and high-resolution CT (HRCT) show patchy or diffuse consolidation or ground-glass opacity in the presence of acute hemorrhage (see Figs. 19-1 to 19-3). Ill-defined centrilobular nodules may be seen and predominate in some patients; these are sometimes visible on radiographs but are easiest

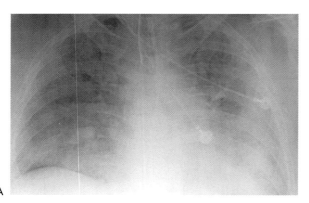
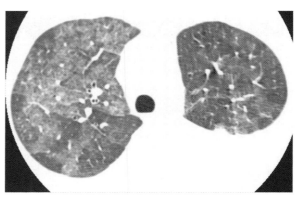

FIG. 19-1. Pulmonary hemorrhage associated with leukemia and thrombocytopenia. **A.** Chest radiograph shows ill-defined increased lung opacity. **B.** HRCT shows patchy areas of ground-glass opacity. The appearance is nonspecific and could also reflect pulmonary edema or infection. A left pleural effusion is also present.

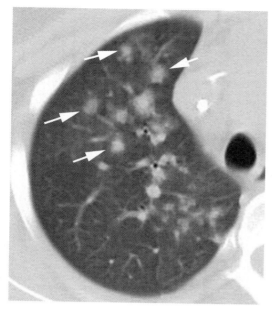

FIG. 19-2. Centrilobular nodules in pulmonary hemorrhage. CT scan in a patient with SLE and pulmonary hemorrhage shows ill-defined centrilobular nodules *(arrows)*.

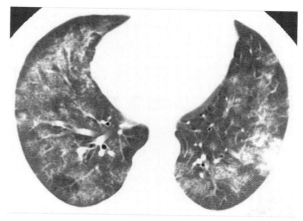

FIG. 19-4. Pulmonary hemorrhage in SLE with a parahilar predominance. Patchy ground-glass opacities and consolidation are visible.

to see on HRCT (see Fig. 19-2). Chest radiographs may be normal or show very subtle abnormalities in patients with pulmonary hemorrhage.

Opacities may be diffuse with uniform lung involvement (see Fig. 19-3) or may show a central and perihilar predominance with relative sparing of the apices, lung periphery, and costophrenic angles (Fig. 19-4). Pleural effusions are not generally associated with pulmonary hemorrhage, although they may be seen in patients with coincident renal failure.

Within a few days of an acute episode of hemorrhage, hemosiderin-laden macrophages begin to accumulate in the interstitium. This occurrence is manifested on chest radiographs by the presence of Kerley's lines, which may be seen in isolation or in conjunction with residual consolidation or ground-glass opacity. On HRCT, interlobular septal thickening may replace or be seen in association with ground-glass opacity (Fig. 19-5). Unless further hemorrhage occurs, complete clearing of air-space and interstitial opacities usually occurs within 10 days to 2 weeks of an acute episode of hemorrhage. This is considerably slower than clearing of pulmonary edema, which hemorrhage may closely resemble.

In patients with recurrent episodes of pulmonary hemorrhage, a persistent reticular abnormality may be seen between episodes of bleeding. This reflects interstitial hemo-

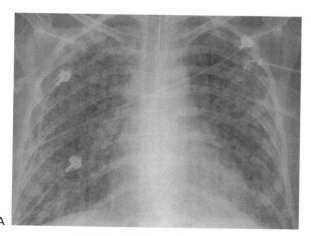

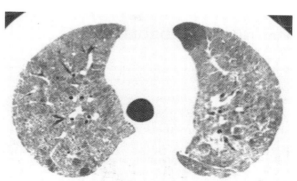

FIG. 19-3. Diffuse pulmonary hemorrhage with diffuse lung involvement. **A.** Interstitial opacities are visible bilaterally. The appearance is nonspecific. **B.** HRCT in a different patient with pulmonary hemorrhage shows diffuse ground-glass opacity.

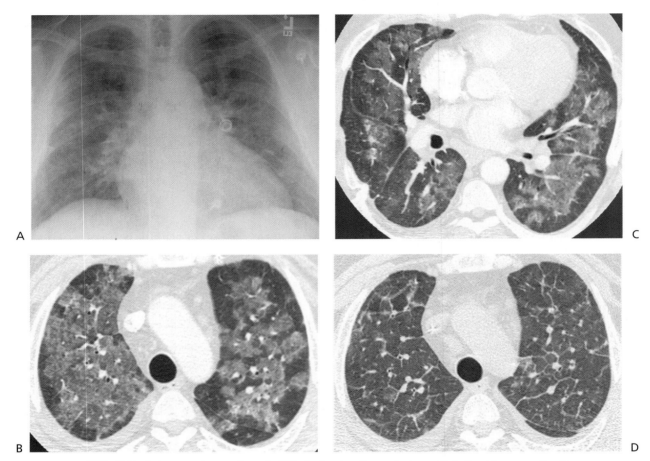

FIG. 19-5. Pulmonary hemorrhage in SLE. **A.** Chest radiograph shows ill-defined lung opacity. **B** and **C.** HRCT shows patchy areas of ground-glass opacity with a parahilar predominance. **D.** Three days after **B** and **C**, ground-glass opacity has resolved. Interlobular septal thickening is now visible.

siderin deposition and mild lung fibrosis and has been termed *pulmonary hemosiderosis.* It may be seen in any cause of recurrent hemorrhage but is particularly common in patients with idiopathic pulmonary hemosiderosis, described below.

GOODPASTURE'S SYNDROME

Anti–glomerular basement membrane disease (Goodpasture's syndrome) most typically occurs in patients aged 20 to 30; men are affected four times as commonly as women (Table 19-1). Hemoptysis, usually mild, and anemia are present in 90%. Other symptoms include cough, dyspnea, and weakness. Findings of renal disease are usually but not always present, including hematuria, proteinuria, and renal failure. Anti–glomerular basement membrane antibodies are almost always (95%) present in the serum. These antibodies are directed against type IV collagen and cross-react with alveolar basement membrane. A pulmonary capillaritis

is present. Renal biopsy shows glomerulonephritis with linear deposition of IgG in the glomeruli.

Although plain radiographs may be normal, they usually show diffuse air-space consolidation or ground-glass opacity, usually bilateral and symmetrical and often with a perihilar predominance (Figs. 19-6A and 19-7). HRCT usually shows consolidation or ground-glass opacity and may be abnormal in the face of subtle plain film findings or normal radiographs (see Fig. 19-6B).

TABLE 19-1. GOODPASTURE'S SYNDROME

Antiglomerular basement membrane antibodies in 95%
Glomerulonephritis
Age 20–30 years
Four times more common in men than women
Hemoptysis and anemia in 90%
Consolidation or ground-glass opacity

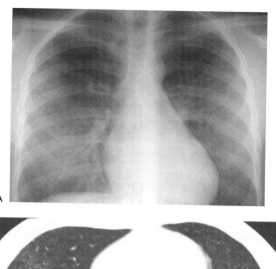

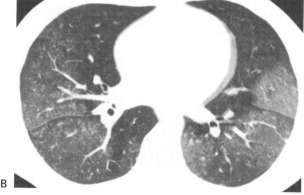

FIG. 19-6. Goodpasture's syndrome. **A.** Chest radiograph shows a subtle increase in lung opacity. **B.** HRCT shows patchy ground-glass opacity.

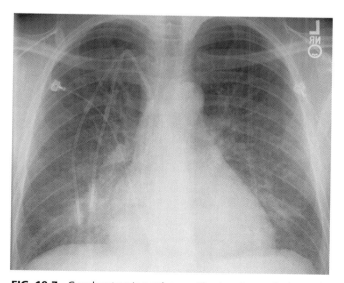

FIG. 19-7. Goodpasture's syndrome. Chest radiograph shows ill-defined parahilar and lower-lobe opacities. The heart appears enlarged because of renal failure and fluid overload, and a dialysis catheter is in place.

After an acute episode of hemorrhage, the air-space opacities tend to resolve, being superseded by an interstitial abnormality or septal thickening.

IDIOPATHIC PULMONARY HEMOSIDEROSIS

Idiopathic pulmonary hemosiderosis (IPH) is a disease of unknown origin characterized by recurrent episodes of diffuse pulmonary hemorrhage without associated glomerulonephritis or a serologic abnormality (Table 19-2). Pathologic findings include alveolar hemorrhage, hemosiderin-laden macrophages, and a variable degree of interstitial fibrosis in longstanding cases. IPH most commonly occurs in children under the age of 10 or young adults. In adults, men are affected twice as often as women. IPH is sometimes associated with cow's milk allergy, thyroid disease, or immunoglobulin A gammopathy has recently been reported in infants with exposure to toxic mold (*Stachybotrys*). Symptoms include cough, hemoptysis, dyspnea, and anemia. The diagnosis is usually made by exclusion. About a quarter of patients die as a result of respiratory insufficiency or cor pulmonale.

Plain radiographic and HRCT findings are similar to those of Goodpasture's syndrome. Predominant findings in the acute phase of disease include diffuse ground-glass opacity. On HRCT ill-defined centrilobular nodular opacities may also be seen. Hemosiderosis and fibrosis may develop with recurrent episodes of hemorrhage.

PULMONARY VASCULITIS

Pulmonary hemorrhage may be associated with vasculitis. Systemic vasculitis syndromes are classified into three groups based on the size of vessels primarily involved (Table 19-3): large vessel vasculitis, medium-sized vessel vasculitis, and small vessel vasculitis. These are briefly reviewed, with emphasis on those associated with pulmonary or intrathoracic abnormalities. Small vessel vasculitis is most important as a cause of pulmonary hemorrhage. Although Goodpasture's syndrome does not result in a systemic vasculitis, it may be classified as a small vessel vasculitis because pulmonary capillaritis is present.

TABLE 19-2. IDIOPATHIC PULMONARY HEMOSIDEROSIS

No serologic abnormalities
No glomerulonephritis
Children or young adults
Associated with exposure to toxic mold

TABLE 19-3. CLASSIFICATION OF PULMONARY VASCULITIS

Large-vessel vasculitis
Giant-cell (temporal) arteritis
Takayasu's arteritis

Medium-sized vessel vasculitis
Polyarteritis nodosa
Kawasaki's disease

Small-vessel vasculitis
Antineutrophilic cytoplasmic antibody (ANCA) associated
   Wegener's granulomatosis
   Churg-Strauss granulomatosis
   Microscopic polyangiitis
Immune complex vasculitis
   Goodpasture's syndrome
   Collagen-vascular diseases
   Behçet's disease
   Henoch-Schönlein purpura
   Antiphospholipid syndrome
   IgA nephropathy
   Mixed cryoglobulinemia

LARGE VESSEL VASCULITIS

Giant Cell (Temporal) Vasculitis

Temporal arteritis is relatively common. Affected patients are generally over 50 years of age. Arteries of the head and neck are typically involved, and the most common symptoms are headache and tenderness in the region of the temporal artery.

Large and medium-sized pulmonary arteries are rarely involved in this disease. Although upper respiratory symptoms such as cough and hoarseness occur in up to 10% of cases, radiographic correlates are lacking. Some patients show nonspecific radiographic abnormalities such as pleural effusion and diffuse reticular opacities, but what these are due to is unclear.

Takayasu's Arteritis

Takayasu's arteritis affects large and medium-sized arteries, most often the aorta and its branches. Women, usually under the age of 40, are affected in 90% of cases. In early disease, pathology shows vessel inflammation and poorly defined necrotizing and nonnecrotizing granulomas; in later lesions, vascular fibrosis and destruction of elastic tissue are present. Pulmonary arteries are involved in 50% of patients. Pulmonary hypertension may occur in late-stage disease but is seldom severe.

Radiographic abnormalities usually reflect aortic involvement, with aortic contour abnormalities, such as dilatation of the arch, a wavy-appearing descending aorta, and prema-

ture aortic calcification. CT and MRI show concentric aortic wall thickening and narrowing of the aortic lumen.

Central pulmonary artery dilatation may be seen on chest radiographs due to pulmonary hypertension but is relatively uncommon. On CT or MRI, stenosis or obstruction of segmental or smaller pulmonary arteries is often seen in late-stage cases. This may be associated with a patchy decrease in the attenuation of peripheral lung parenchyma (i.e., mosaic perfusion), a finding that sometimes is also recognized on chest films. Regional decrease in lung perfusion may be shown using V̇/Q̇ scintigraphy.

MEDIUM-SIZED VESSEL VASCULITIS

Classic polyarteritis nodosa (PAN) typically affects small to medium systemic arteries, resulting in a necrotizing vasculitis. Involvement of arterioles, venules, and capillaries is absent, as is glomerulonephritis. Such abnormalities indicate the presence of microscopic polyangiitis, described below, which may otherwise resemble PAN. Pulmonary artery inflammation is uncommon and seems to be unassociated with specific radiographic abnormalities.

SMALL VESSEL VASCULITIS ASSOCIATED WITH ANCA

Wegener's Granulomatosis

Wegener's granulomatosis is a multisystem disease of unknown cause associated with involvement of the upper respiratory tract (nasal, oral, or sinus inflammation), lower respiratory tract (airway or lung), and kidney. Upper respiratory tract involvement occurs in nearly all patients; lung involvement occurs in 90%; glomerulonephritis occurs in 80% (Table 19-4).

TABLE 19-4. WEGENER'S GRANULOMATOSIS

Multisystem disease
   Upper respiratory tract involved in nearly all patients
   Lung involvement occurs in 90%
   Glomerulonephritis occurs in 80%
Ages 30–60 years
C-ANCA in 90%
Chest radiographs abnormal in 75% at presentation
Multiple nodules and masses
   Usually 2–4 cm
   Cavitation common
   Cavities become thin-walled with treatment
Lung consolidation due to hemorrhage
Tracheobronchial involvement
   Tracheal wall thickening
   Subglottic trachea most often involved
   Luminal narrowing

Lung disease associated with Wegener's granulomatosis is characterized by granulomatous inflammation and necrotizing vasculitis. Limited Wegener's granulomatosis, involving only the lung, may occur.

Wegener's granulomatosis most commonly affects patients between the ages of 30 and 60 years. Most patients have symptoms of sinus disease at presentation (Fig. 19-8). Cough and hemoptysis are also common. Renal disease associated with hematuria, proteinuria, and renal failure is often absent at presentation but develops in most patients. Musculoskeletal symptoms occur in about 30% of patients, usually consisting of arthralgia or arthritis. Neurologic manifestations occur in 20% to 35% of patients. Ocular or skin involvement may also occur.

The presence of C-ANCA is characteristic, being seen in 90% of cases; it is less often present in patients with disease limited to the lung. Lung biopsy is usually more helpful in diagnosis than renal biopsy, which may be nonspecific.

Untreated Wegener's granulomatosis is associated with a poor prognosis, with death usually occurring within 6 months of the onset of renal failure. However, there is a high remission rate following treatment with cyclophosphamide and steroids. Recurrence may be precipitated by infection.

At presentation, chest radiographic abnormalities are visible in 75% of patients with Wegener's granulomatosis.

Lung Nodules and Consolidation

Multiple lung nodules or masses are most common, being visible in more than half of patients at presentation (see Figs. 19-8 and 19-9). Typically, there are fewer than a dozen nodules visible. In most cases, the nodules are bilateral and widely distributed without predominance in any lung region. A solitary nodule or mass may be seen, but this is less common. Masses usually range from 2 to 4 cm in diameter but may be much larger. Masses are round or oval and may be well defined or poorly defined. Calcification of the masses does not occur.

With progression of disease, nodules and masses tend to increase in size and number. With treatment, nodules usu-

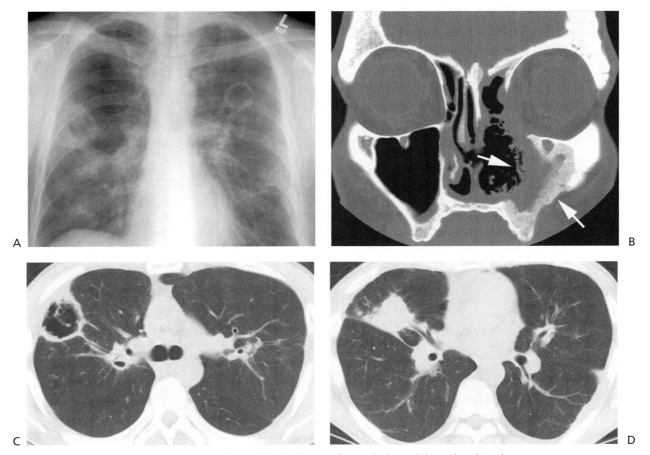

FIG. 19-8. Wegener's granulomatosis. **A.** Chest radiograph shows bilateral cavitary lung masses. **B.** Sinus CT shows soft-tissue thickening in the left maxilla with thickening and poor definition of the maxillary wall *(arrows)*. **C** and **D.** Cavitary mass and solid soft-tissue masses are visible on CT.

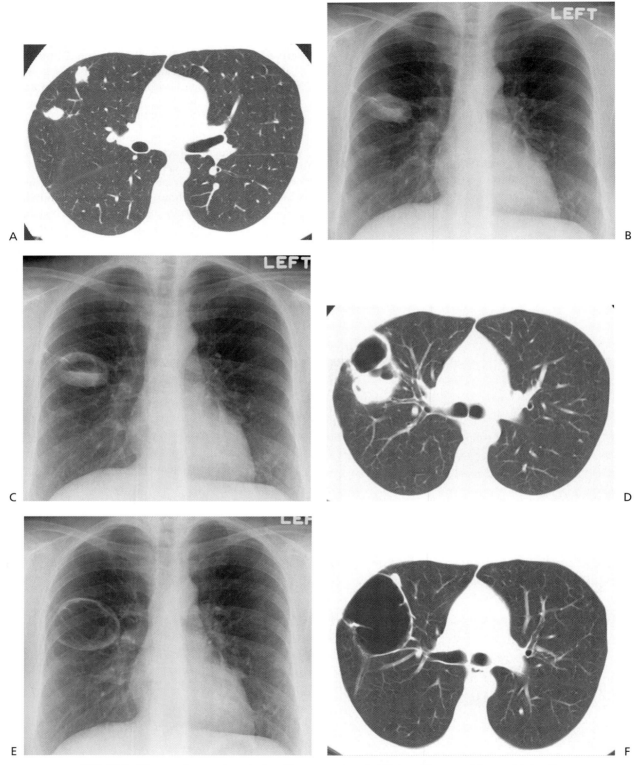

FIG. 19-9. Wegener's granulomatosis with progression. **A.** CT shows two small lung nodules. **B.** Chest radiograph 1 year later shows a right upper-lobe mass containing an air–fluid level. Other ill-defined nodules are also visible. **C.** Two weeks after **B**, there was an increase in the size of the right upper lobe mass with progressive cavitation. The cavity is thin-walled and an air–fluid level is again seen. **D.** CT 2 months after **B** shows an irregular cavitary mass. **E.** Radiograph 3 months after **B** shows a large thin-walled cavity. **F.** CT 5 months after **B** shows a persisting thin-walled cavity.

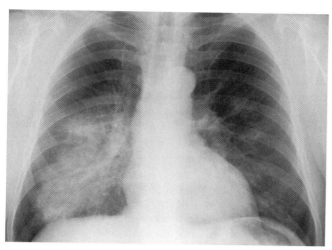

FIG. 19-10. Focal pulmonary hemorrhage in Wegener's granulomatosis. Focal consolidation is visible in the right lower lobe.

ally resolve over a period of months. Complete resolution may occur.

Cavitation occurs in approximately 50% of cases (see Figs. 19-8 and 19-9). Cavities are usually thick-walled, with an irregular inner margin. Air–fluid levels may be present. Typically, cavitary nodules and masses become thin-walled (see Fig. 19-9) and decrease in size with treatment.

Air-space consolidation or ground-glass opacity is the second most common radiographic finding in Wegener's granulomatosis and may occur with or without associated lung nodules or masses. These areas of consolidation usually represent pulmonary hemorrhage. They may be focal, diffuse, or patchy (Figs. 19-10 and 19-11).

Tracheobronchial Involvement

Tracheobronchial lesions occur in approximately 15% to 25% of patients with Wegener's granulomatosis. Concen-

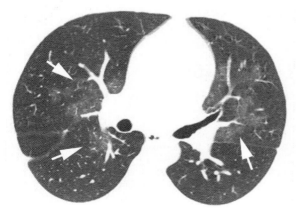

FIG. 19-11. Patchy pulmonary hemorrhage in Wegener's granulomatosis. Patchy ground-glass opacity is visible on HRCT *(arrows)*.

tric airway wall thickening due to inflammation, with narrowing of the airway lumen, is present. Involvement of the subglottic trachea is most typical (see Fig. 22-11 in Chapter 22), with variable involvement of the vocal cords, distal trachea, and proximal mainstem bronchi (see Fig. 22-12 in Chapter 22). Segmental, lobar, or lung atelectasis may result. Abnormalities may be focal or diffuse. They are described in detail in Chapter 22.

Other Findings

Hilar or mediastinal lymph node enlargement may be seen, but this is uncommon and never an isolated finding. Pleural effusions occur in about 10% of cases.

Churg-Strauss Granulomatosis

Churg-Strauss granulomatosis is also associated with ANCA, usually P-ANCA (perinuclear pattern). It is typically manifested by findings of simple pulmonary eosinophilia (i.e., fleeting consolidation), chronic eosinophilic pneumonia (i.e., peripheral areas of consolidation), or pulmonary edema due to cardiac involvement with heart failure. Uncommonly, it results in pulmonary hemorrhage. It is described in Chapter 16.

Microscopic Polyangiitis

Microscopic polyangiitis results in systemic necrotizing small vessel vasculitis. Although the histology is similar to classic PAN, involvement of arterioles, venules, and capillaries distinguishes it from PAN. Also, ANCA (usually P-ANCA) is present in 80%; ANCA is rare in PAN.

Microscopic polyangiitis typically occurs in middle-aged adults; men are more commonly involved. Glomerulonephritis develops in 90% of patients, and other organs may be involved. Pulmonary hemorrhage related to capillaritis occurs in 25%, associated with dyspnea and hemoptysis. Radiographic findings are typical of pulmonary hemorrhage. Pleural effusion and pulmonary edema are seen in about 10%, likely related to renal disease. Progression to pulmonary fibrosis is rare. Treatment with cyclophosphamide and steroids often results in remission.

IMMUNE COMPLEX SMALL VESSEL VASCULITIS

Deposition of immune complexes in the walls of small vessels occurs in several systemic vasculitis syndromes. Diseases associated with small vessel vasculitis and circulating immune complexes include Goodpasture's syndrome, collagen-vascular disease, Behçet's syndrome, Henoch-Schönlein purpura, mixed cryoglobulinemia, antiphospholipid syndrome, IgA nephropathy, and others.

Collagen-vascular Diseases

Diffuse pulmonary hemorrhage may occur with many collagen diseases, probably associated with circulating immune complexes and small vessel vasculitis. SLE is most common (see Figs. 19-2, 19-4, 19-5, and 19-12). Hemoptysis often occurs and may be massive. Radiographic and HRCT findings are similar to other causes of diffuse pulmonary hemorrhage. The pulmonary manifestations of the collagen diseases are described in Chapter 14.

Behçet's Disease

Behçet's disease is a rare systemic small vessel vasculitis likely due to deposition of immune complexes. It is associated with recurrent oral aphthous ulcers, genital ulcers, uveitis, and skin lesions such as erythema nodosum. Other organs and sites are commonly involved, including the joints (arthritis), heart, kidney, gastrointestinal system, and lung.

Behçet's disease is most common in young adults (20 to 35 years) and is particularly common in the Middle East (most notably Turkey) and the Far East (Japan). A familial incidence suggests hereditary factors, including HLA-5. The vasculitis of Behçet's disease results in vessel thrombosis, vascular obstruction, aneurysms, and sometimes vessel rupture. Involvement of the lung or intrathoracic vessels occurs in about 5% to 10% of cases.

Pulmonary artery aneurysms, otherwise an uncommon entity, are frequent in Behçet's disease involving the thorax. These appear as one or more, unilateral or bilateral, rounded hilar or perihilar opacities measuring up to several centimeters in diameter. On CT, these may opacify with contrast, may contain thrombus, or may not opacify because of thrombosis. Poor definition of an aneurysm may be associated with surrounding hemorrhage. Hemoptysis may occur due to leakage or rupture of an aneurysm and may be massive and life-threatening. Pulmonary artery aneurysm is thus associated with a poor prognosis.

Pulmonary artery thrombosis and occlusion may be associated with infarctions or focal pulmonary hemorrhage. Diffuse or patchy consolidation may also be seen, likely related to multiple areas of pulmonary hemorrhage.

Thrombosis of the superior vena cava and brachiocephalic veins may occur, resulting in superior vena cava syndrome, mediastinal edema, and widening of the mediastinum, as seen on chest radiographs. Pleural fluid may be seen, representing (1) effusion associated with pulmonary infarction, (2) hemothorax due to rupture of a pulmonary artery aneurysm, or (3) chylothorax due to great vein obstruction.

Hughes-Stovin syndrome, described in the 1950s, is characterized by pulmonary artery aneurysms and thrombosis, superior vena cava thrombosis, and thrombophlebitis. It likely represents Behçet's disease or a variant of Behçet's disease.

Henoch-Schönlein Purpura

Henoch-Schönlein purpura is characterized by purpura, abdominal pain, gastrointestinal hemorrhage, arthralgia, and glomerulonephritis, although not all are typically present and glomerulonephritis occurs in only 20%. It is usually seen in young children and often follows a respiratory tract infection. Relapses are common, but the prognosis is good. Chronic renal failure develops in a few patients. Diffuse or patchy consolidation may result from capillaritis and pulmonary hemorrhage. Hemoptysis is often associated. Pleural effusion may be seen.

Mixed Cryoglobulinemia

This disease is characterized by purpura, arthralgia, glomerulonephritis, hepatosplenomegaly, and lymph node enlargement. Serum globulins that precipitate with cold are present. Many cases are related to hepatitis C infection; others are associated with other infections, lymphoma, lymphoproliferative disease, or collagen-vascular diseases. Pulmonary disease is uncommon and difficult to characterize. A diffuse reticular pattern may be present, but what this represents is unclear.

SELECTED READING

Aberle DR, Gamsu G, Lynch D. Thoracic manifestations of Wegener granulomatosis: diagnosis and course. Radiology 1990; 174: 703–709.

Cheah FK, Sheppard MN, Hansell DM. Computed tomography of diffuse pulmonary haemorrhage with pathological correlation. Clin Radiol 1993; 48:89–93.

Connolly B, Manson D, Eberhard A, et al. CT appearance of pulmonary vasculitis in children. AJR Am J Roentgenol 1996; 167: 901–904.

Cordier JF, Valeyre D, Guillevin L, et al. Pulmonary Wegener's granulomatosis. A clinical and imaging study of 77 cases. Chest 1990; 97:906–912.

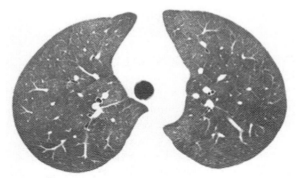

FIG. 19-12. Pulmonary hemorrhage in lupus. Patchy ground-glass opacity is visible on HRCT.

Hoffman GS, Kerr GS, Leavitt RY, et al. Wegener granulomatosis: an analysis of 158 patients. Ann Intern Med 1992; 116:488–498.

Mayberry JP, Primack SL, Müller NL. Thoracic manifestations of systemic autoimmune diseases: radiographic and high-resolution CT findings. Radiographics 2000; 20:1623–1635.

Primack SL, Miller RR, Müller NL. Diffuse pulmonary hemorrhage: clinical, pathologic, and imaging features. AJR Am J Roentgenol 1995; 164:295–300.

Primack SL, Müller NL. Radiologic manifestations of the systemic autoimmune diseases. Clin Chest Med 1998; 19:573–586.

Reuter M, Schnabel A, Wesner F, et al. Pulmonary Wegener's granulomatosis: correlation between high-resolution CT findings and clinical scoring of disease activity. Chest 1998; 114:500–506.

Seely JM, Effmann EL, Müller NL. High-resolution CT of pediatric lung disease: imaging findings. AJR Am J Roentgenol 1997; 168: 1269–1275.

Weir IH, Müller NL, Chiles C, et al. Wegener's granulomatosis: findings from computed tomography of the chest in 10 patients. Can Assoc Radiol J 1992; 43:31–34.

Witte R, Gurney J, Robbins R, et al. Diffuse pulmonary alveolar hemorrhage after bone marrow transplantation: radiographic findings in 39 patients. AJR Am J Roentgenol 1991; 157:461–464.

20

DIFFUSE LUNG DISEASE ASSOCIATED WITH LIPID: EXOGENOUS LIPID PNEUMONIA AND ALVEOLAR PROTEINOSIS

W. RICHARD WEBB

Lipoid pneumonia (lung consolidation containing lipids) may be endogenous or exogenous. Endogenous lipoid pneumonia may occur due to bronchial obstruction with accumulation of lipid-rich cellular debris distal to the obstructing lesion; this is sometimes termed "golden pneumonia" because of its yellow color at gross pathology. The term "postobstructive pneumonia" usually suffices for this condition.

EXOGENOUS LIPOID PNEUMONIA

Exogenous lipoid pneumonia results from the chronic aspiration or inhalation of animal, vegetable, or petroleum-based oils or fats (Table 20-1). Petroleum-based oil (mineral oil) aspiration is most common, usually associated with its use as a laxative. Responsible animal-based oils (e.g., cod-liver and shark-liver oils, clarified butter) and vegetable-based oils are usually aspirated during ingestion or because of esophageal motility abnormalities with reflux.

Acute aspiration results in an aspiration pneumonia. Chronic aspiration results in lipoid pneumonia associated with variable fibrosis and inflammation. The degree of lung inflammation or fibrosis associated with the aspirated oil is related to the amount of free fatty acid present. Animal fats generally result in more inflammation and fibrosis than vegetable or mineral oils because they are hydrolyzed by lung lipases, releasing fatty acids.

A large quantity of oily material must usually be aspirated over a period of time before symptoms develop. Symptoms include cough, mild fever, and chest discomfort; they are least common with mineral oil aspiration. Fat may be identified in the sputum in some patients.

Radiographic and CT Findings

Consolidation, ill-defined masses, or sometimes findings of fibrosis are seen on chest radiographs (Figs. 20-1A, 20-2A, and 20-3A). A lower-lobe distribution is typical but not always present. Opacities may be bilateral or unilateral. The radiographic appearance is nonspecific.

CT shows masses that may be well-defined or ill-defined, or areas of consolidation. As on chest radiographs, these areas tend to have a lower-lobe predominance and are often bilateral. A dependent location is also typical. Bronchi may be seen leading to the abnormal areas.

If a large amount of lipid has been aspirated, CT can show areas of low-attenuation consolidation (-35 to -75 HU) or low-attenuation regions within the visible masses (see Figs. 20-1B–E and 20-2B); this appearance is most common in patients with chronic mineral oil aspiration. Because inflammation or fibrosis may accompany the presence of the lipid material, the CT attenuation of the consolidation or mass need not be low, but often small areas of low-attenuation oil are visible within larger masses (see Figs. 20-1D, 20-1E, and 20-2B). In some patients, necrosis and cavitation are present.

Ground-glass opacity in association with interlobular septal thickening and intralobular lines ("crazy paving") or

TABLE 20-1. EXOGENOUS LIPOID PNEUMONIA

Chronic aspiration of animal, vegetable, or petroleum-based oils or fats
Esophageal dysmotility or reflux
Variable fibrosis and inflammation
Consolidation or masses
Usually dependent or lower lobe
CT
    Well-defined or ill-defined masses
    Variable amounts of low attenuation fat (-35 to -75 HU)
    Necrosis or cavitation
    Patchy ground-glass opacity or crazy paving

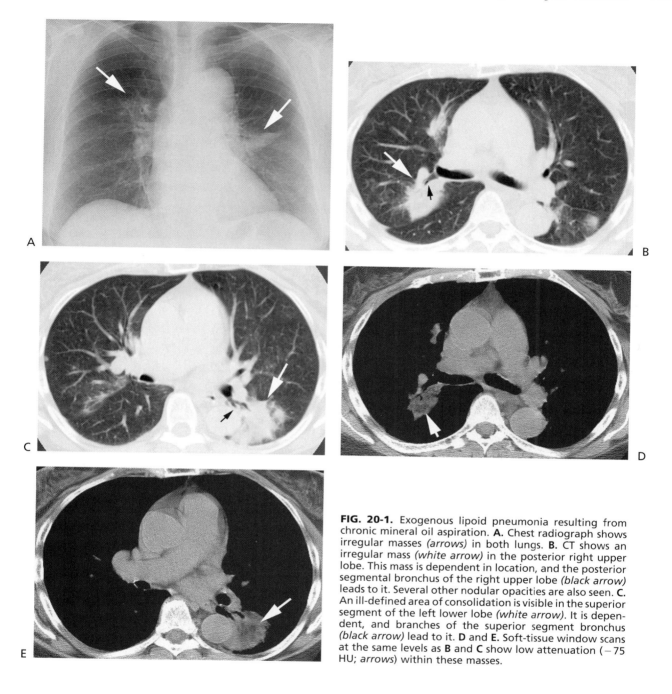

FIG. 20-1. Exogenous lipoid pneumonia resulting from chronic mineral oil aspiration. **A.** Chest radiograph shows irregular masses *(arrows)* in both lungs. **B.** CT shows an irregular mass *(white arrow)* in the posterior right upper lobe. This mass is dependent in location, and the posterior segmental bronchus of the right upper lobe *(black arrow)* leads to it. Several other nodular opacities are also seen. **C.** An ill-defined area of consolidation is visible in the superior segment of the left lower lobe *(white arrow)*. It is dependent, and branches of the superior segment bronchus *(black arrow)* lead to it. **D** and **E.** Soft-tissue window scans at the same levels as **B** and **C** show low attenuation (−75 HU; *arrows*) within these masses.

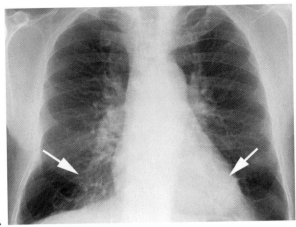
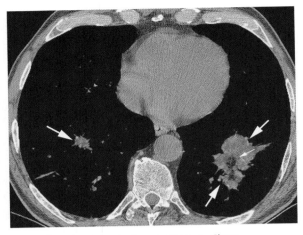

FIG. 20-2. Exogenous lipoid pneumonia resulting from chronic mineral oil aspiration. **A.** Chest radiograph shows irregular consolidation *(arrows)* in both lower lobes. **B.** CT shows irregular masses *(large arrows)* in both lower lobes. The left lower-lobe mass shows low attenuation (−100 HU; *small arrow*) within the mass, although most of the mass appears to be of soft-tissue attenuation.

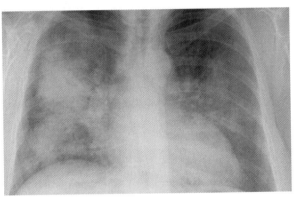
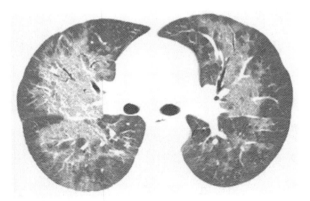

FIG. 20-3. Exogenous lipoid pneumonia resulting from mineral oil aspiration. **A.** Chest radiograph shows patchy parahilar consolidation. **B.** HRCT shows ill-defined parahilar consolidation and ground-glass opacity.

centrilobular nodules may also be seen on CT (see Fig. 20-3B). Subpleural pulmonary fibrosis and honeycombing are occasionally encountered. Some resolution of abnormalities is possible with time.

PULMONARY ALVEOLAR PROTEINOSIS

Pulmonary alveolar proteinosis (PAP) is a disease characterized by filling of the alveolar spaces with a PAS-positive proteinaceous material, rich in lipid; it is associated with an abnormality in the production or clearance of surfactant, although the pathogenesis of PAP is poorly understood (Table 20-2). The lung interstitium is largely normal.

In most cases, PAP is considered idiopathic. Some cases

TABLE 20-2. PULMONARY ALVEOLAR PROTEINOSIS

PAS-positive lipoproteinaceous material fills alveoli
Related to surfactant
Most idiopathic
Also with acute silicosis, immunodeficiency, malignancies, chemotherapy
Symptoms mild and insidious
Superimposed infection with *Nocardia, Mycobacterium avium-intracellulare,* and *Pneumocystis jiroveci* (*P. carinii*)
Treated with bronchoalveolar lavage
Radiographs show ill-defined opacity, consolidation uncommon
HRCT
  Bilateral, patchy, and geographic ground-glass opacity
  "Crazy paving" typical
  Abnormalities decrease after lavage

result from exposure to dusts (particularly silica; see Fig. 20-5) or from immunologic disturbances due to immunodeficiency, hematologic and lymphatic malignancies, or chemotherapy.

Men with PAP outnumber women by the ratio 4:1. Patients range in age from a few months to more than 70 years, with two thirds of patients being between 30 and 50 years old. Symptoms are usually mild and of insidious onset. They include nonproductive cough, fever, and mild dyspnea on exertion. About 30% of patients are asymptomatic.

Radiographic and HRCT Findings

Radiographic manifestations of PAP include bilateral, patchy, diffuse, or parahilar air-space consolidation or hazy ground-glass opacity, which is usually most severe in the lung bases (Fig. 20-4A); dense consolidation and air bronchograms are rare. Although reticular opacities may be seen, they are usually mild. The radiographic appearance often resembles that of pulmonary edema, except for the absence of cardiomegaly and pleural effusion.

High-resolution CT (HRCT) findings (see Figs. 20-4 and 20-5) in patients with PAP include the following:

1. Bilateral areas of ground-glass opacity
2. Smooth interlobular septal thickening in lung regions showing ground-glass opacity (i.e., crazy paving)
3. Consolidation
4. A patchy or geographic distribution

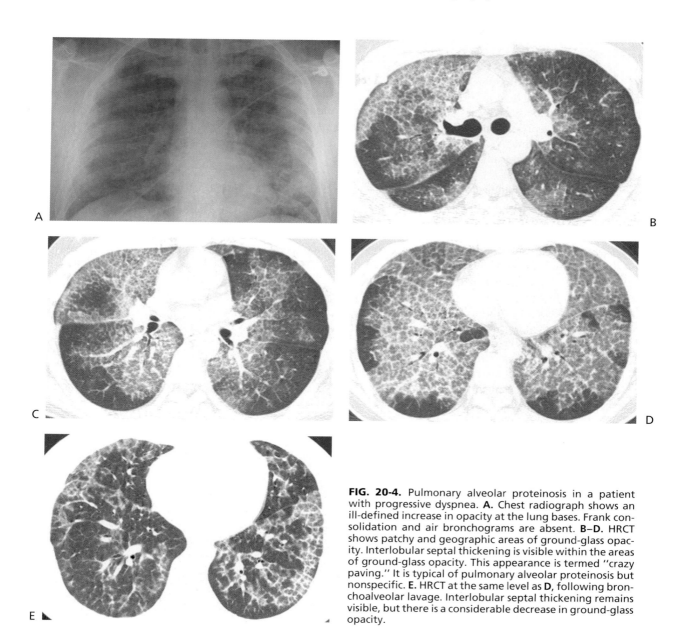

FIG. 20-4. Pulmonary alveolar proteinosis in a patient with progressive dyspnea. **A.** Chest radiograph shows an ill-defined increase in opacity at the lung bases. Frank consolidation and air bronchograms are absent. **B–D.** HRCT shows patchy and geographic areas of ground-glass opacity. Interlobular septal thickening is visible within the areas of ground-glass opacity. This appearance is termed "crazy paving." It is typical of pulmonary alveolar proteinosis but nonspecific. **E.** HRCT at the same level as **D,** following bronchoalveolar lavage. Interlobular septal thickening remains visible, but there is a considerable decrease in ground-glass opacity.

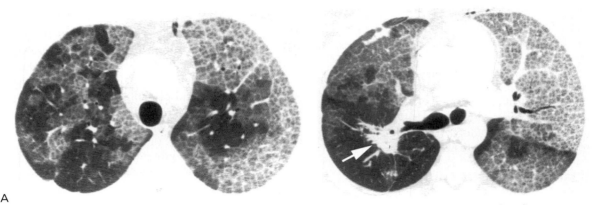

FIG. 20-5. Pulmonary alveolar proteinosis in a patient with severe exposure to silica dust (i.e., acute silicosis). **A.** HRCT shows patchy and geographic ground-glass opacity with crazy paving. **B.** A focal area of consolidation in the right lung *(arrow)* is due to *Nocardia* infection. Crazy paving is evident.

In many patients, areas of ground-glass opacity or consolidation are sharply demarcated from the surrounding normal parenchyma. In some of these cases, sharply marginated lung opacities appear to represent lobules. The distribution of disease is variable, sometimes being mainly central and sometimes peripheral. It is typically bilateral but may be asymmetrical.

The combination of a geographic distribution of areas of ground-glass opacity with smoothly thickened interlobular septa within the areas of air-space disease, resulting in a crazy paving appearance, is strongly suggestive of alveolar proteinosis in patients with subacute or chronic symptoms (see Figs. 20-4B–D and 20-5). However, this appearance can be seen in several other diseases, particularly acute diseases such as pneumonia or pulmonary edema.

Superimposed infection, often by *Nocardia asteroides*, is a common complication of alveolar proteinosis, resulting in focal areas of dense consolidation or abscess formation (see Fig. 20-5B). *Mycobacterium avium-intracellulare* complex (MAC) and *Pneumocystis jiroveci* (formerly *P. carinii*) infections have also been reported in patients with PAP.

Bronchoalveolar lavage is used to wash out the intraalveolar material. Successful treatment is associated with a reduction in the density of ground-glass opacity, although septal thickening may persist, at least temporarily (see Fig. 20-4E). Prior to the advent of bronchoalveolar lavage, about 30% of patients died of respiratory insufficiency or superimposed infection, but the prognosis has improved considerably. After lavage, many patients remain in remission, but others relapse; patients who relapse require retreatment every 6 to 24 months, and a few become refractory to treatment. In occasional cases, interstitial fibrosis develops.

SELECTED READING

Franquet T, Giménez A, Bordes R, et al. The crazy-paving pattern in exogenous lipoid pneumonia: CT-pathologic correlation. AJR Am J Roentgenol 1998; 170:315–317.

Godwin JD, Müller NL, Takasugi JE. Pulmonary alveolar proteinosis: CT findings. Radiology 1988; 169:609–613.

Hugosson CO, Riff EJ, Moore CC, et al. Lipoid pneumonia in infants: a radiological-pathological study. Pediatr Radiol 1991; 21: 193–197.

Johkoh T, Itoh H, Müller NL, et al. Crazy-paving appearance at thin-section CT: spectrum of disease and pathologic findings. Radiology 1999; 211:155–160.

Lee KN, Levin DL, Webb WR, et al. Pulmonary alveolar proteinosis: high-resolution CT, chest radiographic, and functional correlations. Chest 1997; 111:989–995.

Lee KS, Müller NL, Hale V, et al. Lipoid pneumonia: CT findings. J Comput Assist Tomogr 1995; 19:48–51.

Prakash UBS, Barham SS, Carpenter HA, et al. Pulmonary alveolar phospholipoproteinosis: experience with 34 cases and a review. Mayo Clin Proc 1987; 62:499–518.

Wang BM, Stern EJ, Schmidt RA, Pierson DJ. Diagnosing pulmonary alveolar proteinosis. A review and an update. Chest 1997; 111:460–466.

21

DIFFUSE LUNG DISEASES ASSOCIATED WITH CALCIFICATION

W. RICHARD WEBB

A wide variety of lung diseases may be associated with some degree of lung calcification, most notably granulomatous diseases such as sarcoidosis or tuberculosis (Table 21-1).

Several diffuse lung diseases are associated with extensive lung calcification as a common finding or as a primary manifestation of the disease. These are discussed in this chapter.

DIFFUSE PARENCHYMAL AMYLOIDOSIS

The term *amyloidosis* refers to a group of conditions characterized by extracellular deposition of abnormal fibrillar protein. Amyloidosis may be classified according to its etiology, the proteins involved, or its primary manifestation (Table 21-2). The first two of these catgories overlap and are somewhat confusing. The third is most appropriate to the radiologic assessment of amyloidosis, and is easiest to remember.

Classification by Etiology

An etiologic classification of amyloidosis includes (1) *primary amyloidosis* (i.e., that associated with a plasma cell disorder or not associated with underlying disease); (2) *secondary amyloidosis* (i.e., that associated with chronic inflammatory disorders or neoplasms such as Hodgkin's disease); (3) *heredofamilial amyloidosis* (i.e., having a genetic basis); (i.e., having a genetic basis); and (4) *senile amyloidosis*, which usually occurs in patients over the age of 70.

It may be subdivided into systemic forms (i.e., diffuse involvement of multiple organs) or localized forms (i.e., focal involvement largely limited to one organ).

Classification by Specific Proteins

When amyloidosis is classified according to the specific abnormal protein involved, the most important types producing lung disease are amyloid L and amyloid A.

Amyloid L (AL, or light chain amyloidosis) is the most common form of systemic amyloidosis. It may be either idiopathic or associated with plasma cell disorders (about 90% of cases). The lung is involved in 70% to 90% of patients with AL amyloidosis. Cardiomyopathy almost always is present if the lung is involved. Prognosis generally is poor. AL amyloidosis also may result in localized lung involvement. AL typically occurs in patients in their 50s or 60s.

Amyloid A (AA) occurs as secondary amyloidosis in patients with chronic inflammatory diseases (e.g., collagen vascular disease, infections, inflammatory bowel disease, and familial Mediterranean fever) and some neoplasms such as Hodgkin's disease. The lung is commonly involved to some degree, but deposits often are small or clinically insignificant. The prognosis is better than that for AL.

Among patients who have pulmonary involvement by amyloid, about 65% have primary systemic amyloidosis (systemic AL), 30% have localized amyloidosis (localized AL), and 5% have secondary amyloidosis (AA).

TABLE 21-1. DIFFUSE OR MULTIFOCAL LUNG CALCIFICATION

Infectious diseases
  Tuberculosis
  Histoplasmosis
  Healed varicella pneumonia
  Parasitic infections
Sarcoidosis
Silicosis and coal-worker's, pneumoconiosis
Calcified metastases
  Osteogenic and chondrosarcoma
  Mucinous adenocarcinoma
  Thyroid carcinoma
Pulmonary ossification with mitral stenosis
Lung fibrosis with dystrophic calcification
Amyloidosis
Alveolar microlithiasis
Metastatic calcification

TABLE 21-2. CLASSIFICATION OF AMYLOIDOSIS

By etiology
Primary amyloidosis—plasma cell disorder or unassociated with underlying disease
Secondary amyloidosis—associated with chronic inflammatory disorders or neoplasm
Heredofamilial amyloidosis
Senile amyloidosis—usually in patients over 70
Systemic (diffuse involvement of multiple organs)
Localized (focal involvement largely limited to one organ)
By specific proteins
Amyloid L (AL; light-chain amyloidosis)
  Most common
  Usually primary amyloidosis
  Lung involved in 70%–90%, localized or diffuse
  Cardiac involvement
  Poor prognosis
Amyloid A
  Secondary amyloidosis
  Lung involved to a minor degree
  Better prognosis
By manifestation
Diffuse (alveolar septal) amyloidosis
  Usually primary systemic and AL
  Dyspnea due to lung or heart disease
  Small nodules or reticular opacities
  Consolidation
  Lymph node enlargement
  Calcification common
Localized nodular amyloidosis
  Usually primary localized and AL
  Usually asymptomatic
  Lung nodules, often calcified
  Nodules grow slowly
Localized tracheobronchial amyloidosis
  Usually primary localized and AL
  Tracheal and bronchial narrowing or masses
  Calcification common

radiographic abnormality. If radiographs are abnormal, a reticular or reticulonodular pattern typically is seen, usually bilateral and diffuse or with a basal and subpleural predominance (Figs. 21-1 and 21-2A). Focal or patchy areas of consolidation also may be seen. The abnormal areas can calcify or, rarely, show frank ossification. Less often, a small nodular pattern mimicking sarcoidosis or miliary tuberculosis may be seen.

Hilar or mediastinal lymph node enlargement may be seen in patients with AL, either as an isolated finding or in association with interstitial disease. Cardiac infiltration with heart failure may result in pulmonary edema or pleural effusion.

On CT, the most common pulmonary manifestations of diffuse parenchymal amyloidosis consist of multiple small nodules, usually ranging from 2 to 4 mm in diameter (see Fig. 21-2B and C), interlobular septal thickening, fine reticular opacities, focal consolidation, foci of calcification within nodules or areas of consolidation (Fig. 21-3), and traction bronchiectasis. A subpleural and basal predominance may be seen.

Progression of the diffuse parenchymal disease typically occurs with time, with an increase in the reticular opacities, septal thickening, the size and number of nodules and consolidative opacities, and an increase in the size and number of calcifications.

As on chest radiographs, other findings seen on CT include lymphadenopathy, lymph node calcification (Fig. 21-4), and pleural effusion. Lymph node enlargement occurs in up to 75% of cases.

The prognosis of patients usually is related to the underlying disease or to involvement of other organs such as the

Classification by Manifestation

From a radiographic standpoint, it is most useful to classify amyloidosis on the basis of the abnormalities it produces. In general, pulmonary amyloidosis is classified into three types: (1) diffuse or alveolar septal amyloidosis, (2) localized nodular amyloidosis, and (3) tracheobronchial amyloidosis.

Diffuse (Alveolar Septal) Amyloidosis

Primary systemic amyloidosis (systemic AL) with diffuse lung involvement may result in dyspnea and respiratory insufficiency. However, pulmonary symptoms may be related more to associated cardiac involvement. Diffuse lung involvement is much less common and may be incidental with AA amyloidosis or senile amyloidosis. Occasionally, diffuse alveolar septal amyloidosis reflects localized rather than systemic disease.

The lung may be diffusely involved in the absence of a

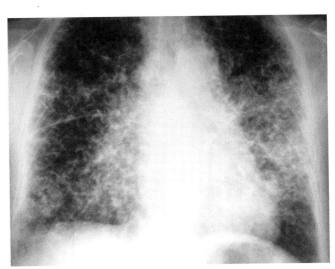

FIG. 21-1. Diffuse alveolar septal amyloidosis. A diffuse reticulonodular pattern is visible, with the abnormality predominating at the lung bases. Lung and lymph node calcification is present, and the heart is enlarged.

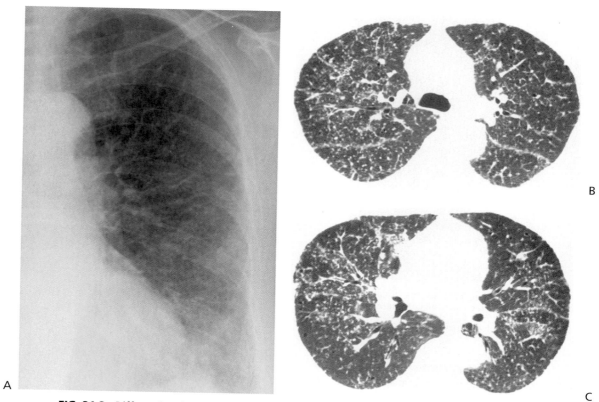

FIG. 21-2. Diffuse alveolar septal amyloidosis. **A.** Coned-down view of a PA radiograph shows a reticular pattern within the left lung, with a basal predominance. **B** and **C.** HRCT shows a diffuse nodular abnormality, with nodules visible in relation to the fissures and interlobular septa.

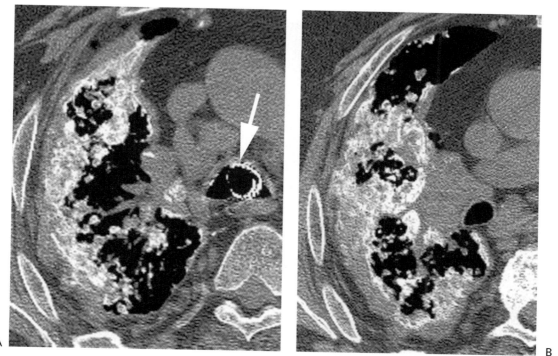

FIG. 21-3. Diffuse alveolar septal amyloidosis. HRCTs at two levels show extensive lung consolidation and calcification. A tracheal stent (*arrow* in **A**) is in place because of airway involvement and narrowing.

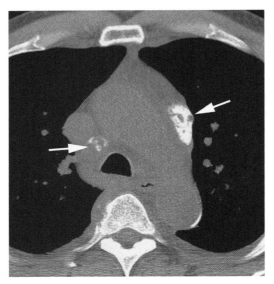

FIG. 21-4. Lymph node enlargement and calcification in amyloidosis. Mediastinal lymph nodes *(arrows)* are densely calcified.

kidney, liver, and heart. In some patients, lung involvement is severe enough to require lung transplantation.

Localized Nodular Amyloidosis

Patients with localized nodular amyloidosis (localized AL) usually are asymptomatic. Localized nodular amyloidosis may manifest as single or multiple lung nodules or masses, usually well-defined and round, ranging from 0.5 to 5 cm in diameter (Fig. 21-5), with stippled or dense calcification in up to 50% of cases on CT and cavitation in a small percentage. Nodules may grow slowly or remain stable over a number of years.

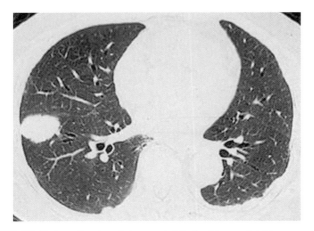

FIG. 21-5. Localized nodular amyloidosis. A large right lung nodule is visible. Small subpleural nodules or focal pleural thickening also are seen.

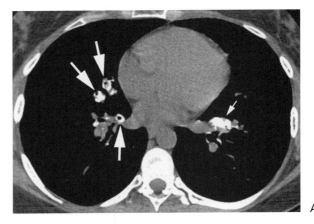

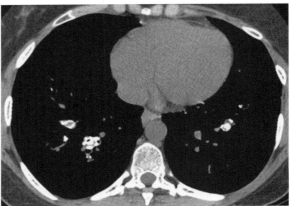

FIG. 21-6. Tracheobronchial amyloidosis. **A.** CT shows extensive bronchial calcifications *(large arrows)*. Hilar lymph node calcification *(small arrow)* also is present. **B.** Airway calcification due to amyloid deposition also is visible more peripherally.

Localized Tracheobronchial Amyloidosis

Localized AL may involve the larynx, trachea, and central bronchi; focal deposits of amyloid within the airway wall or diffuse wall infiltration may be present. Symptoms are common and include hoarseness, stridor, dyspnea, cough, hemoptysis, and recurrent infections. The trachea typically is involved, and concentric or nodular wall infiltration is most common. Calcification is common (Fig. 21-6; also see Fig. 22-13 in Chapter 22).

PULMONARY ALVEOLAR MICROLITHIASIS

Pulmonary alveolar microlithiasis is characterized by the presence of numerous minute calculi (so-called microliths or calcispheres) within alveoli (Table 21-3). It is very rare but has a characteristic radiographic appearance.

Histologically, the calcispheres are located largely within the alveolar lumen, although they probably are formed within the alveolar walls. They consist of concentric layers

TABLE 21-3. PULMONARY ALVEOLAR MICROLITHIASIS

Calcispheres within alveoli (consist of calcium phosphate)
Very rare
20–50 years of age
Familial incidence in half
Often asymptomatic at diagnosis
Abnormalities progress slowly
Radiographs
   Dense lungs
   Basal predominance
   Individual calcified nodules visible
   Black pleural line
HRCT
   Subpleural and perivascular predominance of calcified nodules
   Black pleural line = emphysema

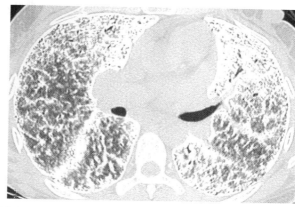

FIG. 21-8. HRCT in alveolar microlithiasis. Extensive lung calcification is present with a subpleural and perivascular predominance.

of calcium phosphate. In the early stages of disease, the alveolar walls appear normal, although fibrosis may occur late in the disease process. Emphysema also may be seen, particularly in the apices and subpleural regions.

Microlithiasis may be seen at any age, but most cases occur in patients from 20 to 50 years of age. Its etiology is unknown, but in about half of cases, the disease also occurs in family members, particularly siblings, suggesting autosomal recessive transmission. Environmental factors also are involved. Abnormalities of calcium metabolism are absent.

Patients typically are asymptomatic at diagnosis, despite spectacular radiographic abnormalities. There is a tendency for the abnormalities to progress slowly over a period of several years, although findings may remain stable. Dyspnea may develop with progression of the disease, with other symptoms including hemoptysis and clubbing. Although lung fibrosis and cor pulmonale may develop, the prognosis generally is good. There is no treatment.

Radiographs show characteristic findings. Despite their small size, the individual calcispheres may be visible as discrete, dense dots, less than 1 mm in diameter (Fig. 21-7). A basal predominance is typical (see Fig. 21-7). When limited in number, the calcispheres predominate in a subpleural location and in relation to vessels, bronchi, and interlobular septa. When myriad, they become confluent and appear very dense, obscuring the hemidiaphragm, heart, and mediastinal contours. If the lungs are sufficiently dense, the heart may appear relatively lucent, a very unusual finding. Another typical finding on chest radiographs, although it is not always seen, is the so-called black pleural line, a stripe of relative lucency at the pleural surface (see Fig. 21-7). Although this feature was thought to be due to sparing of the pleura by the calcispheres, it reflects small subpleural areas of emphysema.

High-resolution CT (HRCT) shows a posterior and lower lobe predominance of the calcifications with a high concentration in the subpleural parenchyma and in association with bronchi and vessels (Figs. 21-8 and 21-9). A peri-

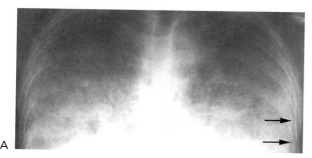

FIG. 21-7. Alveolar microlithiasis. **A.** PA chest radiograph shows diffuse lung involvement with a basal predominance. The lungs appear denser than adjacent ribs. Note a black pleural line on the left *(arrows)*. **B.** Detail view of the left lung in the region of the arrows shown in **A.** Individual dense calcispheres are visible. The subpleural lung appears relatively lucent. This is the black pleural line.

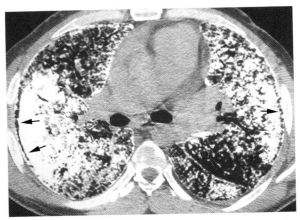

FIG. 21-9. HRCT in alveolar microlithiasis. Lung calcification is confluent in some regions and nodular in others. Small areas of emphysema *(arrows)* in the peripheral lung account for the black pleural line.

TABLE 21-4. METASTATIC CALCIFICATION

Calcification due to abnormal calcium and phosphate metabolism
Hypercalcemia
   Renal failure
   Secondary hyperparathyroidism
   Chronic hemodialysis
Commonly affects lung
Apices most often involved (more alkaline)
Radiographs
   Nodular opacities or consolidation
HRCT
   Opacities often centrilobular
   May be ground-glass opacity
   May or may not appear calcified
Radionuclide bone (^{99m}Tc-diphosphonate) scintigraphy useful
Opacities may resolve with treatment

lobular and centrilobular distribution of the calcifications may be seen, or calcifications may be associated with interlobular septa. Intraparenchymal emphysema may be seen. Subpleural paraseptal emphysema (i.e., the black pleural line) is common (see Fig. 21-9). In children or patients with early disease, ground-glass opacity or reticulation may be the predominant finding; calcifications may be difficult to detect.

Calcification of small interstitial nodules seen on HRCT has a limited differential diagnosis. Multifocal lung calcification, often associated with lung nodules, also has been reported in association with amyloidosis, infectious granulomatous diseases such as tuberculosis, sarcoidosis, silicosis and coal-worker's pneumoconiosis, talcosis, and metastatic calcification.

METASTATIC CALCIFICATION

The term *metastatic calcification* refers to the deposition of calcium in soft tissues due to abnormal calcium and phosphate metabolism (Table 21-4). It is associated with hypercalcemia and is most common in patients with chronic renal failure and secondary hyperparathyroidism and in those undergoing chronic hemodialysis.

Metastatic calcification commonly affects the lung; it typically is interstitial, involving the alveolar septa, bronchioles, and pulmonary arteries, and can be associated with secondary lung fibrosis. Patients may be asymptomatic or may have dyspnea. With appropriate treatment of the underlying abnormality, metastatic calcification may resolve.

Abnormalities typically predominate in the lung apices because they are more alkaline than the lung bases, increasing the likelihood of calcium salt precipitation in this region. A higher ratio of ventilation to perfusion in the apices results

in a decrease in the partial pressure of CO_2 and a corresponding increase in pH.

Plain radiographs are relatively insensitive in detecting metastatic calcification. In some patients, ill-defined nodules or patchy areas of increased opacity may be seen, however, (Figs. 21-10 and 21-11A). Nodules visible on chest

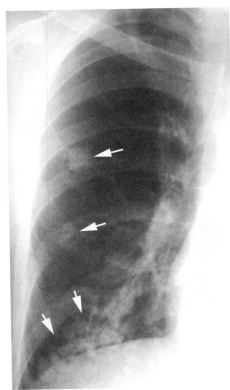

FIG. 21-10. Metastatic calcification in a patient with renal disease and secondary hyperparathyroidism. Dense nodular opacities *(arrows)* are visible in the right lung.

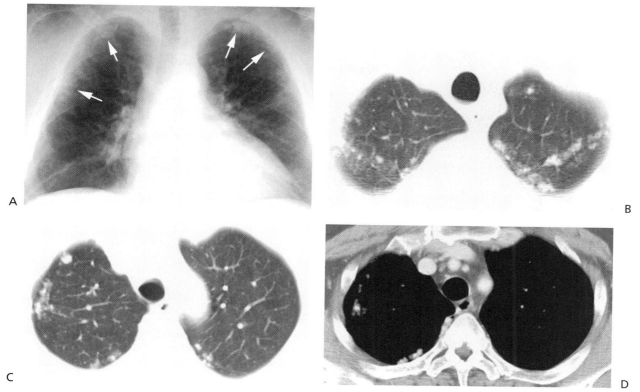

FIG. 21-11. Metastatic calcification in renal failure. **A.** Chest radiograph shows ill-defined nodular opacities *(arrows)* with an apical predominance. **B** and **C.** CT with a lung window setting shows nodular opacities in the peripheral upper lobes. These opacities appear lobular or centrilobular in distribution. **D.** Soft tissue window scan shows evidence of calcification.

films usually appear to be about 1 to 2 cm in diameter. They may or may not appear to be of calcium density. With progressive disease, these opacities become confluent, mimicking pneumonia. An apical predominance of opacities is typical but not invariable (see Fig. 21-11A).

CT can show areas of ground-glass opacity, consolidation, or calcification in the absence of plain film abnormalities. Numerous fluffy and poorly defined nodules, measuring 3 to 10 mm in diameter, are typical, but opacities can appear focal, lobular, patchy, or diffuse (Figs. 21-11 and 21-12). Even with HRCT, these opacities may not appear calcified. An apical predominance is common. Calcification of vessels in the chest wall may also be seen.

Radionuclide bone (^{99m}Tc-diphosphonate) scintigraphy (see Fig. 21-12D) is highly sensitive for the detection of metastatic calcification, and may show lung uptake when

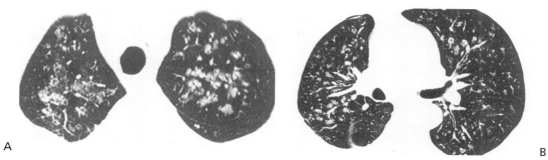

FIG. 21-12. Metastatic calcification in renal failure. **A** and **B.** HRCTs with a lung window setting show nodular opacities in the upper lobes. These opacities appear centrilobular in distribution. They were not obviously calcified on soft tissue windows. *(Figure continues.)*

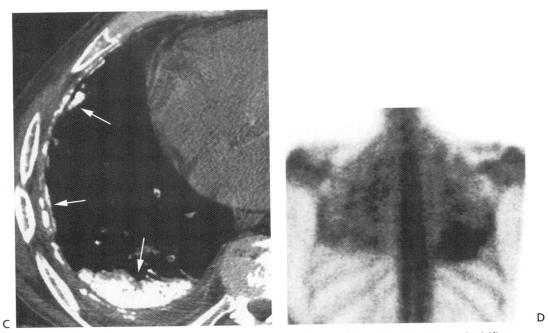

FIG. 21-12. *(Continued)*. **C.** CT at the lung base shows dense subpleural calcification and calcification of consolidated lung *(arrows)*. **D.** Radionuclide bone (^{99m}Tc-diphosphonate) scintigraphy shows extensive isotope uptake within both lungs.

chest films are normal. It may serve to confirm the diagnosis when CT shows typical apical opacities without obvious calcification.

SELECTED READING

Ayuso MC, Gilabert R, Bombi JA, Salvador A. CT appearance of localized pulmonary amyloidosis. J Comput Assist Tomogr 1987; 11:197–199.

Cluzel P, Grenier P, Bernadac P, et al. Pulmonary alveolar microlithiasis: CT findings. J Comput Assist Tomogr 1991; 15: 938–942.

Graham CM, Stern EJ, Finkbeiner WE, Webb WR. High-resolution CT appearance of diffuse alveolar septal amyloidosis. AJR Am J Roentgenol 1992; 158:265–267.

Hartman TE, Müller NL, Primack SL, et al. Metastatic pulmonary calcification in patients with hypercalcemia: findings on chest ra-diographs and CT scans. AJR Am J Roentgenol 1994; 162: 799–802.

Helbich TH, Wojnarovsky C, Wunderbaldinger P, et al. Pulmonary alveolar microlithiasis in children: radiographic and high-resolution CT findings. AJR Am J Roentgenol 1997; 168:63–65.

Johkoh T, Ikezoe J, Nagareda T, et al. Metastatic pulmonary calcification: early detection by high-resolution CT. J Comput Assist Tomogr 1993; 17:471–473.

Korn MA, Schurawitzki H, Klepetko W, Burghuber OC. Pulmonary alveolar microlithiasis: findings on high-resolution CT. AJR Am J Roentgenol 1992; 158:981–982.

Kuhlman JE, Ren H, Hutchins GM, Fishman EK. Fulminant pulmonary calcification complicating renal transplantation: CT demonstration. Radiology 1989; 173:459–460.

Pickford HA, Swensen SJ, Utz JP. Thoracic cross-sectional imaging of amyloidosis. AJR Am J Roentgenol 1997; 168:351–355.

Utz JP, Swensen SJ, Gertz MA. Pulmonary amyloidosis. The Mayo Clinic experience from 1980 to 1993. Ann Intern Med 1996; 124:407–413.

22

THE TRACHEA

W. RICHARD WEBB

THE NORMAL TRACHEA

The trachea extends from the inferior aspect of the cricoid cartilage (at the level of the sixth cervical vertebra) to the carina (at the level of the fifth thoracic vertebra). It measures from 10 to 12 cm in length. The trachea is divided into extrathoracic and intrathoracic portions at the level it passes posterior to the manubrium; the extrathoracic trachea is 2 to 4 cm in length, while the intrathoracic trachea measures 6 to 9 cm in length. From 16 to 22 horseshoe-shaped bands of hyaline cartilage support the anterior and lateral tracheal walls. The incomplete posterior portion of these rings is bridged by a thin band of smooth muscle and fibrous tissue, the *posterior tracheal membrane* (Fig. 22-1).

The plain film appearance of the trachea is described in Chapter 7. On CT, the trachea usually is round or oval in shape, but it can appear horseshoe-shaped, triangular, or like an inverted pear in some normal patients. The tracheal wall is delineated by air in the lumen internally and by mediastinal fat externally and usually is visible as a 1- to 2-mm soft tissue stripe. The posterior tracheal membrane appears thinner than the anterior and lateral tracheal walls, and is variable in shape due to its lack of cartilage; it can appear convex, concave, or flat. The tracheal cartilages may appear calcified or slightly denser than adjacent soft tissue. Calcification of cartilage is most common in older patients, and is particularly common in women (Fig. 22-2). In patients with calcified cartilage, little soft tissue is seen in the tracheal wall internal to the cartilage.

Tracheal diameter varies widely in normal subjects. In normal men, tracheal diameter averages 19.5 mm, with a range of 13 to 25 mm (mean $\pm$ 3 SD) in the coronal plane and 13 to 27 mm in the sagittal plane. In women, tracheal diameter is slightly smaller, averaging 17.5 mm and ranging from 10 to 21 mm in the coronal plane and 10 to 23 mm in the sagittal plane.

On CT performed during or after forced expiration, the posterior tracheal membrane bulges anteriorly, narrowing and, in some cases, nearly obliterating the tracheal lumen (Fig. 22-3). On average, the mean anterior-posterior diameter of the trachea decreases more than 30% during forced expiration due to anterior bulging of the posterior membrane; the transverse diameter decreases by only about 10%.

Tracheal Bronchus

A tracheal bronchus represents the origin of all or part (usually the apical segment) of the right upper lobe bronchus from the trachea; its incidence is about 0.1%. Left tracheal bronchus also occurs but is much less common.

DISEASES ASSOCIATED WITH TRACHEAL NARROWING

Focal tracheal narrowing may be seen with tracheal tumors, tuberculosis, tracheal stenosis or stricture, tracheomalacia, or occasionally with saber sheath trachea, Wegener's granulomatosis, or amyloidosis. Diffuse or generalized tracheal narrowing may be seen with tracheomalacia, saber sheath trachea, Wegener's granulomatosis, amyloidosis, tracheobronchopathia osteochondroplastica, and relapsing polychondritis.

Tracheal Tumors

Tumors of the trachea are rare (Table 22-1). Symptoms often are absent or nonspecific (e.g., cough, dyspnea), and early diagnosis is difficult. Tracheal tumors tend to be inconspicuous on chest radiographs, and may have become quite large before they are detected. CT is highly sensitive in detecting tracheal tumors and the extent of spread. Together, squamous cell carcinoma and adenoid cystic carcinoma account for more than 85% of tracheal tumors. Tumors of many other cell types, both epithelial and mesenchymal, may occur in the trachea but are much less common.

Squamous cell carcinoma is associated with smoking and is multifocal in 10% of cases, often involving the distal trachea; a main bronchus also may be involved (see Figs. 3-19 and 3-20 in Chapter 3). Adenoid cystic carcinoma originates from tracheal mucous glands and most often

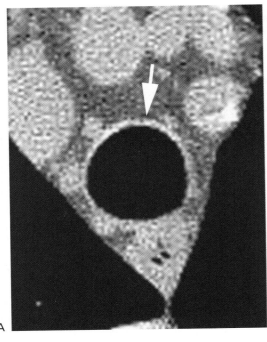
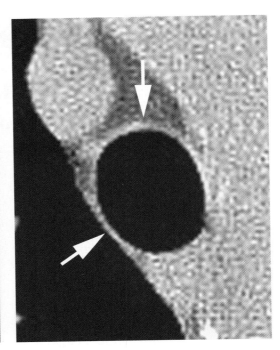

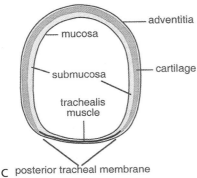

FIG. 22-1. The normal trachea. **A.** HRCT through the normal trachea. The tracheal wall *(arrow)* is outlined by mediastinal fat externally and usually is visible as a 1- to 2-mm soft tissue stripe. The posterior tracheal membrane usually appears thinner than the anterior and lateral tracheal walls, and is variable in shape due to its lack of cartilage. At this level it is partially obscured by the esophagus. **B.** At the level of the aortic arch, the tracheal wall *(arrows)* is outlined by mediastinal fat and the right lung in the region of the right paratracheal stripe. The tracheal wall appears thin. **C.** Diagrammatic representation of the normal components of the tracheal wall.

arises from the posterolateral tracheal wall (Figs. 22-4 and 22-5B). It is slightly less common than squamous cell carcinoma.

On CT, a primary malignant tracheal tumor may appear as a polypoid lesion, a focal sessile lesion, eccentric narrowing of the tracheal lumen, or circumferential wall thickening (see Fig. 22-5; also see Figs. 3-19 and 3-20 in Chapter 3). Attachment to the tracheal wall may be either broad-based or narrow and pedunculated. CT may underestimate the longitudinal extent of the tumor; submucosal spread may be difficult to see on CT. However, CT is superior to bronchoscopy in evaluating extraluminal spread and the trachea distal to an obstructing lesion.

Tracheal metastases may occur via direct extension or by hematogenous spread. Direct extension to involve the trachea most often is secondary to a primary tumor of the lung, larynx, esophagus, or thyroid. These tumors may compress the trachea, displacing tracheal cartilage inward, or

may invade the tracheal lumen, with tumor being seen as abnormal tissue internal to tracheal cartilage (see Fig. 3-37 in Chapter 3). Hematogenous metastases usually originate from melanoma, or from carcinomas of the breast, colon, or kidney. On CT hematogenous metastases may appear as single or multiple, sessile or pedunculated endotracheal lesions (Fig. 22-6).

Squamous cell papilloma is the most common benign tracheal tumor. It represents an abnormal proliferation of squamous epithelium, which may be sessile, papillary, lobulated, or polypoid. Solitary papilloma is associated with smoking and is most common in adults. The condition of multiple papillomas (i.e., papillomatosis) usually begins in childhood with laryngeal involvement and is associated with human papillomavirus infection. On CT a solitary papilloma appears as a well-circumscribed nodule that is confined to the tracheal wall and projects into the tracheal lumen; it often shows acute angles where it contacts the tracheal wall.

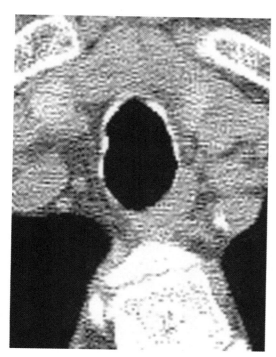

FIG. 22-2. Normal calcification of tracheal cartilage in an elderly woman. Discontinuous calcification of the tracheal wall reflects calcification of individual cartilage rings. The tracheal wall appears thin.

TABLE 22-1. TRACHEAL TUMORS

Primary malignant
Most common (85% of cases)
   Squamous cell carcinoma
   Adenoid cystic carcinoma
Rare
   Other types of bronchogenic carcinoma
   Carcinoid tumor
   Sarcoma
   Lymphoma
Metastatic
Direct invasion most common
   Thyroid carcinoma
   Laryngeal cancer
   Lung cancer
   Esophageal cancer
Hematogenous metastases
   Melanoma
   Breast carcinoma
   Colon carcinoma
   Kidney carcinoma
Benign
Squamous cell papilloma
Papillomatosis
Hamartoma
Mesenchymal tumors

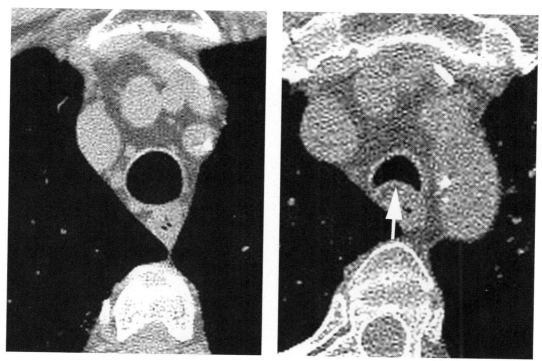

A   B

FIG. 22-3. Normal expiratory CT. **A.** On inspiration, the trachea has a rounded appearance. **B.** During a dynamic forced expiratory scan, there is marked anterior bowing of the posterior tracheal membrane *(arrow)*. This appearance is normal. Little side-to-side narrowing occurs because of the tracheal cartilage.

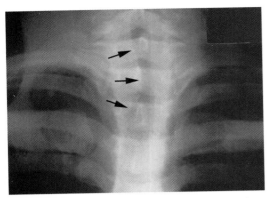

FIG. 22-4. Adenoid cystic carcinoma of the proximal trachea. An eccentric narrowing *(arrows)* of the tracheal lumen is caused by a sessile mass arising from the right tracheal wall.

Tracheal cartilage is unaffected. Papillomatosis is characterized by numerous nodules involving the entire length of the trachea (see Fig. 3-54 in Chapter 3). Other benign tracheal tumors include hamartoma and tumors of mesenchymal origin.

Tracheomalacia

Tracheomalacia refers to weakness of the tracheal wall, usually due to abnormalities of the tracheal cartilage (Table 22-2). It may be congenital and associated with deficient cartilage, but most often is acquired as a result of intubation injuries, tracheal compression by extrinsic masses or vascular lesions (e.g., aortic aneurysm), chronic infection, or chronic obstructive pulmonary disease, or in association with saber-sheath trachea, relapsing polychondritis, or tracheobronchomegaly. It may be localized, or it may involve a long tracheal segment.

Abnormal flaccidity of the tracheal wall may result in inefficient cough, retention of secretions, and chronic airway infection and bronchiectasis. Symptoms include recurrent infection, dyspnea, and stridor.

Radiographs or CT on inspiration may show an increase or decrease in tracheal diameter. The hallmark of tracheomalacia is a significant decrease in the tracheal diameter or collapse of the tracheal walls with expiration. Tracheal collapse may be diffuse or side to side. It should be distinguished from normal invagination of the posterior tracheal membrane; with forced expiration, this phenomenon may result in near-complete obliteration of the tracheal lumen in normal subjects (see Fig. 22-3).

Tuberculosis

Tuberculosis (TB) typically involves both the distal trachea and the proximal main bronchi; isolated tracheal disease is rare. Active inflammation with granulation tissue causes

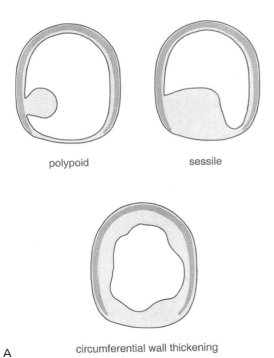

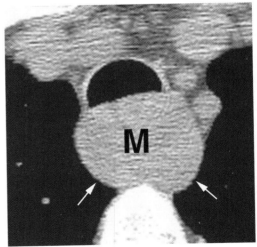

FIG. 22-5. CT appearances of primary tracheal tumor. **A.** Tracheal malignancies may appear polypoid, sessile, or circumferential. **B.** Adenoid cystic carcinoma results in a sessile mass *(M)* arising from the posterior tracheal wall and protruding into the tracheal lumen. The mass extends into the adjacent mediastinum *(arrows)*.

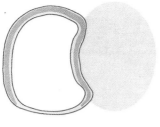

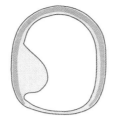
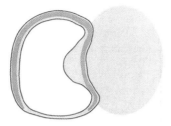

extrinsic compression

endotracheal mass

extrinsic compression
with luminal invasion

A

FIG. 22-6. Tracheal metastasis. **A.** Tracheal metastases may result in tracheal compression with inward displacement of the tracheal wall, an endotracheal mass, or a combination of these findings. **B.** There is narrowing of the trachea with an endoluminal mass *(arrow).* **C.** Soft-tissue window at the same level as **B** shows a mass involving the right tracheal wall and mediastinal soft tissues *(arrows).*

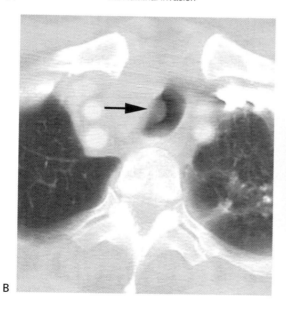

B

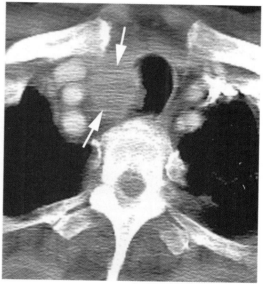

C

irregular circumferential wall thickening with narrowing of the tracheal lumen. In many cases, tracheal infection results from spread from adjacent lymph nodes, and enlarged mediastinal nodes or increased density of mediastinal fat may be seen. Tracheal TB also may occur due to endobronchial spread of infection.

With treatment, wall thickening and tracheal narrowing usually are reversible, although in some patients stricture results, with narrowing of the tracheal lumen in the absence of wall thickening.

Bronchial strictures may be associated with tracheal narrowing. Strictures from TB most often involve the left main bronchus, perhaps because it is longer than the right. CT findings that help to differentiate TB stricture from carcinoma include a long segment of circumferential involvement and the absence of an intraluminal mass.

Tracheal Stenosis

Congenital tracheal stenosis may result from a ring-shaped tracheal cartilage. Acquired tracheal stenosis usually is due to prior intubation or tracheostomy. Progressive dyspnea following extubation typically is present. Inflammation and pressure necrosis of the tracheal mucosa most commonly

TABLE 22-2. NONNEOPLASTIC TRACHEAL DISEASES

Disease	Extent	Appearance	Associations
Tracheomalacia	Focal or diffuse	Collapse of tracheal wall with expiration	Congenital, intubation, extrinsic masses, chronic infection, COPD, saber-sheath trachea, polychondritis, tracheobronchomegaly
Tuberculosis	Distal trachea (and main bronchi)	Early: concentric wall thickening Late: stricture or distortion of cartilage	Mediastinal lymph node disease
Postintubation stenosis	Proximal trachea	Early: concentric wall thickening Late: stricture or distortion of cartilage	Malacia may be present
Saber-sheath trachea	Early: thoracic inlet Late: intrathoracic trachea	Side-to-side narrowing, sagittal diameter normal or increased	COPD, chronic cough; malacia may be present
Wegener's granulomatosis	Focal (subglottic trachea) or diffuse	Concentric wall thickening, cartilage destruction	Occurs in 15%–25% of cases; malacia is not present
Amyloidosis	Focal (nodular) or diffuse	Concentric or nodular wall thickening	Calcification common; malacia is not present
Tracheobronchopathia osteochondroplastica	Diffuse	Calcified submucosal nodules adjacent to tracheal cartilage, nodules spare the posterior membrane	Malacia is not present
Relapsing polychondritis	Diffuse	Thickening of anterior and lateral wall, posterior membrane normal	Arthritis; malacia may be present
Tracheobronchomegaly (Mounier-Kuhn syndrome)	Diffuse	Increased tracheal diameter (>3 cm), tracheal wall normal or appears scalloped, tracheal diverticula	Cystic bronchiectasis often present; COPD, pulmonary fibrosis, Marfan's syndrome, cystic fibrosis, Ehlers-Danlos syndrome, cutis laxa

occur at either the tracheostomy stoma or at the level of the tube balloon, 1 to 1.5 cm proximal to the tube tip; it usually involves 1.5 to 2.5 cm of the tracheal wall. The extrathoracic trachea most often is involved. Focal narrowing may be seen if the tube tip presses on one part of the tracheal wall, usually the anterior wall.

Acute postintubation stenosis results from edema of the tracheal wall or intraluminal granulation tissue. Plain films may show an eccentric or hourglass-shaped tracheal narrowing. On CT, this may be seen as eccentric or concentric soft tissue internal to normal-appearing tracheal cartilage (Fig. 22-7). The outer tracheal wall has a normal appearance, without evidence of deformity or narrowing. Dynamic expiratory images show little change in tracheal dimensions.

In postintubation patients with chronic stenosis or stricture, fibrosis usually is present with deformity of tracheal cartilage. On CT, thickening of the mucosa and submucosa is absent or mild, and deformity of the tracheal cartilage or posterior tracheal membrane, which accounts for narrowing of the lumen (Fig. 22-8), usually is seen. The area of narrowing may be thin and weblike or long. Dynamic expiratory images may or may not show significant malacia. Because of the focal nature of the stenosis, treatment with stenting is useful.

Acute and chronic stenosis may also result from sarcoidosis, histoplasmosis, Wegener's granulomatosis, and ulcerative colitis.

Saber-Sheath Trachea

Saber-sheath trachea is common and almost always is associated with chronic obstructive pulmonary disease. It is characterized by a marked decrease in the coronal diameter of the intrathoracic trachea associated with an increase in its sagittal diameter (Fig. 22-9); the extrathoracic trachea is normal. Although it may involve the entire intrathoracic trachea, in its earliest stages it is visible only at the thoracic inlet. It is thought to be due to chronic injury and malacia of tracheal cartilage due to coughing or increased intrathoracic pressure. The main bronchi are of normal size.

On plain radiographs, a characteristic side-to-side narrowing of the tracheal lumen is visible on the frontal radiograph, beginning at the thoracic inlet (see Fig. 22-9). The right paratracheal stripe, primarily representing tracheal wall, appears normal or slightly increased in thickness. On the lateral radiograph, the tracheal diameter appears normal or slightly increased. If the tracheal diameter on the lateral

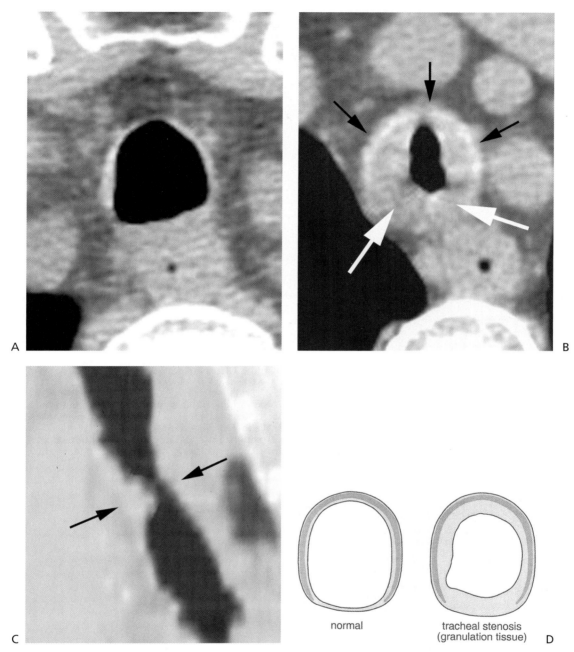

FIG. 22-7. Postintubation tracheal stenosis due to granulation tissue. **A.** Near the thoracic inlet, the trachea appears normal. **B.** Below the level shown in **A**, focal narrowing of the tracheal lumen is associated with increased soft tissue *(white arrows)* within the tracheal lumen. The calcified tracheal cartilage *(black arrows)* appears normal, without evidence of deformity or collapse. **C.** Sagittal reformation shows a focal tracheal narrowing *(arrows)*. **D.** Diagrammatic representation of tracheal stenosis due to granulation tissue, compared to the appearance of a normal trachea. (From Webb EM, Elicker BM, Webb WR. Using CT to diagnose nonneoplastic tracheal abnormalities: appearance of the tracheal wall. AJR Am J Roentgenol 2000; 174:1315–1321.)

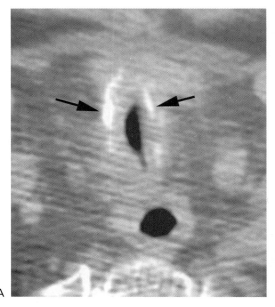
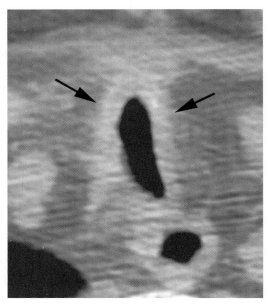

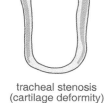

FIG. 22-8. Postintubation tracheal stenosis due to stricture. **A** and **B.** CT at two levels shows side-to-side narrowing of the tracheal lumen resulting from deformity of the tracheal cartilage *(arrows).* **C.** Diagrammatic representation of tracheal stenosis due to cartilage deformity, compared to the appearance of a normal trachea. (From Webb EM, Elicker BM, Webb WR. Using CT to diagnose nonneoplastic tracheal abnormalities: appearance of the tracheal wall. AJR Am J Roentgenol 2000; 174:1315–1321.)

normal   tracheal stenosis (cartilage deformity)

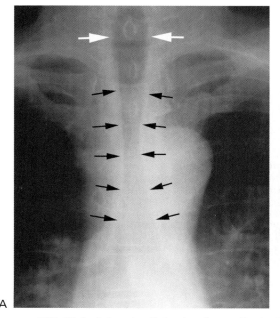
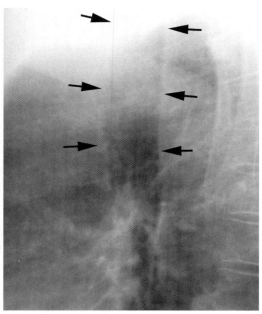

FIG. 22-9. Saber-sheath trachea in a patient with chronic obstructive pulmonary disease. **A.** PA chest radiograph shows hourglass-shaped narrowing of the intrathoracic trachea *(black arrows).* The extrathoracic trachea *(white arrows)* appears normal. **B.** In the lateral projection, the tracheal diameter appears normal or increased *(arrows).*

film measures 1.5 times that seen on the frontal film, saber sheath trachea is considered to be present.

On CT, there is inward bowing of the lateral portions of the tracheal wall and tracheal cartilage with side-to-side narrowing of the tracheal lumen (Fig. 22-10). The tracheal wall usually is of normal thickness. During forced expiration, CT demonstrates further inward bowing of the tracheal walls in many patients.

Wegener's Granulomatosis

Wegener's granulomatosis is a systemic vasculitis. In 90% of cases, serum antineutrophil cytoplasmic antibodies characterized by a diffuse granular cytoplasmic immunofluorescent staining pattern (cytoplasmic antineutrophil cytoplasmic antibody [C-ANCA]) are present.

Tracheobronchial involvement occurs in about 15% to

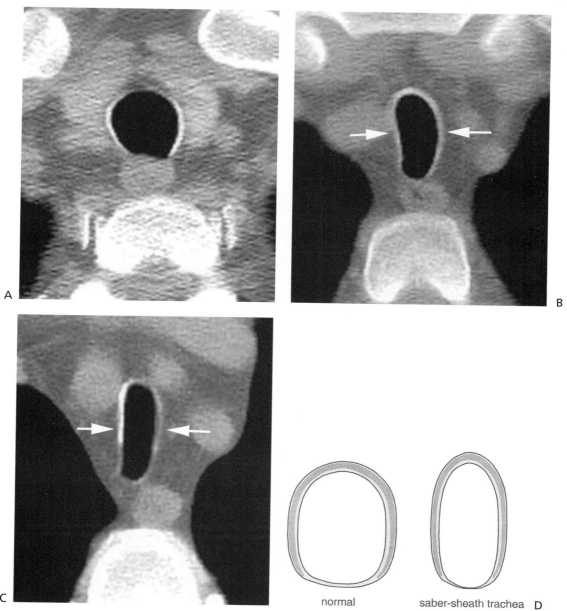

FIG. 22-10. Saber-sheath trachea on CT. **A.** The extrathoracic trachea is normal. The tracheal cartilage is calcified and well seen. **B** and **C.** The intrathoracic trachea at two levels is markedly narrowed from side to side *(arrows)*, associated with deformity of the tracheal cartilage. The sagittal tracheal diameter is increased. The tracheal wall is otherwise normal in appearance. **D.** Diagrammatic representation of saber-sheath trachea. (From Webb EM, Elicker BM, Webb WR. Using CT to diagnose nonneoplastic tracheal abnormalities: appearance of the tracheal wall. AJR Am J Roentgenol 2000; 174:1315–1321.)

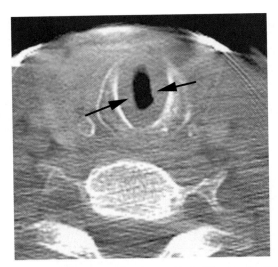

FIG. 22-11. Subglottic tracheal stenosis in Wegener's granulomatosis. Excessive soft tissue *(arrows)* is visible internal to the cricoid cartilage. A tracheostomy is in place below this level.

25% of cases; symptoms are common and include hoarseness, cough, and stridor. Subglottic tracheal involvement is most typical (Fig. 22-11), with variable involvement of the vocal cords, distal trachea, and proximal mainstem bronchi. Abnormalities may be focal or diffuse. Pathologic findings include circumferential airway wall thickening and inflammation, and concentric narrowing of the tracheal lumen; mucosal ulceration and destruction of the cricoid or tracheal cartilage are less common. Tracheal involvement may be life-threatening, but treatment with stents may be helpful.

Plain radiographs show tracheal narrowing on both the frontal and lateral radiographs; this narrowing may be localized or diffuse. Characteristic CT findings include circumferential wall thickening, an increase in the overall tracheal diameter due to wall thickening, and narrowing of the tracheal lumen (Fig. 22-12). Malacia is not typically seen.

Amyloidosis

Tracheobronchial amyloidosis is rare (see Chapter 21). Symptoms are common and include hoarseness, stridor, dyspnea, cough, hemoptysis, and recurrent infections.

Primary tracheobronchial amyloidosis usually is confined to the trachea, with no evidence of concurrent parenchymal disease. Deposits most commonly are diffuse throughout the length of the trachea and are found within the submucosa; the main bronchi also are commonly involved. On plain radiographs and CT, diffuse tracheobronchial amyloidosis usually leads to concentric or nodular thickening of the tracheal wall (Fig. 22-13). Calcification or ossifica-

tion is common. Malacia is not present. Rarely, a single localized submucosal nodule is present, resulting in eccentric wall thickening. Multiple isolated lesions also may be seen. Atelectasis may be associated with bronchial involvement. Progression is typical, and bronchoscopic resection of focal lesions or airway stenting may be helpful in some cases.

Tracheobronchopathia Osteochondroplastica

Tracheobronchopathia osteochondroplastica is a rare, benign disease characterized by development of cartilaginous and osseous nodules within the submucosa of the tracheal and bronchial walls. It is most typical in men older than 50, and usually is detected incidentally. In some patients, dyspnea, cough, hemoptysis, and wheezing may be present.

Nodules tend to be localized to the submucosa directly associated with the tracheal cartilage, sparing the posterior tracheal membrane. The nodules may consist of cartilage or exostoses occurring in relation to the perichondrium of the tracheal cartilage, or they may be metaplastic, arising in elastic tissue.

Plain radiographs show extensive irregular tracheal and central bronchial calcification. CT findings include thickened cartilage with small irregular calcific nodules along their inner aspect, protruding into the tracheal lumen (Fig. 22-14). The nodules typically measure between 3 and 8 mm in diameter. No significant decrease in tracheal diameter is seen with forced expiration. The appearance is much more irregular than that seen with normal cartilage calcification. Similar central bronchial calcification also is seen in many patients.

Relapsing Polychondritis

Relapsing polychondritis is a rare systemic disorder characterized by recurrent episodes of cartilage inflammation most commonly affecting the ear, nose, joints, and the laryngeal and tracheal cartilage. Nonerosive polyarthritis, nasal deformity, and auricular chondritis are characteristic, but need not be present in all cases. The upper airways are affected in more than 50% of cases, and recurrent pneumonia is the most common cause of death. Diffuse tracheal involvement, characterized by a dense inflammatory exudate, is limited to the cartilage and perichondrium, and does not affect the mucosa or submucosa. Histologic findings include edema, granulation tissue, cartilage destruction, and, eventually, fibrosis of the tracheal wall. Both the extrathoracic and intrathoracic portions of the trachea are involved. Treatment often requires the use of tracheal and bronchial stents to maintain airway patency.

Plain radiographs usually show cylindrical narrowing of the extrathoracic and intrathoracic trachea and main

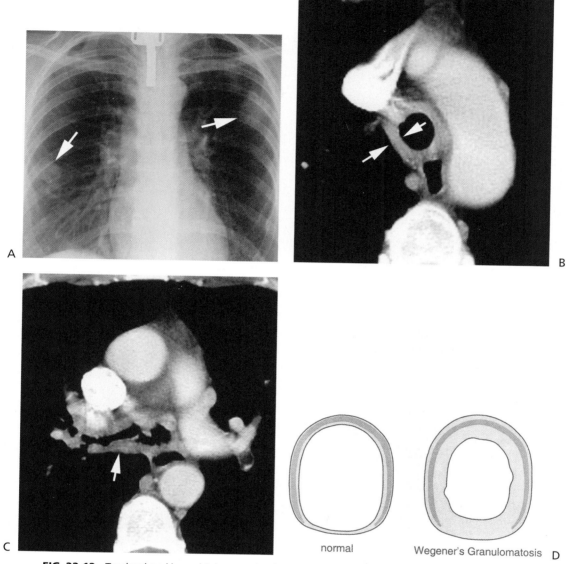

FIG. 22-12. Tracheal and bronchial narrowing in Wegener's granulomatosis. **A.** Chest radiograph shows bilateral lung nodules *(arrows)*. A tracheostomy is in place. **B.** CT shows tracheal narrowing associated with concentric thickening of the tracheal wall *(arrows)*. **C.** At the level of the carina, bronchial wall thickening *(arrow)* also is seen. **D.** Diagrammatic representation of abnormalities in Wegener's granulomatosis. Concentric wall thickening is visible. (From Webb EM, Elicker BM, Webb WR. Using CT to diagnose nonneoplastic tracheal abnormalities: appearance of the tracheal wall. AJR Am J Roentgenol 2000; 174:1315–1321.)

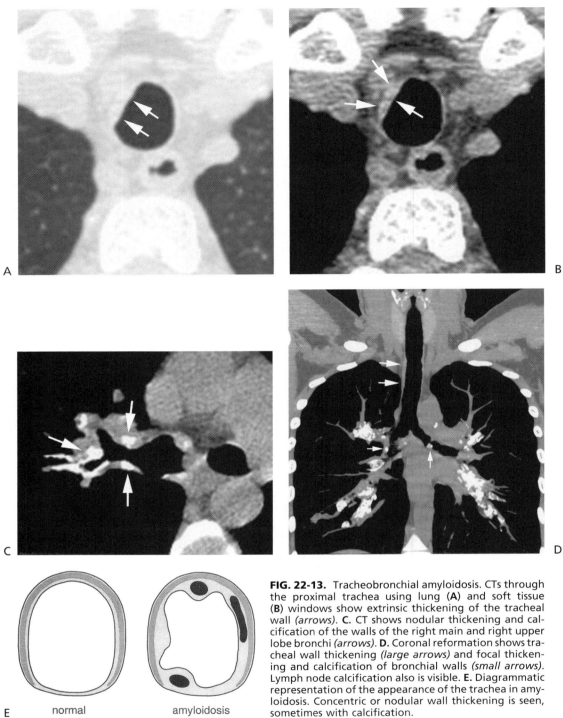

FIG. 22-13. Tracheobronchial amyloidosis. CTs through the proximal trachea using lung (**A**) and soft tissue (**B**) windows show extrinsic thickening of the tracheal wall *(arrows)*. **C.** CT shows nodular thickening and calcification of the walls of the right main and right upper lobe bronchi *(arrows)*. **D.** Coronal reformation shows tracheal wall thickening *(large arrows)* and focal thickening and calcification of bronchial walls *(small arrows)*. Lymph node calcification also is visible. **E.** Diagrammatic representation of the appearance of the trachea in amyloidosis. Concentric or nodular wall thickening is seen, sometimes with calcification.

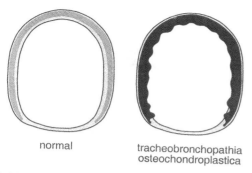

FIG. 22-14. Diagrammatic representation of the appearance of the trachea in tracheobronchopathia osteochondroplastica. Tracheal cartilages are thickened, with small irregular calcific nodules along their inner aspect, protruding into the tracheal lumen. (From Webb EM, Elicker BM, Webb WR. Using CT to diagnose nonneoplastic tracheal abnormalities: appearance of the tracheal wall. AJR Am J Roentgenol 2000; 174:1315–1321.)

bronchi (Fig. 22-15). In most cases, CT shows thickening of the anterior and lateral tracheal walls, but a posterior membrane of normal thickness (Figs. 22-16 and 22-17). Both the inner and outer margins of the thickened tracheal walls are smooth in contour. Collapse of tracheal cartilage may be seen in chronic disease. Narrowing of both the tracheal lumen and the main bronchi is seen. The luminal narrowing may be fixed or may increase with forced expiration (Fig. 22-18).

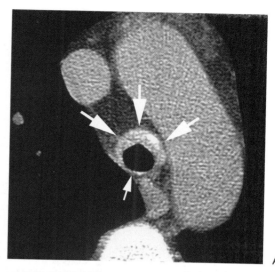

A

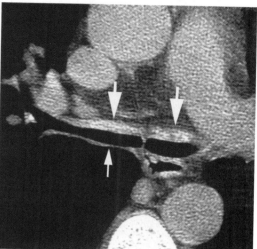

B

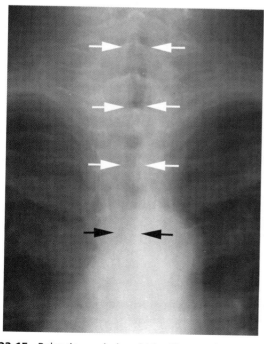

FIG. 22-15. Relapsing polychondritis. Chest radiograph shows cylindrical narrowing of the entire trachea *(arrows).*

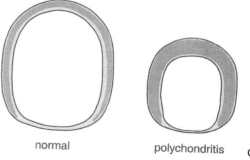

C

FIG. 22-16. Relapsing polychondritis. **A.** CT shows tracheal narrowing. The anterior and lateral tracheal walls (i.e., the cartilaginous portions) are thickened *(large arrows).* The posterior tracheal membrane is of normal thickness *(small arrow).* This appearance is characteristic. **B.** Narrowing of the main bronchi also is seen. The anterior bronchial walls are thickened *(large arrows),* while the posterior wall of the bronchus appears normal *(small arrow).* **C.** Diagrammatic representation of relapsing polychondritis. The anterior and lateral tracheal walls are thickened; the posterior tracheal membrane is of normal thickness. (From Webb EM, Elicker BM, Webb WR. Using CT to diagnose nonneoplastic tracheal abnormalities: appearance of the tracheal wall. AJR Am J Roentgenol 2000; 174:1315–1321.)

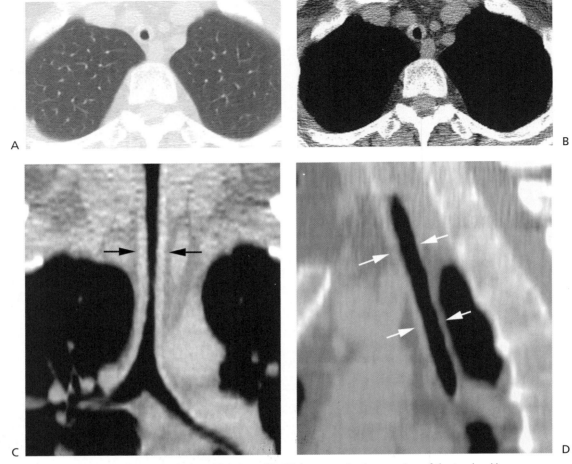

FIG. 22-17. Relapsing polychondritis. **A** and **B.** CT shows marked narrowing of the tracheal lumen, with typical thickening of the anterior and lateral tracheal walls. **C.** Coronal reformation shows diffuse narrowing of the trachea with thickening of its lateral walls *(arrows)*. **D.** Sagittal reformation shows diffuse narrowing of the trachea *(arrows)*.

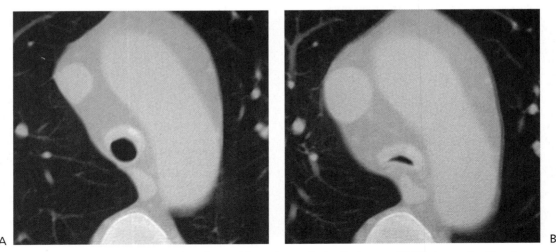

FIG. 22-18. Relapsing polychondritis with tracheomalacia. Expiratory CT (**B**) shows significant collapse of the tracheal lumen compared with an inspiratory scan (**A**).

DISEASES ASSOCIATED WITH INCREASED TRACHEAL DIAMETER

Tracheal Diverticulum

Tracheal diverticulum is a focal herniation of tracheal mucosa through the tracheal wall. Tracheal diverticulum may be seen in normal subjects, although it tends to be associated with chronic obstructive pulmonary disease. It usually is asymptomatic and is detected incidentally.

Tracheal diverticuli almost always occur near the thoracic inlet, along the posterolateral right trachea, between the cartilaginous and muscular portions of the tracheal wall (Fig. 22-19). They can appear as an isolated paratracheal air cyst (Fig. 22-20), usually a few millimeters in diameter, or as an air-filled structure communicating with the tracheal lumen (see Fig. 22-19). They are easily seen on CT, but are rarely visible on plain radiographs.

Mounier-Kuhn Syndrome (Tracheobronchomegaly)

Tracheobronchomegaly, also referred to as *Mounier-Kuhn syndrome,* is characterized by marked dilatation of the trachea and mainstem bronchi, often in association with tracheal diverticulosis, recurrent lower respiratory tract infections, and bronchiectasis (see Table 22-2). Tracheobronchomegaly is diagnosed most often in men in their third and fourth decades; it is much less common in women. There may be a history of recurrent respiratory tract infec-

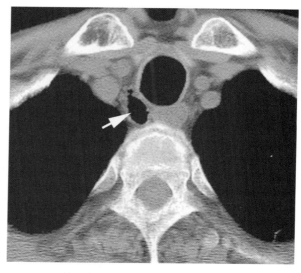

A

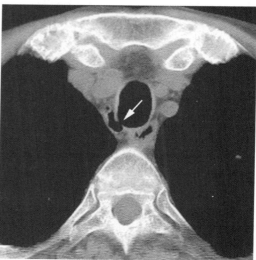

B

FIG. 22-20. Tracheal diverticulum. **A.** A paratracheal air cyst is present in the upper mediastinum, representing a diverticulum *(arrow).* **B.** A defect in the right posterolateral tracheal wall *(arrow)* communicates with the diverticulum.

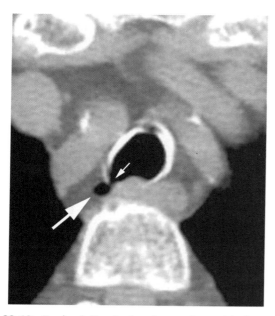

FIG. 22-19. Tracheal diverticulum in a patient with chronic obstructive pulmonary disease. A defect in the right posterolateral tracheal wall *(small arrow)* communicates with a small diverticulum *(large arrow).* This location is characteristic.

tion or chronic cough dating to childhood, but this is not seen in all patients.

Although tracheal enlargement is seen in some patients with chronic pulmonary fibrosis or chronic infection, tracheobronchomegaly most likely is congenital in origin. Histologic examination of the trachea shows a deficiency of smooth muscle and elastic fibers. A cartilage abnormality undoubtedly is present as well, although this abnormality probably is acquired. Tracheomegaly also may occur in association with other congenital disorders such as Marfan's syndrome, cystic fibrosis, Ehlers-Danlos syndrome, and cutis laxa.

The diagnosis is based on radiographic findings of increased tracheal and bronchial diameter. Dilatation usually

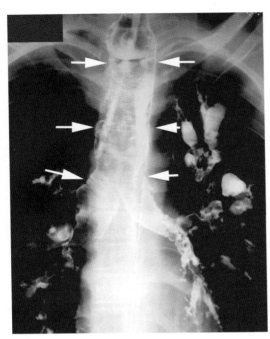

FIG. 22-21. Tracheobronchomegaly. A bronchogram shows tracheal dilatation *(arrows)*, with the tracheal wall having a corrugated or scalloped contour. Central bronchiectasis also is visible.

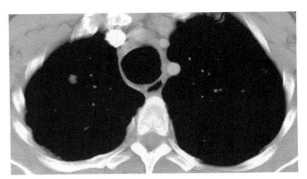

FIG. 22-22. Tracheobronchomegaly. CT above the aortic arch shows marked tracheal dilatation. The trachea measures 37 mm in diameter.

wall. Also common is the finding of a marked tracheal flaccidity or tracheomalacia on expiratory scans.

involves the intrathoracic trachea and the first few bronchial divisions (Fig. 22-21). Tracheobronchomegaly may be suggested in a man if the tracheal diameter measured on the frontal and lateral radiographs exceeds 25 and 27 mm, respectively; in a woman, it may be suggested if these measurements exceed 21 and 23 mm. The trachea tends to have a corrugated or scalloped contour (see Fig. 22-21), because of mucosa protruding between the tracheal cartilage. On the lateral view, this is visible anteriorly. Frank tracheal diverticula also may be present. Bronchiectasis commonly is present and tends to involve the central bronchi; peripheral airways appear normal.

On CT, a tracheal diameter greater than 3 cm (measured 2 cm above the aortic arch) and diameters of 2.4 and 2.3 cm for the right and left main bronchi have been used to make the diagnosis of tracheobronchomegaly (Fig. 22-22), although these measurements are more conservative than those proposed for use on chest radiographs. Tracheal scalloping is more difficult to see in cross section than on chest films. Diverticula, on the other hand, are more easily seen on CT, typically occurring along the posterolateral tracheal

SELECTED READING

Choplin RH, Wehunt WD, Theros EG. Diffuse lesions of the trachea. Semin Roentgenol 1983; 18:38–50.

Gamsu G, Webb WR. Computed tomography of the trachea and mainstem bronchi. Semin Roentgenol 1983; 18:51–60.

Goo JM, Im JG, Ahn JM, et al. Right paratracheal air cysts in the thoracic inlet: clinical and radiologic significance. AJR Am J Roentgenol 1999; 173:65–70.

Im JG, Chung JW, Han SK, et al. CT manifestations of tracheobronchial involvement in relapsing polychondritis. J Comput Assist Tomogr 1988; 12:792–793.

Kwong JS, Müller NL, Miller RR. Diseases of the trachea and mainstem bronchi: correlation of CT with pathologic findings. Radiographics 1992; 12:647–657.

Mariotta S, Pallone G, Pedicelli G, Bisetti A. Spiral CT and endoscopic findings in a case of tracheobronchopathia osteochondroplastica. J Comput Assist Tomogr 1997; 21:418–420.

Pickford HA, Swensen SJ, Utz JP. Thoracic cross-sectional imaging of amyloidosis. AJR Am J Roentgenol 1997; 168:351–355.

Roditi GH, Weir J. The association of tracheomegaly and bronchiectasis. Clin Radiol 1994; 49:608–611.

Screaton NJ, Sivasothy P, Flower CD, Lockwood CM. Tracheal involvement in Wegener's granulomatosis: evaluation using spiral CT. Clin Radiol 1998; 53:809–815.

Shin MS, Jackson RM, Ho KJ. Tracheobronchomegaly (Mounier-Kuhn syndrome): CT diagnosis. AJR Am J Roentgenol 1988; 150:777–779.

Stern EJ, Graham CM, Webb WR, Gamsu G. Normal trachea during forced expiration: dynamic CT measurements. Radiology 1993; 187:27–31.

Webb EM, Elicker BM, Webb WR. Using CT to diagnose nonneoplastic tracheal abnormalities: appearance of the tracheal wall. AJR Am J Roentgenol 2000; 174:1315–1321.

23

AIRWAY DISEASE: BRONCHIECTASIS, CHRONIC BRONCHITIS, AND BRONCHIOLITIS

W. Richard Webb

AIRWAY MORPHOLOGY

Airways divide by dichotomous branching. There are approximately 23 divisions from the trachea to the alveoli.

Bronchi are conducting airways that contain cartilage in their walls. The anatomy of the lobar and segmental bronchi is described in Chapter 6.

Bronchioles are airways not containing cartilage. The largest bronchioles measure about 3 mm in diameter and have walls about 0.3 mm thick. A *terminal bronchiole* is the last purely conducting airway, and does not participate in gas exchange. It is approximately 0.7 mm in diameter, and gives rise to respiratory bronchioles. A *respiratory bronchiole* is the largest bronchiole with alveoli arising from its walls, and, thus, is the largest bronchiole that participates in gas exchange. It gives rise to alveolar ducts and alveoli.

BRONCHIECTASIS

Bronchiectasis is defined as localized, irreversible dilatation of the bronchial tree. Usually this term is used to refer only to cartilage-containing airways, larger than 2 to 3 mm in diameter.

Etiology

Bronchiectasis is associated with a wide variety of causes (Table 23-1), but in up to 40% of cases, the cause cannot be found. Bronchiectasis is commonly associated with acute, chronic, or recurrent infection, particularly infection with bacteria and mycobacteria. Also, bronchiectasis often is present in patients with bronchiolitis obliterans or the Swyer-James syndrome resulting from viral or mycoplasma infection. Immunodeficiency syndromes including AIDS, abnormalities of mucociliary clearance, structural abnormalities of the bronchial wall, and chronic bronchial obstruc-

tion are associated with bronchiectasis, largely because they result in infection.

Noninfectious diseases that result in airway inflammation and mucous plugging also can result in bronchiectasis. These include allergic bronchopulmonary aspergillosis, and, to a lesser extent, asthma. Bronchiectasis also is seen in patients with bronchiolitis obliterans resulting from chronic

TABLE 23-1. CAUSES OF BRONCHIECTASIS

Infection
Bacteria (*Pseudomonas, Staphylococcus, Bordetella pertussis*)
Mycobacteria (tuberculosis, *Mycobacterium avium-intracellulare* [MAC])
Virus
Mycoplasma
Immune deficiency states
Congenital (e.g., hypogammaglobulinemia)
Acquired (e.g., AIDS)
Mucociliary clearance abnormalities
Cystic fibrosis (abnormal mucus)
Dyskinetic cilia syndrome (abnormal cilia)
Young's syndrome
Bronchial obstruction
Congenital bronchial atresia
Endobronchial tumor
Bronchial compression by lymph nodes
Bronchial wall abnormalities
Tracheobronchomegaly
Williams-Campbell syndrome
Immune reactions
ABPA
Asthma
Lung transplant rejection
Graft-versus-host disease
Proteinase-antiproteinase imbalance
Alpha-1-antitrypsin deficiency
Systemic diseases
Collagen-vascular disease
Inflammatory bowel disease

rejection following lung transplantation or chronic graft-versus-host disease (GVHD) in patients with bone marrow transplantation.

Causes of bronchiectasis having a genetic basis include cystic fibrosis; the dyskinetic cilia (Kartagener) syndrome (Fig. 23-1); Young's syndrome; Williams-Campbell syndrome (congenital deficiency of the bronchial cartilage); Mounier-Kuhn syndrome (congenital tracheobronchomegaly); alpha-1-antitrypsin deficiency; immunodeficiency syndromes, including Bruton's hypogammaglobulinemia, IgA, and combined IgA-IgG deficiencies; and the yellow nail lymphedema syndrome (yellow nails, lymphedema, and pleural effusions).

Pathologic Abnormalities

Bronchiectasis usually is associated with bronchial wall thickening, inflammation, destruction of muscular and elastic elements of the bronchial wall, and bronchial and peribronchial fibrosis. Loss of muscular and elastic tissues allows the bronchi to dilate in response to the pull of adjacent tissues (i.e., the normal negative interstitial pressure). Ciliated epithelium is usually replaced by nonciliated or squamous epithelium. These structural abnormalities of the bronchial wall encourage infection, which, in turn, further damages the bronchi.

Inflammation and fibrosis also are associated with oblit-

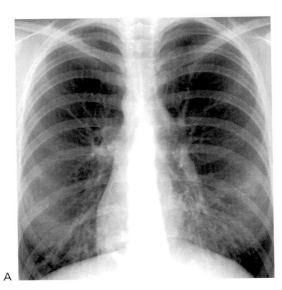

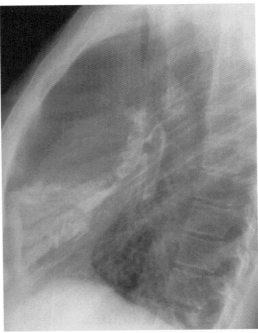

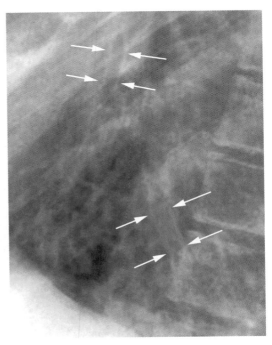

FIG. 23-1. Plain film appearance of bronchiectasis in Kartagener's syndrome. **A.** PA chest radiograph shows situs inversus. Increased linear opacities, visible at both lung bases, represent thickened bronchial walls, or tram tracks. This appearance is characteristic of cylindrical bronchiectasis. **B.** Lateral radiograph also shows this finding. **C.** Detail view of the lateral radiograph shows parallel lines, representing thickened bronchial walls, or tram-tracks *(arrows)*.

eration of small airways and a reduction in the number of bronchial branches, particularly when the disease occurs during childhood, when the lungs are growing.

Volume loss typically is seen within the affected lung. The lung may be air-filled or airless. Pulmonary arteries supplying the abnormal lung usually are reduced in number and size, and regional lung perfusion is decreased accordingly.

Clinical Diagnosis

In general, a clinical diagnosis of bronchiectasis is possible only in the most severely affected patients, and differentiation from chronic bronchitis may be difficult. Most patients present with purulent sputum production, recurrent pulmonary infections, fever, weight loss, and sometimes dyspnea. Hemoptysis also is common, occurring in up to 50% of cases, and may be the only clinical finding. Hemoptysis usually is associated with bronchial artery enlargement related to chronic inflammation. Sputum culture often reveals bacterial infection, with common organisms being *Streptococcus pneumoniae, Pseudomonas, Haemophilus influenzae,* and *Staphylococcus aureus. Aspergillus* species and mycobacteria also may be present.

Pulmonary function tests may show airflow obstruction. However, bronchitis, bronchiolitis, or emphysema often accompanies bronchiectasis and may predominate as the cause of obstructive abnormalities.

Classification

Traditionally, bronchiectasis has been classified into three morphologic types: cylindrical, varicose, and cystic. The severity of bronchial dilatation and anatomic abnormalities, and, to a lesser extent, functional abnormalities, correlate with these three types. Cylindrical bronchiectasis is associated with the least severe abnormalities, and cystic bronchiectasis is associated with the most severe. However, differentiating between them is less important in clinical practice than is a determination of the extent and distribution of the bronchiectasis.

Cylindrical Bronchiectasis

Cylindrical bronchiectasis is characterized by mild bronchial dilatation. The dilated bronchi are of relatively uniform caliber and have roughly parallel walls. Often, smaller bronchi are plugged with purulent secretions. The number of bronchial divisions from the carina to the periphery is slightly reduced.

Varicose Bronchiectasis

With increasingly severe abnormalities of the bronchial wall and increasing bronchial dilatation, the bronchi may assume an irregular, beaded or bulbous configuration, referred to as *varicose bronchiectasis.* Usually, peripheral bronchi are obliterated by fibrous tissue. The number of bronchial divisions is reduced significantly.

Cystic Bronchiectasis

With severe bronchiectasis, airways appear ballooned or "cystic" or "saccular," often exceeding 2 cm in diameter. The typical branching appearance of bronchi in areas of bronchiectasis may be difficult to see. The cysts often appear isolated and are not associated with other abnormal airways. Cysts may be seen in a subpleural location. The number of bronchial divisions from the carina to the periphery is markedly reduced.

Bronchography

Although traditionally considered the gold standard for diagnosing bronchiectasis, bronchography has been replaced by CT. The same findings that were considered classic indicators of bronchiectasis on bronchography still may be used in interpreting CT. These include the following:

1. Proximal or distal bronchial dilatation
2. Abnormal bronchial contours
3. Lack of normal tapering of peripheral airways
4. Reduction in the number of bronchial branches (i.e., "pruning")
5. Luminal filling defects due to mucus.

Plain Radiograph Diagnosis

Plain radiographs are abnormal in 80% to 90% of patients with bronchiectasis, although findings often are nonspecific, and the diagnosis can be suggested in only about 40% of patients. The more severe the abnormality, the easier it is to see, and the more likely it is that an accurate diagnosis will be made.

Tram tracks, parallel line shadows representing thickened bronchial walls, are a common finding in bronchiectasis (see Fig. 23-1). They may be the only finding visible in patients with cylindrical bronchiectasis. However, tram tracks also may be seen with bronchial wall thickening in the absence of bronchiectasis, and thus are nonspecific. When seen in cross section, thick-walled bronchi appear as ring shadows (Fig. 23-2).

Recognizing dilatation of bronchi on plain films is more difficult, unless the dilatation is significant or obvious contour abnormalities are present (e.g., in varicose bronchiectasis). The dilated bronchi may be visible as irregular, oval, or branching tubular air-filled structures (see Fig. 23-2). When seen in cross section, a dilated bronchus may appear larger than the artery adjacent to it. This is known as the "signet-ring" sign, and indicates that bronchial dilatation

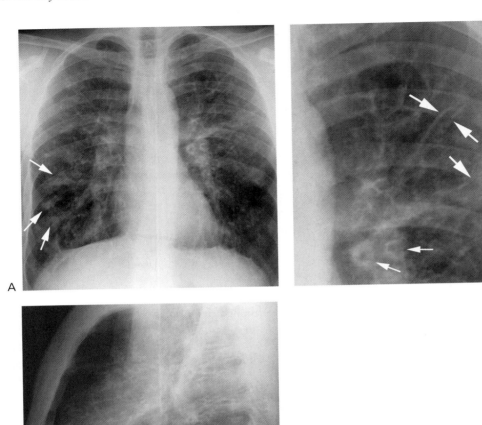

FIG. 23-2. Bronchiectasis in cystic fibrosis. **A.** Chest radiograph shows a number of examples of tramtracks and ring shadows. Mucous plugs *(arrows)* in dilated peripheral bronchi result in nodular and branching opacities. As is typical, lung volumes are large. **B.** Detail view of the left lung shows ring shadows *(small arrows)*, indicative of the signet-ring sign. Dilated bronchi shown by their thickened walls *(large arrows)* have abnormal contours. **C.** Lateral view shows tram tracks and ring shadows. The retrosternal space is increased.

is present (see Fig. 23-2B). Mucous plugs or fluid filling the bronchi sometimes is visible, and may aid in recognizing them as dilated (see Fig. 23-2). Mucous plugs within dilated bronchi may be visible as oval ("finger in glove") or branching ("hand in glove") opacities.

Cystic bronchiectasis results in multiple, air-filled, cystic lesions, which may be thick- or thin-walled, and clustered, lobar, patchy, or diffuse in distribution. Multiple air-fluid levels often are seen because of infection or retained secretions (see Fig. 9-28 in Chapter 9). Because the cysts communicate with each other through the bronchial tree, air-fluid levels tend to be at about the same height in all the affected cysts, but with less fluid present in upper lobe cysts than in lower lobe cysts (i.e., water flows downhill).

Less specific radiographic findings often seen in bronchiectasis include (1) loss of definition of vascular markings in affected lung, presumably secondary to peribronchial inflammation or fibrosis, (2) volume loss in the affected lung or lobe, (3) decreased vessel size in aerated bronchiectatic lung, (4) consolidation of abnormal lung, and (5) compensatory expansion of normal lung.

CT Diagnosis

CT using thick collimation (i.e., 10 mm) is relatively inaccurate in diagnosing bronchiectasis, with a sensitivity of only 60% to 80%. However, the use of HRCT with images spaced at 1 cm intervals or volumetric helical CT using thin collimation (3 cm or less) is very accurate in the diagnosis of bronchiectasis with sensitivity and specificity values exceeding 95%. The use of appropriate and consistent window mean and width settings (-600 to $700/1000$ to 1500

TABLE 23-2. HRCT FINDINGS IN BRONCHIECTASIS

Specific findings of bronchial dilatation
Increased bronchoarterial ratio
  Internal bronchial diameter > adjacent pulmonary artery
  "Signet-ring" sign
Lack of tapering
Contour abnormalities
  Cylindrical bronchiectasis—"tram-tracks"
  Varicose bronchiectasis—"string of pearls"
  Cystic bronchiectasis—"cluster of grapes"
Visibility of airways in peripheral 1 cm of lung

Common nonspecific findings
Bronchial wall thickening
Fluid- or mucus-filled bronchi

Ancillary findings
Volume loss
Mosaic perfusion
Air trapping
Tree-in-bud
Bronchial artery enlargement

HU) is important. Excessively low or narrow window settings exaggerate bronchial wall thickness.

Specific findings of bronchiectasis are those of bronchial dilatation (Table 23-2). Less specific signs include bronchial wall thickening and irregularity and the presence of mucoid impaction. Ancillary findings, commonly seen in bronchiectasis include volume loss, mosaic perfusion visible on inspiratory scans, focal air trapping identifiable on expiration scans, "tree-in-bud," and bronchial artery enlargement.

Bronchial Dilatation

Because bronchiectasis is defined by the presence of bronchial dilatation, recognition of increased bronchial diameter is key to the CT diagnosis of this entity. On high-resolution CT (HRCT), bronchial dilatation may be diagnosed by comparing the bronchial diameter to that of adjacent pulmonary artery branches (i.e., the bronchoarterial ratio), by detecting a lack of bronchial tapering, abnormal bronchial contours, and by identifying airways in the peripheral lung.

Increased Bronchoarterial Ratio

Bronchiectasis is generally considered to be present when the internal diameter of a bronchus is greater than the diameter of the adjacent pulmonary artery branch (i.e., the *bronchoarterial ratio* is greater than 1) when imaged in cross section. This finding not only reflects the presence of bronchial dilatation but also indicates some reduction in pulmonary artery size as a consequence of decreased lung perfusion in the affected lung regions. The association of a dilated bronchus with a much smaller adjacent pulmonary artery

branch has been termed the *signet-ring sign* (Fig. 23-3A and B). This sign is valuable in recognizing bronchiectasis, and in distinguishing it from other cystic lung lesions. It is much easier to see on HRCT than on chest radiographs.

A bronchoarterial ratio *slightly* more than 1 does not always indicate the presence of bronchiectasis, but may be seen in the absence of bronchial wall abnormalities in asthmatic patients, in patients living at high altitudes, and in a small percentage of normal patients. Thus, unless dilatation is obvious, bronchiectasis should not be diagnosed on the basis of an increased bronchoarterial ratio alone. Fortunately, bronchial wall thickening and other abnormalities typically are present in patients with true bronchiectasis.

Lack of Bronchial Tapering

Lack of bronchial tapering may be important in the diagnosis of bronchiectasis, in particular subtle cylindrical bronchiectasis. For this finding to be present, the diameter of the airway should remain unchanged for at least 2 cm distal to a branching point (see Fig. 23-3A and C). Accurate detection of this finding is difficult, however, in the absence of contiguous HRCT sections, especially for vertically or obliquely oriented airways.

Abnormal Bronchial Contours

As stated previously, bronchiectasis may be classified as cylindrical, varicose, or cystic. Recognition of one of these abnormal contours is diagnostic.

Cylindrical bronchiectasis varies in appearance on CT depending on whether the abnormal bronchi lie in the scan plane (see Fig. 23-3A and C) or perpendicular to it. When in the plane of scan, bronchi are visualized along their length and are recognizable as branching tram tracks that fail to taper.

Varicose bronchiectasis results in more irregular bronchial dilatation with a typical varicose appearance (Fig. 23-4A). The bronchial walls often are irregularly thickened. This diagnosis of varicose bronchiectasis can be made easily only when the involved bronchi course horizontally in the plane of scan. This appearance has been likened to a string of pearls. When seen in cross section, the dilated bronchi are visible as thick-walled ring shadows indistinguishable from those of cylindrical bronchiectasis.

Cystic bronchiectasis is characterized by the presence of numerous cysts (see Fig. 23-4B). In general, the dilated airways in patients with cystic bronchiectasis are thick-walled; however, the cysts may be thin-walled. A clear-cut branching appearance of the dilated airways generally is lacking, and it may be difficult to make the distinction from cystic lung disease in some cases. This appearance has been described as similar to a cluster of grapes.

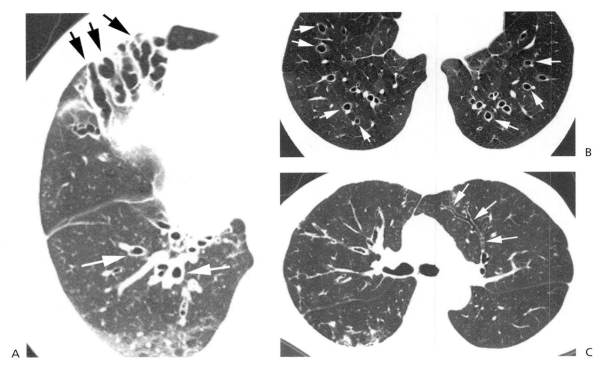

FIG. 23-3. CT findings of bronchiectasis in three patients. **A.** CT shows several examples of the signet-ring sign in the lower lobe *(white arrows)*. Anteriorly, bronchi are seen in the peripheral 1 cm of lung, do not taper, and have a cylindrical appearance *(black arrows)*. Bronchial wall thickening also is visible. **B.** Numerous examples of the signet-ring sign *(arrows)* are visible. Note that the bronchus appears much larger than the adjacent artery. **C.** Cylindrical bronchiectasis with lack of bronchial tapering *(arrows)*. Numerous thick-walled and dilated bronchi are visible, along with mucous plugging in the posterior right lower lobe.

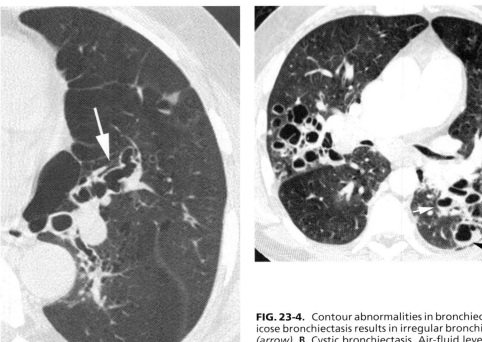

FIG. 23-4. Contour abnormalities in bronchiectasis. **A.** Varicose bronchiectasis results in irregular bronchial dilatation *(arrow)*. **B.** Cystic bronchiectasis. Air-fluid levels are visible within the abnormal bronchi *(arrows)*. The dilated bronchi are visible in the lung periphery.

Visibility of Peripheral Airways

In normal subjects, airways in the peripheral 2 cm of lung are seen uncommonly because their walls are too thin. Peribronchial fibrosis and bronchial wall thickening in patients with bronchiectasis, in combination with dilatation of the bronchial lumen, allow the visualization of small airways in the lung periphery. Bronchi visible within 1 cm of the costal pleural surfaces indicate bronchiectasis (see Figs. 23-3A and 23-4B), but bronchi may be seen within 1 cm of the mediastinal pleural surfaces in normal subjects.

Bronchial Wall Thickening

Although bronchial wall thickening is a nonspecific finding, it usually is present in patients with bronchiectasis (see Fig. 23-3A and C). Identification of bronchial wall thickening is largely subjective. However, because bronchiectasis and bronchial wall thickening often are multifocal rather than diffuse and uniform, a comparison of one lung region to another can be helpful in making this diagnosis. It must be emphasized that using consistent window settings is very important in the diagnosis of bronchial wall thickening; bronchial walls can vary significantly in apparent thickness with different CT window settings.

Mucous Impaction and Air-Fluid Levels

The presence of mucus- or fluid-filled bronchi is nonspecific, but may be helpful in confirming a diagnosis of bronchiectasis (Fig. 23-5). The HRCT appearance of fluid- or mucus-filled airways is dependent on both their size and orientation relative to the scan plane. Larger, mucus-filled airways result in abnormal lobular or branching structures when they lie in the same plane as the CT scan. In cross section, impacted bronchi appear similar to vessels, but on contrast-enhanced scans they may be seen to be low in attenuation.

Patients with cystic bronchiectasis may show fluid levels within the abnormal bronchi (see Fig. 23-4B), due to retained secretions and chronic infection. Air-fluid levels within multiple cystic spaces are typical, and since they tend to communicate with each other through the bronchi, the air-fluid levels appear similar in height.

Mosaic Perfusion and Air Trapping

Many patients with bronchiectasis also show pathologic findings of small airway disease, either bronchiolitis obliterans or infectious bronchiolitis. Consequently, HRCT findings of small airways disease, such as mosaic perfusion (on inspiratory scans) and focal air-trapping (on expiratory scans) are often seen in patients with bronchiectasis.

Tree-in-Bud

The term *tree-in-bud* refers to the presence of nodular and Y-shaped branching structures which resemble a budding tree, in the lung periphery (Fig. 23-6; see also Fig. 10-28 in Chapter 10). This appearance reflects the presence of dilated, mucus- or pus-filled centrilobular bronchioles (the trunk and branches) associated with small nodular areas of bronchiolar dilatation or peribronchiolar inflammation (the buds) at the tips of the branches. This finding is common in patients with airway infection, and, therefore, is common in patients with various causes of bronchiectasis.

Bronchial Artery Enlargement

Enlarged bronchial arteries can be identified pathologically in most cases of bronchiectasis. This condition may result

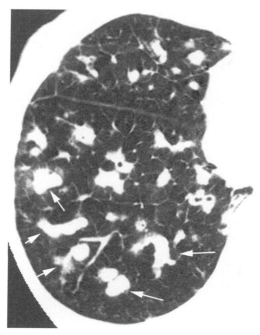

FIG. 23-5. Extensive mucous plugging in bronchiectasis. Numerous dilated, opacified bronchi are visible *(arrows)*, both along their axis and in cross section.

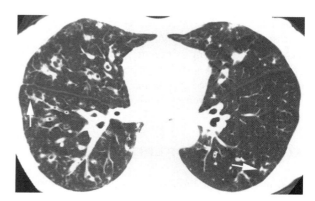

FIG. 23-6. Tree-in-bud in bronchiectasis. Dilated thick-walled bronchi are visible, with areas of mucous plugging. Tree-in-bud is visible in the lung periphery *(arrows)*.

in massive and life-threatening hemoptysis. With multi-detector CT using thin collimation and contrast infusion, abnormally enlarged bronchial arteries may be identified; bronchial arteriograms also may be used for diagnosis in patients with hemoptysis. Bronchial artery embolization may be curative in patients with hemoptysis due to bronchiectasis.

Severity of Bronchiectasis

Systems for grading the severity of bronchiectasis using CT have been developed but are not in common clinical use. However, the severity of bronchiectasis may be related to the diameter of the abnormal bronchi. Also, there is a significant correlation between the extent of bronchiectasis and the forced expiratory volume in 1 sec (FEV_1) and the forced vital capacity (FVC). Furthermore, patients with cystic bronchiectasis are more likely to have infection and purulent sputum than are patients with either cylindrical or varicose bronchiectasis.

Pitfalls in the Diagnosis of Bronchiectasis

Several potential pitfalls in the diagnosis of bronchiectasis should be avoided.

Artifacts due to cardiac or respiratory motion may cause ghosting that can very closely mimic the appearance of tram tracks. Observing other artifacts related to motion helps in identifying them appropriately.

Bronchiectasis is difficult to diagnose with certainty in patients with atelectasis. Normal bronchi dilate in the presence of atelectasis because the collapsed lung results in increased tension on the bronchial wall. Bronchi return to normal size when the collapse resolves. This phenomenon is known as "reversible bronchiectasis" (see Fig. 2-24 in Chapter 2); this term is an oxymoron, since part of the definition of bronchiectasis is that it is irreversible.

Consolidation may obscure vascular anatomy making assessment of bronchoarterial ratios difficult or impossible.

Bronchiectasis may occur in association with fibrotic lung diseases (i.e., "traction" bronchiectasis). Traction bronchiectasis does not represent primary airways disease and is not associated with symptoms of chronic infection. The typical corkscrewed appearance of traction bronchiectasis and its association with obvious fibrosis are diagnostic.

SPECIFIC CAUSES OF BRONCHIECTASIS

In most instances, the radiographic appearance of bronchiectasis is nonspecific, and does not allow a determination of its cause. However, a few diseases, discussed in the following sections, require special attention.

Cystic Fibrosis

Cystic fibrosis (CF) is the most common cause of pulmonary insufficiency in the first three decades of life. It results from an autosomal recessive genetic defect in the structure of the CF transmembrane conductance regulator (CFTR), which leads to abnormal chloride transport across epithelial membranes (Table 23-3). The mechanisms by which this leads to lung disease are not entirely understood, but an abnormally low water content of airway mucus is at least partially responsible, resulting in decreased mucus clearance, mucous plugging of airways, and an increased incidence of bacterial airway infection. Bronchial wall inflammation progressing to secondary bronchiectasis is universal in patients with long-standing disease.

Although a single defect in CFTR is responsible for most cases, more than 100 genetic abnormalities may be associated with CF. These CF genotype variants often cause less severe disease and thus are more likely to be found in adults who first present with symptoms of CF. Individuals who are carriers of the CF gene may have a selective advantage; they appear to be more resistant to typhoid fever than the general population.

TABLE 23-3. CYSTIC FIBROSIS

Autosomal-recessive genetic defect in cystic fibrosis transmembrane conductance regulator
Abnormal chloride transport resulting in abnormal mucus
Bronchiectasis and infection universal
   Pseudomonas (90%)
   Aspergillus (50%)
   Mycobacteria (20%)
Radiographic findings
Increased lung volumes
Small nodular opacities due to impaction of small airways
Bronchial wall thickening or bronchiectasis
Mucoid impaction
Right upper lobe predominance
Atelectasis
Cysts (bronchiectasis, abscess cavities, bullae)
Pneumomediastinum or pneumothorax
Hilar enlargement
HRCT findings
Bronchiectasis
   Central bronchi and upper lobes involved in all cases
   Typically severe (varicose and cystic) and widespread
Bronchial wall thickening
   Central and upper lobe distribution
   Right upper lobe first involved
Mucous plugging
Tree-in-bud
Large lung volumes
Atelectasis
Mosaic perfusion
Air trapping on expiration

Clinical Presentation

Pulmonary abnormalities may be present within weeks of birth, with the earliest abnormalities being retention of mucus in small peripheral airways, mucous gland hyperplasia, and inflammation. The presence of airway infection is fundamental to the development of CF; the first organisms involved are *S. aureus, H. influenzae,* and mucoid *Pseudomonas* species. In adults with CF, *Pseudomonas aeruginosa* predominates (90% of cases), although *Aspergillus* (up to 50% of cases) species and mycobacteria (up to 20% of cases) also may be present. Bronchial wall damage and bronchiectasis occur largely as a result of infection.

Clinical findings of chronic and recurrent infection in a child, associated with abnormal sweat chlorides, usually are diagnostic. Hemoptysis occurs in more than half of cases because of bronchial artery hypertrophy.

Radiographic Findings

Typical radiographic findings (see Figs. 23-2 and 23-7) can help confirm the diagnosis in patients with symptoms or may be suggestive in patients with an atypical presentation (e.g., young adults with CF variants).

Early in the course of disease, plain films are normal. Initial abnormalities include the following:

1. Increased lung volumes due to obstruction of small airways (i.e., increased retrosternal space, flattening of the hemidiaphragms)

2. Impaction of small airways, resulting in small nodular or reticular opacities in the lung periphery
3. Accentuated linear opacities in the central or upper lung regions due to bronchial wall thickening or bronchiectasis.

The earliest abnormalities in patients with CF are in the right upper lobe. Consequently, early findings may include right upper lobe atelectasis or thickening of the wall of the right upper lobe bronchus, best seen on the lateral radiograph.

In older children and adults, bronchiectasis is typical, often involving bronchi in the central lung regions, i.e., *central bronchiectasis.* Dilated bronchi may be cylindrical, varicose, or cystic, depending on the duration and severity of disease. In adult patients and patients with chronic disease, additional abnormalities can include the following:

1. Mucoid impaction
2. Cysts in the upper lobes, representing cystic bronchiectasis, healed abscess cavities, or bullae
3. Atelectasis
4. Pneumothorax (up to 20% of cases)
5. Hilar enlargement due to lymphadenopathy or pulmonary hypertension
6. Pleural thickening (although pleural effusion is uncommon).

In most patients with an established diagnosis of CF, clinical findings and chest radiographs are sufficient for clinical management. A significant exacerbation of symptoms may occur with little visible radiographic change.

HRCT Findings

HRCT can demonstrate morphologic abnormalities in patients with early CF who are asymptomatic, have normal pulmonary function, or have normal chest radiographs. In patients with more advanced disease, HRCT also can show abnormalities not visible on chest radiographs, including bronchiectasis and mucous plugging.

On CT and HRCT, bronchiectasis is seen in all patients with advanced CF (Figs. 23-8 and 23-9). Proximal or parahilar bronchi always are involved when bronchiectasis is present, and bronchiectasis is limited to these central bronchi (i.e., *central bronchiectasis*) in about one third of cases. Typically, all lobes are involved, although early in the disease abnormalities often are predominantly found in the upper lobe, and a predominance in the right upper lobe may be seen in some patients. The differential diagnosis of central bronchiectasis also includes allergic bronchopulmonary aspergillosis, tuberculosis, radiation fibrosis, Mounier-Kuhn syndrome (tracheobronchomegaly), and Williams-Campbell syndrome.

Cylindrical bronchiectasis is most common (95%) on HRCT; varicose and cystic bronchiectasis are visible in as

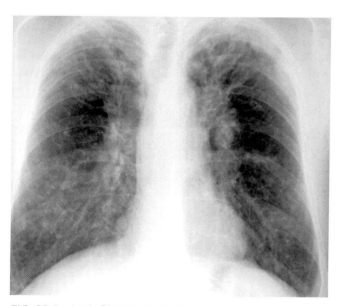

FIG. 23-7. Cystic fibrosis. PA chest radiograph shows increased lung volumes with flattening of the hemidiaphragms. The hilar are enlarged and elevated because of upper lobe volume loss. Bronchiectasis and mucous plugging are visible in the upper lobes.

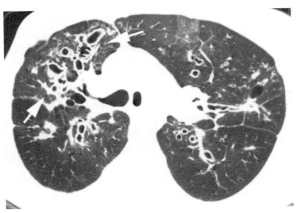

FIG. 23-8. HRCT findings in cystic fibrosis. Parahilar *(central)* bronchiectasis is present *(arrows)*, with a predominance in the right upper lobe. Patchy areas of lucency reflect mosaic perfusion. Some right upper lobe volume loss is apparent.

many as one third of cases. *Cystic lesions* representing cystic bronchiectasis, abscess cavities, or bullae are visible in half of patients and typically predominate in the subpleural regions of the upper lobes.

Bronchial wall or peribronchial interstitial thickening also is commonly present in patients with CF. It usually is more evident than bronchial dilatation in patients who have early disease, and may be seen independent of bronchiectasis. Thickening of the wall of the proximal right upper lobe bronchi often is the earliest abnormal feature visible on HRCT.

Mucous plugging is visible in one quarter to one half of cases, and may be visible in all lobes. Volume loss, collapse, or consolidation can be seen in as many as 80% of patients.

Tree-in-bud (i.e., bronchiolar dilatation with associated infection or mucus impaction) often is visible and can be an early sign of disease in children.

Focal areas of decreased lung opacity, representing *air trapping* or *mosaic perfusion* are common (see Figs. 23-8 and 23-9). These may appear to surround dilated, thick-walled, or mucus-plugged bronchi. Air trapping often is seen on expiratory scans.

Lung volumes may appear increased on CT, although this diagnosis is rather subjective and may be better assessed on chest radiographs.

Hilar or mediastinal lymph node enlargement and pleural thickening also can be seen, largely due to chronic infection. Pulmonary artery dilatation resulting from pulmonary hypertension also can be seen in patients with long-standing disease.

Allergic Bronchopulmonary Aspergillosis

Allergic bronchopulmonary aspergillosis (ABPA) reflects a hypersensitivity reaction to *Aspergillus* organisms and characteristically is associated with eosinophilia, symptoms of asthma such as wheezing, and findings of "central" or "proximal" bronchiectasis, usually with mucoid impaction, atelectasis, and consolidation similar to that seen in patients with eosinophilic pneumonia (Table 23-4). ABPA typically occurs in young adults with a history of asthma or atopy, and in 2% to 10% of patients with CF. Asthma may be present for many years before the diagnosis of ABPA.

ABPA results from both type I (IgE-mediated hypersensitivity) and type III (IgG-mediated antigen-antibody complex reaction) immunologic responses to the endobronchial growth of fungal (e.g., *Aspergillus*) species.

The type I response results in immediate wheezing when the patient is exposed to *Aspergillus* antigens.

The type III reaction results in bronchial inflammation in response to fungi in the airway, which eventually produces bronchiectasis. Bronchiectasis usually is varicose or cystic in appearance, central in location (i.e., central bron-

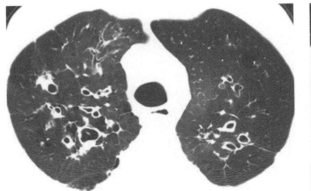
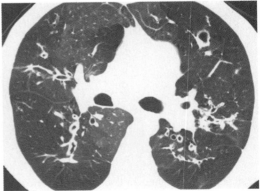

FIG. 23-9. HRCT findings in cystic fibrosis. Central *(parahilar)* bronchiectasis and bronchial wall thickening are present. Mosaic perfusion results in patchy lung opacity with decreased vessel size in the lung periphery.

TABLE 23-4. ALLERGIC BRONCHOPULMONARY ASPERGILLOSIS

Hypersensitivity reaction to *Aspergillus*
History of asthma or atopy, cystic fibrosis
Type I (IgE-mediated) hypersensitivity results in wheezing
Type III (IgG-mediated antigen-antibody complex) reaction results in bronchiectasis
Radiographic findings
Consolidation (i.e., eosinophilic pneumonia)
Central bronchiectasis, upper lobe or widespread
Mucous plugging ("finger in glove")
Increased lung volume
Upper lobe volume loss or scarring
HRCT findings
Central bronchiectasis, widespread
Upper lobe predominance common
Mucous plugging; mucus plugs appear high-density
Tree-in-bud
Atelectasis
Peripheral consolidation or diffuse ground-glass opacity
Mosaic perfusion
Air trapping on expiration

chiectasis), and associated with formation of mucous plugs that contain fungus and inflammatory cells.

Clinical Presentation

The acronym APE TRICS may serve as an aid for remembering the primary criteria for ABPA: which include *A* for asthma; *P* for precipitating antibodies to *A. fumigatus*; *E* for eosinophilia; *T* for positive skin test for *A. fumigatus; R* for radiologic evidence of pulmonary disease; *I* for elevated IgE; *C* for central bronchiectasis; and *S* for elevated *A. fumigatus* serum-specific IgE and IgG. A diagnosis of ABPA is nearly certain when six of these eight criteria are fulfilled. Secondary criteria include the presence of *A. fumigatus* in sputum, a history of expectoration of mucous plugs, and delayed cutaneous reactivity to *Aspergillus* antigen.

Symptoms are similar to those of asthma, including wheezing, cough, and dyspnea. Occasionally, fever, hemoptysis, and chest pain may be associated. Expectoration of mucous plugs containing fungus may occur.

ABPA typically is characterized by repeated exacerbations. Disease progression may be divided into five phases, although these are not invariable: (1) acute presentation; (2) resolution with clearing of pulmonary abnormalities and decline in serum IgE; (3) recurrence; (4) development of dependence on corticosteroids; leading in some cases to (5) pulmonary fibrosis.

Radiographic Findings

Patients presenting with an acute exacerbation of ABPA often show consolidation on chest radiographs. Some con-solidations are patchy, resembling eosinophilic pneumonia. These may be peripheral or parahilar, surrounding abnormal bronchi. Segmental or lobar consolidations may reflect bronchial obstruction by mucus and atelectasis.

Bronchiectasis also is commonly visible with acute or recurrent disease (Figs. 23-10 and 23-11). The abnormal bronchi often are lobar or segmental and, thus, central in location. They may have an oval or branching appearance or may appear round if seen in cross section. Mucous plugs may be seen within the bronchi, outlined by air, or may fill the bronchi, resulting in a finger in glove or hand in glove appearance (see Fig. 23-10). The presence of a dilated, thick-walled bronchus sometimes is termed a *bronchocele*, whereas a bronchocele containing a mucous plug may be referred to a *mucocele*. These tend to have an upper lobe predominance in patients with ABPA. Lung distal to a mucous plug may be collapsed or may be aerated due to collateral ventilation. Aerated lung may appear hyperlucent and hypovascular due to air trapping. Lung volume may be increased because of asthma.

The radiographic findings in ABPA (e.g., central bronchiectasis with an upper lobe predominance (see Figs. 23-10 and 23-11), mucous plugging, consolidation, large lung volumes) may mimic those of CF. In the later stages of disease, upper lobe scarring and volume loss may mimic prior tuberculosis.

CT Findings

HRCT is more sensitive than are plain radiographs in detecting airway abnormalities associated with ABPA. HRCT findings include central bronchiectasis (present in 85% of lobes), usually varicose or cylindrical (see Fig. 23-11B); bronchial occlusion due to mucous plugging (see Figs. 23-10C and D, and 23-11B–D); and bronchial wall thickening. An upper lobe predominance for these abnormalities is common but not invariable. Ectatic airways sometimes may contain an air-fluid level or an aspergilloma.

In about 25% of cases, mucous plugs in ABPA are greater in attenuation than soft tissue (see Figs. 23-10E and 23-11D); these plugs may be quite dense, measuring more than 100 HU. This finding is strongly suggestive of ABPA, and is thought to be due to concentration of calcium oxalate by the fungus. Dense mucous plugs also may be seen with bronchial atresia (see Chapter 1).

A tree-in-bud appearance resulting from mucus filling the bronchioles may be seen, but in most patients with ABPA, the peripheral airways appear normal.

Parenchymal abnormalities including consolidation, collapse, cavitation, and bullae may be identified in as many as 40% of cases, particularly in the upper lobes. Mass-like foci of eosinophilic pneumonia may be seen with acute

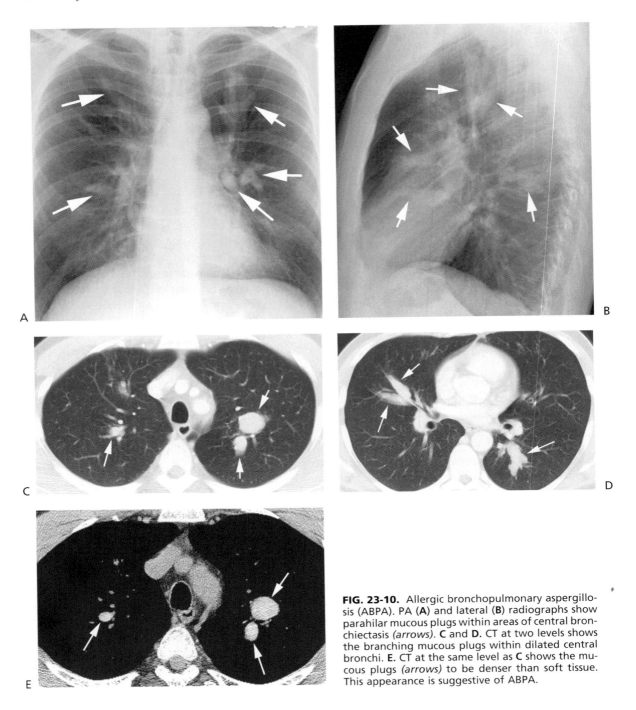

FIG. 23-10. Allergic bronchopulmonary aspergillosis (ABPA). PA (**A**) and lateral (**B**) radiographs show parahilar mucous plugs within areas of central bronchiectasis *(arrows)*. **C** and **D**. CT at two levels shows the branching mucous plugs within dilated central bronchi. **E.** CT at the same level as **C** shows the mucous plugs *(arrows)* to be denser than soft tissue. This appearance is suggestive of ABPA.

exacerbation. Mosaic perfusion and air trapping may be seen.

Asthma

Asthma is characterized by airway inflammation, which is largely reversible (Table 23-5). Pathologically, patients with asthma show bronchial and bronchiolar wall thicken-ing caused by inflammation, infiltration by eosinophils, smooth muscle hyperplasia, and edema, and excess mucus production, which can result in mucous plugging. Bronchiectasis may be seen in some patients with long-standing asthma.

Pulmonary function tests show findings of airway obstruction (e.g., increased airway resistance, increased total lung volume, increased residual volume, and decreased

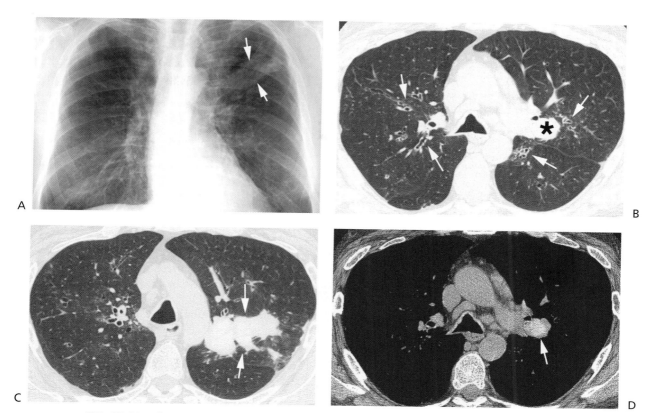

FIG. 23-11. Allergic bronchopulmonary aspergillosis. **A.** PA radiographs show a mucous plug in the central left upper lobe *(arrows)*. **B.** HRCT shows multiple areas of central bronchiectasis and bronchial wall thickening *(arrows)* and a large central mucous plug *(*)*. **C.** HRCT slightly above **B** shows the branching mucous plug *(arrows)*. **D.** CT at the same level as **B** shows the mucous plug *(arrow)* to be denser than soft tissue.

forced vital capacity) during an asthma episode, but typically return to normal between attacks.

Radiographic Findings

Radiographic findings associated with asthma usually are subtle. They include increased lung volume (30% to 40%), increased lung lucency, mild bronchial wall thickening (50%), and mild prominence of hilar vasculature due to transient pulmonary hypertension (10%). Bronchiectasis is not usually recognized, but small mucous plugs sometimes can be seen. Associated complications of asthma, although uncommon, include pneumonia, atelectasis, pneumomediastinum, and pneumothorax. Pneumomediastinum is more common than pneumothorax. Radiographic abnormalities generally are more common and more severe in children with asthma.

Plain radiographs are not commonly used to make a diagnosis of asthma; radiographs often are normal, and visible abnormalities in this disease usually are nonspecific. Radiography also has limited usefulness in patients with an established diagnosis of asthma who suffer an acute attack. Corre-

---

TABLE 23-5. ASTHMA

Reversible airway inflammation and obstruction
Radiographic findings subtle
  Increased lung volume (30%–40%)
  Increased lucency
  Mild bronchial wall thickening (50%)
  Mild hilar prominence
Radiographs most useful in diagnosing complications
  Pneumonia
  Atelectasis
  Pneumomediastinum and pneumothorax
HRCT used to diagnose complications, allergic bronchopulmonary aspergillosis, or emphysema
  Mild bronchial wall thickening or dilatation
  Mucous plugs or tree-in-bud (20%)
  Mosaic perfusion (20%–30%)
  Air trapping on expiration (50%)

lation between the severity of radiographic findings and the severity and reversibility of an asthma attack usually is poor, and radiographs provide significant information that alters treatment in 5% or less of patients with acute asthma. Although it is difficult to generalize regarding the role of radiographs in adults and children with acute asthma, chest films often are used to exclude the presence of associated pneumonia or other complications when significant symptoms or appropriate clinical or laboratory findings are suggestive.

HRCT Findings

CT is not commonly indicated in the routine assessment of patients with asthma, but it sometimes is used when complications, particularly allergic bronchopulmonary aspergillosis (ABPA), are suspected, or in diagnosing emphysema in smokers with asthma.

HRCT shows mild bronchial wall thickening or dilatation of small bronchi (diagnosed by a bronchoarterial ratio slightly greater than 1) in about half of patients with uncomplicated asthma.

Mucoid impaction and tree-in-bud have been reported in as many as 20% of cases, and typically clear following treatment.

Mosaic perfusion or diffuse hyperlucency have been observed on inspiratory scans in 20% to 30% of cases. Expiratory CT can show evidence of patchy air trapping in as many as 50% of asthmatic patients.

Although asthma and ABPA can result in similar abnormalities, patients with ABPA have a higher frequency of bronchiectasis (95%, vs. 30% for asthma), a higher incidence of mucoid impaction, and more severe and extensive abnormalities.

Mycobacterium Avium-Intracellulare Complex Infection

Bronchiectasis in association with lung nodules is characteristic of nontuberculous mycobacterial infection resulting from *Mycobacterium avium-intracellulare* complex (MAC), and is described in detail in Chapter 12. It typically is seen in women older than 60 years.

Dyskinetic Cilia Syndrome and Kartagener's Syndrome

Dyskinetic cilia syndrome (DCS) is characterized by abnormal ciliary structure and movement, resulting in abnormal mucociliary clearance and chronic infection (Table 23-6). Bronchiectasis and sinusitis are common manifestations. About half of patients with DCS also have situs inversus.

TABLE 23-6. DYSKINETIC CILIA SYNDROME AND KARTAGENER'S SYNDROME
Autosomal-recessive defect
Abnormal ciliary structure and movement
Abnormal mucociliary clearance
50% have situs inversus: Kartagener's syndrome
Sinusitis common
Bilateral bronchiectasis, typically lower or middle lobe

The combination of bronchiectasis, sinusitis, and situs inversus is called *Kartagener's syndrome* (see Fig. 23-1).

DCS is an autosomal recessive genetic abnormality with an incidence of about 1 in 20,000 births. Men and women are equally affected. A variety of ultrastructural abnormalities of ciliary microtubules have been reported in association with this syndrome, although in some cases, the cilia appear normal. In men, the syndrome may be associated with immotile spermatozoa and infertility; in women, fertility is not affected. Other congenital abnormalities also may be present. In patients with chronic infections and situs inversus, the diagnosis is not difficult. In the absence of situs inversus, criteria for attributing chronic infection to DCS may include immotile spermatozoa (in men), a family history of DCS, or abnormal cilia on biopsy.

Symptoms of recurrent bronchitis, pneumonia, and sinusitis often date from childhood. Radiographs and CT typically show bilateral bronchiectasis with a basal (lower or middle lobe) predominance. Cylindrical bronchiectasis is most common. Appropriate antibiotic treatment is associated with a normal life expectancy.

Young's Syndrome

Young's syndrome, also referred to as *obstructive azoospermia*, is characterized by male infertility caused by obstruction of the epididymis, bronchiectasis, and sinusitis. It may resemble dyskinetic cilia syndrome clinically, but ciliary abnormalities are absent. The cause is unknown. The radiographic appearance of the bronchiectasis is nonspecific.

Syndrome of Yellow Nails and Lymphedema

The syndrome of yellow nails and lymphedema is characterized by (1) slowly growing nails that are thickened, curved, and yellow-green in color; (2) lymphedema, usually of the lower extremities, due to lymphatic hypoplasia; and (3) exudative pleural effusions associated with pleural lymphatic

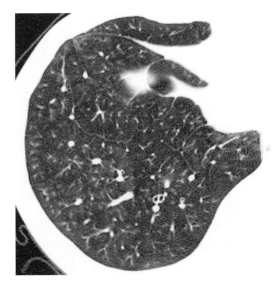

FIG. 23-12. Syndrome of yellow nails. HRCT shows tree-in-bud in the right lower lobe, as a manifestation of airway infection.

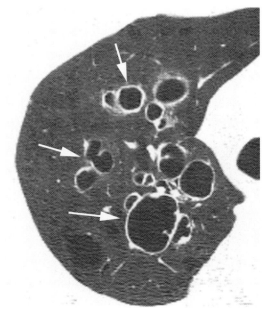

FIG. 23-13. Williams-Campbell syndrome with cystic bronchiectasis. Marked cystic bronchiectasis *(arrows)* is visible in the central lung regions.

dilatation. It is not necessary for all three manifestations to be present; pleural effusion is least common. Chronic sinusitis, airway infection, and bronchiectasis are present in about half of patients (Fig. 23-12). The syndrome typically presents in adulthood.

Tracheobronchomegaly (Mounier-Kuhn Syndrome)

Tracheobronchomegaly, also referred to as *Mounier-Kuhn syndrome,* is characterized by marked dilatation of the trachea and mainstem bronchi, recurrent lower respiratory tract infections, and bronchiectasis (see Fig. 22-21 in Chapter 22). It is most often diagnosed in men in their third and fourth decades; it is much less common in women. The finding of central bronchiectasis associated with dilatation of the trachea is diagnostic. It is described in detail in Chapter 22.

Williams-Campbell Syndrome

Williams-Campbell syndrome is a rare type of congenital cystic bronchiectasis due to defective cartilage in the fourth- to sixth-order (central) bronchi. Radiographs and HRCT may show areas of central cystic bronchiectasis with distal regions of abnormal lucency, probably related to air trapping or bronchiolitis (Fig. 23-13). Ballooning of the central bronchi on inspiration and collapse on expiration may occur. These findings are useful in differentiating Williams-Campbell syndrome from other causes of cystic bronchiectasis.

Alpha-1-Antitrypsin Deficiency

In addition to emphysema, bronchiectasis often (40%) is present in patients with alpha-1-antitrypsin deficiency. This correlates well with the fact that approximately 50% of patients with this deficiency manifest symptoms of airway disease—in particular, chronic sputum production. It is likely that bronchiectasis results from a proteinase-antiproteinase imbalance (also responsible for the emphysema), discussed in Chapter 24.

Bronchiectasis Associated With Systemic Diseases

Bronchiectasis may be an important finding in a number of systemic diseases. Of particular interest is the association between bronchiectasis and collagen-vascular disease and inflammatory bowel disease.

Collagen-vascular Disease

Rheumatoid arthritis (RA) may be associated with a variety of parenchymal abnormalities, including pulmonary fibrosis, organizing pneumonia (OP/BOOP), respiratory tract infections, and necrobiotic nodules. Airway disease, including both bronchiectasis and bronchiolectasis, may also occur in association with RA (see Fig. 14-7 in Chapter 14). One hypothesis suggests that chronic bacterial infections may trigger an immune reaction in genetically predisposed individuals leading to RA; bronchiectasis may precede RA by years. It has also been suggested that steroids or immunosuppressive therapy may lead to an increased incidence of respiratory infections.

On HRCT, bronchiectasis is seen in up to 35% of patients with this disease, even when chest radiographs are normal. Other findings include mosaic perfusion on inspiratory scans (20%) and air-trapping on expiratory scans in (30%). Bronchiectasis may be identified in up to 20% of patients with systemic lupus erythematosus (SLE). A similarly high prevalence of airway pathology has also been noted in patients with primary Sjögren's syndrome.

Ulcerative Colitis and Inflammatory Bowel Disease

A wide range of airway abnormalities has been identified in patients with ulcerative colitis. In addition to OP/BOOP and diffuse interstitial lung disease, these include subglottic tracheal stenosis, chronic bronchitis, and chronic suppurative inflammation of both large and small airways (Fig. 23-14). Similar to what is seen in patients with RA, chronic suppurative airway disease may precede, coexist with, or follow the development of inflammatory bowel disease. Unlike other causes of bronchiectasis, chronic suppurative airway disease associated with ulcerative colitis often responds to treatment with inhaled steroids. Bronchiectasis also is associated with Crohn's disease.

Airway Disease Related to HIV and AIDS

An accelerated form of bronchiectasis may occur in patients with human immunodeficiency virus (HIV) infection and patients with the acquired immunodeficiency syndrome (AIDS). It is likely that bronchiectasis results from recurrent or chronic bacterial airway infection. A wide range of organisms may affect the airways in patients with AIDS, most commonly *H. influenzae, P. aeruginosa, Streptococcus viridans, S. pneumoniae,* mycobacteria, and fungi such as *Aspergillus* organisms.

HRCT findings include bronchial wall thickening, bronchiectasis, bronchial or bronchiolar impaction with tree-in-bud, consolidation, and air trapping (Fig. 23-15). A lower lobe predominance is typical, and both lower lobes usually are involved.

About 10% of all reported cases of aspergillosis in AIDS patients will affect the airways. *Aspergillus* infection typically occurs late in the course of HIV infection and usually is associated with corticosteroid use and granulocytopenia. There are several distinct types of airway aspergillosis, including necrotizing tracheobronchitis, airway invasive aspergillosis, and obstructing bronchopulmonary aspergillosis.

Necrotizing tracheobronchitis and airway invasive aspergillosis are discussed in Chapter 12.

Obstructing bronchopulmonary aspergillosis typically presents with acute fever, dyspnea, and cough associated with the expectoration of fungal casts. It is characterized on

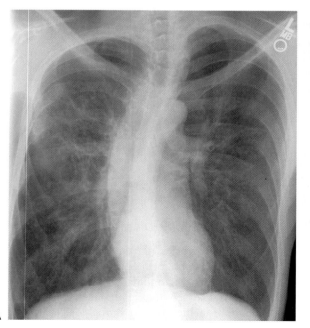
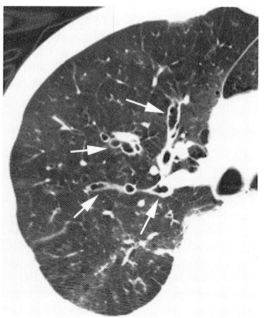

FIG. 23-14. Bronchiectasis in Crohn's disease. **A.** Chest radiograph shows large lung volumes and evidence of bronchial wall thickening, particularly in the upper lobes. **B.** HRCT shows bronchiectasis and bronchial wall thickening *(arrows)*.

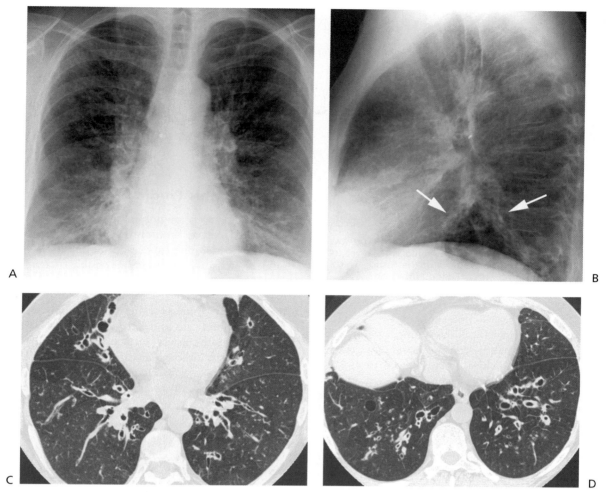

FIG. 23-15. AIDS-related airway disease. **A.** PA chest radiograph shows increased opacities at the lung bases. **B.** Lateral radiograph shows evidence of bronchial wall thickening *(arrows)*. **C** and **D.** HRCT through the lung bases shows evidence of bronchiectasis and bronchial wall thickening typical of AIDS-related airway disease.

CT by the presence of mucoid impaction, typically involving the lower lobe airways. It has been suggested that this form of disease is unique to patients with AIDS.

CT Differentiation of Causes of Bronchiectasis

The reliability of radiographs and CT for distinguishing between different causes of bronchiectasis is limited. However, several general rules apply:

1. Lower lobe bronchiectasis is most typical of childhood infections and syndromes associated with impaired mucociliary clearance (see Figs. 23-12 and 23-16).
2. Bilateral upper lobe bronchiectasis is seen most commonly in patients with CF and ABPA (see Figs. 23-8 to 23-11).

3. Unilateral upper lobe bronchiectasis is most common in patients with tuberculosis (Fig. 23-17).
4. Central bronchiectasis is more common in patients with ABPA and CF (see Figs. 23-8 to 23-11).
5. Severe and extensive bronchiectasis is most common in patients with ABPA and CF (see Figs. 23-8 to 23-11).

CHRONIC BRONCHITIS

Chronic bronchitis is a poorly characterized condition, which, for lack of a better definition, is considered to be present if the patient has chronic sputum production (productive cough on most days of more than 3 months during 2 successive years) that is not caused by a specific disease such as bronchiectasis or tuberculosis.

Morphologic abnormalities in patients with chronic

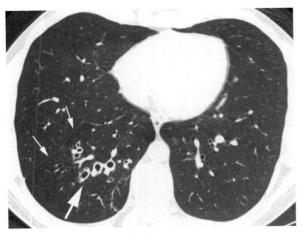

FIG. 23-16. Unilateral lower lobe bronchiectasis. Right lower lobe bronchiectasis *(large arrow)* is associated with lower lobe volume loss and posterior displacement of the fissure. This appearance is most consistent with childhood infection.

bronchitis include bronchial wall thickening, smooth muscle hyperplasia, inflammation, mucous gland enlargement, and bronchiolar abnormalities, often referred to as *small airway disease* or *chronic bronchiolitis.* However, specific pathologic criteria for diagnosing chronic bronchitis have proved elusive, and this entity is best thought of as a clinical syndrome without clear-cut anatomic correlates. Chronic bronchitis is largely related to smoking, air pollution, and infection. There is an increased risk in men and in older patients.

Chronic bronchitis does not necessarily result in pulmonary function findings of airflow obstruction. However, because of its common association with chronic bronchiolitis and emphysema, obstructive disease often is present. The occurrence of functional airway obstruction in patients with some combination of chronic bronchitis, chronic bronchiolitis, and emphysema is termed *chronic obstructive pulmonary disease* (COPD). In some patients with chronic bronchitis and COPD, progressive airway obstruction with hypoxemia leads to pulmonary hypertension and cor pulmonale.

Radiographic Findings

Chest radiographs are normal in 40% to 50% of patients considered to have chronic bronchitis. Plain film abnormalities usually are quite subtle and nonspecific, consisting of mild bronchial wall thickening, visible as tram tracks or ring shadows, and an overall increase in nonspecific lung markings, sometimes referred to as the "dirty chest." Findings of increased lung volume or hyperlucency usually, but not always, indicate associated emphysema. The presence of "saber-sheath trachea" on a chest radiograph may suggest this diagnosis, although it can be seen with other causes of chronic airway obstruction. Central pulmonary artery enlargement indicative of cor pulmonale may be seen.

CT Findings

On HRCT, findings of emphysema often predominate in patients with symptoms of chronic bronchitis. Some bron-

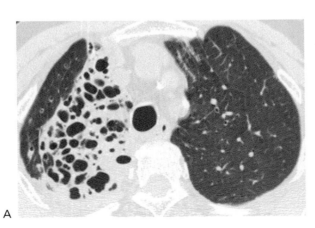

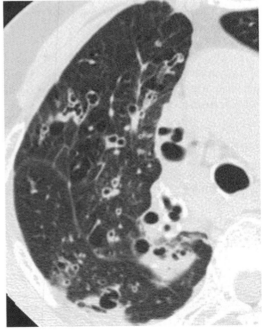

FIG. 23-17. Unilateral upper lobe bronchiectasis in TB. **A.** Right upper lobe bronchiectasis associated with right upper lobe atelectasis is visible on HRCT. The left upper lobe appears normal. **B.** At a lower level, bronchial wall thickening and bronchiectasis are visible.

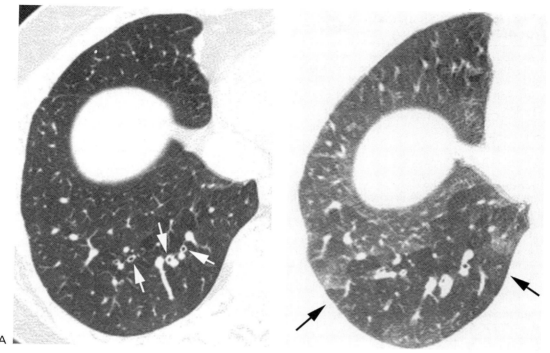

FIG. 23-18. HRCT in a patient with symptoms of chronic bronchitis. **A.** Inspiratory scan shows airway wall thickening *(arrows)* in the lower lobe, without evidence of bronchiectasis (i.e., bronchial dilatation). **B.** Expiratory scan shows air trapping *(arrows)* in this region.

chial wall thickening or centrilobular small airway abnormalities, such as tree-in-bud may be visible on HRCT in patients with clinical findings associated with this entity (Fig. 23-18), but specific HRCT findings usually are lacking. Air trapping may be present.

Neither chest radiographs nor HRCT has much to offer in the diagnosis of patients with chronic bronchitis; these imaging techniques usually are of more value in excluding other causes of chronic sputum production or airflow obstruction, such as bronchiectasis or emphysema. The association of emphysema with chronic bronchitis in patients with chronic airflow obstruction (COPD) is discussed in Chapter 24.

BRONCHIOLITIS

Bronchiolitis is a nonspecific term used to describe inflammation of the small airways. A number of classifications have been proposed to include the wide spectrum of clinicopathologic conditions associated with bronchiolar inflammation.

Bronchiolitis often is classified by its histologic appearance. However, from a diagnostic standpoint, a radiographic classification is more appropriate and easier to use.

Histologic Classification of Bronchiolitis

Histologically, bronchiolitis is classified in different ways by different authors, but several entities are recognized consistently (Table 23-7). These include cellular bronchiolitis, respiratory bronchiolitis, bronchiolitis obliterans (constrictive bronchiolitis), and bronchiolitis obliterans with intraluminal polyps, also known as bronchiolitis obliterans organizing pneumonia (BOOP), and now increasing referred to simply as organizing pneumonia (OP; see Chapter 13).

Cellular Bronchiolitis

Cellular bronchiolitis is seen in a diverse group of diseases characterized by inflammation of the bronchiolar wall or bronchiolar lumen, often associated with fibrosis. This classification most commonly includes the following diseases: (1) infectious bronchiolitis (viral, mycoplasma, bacterial, mycobacterial, and fungal); (2) panbronchiolitis; (3) follicular bronchiolitis; (4) bronchiolitis associated with hypersensitivity pneumonitis; and (5) bronchiolitis associated with asthma. Hypersensitivity pneumonitis (see Chapter 16) and asthma have been discussed;

Infectious Bronchiolitis

Infectious bronchiolitis occurs in somewhat different forms in young children and adults, although the differences be-

TABLE 23-7. HISTOLOGIC CLASSIFICATION OF BRONCHIOLAR DISEASE

Cellular bronchiolitis
Infectious bronchiolitis (viral, mycoplasma, bacteria, mycobacteria, fungus)
Diffuse panbronchiolitis
Follicular bronchiolitis
    Primary in lymphoid interstitial pneumonitis, collagen disease, immunodeficiency, etc.
    Secondary in infection
Hypersensitivity pneumonitis
Asthma
Respiratory bronchiolitis
Bronchiolitis obliterans (constrictive bronchiolitis)
Infection (viral, bacterial, mycoplasma)
Toxic fume inhalation
Drug treatment
Collagen-vascular disease, particularly rheumatoid arthritis
Chronic lung transplant rejection
Bone marrow transplantation with chronic graft versus host disease
Idiopathic
Bronchiolitis obliterans with intraluminal polyps
Synonymous with OP/BOOP

tween these groups represent the two ends of a spectrum rather than distinct entities.

Infectious Bronchiolitis in Children

Acute bronchiolitis typically is a disease of infants and children less than 3 years of age. It is caused by infection, most often by respiratory syncytial virus or adenovirus, *Mycoplasma pneumoniae,* or *Chlamydia* species. Pathologic examination shows necrosis of the bronchiolar epithelium with a bronchiolar and peribronchiolar inflammatory cell infiltrate and bronchiolar edema. Because of the small size of the bronchioles in young children, significant bronchiolar obstruction often results.

Symptoms include those of upper respiratory tract infection followed by dyspnea, tachypnea, wheezing, and sometimes cyanosis and respiratory failure. Severe symptoms persist for a few days, usually followed by prompt recovery.

Radiographic findings in acute bronchiolitis include hyperinflation, patchy areas of consolidation or atelectasis, streaky perihilar opacities or tram tracks due to bronchial wall or interstitial thickening, and reticular or reticulonodular opacities. HRCT may show mosaic perfusion or air trapping.

Hyperinflation is most specific in making the diagnosis of acute bronchiolitis, but its incidence decreases as the age of the patient increases. Hyperinflation is common in children younger than 2 and is uncommon in patients older than 5. In older patients, findings of patchy consolidation, atelectasis, and reticulonodular opacities predominate.

These abnormalities resolve in nearly all cases, but in a small percentage, bronchiolectasis, bronchiolitis obliterans (constrictive bronchiolitis) and bronchiectasis result. This is most common in patients with adenovirus infection.

Infectious Bronchiolitis in Adults

Infectious bronchiolitis in older children and adults may be associated with a variety of organisms, including those already discussed. Additional organisms that may be responsible include bacteria (e.g., *H. influenzae, Bordetella pertussis*), atypical mycobacteria such as MAC, tuberculosis, and fungi. Infectious bronchiolitis also occurs in association with chronic airway disease such as bronchiectasis, chronic bronchitis and COPD (i.e., chronic bronchitis), CF, immunodeficiency syndromes including AIDS, or bronchopneumonia.

In adult patients with infectious bronchiolitis, plain radiographs may show evidence of bronchial wall thickening or bronchiectasis, patchy or ill-defined nodular areas of consolidation due to associated bronchopneumonia, and small nodular or reticulonodular opacities. Hyperinflation and air trapping are less common than in young children.

HRCT commonly shows the finding of tree-in-bud (see Figs. 23-12 and 23-19; see also Fig. 10-28 in Chapter 10). Tree-in-bud is most typical of bacterial or mycobacterial infections, but may sometimes be seen in patients with viral, mycoplasma, or fungal infections. Poorly-defined centrilobular nodules or rosettes of nodules are almost always visible in association with tree-in-bud (see Fig. 23-19B); these may represent dilated bronchioles seen in cross section of nodular areas of peribronchiolar inflammation or pneumonia. Lobular areas of consolidation may accompany the bronchiolar abnormality in patients with "lobular pneumonia" (i.e., bronchopneumonia). Bronchial wall thickening or bronchiectasis may be associated.

It is rarely necessary to obtain a biopsy for diagnosis. The presence of tree-in-bud almost always indicates the presence of infection; this finding means that "the diagnosis is in the sputum." Viral and mycoplasma infections may result in patchy air trapping in the absence of other findings.

As in children, abnormalities resolve with appropriate treatment in the large majority of patients. As in children, in a small number, bronchiolectasis, bronchiolitis obliterans (constrictive bronchiolitis), and bronchiectasis result.

Diffuse Panbronchiolitis

Diffuse panbronchiolitis (DPB) is a disease of unknown etiology that is particularly common in Japan and Eastern Asia. It is thought to be caused by an infection, although the responsible organism has yet to be isolated, in conjunction with genetic susceptibility.

DPB typically affects middle-aged patients, and men are involved twice as often as women. DPB is characterized by symptoms of chronic cough, sputum production, and dyspnea. Nearly three quarters of patients have associated

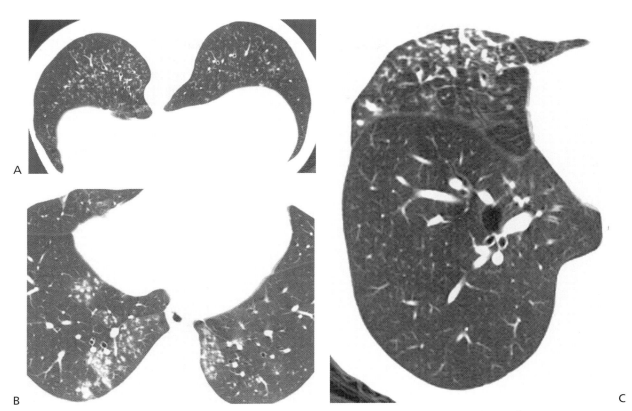

FIG. 23-19. Infectious bronchiolitis in three patients. **A.** Prone scan in a patient with *Pseudomonas* infection shows the appearance of tree-in-bud in the posterior lower lobes. **B.** In another patient with bacterial bronchiolitis, ill-defined centrilobular nodules are visible in both lower lobes. **C.** HRCT through the right lower lobe in a woman with *Mycobacterium avium-intracellulare* complex infection. Tree-in-bud is the primary abnormality.

sinusitis. The disease is progressive and is marked by frequent episodes of superimposed infection, typically with *P. aeruginosa.* Current therapy requires long-term, low-dose administration of erythromycin. Pulmonary function tests show mild to moderate airflow obstruction. Worsening respiratory failure may occur. In nearly 20% of cases, death occurs within 5 years of the onset of the disease with another 30% of patients dying within 10 years.

Histologically, characteristic findings of DPB include centrilobular, bronchiolar, and peribronchiolar infiltrates of acute and chronic inflammatory cells, associated with bronchiolar dilatation, and intraluminal inflammatory exudates. Lymphoid hyperplasia and accumulations of foamy macrophages commonly are seen. This combination of findings has been referred to as the "unit lesion" of panbronchiolitis and is considered unique to this syndrome. DPB characteristically involves respiratory bronchioles. In a minority of patients, there is also evidence of peripheral bronchiectasis.

Chest radiographs in patients with diffuse panbronchiolitis are nonspecific and usually show small nodular or reticulonodular opacities throughout both lungs and increased lung volumes. Bronchial wall thickening may result in perihilar tram tracks.

HRCT findings in patients with diffuse panbronchiolitis are similar to those of infectious bronchiolitis in adults and include centrilobular tree-in-bud; poorly defined centrilobular nodules; dilated, air-filled, thick-walled centrilobular bronchioles; large lung volumes; and mosaic perfusion or air trapping.

Follicular Bronchiolitis

Follicular bronchiolitis is characterized by a proliferation of lymphoid follicles in the walls of bronchioles and the peribronchiolar interstitium, associated with bronchiolar narrowing. Most commonly, it is an incidental finding in patients with chronic airways disease (e.g., bronchiectasis or bronchiolectasis) associated with inflammation or infection (i.e., secondary follicular bronchiolitis; Fig. 23-20). In this setting, it often is associated with clinical and radiographic findings of infection (e.g., bronchiectasis, tree-in-bud), and its distinction from infectious bronchiolectasis is unnecessary.

Follicular bronchiolitis (i.e., primary follicular bronchiolitis) also may occur in patients with rheumatoid arthritis, Sjögren's syndrome, immunodeficiency disorders including

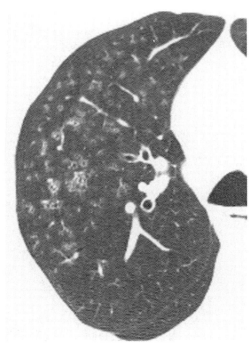

FIG. 23-20. Secondary follicular bronchiolitis in a patient with airway infection. HRCT shows ill-defined centrilobular nodules.

AIDS, and hypersensitivity reactions. Primary follicular bronchiolitis is commonly associated with progressive dyspnea, and response to treatment with corticosteroids is variable. In some cases, infection may be associated.

In patients with follicular bronchiolitis, chest radiographs may appear normal or may show a diffuse reticular or reticulonodular pattern. HRCT typically demonstrates tree-in-bud or small nodular opacities in a centrilobular and peribronchovascular distribution (see Fig. 23-20). In most cases, these measure 1 to 3 mm in diameter. Larger ill-defined centrilobular or peribronchial nodules of ground-glass opacity may also be seen.

Respiratory Bronchiolitis

Respiratory bronchiolitis is part of a spectrum of smoking-related diseases of the airways and lungs, characterized by bronchiolar inflammation, the accumulation of pigmented macrophages within respiratory bronchioles and alveoli, and some degree of fibrosis. This spectrum, in order of increasing severity, includes respiratory bronchiolitis (RB), respiratory bronchiolitis-interstitial lung disease (RB-ILD), and desquamative interstitial pneumonitis (DIP; see Chapter 13).

Respiratory bronchiolitis (RB) often is an incidental finding on biopsy in asymptomatic smokers. Smokers with RB-ILD have signs and symptoms of diffuse interstitial lung disease, and histologically show an exaggerated form of RB,

with evidence of more extensive inflammation and fibrosis. Radiographic and HRCT findings in RB, RB-ILD, and DIP are discussed in detail in Chapter 13.

Chest radiographs are normal in most patients with RB or RB-ILD. HRCT may be normal or may show poorly defined centrilobular ground-glass opacities having a mid- and upper lung predominance, with or without accompanying larger areas of diffuse ground-glass opacity. Multifocal mosaic perfusion or air trapping may be visible in some patients.

Bronchiolitis Obliterans

Bronchiolitis obliterans (constrictive bronchiolitis) is characterized by the presence of concentric fibrosis involving the submucosal and peribronchial tissues of terminal and respiratory bronchioles, resulting in bronchial narrowing or obliteration (Table 23-8). Abnormalities of the large airways such as bronchiectasis may be seen in some cases (see Figs. 10-36 and 10-38 in Chapter 10 and Fig. 14-7 in Chapter 14), Progressive airway obstruction and severe dyspnea, unresponsive to steroid therapy, are typical.

Most commonly, bronchiolitis obliterans (BO) results from (1) infection (viral, bacterial, mycoplasma); (2) toxic fume inhalation (e.g., nitrogen dioxide or silo-filler's lung, sulfur dioxide, ammonia, chlorine, phosgene, smoke); (3) drug treatment (e.g., penicillamine or gold); (4) collagen-vascular disease, particularly rheumatoid arthritis (see Fig. 14-7 in Chapter 14); (5) chronic lung transplant rejection (Fig. 23-21A; see also Fig. 10-38 in Chapter 10); and (6) bone marrow transplantation with chronic graft versus host disease (see Fig. 23-21B). Rarely, it is idiopathic or may be associated with consumption of toxic substances (e.g.,

---

TABLE 23-8. BRONCHIOLITIS OBLITERANS (CONSTRICTIVE BRONCHIOLITIS) AND THE SWYER-JAMES SYNDROME

Concentric fibrosis involving terminal and respiratory bronchioles
Bronchiolar obstruction
Variety of causes
Radiographs often nonspecific
   Large lung volumes
   Increased lucency (60%)
   Reduced size of peripheral vessels
   Central bronchiectasis (35%)
HRCT findings
   Mosaic perfusion, usually patchy in distribution (85%–90%)
   Bronchiectasis
   Air trapping on expiration, usually patchy in distribution
   Air trapping on expiration with normal inspiratory scans
Swyer-James syndrome
   Unilateral radiographic abnormalities
   Affected lung often reduced in volume

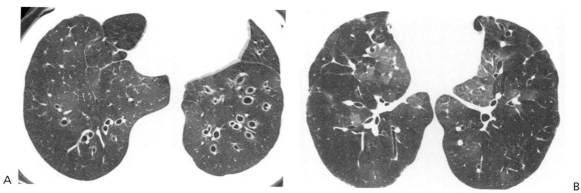

FIG. 23-21. Mosaic perfusion and bronchiectasis in two patients with bronchiolitis obliterans. **A.** A patient with chronic lung transplant rejection shows bronchiectasis and mosaic perfusion on HRCT. **B.** In a patient with graft-versus-host disease following bone marrow transplantation, inhomogeneous lung attenuation represents mosaic perfusion. Note the decreased vessel size in lucent lung regions.

Sauropus androgynus, a plant consumed in Korea) or neuroendocrine hyperplasia with carcinoid tumorlets.

BO results in similar radiographic findings regardless of its cause. Chest radiographs are normal in one third of cases. Visible abnormalities often are subtle, and include hyperinflation, increased lung lucency (60%), peripheral reduction of vascular markings, and findings of central bronchiectasis (35%; see Fig. 10-36 in Chapter 10, and Fig. 14-7 in Chapter 14). Although most patients with BO have bilateral abnormalities, because of the subtle nature of plain film findings in BO, only those with predominantly unilateral disease are easily diagnosed on plain radiographs. This occurrence has been termed the *Swyer-James syndrome* (see Fig. 11-9 in Chapter 11).

HRCT is much more sensitive than chest radiographs in patients with BO. HRCT findings are similar regardless of the cause of disease and include focal or multifocal, sharply defined areas of decreased lung attenuation associated with vessels of decreased caliber (i.e., mosaic perfusion) in 85% to 90% of cases (see Fig. 23-20; see also Fig. 10-36 in Chapter 10). These areas may be lobar, segmental, or may involve individual secondary pulmonary lobules. Air trapping typically is visible in areas of lucency on expiratory HRCT (Fig. 23-22; see also Fig. 10-38 in Chapter 10). In some patients with BO, the presence of air trapping on expiratory scans may be the only abnormal HRCT finding. Bronchiectasis, both central and peripheral, may be present as well, and, when visible, usually occurs in lucent lung regions. Rarely, tree-in-bud or ill-defined centrilobular opacities may be the predominant finding, but recognizable small airway abnormalities usually are inconspicuous in patients with BO.

The *Swyer-James syndrome* (less desirable synonyms include McLeod's syndrome, unilateral emphysema, unilateral lobar emphysema, and unilateral hyperlucent lung) is characterized by predominantly unilateral radiographic findings of BO (Fig. 23-23; see also Fig. 11-9 in Chapter 11). It is the result of lower respiratory tract infection, usually due to viruses, *Mycoplasma* organisms, *B. pertussis,* or tuberculosis, occurring in infancy or early childhood. Damage to the terminal and respiratory bronchioles leads to incomplete development of alveoli. The Swyer-James syndrome was described in the 1950s and has received undeserved attention as a specific entity; nonetheless, it serves to illustrate the typical plain film features of BO. It is characterized radiographically by unilateral hyperlucency of a lung, lobe, or segment, associated with decreased size of associated pulmonary arteries. The volume of the affected lung often is decreased because of abnormal development, but may be normal or increased. Areas of atelectasis and bronchiectasis may be associated. Air trapping is visible on expiratory radiographs. Patients usually are asymptomatic, and the abnormality is detected incidentally. However, dyspnea or recurrent infections may be associated. Ventilation-perfusion scans show matched defects.

Bronchiolitis Obliterans With Intraluminal Polyps

Bronchiolitis obliterans with intraluminal polyps is a process defined by the presence of granulation tissue polyps (Masson bodies) within respiratory bronchioles and alveolar ducts. However, the predominant histologic abnormality usually is an associated organizing pneumonia, and, until recently, the term *bronchiolitis obliterans organizing pneumonia* (BOOP) was more generally used to refer to this entity. The current trend is to ignore the bronchial lesion, and refer to this condition as organizing pneumonia (OP).

OP characteristically results in restrictive rather than obstructive lung disease, and is best considered in the category of interstitial pneumonia (see Chapter 13). HRCT typically shows patchy, nonsegmental, unilateral or bilateral foci of air-space consolidation, ill-defined centrilobular nodules, or

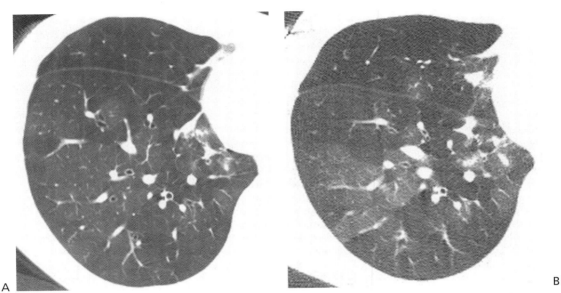

FIG. 23-22. Mosaic perfusion and air trapping in a patient with bronchiolitis obliterans resulting from smoke inhalation. **A.** Inspiratory HRCT shows subtle mosaic perfusion. There is no evidence of bronchiectasis. **B.** Dynamic expiratory scan shows air trapping indicative of bronchiolitis obliterans.

large irregular nodules. The majority of patients respond to treatment with corticosteroids.

Radiographic and HRCT Classification of Bronchiolitis

Chest radiographs in patients with bronchiolitis usually appear normal or show nonspecific abnormalities in patients with bronchiolitis, including ground-glass opacity, poor definition of pulmonary vessels, or ill-defined reticular or nodular opacities. Large lung volumes may be seen, due to air trapping, particularly in patients with bronchiolitis obliterans. Large airway abnormalities such as bronchiectasis may be associated in some cases.

HRCT is of great value in assessing bronchiolar disease (Table 23-9). Abnormal bronchioles may be associated with characteristic abnormalities. Direct HRCT signs of bronchiolar disease result from the presence of bronchiolar dilatation, bronchiolar impaction, bronchiolar wall thickening, or peribronchiolar inflammation. The most important indirect signs of bronchiolar disease are mosaic perfusion on inspiratory scans and air-trapping on expiratory scans.

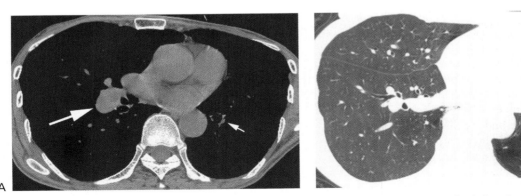

FIG. 23-23. HRCT appearance of the Swyer-James syndrome. **A.** CT shows the left pulmonary artery *(small arrow)* to be much smaller than the right *(large arrow)*. **B.** The left lung is hyperlucent with decreased vessel size. Bronchiectasis also is present, a common finding with bronchiolitis obliterans.

TABLE 23-9. RADIOGRAPHIC (HRCT) CLASSIFICATION OF BRONCHIOLAR DISEASE

Bronchiolar diseases with tree-in-bud
Typical of cellular bronchiolitis
Usually due to infection
  Mycobacterium tuberculosis
  Atypical mycobacterial infections (*Mycobacterium avium-intracellulare*)
  Bacterial infections (e.g., cystic fibrosis; immunosuppressed patients)
  Fungal infections (e.g., airway-invasive *Aspergillus*)
  Viral or mycoplasmal infection
  Asian panbronchiolitis
Other causes
  Follicular bronchiolitis (collagen vascular disease or lymphoid interstitial pneumonitis)
  Asthma
  Allergic bronchopulmonary aspergillosis
  Endobronchial spread of tumor
Bronchiolar diseases with poorly defined centrilobular nodules
Subacute hypersensitivity pneumonitis
Infectious bronchiolitis (viral, *Pneumocystis carinii* pneumonia)
Respiratory bronchiolitis
Follicular bronchiolitis and lymphoid interstitial pneumonitis
OP/BOOP
Bronchiolar disease associated with decreased lung attenuation
Bronchiolitis obliterans (constrictive bronchiolitis)
Hypersensitivity pneumonitis
Respiratory bronchiolitis
Asthma
Bronchiolar disease associated with ground-glass opacity or consolidation
OP/BOOP
Respiratory bronchiolitis
Infectious bronchiolitis

Based on the primary HRCT findings, bronchiolitis may be classified in one of four groups, an approach that is more practical from a diagnostic standpoint than a histologic classification:

1. Bronchiolar disease associated with tree-in-bud
2. Bronchiolar disease associated with poorly defined centrilobular nodular opacities
3. Bronchiolar disease associated with mosaic perfusion
4. Bronchiolar disease associated with focal or diffuse ground-glass opacity or consolidation.

Bronchiolar Diseases Associated With Tree-in-bud

The HRCT finding of tree-in-bud is characterized by the presence of centrilobular, branching or Y-shaped opacities that resemble a budding tree, usually best seen in the lung periphery. A tree-in-bud appearance is most typical of cellu-

lar bronchiolitis, and in clinical practice almost always is the result of acute or chronic infection (e.g., infectious bronchiolitis, CF, bronchopneumonia, TB, MAC). Bacterial and mycobacterial infection is most common in patients with tree-in-bud, but this finding also may be seen with viral, mycoplasmal, and fungal infections.

Occasionally, tree-in-bud occurs without infection in patients with asthma, allergic bronchopulmonary aspergillosis, bronchiolitis obliterans, follicular bronchiolitis, asthma, and endobronchial spread of bronchioloalveolar carcinoma. Mosaic perfusion on inspiratory scans and air trapping on expiratory scan may be present. Abnormalities of the large airways (e.g., bronchiectasis or bronchial wall thickening) also may be seen. Regardless of the associated abnormalities, only a few good examples of tree-in-bud need to be seen in a patient to characterize this pattern.

Bronchiolar Diseases Associated With Poorly Defined Centrilobular Nodules

The hallmark of the bronchiolar diseases associated with poorly defined centrilobular nodules is the finding of ill-defined centrilobular nodules without associated tree-in-bud. This finding usually results from peribronchiolar inflammation or fibrosis, and is associated with a wide range of pathologic entities including cellular bronchiolitis in hypersensitivity pneumonitis, infectious bronchiolitis (particularly in association with viral and *Pneumocystis* pneumonia), respiratory bronchiolitis and respiratory bronchiolitis-interstitial lung disease, LIP and follicular bronchiolitis, and OP. Despite the large number of diseases included in this category, in most cases, the differential diagnosis is simplified by clinical correlation, including occupational and environmental exposure histories.

Bronchiolar Diseases Associated With Mosaic Perfusion

Bronchiolar diseases associated with mosaic perfusion as a predominant abnormality include bronchiolitis obliterans or cellular bronchiolitis in hypersensitivity pneumonia, RB, and asthma. In patients with cellular bronchiolitis, it may be associated with other findings such as tree-in-bud or centrilobular nodules.

Bronchiolar Diseases Associated With Focal Ground-glass Opacity or Consolidation

An association with focal ground-glass opacity or consolidation is characteristic of OP; air trapping and tree-in-bud are characteristically absent. RB or, more often, RB-ILD may be associated with patchy ground-glass opacity; air trapping also may be present. Some causes of infectious bronchiolitis, such as viral or mycoplasmal pneumonia, are associated with patchy consolidation or ground-glass opacity; air trapping and tree-in-bud may be present with these diseases.

SELECTED READING

Akira M, Kitatani F, Lee Y-S, et al. Diffuse panbronchiolitis: evaluation with high-resolution CT. Radiology 1988; 168:433–438.

Aquino SL, Gamsu G, Webb WR, Kee SL. Tree-in-bud pattern: frequency and significance on thin section CT. J Comput Assist Tomogr 1996; 20:594–599.

Arakawa H, Webb WR. Air trapping on expiratory high-resolution CT scans in the absence of inspiratory scan abnormalities: correlation with pulmonary function tests and differential diagnosis. AJR Am J Roentgenol 1998; 170:1349–1353.

Cartier Y, Kavanagh PV, Johkoh T, et al. Bronchiectasis: accuracy of high-resolution CT in the differentiation of specific diseases. AJR Am J Roentgenol 1999; 173:47–52.

Chang AB, Masel JP, Masters B. Post-infectious bronchiolitis obliterans: clinical, radiological and pulmonary function sequelae. Pediatr Radiol 1998; 28:23–29.

Cohen M, Sahn SA. Bronchiectasis in systemic diseases. Chest 1999; 116:1063–1074.

Friedman PJ. Chest radiographic findings in the adult with cystic fibrosis. Semin Roentgenol 1987; 22:114–124.

Garg K, Lynch DA, Newell JD, King TE. Proliferative and constrictive bronchiolitis: classification and radiologic features. AJR Am J Roentgenol 1994; 162:803–808.

Gosink BB, Friedman PJ, Liebow AA. Bronchiolitis obliterans: roentgenographic-pathologic correlation. AJR Am J Roentgenol 1973; 117:816–832.

Gruden JF, Webb WR, Warnock M. Centrilobular opacities in the lung on high-resolution CT: diagnostic considerations and pathologic correlation. AJR Am J Roentgenol 1994; 162:569–574.

Helbich TH, Heinz-Peer G, Eichler I, et al. Cystic fibrosis: CT assessment of lung involvement in children and adults. Radiology 1999; 213:537–544.

Howling SJ, Hansell DM, Wells AU, et al. Follicular bronchiolitis: thin-section CT and histologic findings. Radiology 1999; 212: 637–642.

Kang EY, Miller RR, Müller NL. Bronchiectasis: comparison of preoperative thin-section CT and pathologic findings in resected specimens. Radiology 1995; 195:649–654.

King TE. Overview of bronchiolitis. Clin Chest Med 1993; 14: 607–610.

Lynch DA. Imaging of small airways disease. Clin Chest Med 1993; 14:623–634.

Lynch DA, Newell JD, Tschomper BA, et al. Uncomplicated asthma in adults: comparison of CT appearance of the lungs in asthmatic and healthy subjects. Radiology 1993; 188:829–833.

McGuinness G, Naidich DP, Leitman BS, McCauley DI. Bronchiectasis: CT evaluation. AJR Am J Roentgenol 1993; 160:253–259.

Müller NL, Miller RR. Diseases of the bronchioles: CT and histopathologic findings. Radiology 1995; 196:3–12.

Naidich DP, McCauley DI, Khouri NF, et al. Computed tomography of bronchiectasis. J Comput Assist Tomogr 1982; 6:437–444.

Nishimura K, Kitaichi M, Izumi T, Itoh H. Diffuse panbronchiolitis: correlation of high-resolution CT and pathologic findings. Radiology 1992; 184:779–785.

Padley SPG, Adler BD, Hansell DM, Müller NL. Bronchiolitis obliterans: high-resolution CT findings and correlation with pulmonary function tests. Clin Radiol 1993; 47:236–240.

Park CS, Müller NL, Worthy SA, et al. Airway obstruction in asthmatic and healthy individuals: inspiratory and expiratory thin-section CT findings. Radiology 1997; 203:361–367.

Shah RM, Sexauer W, Ostrum BJ, et al. High-resolution CT in the acute exacerbation of cystic fibrosis: evaluation of acute findings, reversibility of those findings, and clinical correlation. AJR Am J Roentgenol 1997; 169:375–380.

Ward S, Heyneman L, Lee MJ, et al. Accuracy of CT in the diagnosis of allergic bronchopulmonary aspergillosis in asthmatic patients. AJR Am J Roentgenol 1999; 173:937–942.

Wood BP. Cystic fibrosis: 1997. Radiology 1997; 204:1–10.

24

EMPHYSEMA AND CHRONIC OBSTRUCTIVE PULMONARY DISEASE

W. RICHARD WEBB

As defined by the American Thoracic Society, emphysema is "a condition of the lung characterized by permanent, abnormal enlargement of airspaces distal to the terminal bronchiole, accompanied by the destruction of their walls," but "without obvious fibrosis." Currently, it is estimated that 2 million people in the United States suffer from emphysema. It is a significant cause of morbidity and mortality.

It is generally accepted that emphysema results from an imbalance in the dynamic relationship between elastolytic and antielastolytic factors in the lung, usually related to cigarette smoking or enzymatic deficiency. Abnormal or unopposed elastase activity is thought to lead to the tissue destruction that is the primary pathologic abnormality present in patients with this disease.

The proposed mechanisms in development of emphysema in smokers are as follows:

1. Inhaled tobacco smoke attracts macrophages to distal airways and alveoli (referred to as respiratory bronchiolitis).
2. The macrophages, along with airway epithelial cells, release chemotactic substances that attract neutrophils and induce them to release elastases and other proteolytic enzymes. Macrophages also release proteases in response to tobacco smoke.
3. These elastases have the ability to cleave a variety of proteins, including collagen and elastin. Lung elastin normally is protected from excessive elastase-induced damage by alpha-1-protease inhibitors (alpha-1-antiprotease or alpha-1-antitrypsin) and other circulating antiproteinases.
4. Tobacco smoke tends to interfere with the function of alpha-1-antiprotease.
5. In combination, these interactions result in structural damage in the distal airways and alveoli in smokers, leading to emphysema.

Inherited deficiency in alpha-1-antiprotease similarly results in lung destruction and emphysema when neutrophils release elastases and other proteolytic enzymes in response to pulmonary infection.

CLASSIFICATION OF EMPHYSEMA

Emphysema usually is classified into three main subtypes, based on the anatomic distribution of the areas of lung destruction: (1) centrilobular, proximal acinar, or centriacinar emphysema; (2) panlobular or panacinar emphysema; and (3) paraseptal or distal acinar emphysema. The terms *centrilobular, panlobular*, and *paraseptal* are generally accepted and will be used to describe these three types of emphysema in the remainder of this chapter. In their early stages, these three forms of emphysema can be easily distinguished morphologically. However, as the emphysema becomes more severe, distinguishing among the types becomes more difficult.

Centrilobular emphysema predominantly affects the respiratory bronchioles in the central portions of acini, and therefore involves the central portion of secondary lobules. It usually results from cigarette smoking and involves mainly the upper lung zones.

Panlobular emphysema involves all the components of the acinus more or less uniformly, and therefore involves entire secondary lobules. It is associated classically with alpha-1-protease inhibitor (alpha-1-antitrypsin) deficiency, although it also may be seen without protease deficiency in smokers, in elderly persons, distal to bronchial and bronchiolar obliteration, and associated with illicit drug use.

Paraseptal emphysema predominantly involves the alveolar ducts and sacs in the lung periphery, with areas of destruction often marginated by interlobular septa. It can be an isolated phenomenon in young adults, often associated with spontaneous pneumothorax, or can be seen in older patients with centrilobular emphysema.

Bullae can develop in association with any type of emphysema, but they are most common with paraseptal or centrilobular emphysema. A *bulla* is a sharply demarcated area of emphysema measuring 1 cm or more in diameter, and possessing a wall less than 1 mm in thickness. In some patients with emphysema, bullae can become quite large, resulting in significant compromise of respiratory function;

this syndrome is sometimes referred to as *bullous emphysema*. Bullae are most common in a subpleural location, representing foci of paraseptal emphysema associated with air trapping and progressive enlargement.

Irregular air-space enlargement is an additional type of emphysema that occurs in patients with pulmonary fibrosis; this form of emphysema also is referred to as *paracicatricial* or *irregular emphysema*. It commonly is found adjacent to localized parenchymal scars, diffuse pulmonary fibrosis, and in the pneumoconioses, particularly those pneumocarioses associated with progressive massive fibrosis.

EMPHYSEMA AND CHRONIC OBSTRUCTIVE PULMONARY DISEASE

In patients with emphysema, pulmonary function tests usually show findings of chronic airflow obstruction and reduced diffusing capacity. Airflow obstruction in patients with emphysema is due to airway collapse on expiration, resulting largely from destruction of lung parenchyma and loss of airway tethering and support. Abnormal diffusing capacity is due to destruction of the lung parenchyma and the pulmonary vascular bed.

It is important to keep in mind that many patients with emphysema also have chronic bronchitis; both conditions are smoking-related diseases.

The term *chronic obstructive pulmonary disease* (COPD) often is used to describe patients with chronic and largely irreversible airway obstruction, most commonly associated with some combination of emphysema and chronic bronchitis. The term itself indicates some uncertainty as to the exact pathogenesis of the functional abnormalities present; it also may be used to refer to diseases usually associated with airway obstruction, such as emphysema and chronic bronchitis, even if no obstruction is demonstrated on pulmonary function tests.

Respiratory symptoms in patients with COPD usually include chronic cough, sputum production, and dyspnea. Although, cough and sputum production are largely manifestations of chronic bronchitis in patients with COPD, the relative contributions of airways disease and emphysema to respiratory disability often are difficult to determine. Typical pulmonary function abnormalities in emphysema include reductions in the ratio of forced expiratory volume in 1 second (FEV_1) to forced vital capacity (FVC), the FEV_1, and the diffusing capacity.

Radiographic Findings

Radiographic abnormalities in patients with COPD are largely the same as those of emphysema. These include increased lung volume and lung destruction (bullae or reduced vascularity). When both findings are used as criteria for diagnosis, a sensitivity as high as 80% has been reported for chest films, although the likelihood of a positive diagnosis

depends on the severity of disease. When only findings of lung destruction are used for diagnosis, plain films are only about 40% sensitive. Although the accuracy of chest radiographs in diagnosing emphysema is controversial, it can be reasonably concluded from the studies performed that moderate to severe emphysema can be diagnosed radiographically, whereas mild emphysema is difficult to detect.

The presence of increased lung volume, or overinflation, is important in making the diagnosis of emphysema on plain radiographs. However, overinflation is an indirect sign of this disease, and findings of increased lung volume are nonspecific. Such findings can be absent in some patients with emphysema but present in patients who have other forms of obstructive pulmonary disease.

Plain radiographic findings of overinflation (Figs. 24-1 and 24-2; Table 24-1) include the following:

1. Lung height of 29.9 cm or more, measured from the dome of the right diaphragm to the tubercle of the first rib
2. Flattening of the right hemidiaphragm on the lateral projection, with a height of less than 2.7 cm measured from anterior to posterior costophrenic angles
3. Flattening of the right hemidiaphragm on a posteroanterior radiograph, with the highest level of the dome of the right hemidiaphragm less than 1.5 cm above a perpendicular line drawn between the costophrenic angle laterally and the vertebrophrenic angle medially
4. Increased retrosternal air space, measuring more than 4.4 cm at a level 3 cm below the manubrial-sternal junction
5. Right hemidiaphragm at or below the level of the anterior end of the 7th rib
6. Sternodiaphragmatic angle measuring 90 degrees or more

TABLE 24-1. RADIOGRAPHIC FINDINGS IN EMPHYSEMA

Increased lung volume
PA view
  ≥29.9 cm from the dome of the right diaphragm to the first rib
  Flattening of the right hemidiaphragm with a height <1.5 cm
  Right hemidiaphragm at or below the level of the anterior 7th rib
  Blunting of the lateral costophrenic angles
  Visible diaphragmatic slips
Lateral view
  Flattening of the right hemidiaphragm with a height of <2.7 cm
  Increased retrosternal air space, measuring >4.4 cm
  Sternodiaphragmatic angle measuring 90 degrees or more
  Blunting of the posterior costophrenic angle
Lung destruction
Bullae
Lung lucency
Decreased vessel size

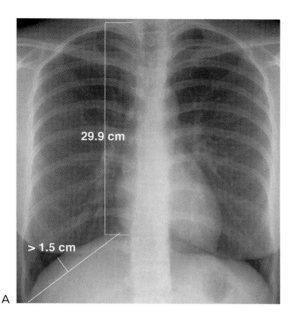

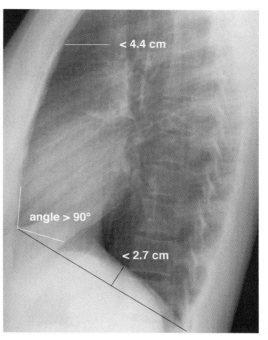

FIG. 24-1. Plain film measurements in emphysema. **A.** Plain radiographic findings of emphysema on the PA radiograph include a lung height of 29.9 cm or more, measured from the dome of the right diaphragm to the tubercle of the first rib and flattening of the right hemidiaphragm on a posteroanterior radiograph, with the highest level of the dome of the right hemidiaphragm less than 1.5 cm above a perpendicular line drawn between the costophrenic angle laterally and the vertebrophrenic angle medially. **B.** Findings of emphysema on the lateral radiograph include flattening of the right hemidiaphragm, with a height of less than 2.7 cm measured from anterior to posterior costophrenic angles; an increased retrosternal air space, measuring more than 4.4 cm at a level 3 cm below the manubriosternal junction; and a sternodiaphragmatic angle measuring 90 degrees or more.

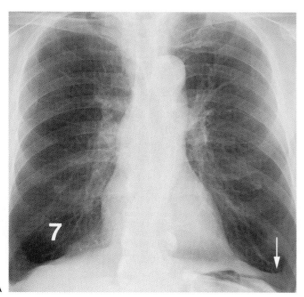

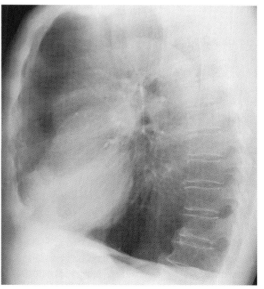

FIG. 24-2. Chest radiographs in emphysema. **A.** PA radiograph shows increased lung height with flattening of the diaphragm. The dome of the right hemidiaphragm is below the level of the anterior right 7th rib *(7)*. Blunting of the costophrenic angles is common in increased lung volumes, as are visible diaphragmatic slips *(arrow)* extending to the chest wall. The lungs appear lucent, and vessel size is reduced. Mild prominence of the hila likely reflects pulmonary hypertension. **B.** The lateral view shows increased depth and lucency of the retrosternal space. The diaphragms are flattened and appear inverted (i.e., their normal curvature is reversed).

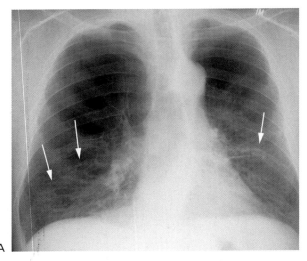

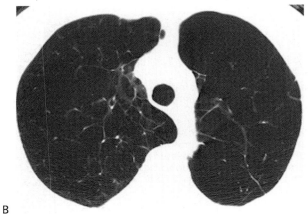

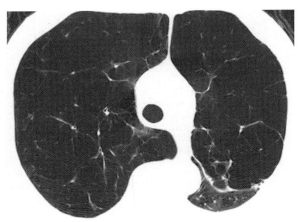

FIG. 24-3. Severe centrilobular emphysema. **A.** Chest radiograph shows lucency in the upper lobes, with vessels being invisible. This appearance is diagnostic of severe emphysema or bullae. Vessels appear displaced inferiorly *(arrows).* This is a common finding with severe emphysema or bullae. **B** and **C.** HRCTs at two levels show severe centrilobular emphysema with marked reduction in vessel size. Areas of emphysema have become confluent, having the appearance of panlobular emphysema.

Blunting of the costophrenic angles or visible diaphragmatic slips on the PA view are common findings in markedly increased lung volume; inversion of the hemidiaphragms may be seen on the lateral view (Fig. 24-2).

The presence of bullae on chest radiographs is the only specific sign of lung destruction caused by emphysema, and usually means that paraseptal or severe centrilobular emphysema is present (Fig. 24-3). However, this finding is uncommon and may not reflect the presence of generalized disease. Bullae usually are visible in the lung periphery, have thin walls, and appear lucent, and lung markings are not seen inside them. Lung lucency may reflect the presence of bullae when they are not visible as discrete structures.

A reduction in size of pulmonary vessels or vessel tapering in the lung periphery also can reflect lung destruction in patients with emphysema (see Fig. 24-2), but this finding lacks sensitivity and can be unreliable. Focal absence or displacement of vessels may reflect the presence of bullae (see Fig. 24-3).

On chest radiographs, centrilobular emphysema usually shows an upper lobe predominance of increased lucency

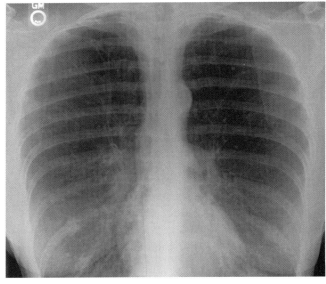

FIG. 24-4. Severe centrilobular emphysema. Chest radiograph shows lucency predominating in the upper lobes with reduced vessel size. Vessels are largest at the bases.

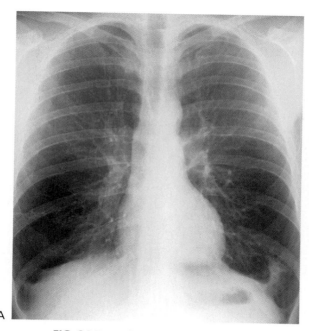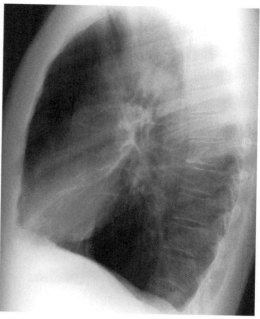

FIG. 24-5. Panlobular emphysema in a 34-year-old man secondary to alpha-1-antitrypsin deficiency. **A.** On the PA view, lung volumes are increased. The lungs appear more lucent at the lung bases, and vessel size is greatest in the upper lobes. **B.** Findings of emphysema, with increased lung volumes and increased lucency, also are visible on the lateral view. Vessels appear small at the lung bases.

and decreased vascularity (see Figs. 24-3 and 24-4). In panlobular emphysema, lucency and decreased vascularity usually appear to involve the lung uniformly or have a basal predominance (Fig. 24-5).

Pulmonary hypertension may develop in patients with emphysema and COPD as a result of destruction of the pulmonary vascular bed. In its early stages, this condition is manifested by dilatation of central pulmonary arteries (see Fig. 24-2). Later, the development of cor pulmonale may result in cardiomegaly and right ventricular enlargement.

HRCT Findings

CT with thick collimation is inadequate for diagnosis of emphysema, but HRCT is highly accurate. On HRCT, emphysema is characterized by the presence of areas of abnormally low attenuation, which can be contrasted easily with surrounding normal lung parenchyma if a sufficiently low window mean (-600 HU to -700 HU) is used. HRCT is highly accurate in diagnosing emphysema, and findings correlate closely with pathology.

In most instances, focal areas of emphysema can be easily distinguished from lung cysts or honeycombing; with the exception of paraseptal emphysema or bullae, focal areas of emphysema lack distinct walls.

Although various CT findings of increased lung volume may also be seen in patients with COPD and emphysema,

their identification is usually secondary to the more direct observation of lung destruction characteristic of the various types of emphysema

Centrilobular Emphysema

Centrilobular emphysema of mild to moderate degree is characterized on HRCT by the presence of multiple small, round areas of abnormally low attenuation, several millimeters to 1 cm in diameter, distributed throughout the lung, but usually having an upper lobe predominance (Fig. 24-6 and Table 24-2). Areas of lucency often appear to be grouped near the centers of secondary pulmonary lobules,

TABLE 24-2. CENTRILOBULAR EMPHYSEMA

Affects the respiratory bronchioles in the central portions of lobules
Cigarette smoking
Upper lobe predominance
Small round areas of low attenuation
Walls usually invisible
Several millimeters to 1 cm in diameter
May be associated with bullae
May become confluent

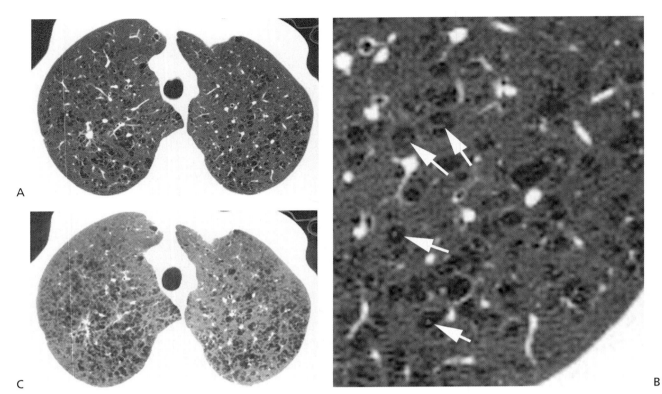

FIG. 24-6. HRCT in centrilobular emphysema. **A.** HRCT through the upper lobes shows multiple small areas of lucency, with a spotty distribution. This is typical of centrilobular emphysema. The individual holes do not have visible walls. A small nodule in the right upper lobe represents a carcinoma. **B.** Coned-down view of the left upper lobe shows the typical appearance of centrilobular emphysema. No walls are visible. Some areas of emphysema are seen to surround small centrilobular arteries *(arrows)*. **C.** Minimum-intensity projection image from a stack of five HRCT images shows the typical distribution of centrilobular emphysema.

surrounding the centrilobular artery branches. Although the centrilobular location of lucencies cannot always be recognized on CT or HRCT, the presence of multiple, small, areas of emphysema, scattered throughout the lung, is diagnostic of centrilobular emphysema. In most cases, the areas of low attenuation lack visible walls (see Figs. 24-6 and 24-7), although very thin and relatively inconspicuous walls are occasionally seen on HRCT, probably related to surrounding fibrosis. In patients with centrilobular emphysema, bullae within the lung may have visible walls (Fig. 24-8), and paraseptal emphysema and subpleural bullae are often seen.

With more severe centrilobular emphysema, areas of destruction can become confluent. When this occurs, the centrilobular distribution of abnormalities is no longer recognizable on HRCT (or on pathology). This appearance can closely mimic the appearance of panlobular emphysema, and a distinction between these is of little clinical significance in this situation (see Fig. 24-3B and C).

Panlobular Emphysema

Panlobular emphysema is characterized by uniform destruction of the pulmonary lobule, leading to widespread areas of abnormally low lung attenuation (Table 24-3). Involved lung appears abnormally lucent, and pulmonary vessels in the affected lung appear fewer and smaller than normal,

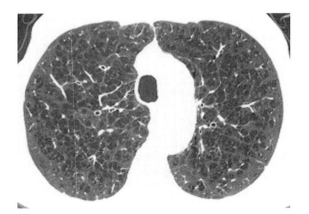

FIG. 24-7. Severe centrilobular emphysema. Multiple focal lucencies are visible in the upper lobes, without visible walls.

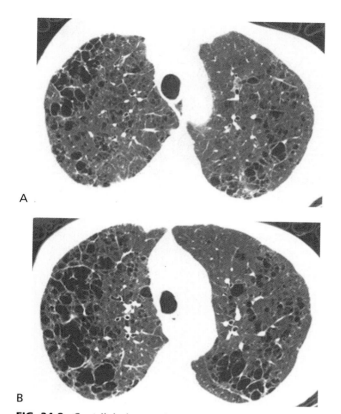

A

B

FIG. 24-8. Centrilobular emphysema with bullae. Centrilobular emphysema is visible in the upper lobes. Areas of emphysema larger than 1 cm are bullae. They often have visible walls. Areas of emphysema in an immediate subpleural location represent paraseptal emphysema.

even moderately severe panlobular emphysema can be very subtle and difficult to detect. Diffuse panlobular emphysema unassociated with focal areas of lung destruction or bullae may be difficult to distinguish from diffuse small airway obstruction and air trapping resulting from bronchiolitis obliterans.

About 40% of patients with alpha-1-antitrypsin deficiency show bronchiectasis or bronchial wall thickening on HRCT. Patients with alpha-1-antitrypsin deficiency are more susceptible to airway damage during episodes of infection than are normal patients because of the same protease-antiprotease imbalance that leads to emphysema.

Paraseptal Emphysema

Paraseptal emphysema is characterized by involvement of the distal part of the secondary lobule and, therefore, is most striking in a subpleural location (Table 24-4). Areas of subpleural paraseptal emphysema often have visible walls, but these walls are very thin and often correspond to interlobular septa (Fig. 24-11). Even mild paraseptal emphysema is easily detected by HRCT.

Areas of paraseptal emphysema larger than 1 cm in diam-

and may be quite inconspicuous (Figs. 24-9 and 24-10). In contrast to centrilobular emphysema, panlobular emphysema almost always appears generalized or most severe in the lower lobes. Focal lucencies, which are more typical of centrilobular emphysema or paraseptal emphysema, and bullae are relatively uncommon but may be seen in less abnormal lung regions.

In severe panlobular emphysema, the characteristic appearance of extensive lung destruction and the associated paucity of vascular markings are easily distinguished from normal lung parenchyma. On the other hand, mild and

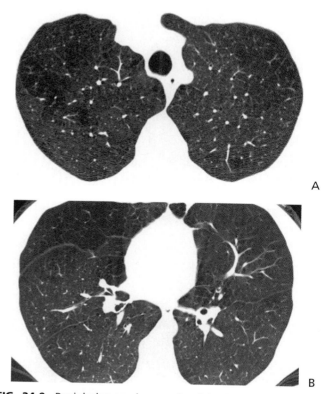

A

B

FIG. 24-9. Panlobular emphysema in alpha-1-antitrypsin deficiency (same patient shown in Fig. 24-5). HRCT scans through the upper (**A**) and lower (**B**) lobes both show a decrease in lung attenuation and vessel size. Focal lucencies, as seen in centrilobular emphysema, are not present.

TABLE 24-3. PANLOBULAR EMPHYSEMA

Affects the entire lobule
Alpha-1-antitrypsin deficiency or cigarette smoking
Diffuse or lower lobe predominance
Diffuse decrease in lung attenuation
Focal areas of destruction or bullae usually absent
Reduction in vessel size
May be subtle in its early stages

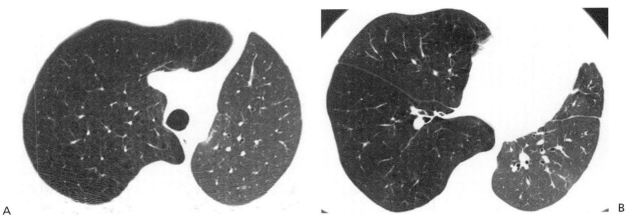

FIG. 24-10. Panlobular emphysema in alpha-1-antitrypsin deficiency (right lung) in a patient with a left lung transplant. HRCT scans through the upper (**A**) and lower (**B**) lobes both show decreased lung attenuation and vessel size. The right lung is considerably larger than the (normal) left lung. The normal left lung attenuation, vascular size, and volume may be contrasted with that of the emphysematous lung.

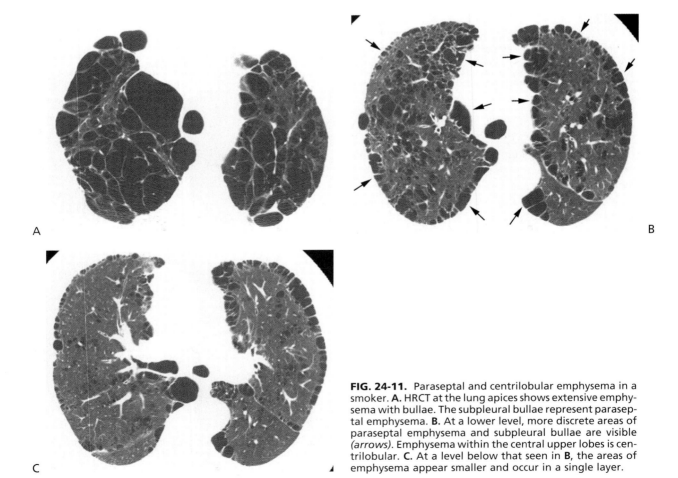

FIG. 24-11. Paraseptal and centrilobular emphysema in a smoker. **A.** HRCT at the lung apices shows extensive emphysema with bullae. The subpleural bullae represent paraseptal emphysema. **B.** At a lower level, more discrete areas of paraseptal emphysema and subpleural bullae are visible *(arrows)*. Emphysema within the central upper lobes is centrilobular. **C.** At a level below that seen in **B**, the areas of emphysema appear smaller and occur in a single layer.

TABLE 24-4. PARASEPTAL EMPHYSEMA

Affects subpleural lobules
Cigarette smoking or idiopathic
Upper lower predominance
May be associated with centrilobular emphysema
Focal subpleural lucencies marginated by interlobular septae
Bullae common

eter are most appropriately termed *bullae* (see Fig. 24-11). Subpleural bullae often are considered to be manifestations of paraseptal emphysema, although they may be seen in all types of emphysema and also as an isolated phenomenon.

HRCT may be useful in the detection of apical subpleural bullae invisible on radiographs in patients with idiopathic spontaneous pneumothorax. This form of pneumothorax occurs most often in tall young adults and is thought to be due to rupture of a subpleural bulla. Apical subpleural emphysema is visible on CT in 80% to 90% of patients with spontaneous pneumothorax.

Although paraseptal emphysema may superficially mimic the appearance of honeycombing, several differences make it possible to distinguish between these entities. Paraseptal emphysema occurs in a single layer at the pleural surface (see Fig. 24-11B and C), whereas honeycombing typically occurs in multiple layers. Paraseptal emphysema is most severe in the apices (see Fig. 24-11); honeycombing is almost always most severe at the bases. Paraseptal emphysema often is associated with cystic spaces larger than 1 cm; such spaces are uncommon with honeycombing.

Bullous Emphysema

The term *bullous emphysema* does not represent a specific pathologic entity, but refers to the presence of emphysema associated with large bullae (Table 24-5). It usually is seen

TABLE 24-5. BULLOUS EMPHYSEMA

Emphysema associated with bullae
May be seen with paraseptal or centrilobular emphysema
Cigarette smoking or idiopathic
"Vanishing lung syndrome"
Large bullae
Often upper lobe
Often asymmetric
Compression of normal lung
Bullae increase or sometimes resolve

in patients with centrilobular or paraseptal emphysema (see Figs. 24-8 and 24-11). A syndrome of bullous emphysema, or *giant bullous emphysema*, has been described based on clinical and radiologic features, and is also known as "vanishing lung syndrome" or "primary bullous disease of the lung." Giant bullous emphysema often is seen in young men, and is characterized by the presence of large, progressive, upper lobe bullae, which occupy a significant volume of a hemithorax, and often are asymmetric (Figs. 24-12 and 24-13). Arbitrarily, giant bullous emphysema is said to be present if bullae occupy at least one-third of a hemithorax. Most patients with giant bullous emphysema are cigarette smokers, but this entity may also occur in nonsmokers.

Typically, bullae increase progressively in size over time. Rarely, bullae may spontaneously decrease in size or disappear, usually as a result of secondary infection or obstruction of the proximal airway. Spontaneous pneumothorax is common.

Quantitative Evaluation of Emphysema

Although routine axial HRCT images usually suffice for evaluating emphysema, minimum-intensity projection (MinIP) images may be used, especially in cases with subtle disease. Coronal reconstructions may be useful in showing the distribution of emphysema.

Emphysema may be quantitated visually or based on CT measurements. Usually visual quantitation of emphysema as mild, moderate, or severe, and a determination of its type and distribution, are sufficient for clinical purposes.

Computer analysis of digital data obtained from HRCT also has been used to determine the severity of emphysema. The simplest method involves the use of a threshold value below which emphysema is considered to be present and a determination of the percentage of lung below that threshold; this is termed the "density mask" or "pixel index" technique. Normal lung density usually varies from -770 HU to -875 HU; on HRCT, emphysema is considered to be present if density measures less than -950 HU.

Complications and Exacerbation of Emphysema and COPD

Acute complications of COPD include pneumonia, infection of bullae, and pneumothorax.

Pneumonia may have a typical appearance with dense consolidation, but in patients with moderate or severe emphysema, and in patients with bullae, lung consolidation may be inhomogeneous with consolidation outlining areas of lung destruction or "holes." In this situation, the lung may have a cystic or "Swiss cheese" appearance; the appearance may mimic cavitation.

The presence of an air-fluid level in a preexisting bulla may indicate infection, hemorrhage, or neoplasm. Thickening of the wall of a bulla may be seen with chronic infection,

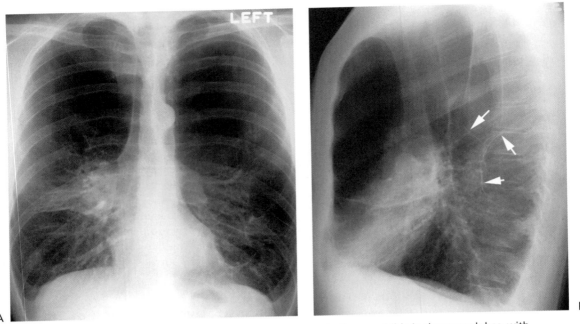

FIG. 24-12. Bullous emphysema in a young man. Large bullae are visible in the upper lobes, with displacement of normal lung to the bases. Bulla walls are visible (*arrows* in **B**).

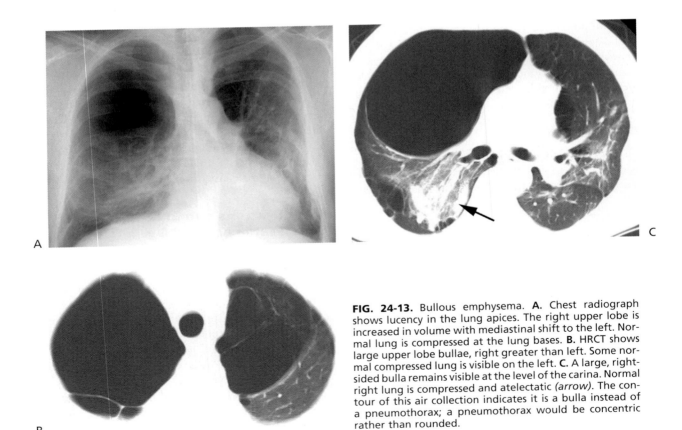

FIG. 24-13. Bullous emphysema. **A.** Chest radiograph shows lucency in the lung apices. The right upper lobe is increased in volume with mediastinal shift to the left. Normal lung is compressed at the lung bases. **B.** HRCT shows large upper lobe bullae, right greater than left. Some normal compressed lung is visible on the left. **C.** A large, right-sided bulla remains visible at the level of the carina. Normal right lung is compressed and atelectatic *(arrow)*. The contour of this air collection indicates it is a bulla instead of a pneumothorax; a pneumothorax would be concentric rather than rounded.

particularly associated with *Aspergillus*, mycetoma, or neoplasm.

Pneumothorax may occur in patients with emphysema, particularly in the presence of paraseptal emphysema and bullae. COPD is the most common cause of secondary spontaneous pneumothorax (pneumothorax associated with a recognized disease). In some patients with emphysema, it may be difficult to distinguish pneumothorax and bullae on chest radiographs. CT may be valuable in this situation.

Exacerbation of symptoms in patients with COPD may be due to one of these complications. However, exacerbations more often are due to abnormalities not associated with distinct radiographic abnormalities, such as worsening airway infection, increased mucous plugging, and obstruction of small airways. Only about 15% of patients with an exacerbation of COPD show significant abnormal radiographic findings and, based on these abnormalities, treatment is changed in only 5%. It has been recommended that chest radiographs be obtained in patients with an exacerbation of COPD only if there is a history of heart disease or congestive heart failure, intravenous drug abuse, seizures, immunosuppression, other pulmonary disease, or an elevated white blood cell count, fever, chest pain, or edema.

Utility of HRCT in the Diagnosis of Emphysema and COPD

HRCT is more sensitive and accurate than plain radiographs in diagnosing the presence, type, and extent of emphysema. Furthermore, HRCT has a high specificity for diagnosing emphysema; emphysema rarely is over diagnosed in normal individuals or in patients with severe hyperinflation due to other causes.

In clinical practice, however, HRCT rarely is used to diagnose emphysema. Usually, some combination of a smoking history, a low diffusing capacity, airway obstruction on pulmonary function tests, and chest radiographs showing large lung volumes or lung destruction is sufficient to make the diagnosis. On the other hand, some patients with early emphysema present with clinical findings more typical of interstitial lung disease or pulmonary vascular disease, namely shortness of breath and low diffusing capacity, without evidence of airway obstruction on pulmonary function tests or emphysema on chest films. In such patients, HRCT can be valuable in making the diagnosis of emphysema, obviating lung biopsy.

HRCT also can be valuable in the preoperative assessment of patients before surgical treatment of emphysema (e.g., bullectomy, lung transplantation, volume reduction surgery). HRCT has become routine in the evaluation of such patients, both before and after operation. It is used to determine the type, severity, and distribution of emphysema (Fig. 24-14). Lung volume reduction surgery, in which areas of emphysematous lung are resected, works best when emphysema predominates in the upper lobes.

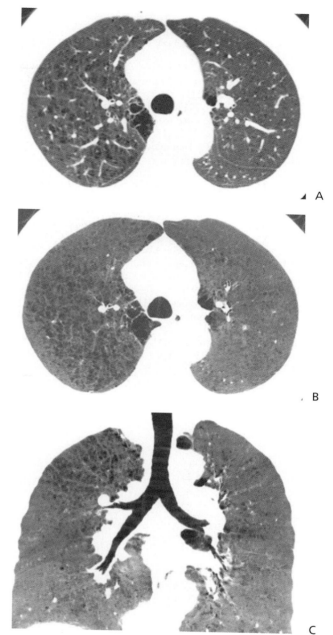

FIG. 24-14. Distribution of centrilobular emphysema shown using volumetric CT reformations. **A.** HRCT in a patient with centrilobular emphysema shows lucencies predominating in the right upper lobe. **B.** Minimum intensity projection image at the same level shows the right upper lobe predominance of disease. **C.** Coronal minimum intensity projection reformation shows the upper lobe predominance typical of centrilobular emphysema.

SELECTED READING

American Thoracic Society. Standards for the diagnosis and care of patients with chronic obstructive pulmonary disease (COPD) and asthma. Am Rev Respir Dis 1987; 136:225–243.

Arakawa H, Kurihara Y, Nakajima Y, et al. Computed tomography measurements of overinflation in chronic obstructive pulmonary disease: evaluation of various radiographic signs. J Thorac Imag 1998; 13:188–192.

Burki NK. Roentgenologic diagnosis of emphysema: accurate or not? Chest 1989; 1178–1179.

Burki NL, Krumpelman JL. Correlation of pulmonary function with the chest roentgenogram in chronic airway obstruction. Am Rev Respir Dis 1980; 121:217–223.

Fishman A, Martinez F, Naunheim K, et al. A randomized trial comparing lung-volume-reduction surgery with medical therapy for severe emphysema. N Engl J Med 2003; 348:2059–2073.

Foster WL Jr, Gimenez EI, Roubidoux MA, et al. The emphysemas: radiologic-pathologic correlations. Radiographics 1993; 13:311–328.

Gevenois PA, de Maertelaer V, De Vuyst P, et al. Comparison of computed density and macroscopic morphometry in pulmonary emphysema. Am J Respir Crit Care Med 1995; 152:653–657.

Gevenois PA, De Vuyst P, de Maertelaer V, et al. Comparison of computed density and microscopic morphometry in pulmonary emphysema. Am J Respir Crit Care Med 1996; 154:187–192.

Guest PJ, Hansell DM. High resolution computed tomography (HRCT) in emphysema associated with alpha-1-antitrypsin deficiency. Clin Radiol 1992; 45:260–266.

Janoff A. Elastases and emphysema. Current assessment of the protease-antiprotease hypothesis. Am Rev Respir Dis 1985; 132:417–433.

Lesur O, Delorme N, Fromaget JM, et al. Computed tomography in the etiologic assessment of idiopathic spontaneous pneumothorax. Chest 1990; 98:341–347.

Pratt PC. Role of conventional chest radiography in diagnosis and exclusion of emphysema. Am J Med 1987; 82:998–1006.

Rationale and design of the National Emphysema Treatment Trial (NETT): a prospective randomized trial of lung volume reduction surgery. J Thorac Cardiovasc Surg 1999; 118:518–528.

Reich SB, Weinshelbaum A, Yee J. Correlation of radiographic measurements and pulmonary function tests in chronic obstructive pulmonary disease. AJR Am J Roentgenol 1985; 144:695–699.

Remy-Jardin M, Remy J, Gosselin B, et al. Sliding thin slab, minimum intensity projection technique in the diagnosis of emphysema: histopathologic-CT correlation. Radiology 1996; 200:665–671.

Sherman S, Skoney JA, Ravikrishnan KP. Routine chest radiographs in exacerbations of chronic obstructive pulmonary disease: diagnostic value. Arch Intern Med 1989; 149:2493–2496.

Slone RM, Gierada DS, Yusen RD. Preoperative and postoperative imaging in the surgical management of pulmonary emphysema. Radiol Clin North Am 1998; 36:57–89.

Stern EJ, Webb WR, Weinacker A, Müller NL. Idiopathic giant bullous emphysema (vanishing lung syndrome): imaging findings in nine patients. AJR Am J Roentgenol 1994; 162:279–282.

Sutinen S, Christoforidis AJ, Klugh GA, Pratt PC. Roentgenologic criteria for the recognition of nonsymptomatic pulmonary emphysema: correlation between roentgenologic findings and pulmonary pathology. Am Rev Respir Dis 1965; 91:69–76.

Thurlbeck WM, Müller NL. Emphysema: definition, imaging, and quantification. AJR Am J Roentgenol 1994; 163:1017–1025.

Thurlbeck WM, Simon G. Radiographic appearance of the chest in emphysema. AJR Am J Roentgenol 1978; 130:429–440.

25

DIFFUSE CYSTIC LUNG DISEASES

W. RICHARD WEBB

A **cyst** is a thin-walled, well-defined, air-containing lung lesion 1 cm or more in diameter. Cysts may be seen in patients with emphysema (i.e., bullae; see Figs. 24-3, 24-8, 24-12, and 24-13 in Chapter 24); honeycombing (i.e., large honeycomb cysts; see Fig. 10-17B in Chapter 10); pneumonia (i.e., pneumatoceles) (Fig. 25-1); cystic bronchiectasis (i.e., dilated bronchi) (Fig. 25-2; see also Fig. 9-28 in Chapter 9); subacute hypersensitivity pneumonitis; trauma with lung lacerations (see Fig. 9-36 in Chapter 9); multiple healing cavities; and some parasitic infections (Table 25-1). The differential diagnosis (see Table 9-6 in Chapter 9) overlaps with that of multiple cavitary masses.

Several rare lung diseases are characterized by cysts as the primary abnormality. These are rare, and include Langerhans cell histiocytosis, lymphangiomyomatosis, tuberous sclerosis, neurofibromatosis, and LIP and Sjögren's syndrome. Another rare disease, tracheobronchial papillomatosis, is discussed in Chapter 3.

PULMONARY LANGERHANS CELL HISTIOCYTOSIS (PULMONARY HISTIOCYTOSIS X)

The term *Langerhans cell histiocytosis* (LCH) refers to a group of diseases of unknown etiology, most often recognized in childhood, in which Langerhans cell accumulations involve one or more body systems, including bone, lung, pituitary gland, mucous membranes and skin, lymph nodes, and liver. This disease also is known as *histiocytosis X* or *eosinophilic granuloma* (Table 25-2). Lung involvement in LCH is common, seen in 40% of patients, and may be an isolated abnormality. In patients with multisystem disease, other commonly affected sites include bone and the pituitary gland.

In the early stage, pulmonary LCH is characterized by the presence of granulomas containing large numbers of Langerhans cells and eosinophils, resulting in destruction of lung tissue. LCH lesions typically are peribronchiolar in distribution. In the later stages of the disease, the cellular granulomas are replaced by fibrosis and lung cysts. Although

LCH is characterized by a clonal proliferation of cells, it is likely that LCH in adults represents an abnormal immune response in response to a unidentified antigenic stimulus rather than a neoplasm.

Over 90% of adult patients are smokers, and LCH is considered to be related to smoking in most cases. Most patients with pulmonary LCH are young or middle-aged adults (average age, 32 years). Common presenting symptoms include cough and dyspnea. Up to 20% of patients present with pneumothorax.

Compared to patients with multisystem disease, the prognosis in patients with isolated pulmonary involvement is good; the disease regresses spontaneously in 25% and stabilizes clinically and radiographically in 50%. In the remaining 25% of cases, the disease follows a progressive downhill course, resulting in diffuse cystic lung destruction. In a small number of cases, death results from either respiratory insufficiency or pulmonary hypertension.

Radiographic Findings

The radiographic findings of LCH include reticular, nodular, and reticulonodular patterns, often in combination

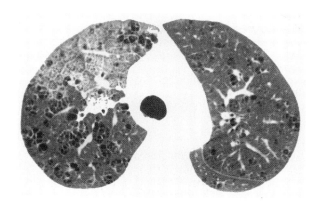

FIG. 25-1. Pneumocystis pneumonia with pneumatoceles. Ground-glass opacity representing acute pneumonia is associated with multiple clustered lung cysts. This appearance is common in pneumocystis pneumonia.

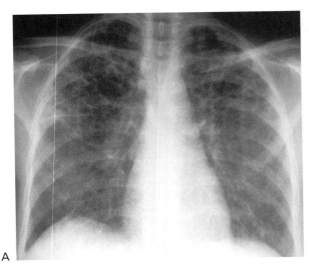

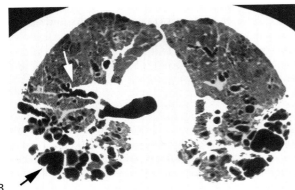

FIG. 25-2. Sarcoidosis with extensive upper lobe cystic bronchiectasis. **A.** Chest radiograph shows a cystic appearance in the upper lobes. **B.** HRCT shows cystic bronchiectasis, possibly associated with areas of emphysema. Abnormal bronchi and branching cysts *(arrows)* are a clue to the correct diagnosis.

TABLE 25-1. MULTIPLE LUNG CYSTS

Bullae
Honeycombing
Pneumonia with pneumatoceles (e.g., pneumocystis)
Cystic bronchiectasis
Hypersensitivity pneumonitis (subacute)
Trauma with lung lacerations
Healing cavities (e.g., abscesses, Wegener's, cavitary rheumatoid nodules)
Langerhans cell histiocytosis
Lymphangiomyomatosis
Tuberous sclerosis
Neurofibromatosis
Lymphocytic interstitial pneumonia
Sjögren's syndrome

TABLE 25-2. LANGERHANS CELL HISTIOCYTOSIS

Lung involvement in 40%; may be an isolated abnormality
90% of adult patients are smokers
Granulomas in early stages
Lung cysts late in course
Cysts irregular in shape
Upper lobe predominance
Spare costophrenic angles
Nodules or cavitary nodules in some

(Figs. 25-3 and 25-4A and B); a cystic appearance may mimic honeycombing. Abnormalities usually are bilateral, predominantly involving the middle and upper lung zones, with relative sparing of the costophrenic angles. Lung volumes are characteristically normal or increased (see Fig. 25-4A and B), an unusual appearance in the presence of reticular opacities or honeycombing.

HRCT Findings

In almost all patients, HRCT demonstrates cystic airspaces, which are usually less than 10 mm in diameter (see Figs. 25-4 to 25-6). The lung cysts have walls, which range from

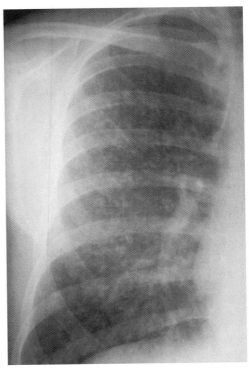

FIG. 25-3. Langerhans cell histiocytosis. Chest radiograph shows a nodular or reticulonodular pattern, predominating in the middle lung zone.

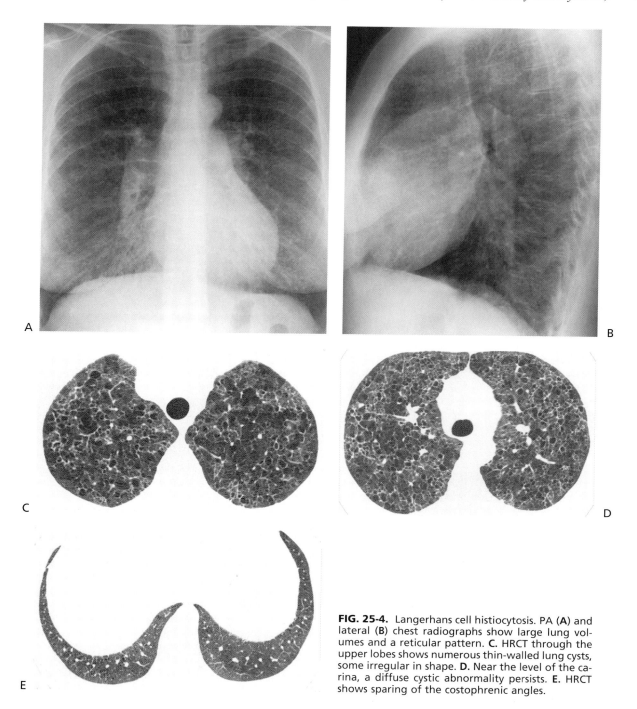

FIG. 25-4. Langerhans cell histiocytosis. PA (**A**) and lateral (**B**) chest radiographs show large lung volumes and a reticular pattern. **C.** HRCT through the upper lobes shows numerous thin-walled lung cysts, some irregular in shape. **D.** Near the level of the carina, a diffuse cystic abnormality persists. **E.** HRCT shows sparing of the costophrenic angles.

being thin and barely perceptible to being several millimeters thick. The presence of distinct walls makes it possible to differentiate these cysts from areas of emphysema. Although many cysts appear round, they can also have bizarre shapes, being bilobed or clover-leaf in appearance (see Figs. 25-4 to 25-6). An upper lobe predominance in the size and number of cysts is common (see Figs. 25-4 and 25-6). Large cysts or bullae (more than 10 mm in diameter) are seen in more than half of cases; some cysts are larger than 20 mm. True honeycombing, often suggested by the chest radiograph, does not occur.

In some patients, cysts are the only abnormality visible on HRCT, but in many cases, small nodules (usually less than 5 mm in diameter) are also present (see Fig. 25-5). Larger nodules, sometimes exceeding 1 cm, may be seen, but are less common (25%). Nodules can vary considerably

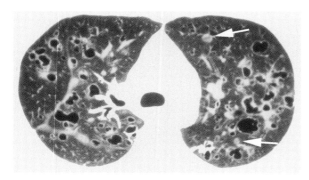

FIG. 25-5. Langerhans cell histiocytosis. HRCT shows numerous irregularly shaped cysts in the upper lobes. Nodules *(arrows)* are visible as well.

in number in individual cases, probably depending on the activity of the disease; nodules can be few in number or myriad. The margins of nodules often are irregular, particularly when there is surrounding cystic or reticular disease. On HRCT, many nodules can be seen to be peribronchial or peribronchiolar, and, therefore, centrilobular in location. Some nodules, particularly those larger than 1 cm in diameter, may show lucent centers, presumably corresponding to small "cavities." These cavities, however, sometimes represent a dilated bronchiolar lumen surrounded by peribronchiolar granulomas and thickened interstitium.

In nearly all cases, the lung bases and the costophrenic sulci are relatively spared (see Fig. 25-4). An upper lobe predominance in size and number of cysts is present in most patients (see Fig. 25-6), and a basal predominance is never observed.

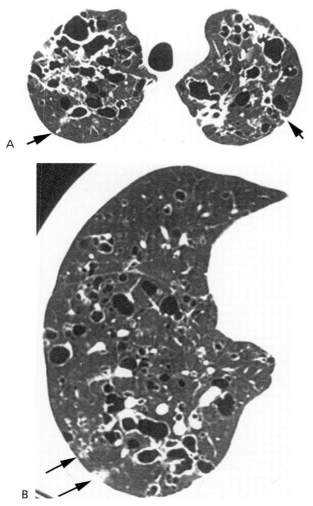

FIG. 25-6. Langerhans cell histiocytosis. **A.** HRCT shows numerous irregularly shaped cysts in the upper lobes. The cysts are thick-walled. This is characteristic of early disease. Nodules *(arrows)* also are visible. **B.** HRCT at the right lung base shows smaller and less numerous cysts as well as nodules *(arrows)*.

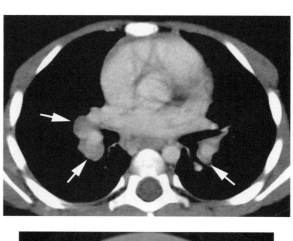

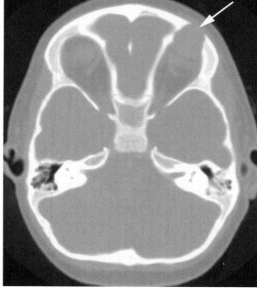

FIG. 25-7. Langerhans cell histiocytosis in a 2-year-old child. **A.** Chest CT shows hilar lymph node enlargement *(arrows)*. **B.** A lytic lesion *(arrow)* in the skull also is visible.

Pulmonary lesions may evolve in a characteristic sequence, beginning with centrilobular nodules, followed by cavitation, the formation of thick-walled cysts, and, finally, thin-walled cysts. Nodular lesions may regress spontaneously or may be replaced by cysts, but cystic lesions, once formed, persist, eventually becoming indistinguishable from diffuse emphysema.

Associated hilar or mediastinal lymph node enlargement or lytic bone lesions also may be present (Fig. 25-7).

LYMPHANGIOMYOMATOSIS

Lymphangiomyomatosis or lymphangioleiomyomatosis (LAM) is a rare disease characterized by progressive proliferation of immature-appearing smooth muscle cells (LAM cells) in relation to bronchioles, small pulmonary vessels, and lymphatics in the chest and abdomen (Table 25-3). Peribronchiolar infiltration eventually leads to bronchiolar obstruction and destruction of lung parenchyma with formation of isolated lung cysts. Very small nodules (1 to 3 mm) also may be present, representing focal proliferations of type II pneumocytes. Renal angiomyolipomas are present in 15% of cases.

Spindle cell proliferation also can involve the hilar, mediastinal, and extrathoracic lymph nodes, sometimes resulting in dilatation of intrapulmonary lymphatics and the thoracic duct. Involvement of the lymphatics can lead to chylous pleural effusions or ascites. Proliferation of cells in the walls of pulmonary veins may cause venous obstruction and lead to pulmonary venous hypertension with resultant hemoptysis.

Lymphangiomyomatosis occurs almost exclusively in women of childbearing age, usually between 17 and 50 years. Occasional cases present in postmenopausal women, probably as a result of slow progression. Although the etiology of LAM remains unclear, a chromosomal abnormality has been reported in some cases.

Most patients present with dyspnea, pneumothorax, or cough. The mean time interval from the onset of symptoms to diagnosis is typically 3 to 5 years. Sixty percent of patients have chylous pleural effusions; up to 80% have pneumothoraces; and 30% to 40% have blood-streaked sputum or frank hemoptysis. Nearly all patients have abnormal pulmonary function at presentation.

Clinical improvement has been reported following treatment with progesterone, tamoxifen, or other antiestrogen agents; radiotherapy; or oophorectomy. Responses to such treatments are variable, however. Progression is typical, and most patients die within 5 to 10 years from the onset of symptoms. As a consequence, LAM is now considered an indication for lung transplantation. The abnormality may recur in the transplanted lung.

Radiographic Findings

On plain radiographs, 80% of patients with LAM show a fine reticular pattern. In patients with advanced disease, a cystic pattern mimicking that of honeycombing may be seen (Figs. 25-8 and 25-9). Lungs usually appear to be diffusely abnormal, with the lung bases involved to the same degree as the apices. As with Langerhans histiocytosis, lung volumes often appear increased despite the presence of reticulation.

Pleural abnormalities may precede, accompany, or be seen after the recognition of lung disease. About 50% of patients have radiographic evidence of pneumothorax at the time of presentation, and unilateral or bilateral pleural effu-

TABLE 25-3. LYMPHANGIOMYOMATOSIS
Proliferation of immature-appearing smooth muscle cells
Women of childbearing age
Identical to the lung disease seen in tuberous sclerosis
Cystic lung destruction
Chylous effusions
Renal angiomyolipomas are present in 15%
Lung cysts
Round in shape
Diffuse distribution
Involve the costophrenic angles
Nodules occasionally seen

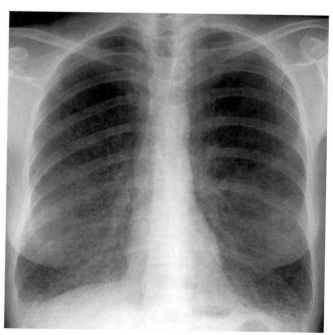

FIG. 25-8. Lymphangiomyomatosis. Chest radiograph shows increased lung volume with reticular opacities at the lung bases. Blunting of the costophrenic angles results from chylous effusions.

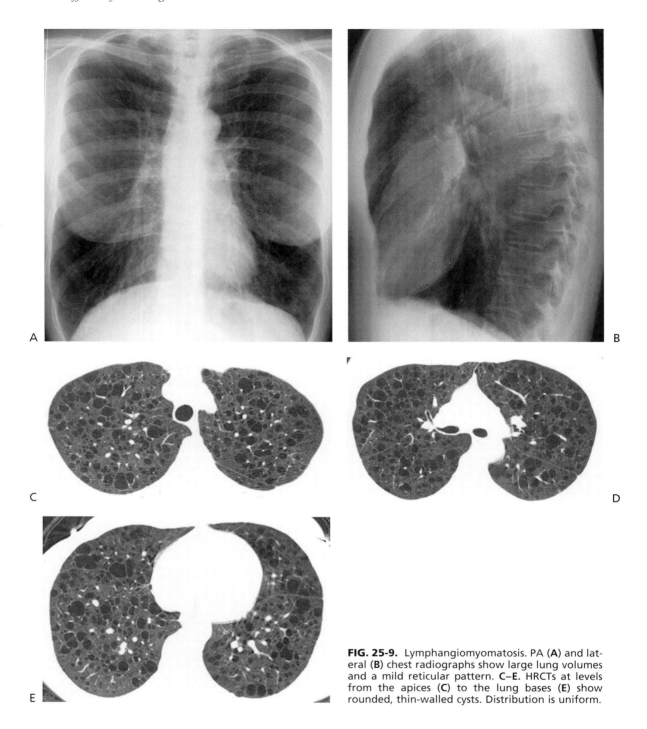

FIG. 25-9. Lymphangiomyomatosis. PA (**A**) and lateral (**B**) chest radiographs show large lung volumes and a mild reticular pattern. **C–E.** HRCTs at levels from the apices (**C**) to the lung bases (**E**) show rounded, thin-walled cysts. Distribution is uniform.

sion is present in 10% to 20% of cases (see Fig. 25-8). About 10% to 25% of patients have normal-appearing radiographs at presentation despite the presence of lung cysts.

HRCT Findings

On HRCT, patients with LAM characteristically show numerous, isolated, thin-walled, rounded lung cysts (see Fig. 25-9). These cysts usually range from 2 to 5 mm in diameter, but may be larger. Their size tends to increase with progression of the disease. In patients with extensive disease in which 80% or more of the lung parenchyma is involved, most cysts are more than 1 cm in diameter. The walls of the lung cysts usually are thin and faintly perceptible. Irregularly shaped lung cysts, as are seen in patients with LCH, are uncommon.

The cysts are most often distributed diffusely throughout the lungs, from apex to base, and no lung zone is spared (see Fig. 25-9); diffuse lung involvement is seen even in patients with mild disease.

In most patients, the lung parenchyma between the cysts appears normal on HRCT. In some cases, however, a slight increase in linear interstitial markings, interlobular septal thickening, or patchy areas of ground-glass opacity also are seen. The latter probably represent areas of pulmonary hemorrhage. Small nodules occasionally are seen, but they are not a prominent feature of this disease as they are with LCH.

In many cases, a specific CT diagnosis may be made when characteristic diffuse, thin-walled, rounded lung cysts are identified in a woman of childbearing age.

On HRCT, as with chest radiography, pneumothorax may be seen to be associated with cysts in patients with LAM. Other features of LAM include pleural effusion and hilar, mediastinal, and retrocrural adenopathy. Renal angiomyolipomas may be visible on scans through the upper abdomen.

TUBEROUS SCLEROSIS

Tuberous sclerosis (TS) is an autosomal-dominant genetic disease of mesoderm associated with the classic triad of seizures, mental retardation, and adenoma sebaceum. It also is associated with abnormalities such as angiomyolipomas of the kidneys, cardiac rhabdomyomas, and retinal phacomas.

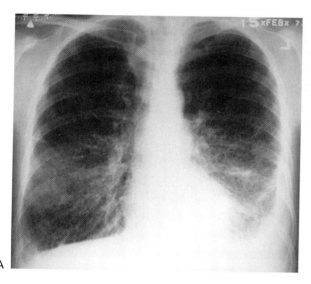

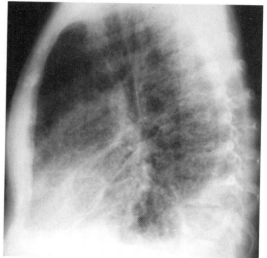

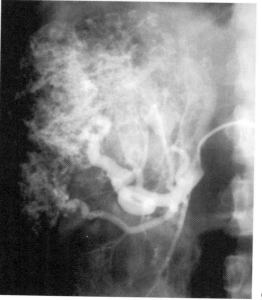

FIG. 25-10. Tuberous sclerosis. PA (**A**) and lateral (**B**) chest radiographs show large lung volumes, a reticular pattern predominant at the lung bases, and bilateral pleural effusions (largest on the left). **C.** Right renal arteriogram shows a mass with abnormal renal artery branches, consistent with angiomyolipoma.

About 1% of patients with TS have lung disease virtually identical to that of LAM, although there may be subtle histologic differences between the two entities. It is not inappropriate to think of the lung disease of TS as a subtype of LAM.

Presenting symptoms are similar. Although TS affects both sexes equally, as with LAM, pulmonary abnormalities have been described almost exclusively in women. Radiographic findings are indistinguishable in individual cases (Figs. 25-10 and 25-11), although the presence of renal angiomyolipomas is more suggestive of TS. However, angiomyolipomas may be seen in LAM in the absence of TS.

NEUROFIBROMATOSIS

Neurofibromatosis is a common genetic disorder, affecting about 1 in 3000 individuals. Thoracic manifestations are protean and include the following:

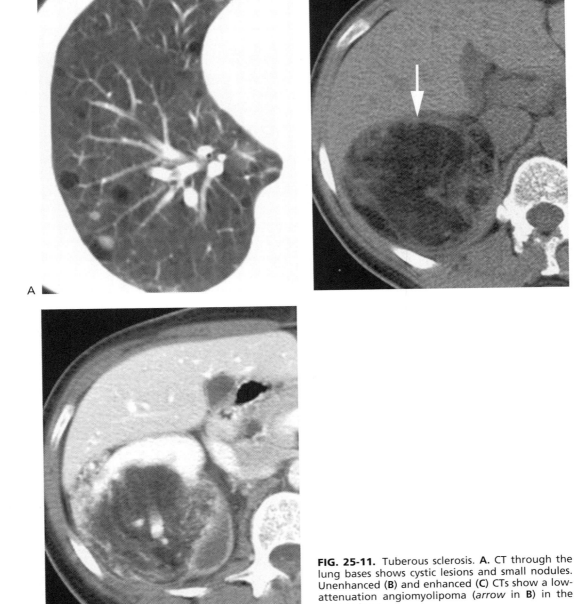

FIG. 25-11. Tuberous sclerosis. **A.** CT through the lung bases shows cystic lesions and small nodules. Unenhanced (**B**) and enhanced (**C**) CTs show a low-attenuation angiomyolipoma (*arrow* in **B**) in the right kidney.

1. Rib abnormalities, including ribbon ribs and rib notching
2. Scoliosis
3. Cutaneous or subcutaneous neurofibromas mimicking the presence of lung nodules on chest radiographs
4. Intercostal or mediastinal neurofibroma or schwannoma (see Figs. 8-65 to 8-68 in Chapter 8)
5. Paraganglioma thoracic meningocele (see Fig. 8-71 in Chapter 8)

Lung disease is present in 10% to 20% of adult patients with neurofibromatosis. It is characterized histologically by bullae in the upper lobes and interstitial fibrosis at the lung bases. Patients typically present with dyspnea.

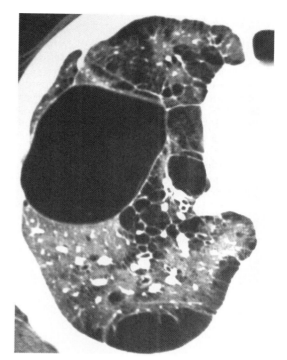

FIG. 25-13. Neurofibromatosis. HRCT shows cysts and bullae indistinguishable from emphysema.

Radiographs usually show upper lobe lucency or bullae, which usually is symmetrical. A reticular pattern, which sometimes is characterized by Kerley's B lines, is seen at the lung bases in 50% of cases (Fig. 25-12). Lung volumes typically are increased, with flattening of the diaphragms. HRCT may show isolated cysts or bullae (Fig. 25-13).

LYMPHOID INTERSTITIAL PNEUMONIA AND SJÖGREN'S SYNDROME

Lymphoid interstitial pneumonia (LIP) is a benign lymphoproliferative disorder characterized by a diffuse interstitial infiltrate of lymphocytes and plasma cells. LIP often occurs in association with collagen-vascular disease and Sjögren's syndrome.

Although both LIP and Sjögren's syndrome may show a variety of radiographic and HRCT abnormalities, including a reticular or reticulonodular pattern and patchy or diffuse ground-glass opacity (see Chapters 13 and 14), multiple thin-walled lung cysts may be the primary manifestation of collagen disease, representing LIP (see Figs. 13-27, 13-29, and 13-30 in Chapter 13). Cysts may be small or large, and may be an isolated abnormality or may be accompanied by other findings of LIP or Sjögren's syndrome, such as ground-glass opacity. The cysts tend to be fewer in number than in patients with LCH or LAM.

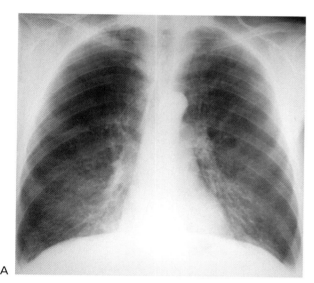

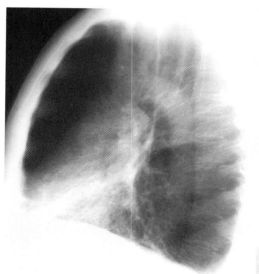

FIG. 25-12. Neurofibromatosis. PA **(A)** and lateral **(B)** chest radiographs show large lung volumes with upper lobe lucency and a reticular pattern predominant at the lung bases.

SELECTED READING

Aberle DR, Hansell DM, Brown K, Tashkin DP. Lymphangiomyomatosis: CT, chest radiographic, and functional correlations. Radiology 1990; 176:381–387.

Brauner MW, Grenier P, Mouelhi MM, et al. Pulmonary histiocytosis X: evaluation with high resolution CT. Radiology 1989; 172:255–258.

Chu SC, Horiba K, Usuki J, et al. Comprehensive evaluation of 35 patients with lymphangioleiomyomatosis. Chest 1999; 115: 1041–1052.

Howarth DM, Gilchrist GS, Mullan BP, et al. Langerhans cell histiocytosis: diagnosis, natural history, management, and outcome. Cancer 1999; 85:2278–2290.

Johkoh T, Müller NL, Pickford HA, et al. Lymphocytic interstitial pneumonia: thin-section CT findings in 22 patients. Radiology 1999; 212:567–572.

Kirchner J, Stein A, Viel K, et al. Pulmonary lymphangioleiomyomatosis: high-resolution CT findings. Eur Radiol 1999; 9:49–54.

Kitaichi M, Nishimura K, Itoh H, Izumi T. Pulmonary lymphangioleiomyomatosis: a report of 46 patients including a clinicopathologic study of prognostic factors. Am J Respir Crit Care Med 1995; 151:527–533.

Lenoir S, Grenier P, Brauner MW, et al. Pulmonary lymphangiomyomatosis and tuberous sclerosis: comparison of radiographic and thin-section CT findings. Radiology 1990; 175:329–334.

Moore AD, Godwin JD, Müller NL, et al. Pulmonary histiocytosis X: comparison of radiographic and CT findings. Radiology 1989; 172:249–254.

Müller NL, Chiles C, Kullnig P. Pulmonary lymphangiomyomatosis: correlation of CT with radiographic and functional findings. Radiology 1990; 175:335–339.

Templeton PA, McLoud TC, Müller NL, et al. Pulmonary lymphangioleiomyomatosis: CT and pathologic findings. J Comput Assist Tomogr 1989; 13:54–57.

26

THE PLEURA AND PLEURAL DISEASE

W. RICHARD WEBB

INTERLOBAR FISSURES

The interlobar fissures represent invaginations of the visceral pleura separating the lobes. Recognizing the fissures is essential in the localization and diagnosis of both pleural and parenchymal abnormalities.

The Major (Oblique) Fissure

On the left, the major fissure separates the lower lobe from the upper lobe. On the right, it separates the lower lobe from the upper and middle lobes (see Figs. 2-29 and 2-30 in Chapter 2).

The major fissures originate posteriorly, above the level of the aortic arch, near the level of the fifth thoracic vertebra, and angle anteriorly and inferiorly, nearly parallel to the sixth rib. Posteriorly the superior aspect of the left major fissure is cephalad to the right in 75%. They terminate along the anterior diaphragmatic pleural surface of each hemithorax, several centimeters posterior to the anterior chest wall.

Portions of one or both major fissures are almost always visible on the lateral radiograph. A thin triangular opacity representing fat is seen in 20% of cases at the point the major fissure contacts the hemidiaphragm. A similar opacity may be seen in the presence of a small amount of pleural fluid.

The major fissures can be distinguished on the lateral radiograph in several ways:

1. The surface of the right hemidiaphragm is visible in its entirety in most patients, while the anterior surface of the left hemidiaphragm is usually obscured by the heart; if a fissure is visible in continuity with the anterior part of a complete diaphragm, it is the right major fissure.
2. The left hemidiaphragm may be identified by its intimate relationship to the stomach bubble; this may in turn allow identification of the left posterior costophrenic angle, the left posterior ribs, and then the left major fissure in continuity with the posterior ribs.
3. The right posterior ribs are usually projected posterior to the left on a well-positioned left lateral radiograph and appear larger than the left ribs because they are far-

ther from the film and more magnified. This is termed the "big rib" sign. A fissure in contiguity with "big ribs" is the right major fissure.
4. The right major fissure may be identified if it is seen contacting the minor fissure.

The major fissures are not clearly seen on frontal radiographs in normal subjects. In 5% to 10% of patients, however, a subtle arcuate opacity may be seen in the upper thorax, extending superiorly and medially from the lateral thorax, representing contact of the superior major fissure with the posterolateral chest wall; this opacity is likely related to a small amount of fat entering the edge of the fissure. Typically, it is sharply margined on its undersurface and ill defined superiorly. A similar but more apparent opacity may be seen with pleural effusion (Fig. 26-1) extending into the posterior part of the major fissure.

On CT, the major fissures are oriented obliquely to the scan plane, and because of volume averaging, their appearance is variable depending on slice thickness.

With a 7- to 10-mm slice thickness, the fissures themselves are visible in only 20% to 40% of cases, although the location of each fissure can usually be inferred because of the presence of an avascular band, several centimeters thick, within the lung parenchyma. These bands appear "avascular" because of the small size of vessels located in the peripheral lung on either side of the fissure. In up to 20% of cases, the major fissures are visible on thick collimated scans as ill-defined bands of opacity, due to volume averaging of the fissure with adjacent lung or hypoinflation of the dependent portions of the upper lobes, adjacent to the fissure. Occasionally the fissure is visible as a linear opacity.

On CT obtained using thin collimation or high-resolution technique, the major fissures usually appear as thin, well-defined lines surrounded by a plane of relatively avascular lung measuring about 1 cm thick. The orientation of the major fissures varies at different levels. In the upper thorax, the major fissures angle posterolaterally from the mediastinum (see Fig. 2-30A in Chapter 2). Within the lower thorax, the major fissures angle anterolaterally from the mediastinum. In nearly 20% of cases, a focal thickening

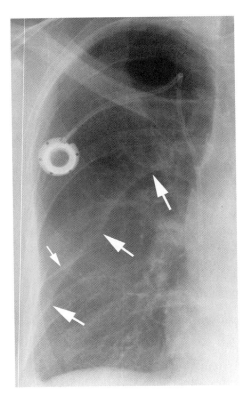

FIG. 26-1. Small pleural effusion outlining the posterior major fissure. The normal location of the major fissure where it contacts the posterolateral chest wall is well shown *(large arrows).* As in this case, it is sharply marginated on its undersurface and ill-defined superiorly. The minor fissure is also visible *(small arrow).*

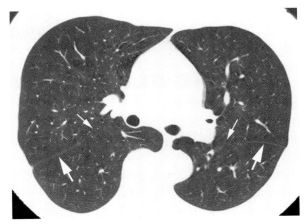

FIG. 26-2. Incomplete major fissures. HRCT shows normal-appearing major fissures laterally *(large arrows).* Medially, the fissures are invisible *(small arrows).*

of the fissure is seen on CT just above its point of contact with the diaphragm; this represents fat extending into the fissure.

If a portion of the fissure is invisible on HRCT, it likely indicates that the fissure is incomplete with partial fusion of the lobes (Fig. 26-2). Incomplete fissures provide a pathway for collateral ventilation or spread of disease from one lobe to another. The right major fissure is incomplete in 70%, and some degree of fusion is present between the lower lobe and the upper lobe in 70% and between the lower lobe and middle lobe in 50%. On the left, the major fissure has been reported to be complete in 30% to 60% of patients.

In some cases, cardiac motion during the scan results in a confusing artifact termed the double-fissure sign; when this artifact is present, the fissure is visible in two locations on the same scan.

The Minor (Horizontal) Fissure

The minor or horizontal fissure separates the superior aspect of the right middle lobe from the right upper lobe. The

minor fissure is incomplete in more than 80% of cases, most often laterally (see Figs. 2-29 and 2-30 in Chapter 2).

On a frontal radiograph, the minor fissure or a portion of the fissure is visible in 50% to 80% of cases, appearing as a roughly horizontal line, generally at or near the level of the anterior fourth rib. Its contour is variable, but its lateral part is often visible inferior to its medial part. Medially, the fissure usually appears to arise at the level of the right hilum and interlobar pulmonary artery.

On the lateral radiograph, the anterior part of the fissure often appears inferior to its posterior part. The posterior part of the fissure may be seen to end at the major fissure or may appear to extend posterior to it.

On conventional CT obtained with 7- to 10-mm collimation, the minor fissure is rarely visible, as its position generally parallels the scan plane. Characteristically, however, the position of the minor fissure can be inferred because of a broad avascular region in the anterior portion of the right lung, anterior to the major fissure, at the level of the bronchus intermedius. This avascular region represents peripheral lung on each side of the fissure, lying in or near the plane of scan. The avascular region is often triangular, with the one corner of the triangle at the pulmonary hilum and the other two corners laterally. However, there is considerable variation in the appearance of the minor fissure due to variations in its orientation and curvature. In some cases, the avascular plane of the minor fissure appears rectangular, round, or elliptical.

The appearance of the minor fissure on HRCT scans is quite variable (Fig. 26-3). Depending on its orientation and contour, the fissure may appear as (1) a linear opacity, directed from anterior to posterior; (2) a linear opacity extending from medial to lateral, paralleling and anterior to the major fissure (see Fig. 26-3A); (3) a circle or ring (see Fig.

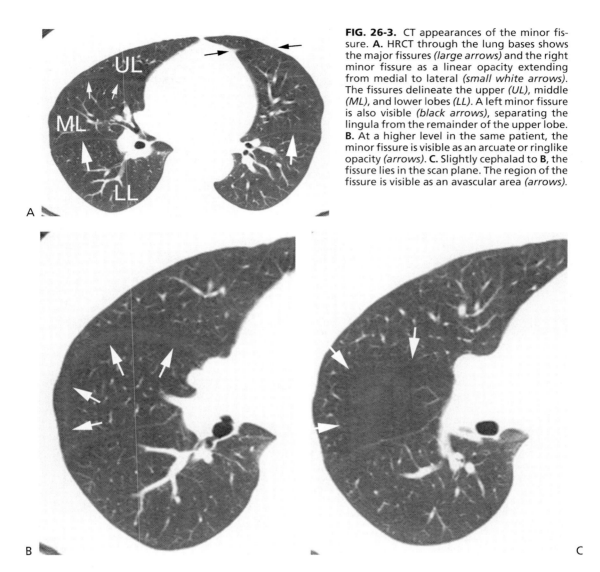

FIG. 26-3. CT appearances of the minor fissure. **A.** HRCT through the lung bases shows the major fissures *(large arrows)* and the right minor fissure as a linear opacity extending from medial to lateral *(small white arrows)*. The fissures delineate the upper *(UL)*, middle *(ML)*, and lower lobes *(LL)*. A left minor fissure is also visible *(black arrows)*, separating the lingula from the remainder of the upper lobe. **B.** At a higher level in the same patient, the minor fissure is visible as an arcuate or ringlike opacity *(arrows)*. **C.** Slightly cephalad to **B**, the fissure lies in the scan plane. The region of the fissure is visible as an avascular area *(arrows)*.

26-3B); or (4) an ill-defined opacity or avascular regions resulting from the fissure lying in the plane of scan (see Fig. 26-3C).

Because the minor fissure often angles caudally, the lower lobe, middle lobe, and upper lobe can all be seen on a single HRCT scan (see Fig. 26-3A). If this is the case, the major and minor fissures can have a similar appearance, with the major fissure being posterior and the minor fissure anterior; in this situation, the lower lobe is most posterior, the upper lobe is most anterior, and the middle lobe is in the middle. If the minor fissure is concave caudally, it can appear ring shaped, with the middle lobe in the center of the ring (see Fig. 26-3B).

Accessory Fissures

Accessory fissures separate a lung segment or a part of a lobe from the remainder of a lobe; numerous accessory fissures have been identified. As many as 50% of lungs show an accessory fissure, but these are less often visible radiographically.

An **azygos fissure** is present in 1 in 200 subjects, defining the presence of an **azygos lobe** (Fig. 26-4). An azygos lobe represents parts of the apical or posterior segments of the right upper lobe. An azygos fissure and azygos lobe are formed when the azygos vein invaginates the right upper lobe during gestation. The azygos fissure consists of four layers of pleura (two parietal and two visceral) and contains the arch of the azygos vein inferiorly. On the frontal radiograph, the azygos fissure has a characteristic curvilinear appearance adjacent to the right mediastinum, convex laterally; the azygos vein has a teardrop appearance at the inferior extent of the fissure. The azygos fissure is identifiable on CT as a thin, curved line. It extends from the right brachiocephalic vein, anteriorly, to a position adjacent to the right posterolateral aspect of the T4 or T5 vertebral

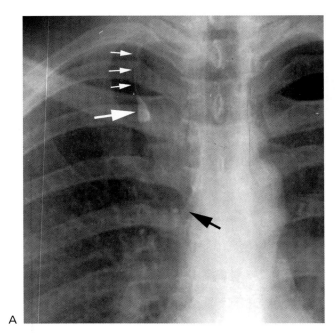

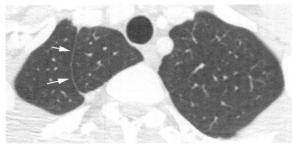

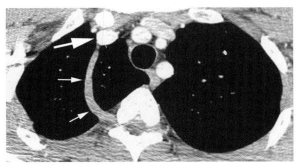

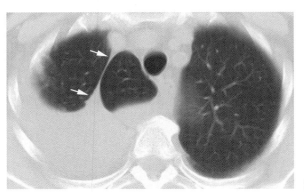

FIG. 26-4. Azygos fissure and azygos lobe. **A.** Chest radiograph shows the characteristic curvilinear appearance of the azygos fissure adjacent to the right mediastinum *(small arrows)*. The azygos arch is visible within the right upper lobe *(large white arrow)* and has a teardrop appearance. The azygos arch is not visible in its normal location *(black arrow)*. **B.** CT shows the typical curved appearance of the azygos fissure *(arrows)*. **C.** At a lower level, the azygos arch *(small arrows)* extends from the right brachiocephalic vein anteriorly *(large arrow)* to a posterior and paravertebral location. **D.** Thickening of the azygos fissure *(arrows)* due to right pleural effusion in a different patient.

body (see Fig. 26-4B and C). A left "azygos" fissure, associated with the left superior intercostal vein, is rarely seen.

The **inferior accessory fissure** separates the medial basal segment of either lower lobe from the remaining basal segments. It is present anatomically in 30% to 45% of lobes. On plain radiographs, this fissure is visible in 10%, extending superiorly and medially from the medial third of the hemidiaphragm. On CT it is seen in 15% of cases extending laterally and anteriorly from the region of the inferior pulmonary ligament to join the major fissure (Fig. 26-5).

The **superior accessory fissure** demarcates the superior segment from the remainder of the lower lobe; it is more common on the right. It is seen at about the same level as the minor fissure.

The **left minor fissure** is present anatomically in approximately 10% of normal lungs, separating the lingula from the remainder of the left upper lobe (Figs. 26-3A and 26-6). It is visible on plain radiographs in about 1%, appearing somewhat higher than the right minor fissure.

INFERIOR PULMONARY LIGAMENTS AND PHRENIC NERVES

The right and left inferior pulmonary ligaments each represent a double layer of pleura that serves to anchor the lung to the mediastinum. They are formed as reflections of the visceral pleura lining the medial surfaces of the lower lobes onto the mediastinal pleural surface. They extend inferiorly and posteriorly from just below the pulmonary hila to the diaphragm. The ligaments can terminate before reaching the diaphragm or extend over the medial diaphragmatic surface. They may divide the medial pleural space below the hila into anterior and posterior compartments. The ligaments may also contain systemic vessels supplying the lung.

The inferior pulmonary ligaments are invisible on chest radiographs. On CT, they are visible as very short, thin, linear or triangular opacities below the level of the right and left inferior pulmonary veins, and often adjacent to the esophagus (Fig. 26-7). Although they do not extend into

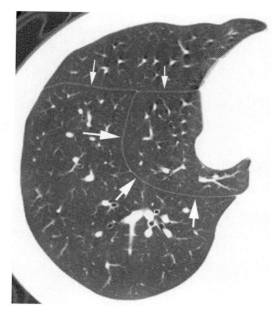

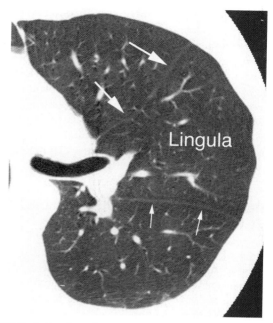

FIG. 26-5. Inferior accessory fissure. The fissure *(large arrows)* separates the medial basal segment of the lower lobe from the remainder of the basal segments. The major fissure *(small arrows)* is noted anteriorly.

FIG. 26-6. Left minor fissure. The minor fissure *(large arrows)* separates the lingular segments from the remainder of the upper lobe. The major fissure *(small arrows)* is also seen.

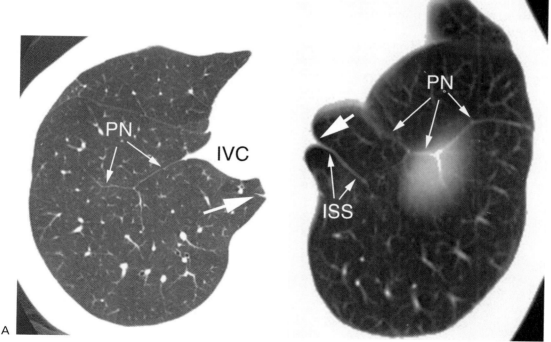

FIG. 26-7. The inferior pulmonary ligaments and pleural reflections over the phrenic nerves. **A.** HRCT on the right shows the inferior pulmonary ligament as a thin triangular opacity *(large arrow)* arising in the region of the esophagus. The pleural reflection overlying the right phrenic nerve *(PN)* is seen lateral to the inferior vena cava *(IVC)*. **B.** CT on the left shows the inferior pulmonary ligament as a triangular opacity *(large arrow)* lateral to the esophagus. A linear opacity extending from the inferior pulmonary ligament into the lung represents the intersublobar septum *(ISS)*. The pleural reflection overlying the left phrenic nerve *(PN)* is seen more anteriorly.

the lung parenchyma, they often appear contiguous with a connective tissue septum in the medial lung, termed the *intersublobar septum* (see Fig. 26-7B). On CT the inferior pulmonary ligaments are visible in 40% to 70% of cases.

Similar thin lines may be seen on CT anterior to the inferior pulmonary ligaments, representing pleural reflections over the right and left phrenic nerves (see Fig. 26-7). On the right, this opacity is usually seen lateral to the inferior vena cava (see Fig. 26-7A). The pleural reflections may be seen to extend over the surface of the diaphragm.

THE PLEURAL SURFACES AND ADJACENT CHEST WALL

A number of structures, arranged in layers, surround the lung and line the inner aspect of the thoracic cavity. Knowledge of their anatomy is helpful in understanding normal radiographic and CT findings and the appearances of pleural diseases (Fig. 26-8).

The combined thickness of the layers of visceral and parietal pleura that surround the lung, and the fluid-containing pleural space, is less than 0.5 mm.

External to the parietal pleura is a layer of loose areolar tissue (extrapleural fat), which separates the parietal pleura from the endothoracic fascia. This fatty layer is very thin in most locations but can be markedly thickened over the lateral or posterolateral ribs, resulting in extrapleural fat pads several millimeters thick.

The thoracic cavity is lined by the fibroelastic endothoracic fascia that covers the surface of the intercostal muscles and intervening ribs, blends with the perichondrium and periosteum of the costal cartilages and sternum anteriorly, and posteriorly is continuous with the prevertebral fascia that covers the vertebral bodies and intervertebral discs.

External to the endothoracic fascia are the three layers of the intercostal muscles. The innermost intercostal muscle passes between the internal surfaces of adjacent ribs and is relatively thin; it is separated from the inner and external

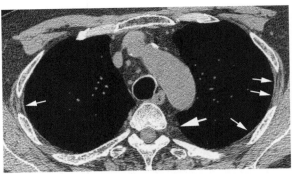

FIG. 26-9. Normal HRCT at the pleural surface. A thin white stripe between adjacent ribs *(small arrows)* represents the intercostal stripe, primarily representing the innermost intercostal muscle. In the paravertebral regions, the innermost intercostal muscle is anatomically absent. In this location *(large arrow)*, no definite line is visible.

intercostal muscles by a layer of fat and the intercostal vessels and nerve.

Although the innermost intercostal muscles are incomplete in the anterior and posterior thorax, other muscles (the transversus thoracis and subcostalis) can occupy the same relative plane. Anteriorly, the transversus thoracis muscle consists of four or five slips that arise from the xiphoid process or lower sternum and pass superolaterally from the second to sixth costal cartilages. The internal mammary vessels lie external to the transversus thoracis. Posteriorly, the subcostal muscles are thin, variable muscles that extend from the inner aspect of the angle of the lower ribs, crossing one or two ribs and intercostal spaces, to the inner aspect of a rib below.

On CT in many normal subjects, a 1- to 2-mm-thick soft tissue stripe is visible in the anterolateral and posterolateral intercostal spaces (the *intercostal stripe*) at the point of contact between lung and chest wall (Fig. 26-9). This line primarily represents the innermost intercostal muscle but also reflects the combined thicknesses of visceral and parietal pleura, the fluid-filled pleural space, the endothoracic fascia,

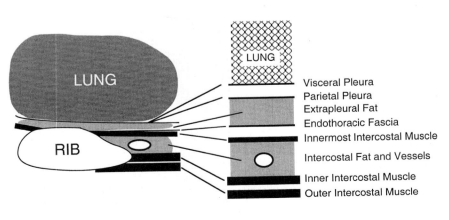

FIG. 26-8. Normal structures at the pleural surface.

and fat layers. Although the pleural layers, fluid-containing pleural space, extrapleural fat, and endothoracic fascia pass internal to the ribs, they are not normally visible in this location. A visible soft tissue stripe passing internal to the ribs or internal to the intercostal stripe (and separated from it by extrapleural fat) usually represents pleural thickening or pleural effusion.

In the paravertebral regions, the innermost intercostal muscle is anatomically absent. In this location, a very thin line (the *paravertebral line*) is sometimes visible on CT at the lung–chest wall interface; this line represents the combined thicknesses of the visceral and parietal pleura and the endo-

thoracic fascia. A visible soft tissue stripe in the paravertebral regions usually represents pleural thickening or pleural effusion.

DIAGNOSIS OF PLEURAL THICKENING

Parietal Pleural Thickening

Most causes of "pleural thickening" visible on radiographs or CT primarily affect the parietal pleura. On CT parietal pleural thickening results in five findings (Fig. 26-10 and Figs. 18-5 and 18-6 in Chapter 18):

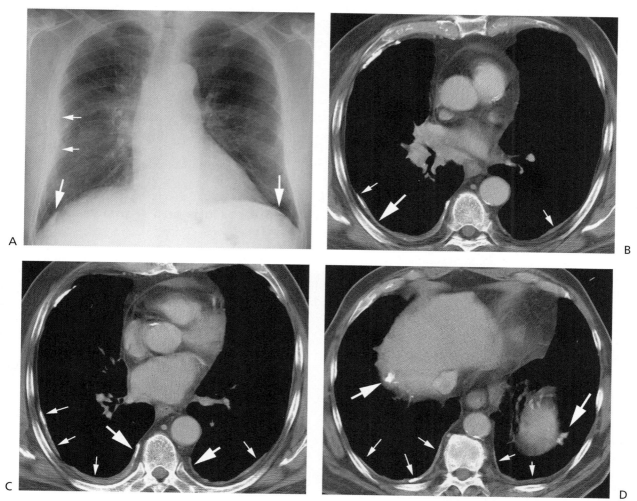

FIG. 26-10. Parietal pleural thickening and calcification in asbestos exposure. **A.** Chest radiograph shows thickened pleura separating aerated lung from the adjacent ribs *(small arrows)*. Pleural calcification *(large arrows)* is visible on the surface of the hemidiaphragms. **B.** CT shows thickened parietal pleura internal to the ribs *(large arrow)* and internal to the intercostal stripe (i.e., innermost intercostal muscle; *small arrows*). In both locations, a layer of thickened extrapleural fat separates the thickened pleura from the chest wall. Pleural calcification is also seen. **C.** Thickened parietal pleura is visible internal to the ribs and internal to the intercostal stripe (i.e., innermost intercostal muscle; *small arrows*). A stripe of density in the paravertebral regions *(large arrows)* indicates pleural thickening. **D.** At the level of the diaphragm, thickened pleura is visible in the paravertebral regions and internal to the ribs *(small arrows)*. Calcified pleura on the surface of the hemidiaphragms *(large arrows)* is typical of asbestos exposure.

1. A stripe of soft tissue density, 1 mm or more in thickness, internal to the ribs (see Fig. 26-10B and C)
2. A stripe of soft tissue density, 1 mm or more in thickness, internal to the innermost intercostal muscle and separated from it by a thin layer of extrapleural fat (see Fig. 26-10C)
3. A distinct stripe of density in the paravertebral region, 1 mm or more in thickness (see Fig. 26-10C)
4. Pleural calcification (see Fig. 26-10B–D)
5. Thickening of the normal extrapleural fat layer (see Fig. 26-10B)

Findings of parietal pleural thickening visible on chest radiographs (see Fig. 26-10) include the following:

1. Blunting of the lateral or posterior costophrenic angle (this may also result from pleural effusion)
2. A stripe of soft tissue density, several millimeters or more in thickness, separating the lung from the adjacent ribs and chest wall, either focal or diffuse (this may also result from pleural effusion)
3. Thickened soft tissue visible internal to the ribs in patients with pneumothorax
4. Pleural calcification
5. An asymmetrical increase in extrapleural fat appearing low in attenuation

Visceral Pleural Thickening

Recognizable visceral pleural thickening almost always occurs in association with parietal pleural thickening and pleural effusion; empyema is the most common cause. Visceral pleural thickening occurring in the absence of parietal pleural thickening is uncommon but may be seen in patients with lung disease, such as lung abscess or diffuse lung fibrosis.

Visceral pleural thickening cannot usually be distinguished from parietal pleural thickening on chest radiographs, although it may appear as any of the following:

1. Thickening of a fissure (this more often reflects pleural effusion)
2. Separation of the lung from the adjacent ribs and chest wall, which may be focal or diffuse, occurring in association with contiguous lung disease (this may also result from parietal pleural thickening or pleural effusion)
3. Thick pleura at the lung surface in patients with pneumothorax

On CT, visceral pleural thickening may appear as either of the following:

1. A distinct stripe of soft tissue at the lung surface in patients with pleural effusion and normal lung parenchyma
2. An enhancing stripe at the lung surface in patients with abnormal lung (thickened visceral pleura often enhances to a greater degree than airless lung)

NORMAL FINDINGS THAT MIMIC PLEURAL THICKENING

Several normal findings can mimic the findings of pleural thickening or effusion.

Normal Fat Pads

Normal extrapleural fat is most abundant over the posterolateral fourth to eighth ribs and can produce fat pads several millimeters thick that extend into the intercostal spaces.

On plain radiographs, the presence of a soft tissue stripe passing internal to the ribs, thus separating the lung from the chest wall, is generally taken to indicate the presence of a pleural thickening or effusion. However, in normal patients with extrapleural fat thickening or fat pads, a similar appearance may be seen. Pleural disease and fat thickening can usually be distinguished; in contrast to pleural thickening or effusion, normal fat thickening is typically symmetrical and smooth in contour, appears low in attenuation, and is unassociated with costophrenic angle blunting.

Normal extrapleural fat can sometimes be seen on CT internal to the ribs. This appears very low in density and is easy to distinguish from thickened pleura.

The Subcostalis and Transversus Thoracis Muscles

These are invisible on chest radiographs. On CT, a 1- to 2-mm-thick line is sometimes seen internal to one or more ribs, along the posterior chest wall at the level of the heart, representing the subcostalis muscle (Fig. 26-11). This may closely mimic the appearance of focal pleural thickening. The subcostalis muscle is visible in only a few patients.

Anteriorly, at the level of the heart and adjacent to the lower sternum or xiphoid process, the transversus thoracis muscles are nearly always visible on CT internal to the anterior ends of ribs or costal cartilages (see Fig. 26-11).

In contrast to pleural thickening, these muscles are smooth, uniform in thickness, and symmetric bilaterally.

Paravertebral Intercostal Veins

These are invisible on chest radiographs. On CT in some normal subjects, segments of intercostal veins seen in the paravertebral regions mimic pleural thickening. Continuity of these opacities with the azygos or hemiazygos veins is sometimes visible, allowing them to be correctly identified (see Fig. 26-11). Also, when viewed using lung window settings, these intercostal vein segments do not indent the lung surface; focal pleural thickening would.

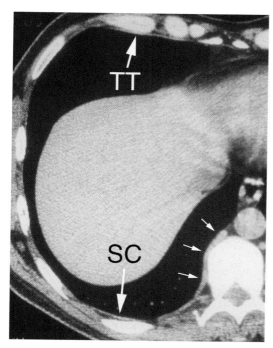

FIG. 26-11. Normal findings mimicking pleural thickening. CT shows the subcostalis muscle *(SC)*, transversus thoracis muscle *(TT)*, and intercostal veins *(small arrows)*.

DIAGNOSIS OF PLEURAL EFFUSION

Plain Radiographs

Pleural effusion cannot be distinguished from pleural thickening on chest radiographs unless high-density calcification or low-density fat is visible in relation to thick pleura or air collections are visible within a pleural fluid collection.

The pleural space extends inferiorly, below the visible lung, in relation to the diaphragm and ribs. In upright subjects, pleural fluid first accumulates in the most inferior portions of the pleural space, including the costophrenic angles and subpulmonic regions. Costophrenic angle blunting is usually the first recognizable plain film finding of pleural fluid (Fig. 26-12A and B).

At least 175 ml of pleural fluid must be present to result in blunting of the lateral costophrenic angle on the frontal radiograph, and as much as 500 ml may be present without recognizable blunting. Blunting of the posterior costophrenic angle on the lateral view requires 75 ml (see Fig. 26-12B). Blunting of the posterior costophrenic angle may sometimes be diagnosed on the frontal view by looking through the shadow of the upper abdominal contents; posterior costophrenic angle blunting results in a sharper lower edge of lung than normally seen. On a properly performed lateral decubitus film, as little as 10 ml of fluid may be seen. Very small pleural fluid collections, either unilateral or bilateral, are seen in a few normal individuals.

With increasing effusion, fluid may be seen lateral to the lower lobes, separating the lung from adjacent ribs. Because the lung is fixed medially by the hilum and inferior pulmonary ligament, medial pleural fluid collections are usually smaller (Fig. 26-13) and more difficult to recognize. Larger effusions result in a typical meniscus appearance with the level of the fluid and its density appearing greater in the lateral hemithorax. The edge separating aerated lung from pleural fluid is often sharp and well defined.

Medial fluid collections may be seen when effusions are large. Most often, these accumulate in the posterior gutters, with thickening of the paravertebral stripes. The collections may be triangular, simulating lower lobe collapse.

Pleural fluid often accumulates in the subpulmonic pleural space (*subpulmonic effusion*), allowing the lung base to float superiorly. Subpulmonic fluid collections may be difficult to recognize on frontal radiographs, although some costophrenic angle blunting, a shallow costophrenic angle, or a hazy costophrenic angle is often present. However, greater superior retraction of the lateral lung (likely because the medial lower lobe is fixed by the inferior pulmonary ligament) results in lateral displacement of what appears to the diaphragmatic dome or peak, with the lung lateral to the peak angling down sharply (Fig. 26-14). On the left side, 2 cm of separation of the lung base from the top of the stomach bubble is typically taken as evidence of a subpulmonic effusion, but this distance is variable in normal individuals.

On the lateral view (see Fig. 26-14B), a subpulmonic effusion often (1) elevates the posterior lung, flattening its undersurface; (2) insinuates itself into the major fissure, resulting in focal triangular thickening of the fissure; and (3) flattens the inferior contour of the lung anterior to the fissure, which then angles sharply downward.

Fluid may extend into the major or minor fissures. This is usually easy to recognize on the lateral radiographs as fissure thickening. On the frontal radiograph, fluid extending into the posterolateral major fissure typically results in an arcuate opacity, sharply defined medially and inferiorly (see Fig. 26-1). Fluid extending into the lateral aspect of the minor fissure and slightly separating the lobes often results in an opacity resembling a rose thorn (the "thorn" sign; see Figs. 26-12A, 26-13A, 26-14B).

Large pleural effusions result in significant or complete lung atelectasis (see Fig. 26-13) and result in a mediastinal shift to the opposite side. Downward displacement or inversion of the hemidiaphragm may be recognized on the left because of downward displacement of the stomach bubble. Supine and semierect radiographs are less sensitive in showing pleural effusion. Signs of effusion on supine radiographs include increased density of a hemithorax due to layering of the effusion posteriorly, blunting of the lateral costophrenic angle, obscuration or poor definition of the hemidiaphragm, and thickening of the paravertebral stripe, usually in the inferior hemithorax, due to accumulation of fluid in the

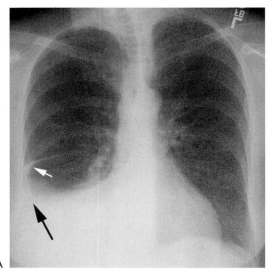

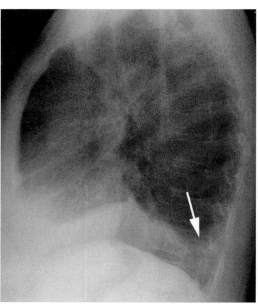

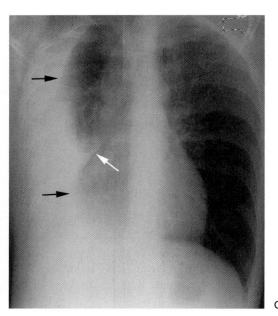

FIG. 26-12. Pleural effusion associated with cirrhosis. **A.** Posteroanterior chest radiograph shows blunting of the right costophrenic angle *(black arrow)*. This usually indicates that 175 ml of pleural fluid is present. Fluid entering the minor fissure *(white arrow)* resembles a rose thorn. This is termed the "thorn" sign of pleural effusion. **B.** Lateral radiograph shows elevation of the lung base by a subpulmonic fluid collection and blunting of the posterior costophrenic angle *(arrow)*. Posterior costophrenic angle blunting occurs with as little as 75 ml of fluid. **C.** Decubitus radiograph shows a large effusion *(black arrows)* separating the aerated lung from the chest wall. Fluid enters the major fissure *(white arrow)*.

posterior gutters. With large effusions, an apical cap may be seen.

On decubitus radiographs, an increase in separation of lung from the chest wall indicates the presence of free pleural effusion (see Fig. 26-12C). Lack in change in thickness indicates pleural thickening or loculated pleural effusion.

CT Findings

Pleural effusion usually appears lower in attenuation than pleural thickening or consolidated or collapsed lung on unenhanced scans, and may be distinguished from them. On contrast-enhanced scans, both airless lung and thickened

pleura enhance, and this difference is accentuated (see Fig. 26-13B).

In the supine position, free pleural effusion first accumulates in the most dependent part of the pleural space, posterior to the lower lobe. The thickness of a free pleural effusion usually decreases in less dependent parts of the thorax, anteriorly and superiorly. As the effusion increases in size, it becomes thicker and wraps around the lung, extending anteriorly and superiorly, and extending into the fissures.

When free pleural fluid accumulates, the lung decreases in volume but tends to maintain its normal shape. Thus, a free pleural effusion generally appears crescent-shaped on CT. Small pleural effusions can be difficult to distinguish

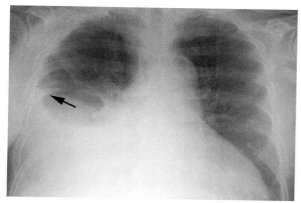 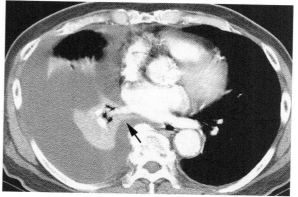

FIG. 26-13. Pleural effusion with liver disease. **A.** Chest radiograph shows a large right pleural effusion with costophrenic angle blunting and a thorn sign *(arrow)*. **B.** A large effusion is visible on CT. The lower lobe is collapsed. Because the lung is tethered medially by the hilar vasculature and inferior pulmonary ligament *(arrow)*, most of the fluid accumulates laterally.

from pleural thickening. Large effusions often extend into the major fissures, displacing the lower lobes medially and posteriorly. Atelectasis is common in patients with large effusions, and atelectatic lung may be seen floating within the fluid.

Pleural Effusion Versus Ascites

Subpulmonic effusion and pleural fluid in the costophrenic angles can be seen below the lung bases on CT and may mimic collections of fluid in the peritoneal cavity. The parallel curvilinear configuration of the pleural and peritoneal cavities at the level of the perihepatic and perisplenic recesses allows fluid in either cavity to appear as a crescentic collection displacing liver or spleen away from the adjacent chest wall.

However, pleural fluid collections and ascites may be distinguished in several ways.

Pleural fluid collections in the posterior costophrenic angle lie medial and posterior to the diaphragm and cause

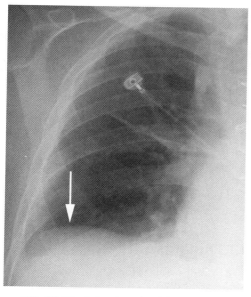 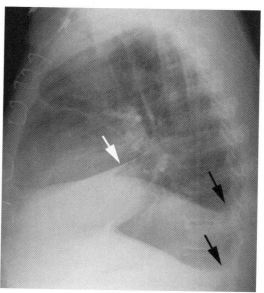

FIG. 26-14. Subpulmonic right pleural effusion. **A.** Posteroanterior chest radiograph shows no evidence of costophrenic angle blunting. There appears to be lateral displacement of the diaphragm dome *(arrow)*. **B.** Lateral radiograph shows blunting of both costophrenic angles *(black arrows)*, and fluid entering the right major fissure, resulting in a thorn sign *(white arrow)*. Flattening of the undersurface of the lobes is also typical of subpulmonic effusion.

lateral displacement of the crus (the "displaced crus" sign). Peritoneal fluid collections are anterior and lateral to the diaphragm; lateral displacement of the crus is not visible.

Pleural fluid can also be distinguished from ascites by the clarity of the interface of the fluid with the liver and spleen (the "interface" sign). With pleural fluid the interface is hazy, whereas with ascites it is sharp.

Fluid seen posterior to the liver is within the pleural space; the peritoneal space does not extend into this region, the so-called bare area of the liver (the "bare-area" sign).

The most reliable method for localizing fluid is to identify its relationship to the diaphragm, if it is visible. In patients with both pleural and peritoneal fluid, the diaphragm often can be seen as a uniform, curvilinear structure of muscle density with relatively low-density fluid both anterior

and posterior to it. Fluid posterior or lateral to the diaphragm is pleural (the "diaphragm" sign).

A large pleural effusion will allow the lower lobe to float anteriorly and lose volume (Fig. 26-15). On CT, the posterior edge of the lower lobe, when surrounded by fluid both anteriorly and posteriorly, can appear to represent the diaphragm (a "pseudodiaphragm"), with pleural fluid posteriorly and ascites anteriorly. Sequential scans at more cephalad levels, however, generally will allow the correct interpretation to be made. Typically, the arcuate density of the atelectatic lower lobe becomes thicker superiorly, is contiguous with the remainder of the lower lobe, and often contains air bronchograms.

LOCULATED FLUID COLLECTIONS

Loculated pleural fluid collections are limited in extent by pleural adhesions. They often occur in association with exudative pleural effusions, high in protein, such as those that occur with empyema. Often they are elliptical or lenticular.

Radiographic Findings

The appearance of loculated pleural fluid on chest radiographs varies with its location and the radiographic projection. Typically, a loculated collection appears sharply marginated when its surface is parallel to the x-ray beam and ill defined when viewed en face (Fig. 26-16A and B). Thus, a collection loculated in the lateral pleural space will appear sharply marginated on the frontal radiograph and ill defined on the lateral film. For a collection loculated anteriorly or posteriorly, the opposite is true.

Localized fluid collections in the fissures may be loculated or may occur in the absence of pleural adhesions. They are most common in patients with congestive heart failure and often are transient. Since they mimic the presence of a focal lung lesion, they have been referred to as "phantom tumor" or "pseudotumor." Typically fluid collections are rounded or lenticular and may show a tapering triangular opacity or "beak" at the point they merge with the fissure itself (Figs. 26-17 and 26-18).

Fluid collections in the minor fissure often appear sharply marginated and lenticular on both posteroanterior and lateral radiographs. Collections in the major fissure may be ill defined on the frontal view.

CT Findings

CT findings of fluid loculation include (1) a localized collection, (2) an elliptical or lenticular shape (rather than crescentic), and (3) a nondependent location (i.e., anterior, lateral, or posterolateral; Figs. 26-16C and 26-18 to 26-20). If air is present within a loculated effusion, multiple septations may be seen, resulting in multiple localized air collections

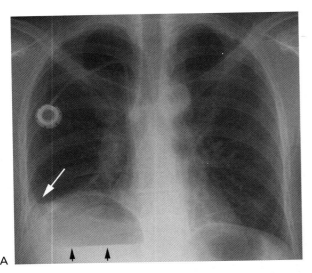

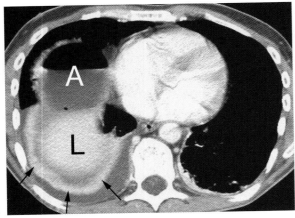

FIG. 26-15. "Pseudodiaphragm" with pleural effusion and lower lobe collapse. **A.** Chest radiograph shows costophrenic angle blunting *(white arrow)* due to right pleural effusion. Air-fluid level represents a subphrenic abscess. **B.** CT shows the abscess cavity *(A)* in a subphrenic location. The liver *(L)* is also visible at this level. The collapsed lower lobe *(arrows)* surrounded by pleural fluid mimics the hemidiaphragm.

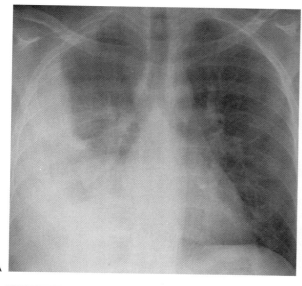

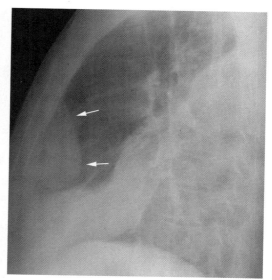

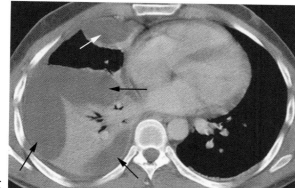

FIG. 26-16. Loculated pleural fluid collections in empyema. **A.** Posteroanterior chest radiograph shows evidence of a large right pleural effusion. **B.** Lateral radiograph shows a lenticular fluid collection anteriorly, with a sharply marginated edge *(arrows)*. A large posterior fluid collection is also present. **C.** Contrast-enhanced CT shows multiple lenticular fluid collections *(arrows)*, indicating the presence of loculation. Some fluid collections are nondependent, also a finding of loculation.

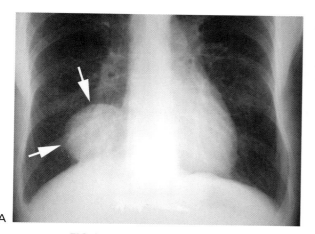

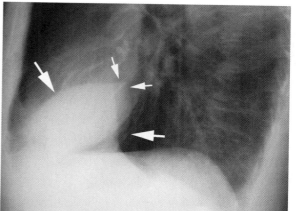

FIG. 26-17. Pseudotumor in congestive heart failure. **A.** Chest radiograph shows a rounded opacity *(arrows)* representing fluid localized to the major fissure. **B.** On the lateral view, the collection appears lenticular *(large arrows)*. A beak *(small arrows)* is seen at its junction with the major fissure. This collection later resolved.

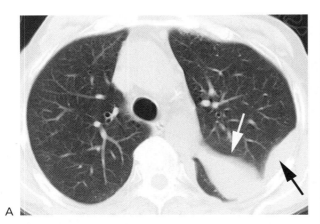

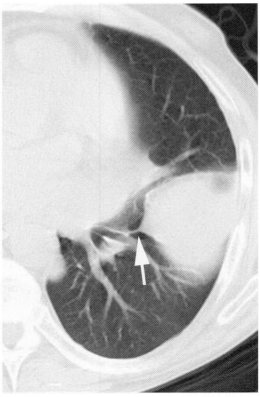

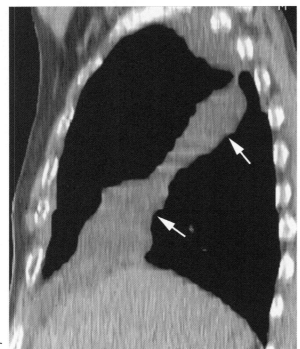

FIG. 26-18. Fluid localized to the major fissure in a patient with cirrhosis and ascites. **A.** A lenticular collection of fluid *(white arrow)* is seen within the fissure. A loculated collection is also present peripherally *(black arrow)*. **B.** At a lower level, a rounded collection is seen within the fissure. A beak *(arrow)* is visible medially. **C.** Sagittal reformation shows fluid thickening the entire major fissure *(arrows)*.

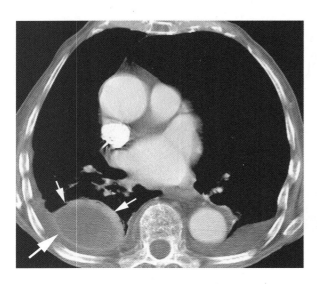

FIG. 26-19. Streptococcal empyema. CT shows a loculated, lenticular fluid collection at the right base, associated with thickening of both the parietal *(large arrow)* and visceral *(small arrows)* pleural layers, the so-called split-pleura sign. The thickened pleura enhances following contrast infusion. The left pleural effusion is unassociated with pleural thickening and may be an exudate or transudate.

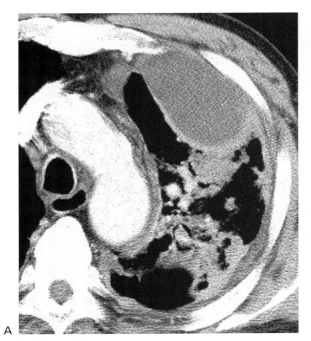 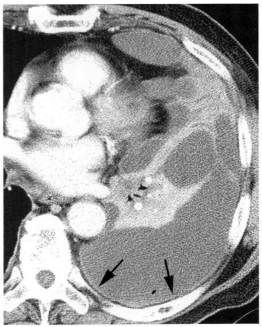

A   B

FIG. 26-20. Empyema with multiple locations. CTs at two levels show multiple loculated fluid collections with thickened parietal pleura *(arrows)*.

or air-fluid levels (Fig. 26-21). Loculated effusions are often associated with pleural thickening, best seen if contrast is infused (see Figs. 26-16C and 26-19). If both the visceral and parietal pleural surfaces are thickened, embracing the fluid collection, the "split-pleura" sign is said to be present (see Fig. 26-19).

A focal or loculated collection of pleural fluid in a major or minor fissure can have a confusing appearance on CT

images and can be misinterpreted as a parenchymal mass. Careful analysis of sequential images usually will confirm the relationship of the opaque mass to the plane of the fissure. If the abnormality is of fluid density, the diagnosis becomes more likely. The edges of the mass may taper to conform to the fissure, forming a "beak," especially if CT with thin collimation is used (see Fig. 26-18). Correlation of CT scans with the plain radiographs can help, particularly for fluid localized in the minor fissure.

TYPES OF EFFUSION: EXUDATES AND TRANSUDATES

Most pleural effusions are classified as exudates or transudates based on their composition. This distinction is usually made at thoracentesis. Other specific causes of pleura effusion are chylothorax and hemothorax.

Exudates

Exudative effusion reflects the presence of a pleural abnormality associated with increased permeability of pleural capillaries (Table 26-1). Exudative effusions have a high protein content. According to generally accepted criteria, an exudative effusion meets at least one of the following criteria:

1. A ratio of pleural fluid protein to serum protein higher than 0.5

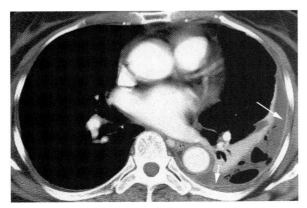

FIG. 26-21. Empyema containing air due to thoracentesis. The parietal pleura is thickened *(arrows)*. Multiple air bubbles indicate a multiloculated proteinaceous effusion. It may be concluded that this effusion is an exudate. The differential diagnosis of an air-containing fluid collection also included bronchopleural fistula and gas-forming organisms.

TABLE 26-1. CAUSES OF EXUDATIVE EFFUSION

Pneumonia (parapneumonic effusion)
Empyema
Tuberculous
Neoplasm
Pulmonary embolism
Collagen-vascular diseases
Abdominal diseases (pancreatitis, abscess, surgery)
Dressler's (post pericardiotomy) syndrome
Asbestos exposure
Meig's syndrome
Uremia
Endometriosis
Drug reactions
Radiation

TABLE 26-2. CAUSES OF TRANSUDATIVE EFFUSION

Congestive heart failure
Pericardial disease
Cirrhosis
Pregnancy and delivery
Hypoalbuminemia
Overhydration
Renal failure
Nephrotic syndrome
Peritoneal dialysis
Myxedema

2. A ratio of pleural fluid lactate dehydrogenase (LDH) to serum LDH that exceeds 0.6
3. A pleural fluid LDH level more than two thirds the upper limits of normal for serum

Less specific criteria used to diagnose an exudate include a pleural fluid specific gravity exceeding 1.016 and a pleural fluid protein level exceeding 3 g/dl.

Common causes of exudative effusion include pneumonia with parapneumonic effusion, empyema, tuberculous pleuritis, neoplasm, pulmonary embolism, collagen diseases such as lupus or rheumatoid arthritis, abdominal diseases (pancreatitis, abscess, surgery), Dressler's (postpericardiotomy) syndrome, asbestos exposure, Meig's syndrome, uremia, endometriosis, drug reactions, and therapeutic radiation.

Transudates

Transudative effusion is unassociated with pleural disease. It usually results from systemic abnormalities causing an imbalance in the hydrostatic and osmotic forces governing pleural fluid formation. They are low in protein and do not meet the criteria for an exudate listed above.

Common causes of a transudative effusion (Table 26-2) include CHF, pericardial disease, cirrhosis, pregnancy and delivery, hypoalbuminemia, overhydration, renal failure, nephrotic syndrome, peritoneal dialysis, and myxedema.

Distinguishing Exudate and Transudate

Distinguishing exudate from transudate is important in differential diagnosis and clinical management. CT numbers cannot be used to reliably predict the protein content or specific gravity of the fluid, and whether it is a transudate or exudate. Most effusions appear to be near water in attenu-

ation on CT, ranging up to 20 to 30 HU regardless of their cause.

The appearance of the parietal pleura on contrast-enhanced CT is of value in predicting the nature of an associated pleural fluid collection. Visibility of the parietal pleura indicates that it is thickened (enhancing pleura is thickened pleura). The presence of thickened parietal pleura in association with a pleural effusion indicates that the fluid collection is an exudate (see Figs. 26-19 to 26-21). This finding is present in about 60% of exudative effusions, and its accuracy in predicting the presence of an exudate is nearly 100%. If pleural thickening is not visible, an associated effusion may be an exudate or a transudate (see Fig. 26-19).

Using sonography, the presence of septation, complex nonseptation, or homogeneous echogenicity may be used to predict the presence of an exudate with a sensitivity and positive predictive value of 65% and 100%, respectively. Anechoic effusions may be either transudative or exudative.

If CT shows air within the fluid collection, for whatever reason (usually thoracentesis), and multiple air bubbles or multiple air-fluid levels are visible (rather than a single air-fluid level; see Fig. 26-21), the presence of proteinaceous and multiloculated effusion may be surmised, as on sonography. An exudate may be confidently diagnosed.

Causes of Exudative and Transudative Pleural Effusion

Abdominal Abscess

Abdominal infections may be associated with ipsilateral pleural effusion. The effusion may be small and a transudate or exudate. Typical findings include small pleural effusion, elevation of the hemidiaphragm, and lower lobe atelectasis. Subphrenic abscess is associated with pleural effusion in 80% of cases; it may occur on either side. Hepatic abscess is associated with effusion in 20%, typically right-sided. Splenic abscess is associated with left-sided effusion in 30%.

Abdominal Surgery

Half of patients who undergo abdominal surgery experience a small pleural effusion within the first 3 postoperative days. Effusions developing after this period likely have another cause. The incidence of pleural effusion is increased in association with upper abdominal surgery, peritoneal fluid, and atelectasis. Orthotopic liver transplantation is almost always associated with right-sided or bilateral effusions.

Asbestos Exposure

Asbestos exposure results in benign exudative pleural effusion in a few exposed individuals. The condition is likely inflammatory in nature and related to the presence of asbestos fibers in relation to the pleural surface. It is dose-related and a relatively early manifestation of disease, usually occurring within 20 years of onset of exposure. Patients are often asymptomatic but may have chest pain. Effusions are usually unilateral and small to moderate in size. They are usually self-limited, lasting a few months, but may be recurrent. Diffuse pleural thickening results in about 20%. Blunting of a costophrenic angle, otherwise unusual with asbestos-related pleural disease, may reflect mild pleural fibrosis. Rounded atelectasis may be associated.

Cirrhosis and Ascites

Cirrhosis is associated with pleural effusion, but the frequency of effusion is much higher if ascites is present. Effusions are typically right-sided or bilateral; isolated left-sided effusions are less common. Most important in the development of effusion is the passage of fluid into the chest through diaphragmatic defects. Reduction in plasma oncotic pressure due to hypoalbuminemia may also contribute to the formation of effusions. The effusions are transudates and may be large.

Collagen-vascular Diseases

Exudative pleural effusion is common in patients with collagen-vascular disease, most commonly systemic lupus erythematosus (SLE) and rheumatoid arthritis (RA).

SLE is associated with pleural effusion in as many as 70% of cases. Arthritis or arthralgia is commonly present. Effusions are usually small and bilateral, and are exudates. Pericardial effusion may also be present. Symptoms include pleuritic pain, fever, and dyspnea.

About 5% to 20% of patients with RA have effusion. Effusions are exudates and have a low glucose, a high LDH, and a high rheumatoid factor. Eighty percent of patients with effusion are men, and 80% have subcutaneous nodules. Effusions in RA may be asymptomatic or associated with chest pain. They are usually small, unilateral, and right-sided. They may be transient, persistent, or recurrent.

Pleural fibrosis may result. Empyema also has an increased incidence in patients with RA.

Congestive Heart Failure

Pleural effusion is present in about half of patients with CHF. CHF is the most common cause of transudative effusion, although exudative effusions may also occur. Pleural fluid accumulates in CHF primarily because pulmonary interstitial (edema) fluid crosses into the pleural space. Bilateral effusions are present in 70% of cases; when unilateral, pleural effusion is more common on the right (20%) than on the left (10%). Although unilateral effusion may be seen, a large unilateral pleural effusion suggests an alternative diagnosis. In a patient with CHF, thoracentesis may be performed if the patient has fever or pleuritic chest pain, the heart is normal in size, and the effusion is unilateral and of sufficient size or bilateral but asymmetrical.

Dressler's Syndrome

Dressler's syndrome (also known as postcardiotomy syndrome, postcardiac injury syndrome, and post–myocardial infarction syndrome) occurs in a few patients with myocardial infarction, pericardial or myocardial injury, or cardiac surgery. It typically occurs 2 or 3 weeks following the precipitating episode and is associated with chest pain, fever, dyspnea, and leukocytosis. Radiographs show pleural effusion (85%), lung consolidation (75%), and findings of pericardial effusion (50%). Pleural effusions are exudative and often bloody. They are usually bilateral and small; when unilateral they are often left-sided. Dressler's syndrome may be self-limited or recurrent. It is thought to be immunologically mediated. Treatment includes aspirin, nonsteroidal antiinflammatory drugs, or steroids.

Drug Reactions

A number of drugs may result in pleural effusion, usually exudative. Effusion may be related to the development of drug-related SLE (see Chapter 14), may reflect allergic reactions, or may be a primary effect of the drug on the pleural surface. Allergic reactions with eosinophilia may be associated with pleural effusion in patients receiving methotrexate or other cytotoxic drugs, nitrofurantoin, propylthiouracil, and muscle relaxants (dantrolene); lung disease is commonly associated. The ergot-based drugs methysergide (migraine treatment) and bromocriptine (Parkinson's disease treatment) may cause pleural effusion and fibrosis.

Meig's Syndrome

Meig's syndrome was originally defined as ascites and pleural effusion associated with ovarian fibroma, but the definition has since extended to refer to other ovarian tumors. Pleural effusions are exudative or transudative and occur on the right side (65%), on the left side (10%), or bilaterally (25%); they may be large. Resection of the ovarian tumor results in resolution of the ascites and pleural effusion.

Myxedema

Pleural effusion occurs in as many as half of patients with myxedema, often associated with pericardial effusion. Associated heart failure or renal disease may be contributory. The effusion may be an exudate or transudate.

Neoplasm

Pleural effusion is common in patients with primary or metastatic pleural tumors. Effusions are usually exudative and may be bloody. Malignant effusions are always exudates, but not all exudative effusions in cancer patients are malignant. Exudative effusions in patients with malignancy may reflect pleura involvement, lymphatic obstruction, or pneumonia. Pleural effusion in patients with malignancy is described in detail below.

Pericardial Disease

Pleural effusion is common in patients with inflammatory pericardial disease. They are left-sided in 70%, bilateral in 20%, and right-sided in 10%. Left-sided effusion likely predominates because of local inflammation. In patients with constrictive pericarditis, effusions may result from elevated left- or right-sided venous pressures; in this setting, as in patients with CHF, effusions are most often bilateral or right-sided.

Pancreatitis

Acute pancreatitis results in effusion in 10% to 20%. Because of the relationship of the pancreatic tail to the left hemidiaphragm, these are usually left-sided (70%) or bilateral. They are exudative and often hemorrhagic and often contain high amylase levels.

Chronic pancreatitis also results in a left-sided effusion in most cases (70%), which contains high amylase. It is most often left-sided or bilateral. Pseudocyst is commonly present. Associated mediastinal pseudocyst with rupture into the pleural space may result in a pancreaticopleural fistula with a large pleural effusion.

Pancreatic abscess may be associated with pleural effusion containing high amylase levels. It is usually left-sided.

Parapneumonic Effusion and Empyema

Pleural effusion is common in patients with pneumonia; this is termed **parapneumonic effusion.** Parapneumonic effusions are typically exudates; they are small and sterile and have normal glucose and pH values. They usually resolve with appropriate antibiotic treatment but may progress to empyema. Empyema is an infected exudative effusion, often requiring tube drainage. These entities are described in detail below.

Pregnancy

Small bilateral transudative pleural effusions are seen in 10% of pregnant women. They are seen for a short time after delivery in up to 25% of women.

Pulmonary Embolism

Pleural effusion occurs in 30% of patients with pulmonary embolism, often associated with infarction. Effusion is more common in patients with the presenting complaint of hemoptysis or pleuritic chest pain (50%) than in those with dyspnea (25%). Exudate is more common (75%) than transudate (25%). They are often unilateral, but this depends on the distribution of emboli. Effusions are usually small and do not increase after 3 days, and the majority resolve within a week. Consolidation is associated in half of cases.

Radiation (Therapeutic)

About 5% of patients having chest radiation develop a small exudative pleural effusion in association with radiation pneumonitis. The effusion occurs on the side of radiation and develops within 6 months of radiation. It resolves slowly with time.

Renal Disease

Several manifestations of renal disease may be associated with pleural effusion:

1. Renal failure with overhydration may result in transudative effusion. Acute glomerulonephritis may be responsible for this occurrence. Effusions are usually bilateral.
2. Nephrotic syndrome may result in transudative effusion because of increased hydrostatic pressure and hypoalbuminemia resulting in decreased plasma oncotic pressure. Effusions are often bilateral and subpulmonic in location.
3. Uremia may result in fibrinous pleuritis and a bloody exudative effusion that is often unilateral and large. Fever, chest pain, and dyspnea are often present. Pericardial effusion is often associated. Chronic fibrotic pleural thickening may result.
4. Hydronephrosis may result in retroperitoneal urinoma and ipsilateral pleural effusion. The effusion is a transudate but contains a high creatinine level.
5. Peritoneal dialysis may result in effusion, usually on the

right side. Fluid likely enters the pleural space via diaphragmatic defects.

CHYLOTHORAX

Chylous effusion or *chylothorax* contains intestinal lymph (i.e., chyle), is high in protein and fatty acid, and is low in cholesterol. It typically appears milky. Chylothorax results from disruption of the thoracic duct (25%) or thoracic lymphatic obstruction by tumor (50% of cases). Simple obstruction of the thoracic duct does not result in chylothorax; it may be tied off without development of chylothorax.

The thoracic duct originates at the cisterna chyli in the upper abdomen and enters the thorax along the right anterior aspect of the spine; it crosses to the left near the level of T6, lying along the left lateral wall of the esophagus, posterior to the descending aorta, and drains into the left brachiocephalic or subclavian vein. Approximately 2 L/day of chyle passes through the thoracic duct, although this volume varies with diet.

Chylous effusion is most common in patients with lymphoma, metastatic neoplasm, or other mediastinal masses (Table 26-3); following thoracic surgery (chylothorax is a complication in about 0.5% of cardiovascular and 4% of esophageal surgeries) or chest trauma (e.g., penetrating or nonpenetrating trauma, thoracic vertebral fracture); inflammatory mediastinal lymph node diseases; mediastinal fibrosis; central vein thrombosis; lymphangiomyomatosis; chylous ascites; and some congenital abnormalities.

Chylous effusions may be small or massive and unilateral or bilateral. They contain protein in addition to fat and appear to be near water in attenuation on CT (Fig. 26-22). Rarely, chylous effusion measures less than 0 HU in attenuation.

Following chest trauma and duct disruption, chyle typically accumulates in the mediastinum before leading to chylothorax. Mediastinal widening or a localized fluid collection may be seen days before development of the

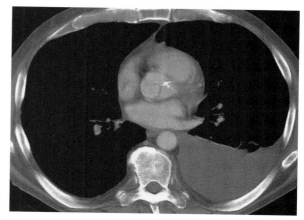

FIG. 26-22. Chylous effusion in lymphoma. The effusion is unassociated with pleural thickening and has no distinguishing characteristics.

chylothorax. Because the location of the thoracic duct is to the right of midline in the lower thorax and to the left in the upper thorax, injury of the lower duct tends to cause right-sided effusion, while injury to the upper duct causes left-sided effusion. Postsurgical chylothorax is often left-sided. Closed trauma usually results in right-sided chylothorax.

Traumatic chylothorax will often resolve over time as the thoracic duct heals. Reduction in lymph flow may be helpful in achieving this result. A pleuroperitoneal shunt may be used. Tube drainage may lead to malnutrition. Ligation of the duct is curative. Chylothorax associated with lymphoma is usually treated with radiation.

Pseudochylous or *chyliform* effusion contains cholesterol but not chyle. It may be seen in patients with chronic inflammatory disease such as tuberculosis or rheumatoid arthritis or in patients with breakdown of cells present within a pleural effusion. Effusions are often chronic, being present for years.

HEMOTHORAX

The term "hemothorax" refers to a pleural fluid collection having a hematocrit over 50% of blood hematocrit. On CT, hemothorax results in fluid with high attenuation (higher than 50 HU), containing relatively dense clot or a fluid-fluid level, with the densest fluid being posteriorly (Fig. 26-23).

Most cases are traumatic, but a select list of entities can result in spontaneous hemothorax. These include rupture of an aneurysm or dissection, pulmonary or pleural neoplasm, pneumothorax, coagulopathy, rupture of a pulmonary arteriovenous malformation, and pulmonary or pleural endometriosis (see below).

TABLE 26-3. CAUSES OF CHYLOTHORAX	
Cause	Prevalence
Tumor	50%
Lymphoma	35%
Other tumor	15%
Trauma	25%
Surgery	20%
Other trauma	5%
Miscellaneous	25%
Congenital	5%
Other	20%

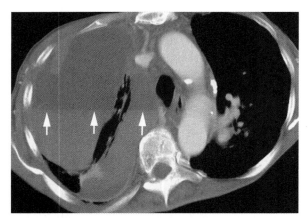

FIG. 26-23. Iatrogenic traumatic hemothorax related to thoracentesis. A large right pleural effusion shows a distinct fluid or hematocrit level *(arrows)*. The dependent fluid measures in excess of 60 HU.

Treatment includes tube drainage or sometimes thoracotomy for control of bleeding. Empyema may complicate hemothorax. Organization of a hemothorax may result in pleural fibrosis and calcification.

FIBRIN BODY

A resolving exudative effusion or hemothorax may deposit a clot of fibrin within the pleural space, termed a *fibrin body* or *pleural mouse*. These usually appear 1 to 2 cm in diameter, mimicking a solitary nodule, but are localized to the pleural space, and are sometimes seen to move with change in patient position (Fig. 26-24). They typically resolve over time but may remain stable or enlarge.

TABLE 26-4. SIMPLE PARAPNEUMONIC EFFUSION
Increased permeability of the visceral pleura
Commonly exudates
Sterile with normal glucose
Small to moderate in size
Dependent in location
No loculation
Meniscus on plain radiographs
Crescentic shape on CT
50% associated with pleural thickening
Resolve with appropriate antibiotic treatment

PARAPNEUMONIC EFFUSION AND EMPYEMA

Pleural fluid accumulates in approximately 40% of patients with pneumonia. The term *parapneumonic effusion* is used to describe this occurrence. Parapneumonic effusions are usually classified in three stages, also known as the three stages of empyema. Progression from one stage to the next does not necessarily occur.

Simple Parapneumonic Effusion (Exudative Stage)

A simple parapneumonic effusion probably results from increased permeability of the visceral pleura occurring in association with pulmonary inflammation in patients with pneumonia (Table 26-4). Effusions in this stage are commonly exudates and are typically small and sterile and have a normal glucose level (more than 40 to 60 mg/dl) and pH (greater than 7.2).

Parapneumonic effusions usually (1) are small to moder-

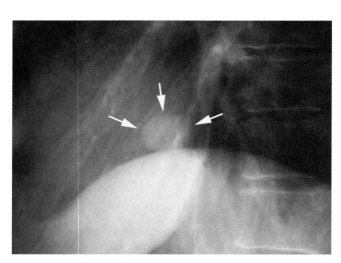

FIG. 26-24. Fibrin ball. Coned-down lateral view shows a well-defined small nodular opacity at the pleural surface *(arrows)*. This moved within the pleural space.

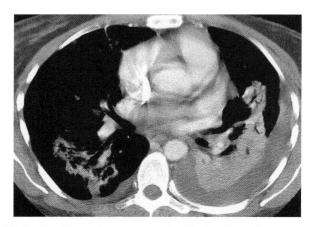

FIG. 26-25. Simple parapneumonic effusion. The left pleural effusion is dependent, crescent-shaped, small, and unassociated with pleural thickening or findings of location. Bilateral pneumonia and a small right pleural effusion are present.

ate in size, (2) are dependent in location, (3) do not show evidence of loculation, (4) show a meniscus on plain radiographs, and (5) appear crescent-shaped on CT (Fig. 26-25). About 50% of parapneumonic effusions are associated with pleural thickening visible on CT. Visceral pleural thickening and the "split-pleura" sign also may be present.

Simple parapneumonic effusion will usually resolve with appropriate antibiotic treatment of the pneumonia and rarely needs tube drainage. A parapneumonic effusion that requires drainage is termed a *complicated parapneumonic effusion*. A complicated parapneumonic effusion is often an empyema.

Empyema (Fibropurulent Stage)

The term **empyema** is generally used when a pleural effusion is infected, although its true definition necessitates the presence of pus in the pleural space (Table 26-5). Although most empyemas occur in association with pneumonia, approximately 10% are unassociated with obvious lung disease.

Up to 75% of bacterial empyemas result from anaerobic infections or mixed anaerobic and aerobic infections. Common anaerobic organisms include *Bacteroides* species, Fusobacterium, anaerobic and microaerophilic cocci, and *Clostridium*. Common aerobic organisms are *Staphylococcus aureus, Streptococcus pneumoniae, Haemophilus influenzae*, and gram-negative enteric bacilli. Tuberculosis may result in empyema.

Empyema is characterized by the presence of infectious organisms in the pleural fluid, increased effusion, increased white blood cells and polymorphonuclear cells in the fluid, fibrin deposition along the pleural surfaces, a tendency for loculation, decreased glucose levels (less than 40 mg/dl) and pH (below 7.2), and increased LDH (over 1,000 IU/L).

In a patient who has pneumonia, the presence of a localized or loculated pleural effusion strongly suggests the presence of an empyema (see Figs. 26-16, 26-19, 26-20, and 26-21). On plain radiographs, empyemas often have a lenticular shape and tend to appear larger or better defined in one projection (e.g., as seen on the posteroanterior radiograph) than in the other (e.g., on the lateral radiograph; see Fig. 26-16). On radiographs, an empyema containing air may be difficult or impossible to differentiate from a peripheral lung abscess abutting the chest wall. This distinction can be an important one to make because empyemas are often treated by tube thoracostomy in addition to systemic antibiotics, whereas most lung abscesses require antibiotics only.

Classical CT findings of empyema (see Figs. 26-16 and 26-19 to 26-21) include an (1) elliptical or lenticular shape, (2) nondependent location, (3) sharp demarcation from the adjacent lung, (4) the split-pleura sign (the enhancing visceral and parietal pleural surfaces split apart by the fluid collection), (5) the thickened pleural layers usually appear smooth and of uniform thickness when enhanced by contrast or outlined by air, and (6) empyemas compress and displace adjacent lung and vessels.

In contrast to empyema, lung abscesses (see Figs. 9-39 and 9-40 in Chapter 9) tend (1) to be round, (2) to be ill-defined, (3) to have shaggy walls of irregular thickness, and (4) to destroy lung without displacing vessels.

In patients with parapneumonic effusion or empyema, it is common (60% to 80% of cases) to see extrapleural fat thickening on CT when parietal pleural thickening is present. Increased attenuation of extrapleural fat representing edema is less common (30% of cases).

Not all empyemas show classical findings. Many empyemas are crescent-shaped and dependent in location, without findings of loculation, being indistinguishable from a simple parapneumonic effusion. Parietal pleural thickening or enhancement is always seen on CT, while visceral pleural thickening or enhancement is seen in half; thus, the split-pleura sign is absent in about half of cases.

Bronchopleural Fistula

Bronchopleural fistula (BPF) results from rupture of the visceral pleura, usually in association with lung abscess and empyema. Unless there has been a recent thoracentesis, gas within a pleural fluid collection is presumptive evidence of empyema and a BPF. The presence of a gas-forming organism is less often associated with gas in the pleural space. Rarely in a patient with lung abscess, the site of BPF (i.e., the point of visceral pleural discontinuity) can be demonstrated on CT. BPF is an indication for chest tube drainage.

Empyema Necessitatis

Empyema (often in association with pneumonia) can involve the chest wall by direct extension; this is termed *empyema necessitatis* or *empyema necessitans*. Tuberculosis accounts for about 70% of cases of empyema necessitatis, but

---

TABLE 26-5. EMPYEMA

"Fibropurulent parapneumonic effusion"
Most empyemas occur with pneumonia
10% unassociated with lung disease
Anaerobic infections or mixed anaerobic and aerobic infections
Polymorphonuclear neutrophils in the fluid
Fibrin deposition along the pleural surfaces
Decreased glucose
Low pH values (<7.2)
Increased LDH (>1000 IU/L)
Elliptical or lenticular shape on radiographs or CT
Nondependent location
Sharp demarcation from the adjacent lung
"Split-pleura" sign
Air = thoracentesis, bronchopleural fistula, gas-forming organism
Empyema necessitates—chest wall involvement
   TB, actinomycosis, etc.

TABLE 26-6. PLEURAL PEEL

Chronic empyema
Pleural fibrosis
Restriction of lung function (i.e., trapped lung)
Smooth pleural thickening
Reduction in size of hemithorax
Pleural calcification

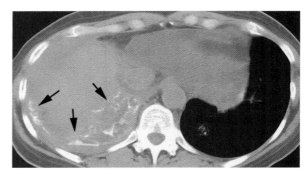

FIG. 26-27. Talc pleurodesis. Pleural thickening and dense talc *(arrows)* are visible.

other organisms such as *Actinomyces, Nocardia,* and other bacteria or fungi can be responsible. Extensive extrapleural fat thickening, edema or extrapleural fat, and subcutaneous collections of pus can be seen on CT.

Tube Drainage of Empyema

Indications for tube placement in patients with a parapneumonic effusion vary depending on the clinical setting, but one of the following criteria is usually sufficient: (1) thick pus on thoracentesis, (2) positive Gram stain from pleural fluid, (3) positive pleural fluid culture, (4) pleural fluid glucose below 60 mg/dl, (5) pleural fluid pH less than 7.2, and (6) LDH greater than 1000 IU/L, or (6) a parapneumonic effusion that does not resolve with antibiotic treatment.

Pleural Peel (Organization Stage)

In patients with chronic empyema, ingrowth of fibroblasts and organization can result in extensive pleural fibrosis and the development of an inelastic fibrotic *pleural peel* or *fibrothorax* (Table 26-6). This can cause lung restriction and decreased lung volume ("trapped lung").

Smooth pleural thickening is typically visible on plain radiographs or CT (Fig. 26-26). Extrapleural fat thickening

is frequently visible on CT, separating the thickened parietal pleura from the intercostal muscle or rib. Calcification, which usually is focal in its early stages, may become extensive. This is most common with tuberculosis.

A very important finding in diagnosing pleural peel on plain film or CT is reduction in volume of the affected hemithorax (see Fig. 26-26). Loculated fluid collections resulting from active infection may be seen on CT in association with the pleural peel.

In addition to chronic empyema, a pleural peel may result from chronic pleural effusion and inflammation in the absence of infection. This may be seen in patients with collagen-vascular diseases, asbestos exposure, uremia, and hemothorax.

Pleural Calcification

Pleural calcification may be associated with pleural fibrosis regardless of its cause. It is seen most commonly with pleural peel in patients with healed tuberculosis or bacterial empy-

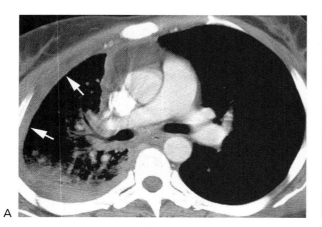
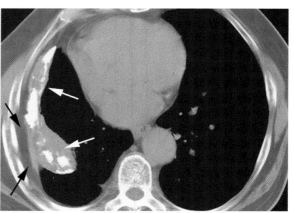

FIG. 26-26. Pleural peel in two patients. **A.** In a patient with chronic empyema, smooth pleural thickening is visible *(arrows)* with reduction in volume of the affected hemithorax. **B.** Following tuberculous empyema, there is right pleural thickening and calcification *(white arrows)*. Extrapleural fat is thickened *(black arrows)*. The volume of the hemithorax is reduced.

ema, hemothorax, or asbestos exposure. When present, it is commonly associated with increased thickness of extrapleural fat.

Talc Pleurodesis

Talc pleurodesis used to treat patients with chronic pleural effusion may mimic the appearance of pleural calcification. Dense accumulations of talc within the pleural space, in association with pleural thickening (Fig. 26-27), are typically seen. Talc is often visible in a clump posteriorly at the lung base.

PLEURAL NEOPLASMS

Radiographic Diagnosis

Neoplasm, either primary or metastatic, is a common cause of pleural mass, pleural effusion, or pleural thickening.

Pleural and Extrapleural Masses

Lesions located in the peripheral thorax, in contact with the chest wall, are generally classified as extrapleural, pleural, or parenchymal and are usually characterized radiographically by the angle (either acute or obtuse) formed by the interface between the lesion and the adjacent pleura.

Extrapleural masses usually displace the overlying parietal and visceral pleura, resulting in an obtuse angle between the lesion and the chest wall. Associated abnormalities including soft tissue mass or rib destruction may help to confirm the mass as extrapleural. Typically, extrapleural masses are sharply marginated at the point they contact lung and displace pulmonary vessels away from them.

Pleural masses, arising from the visceral or parietal pleura, usually remain confined to the pleural space and have an appearance similar to that of extrapleural lesions. The presence of an obtuse angle is common unless the lesion is large (Fig. 26-28). Large pleural lesions may have acute angles where they meet the chest wall, although some pleural thickening is often seen adjacent to them. As with extrapleural masses, pleural lesions are sharply marginated and displace pulmonary vessels away from them.

Pulmonary parenchymal masses, when peripheral, may abut the pleura. A peripheral pulmonary lesion typically results in an acute angle with the pleural surface. Lung masses may result in obtuse angles at the chest wall in the presence of pleural invasion. Pulmonary lesions are often ill defined along their inner aspect and may engulf rather than displace vessels.

Pleural Effusion

Pleural effusion is common in patients with pleural malignancy, either primary or metastatic. Such effusions have a variety of causes but are usually exudates.

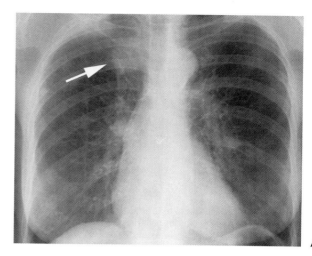

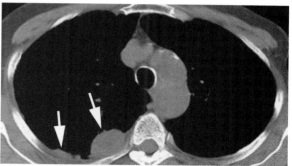

FIG. 26-28. Pleural metastases from chondrosarcoma. **A.** Chest radiograph shows a mass at the right apex. **B.** CT shows pleural masses with obtuse angles. No pleural effusion is associated. This is unusual with pleural metastases and implies a slow-growing lesion.

A **malignant effusion** is one secondary to pleural involvement by tumor and contains malignant cells. The most common causes of malignant effusion are lung cancer and breast cancer. Pleural fluid cytology is positive in 80% to 90% of patients with pleural malignancy, with the highest frequency in patients with adenocarcinoma. Malignant effusions are exudates.

Exudative effusions in patients with malignancy can also reflect lymphatic or pulmonary venous obstruction by tumor or pneumonia. This is particularly true of lung cancer. Only patients with demonstration of tumor cells in the pleural fluid are considered to have unresectable disease.

Malignant effusions may be small or large and unilateral, bilateral, or asymmetrical. A large unilateral effusion suggests malignancy or infection (Figs. 26-29 to 26-31). Regardless of their cause, exudative effusions in cancer patients often require treatment by drainage.

Pleural Thickening

The presence of pleural thickening on CT in a patient with malignancy and pleural effusion indicates the presence of

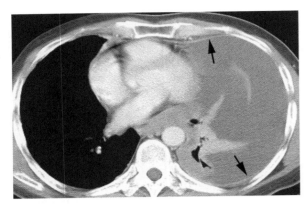

FIG. 26-29. Large unilateral malignant effusion. The effusion is large and the presence of pleural thickening *(arrows)* indicates that it is exudative.

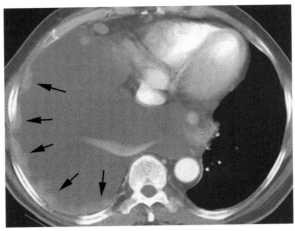

FIG. 26-31. Pleural metastasis in colon carcinoma with nodular pleural thickening. Gross nodular thickening of the parietal pleura is present *(arrows)*. This appearance strongly suggests malignancy.

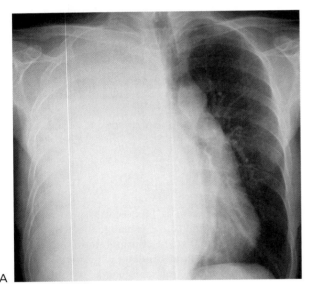

A

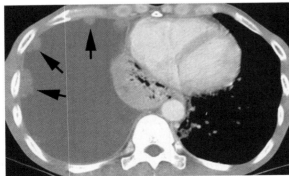

B

FIG. 26-30. Pleural metastases. **A.** Chest radiograph shows a large right pleural effusion with mediastinal displacement to the left. **B.** CT shows nodular pleural thickening *(arrows)* with a large effusion and right lung collapse.

an exudate (see Fig. 26-29) but is of little value in diagnosing malignant effusion. Pleural thickening is seen in 30% cancer patients with a malignant effusion and 40% of those with a benign effusion. Pleural effusion is usually the only abnormality visible on chest radiographs in patients with malignant effusion. In patients with gross pleural involvement by tumor, nodular pleural thickening may be seen (see Figs. 26-30 and 26-31). Metastatic tumor also may involve the pleural space in a concentric fashion.

The CT findings most specific in diagnosing malignant pleural disease are listed below. If one or more of these findings are considered to indicate malignancy, overall diagnostic accuracy is about 75%.

1. Nodular pleural thickening (see Figs. 26-30 and 26-31)
2. Circumferential pleural thickening (pleural thickening surrounding the lung; Fig. 26–32)

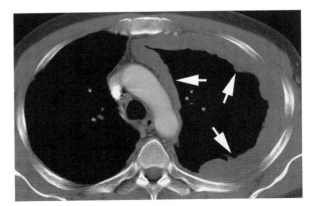

FIG. 26-32. Concentric pleural thickening with metastatic adenocarcinoma. Four findings of malignancy are visible: nodular thickening, circumferential pleural thickening *(arrows)*, parietal pleural thickening greater than 1 cm, and mediastinal pleural thickening.

3. Parietal pleural thickening greater than 1 cm
4. Mediastinal pleural thickening (see Fig. 26-32)

PLEURAL METASTASES

Pleural metastases typically result in pleural effusion. CT may show normal pleura with pleural effusion, smooth pleural thickening (see Fig. 26-29), localized pleural masses (see Figs. 26-28, 26-30, and 26-31), or gross nodular pleural thickening (see Fig. 26-32). Localized pleural masses strongly suggest metastases. Nodular pleural thickening may be seen with metastatic tumor or mesothelioma. In patients with metastases, gross nodular pleural thickening is most typical of adenocarcinoma, but this is seen in a minority of cases.

On chest radiographs, pleural effusion is usually the only visible finding. However, in some patients with pleural metastases, particularly from invasive thymoma, pleural metastases may be unassociated with effusion and visible as rounded or lenticular pleural masses.

LYMPHOMA

In patients with lymphoma, particularly those with Hodgkin's disease, exudative effusions commonly result from mediastinal lymphatic obstruction and resolve following mediastinal radiation; pleural thickening may or may not be present.

Marked thickening of extrapleural soft tissues may be seen with lymphoma or leukemia, often associated with posterior mediastinal lymph node enlargement. This may result in a rind of soft tissue mimicking the appearance of mesothelioma (see Figs. 5-25, 5-30, and 5-37 in Chapter 5). This appearance is associated with effusion.

MESOTHELIOMA

Mesothelioma (also known as malignant or diffuse mesothelioma) is a highly malignant, progressive neoplasm with an extremely poor prognosis (Table 26-7). In most patients,

TABLE 26-7. MESOTHELIOMA

Commonly related to asbestos exposure
Incidence up to 5% in heavily exposed subjects
Latency period of 20–40 years
Arises in relation to the parietal pleura
Epithelial (50%), sarcomatous (25%), or mixed (25%) cell types
Pleural effusion
Concentric and lobulated pleural thickening
Frozen mediastinum sign
Involvement of fissure
Chest wall invasion or distant metastases
Poor prognosis

malignant mesothelioma is related to asbestos exposure. Although mesothelioma is rare in the general population, its incidence in heavily exposed asbestos workers is up to 5%. A latency period of 20 to 40 years between exposure and development of the tumor is typical. Mean age at diagnosis is 60. Symptoms include chest pain, dyspnea, and weight loss.

Mesothelioma arises in relation to the parietal pleura. It is classified pathologically as epithelial (50%), sarcomatous (25%), or mixed (25%). The epithelial type has a slightly better prognosis and tends to be associated with pleural effusion. Pleural effusion is small or absent with sarcomatous tumors. Histologic diagnosis of mesothelioma is difficult using pleural fluid cytology, and biopsy is usually required. Special histologic techniques may be needed to distinguish mesothelioma from adenocarcinoma.

Mesothelioma is characterized morphologically by gross and nodular pleural thickening, which can involve the fissures. Hemorrhagic pleural effusion often occurs. Malignant mesothelioma spreads most commonly by local infiltration of the pleura. Hematogenous metastases are present in 50% of patients, although these are usually insignificant clinically.

Radiographic Findings

Plain radiographs may show pleural effusion as the initial abnormality (Fig. 26-33) or concentric and lobulated pleural thickening (Fig. 26-34). This may reflect nodules of tumor, multiloculated pleural fluid collections, or both. Thickening of the major fissure is common due to tumor.

Because of pleural thickening and mediastinal infiltration, the involved hemithorax may be normal in volume despite the presence of a large effusion (the "frozen mediastinum" sign). The hemithorax may also be reduced in volume because of restriction of lung expansion. Asbestos-related pleural thickening or plaques may also be seen (see Chapter 18).

CT Findings

Pleural fluid collections are visible on CT in 75% (see Fig. 26-33B). Pleural thickening is seen in 90%. Pleural effusion may be visible in the absence of visible pleural thickening in early disease, but this is uncommon.

Nodular concentric pleural thickening is highly suggestive of mesothelioma (Figs. 26-34B and 26-35). However, pleural thickening may also be thin and smooth (Fig. 26-36) or irregular or nodular in contour. Localized pleural masses are uncommon. In early disease, pleural thickening may appear localized and discontinuous. As the disease progresses, pleural thickening becomes continuous, it increases in thickness and nodularity, and the amount of fluid may decrease as the pleural layers become fused.

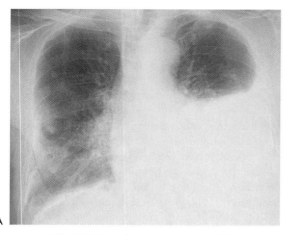
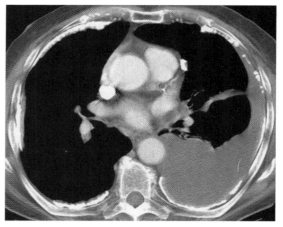

FIG. 26-33. Asbestos exposure with mesothelioma. **A.** Chest radiograph shows pleural plaques and a large left pleural effusion. **B.** CT shows extensive pleural plaques and a left pleural thickening without obvious masses. This reflects left-sided mesothelioma.

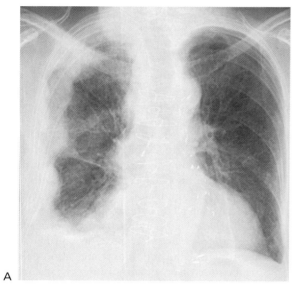
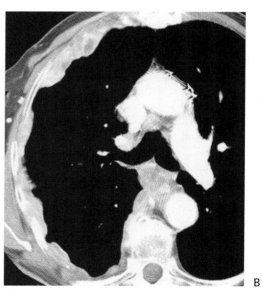

FIG. 26-34. Asbestos exposure with mesothelioma. **A.** Chest radiograph shows lobulated right pleural thickening typical of this tumor. **B.** CT shows extensive nodular pleural thickening.

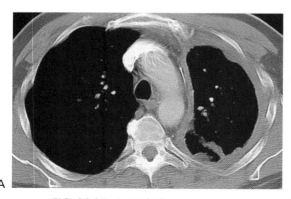
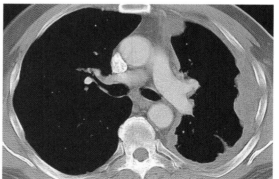

FIG. 26-35. Mesothelioma with concentric nodular pleural thickening. CTs at two levels show concentric nodular pleural thickening typical of mesothelioma. Note reduction in volume of the affected hemithorax because of lung restriction.

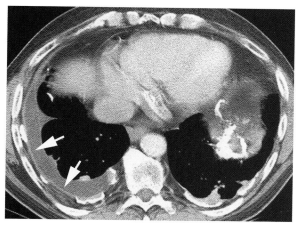

FIG. 26-36. Mesothelioma. CT shows mild pleural thickening *(arrows)* and pleural effusion. Extensive pleural plaques from asbestos exposure are also present.

TABLE 26-8. STAGING SYSTEM FOR MESOTHELIOMA

Stage[a]	Description
T1	Tumor limited to the ipsilateral parietal pleura or associated with scattered foci of visceral pleural involvement.
T2	Ipsilateral parietal pleural tumor with involvement of the diaphragm or confluent involvement of the visceral pleura
T3	Ipsilateral parietal pleural tumor with limited chest wall mediastinal, or pericardial invasion
T4	Extensive chest wall, subdiaphragmatic, mediastinal, or pericardial invasion

[a] T designations describe the extent of local invasion. N and M designations are identical to those used for lung cancer (see Chapter 3).

Fluid can be difficult to distinguish from tumor on CT, since tumor nodules can sometimes appear low in attenuation (Fig. 26-37). However, decubitus scans or scans with the patient prone can help to distinguish underlying tumor from free fluid. Enhancement of the pleura after contrast infusion can also help differentiate tumor from adjacent fluid collections. Calcification usually reflects asbestos exposure, but calcification of tumor may be seen.

Although mesothelioma is visible most frequently along the lateral chest wall, mediastinal pleural thickening or concentric pleural thickening is seen with extensive disease. The abnormal hemithorax can appear contracted and fixed (40%), with little change in size during inspiration (see Fig. 26-35). Thickening of the fissures, particularly the lower part of the major fissures, can reflect tumor infiltration or associated pleural effusion; involvement of the fissures is seen on CT in 85% (see Fig. 26-35A).

Staging

Mesothelioma has a poor prognosis, with a mean survival of about 1 year and a 5-year survival rate of only a few percent. Extrapleural pneumonectomy may be used for treatment, often in combination with chemotherapy and radiation, and survival may be improved in patients with early disease.

Staging systems have been proposed for mesothelioma similar to the TNM system used for lung cancer, but these have limited utility in clinical practice because of the poor prognosis associated with this tumor (Table 26-8; see Fig. 26-37). The stage classifications are similar to those used for lung cancer.

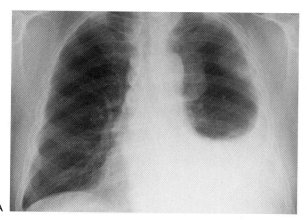
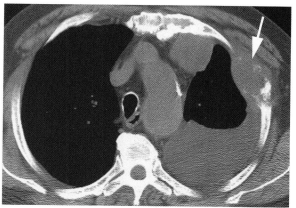

FIG. 26-37. Mesothelioma with chest wall invasion. **A.** Chest radiograph shows a large effusion and a peripheral pleural nodule. **B.** The fluid and nodular areas of tumor are difficult to distinguish except for tumor invasion of the chest wall *(arrows)*.

TABLE 26-9. LOCALIZED FIBROUS TUMOR

No relation to asbestos exposure
Associated with chest pain, hypoglycemia (5%), hypertrophic pulmonary osteoarthropathy (35%)
30% malignant; 70% benign
Arises in relation to the visceral pleura
Pleural effusion rare
Focal pleural mass
Good prognosis

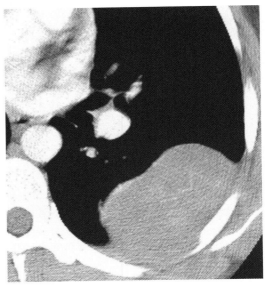

FIG. 26-39. Localized fibrous tumor appearing as a well-defined mass contacting the pleural surface. There is pleural thickening adjacent to the mass.

LOCALIZED FIBROUS TUMOR OF THE PLEURA

Localized fibrous tumor (LFT) of the pleura was formerly known as benign mesothelioma, but it is not mesothelial in origin and is not necessarily benign. Approximately 30% of these tumors are malignant, although they have a good prognosis. It is unassociated with asbestos exposure (Table 26-9).

LFT is usually detected incidentally on chest radiographs. However, it can be associated with hypoglycemia (5% of cases), hypertrophic pulmonary osteoarthropathy (one third of cases), or chest pain. The symptoms resolve with resection.

LFT arises from the visceral pleura in 70%. It typically appears as a solitary, smooth, sharply defined, often large lesion, contacting a pleural surface (Figs. 26-38 and 26-39). When small, LFT tends to have obtuse angles at the pleural surface; when large, angles are usually acute. LFT can be seen within a fissure, mimicking the appearance of loculated fluid. A "beak" or "thorn" sign is often visible on plain

radiographs in patients with an LFT originating in or projecting into a fissure (see Fig. 26-38). They may also arise on a stalk and move with change in patient position. Pleural effusion is not usually present.

On CT, even if acute angles are visible, slight pleural thickening is usually visible adjacent to the mass (see Fig. 26-39). This thickening may reflect a small amount of fluid accumulating in the pleural space at the point where the visceral and parietal pleural surfaces are separated by the mass. Masses may appear homogeneous. Necrosis can result in a multicystic appearance with or without contrast infu-

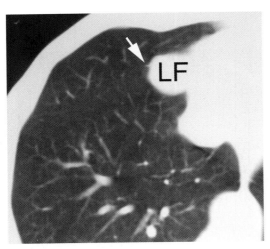

FIG. 26-38. Localized fibrous tumor in the right major fissure. The localized fibrous tumor *(LF)* lies in the plane of the major fissure and shows a small beak *(arrow)* at the point it contacts the fissure. The mass appears smooth and oval.

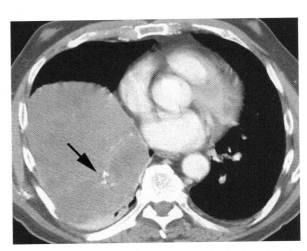

FIG. 26-40. Large localized fibrous tumor in the inferior pleural space. It appears somewhat inhomogeneous in attenuation, and arrow focal calcification is visible.

sion. Large arteries supplying the mass may be seen. Calcification may be present (Fig. 26-40).

PNEUMOTHORAX

Pneumothorax is classified as spontaneous or traumatic.

Spontaneous Pneumothorax

A spontaneous pneumothorax is one occurring without associated trauma. These are classified as primary or secondary.

Primary Spontaneous Pneumothorax

Primary spontaneous pneumothorax occurs without antecedent cause in an otherwise healthy patient. It often occurs at rest and is generally the result of rupture of an apical subpleural bulla (Fig. 26-41). There is an increased inci-

dence of primary spontaneous pneumothorax in young patients (20 to 40 years), men (80% of affected patients are men), tall and thin patients, and smokers (90% are smokers). Pain is common, and a small pleural effusion is present in 10% to 20%, manifested as an air-fluid level. In half of patients, the pneumothorax recurs on the same side; recurrence on the opposite side occurs in 15%.

Secondary Spontaneous Pneumothorax

Secondary spontaneous pneumothorax occurs in patients with underlying lung disease. It is most commonly associated with chronic obstructive pulmonary disease. Other diseases include those associated with lung cysts (e.g., histiocytosis, lymphangiomyomatosis, pneumatocele), cavitation (e.g., tuberculosis, lung cancer, metastases, lung abscess, septic embolism; Fig. 26-42; see also Fig. 3-26 in Chapter 3), air trapping (e.g., asthma, cystic fibrosis), decreased lung compliance (e.g., any cause of fibrosis or honeycombing such as interstitial pneumonitis, radiation, collagen-vascular disease, and sarcoidosis), or diseases of connective tissue (e.g., Ehlers-Danlos syndrome and Marfan syndrome).

Because of underlying lung disease, patients with secondary spontaneous pneumothorax are often symptomatic. Such pneumothoraces have no specific characteristics, but underlying lung appears abnormal. Recurrence rates are higher than for primary spontaneous pneumothorax.

Pneumothorax Ex Vacuo
Pneumothorax ex vacuo is a rare cause of secondary spontaneous pneumothorax occurring in patients with acute lobar atelectasis, usually due to bronchial obstruction (see Fig. 3-27 in Chapter 3). Sudden collapse results in a rapid decrease in intrapleural pressure adjacent to the collapsed lobe. This in turn results in gas entering into the pleural space from tissue and blood. The resulting pneumothorax is seen adjacent to the collapsed lobe.

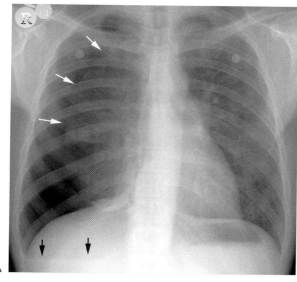

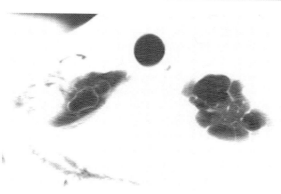

FIG. 26-41. Primary spontaneous pneumothorax in a smoker. **A.** Chest radiograph shows a large right pneumothorax *(white arrows).* An air-fluid level *(black arrows)* is visible at the right base. **B.** Follow-up CT shows apical bullae. Subcutaneous emphysema reflects chest tube drainage.

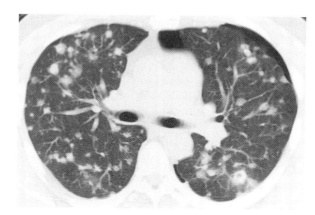

FIG. 26-42. Secondary spontaneous pneumothorax in a patient with cavitary metastatic giant cell tumor. Multiple lung nodules and a small left pneumothorax are visible.

Catamenial Pneumothorax and Pleural Endometriosis

The development of pneumothorax coincident with menstruation, so-called catamenial pneumothorax, is rare. The onset of symptoms is within 48 hours of the onset of menses. It typically occurs in women over 30. Most cases (90%) occur on the right side. Recurrence is typical. Two primary mechanisms have been suggested:

1. Air may reach the peritoneum space during menses via the vagina, uterus, and fallopian tubes. From there it may enter the pleural space through defects in the diaphragm, which are also most common on the right side.
2. Endometrial implants may enter the pleural space by the same route, resulting in pleural endometriosis. If endometrial implants involve the visceral pleura and peripheral lung, their breakdown during menstruation may lead to pneumothorax and/or hemoptysis. This mechanism is more likely than the first.

Pleural endometriosis may also result in catamenial hemothorax. As with catamenial pneumothorax, pleural endometriosis is right-sided in 90%. Enhancing pleural nodules and masses may be seen in addition to pleural effusion, which wax and wane with hormonal changes. These may be seen both within the abdomen and pleural space. The diaphragmatic defects allowing passage of air or endometrium into the pleural space may result from necrotic diaphragmatic endometrial implants.

Traumatic Pneumothorax

Traumatic pneumothorax refers to pneumothorax caused by chest trauma (penetrating or nonpenetrating, accidental or iatrogenic) or mechanical ventilation. Pneumothorax associated with mechanical ventilation is usually the result of high ventilator pressures; pneumothorax with mechanical ventilation usually occurs because of alveolar rupture, which in turn causes interstitial emphysema, pneumomediastinum, and rupture of the pneumomediastinum into the pleural space. Pneumothorax does not cause pneumomediastinum; it is the other way around. Also, interstitial air may track

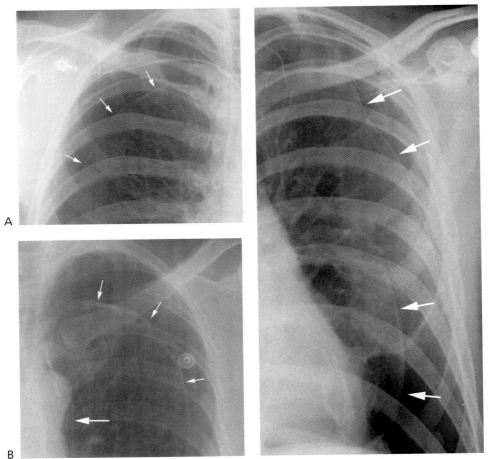

FIG. 26-43. Pleural line in pneumothorax in three patients. A very thin line (*arrows;* thinnest in the patient in **A**) is visible at the edge of the lung. No lung markings are visible peripheral to it. A pleural line may also be seen medially (*large arrow* in **B**).

to a subpleural location, form a subpleural bleb, and rupture directly into the pleural space. Traumatic pneumothorax usually requires chest tube drainage.

Radiographic Findings

Upright Patient

In an upright patient, air usually collects first above the lung apex. The visibility of pneumothorax is accentuated on expiration.

The presence of a visible visceral pleural line is key in making a definite diagnosis of pneumothorax in an erect patient (Fig. 26-43). This is visible as a very thin line at the pleural surface, with black air in the pleura space above or lateral to it, and air in lung below or medial to it. Air may enter the fissure, outlining its pleural surfaces.

In the absence of underlying lung disease or pleural adhesions, the partially collapsed lung maintains its normal shape. Lung markings are not seen peripheral to the pleural line.

A skin fold may mimic pneumothorax, but a pleural line is not visible, and lung markings may be seen peripheral to it (Fig. 26-44). Pneumothorax increases in relative volume on expiration, although significant pneumothoraces are visible on inspiration (Fig. 26-45).

Distinction of a bulla from a pneumothorax is usually based on shape. Pneumothoraces are typically crescent-shaped and taper toward the lung base; bullae are rounded (see Fig. 24-13 in Chapter 24). However, this distinction may be difficult in some cases. Loculated pneumothorax may closely mimic a bulla.

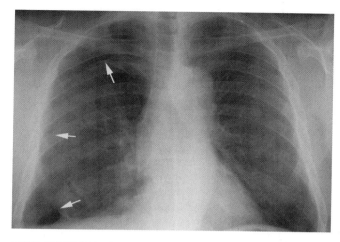

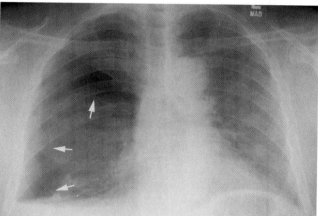

FIG. 26-45. Inspiratory and expiratory radiographs in spontaneous pneumothorax. The relative volume of the pneumothorax *(arrows)* is smaller on inspiration **(A)** than on expiration **(B)**.

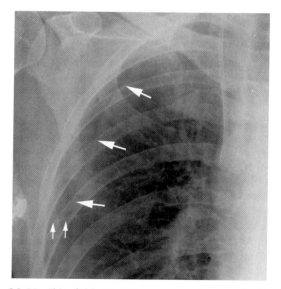

FIG. 26-44. Skin fold mimicking pneumothorax. A skin fold *(large arrows)* mimics pneumothorax, but a distinct pleural line is not visible, and lung markings *(small arrows)* may be seen peripheral to it.

Approximately half of the density of lung is blood, and when lung collapses in the presence of pneumothorax, a significant increase in lung density need not be visible. Reduction in lung volume also results in a reduction in lung perfusion. Until the lung become very small (Fig. 26-46), its density does not significantly increase.

Supine Patient

In supine patients, free pneumothorax usually collects within the anterior pleural space. A visceral pleural line may be seen medially in some patients (see Fig. 26-43B), mimicking pneumomediastinum. A subpulmonic pneumothorax with a visible visceral pleural line may be seen at the lung base. Less specific findings of pneumothorax in supine patients include the following:

1. The costophrenic angle may appear abnormally deep and lucent because of air in the anterolateral pleura space, the "deep sulcus" sign (Fig. 26-47).

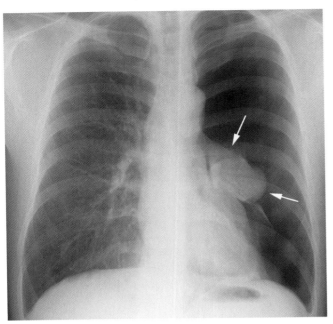

FIG. 26-46. Total spontaneous pneumothorax. The left lung is reduced to the size of a fist *(arrows)*. At this size, compressed lung tissue causes the lung to be dense. No mediastinal shift is present.

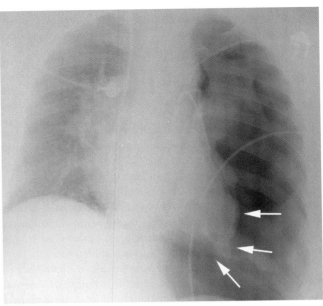

FIG. 26-48. Tension pneumothorax with a deep sulcus sign. Left pneumothorax outlines fat at the cardiac apex, giving it a lumpy appearance *(arrows)*. The left hemidiaphragm is displaced inferiorly and the mediastinum is shifted to the opposite side.

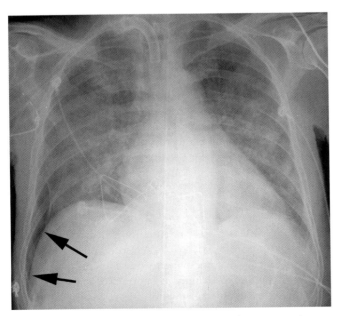

FIG. 26-47. The deep sulcus sign in pneumothorax. A supine radiograph in a patient with pulmonary edema shows a right pneumothorax manifested by a deep sulcus *(arrows)* on the right side. The right diaphragm and right heart borders appear sharp despite lung disease at the lung base.

2. Increased lucency over the chest or upper abdomen
3. Visualization of the anterior costophrenic angle as an edge separate from the diaphragm but parallel to it (the "double-diaphragm" sign)
4. Increased sharpness of the hemidiaphragm (because it is outlined by air), despite lung disease (see Fig. 26-47)
5. Increased sharpness of the cardiac border or mediastinum (because it is outlined by air; see Fig. 26-47)
6. Air in the minor fissure
7. A lumpy appearance at the cardiac apex due to alteration in the shape of the epicardial fat pad in the presence of pneumothorax (Fig. 26-48)

CT Findings

Upright expiratory radiographs and CT are equally sensitive in demonstrating a pneumothorax. CT is considerably more sensitive than supine radiographs in demonstrating pneumothorax.

On CT, a pneumothorax is imaged as air in the pleural space outside the lung and visceral pleura (see Fig. 26-48). Even a very small pneumothorax is visible in the anterior pleural space. Its diagnosis is usually straightforward, although differentiating a medial pneumothorax from pneumomediastinum may be difficult in some cases.

Tension Pneumothorax

Tension pneumothorax means that the pressure of intrapleural air exceeds atmospheric pressure, usually throughout the respiratory cycle; it may be life-threatening. True tension pneumothorax is uncommon. It is most often seen in mechanically ventilated patients or patients with chest trauma. Any pneumothorax in a patient on positive-pressure ventilation should be considered a tension pneumothorax.

Tension pneumothorax is difficult to diagnose on chest radiographs. Shift of the mediastinum away from the pneumothorax is not a reliable finding of tension and can be seen with any large pneumothorax. However, this finding in combination with clinical symptoms of circulatory compromise is usually considered diagnostic. Downward displacement or inversion of the hemidiaphragm also suggests tension (see Fig. 26-48).

In a patient with normal lungs, tension pneumothorax usually results in complete lung collapse. However, in the presence of underlying lung disease such as pulmonary edema, pneumonia, or chronic obstructive pulmonary disease, or in patients receiving positive-pressure ventilation, complete collapse need not occur. Also, complete lung collapse need not indicate tension (see Fig. 26-46).

Hydropneumothorax

Hydropneumothorax, the combination of fluid and air in the pleural space, is readily diagnosed in the upright position because of the presence of an air-fluid level (see Fig. 26-41). In supine or semi-erect patients, a visible pleural line or other findings of pneumothorax may be seen in combination with increased pleural density or findings of pleural fluid. A small amount of fluid is seen in 20% to 40% of patients with pneumothorax, regardless of its cause.

Estimating the Size of a Pneumothorax

There is no precise correlation between pneumothorax size and the need for treatment, although a 30% pneumothorax is generally considered to require treatment. Symptoms are more important in determining which patients require treatment, and this depends on both pneumothorax size and underlying lung disease. Nonetheless, an estimate of pneumothorax size is commonly requested.

The size of a pneumothorax may be estimated by using the average interpleural distance (Table 26-10). The dis-

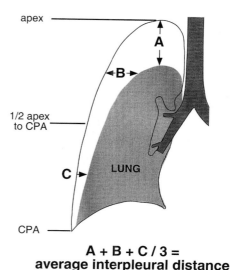

$$A + B + C / 3 =$$
average interpleural distance

FIG. 26-49. Method of calculating average interpleural distance.

tance separating the pleural surface of the lung from the adjacent chest wall (i.e., the depth or thickness of the pneumothorax) is measured in three locations (Fig. 26-49). To make these measurements, divide the hemithorax vertically into two halves, from the apex of the hemithorax to the costophrenic angle. Then measure the distance between lung and the lateral chest at the midpoint of both the upper and lower halves; the third measurement is made vertically above the lung apex. The average of these measurements (i.e., the average interpleural distance) correlates with pneumothorax size in both upright and supine patients (see Table 26-10). Although the accuracy of this estimate is limited, so is the need to accurately determine the size of a pneumothorax. When reviewing Table 26-10, note that the average interpleural distance in millimeters is approximately equal to the pneumothorax percent in an upright patient; in a supine patient, add 9%.

SELECTED READING

Adler BD, Padley SPG, Müller NL. Tuberculosis of the chest wall: CT findings. J Comput Assist Tomogr 1993; 17:271–273.

Alexander E, Clark RA, Colley DP, Mitchell SE. CT of malignant pleural mesothelioma. AJR Am J Roentgenol 1981; 137:287–291.

Aquino SL, Chen MY, Kuo WT, Chiles C. The CT appearance of pleural and extrapleural disease in lymphoma. Clin Radiol 1999; 54:647–650.

Aquino SL, Webb WR, Gushiken BJ. Pleural exudates and transudates: diagnosis with contrast-enhanced CT. Radiology 1994; 192:803–808.

Berkman YM, Auh YH, Davis SD, Kazam E. Anatomy of the minor fissure: evaluation with thin-section CT. Radiology 1989; 170:647–651.

TABLE 26-10. ESTIMATING THE SIZE OF A PNEUMOTHORAX

Average Interpleural Distance (mm)	Percent Pneumothorax	
	Upright Film	Supine Film
10	14%	19%
20	23%	29%
30	32%	39%
40	40%	49%
50	49%	59%

Berkman YM, Davis SD, Kazam E, et al. Right phrenic nerve: anatomy, CT appearance, and differentiation from the pulmonary ligament. Radiology 1989; 173:43–46.

Broaddus VC, Light RW. What is the origin of pleural transudates and exudates? [editorial] Chest 1992; 102:658–659.

Choi BG, Park SH, Yun EH, et al. Pneumothorax size: correlation of supine anteroposterior with erect posteroanterior chest radiographs. Radiology 1998; 209:567–569.

Choi JA, Hong KT, Oh YW, et al. CT manifestations of late sequelae in patients with tuberculous pleuritis. AJR Am J Roentgenol 2001; 176:441–445.

Cooper C, Moss AA, Buy JN, Stark DD. CT appearance of the normal inferior pulmonary ligament. AJR Am J Roentgenol 1983; 141:237–240.

Dynes MC, White EM, Fry WA, Ghahremani GG. Imaging manifestations of pleural tumors. Radiographics 1992; 12:1191–1201.

Federle MP, Mark AS, Guillaumin ES. CT of subpulmonic pleural effusions and atelectasis: criteria for differentiation from subphrenic fluid. AJR Am J Roentgenol 1986; 146:685–689.

Godwin JD, Tarver RD. Accessory fissures of the lung. AJR Am J Roentgenol 1985; 144:39–47.

Godwin JD, Vock P, Osborne DR. CT of the pulmonary ligament. AJR Am J Roentgenol 1983; 141:231–236.

Halvorsen RA, Fedyshin PJ, Korobkin M, et al. Ascites or pleural effusion? CT differentiation: four useful criteria. Radiographics 1986; 6:135–149.

Hulnick DH, Naidich DP, McCauley DI. Pleural tuberculosis evaluated by computed tomography. Radiology 1983; 149:759–765.

Im JG, Webb WR, Rosen A, Gamsu G. Costal pleura: appearances at high-resolution CT. Radiology 1989; 171:125–131.

Kawashima A, Libshitz HI. Malignant pleural mesothelioma: CT manifestations in 50 cases. AJR Am J Roentgenol 1990; 155:965–969.

Lee KS, Im JG, Choe KO, et al. CT findings in benign fibrous mesothelioma of the pleura: pathologic correlation in nine patients. AJR Am J Roentgenol 1992; 158:983–986.

Leung AN, Müller NL, Miller RR. CT in differential diagnosis of diffuse pleural disease. AJR Am J Roentgenol 1990; 154:487–492.

Marks BW, Kuhns IR. Identification of the pleural fissures with computed tomography. Radiology 1982; 143:139–141.

Mirvis S, Dutcher JP, Haney PJ, et al. CT of malignant pleural mesothelioma. AJR Am J Roentgenol 1983; 140:665–670.

Patz EF, Shaffer K, Piwnica-Worms DR, et al. Malignant pleural mesothelioma: value of CT and MR imaging in predicting resectability. AJR Am J Roentgenol 1992; 159:961–966.

Proto AV, Ball JB. Computed tomography of the major and minor fissures. AJR Am J Roentgenol 1983; 140:439–448.

Raasch BN, Carsky EW, Lane EJ, et al. Radiographic anatomy of the interlobar fissures: a study of 100 specimens. AJR Am J Roentgenol 1982; 138:1043.

Rabinowitz JG, Cohen BA, Mendelson DS. The pulmonary ligament. Radiol Clin North Am 1984; 22:659–672.

Rhea JT, DeLuca SA, Greene RE. Determining the size of pneumothorax in the upright patient. Radiology 1982; 144:733–736.

Rost RC Jr, Proto AV. Inferior pulmonary ligament: computed tomographic appearance. Radiology 1983; 148:479–483.

Schmitt WGH, Hübener KH, Rücker HC. Pleural calcification with persistent effusion. Radiology 1983; 149:633–638.

Stark DD, Federle MP, Goodman PC, et al. Differentiating lung abscess and empyema: radiography and computed tomography. AJR Am J Roentgenol 1983; 141:163–167.

Vix VA. Extrapleural costal fat. Radiology 1974; 112:563–565.

Waite RJ, Carbonneau RJ, Balikian JP, et al. Parietal pleural changes in empyema: appearances at CT. Radiology 1990; 175:145–150.

27

PULMONARY THROMBOEMBOLIC DISEASE

MICHAEL B. GOTWAY, GAUTHAM P. REDDY, AND SAMUEL K. DAWN

Deep venous thrombosis (DVT) and pulmonary embolism (PE) represent different ends of the spectrum of a single disease—venous thromboembolism (VTE). VTE is a common problem, yet there are many approaches for establishing the diagnosis, and numerous methods for the investigation of VTE may be employed. Familiarity with risk factors for VTE, the clinical presentations of VTE, laboratory evaluation of VTE, and the imaging evaluation of suspected VTE is extremely important for all physicians, particularly radiologists.

CHEST RADIOGRAPHY

Chest radiographic findings of pulmonary embolism (PE) have been extensively studied. Although chest radiographs in patients with PE may be completely normal, some abnormality usually is present. Among the patients in the Prospective Investigation of Pulmonary Embolism Diagnosis (PIOPED) study who did not have prior cardiopulmonary disease, chest radiographs were abnormal in 84% of patients with proven PE and 66% of those without PE. However, radiographic abnormalities in the setting of PE generally are nonspecific and transient, and usually do not allow a specific diagnosis of PE. In the proper clinical setting, however, certain radiographic findings or combinations of findings may suggest the diagnosis of PE and thus serve to direct further imaging to either establish or exclude this diagnosis.

Pulmonary Vascular Abnormalities

Focal peripheral lucency beyond an occluded vessel, often accompanied by mild dilation of the central pulmonary vessels, known as *Westermark's sign,* (Fig. 27-1), is a very non-specific finding, seen in only 7% to 14% of cases of documented PE in the PIOPED study. Westermark's sign is thought to be caused by embolic obstruction of the pulmonary artery or hypoxic vasoconstriction secondary to ventila-

tion of poorly perfused lung. This sign often is a subtle finding, in many cases not recognized prospectively, and can be mimicked by other common lung diseases, such as emphysema.

Enlargement of the central pulmonary vasculature also may occur with PE and also frequently may be subtle and easily overlooked. This finding may be the result of distention of the vessel by thrombus or by acute rise in pulmonary arterial pressure secondary to the presence of distal emboli. Enlargement of the right descending pulmonary artery, occasionally with a "sausage-like" configuration, may be seen in a number of patients with acute PE, and the size and shape of the artery may normalize following resolution of the embolic event. Enlargement of the right descending pulmonary artery is not specific to PE and may result from pulmonary hypertension of any cause.

Pulmonary edema rarely may occur in association with PE. This finding most often is seen in patients with underlying cardiopulmonary disease, and may be caused by left ventricular failure precipitated by PE.

Focal Parenchymal Opacities

Focal parenchymal abnormalities, particularly atelectasis, were the most common chest radiographic abnormalities in patients with PE in the PIOPED series, occurring in just over two thirds of the patients. Linear opacities often occur near the lung bases and are thought to represent areas of subsegmental atelectasis related to mucous plugging, hypoventilation, or, perhaps, to distal airway closure or focal depletion of surfactant. Such opacities commonly are transient; if they persist, they may represent areas of scarring secondary to prior infarction.

Focal air-space consolidation may occur in patients with PE and may represent pulmonary hemorrhage without infarction or true pulmonary infarction with ischemic necrosis of lung tissue. Estimates of the frequency of pulmonary infarction in patients with PE vary from 10% to 60%. Infarction is most likely to occur when diminished cardiopul-

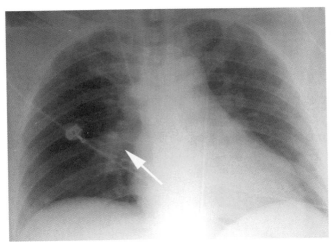

FIG. 27-1. Westermark's sign. Frontal chest radiograph in a 55-year-old woman with acute onset of shortness of breath following surgery shows increased lucency throughout the right lung with enlargement of the right interlobar pulmonary artery *(arrow)*. Acute venous thromboembolism was diagnosed using helical CT shortly after this chest radiograph was obtained.

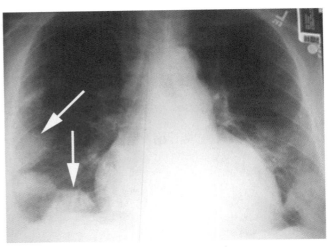

FIG. 27-2. Pulmonary infarction. Frontal chest radiograph in a 36-year-old man with abrupt onset of shortness of breath and hemoptysis shows several wedge-shaped, subpleural opacities in the lower lobes bilaterally *(arrows)*, representing pulmonary infarction. Note that the rounded and truncated medial borders of the opacities face toward the pulmonary hila. Pulmonary embolism was proven at helical CT.

monary reserve is present because both the pulmonary and bronchial arterial systems are impaired. Infarcts often are multiple and occur most frequently in the subpleural regions of the lower lobes, usually within 12 to 24 hours of the onset of symptoms. Infarcts are variable in size and often do not show an air bronchogram, a finding that may favor the diagnosis of infarction over pneumonia. Infarcts typically are ill-defined but may progress over several days to a discrete focal opacity. The classic description of a pulmonary infarct, the "Hampton hump," is a circumscribed, subpleural opacity with a rounded or truncated convex medial border facing toward the pulmonary hilum (Fig. 27-2). This finding is neither common nor specific, however.

Cavitation within a bland (uninfected) infarct is uncommon. Bland infarct cavitation is more likely when the infarct is larger than 4 cm in diameter. When cavitation occurs, it usually is apparent within 2 weeks of the appearance of the air-space opacity.

When air-space opacities are secondary to pulmonary hemorrhage without infarction, resolution of the abnormality usually is rapid; however, true infarction with ischemic tissue necrosis usually takes weeks or months to resolve, leaving linear scars or occasionally associated with pleural thickening. Resolution of pulmonary infarction has been likened to the "melting of an ice cube," implying that an infarct clears by peripheral dissolution whereas pneumonia will gradually clear in an irregular, patchy fashion.

Pleural Effusion and Diaphragmatic Abnormalities

Pleural effusion is detected on chest radiography in about half of patients with PE and usually is unilateral and small.

When pulmonary infarction occurs, pleural effusions may be larger, hemorrhagic, and may take longer to resolve. Diaphragmatic elevation is common in patients with PE, but this finding is nonspecific.

Chest Radiography for the Diagnosis of Pulmonary Embolism

Chest radiographic abnormalities in patients with PE usually are nonspecific and neither establish nor exclude the diagnosis of PE. The sensitivity and specificity of chest radiography for the diagnosis of PE are only 33% and 59%, respectively. The main value of chest radiographs is for the detection of diagnoses that may clinically simulate PE, such as pneumothorax, pulmonary edema, pneumonia, or rib fractures. In addition, a recent chest radiograph is required for the interpretation of ventilation/perfusion (V̇/Ṗ) scintigraphy.

LOWER EXTREMITY VENOUS ULTRASOUND

The primary source of PE is thrombosis within the deep venous system of the lower extremities; about 90% of PEs originate from lower extremity DVT. Less common sources of pulmonary emboli include the deep veins of the pelvis, the renal veins, and the veins of the upper extremities. PE arising from DVT in these less common sites often occurs in a suggestive clinical context, whereas up to 50% of lower extremity DVT episodes may be clinically silent. Additionally, DVT often is asymptomatic, even in the presence of clinical evidence of PE. In nearly one third of patients with PE but without clinical evidence of DVT, contrast venography may reveal the presence of silent DVT. Because the clinical examination is unreliable for the detection of DVT, and the morbidity and mortality related to undiagnosed venous thromboembolism are significant, much effort has been directed toward the development of accurate methods for DVT detection. Traditional methods for DVT detection, such as impedance plethysmography and contrast venography (CV), have been replaced in clinical practice for the most part by laboratory and imaging techniques, including d-dimer assays, contrast-enhanced magnetic resonance venography (MRV), and lower extremity ultrasound. CV traditionally has been considered the gold standard for DVT detection. However, because CV is invasive, expensive, and occasionally can induce venous thrombosis, it is not an optimal screening technique for DVT. During the past two decades, lower extremity ultrasonography has supplanted other imaging and physiologic methods for the initial evaluation of suspected DVT. The noninvasive nature, availability, ease of performance, and accuracy of ultrasonography have resulted in its widespread use as the initial diagnostic study in the evaluation of suspected DVT.

Technique

Ultrasound techniques used in the evaluation of DVT variously include real-time gray scale imaging (with and without compression), continuous wave and pulsed Doppler, color Doppler imaging, and ancillary techniques, such as the Valsalva maneuver and manual blood flow augmentation. A high-frequency linear array transducer is preferred to provide optimal spatial resolution. For larger patients, a lower-frequency transducer may be required to provide adequate tissue penetration to visualize the deep venous system of the lower extremity successfully. The lower extremity veins are imaged in both longitudinal and transverse planes from the level of the inguinal ligament to the popliteal trifurcation, including the common femoral vein, the superficial femoral vein, the popliteal vein, and the saphenous vein at its junction with the common femoral vein. Normal veins appear as tubular, anechoic structures. Although thrombosis occasionally may be seen with gray-scale sonography (Fig. 27-3), real-time imaging alone is not sufficient to exclude DVT, because thrombus may have variable echogenicity and often is anechoic, especially when acute; therefore, compression ultrasonography has become the most reliable maneuver to assess for DVT. With compression ultrasonography, the venous system is visualized in the transverse plane and serially compressed from the inguinal ligament to the popliteal fossa in 1- to 2-cm intervals by exerting gentle pressure with the transducer. The diagnosis of DVT is established by demonstrating lack of venous compression due to intraluminal thrombus (Fig. 27-4).

Additional methods employed during lower extremity

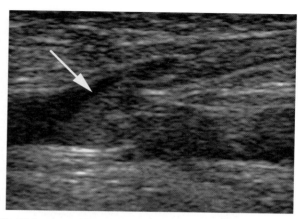

FIG. 27-3. Gray-scale ultrasound demonstration of deep venous thrombosis. Longitudinal image of the common femoral vein at its juncture with the superficial saphenous vein shows echogenic material filling the common femoral vein *(arrow)*, consistent with deep venous thrombosis.

venous ultrasound examinations for suspected DVT include the Valsalva maneuver, spectral Doppler analysis, and color Doppler analysis. In response to a Valsalva maneuver, a normal vein dilates to more than 50% of its original diameter as a result of impaired venous drainage upstream from the area sampled, whereas veins with acute thrombus have pathologic changes in their walls that prevent such dilation. Lack of appropriate response to a Valsalva maneuver also may indicate thrombosis or obstruction of more central veins outside the field of view, such as the inferior vena cava. The Valsalva maneuver requires adequate patient cooperation and generally is limited to assessment of the common femoral vein, which is sufficiently large to demonstrate the caliber changes induced by the altered blood volume caused by the maneuver. Although an abnormal venous response to the Valsalva maneuver supports the diagnosis of DVT when there is a lack of venous compressibility, and a normal response may corroborate the findings of a normal compression ultrasound examination, normal or abnormal Valsalva maneuvers alone are not sufficiently sensitive or specific to establish or exclude the diagnosis of DVT.

Spectral Doppler analysis is particularly useful for vessels that cannot be visualized directly (such as the medial portions of the subclavian veins, the central inferior venous cava [IVC], the superior vena cava [SVC], and brachiocephalic veins). The spectral Doppler waveform of patent central vessels normally shows respiratory phasicity. A monophasic waveform suggests venous obstruction remote from the point of venous interrogation. This abnormal waveform can indicate central DVT, although stenosis or extrinsic compression of the central veins may result in a similar waveform.

Color Doppler imaging is a useful addition to lower extremity compression ultrasonography. Color Doppler is val-

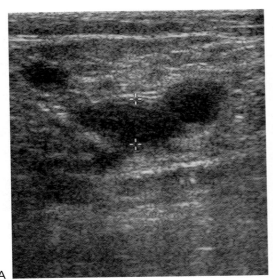 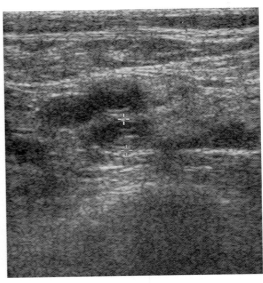

FIG. 27-4. Deep venous thrombosis: compression ultrasonography. **A.** Transverse rest image shows the common femoral vein (indicated by calipers). **B.** Transverse compression image shows that the common femoral vein is not completely compressible (vein marked by calipers), consistent with deep venous thrombosis.

uable for identifying deep venous structures and interrogating deep vessels where the application of direct venous compression is difficult, such as the superficial femoral vein in the adductor hiatus and the iliac veins (Fig. 27-5). In patients who may be difficult to image, such as obese or postoperative patients, or those with swollen extremities, color Doppler imaging is a useful tool for identifying and interrogating venous anatomy. Venous thrombosis is shown on color Doppler imaging as absence of color flow within the vessel lumen (Fig. 27-6) at baseline and with augmentation. In patients with clinically suspected DVT and a technically adequate examination, color Doppler imaging demonstrates high sensitivity (95%) and specificity (98%) for the diagnosis of femoropopliteal DVT. However, for asymptomatic, high-risk patients (e.g., patients who have just undergone orthopaedic surgery or trauma patients), the sensitivity of color Doppler imaging for the detection of femoropopliteal DVT is much lower, perhaps due to the presence of short-segment or nonocclusive thrombus, a relatively high proportion of thrombi limited to the calf veins, or an overall decrease in prevalence of lower extremity DVT in settings where routine DVT prophylaxis is used.

Flow augmentation using spectral Doppler is performed by placing the Doppler gate on the examined vein in the longitudinal plane and manually compressing the calf. A normal response is a rapid rise and fall in blood flow velocity in the interrogated vessel. Such a response implies that the venous system is patent between the point of interrogation and the area of manual compression. Lack of a normal response to flow augmentation may indicate nonocclusive

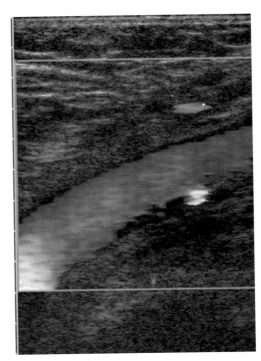

FIG. 27-5. Normal venous color Doppler sonography. Longitudinal image of the external iliac vein shows normal color Doppler signal filling the vessel. Color Doppler is useful for the evaluation of venous segments that are not amenable to compression ultrasonography, such as the external iliac vein.

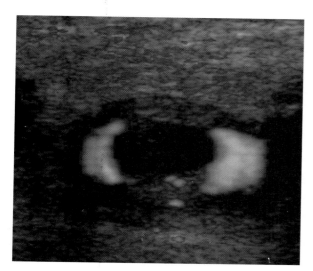

FIG. 27-6. Color Doppler ultrasound demonstration of deep venous thrombosis. Transverse color Doppler image shows exclusion of color Doppler signal from the center of the vein, consistent with deep venous thrombosis.

thrombus, although this observation is not specific for this diagnosis.

Accuracy of Compression Ultrasound

The compression ultrasound examination has been proved to be accurate in multiple studies that compared compression ultrasonography with contrast venography and impedance plethysmography in symptomatic patients. When results of various series are combined, compression ultrasonography demonstrates a sensitivity of at least 93% and a specificity of 98% for femoropopliteal DVT, and these numbers would probably be enhanced some with the routine addition of spectral and color Doppler techniques. The overall diagnostic accuracy of compression ultrasonography in the symptomatic patient is lower, however, when the analysis includes potential calf vein thrombosis.

The reliability of a negative compression ultrasound examination is high. Outcome studies have shown no deleterious effects resulting from withholding anticoagulation therapy in patients with clinically suspected DVT who have negative compression ultrasonography examinations at presentation and at follow-up testing over the next week.

Data on the accuracy of compression ultrasonography in asymptomatic, high-risk patient populations (e.g., following orthopaedic surgery) are conflicting, with some series showing poor sensitivity for lower extremity ultrasound (including spectral and color Doppler techniques), but other studies showing better results. Conflicting data may be the result of differences in study design and study populations.

Calf Veins

The importance of diagnosing isolated calf vein thrombosis is controversial. Although many investigators postulate that clinically significant PE does not originate from calf veins, not all sources agree that calf vein thrombosis is self-limited. Venographic studies have shown that 40% of untreated calf vein thrombi will remain below the knee, 40% will lyse, and 20% may extend into the femoropopliteal system. Once calf vein thrombi extend above the knee, 50% may be associated with abnormal $\dot{V}/\dot{P}$ scintigraphy, indicating possible PE. Many physicians do not treat calf vein thrombosis aggressively, but anticoagulation certainly is warranted for patients with proximal thrombi, so it may be clinically useful to detect calf vein thrombi before proximal migration has occurred. Calf vein thrombosis can be demonstrated with serial imaging by impedance plethysmography or compression ultrasonography, or by direct examination of the veins of the calf. Outcome studies employing compression ultrasonography in symptomatic patients have shown that it is safe to withhold anticoagulation in patients with a negative initial compression ultrasound examination, provided that symptoms prompting the initial compression ultrasound examination do not persist. If lower extremity symptoms persist following the initial examination, a repeat sonogram should be obtained; a small number of patients with an initially negative examination but persistent symptoms will be found to have femoropopliteal DVT on the subsequent compression ultrasound exam. This observation presumably reflects proximal migration of previously undetected calf vein thrombosis.

Another method of addressing suspected calf vein thrombosis is direct examination of the calf veins with ultrasound. The technique of calf vein sonography is not uniformly standardized, and rates of technically adequate examinations vary widely because calf vein sonography is difficult to perform. Several studies have demonstrated encouraging results for calf vein thrombosis detection when examinations are technically satisfactory, though results are variable. Again, color Doppler imaging is a useful adjunct to routine compression ultrasound in the evaluation of symptomatic patients with potential calf vein thrombosis. However, compression ultrasonography, with or without color Doppler, is an insensitive test for calf vein thrombosis for asymptomatic high-risk patients. As with compression ultrasonography in the calf, the utility of color Doppler imaging may be limited by the difficulty in obtaining a technically adequate study.

Upper Extremity Venous Thrombosis

Ultrasound is an excellent screening tool for the assessment of potential upper extremity thrombosis. Routine compression ultrasonography can be utilized in the jugular and brachial venous systems, but the medial aspects of the subclavian veins, the brachiocephalic veins, and the superior vena cava are inaccessible to direct compression. Therefore, interrogation of these vessels requires spectral and color Doppler techniques. Thrombosis may identified by the absence of color Doppler flow within the vessel lumen, occasionally accompanied by echogenic material completely or partially filling the vessel lumen. Spectral Doppler analysis is particularly valuable in the evaluation of potential upper extremity thrombosis. The patency of central venous structures that cannot be visualized directly is inferred by the presence of normal respiratory phasicity. Monophasic flow in the jugular or subclavian veins suggests a central venous abnormality such as DVT, stenosis, or extrinsic compression. Familiarity with these methods is important because the incidence of PE in the setting of upper extremity DVT may be as high as 12%. Furthermore, the incidence of upper extremity DVT is rising, largely due to the increased use of long-term indwelling catheters for total parenteral nutrition, chemotherapy, and other indications.

COMPRESSION ULTRASONOGRAPHY IN THE EVALUATION OF VENOUS THROMBOEMBOLISM

Compression ultrasonography is useful as an initial study in patients presenting with clinical suspicion of PE, particularly when patients present with unilateral DVT symptoms. In such instances, if lower extremity DVT is demonstrated by compression ultrasonography, anticoagulation may be instituted without further testing. This approach is rapid and inexpensive, and avoids the use of ionizing radiation. Although 90% of PEs originate in the lower extremity venous system (making it reasonable to begin the evaluation of VTE here), in one third of patients with proven PE, lower extremity contrast venography is negative for DVT. Nonocclusive thrombus, unrecognized complete embolization of the clot without residua in the legs, and thrombus originating in nonimaged venous segments (e.g., deep pelvic veins), may account for this apparent discrepancy. So, it is clear that a negative lower extremity compression ultrasound examination is insufficiently sensitive to exclude PE in patients with clinical suspicion of PE.

For patients with nondiagnostic, (i.e., intermediate- or low-probability), $\dot{V}/\dot{P}$ scintigraphy results, compression ultrasonography may be obtained in an effort to avoid either CT scanning or pulmonary angiography. In this setting, if the compression ultrasound examination is positive, anticoagulation may be instituted without need for further testing. Compression ultrasonography has been shown to be cost-effective when used in this fashion, because only those patients with normal lower extremity compression ultrasound examinations need further evaluation for suspected PE.

VENTILATION-PERFUSION SCINTIGRAPHY

Scintigraphy has occupied a central role in the evaluation of venous thromboembolism (VTE) for more than three decades. Although CT scanning has emerged as the initial diagnostic test at many institutions for patients suspected of PE, planar $\dot{V}/\dot{P}$ lung scanning still is commonly used for the investigation of suspected PE.

Pulmonary Anatomy and Physiology

A basic understanding of normal pulmonary physiology is required to appreciate the alterations in lung function that occur in patients with PE. Reflex pneumoconstriction may occur in alveoli that are ventilated but not perfused (i.e., abnormally "high" $\dot{V}/\dot{Q}$); abnormally low carbon dioxide tension elicits this response. However, this reflex is not commonly observed and generally is transient, because patients inhale carbon dioxide from tracheal dead space into the poorly perfused alveoli, and bronchial circulation continues to deliver some carbon dioxide to ischemic alveoli, thus moderating this reflex bronchoconstriction. Abnormalities of ventilation may produce regional alveolar hypoxia, which, in turn, induces reflex pulmonary vasoconstriction. Thus alveolar hypoxia (i.e., areas of abnormally low $\dot{V}/\dot{Q}$) causes redistribution of pulmonary blood flow away from hypoventilated alveoli. These pulmonary responses to alterations in regional ventilation and perfusion provide the basis for $\dot{V}/\dot{P}$ scintigraphy.

Technique
Ventilation Scintigraphy

The agent most commonly used for ventilation scintigraphy is xenon-133. Xenon-133 is an inert gas with a principal photon energy of 81 keV and a physical half-life of 5.3 days. The advantages of xenon-133 are that it is relatively inexpensive, is widely available, and allows the acquisition of single-breath, equilibrium, and washout images. A disadvantage of xenon-133 is its low photon energy (81 keV), which generally requires that ventilation scans be obtained before perfusion scans. If technetium perfusion images are acquired prior to the xenon-133 ventilation study, the downscatter from the technetium-99m (^{99m}Tc) photons (140 keV principal photon energy) will be detected in the xenon window of the pulse height analyzer and will degrade the ventilation images. If the ventilation study must be performed or repeated after the perfusion study has been completed, ventilation images can be improved if a ^{99m}Tc background image is obtained using the xenon-133 window. This background image can then be subtracted from the subsequent xenon-133 ventilation images to improve image quality.

Xenon-133 images usually are obtained in the upright

posterior projection to allow evaluation of the largest amount of lung volume. The single-breath image is obtained by having the patient exhale completely and then inhale approximately 5 to 20 mCi (200 to 740 MBq) xenon-133 gas, after which a 15- to 30-second breathhold is performed to obtain a static image. Then, the patient is instructed to breathe a mixture of the exhaled xenon and oxygen for 3 to 5 minutes, as tolerated, while static equilibrium images are obtained; images thus acquired represent the distribution of aerated lung volume. Finally, washout images are acquired by having the patient breathe fresh air while serial 15- to 30-second images are obtained for a period of 3 minutes as xenon clears from the lungs. Normal xenon clearance is bilaterally symmetric and usually is complete in 2 to 3 minutes. Areas of delayed clearance may indicate regional air trapping and are commonly seen in patients with obstructive lung disease.

Xenon-127 has been used for ventilation scintigraphy and has the advantage of higher photon energies (172, 203, and 375 keV), which allow the perfusion study to be performed first. Performing the perfusion study first allows the projection that best shows perfusion defects to be chosen for the ventilation study, thereby allowing a direct comparison between ventilation and perfusion studies and permitting the omission of the ventilation study if the perfusion scan is normal. Xenon-127 also has a relatively long half-life (36.4 days). However, the advantages of xenon-127 are outweighed by the limited availability and expense of this agent. Krypton-81 also has the advantage of a higher photon energies (176 and 192 keV), but krypton is expensive and has a short half-life (13 seconds) which prevents single-breath and washout imaging.

Ventilation imaging also can be performed with aerosols labeled with ^{99m}Tc. Technetium-labeled aerosols have the advantage of the ideal technetium photon energy (140 keV), widespread availability, the optimal half-life of this agent, and they do not require the special exhaust systems that must be employed with xenon studies. Disadvantages of aerosols include the inability to obtain single-breath and washout images and a slightly higher rate of technically inadequate studies compared with xenon imaging. This latter difficulty results from central tracer deposition and inadequate peripheral penetration of the tracer, a problem that is more common in smokers.

The most widely used aerosol is ^{99m}Tc-labeled diethylenetriamine-pentaacetic acid (DTPA). A dose of 25 to 35 mCi (900 to 1300 MBq) of ^{99m}Tc-DTPA is inhaled via nebulizer, and initial images are obtained in the upright position for approximately 200,000 counts. Multiple projections may be obtained. The DTPA aerosol is absorbed across the alveolar-capillary membrane with a clearance time of half-life of 45 to 60 minutes, occasionally faster in smokers. When the aerosol study is performed prior to perfusion imaging, only 1 mCi (37 MBq) of activity related to the aerosol is present in the lungs; thus, the aerosol contributes

little activity to the perfusion image when 4 to 5 mCi (148 to 185 MBq) are used for the latter.

Perfusion Scintigraphy

Pulmonary perfusion scintigraphy is performed with ^{99m}Tc-labeled macroaggregated albumin (MAA). MAA particles range in size from 10 to 40 μm, allowing them to localize in precapillary arterioles by mechanical blockade. The physiologic effect of pulmonary vascular blockade usually is insignificant, because less than 0.1% of precapillary pulmonary arterioles are occluded and the blockage is temporary because the biologic half-life of ^{99m}Tc-MAA particles in the lungs is only 6 to 8 hours.

About 1 to 5 mCi (37 to 185 MBq) of ^{99m}Tc-MAA is injected intravenously during quiet respiration with the patient supine. Supine injections are performed to minimize the normal perfusion gradient between lung apex and base in the upright patient and ensure even tracer distribution. Blood withdrawn into the syringe during venipuncture must not be allowed to remain in the syringe, because small blood clots may form. These will be labeled with tracer, and injection of these labeled clots will result in "hot spots" on the perfusion image. The tracer is injected slowly over several respiratory cycles. The number of particles injected ranges from 200,000 to 700,000, with fewer particles employed in children, pregnant women, or patients with right-to-left shunts or pulmonary hypertension. In such circumstances the number of particles injected should be decreased to 100,000. Any further decrease in the number of particles produces tracer inhomogeneity and result in degraded images.

Imaging is performed immediately after tracer injection, preferably with the patient in the upright position to minimize diaphragmatic motion and maximize lung volume. Imaging may be performed in either the supine or decubitus positions, as needed. Imaging is performed with a large field-of-view camera and either a parallel-hole, all-purpose, or diverging collimator. Planar images are obtained in multiple projections (usually anterior, posterior, both posterior oblique, and both lateral projections). Other specialized projections may be obtained as desired. Each projection is acquired for approximately 500,000 to 750,000 counts. The first lateral view is acquired for 500,000 counts and the opposite lateral view is acquired for the same amount of time needed to obtain the first lateral view.

Interpretation

A normal ventilation scan shows relatively homogeneous pulmonary tracer activity on the single-breath and equilibrium images. During the washout phase, tracer activity slowly clears, with the bases clearing slightly more slowly than the remainder of the lungs. Clearing usually is complete in 2 or 3 minutes. ^{99m}Tc-DTPA aerosols also demonstrate homogeneous tracer activity from lung apex to base but, unlike xenon scans, the trachea and bronchi normally may be seen. Occasionally, swallowed activity may be detected in the esophagus and stomach.

Normal perfusion scans reveal homogeneous pulmonary tracer activity with predictable defects in the expected locations of the heart, pulmonary hila, and aortic arch, depending on the projection obtained.

Various schemes have been devised to interpret $\dot{V}/\dot{Q}$ scintigraphy. These schemes rely on the principle that PE causes decreased or absent pulmonary blood flow in a portion of lung, producing a perfusion defect. Because the alveoli serving these occluded vessels remain ventilated, a $\dot{V}/\dot{Q}$ "mismatch" is created. Unfortunately, many causes of perfusion defects unrelated to PE exist, and PE itself does not always result in a $\dot{V}/\dot{Q}$ mismatch. Hence, PE is neither diagnosed nor excluded by $\dot{V}/\dot{Q}$ lung scanning; rather, the probability of PE in any given patient is generated by interpretation of the lung scan. These probabilities are based on criteria that evaluate the shape, number, location, and size of perfusion defects on the perfusion scan in combination with the findings on the ventilation lung scan and chest radiograph. Perfusion defects are classified as lobar, segmental, or subsegmental; defects that do not conform to segmental lung anatomy are considered nonsegmental defects. The shape of perfusion defects also is important. Perfusion defects resulting from PE usually are wedge-shaped and contact the pleural surface (Fig. 27-7). Defects that do not extend to the pleural surface may show a rim of activity immediately beneath the pleural surface but peripheral to the perfusion defect—a finding known as the "stripe" sign. Such perfusion abnormalities usually are not the result of PE. The number of perfusion defects also may be of some value in determining the likelihood of PE. Solitary perfusion defects usually are not related to PE, whereas multiple subsegmental perfusion defects are associated with PE in up to 50% of cases. The size of a perfusion defect also is significant. Sizes are graded as follows: a small perfusion defect occupies less than 25% of an anatomic lung segment; a moderate perfusion defect represents 25% to 75% of a lung segment; and a large perfusion defect constitutes greater than 75% of an anatomic lung segment. The perfusion scan is interpreted with reference to the chest radiograph, and the size of a perfusion defect is compared to any corresponding chest radiographic abnormality. The chief interpretive schemes (McNeil, Biello, PIOPED, and revised PIOPED classification schemes) have been divided into four diagnostic categories based on the probability of PE at pulmonary angiography: high-probability, intermediate/indeterminate-probability, low-probability, and normal perfusion scintigraphy. In addition to these categories, the original PIOPED criteria included a very-low-probability group in which the prevalence of angiographically documented PE was 9%.

The PIOPED Series

The Prospective Investigation of Pulmonary Embolism Diagnosis (PIOPED) series represents the largest prospective study examining the role of $\dot{V}/\dot{Q}$ scintigraphy in patients with suspected PE. PIOPED scan interpretation criteria were designed to provide diagnostic categories that could be applied to all patients studied with $\dot{V}/\dot{Q}$ scintigraphy. Of 5587 requests for lung scintigraphy in the PIOPED series, 3016 patients were eligible to participate in the trial, and 1493 patients ultimately were enrolled in the study. Among the enrolled patients, 931 were selected for mandatory angiography, and eventually 755 of these patients completed the protocol. Sixty-nine of the patients selected for angiography did not undergo the procedure because their $\dot{V}/\dot{Q}$ lung scans were interpreted as normal, and 107 patients selected for angiography did not undergo the procedure despite the requirement of the study protocol. $\dot{V}/\dot{Q}$ lung scans were compared with pulmonary angiograms, and the interobserver variability for both studies was noted. Patient outcomes were followed for 1 year after study entry. Diagnostic $\dot{V}/\dot{Q}$ scans were obtained in 931 of 933 patients. Among patients with diagnostic scintigraphy, 13% (124 of 931 patients) had high-probability scan interpretations, 39% (364 of 931 patients) had intermediate-probability scan interpretations, 34% (312 of 931 patients) had low-probability scan interpretations, 14% (131 of 931 patients) had normal/near-normal scan interpretations, and 2% had normal scan interpretations. The frequencies of angiographically proven PE for each $\dot{V}/\dot{Q}$ scan category were reported in the PIOPED series, and familiarity with these data are important for any physician dealing with patients suspected of PE. The prevalence of angiographically proven PE in the PIOPED series was 88% for high-probability lung scan interpretations, 33% for intermediate-probability scan interpretations, 16% for low-probability scan interpretations, and 9% for normal/near normal scan interpretations.

On the other hand, only 102 of 251 patients with angiographically documented PE had high-probability scan interpretations, indicating that the sensitivity for a high-probability scan is only 41%. The sensitivity of $\dot{V}/\dot{Q}$ scintigraphy for the detection of PE improves to 82% when high- and intermediate-probability scan interpretations are considered together, and sensitivity increases to 98% when high-, intermediate-, and low-probability scan results are considered together. However, the specificity of $\dot{V}/\dot{Q}$ lung scans falls from 98% when high-probability scans are considered alone to 52% and 10% when high- and intermediate-probability scan results and high-, intermediate-, and low-probability scan interpretations are considered together, respectively.

The interobserver variability for $\dot{V}/\dot{Q}$ interpretation in the PIOPED series was 5%, 8%, and 6%, respectively, for high-probability, very-low-probability, and normal $\dot{V}/\dot{Q}$ scan categories. However, the interobserver variability for intermediate- and low-probability scan categories was higher—25% and 20%, respectively.

The positive predictive value of a high-probability scan interpretation in the PIOPED series in a patient without a prior embolic history was 91%. However, the positive predictive value of a high-probability scan interpretation falls to 74% for patients with prior embolic episodes.

Integration of Clinical Assessment of Pulmonary Embolism Probability With Scan Interpretation

The importance of integration of the clinical pretest probability (i.e., prior probability) of the likelihood of PE with the $\dot{V}/\dot{Q}$ scan interpretation was highlighted by PIOPED (Table 27-1). When a low-probability scan interpretation (angiographically proven PE prevalence of 16%) was combined with a low clinical suspicion for PE (0 to 19% likelihood of PE), the negative predictive value of a low-probability scan increased from 84% to 96% (i.e., the prevalence of PE on angiography decreased from 16% to 4%). Similarly, the negative predictive value of a normal/near-normal scan interpretation rose from 91% to 98% when integrated with a low clinical assessment for the likelihood of PE. The positive predictive value of a high-probability scan interpretation increased from 88% to 96% when combined with a high clinical suspicion (80% to 100% likelihood of PE). In contrast, when a high-probability scan interpretation was integrated with a low clinical suspicion for PE, the positive predictive value of a high-probability scan reading fell from 88% to 56%. Therefore, integration of clinical assessment of the likelihood of PE with scan interpretation results improves the diagnostic accuracy of $\dot{V}/\dot{Q}$ scintigraphy. Unfortunately, most of the PIOPED patients had intermediate-probability $\dot{V}/\dot{Q}$ scan interpretations and intermediate clinical assessments of the likelihood of PE, so most patients did not benefit from this improved diagnostic accuracy, and therefore required further diagnostic evaluation.

Low-Probability Lung Scans

Outcome studies have shown that most patients with low-probability $\dot{V}/\dot{Q}$ scan interpretations do well when anticoag-

ulation is withheld, even though the frequency of angiographically proven PE in this setting is known to range from 14% to 30%. This apparent discrepancy may be explained by subclinical, well-tolerated PE. However, patients with poor cardiopulmonary reserve (e.g., hypotension, coexistent pulmonary edema, right ventricular failure, tachydysrhythmias) and low-probability scan interpretations do not necessarily share the same favorable prognosis, and further diagnostic evaluation is required. Furthermore, patients with low-probability scan interpretations and high-probability pretest clinical assessments or significant risk factors for venous thromboembolism certainly require additional diagnostic evaluation.

Ventilation/Perfusion Scintigraphy and Obstructive Lung Disease

The clinical diagnosis of PE is even more difficult in patients with obstructive lung disease because the clinical manifestations of PE may easily be misinterpreted as a COPD exacerbation, and laboratory values are not sufficiently sensitive or specific to distinguish acute PE from a COPD exacerbation. Unfortunately, $\dot{V}/\dot{Q}$ scintigraphy often is abnormal in patients with moderate or severe COPD. Nevertheless, it has been shown that the diagnostic utility of $\dot{V}/\dot{Q}$ scintigraphy for the evaluation of PE is not diminished in the setting of preexisting cardiopulmonary disease, although intermediate-probability scan interpretations do occur more often in such patients. Furthermore, the diagnostic accuracy of lung scanning in patients with COPD is improved when integrated with the clinical assessment of the likelihood of PE.

Chest Radiography and Ventilation/Perfusion Scintigraphy

The major role of the chest radiograph in the evaluation of suspected PE is the exclusion of diagnoses that clinically simulate PE, such as pulmonary edema, pneumothorax, pneumonia, and pleural effusion. However, the chest radiograph also is essential for the accurate interpretation of $\dot{V}/\dot{Q}$ lung scans. An upright posteroanterior and lateral examination, ideally obtained as close as possible to the $\dot{V}/\dot{Q}$ scan, should be obtained. Perfusion defects substantially larger than corresponding chest radiographic abnormalities are suggestive of PE, whereas perfusion defects substantially smaller than corresponding chest radiographic abnormalities are not commonly associated with PE.

PULMONARY ANGIOGRAPHY IN PATIENTS WITH PULMONARY EMBOLISM

Pulmonary angiography has served as the gold standard for the diagnosis of pulmonary embolism (PE) for decades. An-

TABLE 27-1. SCAN INTERPRETATION AND CLINICAL ASSESSMENT OF PROBABILITY OF PULMONARY EMBOLISM

Scan Probability	High (80%–100%)	Intermediate (20%–79%)	Low (0%–19%)
High	96%	88%	56%
Intermediate	66%	28%	16%
Low	40%	16%	4%
Normal/near-normal	0%	6%	2%
Total	68%	30%	9%

giography traditionally has been indicated whenever a discrepancy between the clinical suspicion for PE and the results of other imaging modalities exists, when V̇/Q̇ scintigraphy is interpreted as high-probability but contraindications to anticoagulation are present, or when conditions that may result in false-positive, high-probability V̇/Q̇ lung scans (e.g., lung carcinoma, pneumonia) coexist with clinical suspicion for PE. Additionally, pulmonary angiography often is obtained before interventions such as mechanical clot fragmentation, catheter-directed pulmonary arterial thrombolysis, peripheral venous thrombolytic therapy, or surgical thromboendarterectomy are initiated. Finally, pulmonary angiography has been used to establish the diagnosis of chronic thromboembolic disease in patients with pulmonary hypertension and for the evaluation of hepatopulmonary syndrome. However, the widespread use of helical CT, especially multislice CT (MSCT) scanning, has largely replaced pulmonary angiography for these indications, unless catheter-directed interventions are anticipated.

Relative Contraindications to Pulmonary Angiography

Iodinated contrast allergy, elevated pulmonary arterial pressure, left bundle branch block, bleeding diatheses, and renal insufficiency are the primary relative contraindications to pulmonary angiography (Table 27-2). Premedication with corticosteroids prior to angiography may be employed for patients who are allergic to iodinated contrast.

Patients with pulmonary arterial pressures higher than 70 mmHg and right ventricular end-diastolic pressures (RVEDP) higher than 20 mmHg have been identified as having a 2% to 3% higher mortality from pulmonary angiography compared to patients with normal or mildly increased pulmonary artery and right ventricular end-diastolic pressures. Despite this, patients with elevated pulmonary arterial pressures often constitute a significant patient population in need of pulmonary angiography. Hence, the presence of increased pressures in the pulmonary circuit is more an indication for selective angiography than an absolute contraindication to the procedure itself.

There is a risk of inducing complete heart block during right heart catheterization in patients with left bundle

branch block. Therefore, preprocedural electrocardiographic evaluation should be performed. If left bundle branch block is identified, a temporary pacemaker may be placed before the procedure is performed.

Bleeding diatheses usually can be managed by administration of the appropriate blood products. Hemostasis at the site of venous entry usually is achieved easily with manual pressure. The risk of postprocedure renal insufficiency may be reduced by maintaining adequate hydration before, during, and following the procedure. Premedication with N-acetylcysteine also may be used for patients with mild insufficiency. Transient elevations in serum creatinine may occur following the procedure, but dialysis rarely becomes necessary.

Minor untoward reactions to contrast material, such as nausea, vomiting, and sensations of warmth, usually require only expectant management. Minor allergic reactions, such as urticaria, may be managed expectantly or with antihistamines, as long as no evidence of laryngeal edema is present. The presence of the latter constitutes a more serious allergic reaction and requires immediate, aggressive management.

Technique

Standard angiographic preparation and technique are used, including continuous cardiac monitoring. A transfemoral venous approach with standard Seldinger technique is employed when possible, although catheterization may be performed through the internal jugular, subclavian, or brachial veins when required. A vascular sheath may be placed, typically 7F. A hand injection through the sheath is performed to confirm patency of the inferior vena cava. A 6.7F Grollman catheter (Cook, Bloomington, IN) or a pigtail catheter with a tip-deflecting wire is used to maneuver across the right heart into the pulmonary arteries. Correlation with prior imaging studies guides which side is the first to be catheterized.

Pulmonary artery pressures should be measured routinely. Right atrial pressure, which approximates right ventricular end-diastolic pressure, also may be measured. For patients with elevated pulmonary arterial pressure or elevated right ventricular end-diastolic pressure, selective catheterization, the use of low osmolar, nonionic contrast agents, balloon occlusion, and lower injection rates may be warranted.

Imaging is obtained in anterior-posterior and oblique projections. Subselective catheterization and magnification imaging may supplement the examination. Injection rates of approximately 20 ml/sec for a total of 40 ml for cut film angiography (CFA) versus 20 to 25 ml/sec for a 1-second injection with digital subtraction angiography (DSA) typically are employed.

DSA is increasingly employed for angiographic techniques, and has largely supplanted cut film methods. DSA image quality has been shown to be equal to that of cut

---

TABLE 27-2. RELATIVE CONTRAINDICATIONS TO PULMONARY ANGIOGRAPHY

Documented contrast material allergy
Elevated right ventricular end-diastolic pressure (>20 mmHg) and/or elevated pulmonary artery pressure (>70 mmHg)
Left bundle branch block
Renal insufficiency/failure
Bleeding diatheses

film, and the interobserver agreement may be higher with DSA. DSA studies are less commonly nondiagnostic than are cut film examinations—3% of angiograms in the PIO-PED study (cut film) were considered nondiagnostic, whereas recent work with DSA techniques indicates that fewer than 1% of DSA examinations are nondiagnostic. Finally, the added benefits of requiring less contrast and less procedural time make DSA an attractive imaging method.

Interpretation

The specificity of pulmonary angiography approaches 100%, for either DSA or CFA, when a filling defect (see Figs. 27-7 and 27-8) or abrupt pulmonary arterial obstruction (Fig. 27-9), with or without outlining of the end of the embolus ("the trailing edge"), is shown in the proper clinical setting. Ancillary criteria that suggest, but are not specific for, the diagnosis of PE include delayed venous return, tortuous vascularity, and decreased pulmonary flow. Angiographic findings in chronic pulmonary thromboembolic disease include pouching, intimal irregularity, tortuosity, webs or bands with poststenotic dilation, abrupt narrowing, and complete vascular obstruction.

Reliability of Pulmonary Angiography for the Diagnosis of Acute Pulmonary Embolism

True false-negative pulmonary angiograms are extremely rare. The reported 5% to 10% frequency of false-positive pulmonary angiography reflects a combination of techni-

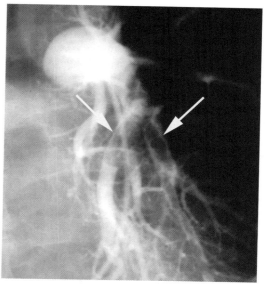

FIG. 27-8. Acute pulmonary embolism: filling defects on pulmonary angiography. Left pulmonary angiogram in a 50-year-old man with indeterminate V̇/Q̇ scintigraphy shows intraluminal filling defects *(arrows)* within the segmental vasculature of the left lower lobe.

cally limited studies and the influence of the timing of the angiogram relative to the embolic event.

A negative pulmonary angiogram interpretation essentially excludes the diagnosis of clinically significant PE. In the PIOPED series, only four patients (0.6%) had clinical evidence, including autopsy information, of PE despite negative angiographic results.

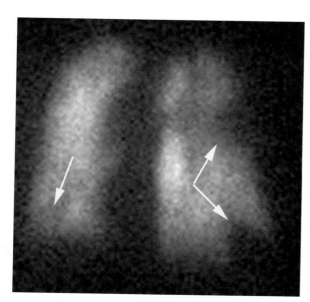

FIG. 27-7. High-probability acute pulmonary embolism seen on V̇/Q̇ scintigraphy. Posterior perfusion image shows numerous, segmental, wedge-shaped perfusion defects *(arrows)*.

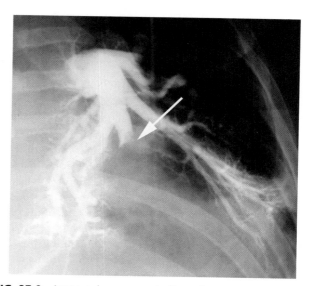

FIG. 27-9. Acute pulmonary embolism: abrupt vascular cutoffs. Left pulmonary angiogram in a 54-year-old man with indeterminate V̇/Q̇ scintigraphy shows abrupt termination of the contrast column *(arrow)* within a segmental left lower lobe artery.

Complications

Procedure-related fatalities occur in approximately 0.2% to 0.5% of patients undergoing pulmonary angiography. The PIOPED study showed no statistically significant relation between pulmonary artery pressure and the frequency of complications, although other investigations have shown that patients with elevated pulmonary arterial or right ventricular end-diastolic pressures are at increased risk for complications while undergoing pulmonary angiography. Recent DSA studies suggest that the incidence of fatal and nonfatal complications with pulmonary angiography is now lower than previously described due to the use of routine cardiac monitoring, modern catheters, low-osmolar, non-ionic contrast agents, and awareness of the potential hazards of nonselective injections in the presence of elevated pulmonary artery pressures.

Major nonfatal complications occur in about 1% to 3% of examinations. These complications include respiratory distress requiring intubation and resuscitation, cardiac perforation (although this complication was not reported in the PIOPED series and has nearly been eliminated since the introduction of pigtail catheters), major dysrhythmias, major contrast reactions, renal failure requiring hemodialysis, and hematomas requiring transfusions.

The incidence of minor complications may occur following pulmonary angiography is about 5%. These complications include contrast-induced renal dysfunction, angina, respiratory distress, contrast reactions that respond promptly to medications and fluids, and transient dysrhythmias.

Helical CT Pulmonary Angiography

The use of CT for diagnosis of PE was first described in 1980, although slow scanning speeds and a lack of dynamic techniques limited its usefulness to occasional patients suspected of having large central emboli. Despite advances in CT technology over the ensuing years, CT was of little value for the diagnosis of PE until the advent of helical CT scanners.

The systematic use of helical single-slice CT (SSCT) for the diagnosis of suspected acute PE was first described in 1992. Because of its reported high accuracy, and distinct limitations in the accuracy or availability of other imaging modalities used for the diagnosis of PE, the use of helical CT has been rapidly embraced, and in many institutions has become the study of choice for suspected pulmonary embolism. Since multislice CT (MSCT) was introduced in 1998, interest in the use of helical CT scanning for suspected PE has become even more widespread. Further experience has clarified the usefulness of helical CT in the diagnosis of PE and has pointed out its limitations, although few data regarding the additional benefit of MSCT scanning are as yet available.

Technical Considerations

When scanning a patient suspected of PE, a specific imaging protocol that is designed to optimize diagnostic information is used. Careful attention to numerous scan parameters is essential to ensure high-quality studies.

Scanning Range and Direction

For SSCT, scans must include the entire range of the visible pulmonary arterial system without necessarily including other areas of the thorax, which would increase radiation dose and possibly adversely affect the timing of the study. SSCT scans should cover the superior portion of the aortic arch to approximately 2 to 3 cm below the inferior pulmonary veins, or about a 10- to 12-cm volume of tissue in the average patient. Scanning should proceed in a caudal-cranial direction. The advantage of scanning in this direction is that respiratory motion is most marked in the lung bases—precisely the area where pulmonary blood flow is maximal and thus where most PEs will be located. Therefore, using a caudal-cranial scanning direction, if the patient were unable to maintain apnea throughout the entire scan, degradation of scan quality would most likely occur in the upper lungs where respiratory motion is minimal and isolated PE less likely.

For MSCT, the scan range need not be limited to a portion of the chest. The scan times are fast enough with these machines that the entire thorax may be imaged, base to apex, in one breathhold.

Duration of Apnea

A single breathhold of approximately 20 seconds is possible in nearly 90% of patients who present for PE imaging. Inspiratory apnea is desirable because it results in increased pulmonary vascular resistance and thus promotes pulmonary arterial contrast enhancement. The patient's ability to maintain apnea may be enhanced by hyperventilation or pre-breathing the patient with oxygen prior to scanning. For patients unable to suspend respiration for the entire scan, quiet breathing during the study usually is not problematic.

Contrast Concentration and Injection Rates

In general, one of three contrast injection protocols may be employed:

High concentration (270 to 320 mg/ml), low rate (2 to 3 ml/sec)

Low concentration (120 to 200 mg/ml), very high rate ($\geq$5 ml/sec)

High concentration (300 to 360 mg/ml) high rate ($\geq$3 ml/sec).

The high concentration, low injection rate protocol has the advantage of being easy to use, even with small-bore IV catheters, but this technique is not in general use. The low concentration, very high injection rate protocol enjoys the advantage of reduced streak artifacts in the superior vena cava when upper extremity veins are injected and may improve visualization of small pulmonary arteries. However, the contrast usually must be diluted manually, thus incurring the risk of contamination of the otherwise sterile solution. Most institutions inject undiluted nonionic contrast intravenously at a rate of 3 ml/sec or higher for helical CT pulmonary angiograms (hCTPA). High concentration, high injection rates maximize pulmonary arterial opacification and allow the use of preloaded syringes, and are therefore convenient as well as effective.

Some institutions inject saline after the contrast medium has been injected. Saline injections, often referred to as "saline chasers," permit the use of less intravenous contrast while maintaining excellent image quality. The use of saline chasers requires a dual-power injector, capable of first injecting contrast and then immediately injecting saline at the end of the contrast injection. Given the widespread use of hCTPA, even small reductions in the amount of intravenous contrast required for these studies may produce significant cost savings.

Regardless of the injection protocol used, the contrast injection must be maintained throughout the scan acquisition to avoid contrast washout and consequent flow artifacts in the pulmonary arteries.

Collimation and Reconstruction Increment

On SSCT systems, 2- to 3-mm collimation imaging with narrow overlapping reconstruction (typically 1 to 2 mm) provides excellent image quality. To image a given volume of tissue, narrower collimation with faster table transport speeds (increased pitch) is favored over wider collimation with slower table transport speeds. Doubling the pitch results in only about a 30% increase in effective slice thickness, so larger volumes of tissue may be scanned with narrow collimation, improving spatial resolution.

The incredible speed of MSCT systems allows the entire chest to be scanned rapidly using very narrow collimation, thus maximizing resolution. Typically, 1- or 2-mm collimation is employed with MSCT scanning (with or without overlapping reconstruction). Overlapping reconstructions do improve the quality of image post-processing, but at the expense of increased data storage requirements.

Contrast Bolus Timing

Proper timing of pulmonary arterial opacification is critical for adequate study quality. Although only the pulmonary arterial system requires examination, it may be desirable to opacify the pulmonary veins and left atrium as proof that the scan was not initiated before complete pulmonary arterial system enhancement. For most patients, a presumptive scan delay of 20 seconds for an upper extremity injection results in adequate pulmonary arterial system enhancement. Longer delays are required with lower extremity injections or if the patient has poor right ventricular function. Alternatively, manual bolus timing may be performed. A limited amount of contrast may be injected while scanning once per second over the main pulmonary arterial segment after a delay of 10 seconds. The time to peak enhancement may be determined visually or by measuring CT attenuation values. Once the time to peak enhancement is known, the proper scan delay may then be programmed. Finally, bolus timing software programs take the guesswork from proper scan timing. Such programs allow the user to place region-of-interest cursors over the vessel or vessels used for timing purposes, and the scanner automatically plots a time-attenuation curve as images of the region selected for timing are acquired once per second after a short delay (typically 8 to 10 seconds). The scan is triggered manually once the proper timing has been achieved. Using this method, proper timing is ensured without requiring the additional step of a manual timing bolus.

Pitch

For SSCT systems, the proper pitch to be used depends on the collimation employed. It is preferable to employ larger pitch values with narrower collimation than the reverse. Thus, the pitch should be increased to the value that is required to acquire the scan volume in a single breathhold. With subsecond SSCT, pitch values of 1.7 to 2 usually are used.

Rapid table transport speed should be used for MSCT pulmonary angiography. It is not necessary to use the fastest possible table transport speed for hCTPA, particularly with 16-slice systems. Rather, a balance among the collimation, table transport speed, and imaging time is required.

Image Review and Postprocessing

Viewing scans at the scanner monitor or using a work station is recommended for diagnosis. The ability to view contiguous scans rapidly in sequence and change window settings rapidly can be very useful in clinical practice.

Multiplanar reformatted images sometimes may be valuable for identifying abnormalities of small arteries that have an oblique course, and may be particularly useful for demonstrating chronic pulmonary emboli. Three-dimensional reconstructions may be performed, including volume rendering, and occasionally are useful for displaying complex anatomic relationships.

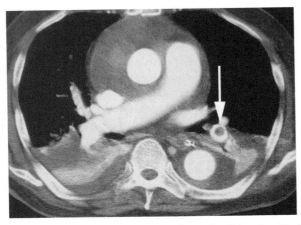

FIG. 27-10. Acute pulmonary embolism: the "doughnut" sign on helical CT pulmonary angiography. Axial CT pulmonary angiogram in a 60-year-old man with shortness of breath following aortic dissection repair shows a round intraluminal filling defect *(arrow)* within the left lower lobe pulmonary artery. High-attenuation material surrounding the ascending aorta represents postsurgical hemorrhage.

Helical CT Pulmonary Angiography Findings in Pulmonary Embolism

Acute PE is diagnosed when an intraluminal filling defect is seen, surrounded to a variable degree by contrast. An acute thrombus may appear to be central within a pulmonary artery when seen in cross section (the "doughnut" sign) (Fig. 27-10), or may be outlined by contrast when imaged along its axis (the "railroad track" sign) (Fig. 27-11); these

are the only absolutely reliable signs of acute PE. In some patients with acute emboli, an eccentric thrombus adherent to the vessel wall may be seen, but this finding is more typical in patients with chronic PE. An obstructed artery can be seen as an unopacified vessel, but this finding also may be seen with chronic emboli.

Ancillary Findings in Patients With Pulmonary Embolism

Ancillary findings on helical CT pulmonary angiography that suggest PE include mosaic perfusion, peripheral consolidations, and pleural effusions.

More than 50% of lung parenchymal attenuation on CT is due to pulmonary blood flow. Therefore, any process that alters pulmonary blood flow has the potential to produce visible changes in parenchymal attenuation. Inhomogeneous lung opacity resulting from alterations in pulmonary blood flow has been referred to as *mosaic perfusion*. Although mosaic perfusion often is related to airway-induced alterations in pulmonary blood flow, vascular causes, including emboli, also may produce mosaic perfusion (Fig. 27-12).

Peripheral consolidations may represent pulmonary hemorrhage with or without pulmonary infarction, particularly when such opacities are wedge-shaped and located in the subpleural regions of lung (Fig. 27-13). Among patients who undergo hCTPA, there is a higher incidence of parenchymal opacities in patients found to have emboli than in those without visible emboli. Unfortunately, peripheral consolidations, even in the setting of suspected PE, rarely are diagnostic by themselves.

Pleural effusions often are present in patients with PE, but they also are commonly seen in patients in whom PE is excluded. There are no CT features of pleural effusion that allow the specific diagnosis of PE.

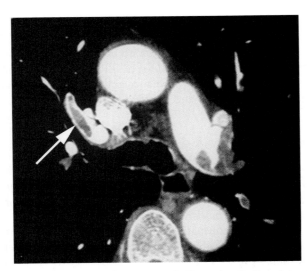

FIG. 27-11. Acute pulmonary embolism: the "railroad track" sign on helical CT pulmonary angiography. Axial CT pulmonary angiogram in a 45-year-old man with shortness of breath shows a linear intraluminal filling defect *(arrow)* within the anterior segmental right upper lobe pulmonary artery.

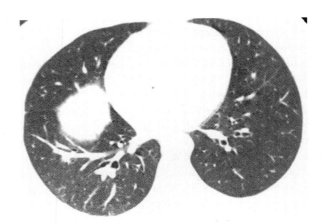

FIG. 27-12. Acute pulmonary embolism: oligemia. Axial CT pulmonary angiogram in a previously healthy 26-year-old man who developed syncope after a neurosurgical procedure shows decreased pulmonary parenchymal attenuation associated with diminished vascular size throughout the left lower lobe.

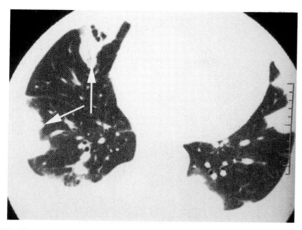

FIG. 27-13. Acute pulmonary embolism: pulmonary infarction. Lung windows from a helical CT pulmonary angiogram in a 36-year-old man with proven pulmonary embolism (same patient as Fig. 27-2) shows bilateral wedge-shaped subpleural opacities *(arrows)* representing pulmonary infarction.

CT Venography

Following a CT study for diagnosis of possible PE, CT venography of the lower extremities, pelvis, and inferior vena cava may be performed without the injection of additional contrast. The entire abdomen, pelvis, and lower extremities, from the symphysis pubis to the tibial plateaus, may be scanned, or the scans may be limited to the pelvic veins and femoropopliteal venous segments. Scans obtained at 3 minutes after the start of contrast injection show opacified veins in the legs and pelvis; thrombi are visible as filling defects within the veins (Fig. 27-14). The addition of CT

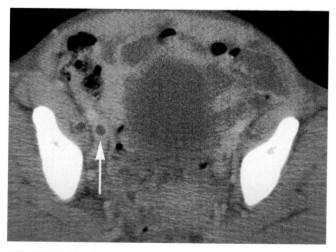

FIG. 27-14. Deep venous thrombosis demonstrated on indirect CT venography. Axial image through the pelvis obtained 3 minutes after the injection of intravenous contrast medium for the thoracic portion of a helical CT pulmonary angiogram shows a filling defect with the right external iliac vein *(arrow)* representing deep venous thrombosis.

venography to helical CT pulmonary angiography allows for the assessment of venous thromboembolism in general in addition to PE. Several studies have shown that the addition of CT venography improves the diagnostic yield for VTE compared to helical CT pulmonary angiography alone.

Accuracy of CT in Diagnosing Acute Embolism

The accuracy of hCTPA for diagnosing pulmonary emboli depends on the size of the artery affected and the size of the emboli. Acute emboli in large pulmonary arteries can be diagnosed with an accuracy of 100%. In patients suspected of having massive embolism, hCTPA should be diagnostic.

Overall, pooled data from a number of studies suggest sensitivity values of about 90% and specificity values exceeding 90% for the SSCT diagnosis of pulmonary emboli involving main to segmental artery branches in unselected patients with suspected PE, although reported values of sensitivity range from 53% to 100% in different studies, with specificity values ranging from 78% to 96%.

For small, subsegmental emboli, the sensitivity and accuracy of SSCT decreases, with reported sensitivity rates of 53% to 63%. However, thrombi limited to small vessels are uncommon in patients with PE. Overall, 6% to 30% of patients with PE have subsegmental emboli only. It should be noted that the highest frequency of isolated subsegmental emboli (30%) and the lowest sensitivity of SSCT (53%) have been reported in patients with nondiagnostic (intermediate- or low-probability) V̇/Q̇ scans, whereas the lowest frequency of subsegmental emboli (6%) and the highest accuracy of SSCT are found when unselected patients with suspected PE are studied. Among studies showing the lowest sensitivity rates for SSCT (53% to 63%), a significant number of patients had small thrombi. In such studies, patients had both SSCT and pulmonary arteriography, most likely because of nondiagnostic V̇/Q̇ radionuclide scans; patients with nondiagnostic scans have a comparatively high prevalence of small emboli.

It is questionable if emboli limited to subsegmental vessels, which are the ones most likely to be missed on hCTPA, are clinically significant. Some evidence supports the contention that small emboli are clinically insignificant in patients who do not have evidence of deep venous thrombosis and have normal cardiopulmonary reserve. On the other hand, as many as 8% of patients suspected of PE who have underlying cardiac or pulmonary disease and nondiagnostic radionuclide lung imaging die of untreated PE. These data imply that small thrombi are potentially significant in patients with limited cardiopulmonary reserve.

The controversies regarding the accuracy hCTPA for the diagnosis of PE are complex, and reflect in part the different populations studied as well as different study methodologies. When interpreting these data, it is important to recognize that pulmonary angiography, the gold standard used for comparison in many studies examining hCTPA for PE, is imperfect, particularly for the diagnosis of small thrombi. Several investigators have shown that pulmonary angiography has high interobserver variability for the diagnosis of small thrombi, and this should be kept in mind when evaluating the results of hCTPA studies. Furthermore, the improved resolution provided by MSCT scanning could translate into improved detection of small thrombi, but such data are not yet available.

Finally, perhaps the most important question to answer regarding hCTPA for PE is whether or not anticoagulation may be withheld safely in patients with hCTPA scans interpreted as negative for PE. Several variably sized outcome studies detailing such information have been reported, all indicating that the negative predictive value of hCTPA equals or exceeds 98%, and provides reliability equivalent to negative pulmonary angiography or normal perfusion scintigraphy results.

Comparison With Other Modalities

The accuracy of hCTPA for diagnosing PE has been compared to that of V̇/Q̇ scintigraphy in several studies, and hCTPA has been shown to have a higher sensitivity with similar specificity compared to V̇/Q̇ scintigraphy. Furthermore, hCTPA provides the additional benefit of suggesting or confirming alternate clinical diagnoses in patients with hCTPA scans interpreted as negative. When together considering positive scans and scans interpreted as negative, but with alternative diagnoses present on scans interpreted as negative, a confident diagnosis may be obtained with hCTPA in 90% or more patients.

Several studies have evaluated the accuracy of transthoracic and transesophageal echocardiography with hCTPA for the detection of acute PE. Predictably, transthoracic and transesophageal echocardiography were found to have a limited accuracy for detecting PE. The major role of echocardiography in the evaluation of patients with PE is for risk stratification for those patients with proven PE. Several investigators have shown that patients with PE and echocardiographic evidence of right ventricular strain (e.g., right ventricular enlargement, right ventricular wall motion abnormalities, and leftward bowing of the interventricular septum) are at higher risk for death, and therefore may be candidates for more aggressive interventions, such as pharmacologic or mechanical thrombolysis.

Chronic Pulmonary Embolism

hCTPA is an excellent study for the evaluation of patients with suspected chronic PE, and several hCTPA findings are specifically suggestive of chronic thromboembolic disease. Histopathologically, chronic pulmonary emboli usually are organizing thromboemboli, and typically are adherent to

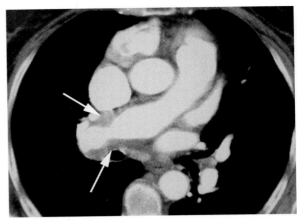

FIG. 27-15. Chronic thromboembolic disease: adherent, organizing thrombus. Axial helical CT pulmonary angiogram image shows organizing thrombus along the lateral walls of the right pulmonary artery *(arrows)*, consistent with chronic pulmonary embolism.

the vessel wall. Therefore, chronic emboli are eccentric in location and usually appear as a smooth or sometimes nodular thickening of the vessel wall on hCTPA studies (Fig. 27-15). When an artery is seen in cross section, the chronic emboli may appear to involve one wall of the vessel, may be horseshoe-shaped, or may occasionally appear concentric, with contrast in the vessel center, an appearance that likely reflects recanalization of a previously occluded vessel. Chronic emboli occasionally may calcify, and the main pulmonary arteries may be dilated because of associated pulmonary hypertension. Additionally, small linear filling defects, or "webs" (Fig. 27-16), are indicative of chronic PE. Geographic regions of mosaic perfusion (oligemia) also may be encountered in patients with chronic PE (Fig. 27-17), either

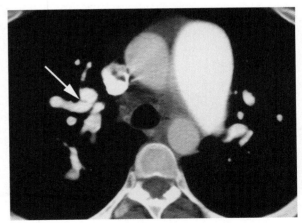

FIG. 27-16. Chronic thromboembolic disease: intravascular webs. Axial helical CT pulmonary angiogram image shows a linear filling defect within a right upper lobe segmental pulmonary artery *(arrow)*, consistent with chronic pulmonary embolism.

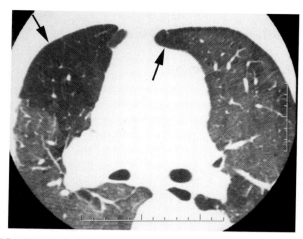

FIG. 27-17. Axial helical CT pulmonary angiogram photographed in lung windows shows bilateral inhomogeneous lung opacity, with abnormally small-appearing vessels in the regions of decreased lung attenuation *(arrows)*. This finding is consistent with mosaic perfusion due to chronic thromboembolic disease.

with or without central findings of chronic PE. Often pulmonary vessels appear smaller in the regions of hypoattenuation, a finding that aids in suggesting a vascular cause for inhomogeneous lung opacity over an airway etiology. Overall, hCTPA has a sensitivity of 94% to 100% and a specificity of 96% to 98% for diagnosing chronic PE.

PITFALLS IN THE DIAGNOSIS OF PULMONARY EMBOLISM

Awareness of several pitfalls in the diagnosis of acute pulmonary embolism is required for accurate diagnosis. Pitfalls in the hCTPA diagnosis of PE may be divided into anatomic and technical etiologies. Anatomic pitfalls include lymph nodes, pulmonary veins, volume averaging of pulmonary arteries, impacted bronchi, pulmonary arterial catheters, cardiac shunts, and pulmonary arterial sarcoma. Technical causes of pitfalls on helical CT pulmonary angiography include respiratory and cardiac motion, improper contrast bolus timing, and quantum mottle. A detailed knowledge of normal bronchovascular anatomy is required for accurate interpretation of hCTPA studies.

Anatomic Pitfalls

Lymph Nodes

Normal hilar lymph nodes commonly simulate acute PE on hCTPA imaging. Normal nodes appear as soft tissue structures which typically are lateral to upper lobe anterior segmental pulmonary arteries but medial in relation to the lower lobe pulmonary arteries. Knowledge of the typical

location of lymph nodes makes it possible to discriminate between them and true PE.

Pulmonary Veins

Pulmonary veins course within connective tissue septa, separate from pulmonary arteries and bronchi, which run together. Knowledge of this anatomic relationship allows one to avoid diagnosing an artifact within a pulmonary vein as acute PE. When a filling defect is encountered, particularly in the peripheral aspects of the lung, if the vessel showing the filling defect is immediately adjacent to a bronchus, the filling defect resides within a pulmonary artery and PE may be diagnosed. If the vessel showing the potential filling defect is not accompanied by a bronchus, it is likely a pulmonary vein and therefore PE should not be diagnosed. Additionally, pulmonary veins may be followed sequentially to their confluence at the left atrium, allowing one to distinguish veins from arteries easily.

Partial Volume Averaging of Pulmonary Arteries

Vessels oriented in the transverse plane are the most difficult to image. Occasionally, particularly in the left upper lobe, partial volume averaging of the anterior segmental pulmonary artery may create the appearance of an intraluminal filling defect. The true nature of the abnormality may be recognized by the characteristic location and orientation of the vessels affected, particularly when the image just caudal to the image showing the potential filling defect reveals only lung—this implies that the image in question represents volume averaging of the undersurface of a pulmonary artery with adjacent lung parenchyma. Volume averaging artifacts are much less common on MSCT studies than SSCT examinations.

Impacted Bronchi

Rarely, a calcified bronchus with mucoid impaction creates the appearance of an intraluminal filling defect surrounded by contrast. Review of lung windows at the appropriate location demonstrates absence of an air-filled bronchus, and review of images with a wider window width may reveal calcification within the bronchial walls, which may superficially simulate intravenous contrast within a pulmonary artery surrounding an intraluminal filling defect. Again, there is no substitute for a detailed knowledge of pulmonary bronchovascular anatomy for the proper interpretation of hCTPA studies.

Intracardiac and Extracardiac Vascular Shunts

Intracardiac shunts, such as atrial and ventricular septal defects, may result in either left-to-right or, eventually, right-to-left shunting of blood. One of the more common causes of an extracardiac, left-to-right shunting of blood is bronchial arterial hypertrophy induced by chronic pleural and parenchymal pulmonary inflammatory disease. In this circumstance, flow is directed from the bronchial arteries into the pulmonary arteries; such retrograde flow potentially may induce flow artifacts that could create the appearance of low-attenuation defects within the pulmonary arterial system.

The presence of a patent foramen ovale has been associated with diminished pulmonary arterial opacification and poor-quality hCTPA studies. When right-to-left shunts occur, poor opacification of pulmonary arteries may result from shunting of contrast-enhanced blood across atrial or ventricular septal defects, producing early, intense enhancement of the left cardiac chambers and aorta and diminished pulmonary arterial enhancement. Because a patent foramen ovale may be present in 15% to 25% of the general population, the potential for shunting in patients undergoing hCTPA, and the potential for producing suboptimal hCTPA studies, may be significant.

Pulmonary Arterial Catheters

The tip of a pulmonary arterial catheter may create a small filling defect within a pulmonary artery. This artifact probably will be encountered more often as hCTPA is increasingly employed for the investigation of suspected acute PE in critically ill patients; such patients are practically by definition at increased risk for venous thromboembolism. The artifact is easily recognized if the catheter is seen; however, the dense contrast bolus occasionally may obscure visibility of the catheter. In such circumstances, review of the scout image will show the location of the catheter tip.

Pulmonary Artery Sarcoma

Pulmonary arterial sarcoma probably is the rarest pitfall in the diagnosis of suspected PE. These tumors are visualized as intraluminal filling defects within the central pulmonary arteries. If recognized preoperatively, the tumor often is mistaken for PE. The polypoid nature of tumor growth, enhancement of the intravascular tumor itself, and ipsilateral lung nodules may reveal the true nature of the abnormality.

Technical Pitfalls

Respiratory and Cardiac Motion Artifacts

Motion artifacts often result in apparent low attenuation defects within pulmonary arteries; recognition of the artifact depends on identifying the presence of motion effects on other structures on the same image. Because motion artifacts can be severe and can render a scan nondiagnostic in quality, every attempt to limit motion degradation should be made.

Occasionally it may be appropriate to repeat a scan after correctable factors have been identified.

Improper Bolus Timing

Accurate evaluation of helical CT pulmonary angiography requires adequate enhancement of the pulmonary arterial system. Methods for achieving proper bolus timing have been discussed previously. Because laminar flow within vessels dictates that blood flowing within the center of the vessel flows faster than blood at the periphery of the vessel, scanning after the delivery of the contrast bolus may, rarely, create the appearance of a filling defect, simulating PE (Fig. 27-18). If the bolus arrives too late (as may occur in a patient with venous stenosis within the injected extremity) no contrast will be present within the pulmonary arterial system once the scan is initiated. Once improper timing is recognized, it usually is corrected easily; the scan may then be performed again with the proper timing.

Quantum Mottle

Quantum mottle, or image noise, may result in unsatisfactory study quality. Mottle is more likely to be encountered

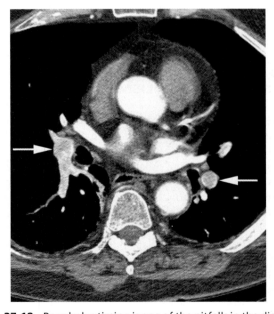

FIG. 27-18. Poor bolus timing is one of the pitfalls in the diagnosis of pulmonary embolism. Axial CT pulmonary angiogram initiated too late following the beginning of the intravenous contrast injection shows apparent filling defects with the right and left lower lobe pulmonary arteries *(arrows)*. This artifact is created by laminar flow, which dictates that flow within the center of the vessel is faster than flow at the vessel periphery. In this case, contrast along the periphery of the vessel transited the vessel at a slower pace than blood at the center of the vessel, allowing contrast-enhanced blood at the center of the vessel to wash out before imaging begins. Repeat scanning with the proper contrast injection delay showed no evidence of PE.

if the field of view is small and the collimation is very narrow (as with MSCT). To reduce mottle, the field of view should be set properly, and the mA must be increased appropriately; these maneuvers obviously come at the expense of increased radiation dose.

Incidental Pulmonary Emboli

Incidental pulmonary emboli may be detected in nearly 1% to 2% of patients undergoing contrast-enhanced thoracic CT for non–embolic-related reasons, often oncologic indications; such patients almost always are at high risk for thromboembolism. This finding may be extremely important, and often results in significant changes in patient management.

MAGNETIC RESONANCE IMAGING

MR imaging of the chest presents significant challenges, including the relative lack of signal due to the paucity of protons within the chest, susceptibility artifacts resulting from air and soft tissue interfaces within the thorax, and image degradation from respiratory and cardiac motion. In recent years, the development of faster and stronger gradients and the evolution of contrast-enhanced magnetic resonance angiography (MRA) have made rapid high-resolution imaging of the thorax and pulmonary vascular system possible, and MR imaging of the pulmonary vascular system has evolved significantly. Additional techniques for cardiopulmonary imaging—lung perfusion MRI and hyperpolarized 3-helium—also have been investigated and may provide unique diagnostic information. MR venography of the pelvis and lower extremities has been shown to be an accurate technique for the diagnosis of DVT, and may be combined with the thoracic examination to provide a comprehensive evaluation for patients with suspected VTE.

Techniques

Conventional MR angiography techniques, such as two- (2D) or three-dimensional (3D) time-of-flight, depend on blood flow to produce contrast between the vessels and the surrounding tissues. Early investigation with these methods yielded promising results for imaging of the pulmonary arteries, especially for evaluation of PE. However, time-of-flight methods suffer from several limitations, including insensitivity to slow flow, excessive respiratory and pulsation motion artifacts, and relatively poor spatial resolution. The introduction of 3D MR angiography techniques using intravenous gadolinium chelate contrast agents represents a major advance in MR imaging of PE. Because of the T1-shortening effect of gadolinium, contrast-enhanced 3D MR angiography does not rely on blood flow to produce images of vessels. Therefore, high-quality vascular imaging can be performed without artifacts due to flow phenomena. Single-breathhold monophasic protocols, with scan times between 20 and 30 seconds, or time-resolved multiphasic protocols, with scan times under 10 seconds, now are routinely possible and allow high-quality imaging, even in severely dyspneic patients.

The protocol for 3D MR angiography varies from institution to institution. Phased array coils are used to optimize the signal-to-noise ratio. A gradient-recalled echo (GRE) localizing sequence is obtained in the transverse plane. The coronal 3D spoiled gradient echo (SPGR) MR angiography acquisition may then be prescribed from the transverse images. Twenty-eight images are obtained using a slice thickness of 2.6 to 3 mm, repetition time (TR) of 4 to 7 msec, echo time (TE) of 1 to 2 msec, and flip angle of 45 degrees.

The angiographic (SPGR) sequence is completed during a breathhold of 20 to 25 seconds. To aid in breath holding, the patient can be provided with oxygen by nasal cannula, at a rate of 2 L/min. Gadolinium contrast (approximately 0.1 to 0.2 mmol/ml) is administered via an antecubital vein with use of a power injector (2 ml/sec, 40 ml total), often followed by a saline chaser. The scan begins approximately 5 to 10 seconds after the start of the injection of contrast medium when imaging the pulmonary arteries. Timing of the acquisition can be optimized with bolus-detection software or by performing a preliminary acquisition with use of a test bolus to estimate circulation time.

The complete sequence is performed in approximately 20 to 30 seconds, and the entire study can be completed in 30 to 45 minutes. Multiplanar maximum intensity projection reconstructions of the 3D MR angiography, performed on an off-line workstation, often are invaluable for interpretation of the study.

For optimal assessment of the vessels, 3D MR angiography can be supplemented in some cases by a sequence in the transverse plane, such as segmented k-space ("breathhold") cine acquisition. This sequence requires electrocardiographic gating to produce multiple images at each location, one image per phase of the cardiac cycle.

Recently, blood-pool MR contrast agents have been developed. Some of these agents are large particles, such as dextran or iron oxide complexes, whereas others bind to serum proteins, allowing them to remain in the vascular system for several hours. Because such agents circulate for a prolonged period of time, they allow for repeated image acquisitions, making possible combined pulmonary arterial and pelvic/lower extremity venous imaging.

Advantages and Disadvantages of MR for Diagnosis of Pulmonary Embolism

Gadolinium-enhanced 3D MR angiography has proved its utility for a number of thoracic applications, including diagnosis of PE. Advantages of MRA over hCTPA and pulmonary angiography include the use of gadolinium-chelate contrast agent and the lack of ionizing radiation. Unlike iodinated contrast media, gadolinium chelates are not nephrotoxic, and the risk of contrast reaction is very low. Limitations of MR angiography include a relatively long breathhold time and the fact that MR is contraindicated in selected patients who may be at risk for PE, including those with pacemakers.

Pulmonary Embolism Findings on MRI and MRA

MRI and MRA findings of PE depending on the imaging sequence employed. The short T1 signal of methemoglobin in pulmonary emboli produces high signal on T1-weighted imaging. On breathhold cine acquisition sequences, pulmonary emboli usually appear as very-low-signal-intensity filling defects within high-signal blood pool, whereas on 3D contrast-enhanced MRA sequences, emboli appear as very-low-signal foci surrounded by high-signal intraluminal contrast.

Much like hCTPA, acute PE is diagnosed when an intra-arterial filling defect is identified. Expanded, unenhanced pulmonary arteries also may suggest acute pulmonary embolization. Chronic thromboembolic disease may be suggested when eccentric filling defects (Fig. 27-19) or intravascular webs are identified, often in the presence of an enlarged main pulmonary arterial segment, reflecting pulmonary hypertension.

Accuracy of MRI and MRA for the Diagnosis of Pulmonary Embolism

Studies examining the utility and accuracy of MR techniques for the diagnosis of PE are smaller and far less numer-

ous than studies detailing other imaging methods used to evaluate patients suspected of pulmonary embolism, including hCTPA. Nevertheless, data are available from both experimental and clinical studies utilizing MR for the diagnosis of PE. Pooled analysis of the results of several studies shows that the sensitivity for MR techniques for the detection of PE ranges from 75% to 100%, with specificity usually exceeding 90%. Reports of the interobserver agreement of MR examinations for PE have shown good results, although the rate of technically inadequate studies has been slightly higher for MR than for hCTPA. Predictably, MRI/MRA techniques show their highest sensitivity for central emboli, with diminishing sensitivity for smaller emboli, especially for subsegmental PE.

MR Perfusion and Ventilation Imaging of the Lung

Perfusion and ventilation imaging of the lung is now possible. Several methods for pulmonary perfusion imaging exist. Pulmonary perfusion may be performed in combination with 3D MRA, using gadolinium-based contrast agents and a sequence with short TR and TE, in a time-resolved fashion, by employing the first-pass effect. As contrast enters the imaging volume, regions of diminished perfusion become increasingly apparent as first the vessels and then the pulmonary parenchyma enhance. This technique may allow the demonstration of pulmonary parenchymal perfusion defects as well as the intraluminal emboli producing the perfusion abnormalities. MR pulmonary perfusion may also be performed using blood pool agents. Because these agents circulate for a prolonged period of time, perfusion imaging of the lung may be followed by lower extremity and pelvic

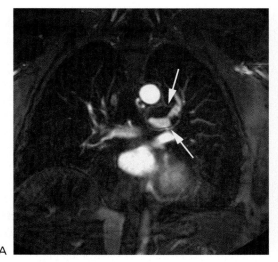
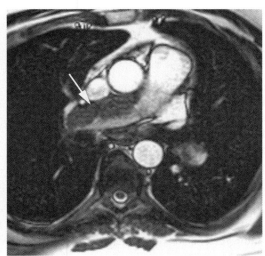

A   B

FIG. 27-19. Chronic thromboembolic disease on MRA imaging. **A.** Coronal MRA image shows a peripheral, low-signal filling defect in the main pulmonary artery *(arrows)*, representing chronic thromboembolic disease. **B.** Axial cine image shows low signal along the anterior wall of the right pulmonary artery *(arrow)*.

imaging for potential DVT. Finally, MR pulmonary perfusion may be performed with noncontrast methods, such as arterial spin labeling; this technique is capable of distinguishing stationary from moving tissue, and thus may provide information on pulmonary blood flow.

Preliminary techniques for MR ventilation imaging have been studied in recent years. Using hyperpolarized noble gases or molecular oxygen, MR ventilation imaging is now possible. MR ventilation techniques may be combined with MR pulmonary perfusion methods to create a map of pulmonary ventilation and perfusion in a fashion similar to $\dot{V}/\dot{Q}$ scintigraphy. However, experience with these techniques currently is limited, and, although promising, further technical refinements will be required.

SELECTED READING

Fraser RS, Müller NL, Colman N, Paré PD. Diagnosis of Diseases of the Chest. Philadelphia: WB Saunders, 1999, pp 1897–1945.

Frazier AA, Galvin JR, Franks TJ, Rosado-De-Christenson ML. From the archives of the AFIP: pulmonary vasculature: hypertension and infarction. Radiographics 2000; 20:491–524.

Gotway MB, Edinburgh KJ, Feldstein VA, et al. Imaging evaluation of suspected pulmonary embolism. Curr Probl Diagn Radiol 1999; 28:129–184.

Gotway MB, Patel RA, Webb WR. Helical CT for the evaluation of suspected acute pulmonary embolism: diagnostic pitfalls. J Comput Assist Tomogr 2000; 24:267–273.

Remy-Jardin M, Remy J. Spiral CT angiography of the pulmonary circulation. Radiology 1999; 212:615–636.

Remy-Jardin M, Remy J, Wattinne L, Giraud F. Central pulmonary thromboembolism: diagnosis with spiral volumetric CT with the single-breath-hold technique—comparison with pulmonary angiography. Radiology 1992; 185:381–387.

Tapson VF, Carroll BA, Davidson BL, et al. The diagnostic approach to acute venous thromboembolism. Clinical practice guideline. Am J Respir Crit Care Med 1999; 160:1043–1066.

van Beek EJR, Wild JM, Fink C, et al. MRI for the diagnosis of pulmonary embolism. J Magn Res Imag 2003; 18:627–640.

28

PULMONARY ARTERIAL HYPERTENSION

MICHAEL B. GOTWAY, GAUTHAM P. REDDY, SAMUEL K. DAWN, AND AKHILESH SISTA

ANATOMY AND PHYSIOLOGY OF THE PULMONARY CIRCULATION

The pulmonary circulation consists of two parallel networks: the pulmonary arterial circulation and the bronchial arterial circulation. Pulmonary arteries course along the lobar, segmental, and subsegmental airways to the level of the terminal bronchioles. Small pulmonary arteries from the subsegmental level to the terminal bronchioles possess a thick muscular media, and range from 50 to 1000 μm in size. These small pulmonary arteries progressively lose much of their muscle within the arteriolar media as well as their external elastic membrane. By the level of the respiratory bronchioles and alveolar ducts they are termed *pulmonary arterioles,* and range in size from 10 to150 μm. These vessels ramify further within the alveolar walls to form a rich capillary network. Capillary blood collects in venules, which coalesce progressively to form veins, which course within the interlobular septa, eventually to empty into the left atrium.

The bronchial circulation, accounting for about 1% of the systemic cardiac output, originates from the thoracic aorta or intercostal arteries. Bronchial arteries, averaging two per lung, course within the pulmonary hila along the mainstem bronchi to the level of the terminal bronchiole, and form a plexus that extends from the adventitia through to the submucosa of the associated airway. Bronchial arteries freely form anastomoses with pulmonary arteries, primarily at the capillary and postcapillary levels.

Unlike the tracheobronchial system, in which the major component to air-flow resistance is located within the large airways, the major site of resistance to pulmonary arterial blood flow is located at the small muscular pulmonary arterial and arteriolar level. Caliber changes in the vessels at this level regulate pulmonary arterial pressure and are critical for optimizing ventilation and perfusion matching.

The pulmonary circulation is a low pressure system—the mean arterial pressure is approximately one sixth that of the systemic circulation. This low pressure is maintained at a relatively consistent level even with large increases in pulmonary blood flow such as may occur with exercise. This is possible because when the body is at rest, numerous pulmonary capillaries normally are not perfused; these capillaries are "recruited" when increased pulmonary blood flow must be accommodated.

PATHOGENESIS

Pulmonary hypertension is defined as a pulmonary systolic arterial pressure equal to or exceeding 25 mmHg at rest or 30 mmHg with exercise, or a mean pulmonary arterial pressure equal to or exceeding 18 mmHg. Pulmonary venous hypertension is present when pulmonary venous pressure, usually approximated by measurement of the pulmonary capillary wedge pressure, is equal to or exceeds 18 mmHg. Several mechanisms may produce a decrease in the total number of small pulmonary arteries, thereby increasing pulmonary vascular resistance and producing elevated pulmonary arterial pressure. These mechanisms include intraluminal arterial occlusion, muscular contraction of small pulmonary arteries, vascular remodeling with wall thickening, or conditions that produce pulmonary venous hypertension. Several of these mechanisms may be operative simultaneously in a patient with pulmonary hypertension.

The pulmonary vascular endothelium responds to changes in oxygen tension, transmural pressure, and pulmonary blood flow, and participates actively in the regulation of pulmonary arterial pressure through the elaboration of various vasoactive substances, such as prostacyclin, nitrous oxide, and endothelin. The agents have a direct effect on pulmonary vascular smooth muscle tone (promoting relaxation and vasodilation), and also may directly affect platelet function. Abnormalities in endothelial cell function or injuries to these cells may be the fundamental derangement that ultimately produces the structural vascular changes observed in patients with pulmonary hypertension.

Various histopathological abnormalities may be observed in patients with pulmonary hypertension, varying somewhat depending on the cause of hypertension. In general, regardless of the specific cause of the pulmonary hypertension, the pulmonary arteries become dilated, occasionally to the point of being considered aneurysmal. Pulmonary arterial atherosclerosis, although occasionally present to a mild degree in the larger pulmonary arteries of normal adults, often is extensive in patients with pulmonary hypertension and commonly involves small arteries. Pulmonary hypertension–related pulmonary arterial atherosclerosis pathologically appears similar to atherosclerosis in systemic arteries, although complicating features, such as necrosis, ulceration, and calcification, are relatively uncommon. Thickening of the muscular media of small pulmonary arteries is a common feature in many causes of pulmonary hypertension, and usually results from a combination of muscular hyperplasia and hypertrophy. Often, extension of muscular tissue into arterioles that normally contain no muscle, or "arterialization," may be observed in patients with pulmonary arterial hypertension.

The term *pulmonary plexogenic arteriopathy* refers to a constellation of histopathological vascular changes that often is encountered in patients with primary pulmonary hypertension, but it also may be seen in patients with pulmonary hypertension of other etiologies, such as hepatic disease, connective tissue disorders, congenital cardiovascular disease, and some medication prescribed for weight loss. Histopathological features present in pulmonary plexogenic arteriopathy include a combination of fibrinoid necrosis, dilation lesions, plexiform lesions, intimal fibrosis, and vasculitis. Plexiform lesions affect small muscular arteries ranging in size from 100 to 200 μm, usually near vascular branch points, and consist of a focally dilated muscular vessel with a disrupted internal elastic membrane that contains very narrow vascular channels interspersed with fibroblasts and connective tissue. Plexiform lesions are characteristic of prolonged severe pulmonary hypertension.

GENERAL IMAGING MANIFESTATIONS

The characteristic finding of pulmonary arterial hypertension on chest radiography, CT, or MRI is dilation of the central pulmonary arteries with rapid tapering of the pulmonary vessels as they course peripherally (Fig. 28-1A). This pattern is present regardless of the etiology of the pulmonary hypertension.

Chest radiography may reveal enlargement of the main pulmonary artery segment and dilation of the right and left interlobar pulmonary arteries in patients with pulmonary hypertension of any etiology. It has been suggested that pulmonary arterial hypertension may be diagnosed on chest radiography if the transverse diameter of the right interlobar pulmonary artery, measured from the lateral aspect of the

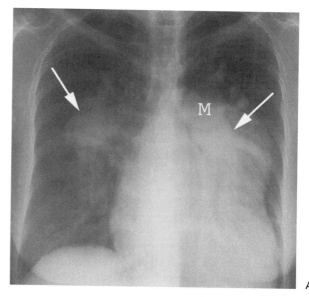

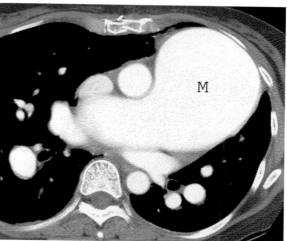

FIG. 28-1. Pulmonary arterial hypertension: pulmonary arterial enlargement. **A.** Frontal chest radiograph shows massive enlargement of the main pulmonary artery *(M)* and bilateral interlobar pulmonary arteries *(arrows)*. **B.** CT shows massive enlargement of the main pulmonary artery *(M)*.

vessel to its medial portion adjacent to the bronchus intermedius, exceeds 15 mm in women and 16 mm in men. Similarly, an enlarged left pulmonary artery also may indicate the presence of pulmonary hypertension. The left pulmonary artery is best measured on the lateral radiograph from the orifice of the left upper lobe bronchus to the posterior aspect of the vessel; when this measurement exceeds 18 mm, pulmonary hypertension probably is present.

The main pulmonary arterial segment cannot be measured on chest radiography, but it is measured easily on CT or MRI. The upper size limit for a normal main pulmonary arterial segment on axial CT or MR images is 29 mm. When the main pulmonary artery segment exceeds this size (see Fig. 28-1B), pulmonary hypertension is usually, but not invariably, present. Furthermore, pulmonary hypertension may be present in patients with a main pulmonary arterial segment that is normal in size. Rather than measure the main pulmonary artery, one may compare the size of the main pulmonary artery with the ascending aorta near the base of the heart. If the main pulmonary artery is visibly larger than the aorta, elevated pulmonary pressures usually are present.

When pulmonary hypertension is prolonged and severe, calcification of the pulmonary arteries, usually affecting the main, right, or left pulmonary arteries, and, less commonly, the lobar pulmonary arteries, may be present. This finding usually, but not invariably, is associated with irreversible vascular disease.

Although chest radiography and CT scanning often may suggest the presence of pulmonary hypertension, echocardiography is the examination most commonly used for noninvasive assessment of possible pulmonary hypertension. Echocardiography, using continuous wave or pulsed Doppler, provides noninvasive measurement of pulmonary arterial pressures and also allows detailed morphologic evaluation of the right ventricle. Echocardiography also is used for assessment of the hemodynamic changes in the pulmonary arterial circulation in response to a variety of challenges, such as exercise or pharmacologic agents; this technique is termed *stress echocardiography*.

MRI can provide functional information equivalent to that available from echocardiography (including stress echocardiography), such as direction and velocity of blood flow, in addition to specific anatomic information. MR techniques are well suited to the evaluation of patients with pulmonary hypertension because they allow both a detailed anatomic and an extensive functional examination of the cardiovascular system.

CLASSIFICATION

Numerous classification schemes have been developed to categorize the causes of pulmonary hypertension. One method has been to examine the disease from a physiologic perspective, using the relations among pressure, pulmonary vascular resistance, and pulmonary flow. In this type of classification, diseases that cause increased resistance, increased flow, or increased pulmonary vascular pressure are grouped separately. The World Health Organization has classified pulmonary hypertension into pulmonary arterial hypertension, pulmonary venous hypertension, pulmonary hypertension secondary to hypoxemia/respiratory disease, pulmonary hypertension secondary to thromboembolic disease, and pulmonary hypertension secondary to processes affecting the pulmonary vasculature directly. Other investigators have classified pulmonary arterial hypertension into pre- and postcapillary etiologies (Table 28-1). This classification

TABLE 28-1. CLASSIFICATION OF PULMONARY ARTERIAL HYPERTENSION

Precapillary Etiologies	Postcapillary Etiologies
Primary pulmonary hypertension	Left-sided cardiovascular disease
	Mitral stenosis
	Cor triatriatum
	Aortic valvular disease
	Cardiac tumors
Pulmonary hypertension associated with:	Extrinsic pulmonary venous compression
Hepatic disease	Fibrosing mediastinitis
HIV infection	
Drugs and toxins	
Congenital cardiovascular disease	Pulmonary venoocclusive disease
Chronic thromboembolic disease	
Nonthrombotic embolization	
Neoplastic emboli	
Particulates and foreign material	
Parasites	
Chronic alveolar hypoxia	
COPD	
Interstitial lung disease	
Hypoventilation syndromes	
Pulmonary capillary hemangiomatosis	

scheme is in common use, and is the one used in this chapter, although further delineations are drawn from the other classification systems described.

Precapillary Pulmonary Hypertension

Possible causes of precapillary pulmonary hypertension include primary pulmonary arterial hypertension, congenital cardiovascular left-to-right shunts, pulmonary thromboembolism, nonthrombotic pulmonary arterial embolization (including tumor, particulate, and parasitic thromboemboli), and chronic alveolar hypoxia.

Primary Pulmonary Hypertension

Etiology and Pathogenesis

The etiology of primary pulmonary hypertension (PPH) is unknown. The disease affects females more commonly than males. There are two forms of primary pulmonary hypertension—familial and sporadic. Familial forms, which account for about 10% of cases of PPH, show autosomal dominant inheritance with incomplete penetrance and have been localized to chromosome 2.

PPH usually can be attributed to an imbalance between vasodilating agents and vasoconstricting agents, with a relative paucity of prostacyclin and nitric oxide synthase expression and an increase in expression of endothelin-1.

The inciting factors are unknown, but the pathological progression of the disease has been well characterized. Arterial medial hypertrophy, intimal proliferation and fibrosis, necrotizing arteritis, and plexiform lesions are manifestations of the progressive proliferation and destruction of the pulmonary arterial circulation. Superimposed organized thrombi may be present, making the distinction between chronic thromboembolic pulmonary hypertension and PPH difficult.

Several conditions that are associated with pulmonary arterial hypertension are characterized histopathologically by plexogenic pulmonary arteriopathy. These conditions include connective tissue disorders (particularly systemic lupus erythematosus and progressive systemic sclerosis), pulmonary arterial hypertension associated with hepatic disease, the acquired immunodeficiency syndrome (AIDS), and effects of certain drugs prescribed for weight loss, such as fenfluramine. The proposed mechanism in portal hypertension is thought to be the incomplete hepatic degradation of humoral factors that exert vasoconstricting and inflammatory effects on the pulmonary circulation. The human immunodeficiency virus (HIV) has been shown to infect endothelial cells of the pulmonary circulation directly, giving rise to the theory that endothelial damage plays a role in the pathogenesis of PPH, although there is little evidence for a direct cytotoxic effect by HIV on the pulmonary vascular endothelium. Pulmonary hypertension in these settings is similar histopathologically to PPH; it is the clinical scenario that defines these syndromes as distinct from PPH.

Clinical Presentation

Patients with PPH usually present with dyspnea on exertion. Other presenting symptoms include fatigue, syncope, chest pain, and, occasionally, cough. Raynaud's phenomenon may be present in certain patients, particularly those with pulmonary hypertension associated with connective tissue diseases such as systemic lupus erythematosus and progressive systemic sclerosis.

Pulmonary hypertension associated with liver disease usually occurs in the setting of cirrhosis, and very rarely in patients with noncirrhotic portal hypertension due to portal fibrosis or multifocal nodular hyperplasia. Most patients with cirrhosis do not develop pulmonary arterial hypertension; pulmonary hypertension occurs in fewer than 1% of cirrhotic patients. However, the rate may be higher when considering patients with severe cirrhosis, such as those awaiting liver transplantation. Pulmonary arterial hypertension associated with cirrhosis improves slowly following liver transplantation.

Patients with AIDS-related pulmonary hypertension have a presentation similar to that of patients with PPH, except that it occurs at a slightly earlier age. Patients usually

are still relatively immunocompetent—in most, the CD4 count is above 200 cells/μL at presentation.

The prognosis of PPH is dismal, with most patients dying within 2 to 5 years of diagnosis.

Imaging Manifestations

Chest radiography in patients with PPH shows enlargement of the main, right, and left pulmonary arteries, often with enlargement of the right ventricle and right atrium. High-resolution CT (HRCT) may show that the peripheral pulmonary arteries are substantially larger than usual (Fig. 28-2). CT and black blood MR techniques will show these same findings to advantage. Occasionally black blood MR imaging will show increased signal within the pulmonary arteries as a result of slow flow.

High-resolution CT may demonstrate inhomogeneous lung opacity, representing the presence of differential pulmonary parenchymal perfusion. The regions of decreased pulmonary parenchymal attenuation represent areas of mosaic perfusion, and the vessels in these regions of lung often are visibly smaller than their counterparts in regions of increased lung attenuation. Although airway diseases may result in a similar pattern of mosaic perfusion, vascular and airway causes of mosaic perfusion may be distinguished using postexpiratory imaging. When due to airway diseases, differences in lung attenuation become accentuated with postexpiratory imaging, whereas a proportional increase in attenuation in areas of both increased and decreased attenuation is expected for patients with pulmonary vascular disease.

Occasionally HRCT shows centrilobular ground-glass opacities in patients with PPH, representing foci of hemorrhage or cholesterol granulomas.

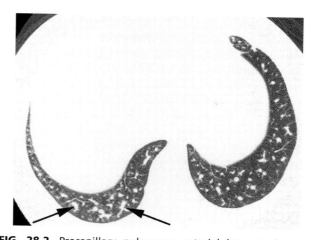

FIG. 28-2. Precapillary pulmonary arterial hypertension: enlargement of peripheral pulmonary arteries. Axial CT through the lung bases in a patient with fenfluramine-induced pulmonary hypertension shows that the peripheral pulmonary arteries are abnormally large *(arrows)*.

Ventilation/perfusion (V̇/Q̇) scintigraphy commonly is abnormal in patients with PPH, and often is interpreted as having low probability for pulmonary thromboembolism.

Pulmonary arteriography in patients with pulmonary arterial hypertension shows tapering peripheral vessels with a "corkscrew" appearance, occasionally with visualization of subpleural collateral vessels.

In general, non-PPH precapillary pulmonary hypertension due to conditions associated with pulmonary plexogenic arteriopathy is indistinguishable radiographically from PPH. Patients with connective tissue disease–associated pulmonary hypertension may show evidence of fibrotic lung disease.

Congenital Cardiovascular Diseases: Left-to-Right Shunts

Etiology and Pathogenesis

Intracardiac and extracardiac left-to-right shunts, such as ventricular septal defects, atrial septal defects, partial anomalous pulmonary venous return, and patent ductus arteriosus, produce increased blood flow through the pulmonary arterial bed. This increased pulmonary arterial flow produces persistently increased vasomotor tone within the pulmonary arteries, and eventually may lead to the development of pulmonary plexogenic arteriopathy and irreversible vasculopathy. Eventually, the left-to-right shunting may reverse, producing a right-to-left shunt—this situation represents the development of Eisenmenger's syndrome.

Most patients with congenital left-to-right shunts have corrective surgery during infancy or early childhood, before the onset of severe pulmonary hypertension. For the rare patient in whom childhood surgical repair is not done, lung biopsy may be performed to assess the potential success of surgical intervention for reversing the vasculopathy. This histopathological grading system is called the *Heath-Edwards grading system,* and originally was described using a six-point scale; recently, a three-point system has been proposed. The Heath-Edwards grading system allows prediction of disease reversibility. Grades I and II (medial hypertrophy, intimal proliferation, and neomuscularization) represent mild, reversible disease. Grade III, characterized by intimal fibrosis and luminal obliteration, is considered borderline. Higher grades, corresponding with plexiform lesions, aneurysm, and necrotizing arteritis, are considered to represent irreversible changes, and surgical correction of the abnormality would not reverse the pulmonary hypertension.

Clinical Presentation

Many patients with congenital cardiovascular disease and left-to-right shunts are asymptomatic. Among patients who do experience symptoms, palpitations, fatigue, shortness of breath, and dyspnea on exertion commonly are reported. Cardiac failure may ensue in some patients. Physical examination may reveal suggestive cardiac murmurs.

Imaging Manifestations

The chronic increase in pulmonary flow causes the stereotypical radiographic changes associated with pulmonary hypertension—increased size of the pulmonary trunk and central pulmonary arteries, diminished peripheral vessel caliber, and right ventricular chamber dilatation. It is important to note, however, that normal chamber size may represent increasing pulmonary pressures with progression toward Eisenmenger's physiology.

CT may display calcification (Fig. 28-3) and thrombus within the main pulmonary arteries secondary to high pressure and turbulent flow within the affected vessels. CT, particularly helical CT pulmonary angiography (hCTPA), also may provide a direct view of abnormal vascular connections such as atrial septal defects (Fig. 28-4), partial anomalous pulmonary venous return (Fig. 28-5), and patent ductus arteriosus.

MR imaging, in addition to revealing dilated pulmonary arteries and enlargement of the right ventricle, also may show abnormal atrial or ventricular connections (Fig. 28-6A) as well as abnormal intravascular signal, such as flow jets between vascular chambers of different pressure (see Fig. 28-6B).

CT or MR imaging may reveal dilation of the patent

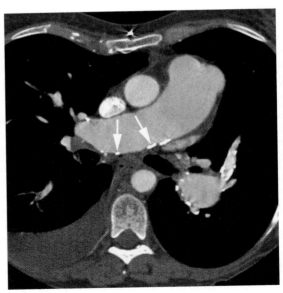

FIG. 28-3. Calcification of the pulmonary arteries in precapillary pulmonary hypertension due to congenital cardiovascular disease. Axial CT pulmonary angiogram shows calcification of the pulmonary artery walls *(arrows)*, diagnostic of pulmonary arterial hypertension.

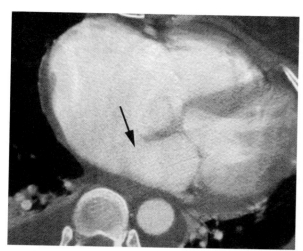

FIG. 28-4. Precapillary pulmonary hypertension due to congenital cardiovascular disease. Axial hCTPA shows discontinuity of the interatrial septum *(arrow)*, representing an atrial septal defect.

ductus, possibly with aneurysm formation or mural calcification.

Chronic Pulmonary Thromboembolism

Etiology and Pathogenesis

Thromboemboli have numerous sources, including the deep veins of the pelvis and thigh, the right atrium, indwelling catheters, or septic thromboemboli in patients with endocarditis involving the tricuspid or pulmonic valves.

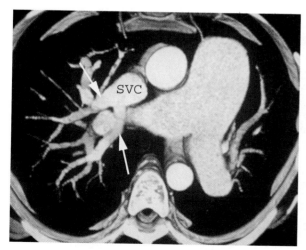

FIG. 28-5. Precapillary pulmonary hypertension due to congenital cardiovascular disease. Axial volume-rendered image from an hCTPA examination shows right upper lobe pulmonary veins *(arrows)* draining into the posterior aspect of the superior vena cava *(SVC)*, representing partial anomalous pulmonary venous return. Note the enlarged main pulmonary artery.

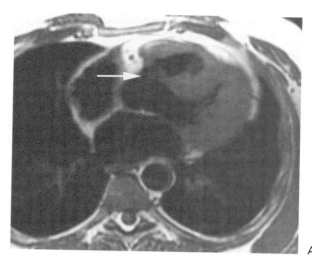

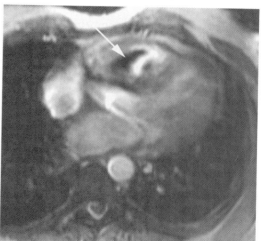

FIG. 28-6. Precapillary pulmonary hypertension due to congenital cardiovascular disease. **A.** Axial T1-weighted spin echo image shows a supracristal ventricular septal defect *(arrows)*. **B.** Axial cine image shows a low-signal flow jet within the right ventricle *(arrow)*, confirming left-to-right shunting through the ventricular septal defect.

Emboli commonly are multiple and bilateral, with a predilection for the right pulmonary circulation. Acute thromboembolic disease can produce transient pulmonary arterial pressure elevations, but sustained elevations are more likely to be a consequence of chronic thromboembolic disease, which occurs in less than 1% of patients with acute emboli.

Thromboemboli induce pulmonary arterial hypertension by occluding the pulmonary vascular bed. This occlusion may develop as a result of numerous repeated small thromboembolic episodes, a few large embolic episodes that fail to resolve completely, or the development of in situ thrombosis within small vessels and proximal migration of thrombosis, without actual embolization from deep venous sources. There are data to suggest that the latter mechanism plays a major role in the development of chronic thromboembolic pulmonary hypertension. The final common event leading to the development of elevated pulmonary hypertension is cytokine-mediated pulmonary arterial scarring resulting from lysis of pulmonary thromboemboli, and this scarring may occur after only one thromboembolic episode.

Pathologically, chronic emboli may organize, forming vascular channels interspersed with connective tissue. Fibrous bands and webs, representing organizing thrombi, are seen, often in association with fresh thrombi. The elevated pulmonary pressures also produce the characteristic histopathological changes of medial hypertrophy and intimal proliferation and luminal obliteration, often in association with atherosclerosis. Plexogenic lesions are not present.

Clinical Presentation

Patients at high risk for the development of chronic thromboembolic disease include patients with cancer, chronic cardiac or pulmonary disease, and clotting disorders. Patients with chronic thromboembolic pulmonary hypertension often complain of dyspnea on exertion, chest pain, cough, and syncope. Lupus anticoagulant may be found in 20% of patients with chronic thromboembolic pulmonary hypertension. The onset of pulmonary hypertension in patients with chronic thromboembolic disease indicates a poor prognosis.

The treatment of chronic thromboembolic pulmonary hypertension depends on the extent of clot burden within the pulmonary circulation. If thromboemboli are shown within the lobar arteries or more proximally, the patient may be a candidate for surgical thromboembolectomy.

Thromboemboli distal to the proximal segmental vessels usually are not amenable to surgical resection, and oral anticoagulation is the preferred treatment.

Imaging Manifestations

Chest radiography may be normal early in the course of the development of chronic thromboembolic hypertension. Later, the characteristic findings of pulmonary arterial hypertension, including enlargement of the main, right, and left pulmonary arteries, is seen. Subpleural opacities representing recent or remote pulmonary infarction may be encountered.

Helical CT pulmonary angiography is the study of choice for the evaluation of central chronic thromboembolic pulmonary hypertension. Eccentric filling defects adjacent to the vessel wall, representing organizing thrombi, are characteristic of chronic thromboembolic disease. These thrombi may calcify. The eccentric nature of organizing thrombi may be shown to advantage with multiplanar reformatted imaging (Fig. 28-7). Organizing thrombi may undergo recanalization, in which case CT will show small foci of contrast within an occluded vessel. Linear intraluminal filling defects representing intravascular webs also may be seen. Abrupt narrowing of pulmonary arteries with reduction in arterial diameter is common in patients with chronic thromboembolic pulmonary hypertension, and hCTPA also may show markedly hypertrophied bronchial arteries in these patients.

HRCT may show bilateral, geographically distributed inhomogeneous lung opacity in patients with chronic thromboembolic pulmonary hypertension, representing

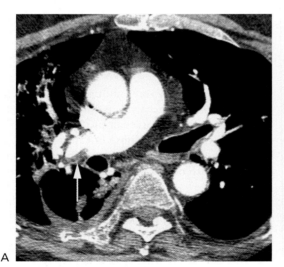
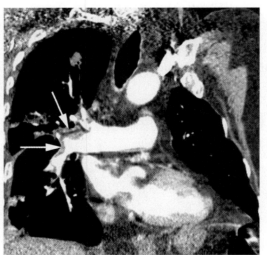

FIG. 28-7. Reformatted imaging provides added value for imaging of chronic thromboembolic disease. **A.** Axial CT pulmonary angiogram shows an eccentric filling defect *(arrow)* in the distal right pulmonary artery, consistent with chronic thromboembolic disease. **B.** Coronal reformatted image show the eccentric nature of the filling defect *(arrows)* to advantage.

mosaic perfusion. The vessels within the regions of decreased pulmonary parenchymal attenuation often are visibly smaller than their counterparts in the areas of normal or increased parenchymal attenuation. Small foci of subpleural consolidation, representing areas of prior pulmonary infarction, also may be evident.

V̇/Q̇ scanning often is interpreted as high-probability in patients with chronic thromboembolic pulmonary hypertension, although scintigraphy may underestimate the degree of hemodynamic derangement associated with chronic thromboembolic pulmonary hypertension. Furthermore, in the Prospective Investigation of Pulmonary Embolism Diagnosis (PIOPED) series, the positive predictive value of a high-probability V̇/Q̇ scan interpretation fell from 91% to 74% for patients with a prior history of thromboembolic disease, representing a loss of specificity in the high-probability scan interpretation. Other studies have shown high sensitivity and specificity for V̇/Q̇ scintigraphy for the detection of chronic thromboembolic pulmonary hypertension, but the limitations of this technique usually favor hCTPA as the first step in the diagnostic evaluation of these patients.

Findings of central chronic thromboembolic pulmonary hypertension on MRI and magnetic resonance angiography (MRA) are similar to those on CT. Chronic, organized thrombi appear as very-low-signal foci adjacent to the vascular wall on T1-weighted images. Vascular webs and stenoses and hypertrophied bronchial arteries may be visible.

Pulmonary angiography typically shows vascular tortuosity, webs, bands, stenoses, "pouching defects," and abrupt vascular cutoffs or occlusions in patients with chronic thromboembolic pulmonary hypertension.

NONTHROMBOTIC PULMONARY ARTERIAL EMBOLIZATION

Nonthrombotic emboli to the pulmonary arterial circulation may produce precapillary pulmonary arterial hypertension. Potential etiologies include tumor emboli, particulates such as mercury and talc, and parasites.

Tumor Embolization

Etiology and Pathogenesis

As many as 25% of patients with a solid malignancy may have microemboli that lodge in the pulmonary circulation. The most common etiology of tumor microembolization is gastric cancer, but breast, lung, ovarian, renal, hepatocellular, and prostate cancers also may produce tumor emboli. Most emboli preferentially occlude small arteries and arterioles, with the exception of atrial myxomas and renal carcinomas, which may form larger, more centrally located, thromboemboli.

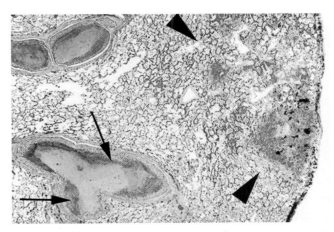

FIG. 28-8. Pulmonary arterial tumor embolism in a patient with carcinoma. This histopathological specimen shows tumor filling small pulmonary arterioles *(arrows)*, producing a branching configuration. Hemorrhagic infarction also is present *(arrowheads)*.

Histopathological specimens in patients with pulmonary tumor embolization show visible tumor within pulmonary arteries, often accompanied by lymphangitic tumor, organizing thrombi, pulmonary infarction, and intimal fibrosis (Fig. 28-8). Larger vessels may be affected, although small, peripherally located pulmonary arteries (at the centrilobular artery level) may be affected as well. Occasionally, myxoid intimal hyperplasia may be present and may induce arteriolar obliteration. This situation has been referred to as *thrombotic tumor microangiopathy*.

Clinical Presentation

Because tumor emboli are quite small, symptoms related to tumor embolization are uncommon. If the embolic load is great enough, patients may present with dyspnea on exertion, hypoxemia, chest pain, cough, syncope, and even right-sided heart failure.

Imaging Manifestations

Chest radiographs in patients with intravascular tumor embolization often are normal, but sometimes they may resemble pulmonary lymphangitic carcinomatosis.

In addition to the characteristic findings of pulmonary hypertension and thromboembolism described previously, CT scans of patients with tumor emboli may reveal lymphadenopathy, lymphangitic carcinomatosis, and peripheral, wedge-shaped opacities representing infarction. When emboli affect larger vessels, such as subsegmental arteries, CT may reveal a "beaded" appearance of these vessels. When smaller vessels are affected (at the centrilobular level), beading and nodularity may be observed, and the affected vessels may assume a branching configuration, resembling "tree-in-bud."

Lung scintigraphy may reveal subsegmental unmatched perfusion defects, indistinguishable from thromboembolic disease. Pulmonary angiography may show a delayed arterial phase, intravascular filling defects with a beaded appearance, and peripheral pruning.

Particulate Embolization

Etiology and Pathogenesis

Intravascular mercury embolization may produce pulmonary hypertension. After injection, mercury embolizes small vessels and eventually migrates from the vessel into the surrounding pulmonary interstitium, where the metal elicits an inflammatory, granulomatous response that produces vascular obstruction and, eventually, pulmonary hypertension.

Pulmonary talcosis results from the intravascular injection of talc. Talc is an insoluble filler used as a binding agent in several medications. When intravenous drug users abuse medications containing talc, they intravenously inject a suspension containing crushed tablets intended for oral use, thereby embolizing small pulmonary arterioles with talc. The talc may migrate from the vessels into the surrounding pulmonary interstitium, where its presence elicits a foreign body granulomatous response. Vascular thrombosis with recanalization, medial arterial hypertrophy, fibrosis, and refractile talc particles are present in histopathological specimens.

Clinical Presentation

Mercury may be injected into the vascular system accidentally or intentionally. Intentional mercury injection most often represents a suicide attempt.

Pulmonary talcosis usually produces few symptoms, but patients may present with chronic, progressive shortness of breath, dyspnea on exertion, and cough. Symptoms may progress even after cessation of drug abuse.

Imaging Manifestations

On chest radiography, mercury embolization appears as fine, branching, symmetric, very dense nodules representing intra-arterial mercury deposits. Metal deposits also may collect within the heart, particularly at the apex of the right ventricle.

Chest radiographs in patients with talc embolization show diffuse, bilateral, small nodular opacities about 1 to 2 mm in diameter throughout the lung parenchyma. Perihilar conglomerate masses associated with fibrosis, producing retraction of lung parenchyma and relative hyperlucency in the lower lung, may be seen in some patients.

CT may demonstrate numerous, small micronodules with or without patchy ground-glass opacity. Upper lobe fibrotic opacities, resembling progressive massive fibrosis, may be present. These fibrotic opacities may show high attenuation due to the presence of talc.

Parasitic Embolization

Etiology and Pathogenesis

Cardiopulmonary schistosomiasis most often is the result of infection with *Schistosoma mansoni,* which is endemic in the Middle East, Africa, and South America. There usually is a latency period of 5 years or more after the onset of infection before cardiopulmonary disease develops. Secreted ova migrate to the lungs via portal-systemic collaterals and lodge within medium-sized muscular arteries and arterioles. Within the pulmonary circulation, the eggs elicit an inflammatory reaction that results in medial hypertrophy, granuloma formation, intimal hyperplasia, collagen deposition and fibrosis, and obliterative arteritis. An associated eosinophilic alveolitis may be present.

Clinical Presentation

Presenting symptoms of parasitic embolization include hepatosplenomegaly, symptoms of right heart failure, dyspnea, and cough. Patients with cardiopulmonary schistosomiasis always have cirrhosis and portal hypertension.

Imaging Manifestations

Chest radiography in patients with parasitic embolization shows findings consistent with pulmonary arterial hypertension. Small nodules, representing parasitic granulomas, may be evident. Pulmonary infarction rarely is seen with parasitic embolization.

HRCT may demonstrate nodules, interstitial prominence and thickening, and ground-glass opacity associated with the classic findings of pulmonary hypertension.

CHRONIC ALVEOLAR HYPOXIA

Etiology and Pathogenesis

Etiologies of chronic alveolar hypoxia that may produce pulmonary arterial hypertension include chronic obstructive pulmonary disease (COPD), interstitial lung diseases, and hypoventilation syndromes, such as sleep apnea. These disorders produce hypoxia, with or without associated acidosis, through $\dot{V}/\dot{Q}$ mismatching, shunt, or alveolar hypoventilation. Other associated conditions, such as polycythemia, destruction of the alveolar-capillary membrane, systemic arterial flow through bronchial artery-pulmonary artery anastomoses, and pulmonary thromboemboli also may play a role in chronic alveolar hypoxia-induced pulmonary arterial hypertension.

Chronic Obstructive Pulmonary Disease

Chronic obstructive pulmonary disease is a constellation of four diseases—emphysema, chronic bronchitis, asthma, and bronchiectasis—that share the common characteristic of airflow obstruction on forced expiration. $\dot{V}/\dot{Q}$ mismatching is the primary mechanism of hypoxemia in COPD, and regional alveolar hypoxia physiologically results in hypoxic vasoconstriction and increased resistance in the pulmonary arterial vasculature. The pulmonary arterial hypertension that results from this sequence of events is exacerbated by the alveolar capillary destruction present in patients with COPD.

The onset of pulmonary hypertension in the patient with COPD is associated with a poor prognosis, with a 5-year survival of 10% in patients with pulmonary artery pressures greater than 45 mmHg.

Interstitial Lung Disease

Pulmonary arterial hypertension associated with interstitial lung diseases is produced in part by chronic hypoxemia. Fibrotic restriction of pulmonary vessels, limiting their distensibility, and reduction of the vascular surface area also may play a role. As mentioned earlier, in the case of connective tissue diseases, the development of pulmonary hypertension may be related to immunologic mechanisms.

Progressive systemic sclerosis produces changes in the vasculature more commonly than rheumatoid arthritis or systemic lupus erythematosus, and, therefore, has a higher association with pulmonary hypertension. The onset of pulmonary hypertension carries a poor prognosis in patients with progressive systemic sclerosis—the 5-year survival for patients with progressive systemic sclerosis associated with pulmonary hypertension is only 10% compared with a 75% 5-year survival for patients with progressive systemic sclerosis and interstitial lung disease without pulmonary hypertension.

Alveolar Hypoventilation Syndromes

Alveolar hypoventilation syndromes, such as obesity-hypoventilation syndrome or obstructive sleep apnea, results in chronically depressed Po_2 and elevated Pco_2. The chronic hypoxemia produces pulmonary arterial vasoconstriction and increased pulmonary arterial resistance, resulting in pulmonary hypertension.

Clinical Presentation

The clinical presentation of both COPD and interstitial lung diseases is dominated by the presence of the lung disease, and pulmonary hypertension may not be recognized until cor pulmonale develops.

Imaging Manifestations

The appearance of pulmonary hypertension caused by COPD and chronic alveolar hypoxia on chest radiography is similar to that of pulmonary hypertension from any other cause. The presence of abnormally large lung volumes and other stigmata of COPD are key to diagnosing obstructive lung disease as the cause of pulmonary hypertension. Basilar reticulation and diminished lung volumes suggest interstitial lung disease in patients with precapillary pulmonary hypertension. HRCT is more sensitive and specific than chest radiography for the diagnosis of pulmonary hypertension associated with either COPD or interstitial lung disease.

POSTCAPILLARY PULMONARY HYPERTENSION

Postcapillary pulmonary hypertension results from any process that elevates pulmonary venous pressure. As the pressure in the pulmonary venous system rises, there is a concomitant increase in pressure in the arterial system to maintain flow across the pulmonary capillary bed. As the pressure in the pulmonary arterial bed rises, the histologic changes of medial expansion, intimal proliferation, and progressive fibrosis take place as they do in precapillary pulmonary hypertension.

The etiologies that most commonly produce postcapillary pulmonary hypertension are diseases affecting the left side of the heart, such as left ventricular failure, systemic hypertension, and mitral valvular disease. Unusual left-sided obstructive lesions that may produce postcapillary pulmonary hypertension include atrial myxoma, cor triatriatum, and other left-sided congenital cardiac anomalies. Pulmonary venous obstruction, such as may occur with fibrosing mediastinitis, also may produce postcapillary pulmonary hypertension. Finally, pulmonary veno-occlusive disease is a very rare cause of postcapillary pulmonary hypertension.

Left-Sided Cardiovascular Disease

The most commonly encountered left-sided cardiovascular causes of pulmonary venous hypertension are left ventricular dysfunction, aortic stenosis, aortic regurgitation, mitral stenosis, or an obstructing intra-atrial tumor or thrombus. In patients with left-sided tumor or thrombus, the size of the obstructing lesion correlates with the degree of pulmonary hypertension.

Secondary pulmonary hypertension arises when increased venous pressure requires elevated arterial pressure to promote forward flow. The histopathologic changes in the arterial system, therefore, are caused secondarily by the increased venous pressure. Histopathological specimens from the venous system show medial hypertrophy, interstitial thickening and edema, hemosiderosis, and, occasionally, venous infarction.

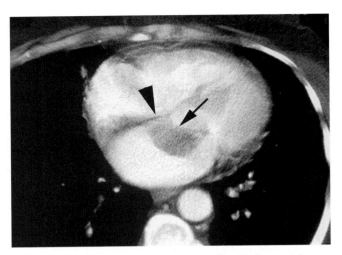

FIG. 28-9. Left atrial myxoma in postcapillary pulmonary hypertension. This axial CT image shows a filling defect within the left atrium attached to the anterior mitral valve leaflet *(arrow)* and a portion of the interatrial septum *(arrowhead).*

The clinical presentation of left-sided cardiovascular disease is variable and depends on the specific disorder under consideration. Chronic left-sided cardiac diseases often present with progressive shortness of breath and exercise intolerance; chest pain, syncope, cough, and lower extremity edema may also be present. Atrial myxomas may present with the same symptoms, or they may produce symptoms of systemic embolization or constitutional symptoms, such as fever and weight loss.

Chest radiographs and CT scanning show the characteristic findings of venous hypertension, including interlobular septal thickening (Kerley A and B lines) and pleural effusion, with or without air-space opacity representing alveolar edema. If secondary pulmonary hypertension has developed, central pulmonary artery prominence will be superimposed.

Some left-sided cardiovascular diseases have radiographic features that may allow a specific diagnosis with chest radiography or CT. Mitral stenosis may result in ossific micronodules within the pulmonary parenchyma. Atrial myxomas, if calcified, occasionally may be seen within the left atrium on chest radiographs. On contrast-enhanced CT, myxomas appear as filling defects within a cardiac chamber (usually the left atrium), often attached to the interatrial septum or anterior leaflet of the mitral valve (Fig. 28-9).

Echocardiography is the imaging method most commonly chosen for the evaluation of left-sided cardiac disease or suspected cardiac tumors. Echocardiography provides useful functional cardiac information, such as estimates of chamber volume and pressure and stroke volume. Echocardiography also has the ability to determine the degree of functional impairment due to the size of a cardiac mass

lesion, the degree of valvular dysfunction caused by the lesion, and the lesion's mobility.

MRI also shows the location and morphology of cardiac masses, such as atrial myxomas, to advantage. In addition, it provides valuable functional data analogous to that obtained with echocardiography.

Fibrosing Mediastinitis

Fibrosing mediastinitis represents a progressive proliferation of collagenous and fibrous tissue throughout the mediastinum, producing encasement and compression of mediastinal structures. Granulomatous infections, particularly *Histoplasma capsulatum* and *Mycobacterium tuberculosis*, are among the most common causes of fibrosing mediastinitis.

The deposition of fibrous tissue in fibrosing mediastinitis commonly affects relatively deformable structures, such as the superior vena cava, the trachea and central airways, the pulmonary arteries, the pulmonary veins, and the esophagus. Pulmonary hypertension may be produced by fibrous encasement of either the pulmonary arteries or draining pulmonary veins. The former produce precapillary pulmonary hypertension, which often is mistaken for chronic thromboembolic disease, and the latter produces post-capillary pulmonary hypertension. Pulmonary venous obstruction is patchy in distribution, producing wide variations in pulmonary capillary wedge pressure measurements, although the wedge pressure usually is elevated. Cardiac catheterization reveals normal left heart size and pressures.

Fibrosing mediastinitis produces histopathological changes characteristic of venous hypertension, including medial hypertrophy, septal thickening secondary to edema, hemosiderin-laden macrophages, venous infarction, and the typical vascular changes of pulmonary arterial hypertension. Thrombi may be found within affected veins.

The predominant symptoms of fibrosing mediastinitis depend on the structures most severely involved. Patients often present with nonspecific symptoms of pulmonary venous hypertension such as dyspnea and hemoptysis. The treatment for the disorder is limited; if focal fibrosis of a pulmonary vein is diagnosed, surgical treatment may be effective. Corticosteroids have shown limited efficacy in reversing the disease.

Chest radiographs often show a widened mediastinum with hilar prominence and calcified lymph nodes. Findings of pulmonary venous hypertension, including interlobular septal thickening and alveolar edema, may be present. Fibrosing mediastinitis may result in airway stenoses which may cause lobar volume loss.

CT reveals extensive infiltration of the mediastinum with abnormal soft tissue. Fibrosing mediastinitis due to *Histoplasma capsulatum* usually produces extensive lymph node calcification, which is readily identified with CT. Contrast-enhanced CT may show extensive collateral vein formation due to fibrotic involvement of systemic thoracic veins such as the superior vena cava or azygos vein. Pulmonary artery compression may be visualized directly (Fig. 28-10). Pulmonary venous infarcts, appearing as subpleural, wedge-shaped consolidations, may be seen in patients with pulmonary venous involvement. V̇/Q̇ scintigraphy may show focal unmatched perfusion defects. Unilateral lack of perfusion of one lung has been reported in patients with fibrosing mediastinitis.

Pulmonary angiography findings vary depending on the location of obstruction. If the arterial circulation is affected primarily, asymmetric narrowing of the pulmonary arteries will be present. When pulmonary veins are affected primarily, venous phase angiography will show stenoses, dilation, or obstruction, often near the junction of the affected vein and the left atrium.

Pulmonary Veno-occlusive Disease

Pulmonary veno-occlusive disease (PVOD) is an idiopathic condition, similar to primary pulmonary hypertension, but affecting the pulmonary venous circulation. It has been seen in connection with pregnancy, drugs (bleomycin, carmustine, oral contraceptives), toxic ingestions, and bone marrow transplantation, and both immunologic mechanisms and viral infections have been implicated as potential etiologies as well. The characteristic hemodynamic feature of PVOD is normal or only mildly elevated pulmonary capillary wedge pressures with normal left atrial and ventricular function and pressures. PVOD affects the venous bed in a patchy distribution, accounting for some variability in wedge pressure measurements.

Histopathological specimens in patients with PVOD show obliteration of small pulmonary veins and venules by fibrosis. Plexiform lesions are absent, but capillary proliferation may be seen, implying the presence of angiogenesis. Prior episodes of infraction and alveolar hemorrhage may be found.

Patients present with chronic, progressive dyspnea, hemoptysis, and malaise, usually during childhood and adolescence. It is important to distinguish between patients presenting with PVOD and those with interstitial lung disease. This distinction is important because therapy for interstitial lung disease–induced pulmonary hypertension is vasodilation, which could precipitate pulmonary edema in patients with PVOD. The prognosis for PVOD is poor, with most patients dying within 3 years of diagnosis.

Chest radiography in patients with PVOD shows features typical of pulmonary hypertension, but evidence of

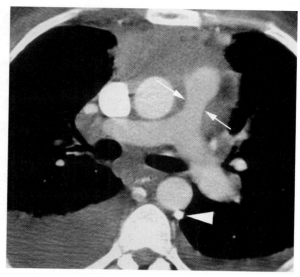

FIG. 28-10. Postcapillary pulmonary hypertension. CT scan shows abnormal soft tissue within the anterior mediastinum and compression of the main pulmonary artery *(arrows)*. Note the presence of an intensely enhanced hemiazygos vein *(arrowhead)*. Multiple biopsies revealed fibrous tissue, consistent with fibrosing mediastinitis.

pulmonary edema often is present as well. Left atrial enlargement and redistribution of blood flow into the upper lobes are absent, making it possible to distinguish PVOD from mitral stenosis. HRCT shows small central pulmonary veins, patchy, dependent ground-glass opacity, smoothly thickened interlobular septa, and pleural effusions.

V̇/Q̇ scintigraphy shows patchy perfusion, most likely secondary to superimposed arterial hypertension. Pulmonary angiography shows stigmata of pulmonary hypertension, including enlarged pulmonary arteries with peripheral pruning, but with delayed filling of the central pulmonary veins and a prolonged parenchymal enhancement phase. These latter findings are secondary to the obstruction present in the venous system.

SELECTED READING

Fraser RS, Müller NL, Colman N, Paré PD. Diagnosis of Diseases of the Chest. Philadelphia: WB Saunders, 1999: 1897–1945

Frazier AA, Galvin JR, Franks TJ, Rosado-DeChristenson ML. From the archives of the AFIP: pulmonary vasculature: hypertension and infarction. Radiographics 2000; 20:491–524.

Remy-Jardin M, Remy J. Spiral CT angiography of the pulmonary circulation. Radiology 1999; 212:615–636.

29

COMPUTED TOMOGRAPHY AND MAGNETIC RESONANCE IMAGING OF THE THORACIC AORTA

GAUTHAM P. REDDY, MICHAEL B. GOTWAY, AND CHARLES B. HIGGINS

The aorta can be imaged directly with a number of modalities: x-ray angiography, transesophageal echocardiography (TEE), multislice computed tomography (MSCT), and magnetic resonance imaging (MRI). Because some diseases of the thoracic aorta are life-threatening, the aorta must be evaluated fully when pathology is suspected. For comprehensive diagnostic assessment of the thoracic aorta, the lumen, aortic wall, and periaortic region must be viewed to assess intraluminal, mural, and extramural disease. Aortic pathology can involve any or all of these three locations. Imaging techniques must have the capability of evaluating the entire thoracic aorta as well as the origins of the arch vessels to define the extent of involvement. In some patients the status of the aortic valve and annulus also must be delineated. Imaging studies are needed for the initial diagnosis and, in some instances, for surveillance of disease progression over time.

MSCT and MRI are the mainstays of evaluation of the thoracic aorta. The choice of when to use MSCT and MRI varies from institution to institution. At many centers, MSCT is preferred for acutely ill patients, and MRI for patients who are stable.

The advantages of MSCT are its speed, ease of use, and lack of operator dependence. At many institutions, MSCT is the examination of choice for evaluation of acute aortic pathology, including dissection, intramural hematoma, aneurysm rupture, penetrating ulcer, and acute traumatic injury. MSCT can image the lungs and pleura, which can be especially important in the acute setting, because vascular and nonvascular diseases can have similar clinical presentations and may be difficult to differentiate on the basis of signs and symptoms.

MRI is valuable for comprehensive noninvasive morphologic and functional evaluation of the thoracic aorta. MRI has several advantages, including multiplanar imaging, intrinsic contrast between the blood pool and vessel wall, a wide range of soft tissue contrast that allows the delineation of the vascular and perivascular structures, the ability to evaluate both morphology and function of the vascular system, avoidance of iodinated contrast agent, and absence of ionizing radiation. Because of these capabilities, MRI remains the optimal method of evaluating aortic disease in patients who are not acutely ill. MRI can serve as a complementary imaging modality in acute aortic syndromes when CT is contraindicated (such as in patients with renal failure) or when CT does not provide complete evaluation of the disease process.

TECHNIQUES

Multislice Computed Tomography

MSCT techniques have evolved rapidly as scanners with additional detector rows have become available. Nonetheless, certain variables must be optimized to yield the highest image quality: collimation, pitch, field-of-view, reconstruction increment, amount, rate and timing of contrast administration, distance to be scanned, milliamperage, and tube rotation time. Occasionally, a compromise among these parameters is necessary to optimize the scan.

MSCT of the thoracic aorta should begin with a noncontrast series to assess the possibility of intramural hematoma. Slice thickness of 5mm is sufficient. This series is followed by the contrast-enhanced scan.

Optimal MSCT requires a post-patient collimation of 1 to 2.5 mm, which provides excellent spatial resolution and allows for high-quality reconstructed images. The entire chest, abdomen, and pelvis can be scanned rapidly. A pitch of 1.5 to 2 allows a large volume of coverage to be obtained in a reasonable time. The field of view should include at least outer rib to outer rib at the widest portion of the thorax. A reconstruction interval that provides an overlap of nearly 50% in slice thickness can be used to generate excellent quality images.

There is no consensus regarding the iodine concentration that should be used for MSCT. Undiluted (300 or 360 mg I/ml) contrast agent usually is appropriate. About 100 to 140 ml of contrast agent is injected at a rate of 3 to 5 ml/sec. These rates can be achieved using a 20-gauge intravenous catheter. A standard scan delay of 25 seconds after start of injection usually suffices for MSCT. However, patients with diminished cardiac function or an unsuspected stenosis of the injected vein may require longer delays to achieve optimal opacification of the vessel. A test bolus can be used to determine circulation time, but the preferred method involves the use of a bolus tracking software program, which is built into most MSCT scanners.

The contrast-enhanced MSCT should extend from the thoracic inlet to below the aortic bifurcation in the pelvis to assess the possibility of pathology extending into the arch vessels and iliac arteries.

The mA used is critical for obtaining high quality studies. Values of 120 to 150 mA per tube rotation usually suffice for most patients, but patients who weigh more will require an upward adjustment in the mA. MSCT of the aorta is best achieved with the shortest available tube rotation time, as low as 400 msec with currently available machines.

MRI

Several MRI techniques are useful for imaging the thoracic aorta. The most important sequences are electrocardiogram (ECG)-gated spin-echo (SE) and gradient-echo (GRE) sequences as well as contrast-enhanced three-dimensional (3D) MR angiography (MRA). With respect to the long axis of the aorta, images can be acquired parallel (sagittal oblique or sagittal) or perpendicular (transverse). Use of orthogonal planes helps to distinguish among intraluminal, mural, and extramural pathologies and reduces partial volume averaging. ECG gating is used for SE and GRE acquisitions but not for MRA.

A typical protocol for imaging of the thoracic aorta consists of SE, GRE, and MRA sequences. Transverse images are acquired from a level 1 cm above the aortic arch to the level of the diaphragm, using a slice thickness of 5 to 8 mm. Transverse breathhold fast GRE (true fast imaging with steady-state precession [FISP] or balanced fast-field echo [FFE]) cine MRI is performed in the same anatomic region. A slice thickness of 10 mm is used for the cine sequence. An SE sequence is acquired in the oblique sagittal or sagittal plane (slice thickness 3 to 5 mm) to display the entire length of the aortic arch, along with the ascending aorta and proximal descending aorta, on the same image. This sequence may be useful to visualize the origins of the arch vessels, which is important when aortic dissection is suspected. The oblique sagittal imaging sequence is prescribed from the transverse image at the level of the aortic arch. Contrast-enhanced 3D MRA is performed in the sagittal or oblique sagittal plane.

With the SE technique, double inversion recovery technique is used to suppress the signal of the intraluminal blood. The aortic lumen, therefore, is homogeneously black. Although this technique can be valuable, the lumen signal is not completely black when flow is inordinately slow. The repetition time (TR) is equal to the time of one heartbeat, usually 400 to 1100 msec, and the echo time (TE) is 30 to 40 msec.

GRE sequences render the blood pool homogeneously bright. These sequences are especially useful for aortic evaluation because they demonstrate intraluminal pathology as a filling defect in the bright blood pool. The bright signal of the blood on GRE images is secondary to flow-related enhancement. With GRE imaging radiofrequency (RF), pulses are applied to saturate a volume of tissue. Because the TR is short, there is little time for signal recovery from stationary tissue. The maximum signal is emitted by blood flowing into the volume of tissue, therefore, because this blood contains the only protons that have not been saturated by the RF pulses. Slow blood flow, which results in decreased flow enhancement, is the primary factor that causes signal depression on GRE images. Signal loss on GRE imaging also can occur as a consequence of disturbed flow caused by intravoxel phase dispersion, such as occurs with turbulence from a flow jet.

In the thorax, GRE sequences often are performed as breathhold cine acquisitions. GRE cine images are acquired at multiple contiguous slice locations. An ECG signal is acquired along with the imaging data so that images can be reconstructed at multiple phases (frames) of the cardiac cycle. Usually 16 to 32 frames are acquired at each anatomic level. The TR is in the range of 20 to 30 msec and the TE usually is 3 to 5 msec.

Three-dimensional MRA with intravenous gadolinium chelate contrast agent relies on the T1-shortening effect of gadolinium to produce high signal intensity in blood vessels, thereby avoiding flow-related artifacts. The protocol for 3D MR angiography varies from institution to institution. One of the most effective protocols prescribes MRA in the sagittal or oblique sagittal planes. ECG gating is not required to perform this sequence. From 28 to 40 images are obtained using a slice thickness of 1.2 to 2.0 mm, TR of 3 to 5 msec, TE of 1 to 2 msec, and flip angle of 45 degrees.

The MRA sequence is performed during a breathhold of 20 to 25 seconds. The patient can be provided with oxygen by nasal cannula, at a rate of 2 L/min, to aid in breathholding. The contrast agent is administered via an antecubital vein with use of a power injector (2 ml/sec, 20 to 40 ml [0.1 to 0.3 mmol/kg] total in adults). Timing of the acquisition can be optimized by using real-time imaging for bolus detection or by performing a preliminary acquisition employing a test bolus to estimate circulation time. Multiplanar maximum intensity projection reconstructions can be valuable for interpretation of the study and for display of images.

NORMAL DIMENSIONS OF THE THORACIC AORTA

Normal sizes of the thoracic aorta (mean and standard deviation) have been determined in a population of young adults, and should be as follows when measured on axial MR or CT images:

Sinus of Valsalva: 3.3 ± 0.4 cm
Mid ascending aorta: 3.0 ± 0.4 cm
Proximal descending aorta: 2.4 ± 0.4 cm

A diameter exceeding 4 cm is considered to indicate a dilated thoracic aorta.

PSEUDOCOARCTATION

Pseudocoarctation is caused by elongation of the aortic arch and kinking at the site where the aorta is tethered by the ligamentum arteriosum (Fig. 29-1). Although the appearance of the aorta in pseudocoarctation is similar to that of true coarctation, collateral circulation does not develop because there is no pressure gradient across the site of kinking.

AORTIC DISSECTION

Aortic dissection is a separation of the aortic wall that results from a tear in the intima. Blood can enter the aortic wall through an intimal disruption and extend proximally and distally in the media, displacing the intima inward. The dissection may reenter the lumen at one or more sites of fenestration. Typically, blood flows in both the true and false channels, although the false channel sometimes is thrombosed. The dissection may disrupt the adventitia and cause pericardial tamponade, exsanguination, pleural hemorrhage, or periaortic hematoma. If the dissection involves or occludes branches of the aorta, cerebral ischemia, myocardial infarction, renal insufficiency, or mesenteric infarction can ensue.

Aortic dissection can result from an intramural hematoma, which is caused by rupture of the vasa vasorum, the arteries that supply the aortic wall. The ruptured vasa vasorum bleed into the aortic wall, which can result in an intimal tear and separation of the wall. If the intima does not separate, causing a frank dissection, then an intramural hematoma remains. The intramural hematoma may be localized, or it can extend along the wall in antegrade or retrograde direction or sometimes rupture through the adventitia. An intramural hematoma can be considered to be a form of dissection, and management is similar to that of a frank dissection.

The most common predisposing factor for aortic dissection is hypertension. Other etiologies include connective tissue disorders such as Marfan syndrome or Ehlers-Danlos syndrome, bicuspid aortic valve, aortic aneurysm, and arteritis.

The longitudinal extent of the dissection or intramural hematoma is an important factor in determining management. A dissection can begin at any location in the aorta. The most common sites of origin are just above the sinuses of Valsalva or just beyond the origin of the left subclavian artery. Dissections typically progress in the direction of blood flow (antegrade dissection), although on occasion they can proceed opposite to the blood flow (retrograde

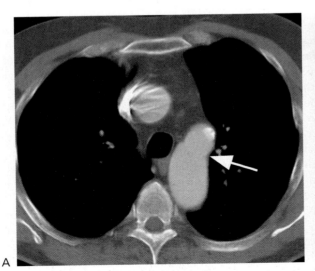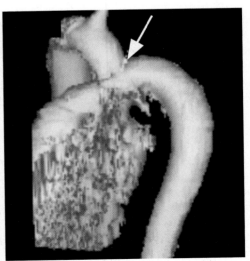

FIG. 29-1. Pseudocoarctation. Axial image (**A**) and volume-rendered reformation (**B**) of a contrast-enhanced CT scan demonstrate kinking *(arrows)* of the distal aortic arch.

dissection). Depending on the site and extent of aortic involvement, aortic dissection can be classified as Stanford type A (involving the ascending aorta) or type B (involving the descending aorta only, beyond the left subclavian artery origin). Another classification, the DeBakey system, divides dissections into three types: type I involves the ascending aorta and extends into the descending aorta; type II involves the ascending aorta only; and type III involves the descending aorta only, distal to the origin of the left subclavian artery.

There are four life-threatening complications of type A (I and II) dissection: pericardial hemorrhage and tamponade; aortic valve rupture and acute aortic insufficiency; coronary artery dissection and myocardial infarction; and carotid artery dissection and stroke. Therefore, patients with type A dissection usually undergo immediate surgery. Type B usually can be managed medically. Intramural hematoma also can be classified as type A and B. The natural history of type A and B intramural hematoma is similar to that of other type A and B dissections. However, the prognosis of type A intramural hematoma with medical therapy is better than that of type A dissection. The dissection is not completely eradicated with either surgical or medical management, so close monitoring is necessary to assess progression or complications.

Approach to Evaluation

Because it is life-threatening, aortic dissection must be diagnosed rapidly and definitively. The primary goals of imaging examinations are to establish the diagnosis by demonstrating the intramural hematoma or the intimal flap and false channel and to identify the extent of dissection. Involvement of the arch vessels and coronary arteries must be assessed. It also is vital to identify pericardial hematoma, which can result in tamponade and is an indication for immediate surgery. Other findings that should be identified are periaortic or mediastinal hematoma, as well as pleural hemorrhage.

Because of the noninvasive nature of MSCT and MRI, they are ideal techniques for the initial evaluation of aortic dissection and for surveillance of patients treated for dissection.

Imaging

The MSCT diagnosis of aortic dissection is based on evaluation of both unenhanced and enhanced images. Unenhanced scans are useful for demonstrating high-attenuation intramural hematoma or thrombosis of the false lumen (Fig. 29-2). Unenhanced images also may show inward displacement of intimal calcification. The most reliable finding for the diagnosis of dissection on MSCT is the presence of an intimal flap separating the true and false channels (Figs. 29-3 and 29-4). Contrast-enhanced scans also can reveal the patency of branch vessels and can demonstrate differential flow rates between the true and false channels.

Intramural hematoma appears as crescentic or circumferential area of high-density thickening of the aortic wall on noncontrast MSCT. Although the hyperattenuation may be appreciated on postcontrast images, the findings usually are more easily seen on noncontrast images (see Fig. 29-2).

On MRI examinations, definitive diagnosis of dissection requires the identification of the intimal flap or an intramural hematoma. The intimal flap often appears as a linear structure within the aorta (Fig. 29-5). When there is rapid flow in the true and false channels, the intimal flap is discerned between the flow void in both channels on SE images. The dissection usually extends over a long region of the aorta; however, focal dissection can occur (see Fig. 29-5). Blood flow often is slower in the false channel, resulting

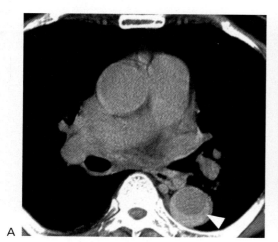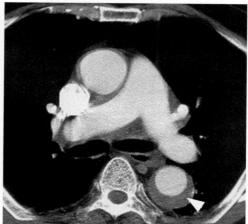

FIG. 29-2. Noncontrast (**A**) and contrast-enhanced (**B**) CT images demonstrate a type B intramural hematoma *(arrowheads)* in the descending aorta. The intramural hematoma manifests as eccentric, high-density thickening of the aortic wall on noncontrast CT.

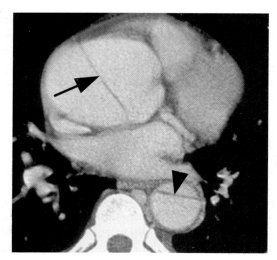

FIG. 29-3. Type A dissection. Contrast-enhanced CT reveals an intimal flap in the ascending *(arrow)* and descending *(arrowhead)* aorta.

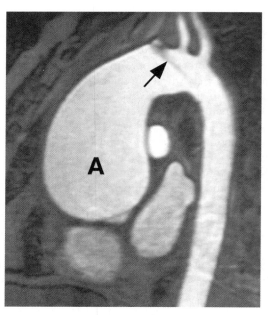

FIG. 29-5. Focal dissection in a patient with annuloaortic ectasia. Oblique sagittal maximum intensity projection of a gadolinium-enhanced MR angiogram demonstrates an intimal flap *(arrow)* in the aortic arch. Note the aneurysm of the aortic root and ascending aorta *(A)*, consistent with annuloaortic ectasia.

in partial or complete filling of this lumen with signal of variable intensity, thereby allowing differentiation between the true and the false channels. GRE cine MRI or MRA may be used to distinguish between slow flow and thrombus in the false lumen.

MRI can be used to determine whether aortic branches (the arch arteries or celiac, superior mesenteric, and renal arteries) arise from the true or false channel (Fig. 29-6).

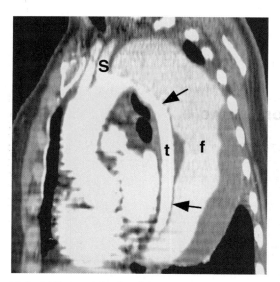

FIG. 29-4. Oblique sagittal reformation image of a contrast-enhanced CT scan demonstrates a type B dissection beginning just distal to the origin of the left subclavian artery *(s)*. The intimal flap *(arrows)* separates the true lumen *(t)* from the dilated false lumen *(f)*. Note the relatively mild enhancement of the false lumen, indicating relatively slow flow.

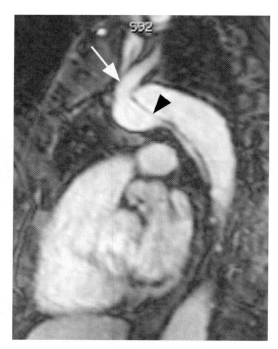

FIG. 29-6. Type B dissection sparing the arch vessels. Sagittal source image of a contrast-enhanced MR angiogram demonstrates an intimal flap *(black arrowhead)* beginning just distal to the origin of the left subclavian artery *(white arrow)*. The dissection does not extend into the left subclavian artery.

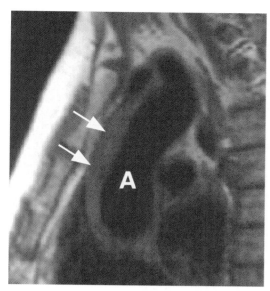

FIG. 29-7. Type A intramural hematoma. ECG-gated sagittal spin-echo MR images shows intermediate to high signal thickening *(arrows)* of the wall of the ascending aorta *(A)*, consistent with an intramural hematoma.

MRI also can identify extension of the intimal flap into the aortic arch branches. Intramural hematoma is diagnosed on SE images by the presence of intermediate- or high-signal-intensity material within the wall of the aorta (Fig. 29-7). The wall is thickened eccentrically or circumferentially.

MSCT and MRI can assess the most critical complication of dissection, which is blood leaking from the aorta into the pericardium, mediastinum, or pleura (Fig. 29-8). Within the first few hours after hemorrhage, blood usually has high signal intensity on SE images.

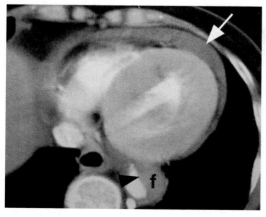

FIG. 29-8. Complication of type A dissection. Contrast-enhanced CT reveals a high-density pericardial effusion *(white arrow)*, indicating hemopericardium. Note the thrombosis of the false lumen *(f)*, separated from the true lumen by an intimal flap *(black arrowhead)*.

Occasionally it can be difficult to differentiate between the true and false channels. The true lumen usually is located along the left posterolateral aspect of the descending thoracic aorta and abdominal aorta. In many cases the true lumen is compressed by the false lumen. When the dissection flap appears as a circular or oval structure within the center of the aorta, the center of the circular or oval structure represents the true lumen.

For assessment of dissection, the diagnostic accuracy of both MRI and helical CT is high. Sensitivity and specificity are over 95%. The diagnostic accuracy of MRI and CT has been compared to that of TEE. Whereas the sensitivities of the three techniques are almost 100%, some studies have shown that the specificity of MRI and CT may be significantly better than that of TEE. The accuracy of gadolinium-enhanced MRA is similar to that of SE and GRE MRI. However, MRA is less sensitive for intramural hematoma and periaortic pathology. Because the diagnostic accuracies of MRI and CT are similar, they can be used interchangeably for evaluation of aortic dissection. At some institutions, MSCT may be preferred in the acute setting and MRI when the situation is not acute.

Patient Follow-up

Type A dissections are treated by surgery, whereas type B dissections usually are managed medically. In both groups of patients, MSCT and MRI can be used to monitor the progression of disease and to identify complications such as aneurysm formation in the false lumen (Fig. 29-9); compression and occlusion of branch vessels; and recurrent, progressive dissection. MRI has shown aneurysmal dilatation of the false channel in type A and type B dissections and persistent patency of the false lumen in most patients after repair of the ascending aorta. Thrombosis of the false channel and remodeling of the thoracic aorta can occur in some patients.

THORACIC AORTIC ANEURYSM

Aortic diameter exceeding 4 cm is called *dilatation,* and a diameter over 5 cm is termed an *aneurysm.* The maximum diameter of the aorta is an important determinant of the risk of rupture. When the aortic diameter is more than 6 cm, the risk of rupture in the short term is greater than 30%.

Thoracic aortic aneurysms vary in shape and size. Saccular aneurysms are localized and do not involve the entire circumference of the aorta (Fig. 29-10). Fusiform aneurysms involve the entire aortic circumference and may extend over a great length of the vessel (Fig. 29-11). Annuloaortic ectasia results from cystic medial necrosis, which is associated with Marfan syndrome, although it can be idiopathic. In annuloaortic ectasia the aortic root, and often the

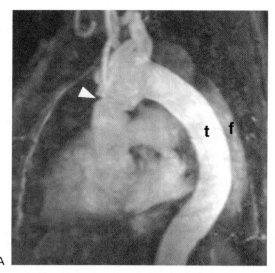

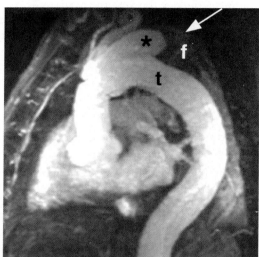

FIG. 29-9. Aneurysm of the false lumen. **A.** Sagittal maximum-intensity projection *(MIP)* of a contrast-enhanced MR angiogram about 1 month after repair of a type A dissection with a graft in the ascending aorta. Note the suture artifact at the anastomotic site *(arrowhead)*, giving the misleading appearance of slight narrowing. The false lumen *(f)* is largely thrombosed and therefore poorly opacified. **B.** Sagittal MIP of a contrast-enhanced MR angiogram 9 months later shows an aneurysm *(arrow)* of the false lumen *(f)*, as well as outpouching *(*)* of the true lumen *(t)* in the aortic arch.

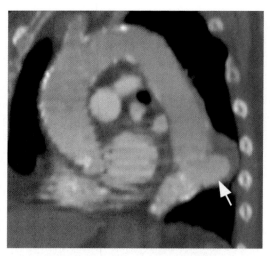

FIG. 29-10. Saccular aneurysm. Oblique sagittal reformation of a contrast-enhanced CT demonstrates a saccular aneurysm *(arrow)* in the descending aorta.

rosis. Other etiologies of true aneurysms include connective tissue disorders such as Marfan syndrome, arteritis (Takayasu or giant cell arteritis), idiopathic cystic medial necrosis, complications of aortic valve disease, and aneurysm of the ductal remnant.

Mycotic aneurysms result from infection of the aortic wall and occlusion of the vasa vasorum by septic emboli;

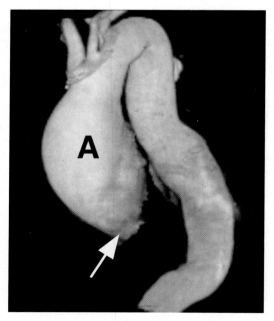

FIG. 29-11. Fusiform aneurysm. Volume-rendered reconstruction of a contrast-enhanced MR angiogram shows a large fusiform aneurysm of the ascending aorta *(A)*. This is not annuloaortic ectasia, because the aortic root *(arrow)* is not enlarged.

entire ascending aorta, is enlarged (Fig. 29-12; see also Fig. 29-5). Many aneurysms involving the thoracic aorta also involve the abdominal aorta.

In a true aneurysm, all three layers of the aortic wall are intact, whereas a false aneurysm results from a focal disruption of the aortic wall contained by the adventitia and surrounding fibrous tissue. Common causes of false aneurysm are trauma (Fig. 29-13) and infection (Fig. 29-14). True aneurysms most often are secondary to atheroscle-

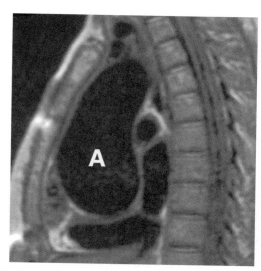

FIG. 29-12. Annuloaortic ectasia in a patient with Marfan syndrome. Note the marked, diffuse enlargement of the aortic root and ascending aorta *(A)*.

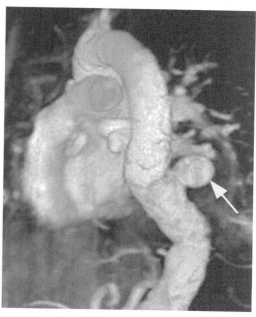

FIG. 29-14. Mycotic pseudoaneurysm. Volume-rendered reformation of a gadolinium-enhanced MR angiogram reveals a pseudoaneurysm *(arrow)* of the descending aorta.

this causes weakening of the wall, resulting in aneurysm formation. Etiologies of mycotic aneurysm include septic emboli from intravenous drug use and indwelling catheters, infection of prosthetic valves, or infection of atherosclerotic plaque. Common infectious agents include *Salmonella,*

Staphylococcus aureus, streptococci, tuberculosis, and fungi, such as *Candida* and *Aspergillus*. Mycotic aneurysms usually are saccular, and they may grow quickly (see Fig. 29-14). Mycotic aneurysms can be associated with periaortic fat infiltration and inflammation or gas formation. Mycotic aneurysms are at high risk for rupture.

Imaging

In the imaging evaluation of thoracic aortic aneurysm, the primary goals are measurement of the maximum diameter of the aorta, demonstration of the extent of the aneurysm, identification of branch vessel involvement, and detection of periaortic hematoma. The demonstration of mural thrombus is important in patients who present with peripheral embolization.

MSCT can demonstrate the extent and diameter of a thoracic aortic aneurysm accurately. MSCT readily delineates the aortic lumen, associated thrombus, and calcification. Branch vessel involvement and the local effect of the aneurysm, such as bronchial compression, also are clearly depicted with MSCT.

MSCT findings of aortic aneurysm rupture include high-density fluid in the wall of the aorta, pleural space, or pericardium (Fig. 29-15). Mediastinal hematoma also suggests the possibility of aneurysm rupture. The "draped aorta" sign may indicate an early, contained rupture. This sign manifests as indistinctness of the posterior wall or close alignment of the posterior wall with the contour of the adjacent vertebral bodies.

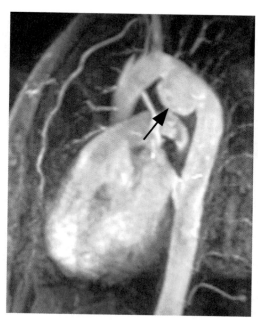

FIG. 29-13. Chronic pseudoaneurysm secondary to deceleration injury. Oblique sagittal maximum intensity projection of an MR angiogram demonstrates a pseudoaneurysm *(arrow)* in the ductal region, a classic location for a traumatic pseudoaneurysm. The patient had been involved in a high-speed motor vehicle accident several years earlier.

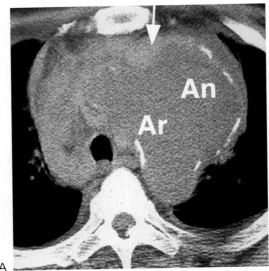 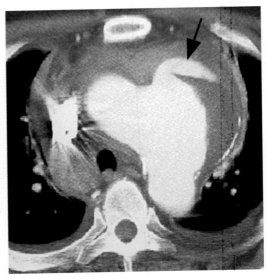

FIG. 29-15. Aneurysm rupture. **A.** Noncontrast CT at the level of the aortic arch *(Ar)* demonstrates a large saccular aneurysm *(An)* with a partially calcified rim. The high-density material *(white arrow)* in the mediastinum represents hematoma secondary to aneurysm leak. **B.** Postcontrast CT shows the penetrating aortic ulcer *(black arrow)* thought to be responsible for the rupture.

MRI also readily depicts the size and extent of an aneurysm of the ascending or descending thoracic aorta. The outer dimension of the aneurysm and the size of the patent lumen can be seen. Because MRI, unlike angiography, can demonstrate the outer wall of the aorta, it allows accurate measurement of the aneurysm diameter even when there is wall thickening or mural thrombus. Mural thrombus and atherosclerotic plaque are depicted as eccentric or concentric thickening of the aortic wall. The patent lumen usually can be determined by the flow void on SE MRI. However, slow flow can produce intraluminal signal on SE images. Slow flow can be differentiated from thrombus with GRE cine MRI or contrast-enhanced MRA. MRA is especially effective for demonstrating the extent of thoracic aortic aneurysm, the relation to the aortic branches, and the precise dimensions, especially in the aortic arch.

Identification of periaortic or mediastinal hematoma is vital in the evaluation of aneurysm rupture. On SE images, hematoma usually appears as an area of high signal intensity, although it may produce intermediate signal intensity during the first few hours after bleeding. MRI can delineate the extent of the hemorrhage, which may spread through the mediastinum or be localized to the periaortic region, pleural space, subpleural space, or pericardium.

MRI is an effective noninvasive means of monitoring the progression of thoracic aortic aneurysms. If the aortic diameter is greater than 6.0 cm or if there is a rapid increase in diameter, surgical repair usually is necessary. Because MRI is noninvasive and accurate, it also is the optimal method for sequential follow-up of the aorta in patients

with a high risk for developing dissection, such as those with Marfan or Ehlers-Danlos syndromes (see Fig. 29-5).

False aneurysms can be revealed by MSCT, contrast-enhanced MRA, or a combination of transverse and sagittal or sagittal oblique MR images. MRI is useful for depiction of the longitudinal extent of the false aneurysm. Posttraumatic false aneurysms seen on MSCT and MRI most often are located at the site of the ligamentum arteriosum and involve either the entire aortic circumference or only the anterior wall (see Fig. 29-13).

ATHEROSCLEROSIS AND PENETRATING AORTIC ULCER

Aortic thrombus often is present in the wall of aneurysms and sometimes in regions of atherosclerosis. Aortic thrombus may lead to peripheral embolization. In a patient with peripheral embolization, the left atrium, left ventricle, and aorta are evaluated for the source of the embolus. The most common sources are the left atrium, in patients with atrial fibrillation, or the left ventricle, in patients with dilated cardiomyopathy or recent myocardial infarction. Embolization from aortic thrombus is less common.

Cine MR images are useful because they depict the motion of the clot within the aortic lumen and can distinguish the thrombus from signal due to slow blood flow. MRA also is effective for differentiating thrombus from slow flow (Fig. 29-16). SE images also are useful (see Fig. 29-16B), but may be difficult to interpret if slow flow produces intra-

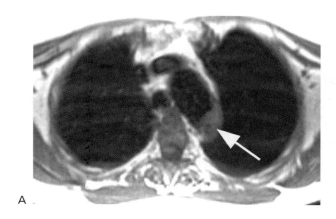

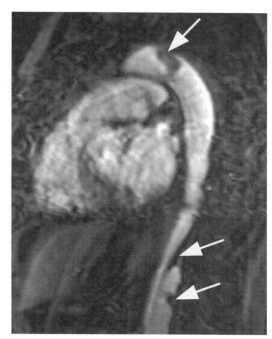

FIG. 29-16. Aortic thrombus. ECG-gated axial spin-echo MR image (**A**) and sagittal source image (**B**) from a gadolinium-enhanced MR angiogram demonstrate multiple areas of aortic thrombus *(arrows)*, thought to be the source of peripheral emboli.

luminal signal. By evaluating the heart and aorta in a single examination, MRI can be used to provide comprehensive investigation of the possible sources of peripheral embolization.

MSCT readily depicts the location and morphology of aortic thrombus and atherosclerotic plaque. Thrombus and plaque typically appear as low-density material adjacent to the aortic wall, on the luminal side of intimal calcifications. Although TEE is used more commonly for the specific investigation of aortic thrombus, disease in the cranial aspect of the ascending aorta and arch may be more effectively identified with MSCT.

PENETRATING AORTIC ULCER

Penetrating aortic ulcer occurs when atherosclerotic plaque ulcerates, disrupts the intima, and extends into the media. This can result in mural hemorrhage (intramural hematoma) and extension along the media, or, rarely, frank dissection or rupture through the adventitia. The most common location is the mid–descending thoracic aorta. The clinical presentation of aortic ulcer is similar to that of dissection, usually with sudden onset of chest or back pain. Penetrating ulcer involving the ascending aorta is treated surgically, whereas ulcers in the descending aorta usually can be managed medically.

Penetrating aortic ulcer appears on unenhanced MSCT as an intramural hematoma. Contrast-enhanced MSCT shows a focus of contrast agent projecting beyond the confines of the lumen (Fig. 29-17). Aortic mural enhancement and, rarely, active contrast extravasation may be seen. Com-

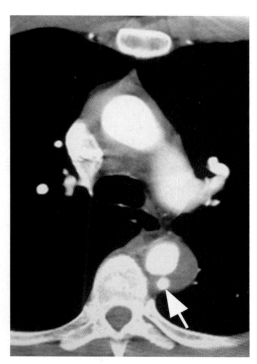

FIG. 29-17. Penetrating aortic ulcer. Contrast-enhanced CT scan demonstrates a penetrating ulcer *(arrow)* in the descending aorta.

plications such as dissection, pseudoaneurysm, or aortic rupture may be present (see Fig. 29-15B).

MRA may be especially effective for demonstration of a penetrating ulcer. SE or GRE sequences are valuable for showing an intramural hematoma associated with an ulcer, as well as pseudoaneurysm caused by extension through the adventitia.

ACUTE TRAUMATIC AORTIC INJURY

Acute traumatic aortic injury (ATAI) usually is the result of severe deceleration, such as a high-speed motor vehicle accident or a fall from a great height. ATAI results in exsanguination and immediate death in 80% to 90% of patients. Among patients with ATAI who survive the initial trauma, the mortality of untreated ATAI may be as high as 1% per hour for the first 48 hours. Therefore, it is essential that ATAI be diagnosed expeditiously and repaired surgically or with placement of an endovascular stent graft. If ATAI is not diagnosed and treated, and the patient survives, in the long term chronic pseudoaneurysm may develop.

The most common sites of injury are the aortic isthmus (90%), the ascending aorta (5% to 10%), and the descending aorta near the diaphragmatic hiatus (1% to 3%). A nearly circumferential laceration often is present, although partial tears of the aorta may occur. Arch vessel injuries may coexist.

MSCT can be used in conjunction with angiography or can avert angiography altogether. MSCT findings of ATAI can be classified as direct or indirect. The most common direct finding of ATAI is a pseudoaneurysm (Fig. 29-18). Other direct signs include an abnormal aortic contour or abrupt change in caliber, kinking of the aorta (pseudocoarctation), occlusion of a segment of aorta, and an intimal flap. Extravasation of contrast agent is rare. Patients with direct findings of ATAI can be taken to surgery immediately.

Indirect signs of ATAI include mediastinal and retrocrural hematomas (Fig. 29-19). Although mediastinal or retrocrural hematoma raises the possibility of ATAI, it is not specific because it may result from mediastinal venous bleeding. When a mediastinal hematoma is noted, its relation to the aorta is paramount. A hematoma that obscures the fat plane surrounding the aorta or arch vessels is suspicious for occult ATAI or branch vessel injury and may be assessed further with aortography. If a mediastinal hematoma does not directly contact the aorta or great arteries, then the cause is mediastinal venous bleeding, and aortography is not required.

For the diagnosis of ATAI, the sensitivity of helical CT approaches 100%, and the specificity is more than 80%. Data regarding the use of MSCT for ATAI are not yet available, but it is expected that MSCT is at least as accurate as single-detector helical CT.

PERIAORTIC ABSCESS

In patients with bacterial endocarditis, MRI can be used to identify complications such as a periaortic abscess. The

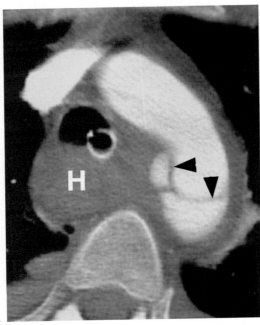
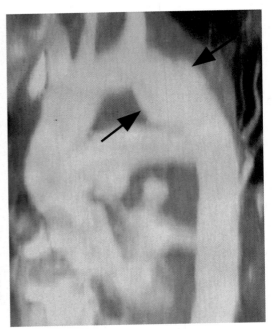

FIG. 29-18. Acute traumatic aortic injury. **A.** Contrast-enhanced CT shows a hematoma (H) adjacent to the aortic arch, with intimal disruption (*arrowheads*) in the distal arch. **B.** Oblique sagittal reformation demonstrates a pseudoaneurysm (*arrows*) at the site of injury.

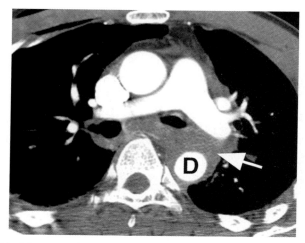

FIG. 29-19. Mediastinal hematoma. Contrast-enhanced CT scan in a patient who fell from a great height demonstrates a mediastinal hematoma *(arrow)* adjacent to the descending aorta *(D)*. Mediastinal hematoma is an indirect but nonspecific sign of aortic injury.

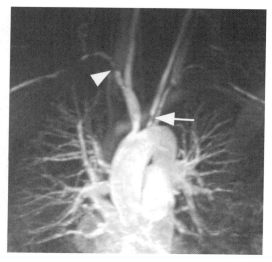

FIG. 29-21. Takayasu arteritis. Coronal oblique maximum-intensity projection of a contrast-enhanced MR angiogram of the aortic arch. Note multiple stenoses in the arch vessels, most severe in the proximal left common carotid *(arrow)* and right subclavian *(arrowhead)* arteries.

abscess cavities may be similar to a false aneurysm, with a cavity communicating with the aorta. MRI may show a flow void in the cavity, which implies communication with the aortic lumen (Fig. 29-20). MRI can be used to monitor progression of these abscess cavities.

AORTITIS

In aortitis, MRI and MSCT can demonstrate mural thickening, as well as stenosis, occlusion, or dilatation of the aorta and its branches (Fig. 29-21). Takayasu arteritis is characterized by wall thickening of the aorta or arch vessels along with stenosis of the lower thoracic or abdominal aorta, best depicted with MRI. In patients in the active phase of aortitis, contrast-enhanced SE MRI demonstrates thickening and enhancement of the aortic wall (Fig. 29-22). MRI and MSCT may be especially valuable in patients with severe stenosis or occlusion of arch vessels or of the abdominal aorta, because passage of an angiography catheter into the thoracic aorta may be particularly difficult. Contrast-enhanced MRA and MSCT play an important role in evalu-

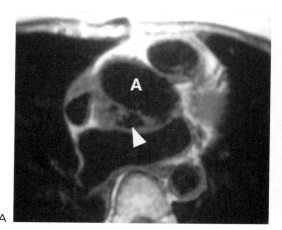

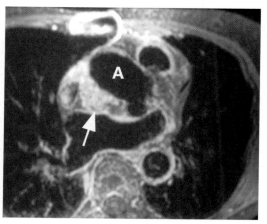

FIG. 29-20. Periaortic abscess and pseudoaneurysm. **A.** ECG-gated axial MR image shows a pseudoaneurysm *(arrowhead)* of the ascending aorta *(A)* secondary to a periaortic abscess. **B.** Gadolinium-enhanced ECG-gated axial MR image demonstrates periaortic enhancement *(arrow)* at the site of the abscess.

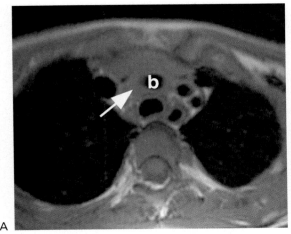
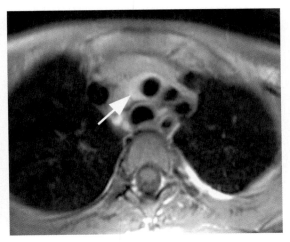

FIG. 29-22. Takayasu arteritis: active phase. Noncontrast (**A**) and contrast-enhanced (**B**) ECG-gated axial spin-echo MR images show thickening and enhancement *(arrows)* of the wall of the brachiocephalic artery *(b)*.

ation of patients with aortitis because SE and GRE MRI sequences have limited accuracy for identifying stenoses of aortic branch arteries and more peripheral vessels.

THORACIC AORTIC NEOPLASM

Secondary involvement of the aorta by a mediastinal tumor or bronchogenic carcinoma can occur. Staging CT and MRI can show involvement of the aorta, which renders the tumor inoperable. Primary aortic neoplasms are rare and include angiosarcoma or spindle cell sarcoma.

Aortic neoplasm can manifest as an irregular mass projecting into the vessel lumen. MSCT and MRI can define the intraluminal and perivascular extent of the neoplasm. Findings that suggest secondary tumor involvement are irregular thickening of the aortic wall, intraluminal mass, and tumor extending around more than 180 degrees of the aortic circumference.

COMPLICATIONS OF AORTIC GRAFTS

MRI and MSCT can be used to demonstrate complications of grafts placed in the thoracic aorta. Serious postoperative complications include dehiscence of the surgical suture line, more commonly at the proximal anastomosis. Dehiscence may cause pseudoaneurysm formation; pseudoaneurysm at the site of coronary artery reimplantation may cause myocardial ischemia and infarction. Aneurysm and dissection also may occur, especially in patients with cystic medial necrosis.

MRI and MSCT are useful for identifying pseudoaneu-

rysms, periaortic hemorrhage in the early or late postoperative period, and graft infection. The ability of MRI to depict extraluminal as well as luminal pathology is a definite advantage over angiography. On transverse MR or MSCT images, a saccular pseudoaneurysm is easily recognized. However, a fusiform pseudoaneurysm may not be identified so readily, because it may cause only mild aortic dilatation. Thus, a fusiform aneurysm may be displayed more effectively by MRA in the sagittal or oblique sagittal planes or by MSCT reconstructions.

SELECTED READING

Chung JW, Park JH, Im JG, et al. Spiral CT angiography of the thoracic aorta. Radiographics 1996; 16:811–824.

Dyer DS, Moore EE, Mestek MF, et al. Can chest CT be used to exclude aortic injury? Radiology 1999; 213:195–202.

Ganaha F, Miller DC, Sugimoto K, et al. Prognosis of aortic intramural hematoma with and without penetrating atherosclerotic ulcer: a clinical and radiological analysis. Circulation 2002; 106:342–348.

Khan IA, Nair CK. Clinical, diagnostic, and management perspectives of aortic dissection. Chest 2002; 122:311–328.

Krinsky GA, Rofsky NM, DeCorato DR, et al. Thoracic aorta: comparison of gadolinium-enhanced three-dimensional MR angiography with conventional MR imaging. Radiology 1997; 202:183–193.

Laissy JP, Blanc F, Soyer P, et al. Thoracic aortic dissection: diagnosis with transesophageal echocardiography versus MR imaging. Radiology 1995; 194:331–336.

Levy JR, Heiken JP, Gutierrez FR. Imaging of penetrating atherosclerotic ulcers of the aorta. AJR Am J Roentgenol 1999; 173:151–154.

Prince MR, Narasimham DL, Jacoby WT, et al. Three dimensional gadolinium-enhanced MR angiography of the thoracic aorta. AJR Am J Roentgenol 1996; 166:1387–1397.

Winkler ML, Higgins CB. Magnetic resonance imaging of perivalvular infectious pseudoaneurysms. AJR Am J Roentgenol 1986; 147:253–256.

30

RADIOGRAPHY OF ACQUIRED HEART DISEASE

CHARLES B. HIGGINS

The thoracic radiograph is one of the earliest points of departure in the evaluation of heart disease. It may provide the first indication that cardiac disease is present, but more frequently it is used to determine the severity of known or suspected disease. The severity of some cardiac diseases is readily reflected on the thoracic radiograph, while other significant diseases cause little or no alterations in the pulmonary vessels or cardiac silhouette. Consequently, the thoracic radiograph may have only limited value in the assessment of some diseases, while in others it may serve as one of the most sensitive and reliable gauges of the course of the disease. The propensity of various cardiac diseases to cause substantial cardiomegaly serves as the major dividing line in our system for cataloging acquired heart disease.

APPROACH TO THE CHEST X-RAY IN ACQUIRED HEART DISEASE

A systematic approach is directed toward discerning the pertinent findings from the radiograph and, for each finding, narrowing the array of diagnostic considerations. A free-floating approach places one into the unnecessary jeopardy of failing to examine salient features of the cardiovascular anatomy.

A five-step systematic approach permits the orderly examination of the thoracic radiograph, and at each step it is possible to narrow the diagnostic possibilities (Figs. 30-1 and 30-2). A radiographic classification of acquired heart disease is used in association with this five-step examination (see Fig. 30-2; Table 30-1).

The five steps in the examination of the thoracic radiograph in patients with suspected cardiac disease are (1) thoracic musculoskeletal structures, (2) pulmonary vascularity, (3) overall heart size, (4) specific chamber enlargement, and (5) great arteries (ascending aorta, aortic knob, main pulmonary arterial segment).

Thoracic Musculoskeletal Structures

Examination of the thoracic wall discloses evidence of prior operations, such as rib or sternal deformities or sternal wire sutures. Sternal deformities such as pectus may serve as a clue to cardiac lesions associated with it, such as Marfan syndrome and mitral valve prolapse; or perhaps the deformity is responsible for a cardiac murmur or even symptoms caused by cardiac compression. Narrow anteroposterior diameter of the thorax can be caused by a straight thoracic spine (straight-back syndrome) or pectus excavatum. A narrow anteroposterior diameter is defined as a distance between the sternum and the anterior border of the vertebral body that measures less than 8 cm and a ratio of the transverse diameter (determined by frontal view) to the anteroposterior diameter (determined by lateral view) exceeding 2.75. The anteroposterior diameter is the maximum diameter from the undersurface of the sternum to the anterior border of the vertebral body.

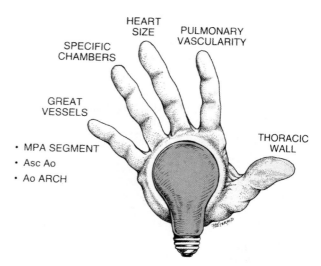

FIG. 30-1. Five-step approach to analysis of the thoracic radiograph in cardiac disease.

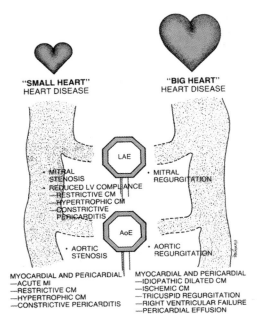

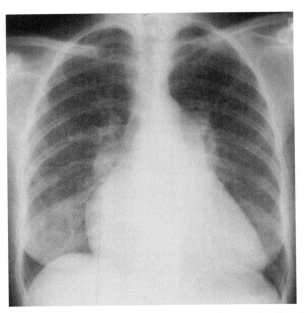

FIG. 30-2. Diagnostic pathway for the identification of the hemodynamically predominant cardiac lesion. Signposts gleaned from the thoracic radiograph guide the analysis.

FIG. 30-3. Pulmonary venous hypertension in mitral valve disease. Radiograph demonstrates redistribution of pulmonary blood flow (upper lobe vessels larger than lower lobe vessels) indicating grade I pulmonary venous hypertension. There is cardiomegaly and straightening of the upper left cardiac border indicative of left atrial enlargement.

Pulmonary Vascularity (Pulmonary Edema)

There are three steps in assessing pulmonary vascularity: the type of abnormality (pulmonary arterial overcirculation versus pulmonary venous hypertension); the severity of the pulmonary vascular abnormality; and determination of the symmetry, asymmetry, or even focal nature of the abnormality. In patients with acquired heart disease, the type of abnormality is usually pulmonary venous hypertension (PVH). The major signs of PVH are equalization or larger diameter of the upper compared to the lower lobe vessels; loss of prominence or clear visualization of the right lower lobe pulmonary artery; prominence of the interstitial mark-

ings, especially the appearance of Kerley A and B lines; indistinctness of the pulmonary vascular margins and/or hilar vessels; loss of the right hilar angle; and alveolar filling (Figs. 30-3 to 30-6). After repeated episodes of pulmonary edema in longstanding cases of mitral valve disease, perma-

TABLE 30-1. RADIOGRAPHIC CLASSIFICATION OF ACQUIRED HEART DISEASE

Small Heart (C/T <0.55)	Large Heart (C/T >0.55)
Aortic stenosis	Aortic regurgitation
Arterial hypertension	Mitral regurgitation
Mitral stenosis	Tricuspid regurgitation
Acute myocardial infarction	High-output states
Hypertrophic cardiomyopathy	Congestive cardiomyopathy
Restrictive cardiomyopathy	Ischemic cardiomyopathy
Constrictive pericarditis	Pericardial effusion
	Paracardiac mass

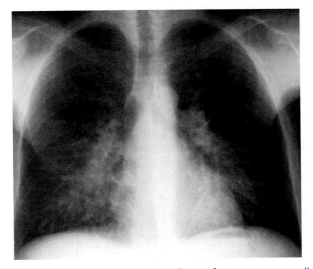

FIG. 30-4. Interstitial pulmonary edema after acute myocardial infarction. Radiograph demonstrates interstitial pulmonary edema with Kerley B lines, indistinct vascular margins, and peribronchial cuffing.

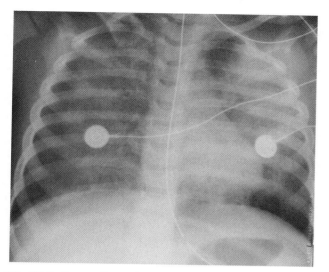

FIG. 30-5. Noncardiac pulmonary edema. Alveolar pulmonary edema with normal heart size in a child after drowning.

TABLE 30-2. SIGNS OF PULMONARY VENTRICULAR HYPERTENSION BY GRADE OF SEVERITY

Grade I: vascular redistribution
Equal upper and lower lobe vessels
Larger upper lobe vessels
Grade II: interstitial edema
Kerley A or B lines
Increased prominence of "interstitial markings"
Peribronchial cuffing
Loss of the hilar angle
Enlargement and indistinctness of hila
Subpleural edema (increased thickness of pleura)
Loss of visibility of much of the descending branch of the right
   pulmonary artery
Grade III
Confluent acinar shadows (pulmonary alveolar edema)
Perihilar alveolar filling
Lower lobe or more generalized alveolar filling

nent interstitial lines or ossific nodules may appear. Ossific nodules are small foci of bony metaplasia that appear in the lungs only after multiple episodes of edema and chronic PVH. Foci of hemosiderin may form fibrotic nodules in patients with multiple episodes of edema as well as after multiple episodes of pulmonary hemorrhage.

The severity of PVH can be gauged by the signs observed. The radiographic severity of PVH can be divided into three grades: grade I (redistribution of pulmonary blood volume); grade II (interstitial pulmonary edema); and grade III (alve-

olar pulmonary edema; Table 30-2). The pulmonary venous pressure (or mean left atrial wedge pressure) associated with edema varies depending on whether the cardiac dysfunction is acute or chronic (Table 30-3). The venous pressure in chronic disease is approximately 5 mm Hg greater for each grade of PVH compared to that in acute disease.

Asymmetric PVH

Asymmetric distribution of PVH or pulmonary edema raises a number of diagnostic possibilities (Table 30-4, Fig. 30-7). The most frequent cause of such asymmetry is probably gravitational; patients with heart disease frequently sleep lying on their right side because of consciousness of the prominent left-sided pulsation (prominent point of maximum impulse in the presence of cardiomegaly). The next most frequent cause is underlying lung disease such as

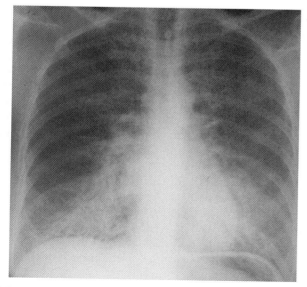

FIG. 30-6. Alveolar pulmonary edema with normal heart size in a patient with left atrial myxoma obstructing the mitral valve.

TABLE 30-3. CORRELATES OF LEFT ATRIAL PRESSURE (MEAN)ª AND PULMONARY VASCULAR HYPERTENSION GRADE

	Left Atrial Pressure	
	Acute Disease (Myocardial Infarction)	Chronic Disease (Mitral Stenosis)
Grade I	12–19 mm Hg	15–25 mm Hg
Grade II	20–25 mm Hg	25–30 mm Hg
Grade III	>25 mm Hg	>30 mm Hg

ª Left atrial mean pressure is usually inferred from the mean pulmonary wedge pressure. Correlation between left atrial pressure and radiographic signs of pulmonary edema is only fair because of phase lag between rapid pressure changes and slower changes in radiographic alterations.

TABLE 30-4. UNILATERAL PULMONARY EDEMA

Gravitational
Chronic lung disease (emphysema)
Unilateral pulmonary arterial obstruction
   Thromboembolic disease
   Extrinsic obstruction of pulmonary artery
   Lung cancer, thoracic aortic aneurysm, mediastinal fibrosis
Unilateral pulmonary venous obstruction
   Left atrial tumor
   Mediastinal tumor encasing pulmonary veins
   Mediastinal fibrosis
Reexpansion pulmonary edema
   Postpneumothorax, postthoracentesis

TABLE 30-5. NONCARDIOGENIC PULMONARY EDEMA

Drowning
Asphyxia
Upper airway obstruction
High altitude
Increased intracranial pressure
Reexpansion pulmonary edema
Noxious gases
   Smoke inhalation
   Nitrous dioxide (silo filler's disease)
   Sulfur dioxide
   Others
Drugs
   Aspirin
   Valium, librium, barbiturates, heroin, cocaine, methadone
Poisons—parathion
Blood transfusion reaction
Contrast media reaction
Adult respiratory distress syndrome

chronic obstructive pulmonary disease, which obliterates portions of the pulmonary vascular bed. Edema or pulmonary venous distention appears in the normal or less severely abnormal portions of the lungs. Unilateral pulmonary edema may occur contralateral to an occluded or severely stenotic pulmonary artery. Such unilateral edema might appear contralateral to a pulmonary embolism, or a pulmonary artery stenosis caused by congenital anomalies (branch pulmonary arterial stenosis, proximal interruption or agenesis of a pulmonary artery) or acquired diseases (bronchogenic carcinoma, Takayasu's arteritis, fibrosing mediastinitis, mediastinal tumors). Unilateral edema is infrequently used by unilateral obstruction of pulmonary veins caused by medias-

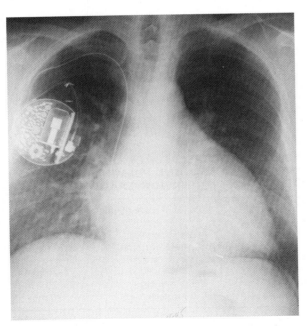

FIG. 30-7. Asymmetric pulmonary edema. Unilateral pulmonary edema in a patient with a metastatic tumor selectively obstructing the right pulmonary veins. Note the increased density of the right lower lung field.

tinal or lung tumors, primary and secondary tumors of the heart and pericardium, mediastinal fibrosis, and complications of the Mustard procedure and other procedures used in congenital heart disease. Finally, pulmonary edema induced by reinflation of a collapsed lung or after thoracentesis must be considered.

Pulmonary edema may occur in the absence of underlying cardiac disease. Such noncardiogenic edema is usually due to damage to the alveolar-capillary membrane, causing a leak of fluid into the lung at normal or near-normal pulmonary venous pressure and capillary oncotic pressure. A partial list of the many settings in which this occurs is shown in Table 30-5.

Overall Heart Size

Acquired heart disease can be divided into two groups, depending on the presence or absence of substantial cardiomegaly. "Small heart" heart disease is associated with a normal heart size or only mild cardiomegaly. For the sake of our discussion, we will set a cardiothoracic (CT) ratio of less than 0.55 as consistent with this group of lesions. The choice of 0.55 is obviously somewhat arbitrary. The CT ratio is calculated using the convention of measuring the thoracic diameter as the distance from the inner margin of the ribs at the level of the dome of the right hemidiaphragm and the cardiac diameter as the horizontal distance between the most rightward and most leftward margins of the cardiac shadow. The second group, called "big heart" heart disease, is characterized by substantial cardiomegaly (CT ratio greater than 0.55).

The pathophysiologic factors associated with "small heart" heart disease are pressure overload and reduced ventricular compliance. The pathophysiologic factors associated with "big heart" heart disease are volume overload and myocardial failure. Pericardial effusion also is included in this group.

The cardiac lesions included in the two groups are listed in Table 30-1. The major pressure overload types of acquired lesions are aortic and mitral stenosis and hypertension. The major volume overload types of acquired lesions are aortic, mitral, and tricuspid regurgitation and high output states. Cardiac diseases that cause reduced left ventricular (LV) compliance or resistance to full expansion of the ventricles are acute myocardial infarction (MI), hypertrophic cardiomyopathy, restrictive cardiomyopathy, and constrictive pericardial disease.

Specific Chamber Enlargement

It is not until the fourth step in the examination of the chest x-ray that attention should be directed to determining specific chamber enlargement. A critical observation is the identification of left atrial enlargement. It is also useful to determine which ventricle is enlarged or if both ventricles are enlarged. It is sometimes not possible to clearly determine the type of ventricular enlargement on the thoracic radiograph. The radiographic signs observed with enlargement of each of the cardiac chambers are given below.

Left Atrial Enlargement

1. Right retrocardiac double density. Distance from the middle of the double density (lateral border of left

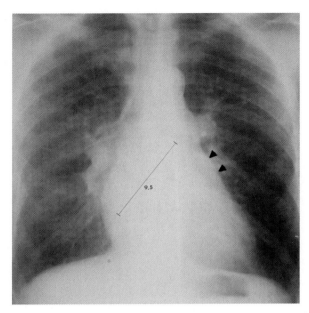

FIG. 30-9. Left atrial double intensity in mitral regurgitation. The left atrial dimension is the length of a line from the middle of the double density to the medial border of the left bronchus. A value greater than 7 cm indicates left atrial enlargement. Note also enlargement of the left atrial appendage *(arrowheads)*.

atrium) to the middle of the left bronchus is less than 7 cm in greater than 90% of normal subjects and greater than 7 cm in 90% of patients with left atrial enlargement, proven by echocardiography (Figs. 30-8 and 30-9). In cases of severe left atrial enlargement, the right atrial border may extend further to the right than the right atrial border (Fig. 30-10).

2. Enlargement of the left atrial appendage. This is seen as a bulge along the left cardiac border just beneath the main pulmonary artery segment (see Figs. 30-8 to 30-10). Using the left bronchus as an orientation point, the bulge above it is the main pulmonary artery segment, while the bulge at the level of and/or just below the left bronchus is the left atrial appendage.

3. Splaying of the carina and/or elevation of the left bronchus (see Figs. 30-10 and 30-11)

4. Horizontal orientation of the distal portion of the left bronchus

5. Posterior displacement of the left upper lobe bronchus (see Fig. 30-11). On the lateral radiograph, the circular shadow of the right upper lobe and left bronchi is located within the tracheal air column. Left atrial enlargement causes displacement of the left bronchus posterior to this level and beyond the plane of the trachea.

Right Atrial Enlargement

1. Lateral bulging of the right heart border on the posteroanterior radiograph (see Fig. 30-11)

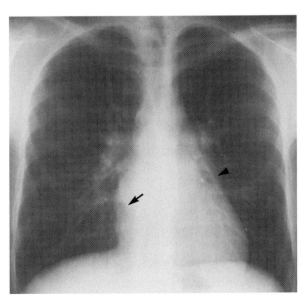

FIG. 30-8. Mitral stenosis causing left atrial enlargement. Subtle convexity along the upper left cardiac border is caused by enlargement of the left atrial appendage *(arrowhead)*. Note right retrocardiac double density *(arrow)* caused by enlargement of the left atrial chamber.

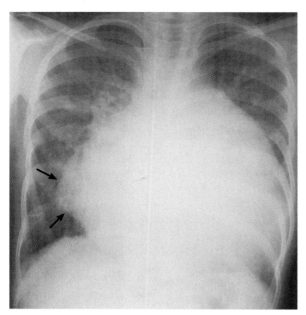

FIG. 30-10. Mitral regurgitation. There is cardiomegaly and marked left atrial enlargement with pulmonary ventricular hypertension. The left atrium is enlarged to the extent that it forms the right heart border on the frontal view *(arrows)*.

2. Elongation of the right heart border on the posteroanterior view. A rough rule is that a right atrial border exceeding 60% in length of the mediastinal cardiovascular shadow is a sign of substantial right atrial enlargement (Fig. 30-12).

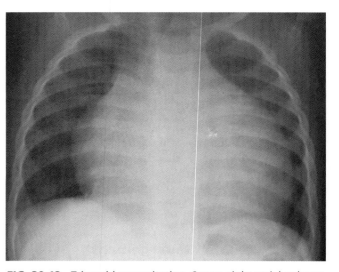

FIG. 30-12. Tricuspid regurgitation. Severe right atrial enlargement is evident by the elongation of the right atrial shadow. The length of the right atrial border exceeds 60% of the height of the mediastinal cardiovascular structures.

Left Ventricular Enlargement

1. On the posteroanterior view, leftward and downward displacement of the cardiac apex. The vector of enlargement of the LV is leftward and downward compared with the vector of right ventricular enlargement, which is leftward only or perhaps leftward plus upward (Figs. 30-13 and 30-14).

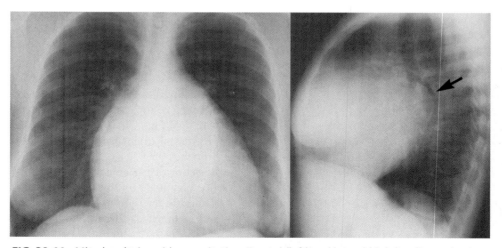

FIG. 30-11. Mitral and tricuspid regurgitation. Frontal **(left)** and lateral **(right)** radiographs show prominent double densities on both sides of the spine due to marked left atrial enlargement. Right atrial enlargement is shown by the elongation of the right-sided convexity on the front view. Prominent upper left cardiac border on frontal view is caused by dilatation of the right ventricular outflow region. Lateral view shows posterior displacement of the left bronchus *(arrow)* by the enlarged left atrium and obliteration of the retrocardiac space by right ventricular enlargement.

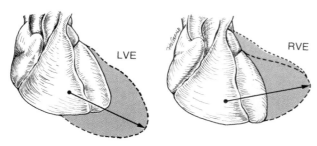

FIG. 30-13. "Vectors of enlargement" for the left and right ventricles. For left ventricular enlargement *(LVE)*, the vector is directed leftward and caudal. For right ventricular enlargement *(RVE)*, the vector is directed leftward or leftward and slightly cranial.

2. On the lateral view, the posterior border of the heart is displaced posteriorly. The Hoffman-Rigler sign is measured 2.0 cm above the intersection of the diaphragm and the inferior vena cava. A positive measurement for LV enlargement is a posterior border of the heart extending more than 1.8 cm behind the inferior vena caval shadow at this level.

Right Ventricular Enlargement

1. On the posteroanterior view, the left border of the heart is enlarged directly laterally or laterally and slightly supe-

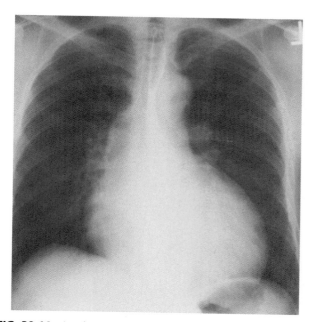

FIG. 30-14. Aortic regurgitation. The ventricular contour is enlarged along a left inferolateral vector, causing the apex to droop over the left hemidiaphragm. Concavity along the upper left cardiac border indicates that the right ventricle is not enlarged. There is enlargement of the thoracic aorta.

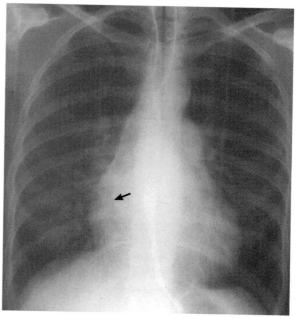

FIG. 30-15. Mitral stenosis with pulmonary arterial hypertension and interstitial pulmonary edema. Cardiomegaly is caused by right ventricular enlargement. The vector of enlargement of the ventricle is directly lateral, indicating right ventricular enlargement. The most lateral portion of the apex is located above the diaphragm. Left atrial enlargement is indicated by double density *(arrow)*. Pulmonary arterial hypertension is indicated by pulmonary arterial enlargement.

riorly (see Fig. 30-13). In some instances, this causes the apex to be displaced superiorly ("upward tipped apex"; Fig. 30-15); in the extreme form this causes a "boot shape" (Fig. 30-16).

2. On the lateral view, the retrosternal space is encroached upon by the enlarged right ventricle. Right ventricular enlargement is inferred by contact of the right heart border over greater than one third of the sternal length. A prominent convexity to the anterior border rather than the usual straight surface is an early sign of right ventricular enlargement.

Signposts for Cardiac Valvular Lesions

There are three signposts on the thoracic radiograph that direct attention to a certain cardiac valve:

1. Left atrial enlargement
2. Ascending aortic enlargement
3. Right atrial enlargement

These signs point specifically to the following:

1. Mitral valve (left atrium)
2. Aortic valve (ascending aorta)
3. Tricuspid valve (right atrium)

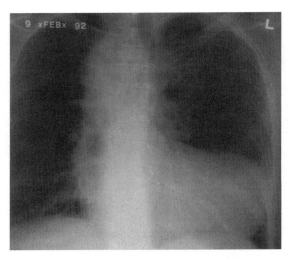

FIG. 30-16. Tetralogy of Fallot after total correction with severe pulmonary regurgitation. Substantial right ventricular enlargement is evident. The vector of enlargement of the ventricle is leftward and cranial, causing uplifting of the apex in relation to the diaphragm. Note the right aortic arch.

Using our classification system ("big heart" versus "small heart" heart disease) and applying the signpost, we can analyze the thoracic radiograph in accordance with the flow diagram shown in Figure 30-2. This schema obviously works well for diseases causing typical alterations in the chest x-ray. Of course, a specific cardiac lesion does not always cause typical features because of other associated abnormalities or because the lesion is very mild or has been present for insufficient time to alter the cardiac morphology to a degree discernible on the thoracic radiograph.

The schema can be briefly described by considering the chest x-ray that shows a normal heart size or mild cardiomegaly in a patient with significant heart disease. This means that the lesion likely causes pressure overload (hypertension, aortic stenosis, or mitral stenosis) or reduced LV compliance. If the left atrial signpost is present, then attention is directed to the mitral valve (see Fig. 30-8). The diagnosis should be either mitral valvular stenosis or resistance to left atrial emptying. Diseases that significantly reduce LV compliance (and increase LV diastolic pressure) cause resistance to left atrial emptying and thereby induce left atrial enlargement. Diseases that may reduce LV compliance are hypertrophic cardiomyopathy, restrictive cardiomyopathy, and constrictive pericardial disease. Acute MI may also reduce LV compliance, but usually this has not been present for a sufficient time to cause left atrial enlargement. LV hypertrophy from any cause can reduce LV compliance if it is sufficiently severe.

If the ascending aorta is enlarged, then this signpost points to the aortic valve, indicating aortic stenosis (Fig. 30-17). Systemic hypertension can produce a similar appearance, although it usually causes enlargement of the entire thoracic aorta rather than the ascending aorta alone. If no signposts are present, then the diagnosis is unlikely to be a valvular lesion. The absence of signposts should direct attention to a disease directly afflicting the myocardium or pericardium, such as acute MI, hypertrophic cardiomyopathy, restrictive cardiomyopathy, and constrictive pericardial disease. However, even these latter diseases sometimes induce left atrial enlargement, as stated above.

The schema for a patient with substantial cardiomegaly proceeds along the following path. The big heart suggests

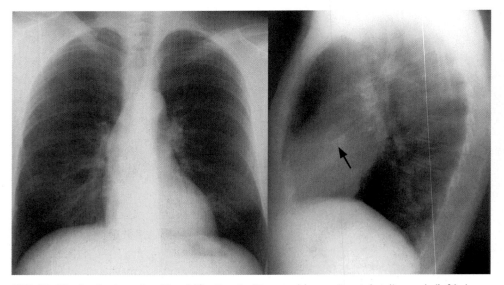

FIG. 30-17. Aortic stenosis with calcification in 43-year-old man. Frontal radiograph (**left**) shows a nearly normal appearance except for enlargement of the ascending aorta. Lateral view (**right**) demonstrates heavy calcification *(arrow)* of the aortic valve.

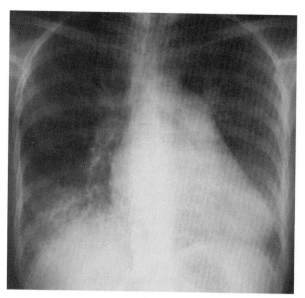

FIG. 30-18. Mitral regurgitation with pulmonary arterial hypertension. There is cardiomegaly and left ventricular and left atrial enlargement. The pulmonary arterial enlargement indicates pulmonary arterial hypertension. There is also right lower lobe pneumonia.

that there is either a volume overload lesion (valvular regurgitation) or myocardial failure or pericardial effusion. High output states are certainly a volume overload and can cause substantial cardiomegaly, but sometimes they cause only mild cardiomegaly. If left atrial enlargement is noted, then the signpost points to mitral regurgitation (Figs. 30-18 and

30-19). If the ascending aorta is enlarged in "big heart" heart disease, then this signpost points to aortic regurgitation (see Fig. 30-14). If the right atrium is enlarged, then this signpost points to tricuspid regurgitation (see Fig. 30-11). Acquired pulmonic regurgitation is rare, except as a consequence of operation for right ventricular outflow obstruction, and is not considered in this schema. If no signposts are present, then the favored diagnostic considerations are congestive (dilated) cardiomyopathy or pericardial effusion.

RADIOGRAPHIC FEATURES OF SPECIFIC CARDIAC LESIONS

Aortic Stenosis

Aortic stenosis is a pressure overload lesion for which the compensatory mechanism is concentric LV hypertrophy (Table 30-6). Concentric LV hypertrophy causes a slight reduction in the volume of the LV but little increase in the overall cardiac size. Consequently, aortic stenosis, for much of its natural history, is a disease that is clearly "small heart" heart disease. There is little or no cardiac enlargement. The characteristic radiographic feature is enlargement of the ascending aorta (see Figs. 30-17, 30-20, and 30-21). The pulmonary vascularity is also generally normal for much of the course of aortic stenosis. However, in the decompensated phase of aortic stenosis, there may be evidence of PVH due to LV failure. Occasionally, when LV hypertrophy has reduced LV compliance considerably, there may also be signs of PVH even in the absence of LV enlargement.

Hypertension

Hypertensive heart disease is a pressure overload lesion and consequently is associated with a normal heart size for much of the compensated phase of this disease (Table 30-7; Fig. 30-22). The severity or even the presence of LV hypertrophy cannot be reliably determined from the thoracic radiograph.

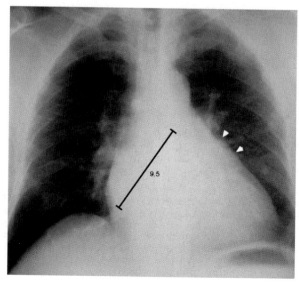

FIG. 30-19. Mitral regurgitation causing cardiomegaly and left ventricular and left atrial enlargement. Note the enlarged left atrial appendage *(arrowheads)*. Left atrial dimension is 9.5 cm.

TABLE 30-6. SALIENT RADIOGRAPHIC FEATURES OF AORTIC STENOSIS

Enlargement of the ascending aorta due to poststenotic dilatation (see Figs. 30-17 and 30-20)
Mild or no cardiomegaly in compensated stage
Substantial cardiomegaly occurs only after myocardial failure has ensued
No pulmonary venous hypertension or pulmonary edema is seen during most of the course of this disease
Calcification of aortic valve may be discernible on radiograph but is more readily shown on CT (see Fig. 30-21)

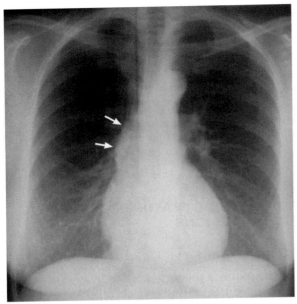

FIG. 30-20. Aortic stenosis. Frontal radiograph shows normal cardiac size and normal pulmonary vascularity. The sole abnormality in this 40-year-old subject is enlargement of the ascending aorta *(arrows)*. The posterior aortic arch is normal in size.

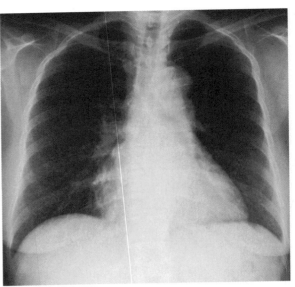

FIG. 30-22. Systemic hypertension. Frontal view shows borderline cardiomegaly and prominence of the entire thoracic aorta.

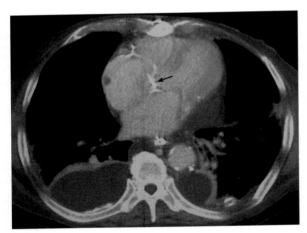

FIG. 30-21. CT scan shows calcification of the aortic valve *(arrow)* in a patient with valvular aortic stenosis.

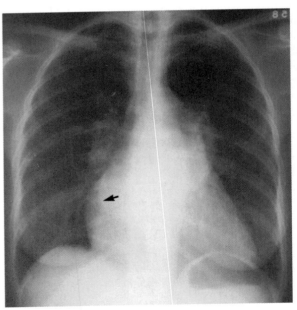

FIG. 30-23. Mitral stenosis. Frontal thoracic radiograph demonstrates left atrial and right ventricular enlargement. Left atrial enlargement is indicated by right retrocardiac double density *(arrow)* on the frontal view. There is pulmonary arterial hypertension as shown by enlargement of the main and central pulmonary arteries. The thoracic aorta is inconspicuous. Right ventricular enlargement is indicated by lateral displacement of the ventricular margin (apex uplifted) on the frontal view.

TABLE 30-7. SALIENT RADIOGRAPHIC FEATURES OF ARTERIAL HYPERTENSION

Enlargement of the thoracic aorta—ascending, arch, and descending aorta (see Fig. 30–22)
Mild or no cardiomegaly until the onset of myocardial failure
No pulmonary edema or pulmonary venous hypertension until the occurrence of diastolic dysfunction due to severe left ventricular hypertrophy or myocardial failure

Mitral Stenosis

The features of a thoracic radiograph are frequently diagnostic for mitral stenosis (see Figs. 30-8, 30-15, 30-23, and 30-24). Likewise, the radiograph provides considerable insight into the severity of mitral stenosis. While mitral stenosis is a pressure overload lesion that causes little increase in overall heart size during the early phase of the disease, it does produce characteristic enlargement of the left atrium and the left atrial appendage and produces signs of PVH (Table 30-8).

Hypertrophic Cardiomyopathy

The chest radiograph is neither specific nor sensitive for the diagnosis of hypertrophic cardiomyopathy. More than 50% of patients with hypertrophic cardiomyopathy have a normal chest x-ray. In a few patients there is some abnormality of the chest x-ray, which is usually relatively vague and not particularly indicative of this disease. Since some patients with hypertrophic cardiomyopathy have a reduction in LV compliance, the radiograph sometimes demonstrates PVH. The PVH is usually relatively mild. The overall heart size is generally normal. In patients with reduced LV compliance, left atrial size may be increased. Approximately 30% of patients with symptomatic hypertrophic cardiomyopathy have associated mitral regurgitation. Because of the mitral regurgitation, there again is a proclivity to left atrial enlargement. A few patients have a squared appearance of the left

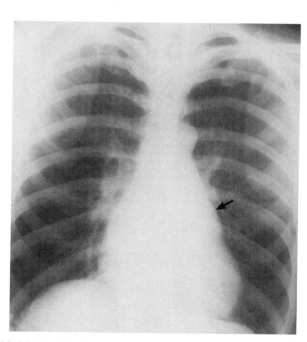

FIG. 30-24. Mitral stenosis causing moderate enlargement of the left atrium and appendage. The wall of the appendage is calcified *(arrow).*

TABLE 30-8. SALIENT RADIOGRAPHIC FEATURES OF MITRAL STENOSES

Pulmonary venous hypertension or edema is present (see Fig. 30-15).

Pulmonary edema may be observed intermittently.

Mild cardiomegaly is seen in isolated mitral stenoses (see Figs. 30-8, 30-15, and 30-24).

Enlargement of the left atrium is characteristic (see Figs. 30-8, 30-15, 30-23, and 30-24).

Enlargement of the left atrial appendage is frequent and suggests a rheumatic etiology (see Figs. 30-8 and 30-24).

Right ventricular enlargement indicates some degree of pulmonary arterial hypertension or associated tricuspid regurgitation.

Enlargement of the pulmonary arterial segment is indicative of associated pulmonary arterial hypertension (see Fig. 30-23).

Right ventricular enlargement in the absence of prominence of the main pulmonary artery suggests associated tricuspid regurgitation. The right atrium is also enlarged with tricuspid regurgitation (see Fig. 30-11).

The ascending aorta and aortic arch are usually inconspicuous in isolated mitral stenosis. Even slight enlargement of the thoracic aorta raises the question of associated aortic valve disease.

---

cardiac border. This is caused by a prominent evagination on the upper left cardiac border. This focal enlargement is a consequence of extreme enlargement of the upper or outflow portion of the ventricular septum (Table 30-9).

Restrictive Cardiomyopathy

Restrictive cardiomyopathy is a relatively rare disease that may occur in an idiopathic form or may be the form of cardiomyopathy that is a consequence of various infiltrative diseases of the left ventricle. Types of infiltrative processes of the left ventricle that may produce restrictive cardiomyopathy include sarcoidosis, hemochromatosis, and amyloidosis.

During the early stage of restrictive cardiomyopathy the cardiac size is within normal limits. Restrictive cardiomyopathy has as its main physiologic deficit a reduction of LV

TABLE 30-9. SALIENT RADIOGRAPHIC FEATURES OF HYPERTROPHIC CARDIOMYOPATHY

Normal in most patients

Mild cardiomegaly and pulmonary venous hypertension in a minority of patients

Left atrial enlargement can be caused by associated mitral insufficiency or reduced left ventricular compliance.

In the obstructive form (subaortic stenosis), ascending aortic enlargement is infrequent.

Left ventricular enlargement may occur in end-stage disease.

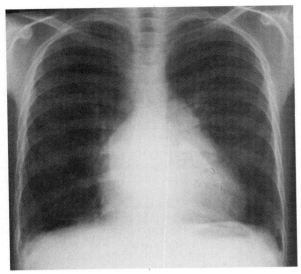

FIG. 30-25. Restrictive cardiomyopathy. Normal cardiac size with left atrial enlargement.

TABLE 30-10. SALIENT RADIOGRAPHIC FEATURES OF RESTRICTIVE CARDIOMYOPATHY

Pulmonary venous hypertension is typical.
Pulmonary edema may occur intermittently.
Normal heart size or mild cardiomegaly in most patients (see Figs. 30-25 and 30-26)
Left atrial enlargement (see Fig. 30-26)
Left atrial appendage is typically not enlarged.
Moderate to severe cardiomegaly can ensue in end-stage disease.

the plain radiograph may mimic the appearance of mitral stenosis. In advanced disease there is frequently some degree of LV enlargement, which along with the left atrial enlargement usually results in a mild to moderate cardiomegaly (see Fig. 30-26). However, in some patients the restrictive cardiomyopathy may progress to congestive cardiomyopathy, which is associated with considerable cardiomegaly and LV enlargement (Table 30-10).

Acute Myocardial Infarction

The plain radiograph is obtained in the emergency room in most patients with an acute MI. The initial chest x-ray or a chest x-ray within the first 24 hours after the onset of acute MI is normal in approximately 50% of patients with initial acute MI. In the other 50% of patients, the most frequent finding is some degree of PVH or pulmonary

compliance. Because of the reduced compliance, there is frequently an elevation in pulmonary venous pressure, which of course is reflected on the chest radiograph as various degrees of PVH (Figs. 30-25 and 30-26). Likewise, because of the reduced LV compliance, there is a rise in left atrial pressure, which may cause a left atrial enlargement to be visible on the radiograph. Because the major radiographic features of this disease are PVH and left atrial enlargement,

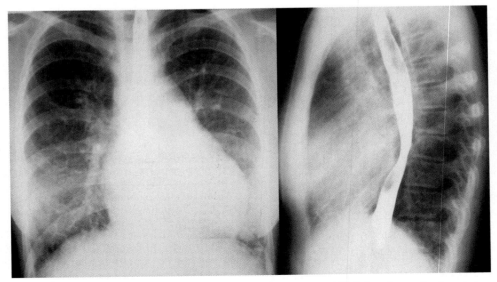

FIG. 30-26. Restrictive cardiomyopathy. Frontal (**left**) and lateral (**right**) radiographs show interstitial pulmonary edema and left atrial and right ventricular enlargement.

edema, along with a normal heart size (Fig. 30-27). The major physiologic deficit in the early phase of acute MI is an abrupt decrease in LV compliance, which results in an increase in pulmonary venous pressure. The increase in pulmonary venous pressure is reflected on the chest x-ray by varying degrees of PVH or pulmonary edema. It is unusual for the patient with a first acute MI, even when the infarction is severe and eventually lethal, to have cardiomegaly or perceptible LV enlargement.

The plain chest x-ray does provide some insight into the severity of the acute MI. The gauge of severity is the degree of PVH. Indeed, a relationship has been shown between the degree of PVH on the plain radiograph within the first 24 hours and the early and late survival rates after the initial MI (Fig. 30-28). The plain radiograph may also be useful in demonstrating complications of acute MI, such as cardiac rupture; pericardial effusion; LV aneurysm, both true and false; papillary muscle rupture; and intractable congestive heart failure.

Some patients with a true LV aneurysm demonstrate a normal chest x-ray. However, in many patients there is evidence of an abnormal cardiac configuration, especially an abnormal evagination along the midportion of the left cardiac border or in the region of the cardiac apex (Fig. 30-29). The abnormal contour generally occurs in these sites because the most frequent location of a true LV aneurysm is the anterolateral wall or the apical wall of the LV. Calcification of the anterolateral region of the LV is suggestive of LV aneurysm (Fig. 30-30). Calcification of an infarct is more readily displayed on CT (Fig. 30-31).

An abnormal evagination that is localized to the posterior wall or the diaphragmatic wall of the LV should raise the

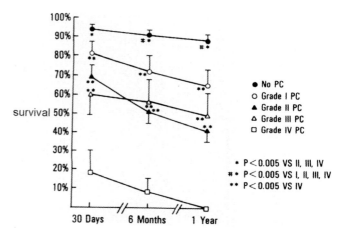

FIG. 30-28. Thirty-day, 6-month, and 12-month survival rates in relation to the severity of pulmonary ventricular hypertension (PVH) on the initial chest x-ray of patients after acute MI. With any degree of PVH, survival is decreased compared to patients with no PVH. (From Battler A, Karliner JS, Higgins CB, et al. The initial chest x-ray film in acute myocardial infarction: prediction of early and late mortality and survival. Circulation 1980; 61:1004.)

possibility of a false LV aneurysm (Fig. 30-32). While only approximately 5% of true LV aneurysms involve the upper diaphragmatic and posterior wall, these sites are the most frequent ones for false LV aneurysm. Consequently, an abnormal contour or a double density localized to these sites should raise the consideration of this diagnosis. The differentiation of a false aneurysm from a true aneurysm becomes important because of the known propensity of false aneurysms to be complicated by late rupture. Other plain radiographic signs of a false aneurysm are an aneurysm that is extremely large with a prominent projection off the posterior or diaphragmatic surface of the heart (see Fig. 30-32), and an increase in the size of the aneurysm on sequential studies. A false aneurysm is more frequently associated with occlusion of either the circumflex or right coronary artery, while a true aneurysm is most frequently associated with occlusion of the left anterior descending coronary artery.

Papillary muscle rupture is a dramatic event that usually induces severe and many times intractable pulmonary edema. Partial rupture of the papillary muscle, resulting in less severe mitral regurgitation, may produce a moderate degree of mitral regurgitation and less severe or even no evidence of pulmonary edema. The dramatic radiographic findings in acute papillary muscle rupture are pulmonary edema with little increase in left atrial size or cardiomegaly. If the patient survives beyond several weeks or months, then varying degrees of left atrial enlargement and cardiomegaly may be present.

Postinfarction rupture of the ventricular septum may produce a radiographic appearance very similar to that of acute mitral regurgitation. The radiographic signs of acute ventricular septal defect include an increase in the promi-

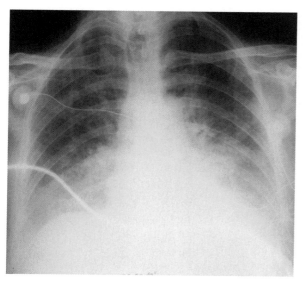

FIG. 30-27. Acute MI with alveolar pulmonary edema. Note alveolar filling in perihilar regions and lower lobes with normal heart size.

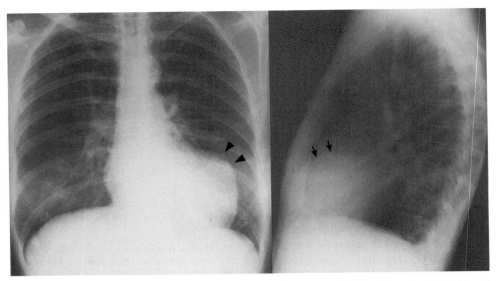

FIG. 30-29. True left ventricular aneurysm complicating myocardial infarction. Frontal **(left)** and lateral **(right)** views. Abnormal evagination of left cardiac border *(arrowheads)* is typical for an aneurysm involving the anterolateral and/or apical segment of the left ventricle. Lateral view demonstrates an anterior double density *(arrows)*, characteristic of an anterolateral aneurysm.

nence of the pulmonary arteries (i.e., pulmonary arterial overcirculation), usually pulmonary edema, and mild degrees of cardiomegaly. Again, if the patient tolerates the episode and survives for several weeks to months, then the degree of cardiomegaly may be more considerable, and there may even be signs of left atrial enlargement.

Dressler's syndrome, another complication of acute MI, occurs within the first weeks to months after an acute MI. This is an autoimmune response to various antigens that are released during the acute MI. This autoimmune response involves the pericardial and pleural surfaces, eventuating in pericardial and pleural effusions. Chest radiographs in this syndrome demonstrate an increase in cardiac size as a consequence of the pericardial effusion, along with evidence of unilateral or bilateral pleural effusions (Table 30-11).

FIG. 30-30. Calcified apical left ventricular aneurysm. Lateral thoracic radiograph shows calcification *(arrows)* on the anteroapical region of the left ventricle.

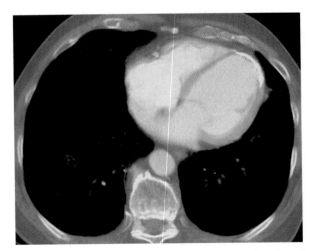

FIG. 30-31. CT scan shows mural calcification at the site of an old apical myocardial infarction.

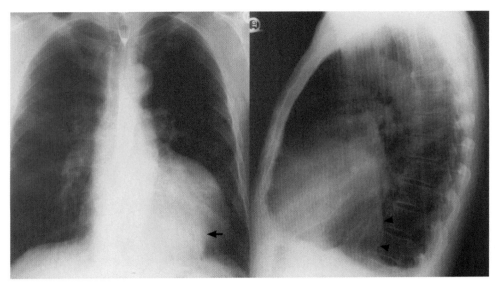

FIG. 30-32. False left ventricular aneurysm complicating myocardial infarction. Frontal (**left**) and lateral (**right**) radiographs show left retrocardiac density (*arrow*) on the frontal view and large posterior evagination (*arrowheads*) of left ventricular contour on the lateral view. Large size and posterior location are characteristics of false aneurysm.

Constrictive Pericarditis

Constrictive pericarditis is a disease that is being encountered with increasing frequency. Currently, the major causes are iatrogenic. The most frequent inciting factor is postoperative bleeding associated with cardiac surgery, especially coronary revascularization procedures. The second most frequent inciting factor is mediastinal irradiation; the third most common cause is repeated episodes of viral pericarditis. Uremic pericardial disease may also eventuate in constrictive pericarditis, but usually this disease produces an effusive/constrictive type of pericardial disease. In Third World countries, tuberculosis continues to be a major cause of constrictive pericarditis.

The plain radiograph is frequently but not always abnormal in patients with hemodynamically significant constrictive pericarditis. Because of pericardial constriction there is restriction to left atrial emptying during diastole, with a subsequent rise in left atrial and pulmonary venous pressures. The rise in pulmonary venous pressure is reflected on the chest radiograph by signs of PVH, such as redistribution and interstitial or alveolar pulmonary edema. The overall cardiac size is usually normal or there is only mild cardiomegaly (Fig. 30-33). There is frequently left atrial enlargement but normal ventricular size. Recognition of pericardial calcification supports or may initially suggest the diagnosis of constrictive pericarditis (Fig. 30-34; Table 30-12).

TABLE 30-11. SALIENT RADIOGRAPHIC FEATURES OF ACUTE MYOCARDIAL INFARCTION

Normal chest x-ray in about 50% of first acute infarctions.
Normal heart size with pulmonary venous hypertension or pulmonary edema in about 50% of first acute infarctions (see Fig. 30-27).
Cardiomegaly is usually indicative of acute infarction in a patient with history of previous infarctions.
Cardiomegaly may be indicative of ischemic cardiomyopathy.
Signs of complication of acute myocardial infarction
Intractable pulmonary edema may occur with papillary muscle rupture (mitral regurgitation) or ventricular septal rupture (left to right shunt).
Enlarged cardiac silhouette may be caused by pericardial effusion.
Abnormal cardiac contour may be a sign of true (bulge of the anterolateral or apical regions) (see Fig. 30-29) or false (bulge of the posterior or diaphragmatic regions) aneurysms (see Fig. 30-32).

TABLE 30-12. SALIENT RADIOGRAPHIC FEATURES OF CONSTRICTIVE PERICARDITIS

Pulmonary venous hypertension
Normal heart size or mild cardiomegaly
Left atrial enlargement may be discernible.
Flattened cardiac contours are pathognomonic but infrequently observed (see Fig. 30-33).
Calcification of the cardiac margin, especially the atrioventricular and interventricular grooves (see Figs. 30-33 and 30-34)

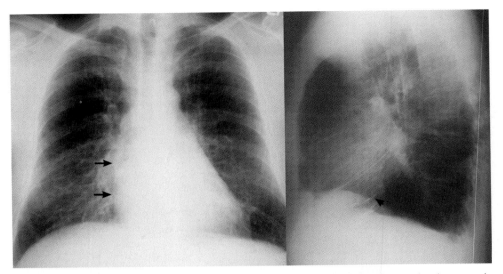

FIG. 30-33. Constrictive pericarditis. Frontal **(left)** and lateral **(right)** radiographs show grade I pulmonary ventricular hypertension and flattened right cardiac contour *(arrows)*, which are characteristics of constrictive pericarditis. Lateral view demonstrates calcification *(arrowhead)* in the posterior interventricular groove.

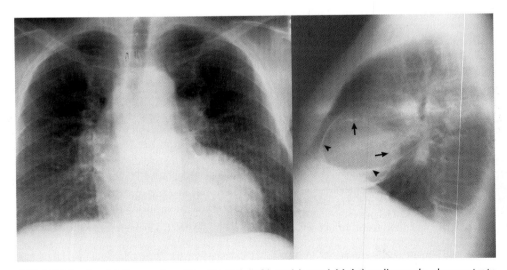

FIG. 30-34. Constrictive pericarditis. Frontal **(left)** and lateral **(right)** radiographs demonstrate pericardial calcification. The calcification involves the atrioventricular *(arrows)* and the interventricular *(arrowheads)* grooves.

"BIG HEART" HEART DISEASE

Aortic Regurgitation

Aortic regurgitation is characterized on the plain radiograph by a substantial degree of cardiomegaly, which is due predominantly to LV enlargement (see Figs. 30-14 and 30-35). A signpost pointing to the aortic valve is present in this disease, consisting of enlargement of the ascending aorta, aortic knob, and usually the descending thoracic aorta. As opposed to aortic stenosis, the enlargement of the thoracic aorta involves the aortic knob as well as the ascending aorta. Consequently, "big heart" heart disease with the aortic signpost is indicative of aortic regurgitation.

The severity of aortic regurgitation is reflected on the plain radiograph. Since this is a volume overload lesion, the extent of the increase in volume of the heart is related to the severity and the duration of aortic regurgitation. For most of the course of aortic regurgitation, the pulmonary vascularity is normal. Consequently, the presence of PVH in a patient with aortic regurgitation is indicative of LV failure and is frequently associated with end-stage aortic valve disease (Table 30-13).

Mitral Regurgitation

The plain radiograph in mitral regurgitation shows variable degrees of PVH, cardiomegaly, left atrial enlargement, and LV enlargement (see Figs. 30-9 to 30-11, 30-18, and 30-

TABLE 30-13. SALIENT RADIOGRAPHIC FEATURES OF AORTIC REGURGITATION

Absence of pulmonary venous hypertension or pulmonary edema until late in the course of this lesion
Moderate to severe cardiomegaly (see Figs. 30-14 and 30-35)
Left ventricular enlargement (see Figs. 30-14 and 30-35)
Enlargement of ascending aorta and aortic arch (see Figs. 30-14 and 30-35)

19) and sometimes signs of right-sided chamber enlargement (see Figs. 30-10 and 30-11). In the presence of isolated mitral regurgitation the ascending aorta is relatively small. Consequently, recognition of prominence of the ascending aorta in a patient with isolated mitral valve disease raises the prospect of associated aortic valve disease.

The left atrial appendage is generally enlarged in patients who have a rheumatic etiology of the mitral regurgitation (see Figs. 30-10 and 30-19). On the other hand, the left atrial appendage is frequently not enlarged in patients who otherwise have left atrial enlargement of nonrheumatic etiology.

The severity of PVH in mitral regurgitation is generally less than in isolated mitral stenosis. Most patients with compensated mitral regurgitation have minimal or no signs of PVH. A practical axiom is that mitral stenosis causes PVH that is prominent in relation to the degree of left atrial enlargement, whereas mitral regurgitation is associated with left atrial enlargement that is out of proportion to the expected severity of PVH. Patients with mixed mitral stenosis and mitral regurgitation may have both very substantial left atrial enlargement as well as prominent signs of PVH. The giant left atrium can be associated with either mitral stenosis or regurgitation but is more frequently caused by the latter. The right border of the left atrium may even extend beyond the border of the right atrium rather than causing a right retrocardiac double density (see Fig. 30-10).

The plain radiograph may be useful in assessing the severity of mitral regurgitation. Because this is a volume overload lesion, the overall heart size may be a reasonable indicator of the severity of regurgitation. Likewise, the overall heart size may be of some prognostic use in patients undergoing mitral valve replacement. In general, patients with lesser degrees of cardiomegaly demonstrate a greater 5-year survival rate after replacement of the mitral valve (Table 30-14).

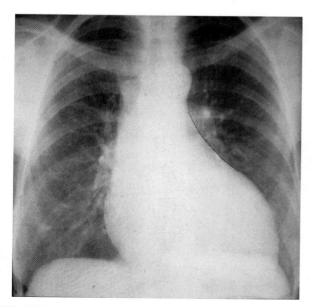

FIG. 30-35. Aortic regurgitation. Frontal radiograph shows marked cardiomegaly with displacement of the ventricular contour laterally and caudally, indicating left ventricular enlargement. The ascending aorta and the contour of the posterior aortic arch are enlarged. Concavity *(broken line)* along the upper left cardiac border indicates no right ventricular enlargement.

Tricuspid Regurgitation

The signs of tricuspid regurgitation may be difficult to discern on the plain radiograph. Signs of right atrial enlargement are frequently dubious and not sharply discriminated from normal. Indeed, there must be substantial right atrial

TABLE 30-14. SALIENT RADIOGRAPHIC FEATURES OF MITRAL REGURGITATION

Variable degree of pulmonary venous hypertensive or pulmonary edema (less severe than with mitral stenosis)
Moderate to severe cardiomegaly (see Figs. 30-9 to 30-11, 30-18, and 30-19)
Left ventricular enlargement (see Figs. 30-9 and 30-10)
Left atrial enlargement (see Figs. 30-9 and 30-10)
Enlargement of left atrial appendage (rheumatic etiology; see Figs. 30-10 and 30-19)

TABLE 30-15. SALIENT RADIOGRAPHIC FEATURES OF AORTIC REGURGITATION

No pulmonary venous hypertension or pulmonary edema (isolated tricuspid regurgitation)
Pulmonary venous hypertension or edema indicates associated mitral valve disease
Moderate to severe cardiomegaly (see Figs. 30-11, 30-12, 30-36)
Right ventricular enlargement
Right atrial enlargement (see Figs. 30-11, 30-12, 30-36)

enlargement before it is possible to recognize its occurrence. In general, the best sign of right atrial enlargement is elongation of the right atrial border (see Fig. 30-12). The radiographic signs of tricuspid regurgitation are normal or perhaps reduced prominence of the pulmonary vascularity, cardiomegaly, right atrial enlargement, and occasionally signs of superior vena caval and especially inferior vena caval enlargement (see Figs. 30-11 and 30-12).

Cardiomegaly, with the signpost of right atrial enlargement, would indicate the likely diagnosis of tricuspid regurgitation. The cardiac contour in patients with tricuspid regurgitation may be similar to that of congestive cardiomyopathy and pericardial effusion. The most extreme cardiomegaly is seen with severe tricuspid regurgitation of long duration; it can cause the "wall-to-wall" heart (Fig. 30-36 and Table 30-15).

Congestive Cardiomyopathy

The radiographic appearance in congestive cardiomyopathy is relatively nonspecific. There is usually some degree of PVH and substantial cardiomegaly (Figs. 30-37 and 30-38). Characteristically, the cardiomegaly exists without the presence of signposts to the aortic, mitral, or tricuspid valve. Consequently, substantial cardiomegaly ("big heart" heart disease), without radiographic signposts, should raise the diagnostic consideration of congestive cardiomyopathy. Of course a similar appearance can exist with pericardial effusion. At the current time, the most frequent cause of congestive or dilated cardiomyopathy is ischemic heart disease. However, from a strict classification point of view, ischemic heart disease should not be considered as part of the group of congestive cardiomyopathies. Congestive cardiomyopathy is actually defined by the International Conference on

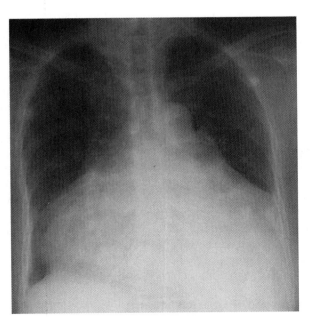

FIG. 30-36. Tricuspid regurgitation. The features of this lesion are diminished pulmonary vascularity, marked cardiomegaly, and right atrial and right ventricular enlargement. The severe enlargement of the right-sided chamber produced the "wall-to-wall" heart."

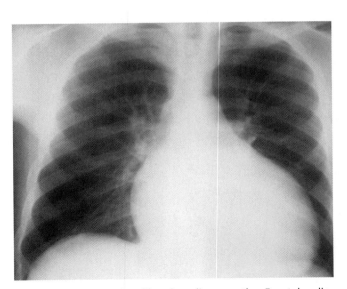

FIG. 30-37. Congestive dilated cardiomyopathy. Frontal radiograph shows biventricular enlargement and mild pulmonary ventricular hypertension (grade I). Enlargement of the left ventricle is indicated by a vector of ventricular enlargement directed laterally and caudally on the frontal view. Right ventricle enlargement is indicated by the prominent convexity of the upper left cardiac border on the frontal view.

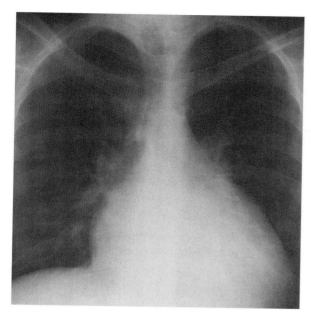

FIG. 30-38. Congestive dilated cardiomyopathy. Frontal radiograph shows moderate cardiomegaly with biventricular but no discernible left atrial enlargement.

TABLE 30-16. SALIENT RADIOGRAPHIC FEATURES OF CONGESTIVE (DILATED) CARDIOMYOPATHY

Pulmonary venous hypertension or pulmonary edema may be but is not invariably present.
Moderate to severe cardiomegaly (see Figs. 30-37 and 30-38)
Left ventricular enlargement
Left atrial enlargement is infrequently evident but can be caused by mitral regurgitation caused by left ventricular enlargement.

Myocardial Disease as a dilated cardiomyopathy without known etiologic identification (Table 30-16).

Pericardial Effusion

The cardiac configuration in pericardial effusion is relatively nonspecific. It has been assumed that the presence of substantial cardiomegaly in the absence of signs of PVH should be a clue to the presence of pericardial effusion (Figs. 30-39 and 30-40). This radiographic appearance is actually quite nonspecific. Similar to the appearance of congestive cardiomyopathy, the cardiac configuration is that of cardiomegaly without a radiographic signpost. A specific appearance providing a diagnosis of pericardial effusion is relatively infrequent in this entity. The so-called water-bottle appearance of the heart is nonspecific and difficult to recognize. The "fat pad" sign seen on the lateral radiograph does permit identification but occurs in only a few patients (see Fig. 30-39). The varying density sign is also sometimes present on the frontal radiograph (see Fig. 30-40). This consists of a lesser density at the periphery of the cardiac contour compared to the central portion of the cardiac contour. The cause of this varying density is that the x-ray beam encounters only fluid toward the periphery of the pericardial effusion, while in the center of the pericardial effusion the radiographic beam must pass through both water anteriorly and the cardiac substance more centrally.

With the frequent use of echocardiography, large pericardial effusions are being encountered less frequently. The presence of any degree of pericardial effusion can be easily recognized by echocardiography (Table 30-17).

Paracardiac Masses

Enlargement of the cardiac contour may not always be indicative of cardiac enlargement itself or pericardial effusion.

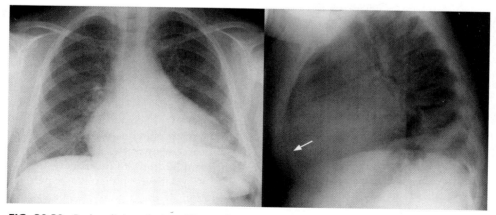

FIG. 30-39. Pericardial perfusion. "Fat pad" sign is shown on lateral view (**right**). A stripe of water density (*arrow*) separates two fat layers on the outer surface of the parietal pericardium and beneath the visceral pericardium.

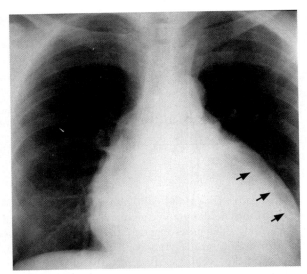

FIG. 30-40. Pericardial perfusion. Varying cardiac density sign caused by transition of density near the margin of the cardiac silhouette *(arrows)*.

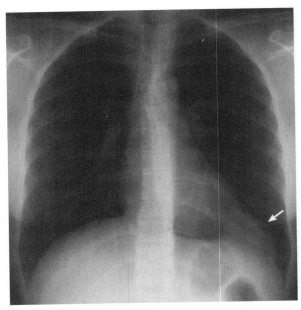

FIG. 30-42. Pericardial cyst. Frontal radiograph shows a mass *(arrow)* adjacent to the cardiac apex.

TABLE 30-17. SALIENT RADIOGRAPHIC FEATURES OF PERICARDIAL EFFUSION

No pulmonary venous hypertension or pulmonary edema
Moderate to severe enlargement of cardiac silhouette
Associated pleural effusion is not uncommon
Specific features, such as "fat pad" and/or "variable density" signs, are infrequently evident (see Figs. 30-39 and 30-40)

One must also consider the infrequent possibility that the enlargement represents a cardiac or paracardiac mass (Figs. 30-41 and 30-42). Such consideration should be prompted by recognition of an unusual cardiac contour. The various causes of paracardiac masses are legion, but considerations are pericardial cysts, paracardiac tumors such as lymphoma and germinal cell tumor, cardiac tumors such as rhabdomyoma or various sarcomas, metastasis to lymph nodes within the pericardiophrenic angle, eventration or hernia of the diaphragm, neural tumors of the phrenic nerve, and various types of skeletal muscle tumors arising from the diaphragm. The diagnosis of the paracardiac mass can be readily made by CT and even more precisely with gated MRI.

ABNORMAL CARDIAC CONTOURS

Enlargement of the Main Pulmonary Arterial Segment

Enlargement of the main pulmonary arterial segment is usually due to enlargement of the main pulmonary artery itself (Fig. 30-43). There are a number of causes of enlargement of the main pulmonary artery (Table 30-18).

Enlargement of the main pulmonary artery segment is the main indicator of pulmonary arterial hypertension (see Fig. 30-43). Severe pulmonary hypertension may cause calcification of the central pulmonary arteries (Fig. 30-44). Whenever one recognizes enlargement of the main pulmonary artery segment in a patient with no known pulmonary valvular disease, the differential diagnosis of pulmonary ar-

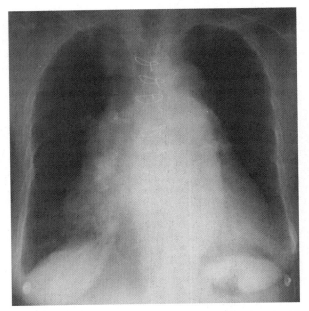

FIG. 30-41. Right paracardiac mass caused by loculated pericardial hematoma after cardiac surgery.

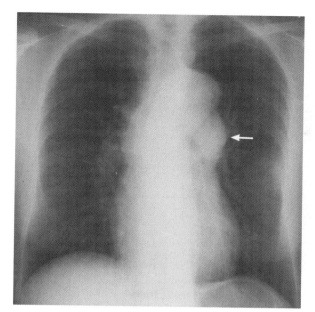

FIG. 30-43. Marked dilatation of the pulmonary artery *(arrow)* due to Eisenmenger's syndrome caused by patent ductus arteriosus. The main pulmonary artery and aortic arch are moderately enlarged.

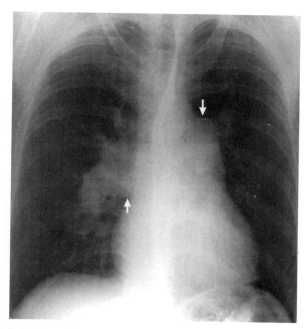

FIG. 30-44. Pulmonary arterial hypertension due to Eisenmenger's complex; the underlying lesion was an atrial septal defect. Frontal view shows the markedly enlarged main *(arrow)* and right pulmonary arterial segments. There is calcification *(arrow)* in the pulmonary arteries consistent with a systemic arterial pressure level in the pulmonary circulation.

terial hypertension must be considered. The differential diagnosis of pulmonary hypertension should lead to a systematic organization of the diagnostic possibilities. There are five diagnostic categories for pulmonary arterial hypertension: (1) pulmonary arterial hypertension resulting from pulmonary venous hypertension; (2) pulmonary arterial hypertension resulting from left-to-right shunts resulting in pulmonary arteriolar disease (arteriolopathy); (3) pulmonary arterial hypertension resulting from obliteration of the pulmonary vascular bed from chronic lung disease; (4) pulmonary arterial hypertension resulting from obliteration of the pulmonary vascular bed as a consequence of pulmonary embolic disease or schistosomiasis; and (5) primary pulmonary hypertension. Radiographic signs that permit the differential diagnosis of the various causes include recognition of the following:

1. Signs of PVH would indicate the likelihood that the pulmonary arterial hypertension is secondary to PVH.
2. Signs of chronic lung disease such as chronic obstructive pulmonary disease or interstitial lung disease would indicate this as the etiology.
3. Asymmetric pulmonary vascularity or signs of pulmonary scarring might indicate the presence of chronic thromboembolic disease.
4. Marked enlargement of the central pulmonary arteries or signs of enlargement of the specific cardiac chambers may indicate the presence of a previous left-to-right shunt that has resulted in Eisenmenger's syndrome.

TABLE 30-18. ENLARGEMENT OF MAIN PULMONARY ARTERY: ETIOLOGY

Pulmonary arterial hypertension
Excess pulmonary blood flow (left to right shunts, chronic high output states)
Valvular pulmonic stenosis
Pulmonary regurgitation
Congenital absent pulmonary valve (aneurysmal pulmonary artery)
Absence of left pericardium
Aneurysm of pulmonary artery
Idiopathic dilatation of pulmonary artery

Enlargement of Left Atrial Appendage Region or Middle Segment of Left Heart Border

An evagination ("mogul") in the region of the left atrial appendage on the frontal view should lead to a series of differential diagnostic considerations. The left atrial appendage region is considered to be the region immediately adjacent to and below the left bronchus (see Figs. 30-8, 30-10, 30-18, and 30-19). This is in contradistinction to the

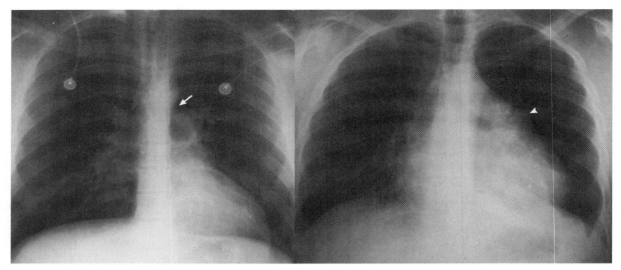

FIG. 30-45. Complete **(left)** and partial **(right)** absence of left pericardium. Complete absence causes a shift of the heart to the left without a shift of the mediastinum (note the central position of the trachea) and a prominent convexity of the upper left cardiac margin. Lung *(arrow)* is insinuated between the aorta and pulmonary artery, indicating an absence of the pericardium at this site. Partial absence causes a prominent convexity *(arrowhead)* of the mid-left cardiac margin, especially in the region of the left atrial appendage segment.

region of the main pulmonary artery segment, which is above the left bronchus. The two normal structures that reside within this area are the left atrial appendage and the right ventricular outflow tract; the left atrium is situated posterior to the right ventricular outflow region. The outflow portion of the ventricular septum is also located within this region. The pericardium covers the left atrial appendage and the right ventricular outflow tract in this region as in other parts of the heart. Other structures are occasionally abnormally positioned at this site. The abnormally positioned structures that can lie within this site are a juxtaposed right atrial appendage and a transposed ascending aorta with the associated inverted right ventricular outflow region.

The differential diagnoses of an enlargement or evagination of the middle segment of the left heart border are multiple (Table 30-19; Fig. 30-45).

Enlargement of the Left Lower Cardiac Border–ventricular Region

Enlargement along the lower left cardiac border in the region of the ventricles is most frequently caused by enlargement of either the right or left ventricle (see Fig. 30-13). An abnormal convexity evagination within this region has a limited differential diagnosis (Table 30-20).

Enlargement of the Right Heart Border

Enlargement of the right heart contour in the frontal view is generally ascribed to right atrial enlargement. There are

TABLE 30-19. ENLARGEMENT OF THE MIDDLE SEGMENT OF LEFT HEART BORDER: ETIOLOGY

Dilated left atrial appendage (rheumatic mitral valve disease)
Partial absence of left pericardium (see Fig. 30-45)
Enlargement of right ventricular outlet region such as occurs with left-to-right shunts
Asymmetric form of hypertrophic cardiomyopathy (occurs in small minority of cases)
Levo transposition of the great arteries
Juxtaposition of atrial appendages (rare anomaly usually associated with tricuspid atresia)
Left ventricular aneurysm
Cardiac tumor
Aneurysm or pseudoaneurysm of left circumflex coronary artery
Pericardial cyst or tumor
Mediastinal tumor

TABLE 30-20. EVAGINATION OF LEFT LOWER HEART BORDER: ETIOLOGY

Ventricular aneurysm
Ventricular tumor
Pericardial cyst, diverticulum or tumor
Left ventricular diverticulum
Mediastinal or lung tumor
Pericardial fat pad

TABLE 30-21. ENLARGEMENT OF RIGHT HEART AND BORDER

Right atrial enlargement
Pericardial fat pad
Eventration or hernia of diaphragm
Pericardial cyst or diverticulum
Pericardial tumor
Cardiac tumor
Diaphragmatic tumor
Mediastinal tumor

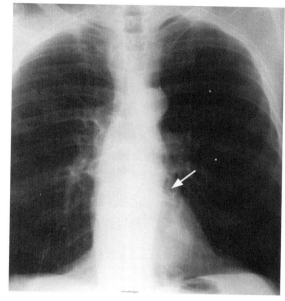

FIG. 30-47. Calcification in the left anterior descending coronary artery *(arrow)*. This is the most frequent site where coronary arterial calcification is observed on the frontal radiograph.

a few other abnormalities that can also enlarge this contour and produce an abnormality in the contour (Table 30-21).

Cardiac Calcification

Calcification in the central cardiovascular structures is frequent and is an important diagnostic sign. In a few instances, calcification of a specific shape and location is pathognomonic for a disease. The various cardiovascular calcifications include the following:

1. Ascending aortic calcification. This is most frequently observed on the right anterolateral margin of the ascending aorta in elderly individuals, especially in the presence of aortic valve disease. In the past, it was considered to be a characteristic of luetic aortitis.
2. Mitral annular calcification (Fig. 30-46). This is a dense C-shaped calcification in the region of the mitral valve. It may be a causative factor of mitral regurgitation. It is frequently observed in apparently normal elderly patients.

3. Aortic annular calcification, a circular calcification in the region of the aortic valve. Extension of this calcification into the region of the conducting system can produce complete heart failure.
4. Valvular calcification (aortic and mitral). Calcification of the aortic valve of sufficient density and extent to be visualized on the radiograph (see Fig. 30-17) is nearly always associated with hemodynamically important aortic stenosis (gradient more than 50 mm Hg).

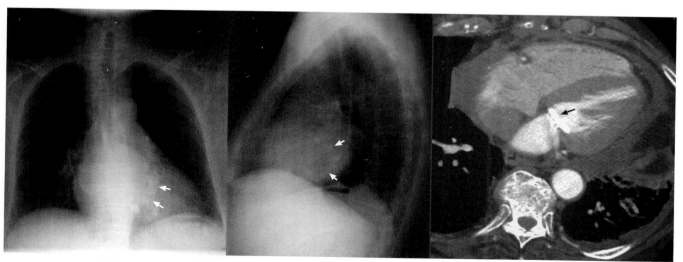

FIG. 30-46. Mitral annular calcification. Frontal **(left)** and lateral **(middle)** views and CT scan **(right)** show a C-shaped calcification *(arrows)* in the mitral annulus.

5. Coronary arterial calcification. Coronary arterial calcification is frequently observed by fluoroscopy or CT. It must be both dense and extensive to be recognized on the thoracic radiograph (Fig. 30-47).

6. Left ventricular mural calcification. This is most frequently located in the anterolateral or apical regions of the left ventricle and marks the site of a transmural MI or aneurysm (see Figs. 30-30 and 30-31).

7. Pericardial calcification is indicative of constrictive pericarditis. It is located usually in the interventricular or atrioventricular grooves of the heart (see Figs. 30-33 and 30-34).

8. Unusual sites of calcification may represent intracardiac tumor (left atrial myxoma), pericardial tumor (dermoid), or healed granulomas (myocardial tuberculoma). An extremely rare process of the left ventricle, Loeffler's eosinophilic fibroplasia, can cause calcification of the left ventricular wall.

SELECTED READING

Higgins CB. Essentials of Cardiac Radiology and Imaging. Philadelphia: JB Lippincott, 1992.

Miller SW. Cardiac Radiology: The Requisites. Boston: Mosby-Year Book, 1996.

Skorton DJ, Shelbert HR, Wolf GL, Brundage BH. Cardiac Imaging. Philadelphia: WB Saunders, 1996.

Steiner RM. Radiology of the heart and great vessels. In: Braunwald E, Zipes DP, Libby P. Heart Disease. Ed 16. Philadelphia: WB Saunders, 2001.

31

RADIOGRAPHY OF CONGENITAL HEART DISEASE

CHARLES B. HIGGINS

The radiographic diagnosis of congenital heart disease can be a confusing and difficult topic because of the myriad of congenital heart lesions that exist. Assessment of the plain radiograph can usually provide only a notion of the generic type of congenital heart lesion rather than a clear indication of specific lesions. An approach that is cognizant of the realistic insights possible from the plain radiograph must be pursued. Such an approach should be based on the observations on the radiograph that can be made with some degree of certitude and in which there is minimal ambiguity. Such an approach should also take advantage of the clinical information upon which one can rely. The current classification system depends on a few clinical observations and a few findings on the radiograph that can be made with reasonable reliability.

CLINICAL-RADIOGRAPHIC CLASSIFICATION OF CONGENITAL HEART DISEASE

This classification depends on two pieces of clinical data: (1) whether it is cyanotic or noncyanotic and (2) symptoms of congestive heart failure, such as dyspnea, tachypnea, tachycardia, and frequent respiratory infections. The salient radiographic findings are (1) increased or decreased pulmonary arterial vascularity and (2) cardiomegaly or nearly normal heart size.

This classification system permits most major lesions involving right-to-left or left-to-right shunts to be classified into four categories (Table 31-1). A fifth group consists of patients with primarily pulmonary venous congestion (Table 31-2). Therefore, when interpreting the chest x-ray, the physician attempts to decide which class or category of congenital heart lesions exists. The decision on the specific lesion is usually based on the statistical frequency of a particular cardiac lesion within one or more groups. Based on the clinical and radiographic findings, there are five groups of congenital heart lesions. The groups and criteria as used in this classification system are as follows:

Group I: left-to-right shunts
  Noncyanotic: Sometimes symptoms of pulmonary congestion or congestive heart failure
  Radiographic signs of pulmonary arterial overcirculation (Fig. 31-1)

Group II: right-to-left shunts with little or no cardiomegaly
  Cyanosis
  Decreased or normal pulmonary arterial vascularity and little or no cardiomegaly (Fig. 31-2)

Group III: right-to-left shunts with cardiomegaly
  Cyanosis
  Radiographic evidence of normal or decreased pulmonary blood flow and cardiomegaly (Fig. 31-3)

Group IV: admixture lesions (i.e., both right-to-left and left-to-right shunts)
  Cyanosis
  Radiographic evidence of increased pulmonary arterial vascularity and usually cardiomegaly (Fig. 31-4)

It is frequently difficult to distinguish between normal and diminished pulmonary vascularity. This observation can be greatly simplified, however, when one remembers that normal pulmonary vascularity, as gleaned from the radiograph in a patient with cyanosis, can be equated with decreased pulmonary vascularity. Consequently, the major observation on the radiograph in terms of pulmonary vascularity in the cyanotic patient is to determine whether the pulmonary vascularity is increased. Normal or diminished pulmonary vascularity in a patient with cyanosis indicates that the lesion produces a right-to-left shunt. Increased pulmonary vascularity in a cyanotic patient indicates that there is an admixture lesion; the cyanosis is indicative of right-to-left shunting, and increased pulmonary vascularity is a sign of left-to-right shunting.

Groups of Congenital Heart Lesions

Group I

Group I contains all of the left-to-right shunts; consequently, this is the group into which most patients with

TABLE 31-1. CLASSIFICATION OF SHUNT LESIONS

Group I lesions: acyanotic; pulmonary arterial overcirculation
Atrial septal defect
Partial anomalous pulmonary venous connection
Atrioventricular septal defect (endocardial cushion defect)
Ventricular septal defect
Patent ductus arteriosus
Other aortic level shunts (e.g., ruptured sinus of Valsalva aneurysm, aorticopulmonary window)
Group II lesions: cyanotic; decreased pulmonary vascularity, no cardiomegaly
Tetralogy of Fallot
Transposition with pulmonic stenosis and VSD
Double-outlet right ventricle with pulmonic stenosis and VSD
Double-outlet left ventricle with pulmonic stenosis and VSD
Single ventricle (univentricular atrioventricular connection) with pulmonic stenosis
Corrected transposition with pulmonic stenosis and VSD
Pulmonic atresia with intact ventricular septum, type I
Pulmonic stenosis with atrioventricular septal defect
Hypoplastic right ventricle syndrome
Some types of tricuspid atresia (large ASD and pulmonary stenosis or atresia)
Group III lesions: cyanotic; decreased pulmonary vascularity; cardiomegaly
Ebstein's anomaly
Pulmonary stenosis (critical) with ASD or patent foramen ovale
Some types of tricuspid atresia (restrictive ASD)
Pulmonary atresia with intact ventricular septum, type II
Transient tricuspid regurgitation of the newborn
Group IV lesions: cyanotic; pulmonary arterial overcirculation
Transposition of great arteries
Truncus arteriosus
Total anomalous pulmonary venous connection
Tricuspid atresia
Single ventricle (univentricular atrioventricular connection)
Double outlet right ventricle
Double outlet left ventricle
Atrioventricular septal defect (complete form)
Hypoplastic left heart syndrome
Pulmonary arteriovenous fistulae

ASD, atrial septal defect; VSD, ventricular septal defect.

TABLE 31-2. GROUP V LESIONS

Pulmonary venous hypertension (congestion)
Cardiomegaly disproportionate to pulmonary vascularity
Nonstructural heart disease in newborns
Asphyxia
Hypervolemia, hyperviscosity
Overhydration
Twin-twin transfusion
Maternal-fetal transfusion
Excess stripping of the cord
Paroxysmal atrial tachycardia
Heart block
Hypoglycemia
Hypocalcemia
Hydrops fetalis
Systemic hypertension
Structural heart disease in newborns
Hypoplastic left heart syndrome
Total anomalous pulmonary venous connection, type III
Coarctation of the aorta
Critical aortic stenosis
Endocardial fibroelastosis
Anomalous origin of the coronary artery from the pulmonary artery
Intrauterine myocarditis

of the possibilities is that the left-to-right shunt is diminishing in size because of a decrease in the size of the ventricular septal defect (VSD). Another consideration is the coexistence of additional cardiac lesions, such as primary myocardial disease or coarctation of the aorta.

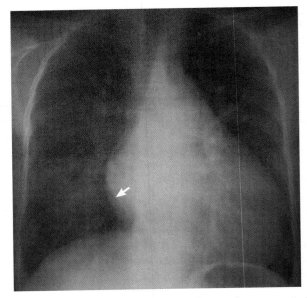

FIG. 31-1. Patent ductus arteriosus. Note pulmonary arterial overcirculation and cardiomegaly. Pulmonary arterial overcirculation is indicated by prominent hilar vessels. There is a left atrial double density *(arrow)* and enlarged aortic arch.

congenital heart disease are classified. The criteria that place a patient within this category are for the most part dependent on the clinical recognition of the absence of cyanosis with the subsequent demonstration on the chest radiograph of increased pulmonary arterial vascularity (see Figs. 31-1 and 31-5 to 31-9). The degree of cardiomegaly is usually in proportion to the increase in pulmonary vascularity. The left-to-right shunts are volume overload lesions. Consequently, there is frequently cardiomegaly, and this cardiomegaly should in general be in proportion to the prominence of the pulmonary vascularity. When cardiomegaly exists out of proportion to the pulmonary arterial vascularity, then one must consider a number of possibilities. One

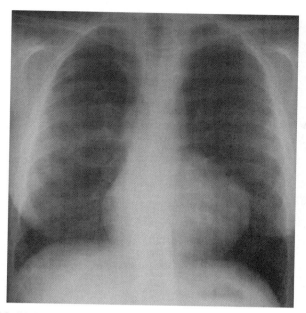

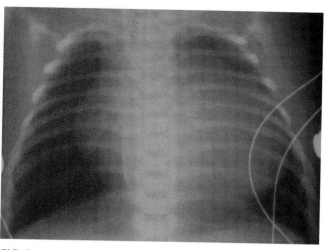

FIG. 31-3. Ebstein's anomaly. Note decreased pulmonary vascularity with cardiomegaly. Hilar vessels are small and segmental pulmonary arteries are hardly visible, especially in the upper lobes. Vector of enlargement of the apex of the heart is directly lateral, indicating right ventricular enlargement.

FIG. 31-2. Tetralogy of Fallot. Note decreased pulmonary vascularity without cardiomegaly. The main pulmonary arterial segment is concave and the hilar vessels are small. The apex is situated high above the diaphragm.

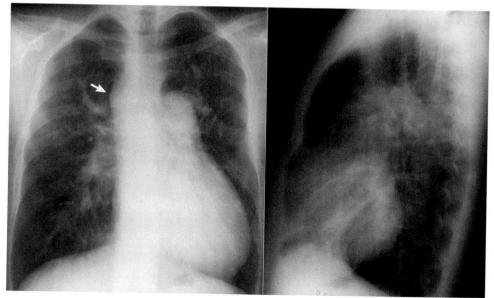

FIG. 31-4. Truncus arteriosus, type I. Note pulmonary arterial overcirculation in the presence of cyanosis and cardiomegaly. There is an enlarged aorta with right arch *(arrow)*.

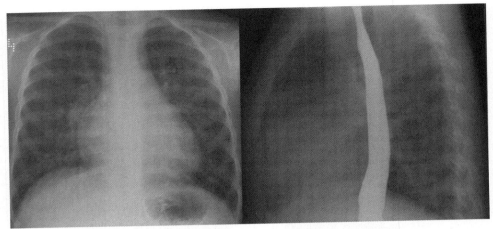

FIG. 31-5. Atrial septal defect. Frontal **(left)** and lateral **(right)** views. Pulmonary arterial overcirculation is shown by large hilar and segmental pulmonary arteries. The absence of left atrial enlargement, indicated by no impression on the barium-filled esophagus, is characteristic for an atrial-level shunt.

Two signposts can be used to help distinguish among the various types of left-to-right shunts (see Fig. 31-8). The first of these is the left atrium. Left atrial enlargement indicates that the predominant lesion is not an atrial level shunt but rather a VSD or a patent ductus arteriosus (PDA). The atrial septal defect and partial anomalous pulmonary venous connection lack both of these signposts (see Fig. 31-5). The next signpost is the aortic arch. A prominent aortic arch distinguishes between the PDA and the VSD. The aortic arch usually has a normal dimension or is small in VSD

(see Fig. 31-6). PDA is associated with left atrial enlargement and a prominent aortic arch (see Figs. 31-1, 31-7). In infants, prominence of the aortic arch may be difficult to recognize, so this signpost may not always be available. Consequently, since a VSD is a more frequent lesion, this should be the diagnosis when there is left atrial enlargement and no clearly discernible enlargement of the aortic arch. An exception to this rule is in the premature infant, where a PDA is statistically by far the most frequent congenital heart lesion. The radiograph of the premature infant with

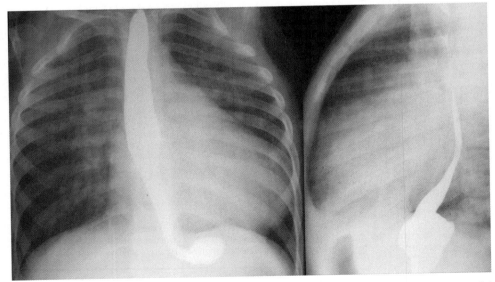

FIG. 31-6. Ventricular septal defect. Frontal **(left)** and lateral **(right)** views. Pulmonary arterial overcirculation is evidenced by shunt vessels and prominent hilar vessels. Heart size is increased in proportion to overcirculation. Left atrial enlargement produces impression on and displacement of the barium-filled esophagus, as shown on the lateral view.

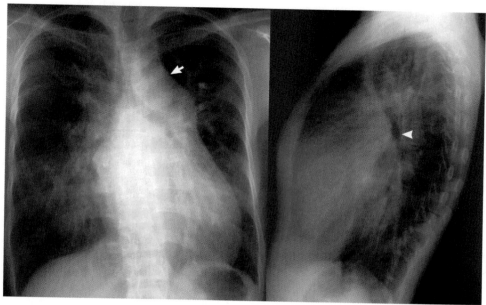

FIG. 31-7. Patent ductus arteriosus. Frontal **(left)** and lateral **(right)** views. Note pulmonary arterial overcirculation and cardiomegaly. The prominent aortic arch *(arrow)* and descending aorta are diagnostic signs of patent ductus arteriosus. On the lateral view, the enlarged left atrium causes posterior displacement of the left bronchus *(arrowhead).*

PDA usually does not disclose signs of left atrial and aortic arch enlargement.

The plain radiograph may be useful in determining the severity and progression of left-to-right shunts. The severe volume overload with large left-to-right shunts causes pulmonary venous congestion or pulmonary edema in addition

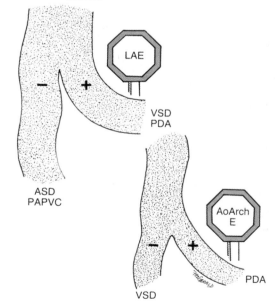

FIG. 31-8. Signposts on the diagnostic pathway of left-to-right shunts.

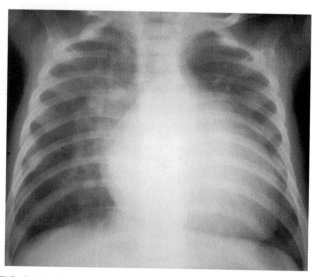

FIG. 31-9. Ventricular septal defects. Large-volume left-to-right shunt causing pulmonary edema, severe pulmonary arterial overcirculation, and cardiomegaly. Indistinct hilar and segmental arteries on the right side are caused by interstitial edema.

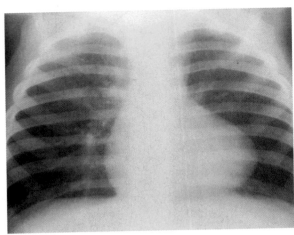

FIG. 31-10. Tetralogy of Fallot. Note pulmonary oligemia with more diminished vascularity on the left, especially the left upper lobe. Normal heart size and concave pulmonary artery segment are characteristic features in the infant.

to pulmonary arterial overcirculation (see Fig. 31-9). In individuals with large left-to-right shunts, there should also be substantial cardiomegaly.

Group II

A lesion is included in group II when there is cyanosis and the plain radiograph demonstrates diminished or normal pulmonary vascularity and the absence of substantial cardiomegaly (see Figs. 31-2, 31-10, and 31-11). The pathophysi-

ology that produces this constellation of findings involves a nonrestrictive intracardiac shunt and a severe obstruction to pulmonary blood flow. The nonrestrictive intracardiac shunt permits equalization of the pressures between two chambers, and this prevents substantial enlargement of the right ventricle. Consequently, there is usually little or no cardiomegaly. An example of the importance of the size of the intracardiac defect is in patients with tricuspid atresia. The patient with tricuspid atresia with a large atrial septal defect demonstrates little or no cardiomegaly (Fig. 31-12). On the other hand, the patient with tricuspid atresia with a restrictive atrial septal defect experiences substantial right atrial enlargement, which results in cardiomegaly. Consequently, the former patient would be classified in group II, the latter patient in group III. Tricuspid atresia can be classified in group IV when there is an associated increase in pulmonary blood flow, which is caused by either a large left-to-right shunt at the ventricular septal level or the concurrence of transposition of the great vessels. Transposition of the great arteries (TGA) occurs in approximately 30% of patients with tricuspid atresia.

Statistically, the most frequent lesion in group II is tetralogy of Fallot. The remaining diagnostic considerations are, for the most part, variants of tetralogy of Fallot. Some examples of these lesions are TGA with severe pulmonary stenosis and unrestrictive VSD and double-outlet right ventricle with severe pulmonic stenosis and an unrestrictive VSD. Table 31-1 provides a reasonably complete list of the differ-

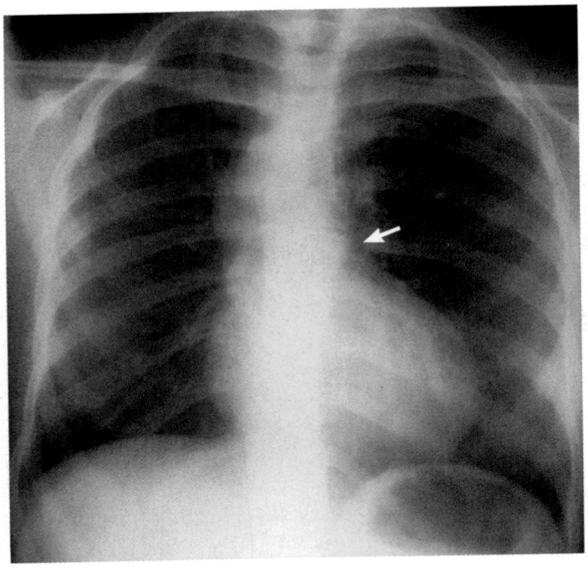

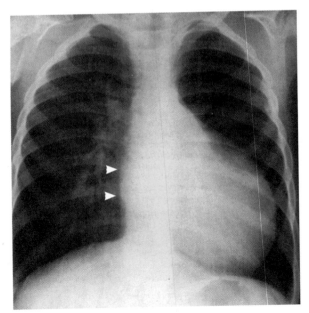

FIG. 31-12. Tricuspid atresia with large (nonrestrictive) atrial septal defect. There is decreased pulmonary vascularity and only mild cardiomegaly. Note the flattened right atrial border *(arrows)*, which is characteristic for this lesion when there is a large nonrestrictive atrial septal defect.

FIG. 31-11. Pulmonary atresia with ventricular septal defect (severe tetralogy of Fallot). Pulmonary oligemia, absent main pulmonary artery segment *(arrow)*, and normal heart size are characteristic features. There is a right aortic arch.

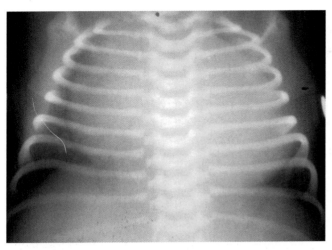

FIG. 31-13. Pulmonary atresia with intact ventricular septum, type II. Substantial tricuspid regurgitation in association with this anomaly (type II) causes right-sided chamber enlargement, especially right atrial enlargement.

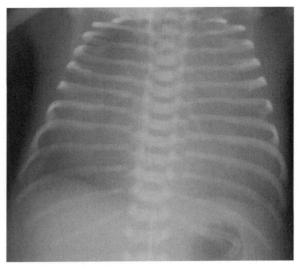

FIG. 31-15. Tricuspid regurgitation of the newborn. Pulmonary vascularity is decreased and marked cardiomegaly is present due to right-sided chamber enlargement. Extreme cardiomegaly producing the "wall-to-wall" heart is usually due to severe tricuspid regurgitation.

ential diagnostic considerations in group II. However, the plain radiograph infrequently permits a specific diagnosis to be chosen from among this myriad of lesions.

Group III

Group III lesions differ from group II lesions by the radiographic observation of cardiomegaly (see Figs. 31-3 and 31-13 to 31-15). These patients have cyanosis, normal or de-

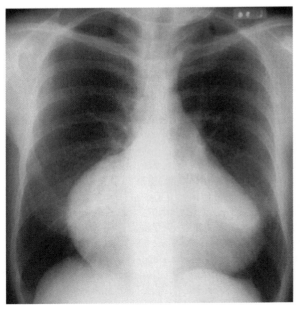

FIG. 31-14. Ebstein's anomaly in an adult. Note decreased pulmonary vascularity and marked cardiomegaly. The prominent bulging and elongation of the right heart border are indicative of severe right atrial enlargement.

creased pulmonary vascularity, and a substantial degree of cardiomegaly. The cardiac chamber that is frequently enlarged in this lesion is the right atrium. Many of the patients in this category have substantial tricuspid regurgitation, which is a major pathogenetic mechanism of the right atrial enlargement and cardiomegaly. The "wall-to-wall" heart (extension from the right to the left chest wall) should prompt the diagnostic consideration of a lesion causing tricuspid regurgitation.

There is no statistically dominant diagnostic consideration in this category, but the following lesions must be considered in the differential diagnosis: severe ("critical") pulmonary stenosis with an atrial septal defect or patent foramen ovale; type II pulmonary atresia with intact ventricular septum; tricuspid atresia with a restrictive atrial septal defect; and Ebstein's anomaly. In the older child and adult with this constellation of findings, the most likely diagnosis is Ebstein's anomaly (see Fig. 31-14). Uhl's anomaly is a rare cause of a cardiac configuration similar to Ebstein's anomaly. Another unusual diagnosis in this category, which appears only in the neonatal period, is tricuspid regurgitation of the newborn (see Fig. 31-15). In this entity there is frequently substantial cardiomegaly, diminished pulmonary blood flow, and cyanosis within the first few days of life. However, with reduction in pulmonary vascular resistance over time, the amount of tricuspid regurgitation decreases and the cardiomegaly may resolve.

Group IV

A lesion is included in this group when the radiograph displays pulmonary arterial overcirculation in the presence of

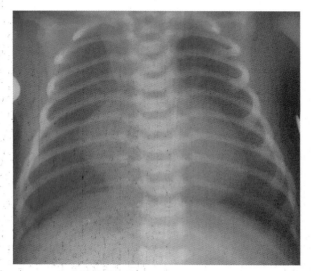

FIG. 31-16. Transposition of the great arteries. Pulmonary arterial overcirculation and an ovoid heart with a narrow base (vascular pedicle) of the heart are characteristic features.

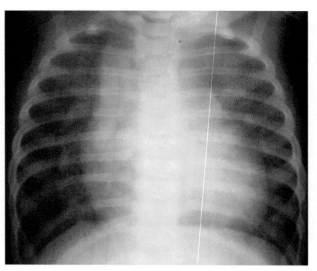

FIG. 31-18. Total anomalous pulmonary venous connection, supracardiac type (type I). Note pulmonary arterial overcirculation and cardiomegaly. Enlargement of supracardiac region is caused by an enlarged left-sided vertical vein and a dilated right superior vena cava; it is characteristic of this anomaly.

cyanosis. The heart size is usually increased. The observation of increased pulmonary vascularity in a patient with cyanosis is an incongruous finding and should alert the observer to the presence of an admixture lesion rather than a strictly left-to-right shunt. An aid to remembering the major diagnoses in this category is the letter T. The most common diagnosis in this category is TGA, which is the most frequent cyanotic congenital heart lesion at birth (Fig. 31-16). The other diagnostic considerations are truncus arteriosus (Fig. 31-17), total anomalous pulmonary venous connection (Fig. 31-18), tricuspid atresia, and single ("tingle") ventricle. Double-outlet right ventricle and double-outlet

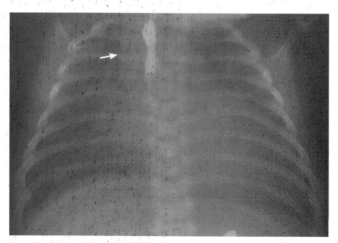

FIG. 31-17. Truncus arteriosus. Pulmonary arterial overcirculation and right aortic arch *(arrow)* are characteristics of truncus arteriosus.

left ventricle are also considered in this category, but these can be brought to mind when one thinks of TGA, since these lesions are essentially hybrids of TGA. The lesion that is frequently forgotten in this group is multiple pulmonary arterial venous malformations. The patient with multiple pulmonary arterial venous malformations is frequently mildly or even moderately cyanotic, and because of the several malformations within the lung, there is the appearance of increased pulmonary arterial vascularity.

Pulmonary Venous Congestion or Pulmonary Edema

A fifth group of congenital lesions are those that produce predominantly pulmonary venous congestion and alter the pulmonary venous vascularity rather than the pulmonary arterial vascularity. Patients with these lesions may have shunts, but inclusion in group V requires that the predominant pathophysiologic event is pulmonary venous congestion (Figs. 31-19 to 31-21; see Table 31-2).

The clinical features of the group V lesions are lack of cyanosis and frequently severe symptoms of heart failure. These usually consist of dyspnea, tachypnea, and tachycardia. The salient radiographic findings are indistinctness of the pulmonary vascularity, especially in the perihilar area, or interstitial pulmonary edema (see Figs. 31-19 and 31-21). Another observation that places a lesion into this group is disproportionately prominent cardiomegaly in comparison to the prominence of pulmonary vascularity (see Figs. 31-19 and 31-20).

The lesions included in this category are listed in Table

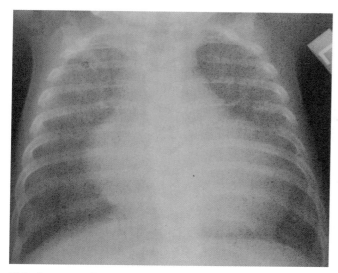

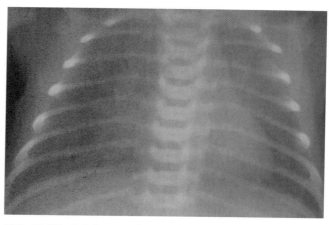

FIG. 31-21. Total anomalous pulmonary venous connection, type III. Radiograph shows pulmonary edema and normal heart size.

FIG. 31-19. Endocardial fibroelastosis. Pulmonary edema and cardiomegaly are characteristic features of group V lesions.

31-2. The statistical frequencies of the lesions in this category are also important in deciding on the diagnosis. Diagnosis in this category includes conditions that produce reversible stresses upon the heart of the newborn as well as structural cardiac lesions. Lesions in this category tend to present at certain times after birth; for instance, the nonstructural causes of pulmonary venous congestion or edema usually present within the first day or two of life. Abnormalities that may be encountered within the first day of life

include severe anemia (hydrops fetalis), asphyxia, hypocalcemia, hypoglycemia, abnormalities of heart rate and rhythm, hypervolemia, and intrauterine myocarditis. Pulmonary venous congestion with substantial cardiomegaly presenting in the first day or so of life is a feature of hypoplastic left heart (Fig. 31-22). Pulmonary venous congestion with an essentially normal heart size presenting within the first day or so of life is the feature of total anomalous pulmonary venous connection, infradiaphragmatic type, with obstruction (see Fig. 31-21). In the infant presenting with these features between 1 week and 3 weeks of age, statistically the most frequent diagnosis is coarctation of the aorta

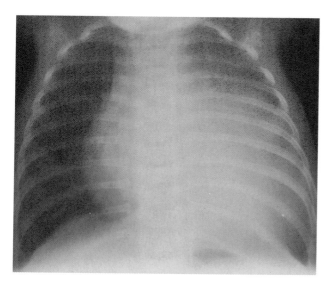

FIG. 31-20. Anomalous origin of the left coronary artery from the pulmonary artery. Cardiomegaly is disproportionate to pulmonary vascularity in a noncyanotic infant. Left atrial enlargement (right retrocardiac double density) is caused by mitral regurgitation from papillary muscle infarction.

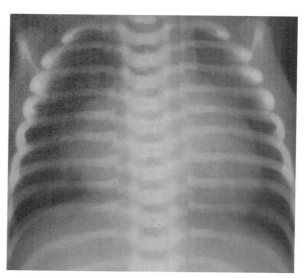

FIG. 31-22. Hypoplastic left heart. Note pulmonary venous congestion and edema and cardiomegaly. Prominent right atrium and ventricle and posterior aortic arch are characteristic features of this lesion.

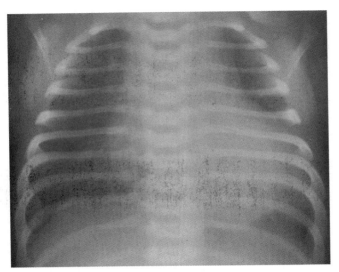

FIG. 31-23. Severe coarctation of the aorta in a newborn. There is marked cardiomegaly with pulmonary edema.

(Fig. 31-23). Rib notching is not evident in infants with coarctation.

Salient Radiographic Features of Specific Lesions

Acyanotic

Atrial Septal Defect and Partial Anomalous Pulmonary Venous Connection

There are four types of atrial septal defects: secundum (most frequent); primum; sinus venosus (superior and inferior vena caval locations); and coronary sinus (least frequent). The primum type is usually part of an atrioventricular septal defect, which was formerly called endocardial cushion defect. In addition, a patent foramen ovale exists in many children with congenital heart disease, and the foramen may

be stretched in the setting of elevated right-sided pressures. An aneurysm may also form at the site of the thin fossa ovalis; this may occur as an isolated anomaly or may exist in association with a septal defect or patent foramen ovale. The defects are named according to their position in the atrial septum: ostium secundum in the region of the fossa ovalis, which is approximately the middle of the septum; primum in the lower part of the septum and bordering on the atrioventricular valves; sinus venosus in either the upper part of the septum and bordering on the ostium of the superior vena cava or in the lower septum and bordering on the ostium of the inferior vena cava. A rare type of defect occurs at a site normally occupied by the coronary site and coexists with absence of the wall separating the coronary sinus from the left atrium so that the associated left superior vena cava enters into the left atrium. The coexistence of large primum and secundum defects constitutes a common atrium.

The isolated atrial septal defect and partial anomalous pulmonary venous connection conduct left-to-right shunts. A stretched foramen ovale or atrial septal defect may permit predominant right-to-left shunting in complex lesions with

---

TABLE 31-4. SALIENT RADIOGRAPHIC FEATURES OF ATRIAL SEPTAL DEFECT WITH PULMONARY ARTERIAL HYPERTENSION

Enlarged main and central pulmonary arteries (see Fig. 31-24)
Disparity in enlargement of central and lobar arteries to peripheral arteries
Calcification of main or central pulmonary arteries
Onset of severe pulmonary arterial hypertension may be associated with reduction in degree of cardiomegaly or normal heart size.
Cardiomegaly may be persistent because of tricuspid insufficiency caused by severe pulmonary hypertension.

TABLE 31-3. SALIENT RADIOGRAPHIC FEATURES OF ATRIAL SEPTAL DEFECT

Pulmonary arterial overcirculation: Generally a 2:1 shunt must exist before pulmonary plethora is universally present. About 50%–60% of patients with less than 2:1 shunt have only mild or no evident pulmonary plethora. Pulmonary edema rarely occurs in the simple atrial septal defect.
Enlargement of right atrium (see Fig. 31-5)
Enlargement of right ventricle
Enlargement of main and hilar pulmonary arterial segments: In older subjects, the right pulmonary artery is sometimes especially prominent (see Fig. 31-24).
Small ascending aorta and aortic arch
Small superior vena caval shadow

TABLE 31-5. SALIENT RADIOGRAPHIC FEATURES OF PARTIAL ANOMALOUS PULMONARY VENOUS COARCTATION

Pulmonary arterial overcirculation: This may be apparent or more severe only in the lung with anomalous drainage.
Enlargement of right atrium
Enlargement of right ventricle
Enlargement of main and hilar pulmonary arterial segments
Small ascending aorta and aortic arch
Enlargement of superior vena cava, azygous vein, coronary sinus or other systemic veins, depending on site of connection
Prominent left superior vena cava
Abnormal course of pulmonary veins through the lung or in relation to mediastinal margins (see Fig. 31-25)

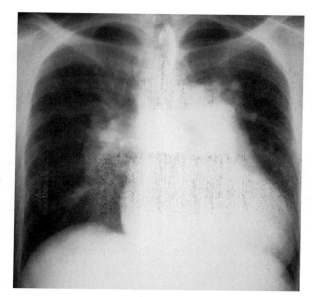

FIG. 31-24. Atrial septal defect in an adult. The radiograph shows pulmonary arterial overcirculation and cardiomegaly due to right-sided chamber enlargement. Severe dilatation of the central pulmonary arteries is a feature of this anomaly in the adult. The right pulmonary artery is very prominent.

of the right ventricle can reverse this pattern. A large atrial septal defect is defined as one that results in equalization of pressure between the atria (Tables 31-3 to 31-6; Figs. 31-24 and 31-25).

Atrioventricular Septal Defect (Endocardial Cushion Defect)

The embryonic endocardial cushions contribute to the development of the medial portions of the mitral and tricuspid valves, the primum atrial septum, and the inlet portion of the ventricular septum (Fig. 31-26). Defects in this region have been called endocardial cushion defects but more recently have received the name **atrioventricular septal defects** (AVSDs). The fundamental lesion is a common atrioventricular valve and variable deficiency of the primum atrial septum and the inlet ventricular septum. The atrioventricular valve in this anomaly has five leaflets, with two of the leaflets spanning the ventricular septum and the opening to both ventricles. The spanning leaflets are the anterior and posterior bridging leaflets. If there is a tongue of tissue connecting the anterior and posterior bridging leaflets and

severe right-sided obstruction (i.e., tricuspid atresia). The volume of shunting across an interatrial communication usually depends on the size of the defect and the relative distensibility of the two ventricles. The wall of the right ventricle is more distensible than the left ventricle during diastole, so blood preferentially flows toward the right ventricle at this time. However, obstruction of flow into or out

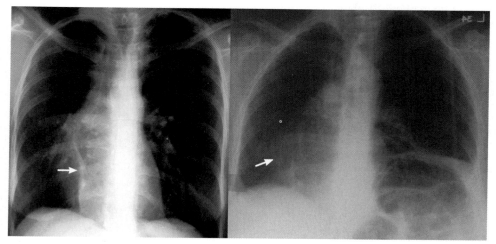

FIG. 31-25. Two patients with scimitar syndrome. **Left.** Radiograph showing a scimitar vein near the right diaphragm, a dextroposed heart, and a small right lung. The scimitar vein *(arrow)* enlarges in its course toward the diaphragm. **Right.** Radiograph showing multiple anomalous veins *(arrow)* arching toward the right hemidiaphragm. The increased diameter of the veins from superior to inferior indicates that they are anomalous veins rather than pulmonary arteries. The heart is dextroposed. There is an incidental eventration of the left hemidiaphragm.

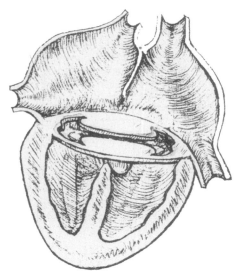

FIG. 31-26. Diagram of complete form of atrioventricular septal defect. The defect consists of a primum atrial septal defect, an inlet ventricular septal defect, and a single atrioventricular valve spanning the ventricular septal defect.

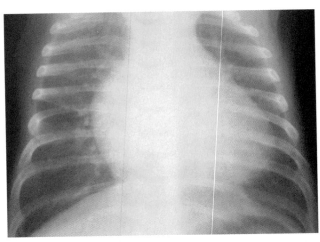

FIG. 31-27. Atrioventricular septal defect/primum atrial septal defect. Radiography shows pulmonary arterial overcirculation and cardiomegaly due to right atrial and ventricular enlargement. The vector of ventricular enlargement is laterally and superiorly, causing the apex to be located high above the diaphragm. Prominent bulging of the upper right atrial border is a feature of primum atrial septal defects.

this tongue is attached to the crest of the inlet ventricular septum, then incomplete forms of the defect result. The anomaly exists in a complete form with a single atrioventricular valve, primum atrial septal defect, and inlet VSD. In the complete form, no connecting tissue exists between the bridging leaflets. Incomplete forms are said to exist when there are two atrioventricular valves; the individual valves are formed by the connecting tongue of tissue. Portions of the valves are frequently deficient, such as underdevelopment of the septal leaflet of the tricuspid valve and a cleft in the anterior leaflet of the mitral valve. Actually, this "cleft" is the commissure between the anterior bridging leaflet and

the mural leaflet of the left-sided portion of the atrioventricular valve.

The most common incomplete lesion is a primum atrial septal defect and a "cleft" in the mitral valve, causing varying degrees of mitral regurgitation. Because the primum atrial septal defect is situated immediately above the cleft, mitral regurgitation may traverse the defect and enter the right atrium. Consequently, the left atrium may not be enlarged even in patients with substantial mitral regurgitation (Table 31-7; Figs. 31-27 and 31-28).

TABLE 31-7. SALIENT RADIOGRAPHIC FEATURES OF ATRIOVENTRICULAR SEPTAL DEFECT

Skeletal features of trisomy 21, such as 11 ribs, double manubrial ossification center, and tall vertebral bodies
Pulmonary arterial overcirculation: This is severe in the complete forms and may be associated with pulmonary edema. Concurrent pneumonia is frequent in the complete form, especially in the child with mongolism.
Enlargement of right atrium: The superior margin of the right atrium is frequently prominent (see Figs. 31-27 and 31-28).
Enlargement of right ventricle (see Fig. 31-28)
Enlargement of main and central pulmonary arterial segments
Left atrial enlargement may be present but is generally not severe and may be absent despite mitral regurgitation.
Small thoracic aorta
A cleft mitral valve without a primum defect (rare) produces the radiographic configuration of mitral regurgitation.

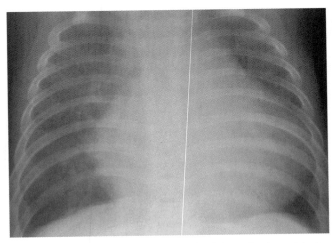

FIG. 31-28. Atrioventricular septal defect (atrioventricular canal). Pulmonary arterial overcirculation and cardiomegaly due to right atrial and ventricular enlargement are present. There is elongation of the right atrial border, indicating substantial right atrial enlargement.

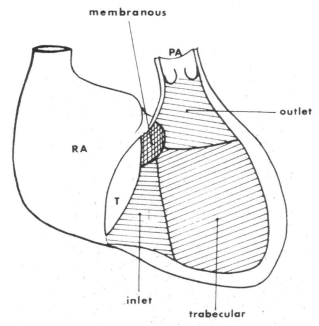

FIG. 31-29. The regions of the ventricular septum. The types of defect are named according to the region of the septum that is completely or partially defective. *PA*, pulmonary artery; *RA*, right atrium; *T*, tricuspid valve. (From Higgins CB, et al. Congenital Heart Disease: Echocardiography and Magnetic Resonance Imaging. New York: Raven Press, 1990.)

Ventricular Septal Defect

VSDs have been characterized by their location in the septum: perimembranous, outlet, inlet, and trabecular (Fig. 31-29). Defects in the perimembranous and outlet regions have also been described in relation to the crista supraventricularis of the right ventricle as infracristal (more frequent) and supracristal types. While any perimembranous or outlet VSD can cause aortic regurgitation, the supracristal type frequently causes prolapse of the right sinus of Valsalva and aortic regurgitation. Prolapsed sinus tissue may reduce the size or obliterate the septal defect. The outlet defect may be caused by malposition of the outlet septum, resulting in a small right ventricular outflow region and an aorta overriding the septal defect (tetralogy of Fallot). VSDs are not uncommonly multiple. Multiple defects in the trabecular septum may produce a "Swiss cheese septum."

A small VSD is one in which the diameter or cross-sectional area is less than that of the aortic annulus. A large or nonrestrictive defect has a diameter or cross-sectional area exceeding the aortic annulus. A nonrestrictive defect permits equalization of pressures in the two ventricles. Isolated VSD causes a left-to-right shunt in which the volume is determined by the cross-sectional area of the defect and pulmonary vascular resistance. With large defects, shunting is not restricted by the defect but is controlled only by pulmonary vascular resistance. With low pulmonary vascular resistance

the volume of the shunt is great, causing severe pulmonary overcirculation and eventually pulmonary edema and elevated left ventricular end-diastole pressure. With higher resistance the flow is less severe and there is pulmonary arterial hypertension. Increased pulmonary vascular resistance and pulmonary arterial hypertension may be due to pulmonary arteriolar constriction (reversible) or arteriolopathy (irreversible).

Most isolated VSDs close spontaneously. The process of closure is frequently marked by a ventricular septal aneurysm. The aneurysm usually consists of portions of the septal leaflet of the tricuspid valve adherent to the rim of the defect; a hole may develop in the adhesed leaflet. Although the supracristal defect may be obstructed by the prolapsed sinus of Valsalva, it does not actually close. The inlet VSD (part of the AVSD) rarely closes spontaneously.

In the early postpartum period, pulmonary vascular resistance has not declined completely to adult levels, and the elevated resistance limits the left-to-right shunting through large defects. Pulmonary arteriolar resistance tends to reach a nadir 4 to 6 weeks postnatally and pulmonary overcirculation peaks. Because of the process of gradual closure and a relative decrease in the defect due to cardiac growth, the defect is physiologically maximal during the first year of life. Since VSD is a volume overload lesion and the volume overload is directly related to the excess pulmonary blood flow, cardiac enlargement is proportional to the degree of overcirculation (Table 31-8; see Figs. 31-6, 31-9, and 31-30).

Patent Ductus Arteriosus

The ductus arteriosus connects the proximal descending aorta to the proximal left pulmonary artery just beyond the pulmonary arterial bifurcation. With mirror-image right aortic arch, the ductus usually connects the distal left innominate artery to the left pulmonary artery. With non–mirror-image right arch (retroesophageal left subcla-

---

TABLE 31-8. SALIENT RADIOGRAPHIC FEATURES OF HEMODYNAMICALLY SIGNIFICANT VENTRICULAR SEPTAL DEFECT

Pulmonary arterial overcirculation (see Figs. 31-6 and 31-9): With large shunts pulmonary edema is frequent during infancy.

Enlargement of the left atrium (see Figs. 31-6 and 31-30): This may not be easy to identify during infancy.

Enlargement of either or both ventricles

Enlargement of main and central pulmonary arterial segments (see Fig. 31-9)

Disproportionate enlargement of central pulmonary arteries compared with peripheral vasculature suggests the Eisenmenger's complex but can also be observed with very large shunts. Pulmonary arterial calcification can occur in Eisenmenger's complex.

Small thoracic aorta: Right aortic arch is alleged to occur in about 2% of ventricular septal defects.

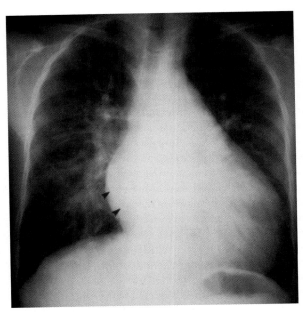

FIG. 31-30. Ventricular septal defect. Radiograph shows increased pulmonary blood flow and cardiomegaly. A right retrocardiac double density *(arrowheads)* indicates left atrial enlargement. Aortic arch is normal in size.

TABLE 31-9. SALIENT RADIOGRAPHIC FEATURES OF HEMODYNAMICALLY SIGNIFICANT PDAs

Pulmonary arterial overcirculation (see Figs. 31-1 and 31-7)
Enlargement of left atrium (see Fig. 31-7)
Enlargement of left ventricle (see Figs. 31-1 and 31-7)
Enlargement of aortic arch (see Figs. 31-1 and 31-7): While this may not be evident with infants, it is an invariable feature in the older child and adult. It may also be possible to identify prominence of the ascending aorta and lateral displacement of the descending aorta.
Enlargement of the main and central pulmonary arterial segments: This tends to be less prominent than in atrial septal defect.
Abnormal contour of the posterior aortic arch and proximal descending aorta: In many normal subjects, there is a localized dilatation of the aorta at the site of attachment of the ligamentum arteriosus, the aortic spindle (also called infundibulum). This aortic spindle is enlarged in patients with patent ductus arteriosus. The combined shadows of the posterior arch and aortic spindle cause apparent elongation, prominence or atypical contour of the aortic knob. The aorticopulmonary window may be obliterated or convex due to the patent ductus arteriosus.
Calcification in the aorticopulmonary window due to calcification of the walls of the ductus in older individuals (see Fig. 31-32)

vian artery), the ductus connects the proximal right descending aorta to the proximal left pulmonary artery and causes a vascular ring.

PDA closes within the first day of life in full-term neonates, but persistent PDA is frequent in the premature infant. Significant left-to-right shunting in a premature infant during the early neonatal period is nearly always due to PDA. The shunt is predominantly left to right and causes pulmonary overcirculation and, if severe, pulmonary edema. However, right-to-left shunting across a PDA may be encountered in neonates if the pulmonary vascular resistance fails to decline from fetal levels (persistent fetal circulation).

PDA occurs as an isolated anomaly but also frequently in association with other simple and complex anomalies. There is a propensity for the triplex of PDA, coarctation of the aorta, and VSD to occur. PDA is also frequently present in cyanotic lesions with severe obstruction to pulmonary blood flow, such as pulmonary atresia. The PDA is life-sustaining in these instances but cannot be relied upon to maintain pulmonary blood flow because it may severely constrict or obliterate over time.

The large-caliber PDA may conduct a large left-to-right shunt because a gradient exists between the aorta and pulmonary artery throughout the cardiac cycle. Flow through the PDA is controlled by the caliber of the ductus and pulmonary vascular resistance. The volume overload (excess pulmonary blood flow) causes enlargement of the left atrium and left ventricle. The left-to-right shunt continually recirculates to the lungs, left atrium, left ventricle, ascending aorta, and aortic arch. The volume experienced by the left-sided chamber causes an elevated left ventricular diastolic pressure. With large shunts, the excess blood flow and elevated left ventricular diastolic pressure eventuates in pulmonary edema. The excess flow and elevated pulmonary venous pressure may cause considerable pulmonary arterial hypertension, which induces right ventricular hypertrophy. The eventual outcome of the process is pulmonary arteriolopathy and Eisenmenger's syndrome (Tables 31-9 and 31-10; Figs. 31-31 and 31-32).

TABLE 31-10. SALIENT RADIOGRAPHIC FEATURES OF PATENT DUCTUS ARTERIOSUS WITH PULMONARY ARTERIAL HYPERTENSION

Enlarged main and central pulmonary arteries (see Fig. 31-31)
Disparity in enlargement of central and lobar arteries compared with peripheral arteries
Calcification of main or central pulmonary arteries
Calcification of the ductus (track-like calcification in the aorticopulmonary window (see Figs. 31-31 and 31-32).
Onset of pulmonary arterial hypertension is usually accompanied by a decrease in cardiomegaly or normal heart size (see Fig. 31-31).
Enlargement of the aortic arch and proximal descending aorta (see Fig. 31-31)

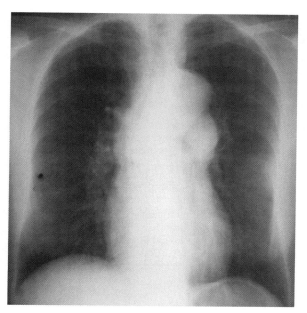

FIG. 31-31. Eisenmenger's complex caused by patent ductus arteriosus. Thoracic radiograph shows no pulmonary arterial overcirculation but instead reveals attenuated peripheral vessels, normal heart size, and markedly enlarged main pulmonary arterial segment and aorta.

Aorticopulmonary Window

This rare anomaly is a large connection between the ascending aorta and the main pulmonary artery. Both semilunar valves are present, and this feature distinguishes the lesion from truncus arteriosus. This lesion usually causes a large left-to-right shunt and pulmonary edema in early infancy.

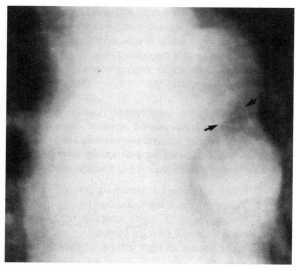

FIG. 31-32. Coned-down view of the aorticopulmonary window of the patient in Figure 31-31 shows parallel lines of calcification (*arrows*) in the wall of the patent ductus.

The physiology of this lesion is similar to PDA but is invariably severe, so nearly all cases present during early infancy. This lesion is almost never encountered in childhood or adult life. If an untreated patient is rarely encountered beyond infancy, irreversible pulmonary arterial hypertension is present.

The radiographic features should resemble PDA if the patient survives beyond infancy. The usual radiographic appearance is severe pulmonary overcirculation and pulmonary edema. The ascending aorta and main pulmonary arterial segment are more prominent than for PDA in the infant.

Congenital Sinus of Valsalva Aneurysm and Fistula

The aneurysm begins as a funnel-shaped outpocketing at a congenital weakness at the junction of the aortic media and annulus fibrosis of the aortic valve. Congenital aneurysm arises from the right coronary sinus and noncoronary sinus. Aneurysms of the right coronary sinus rupture into the right ventricle or right atrium, while those of the noncoronary sinus rupture into the right atrium. This entity should be distinguished from diffuse aneurysmal dilatation of the sinuses, which occurs in Marfan's syndrome. A large acute rupture may cause intractable pulmonary edema. All fistulas to the right heart cause volume overload of the left heart since there is volume overload of the downstream chambers. Depending on the site of rupture, volume overload of the right ventricle, right atrium, or both also occurs. These lesions may also be associated with aortic regurgitation and perimembranous or supracristal VSD (Table 31-11).

Coronary Arteriovenous Fistula

This is a fistula or angiodysplasia from a coronary artery to a coronary vein, coronary sinus, right atrium, right ventricle, or pulmonary artery. There may be multiple sites of communication. The involved coronary artery is usually dilated and tortuous. The right coronary artery is involved more frequently and most frequently enters the right atrium or ventricle. The shunt is usually small and does not produce recognizable pulmonary overcirculation or volume overload enlargement of the heart.

TABLE 31-11. SALIENT RADIOGRAPHIC FEATURES OF CORONARY SINUS FISTULA

Pulmonary arterial overcirculation or edema
Enlargement of left-sided cardiac chambers
Enlargement of right ventricle (rupture into right ventricle or right atrium)
Enlargement of right atrium (rupture into right atrium)
Enlargement of main pulmonary and central pulmonary arterial segments
Rarely, the aneurysm is sufficiently large so that there is asymmetric dilatation at the base of the aorta.
Curvilinear calcification of the aneurysm (infrequent)

Pulmonary arterial overcirculation and cardiomegaly are usually not evident. The ectatic coronary artery is infrequently discernible on the thoracic radiograph. Ectasia of the circumflex coronary artery may cause a localized bulge in the upper left cardiac margin in the region near the site of the left atrium on the frontal radiograph. Calcification rarely occurs in the ectatic coronary artery.

Cyanotic

Tetralogy of Fallot

The major components of this anomaly are caused by a displacement of the outlet septum (conal septation) toward the right ventricle, resulting in a diminutive right ventricular outflow region and failure of alignment of the outlet portion with the remainder of the ventricular septum. The latter abnormality causes a large VSD (infracristal), and the aorta is located immediately over the defect. Consequently, right ventricular blood is ejected directly into the aorta. There is a reciprocal relationship between the aortic and pulmonary arterial diameters; the ascending aorta is substantially enlarged in the presence of severe pulmonic stenosis and pulmonic atresia. The VSD is nonrestrictive, so pressures are equal in the ventricles. Multiple VSDs may occur in this anomaly.

The obstruction to pulmonary blood flow is frequently diffuse and exists at multiple levels, causing subvalvular, valvular, and supravalvular stenoses. There is invariably infundibular stenosis. The annulus and proximal pulmonary artery are usually hypoplastic. The stenosis may involve the entire outflow region and may include severe hypoplasia of the segmental and intraparenchymal pulmonary arteries. The extreme form of tetralogy is pulmonary atresia with a nonrestrictive VSD. Branch pulmonary arterial stenosis, especially at the origin of the left pulmonary artery, may cause asymmetric pulmonary blood flow. However, even in the absence of branch stenosis, preferential flow occurs to the right lung due to the orientation of the right ventricular outflow tract. A right aortic arch is present in about 20% of patients with tetralogy; the incidence is about 25% with pulmonary atresia and VSD (extreme form of tetralogy).

The physiology of the anomaly consists of reduced pulmonary blood flow and arterial desaturation. Because of the reduced blood flow through the lungs, the left-sided cardiac chambers are small. Radiographic features are shown in Tables 31-12 and 31-13 and Figs. 31-2, 31-10, 31-11, 31-33, and 31-34.

Early in life the thoracic radiograph may not be typical, but it becomes characteristic later. Regression of the thymus reveals the concave main pulmonary artery segment, which is characteristic for tetralogy of Fallot.

After surgical repair of tetralogy, a number of radiographic findings may be identified, such as aneurysm of a right ventricular outflow patch; asymmetry of pulmonary vascularity due to persistent branch pulmonary arterial ste-

TABLE 31-12. SALIENT RADIOGRAPHIC FEATURES OF TETRALOGY OF FALLOT

Decreased pulmonary vascularity (see Figs. 31-2, 31-10, 31-11 and 31-33): Normal vascularity in a cyanotic individual is equated with decreased vascularity since the distinction between normal and mildly decreased vascularity is frequently difficult.
Normal or nearly normal cardiac size
Right ventricular enlargement or prominence: This may cause an uplifted cardiac apex (see Figs. 31-2, 31-10, and 31-33).
Concave or absent main pulmonary arterial segment (see Figs. 31-11 and 31-33)
Small hilar pulmonary arteries: This may be most evident on the lateral view.
Asymmetric pulmonary vascularity is frequent, especially because of associated branch pulmonary artery stenosis.
Prominent ascending aorta and aortic arch
Right aortic arch (20%-25% of cases; see Figs. 31-11 and 31-33)

TABLE 31-13. SALIENT RADIOGRAPHIC FEATURES OF TETRALOGY OF FALLOT WITH ABSENT PULMONARY VALVE

Decreased distal pulmonary vascularity
Aneurysmal enlargement of main and central pulmonary arteries (see Fig. 31-34)
Cardiac size variable, depending on severity of pulmonary regurgitation

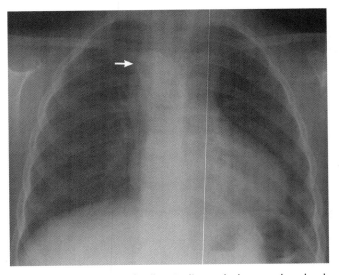

FIG. 31-33. Tetralogy of Fallot. Radiograph shows reduced pulmonary vascularity, normal heart size, right ventricular prominence, concave main pulmonary arterial segment, and right aortic arch *(arrow)*.

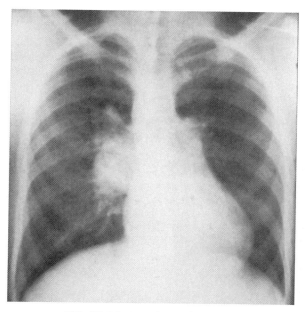
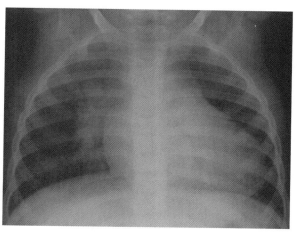

FIG. 31-34. Tetralogy of Fallot with absent pulmonary valve in an adult (**left**) and an infant (**right**). Aneurysmal dilatation of main and right pulmonary arterial segments is diagnostic of this anomaly. Note the disparity in size of the right hilar arterial region and the peripheral segments of the pulmonary arteries.

nosis; and progressive right ventricular enlargement due to pulmonary regurgitation complicating a transannular patch (Fig. 31-35). Pulmonary arterial overcirculation can develop when a hemodynamically significant residual VSD exists after successful repair of outflow stenosis.

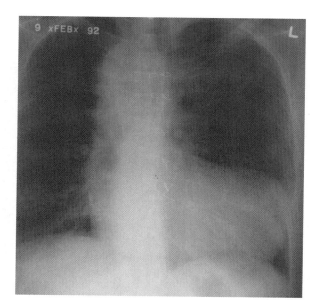

FIG. 31-35. Tetralogy of Fallot with severe pulmonary regurgitation several years after repair. The cardiomegaly is caused by marked right ventricular enlargement, as indicated by the uplifted apex.

Transposition of Great Arteries

TGA is one of several abnormalities of arterioventricular connection. The others are double-outlet right ventricle, double-outlet left ventricle, and truncus arteriosus. All of these anomalies are admixture lesions, all produce cyanosis, and in the absence of obstruction to blood flow, all are associated with pulmonary arterial overcirculation.

In TGA, the aorta arises from the right ventricle and the pulmonary artery arises from the left ventricle. The base of the aorta is positioned anterior to pulmonary artery. If the aorta lies to the right of the pulmonary artery, the name d-TGA (dextro-TGA) applies, while if the aorta lies to the left of the pulmonary artery, the name l-TGA (levo-TGA) applies. If the aorta is directly anterior to the pulmonary artery, the term a-TGA (antero-TGA) is sometimes used.

The physiologic consequence of TGA is pulmonary arterial overcirculation and cyanosis due to the combination of left-to-right and right-to-left shunts (admixture lesion). Because the pulmonary and systemic circulations are parallel, most of the blood ejected by the left ventricle into the pulmonary artery is recirculated. The severity of overcirculation is usually greater in the presence of VSD and reduced in the presence of pulmonic stenosis. Cardiac size increases in relation to the pulmonary overcirculation. Pulmonary arterial hypertension and arteriolopathy tend to ensue early in life in children with TGA. Pulmonary arteriolopathy and fixed hypertension not uncommonly develop at 6 to 12 months of age in children with TGA with VSD.

TGA is the most frequent cyanotic heart lesion. Without

surgical intervention, most of the infants would die in the first year of life.

The radiographic appearance is influenced a great deal by the associated lesions. TGA is the most frequent anomaly causing pulmonary overcirculation in a cyanotic infant (see Fig. 31-16). The presence of significant pulmonic stenosis produces a radiographic appearance similar to tetralogy of Fallot (i.e., decreased pulmonary vascularity and normal heart size in a cyanotic infant). The radiographic appearance during the first day or first few days of life may not be characteristic, since a prominent thymus conceals the narrow great vessel region and pulmonary blood flow is still limited by high pulmonary vascular resistance persisting from intrauterine life. After thymic involution in the stressed newborn, the narrow base of the heart becomes evident (Table 31-14; see Fig. 31-16).

Corrected Transposition (l-TGA)

Corrected transposition consists of arterioventricular transposition and atrioventricular discordance. The aorta originates from the right ventricle and the right ventricle is inverted with connection to the left atrium. There is an L-ventricular loop with the morphologic right ventricle to the left of the morphologic left ventricle. Thus, blood flow in the central circulation is corrected; pulmonary venous blood flows to the left atrium, to the right ventricle, and into

TABLE 31-14. SALIENT RADIOGRAPHIC FEATURES OF TRANSPOSITION

Pulmonary arterial overcirculation: Asymmetry of pulmonary flow, greater on the right side, is sometimes apparent.

Pulmonary edema is frequent, especially in the presence of a VSD or PDA.

Cardiomegaly: A cardiothoracic ratio exceeding 0.58 constitutes cardiomegaly in the neonatal period.

In newborns, specific chamber enlargement is difficult to identify. In older children, there is left atrial and right ventricular enlargement.

Narrow vascular pedicle: The great vessels are usually but not invariably inconspicuous (see Fig. 31-16). The ascending aorta occupies a more medial position than normal and is hidden in the mediastinum. Likewise, the pulmonary artery lies medially within the mediastinum, so a typical main pulmonary arterial segment is not present. Thus, there is the incongruity of pulmonary arterial overcirculation with a small or absent main pulmonary arterial segment. Infrequently, even in complete TGA, the aorta lies to the right or left of the pulmonary artery, causing a normal or even increased width of the pedicle.

Right aortic arch occurs in about 5% of patients with TGA, usually in association with pulmonic stenosis and VSD.

In the presence of pulmonic stenosis and VSD, there is decreased pulmonary vascular size and normal heart size, producing an appearance similar to tetralogy of Fallot.

ASD, atrial septal defect; TGA, transposition of the great arteries; VSD, ventricular septal defect.

TABLE 31-15. SALIENT RADIOGRAPHIC FEATURES OF CORRECTED TRANSPOSITION

Prominent convexity of upper left cardiac border (see Fig. 31-36): The convexity may extend nearly to the arch or merely involve the base of the heart.

Ascending aortic shadow on the right is not visible (see Fig. 31-36).

Crossing of the edge of the ascending aorta and the lateral edge of the proximal descending aorta

Conspicuous absence of a convex main pulmonary arterial segment even in the presence of pulmonary arterial overcirculation: Sometimes there is upward tilt of the right and downward tilt of the left pulmonary artery.

Left atrial enlargement can be caused by pulmonary overcirculation caused by the ventricular septal defect or by tricuspid regurgitation caused by Ebstein's anomaly.

the aorta. Most patients with corrected transposition have significant additional cardiac anomalies. The most frequent ones are pulmonic stenosis, VSD, Ebstein's anomaly (tricuspid regurgitation into the left atrium), and complete heart block (Table 31-15; Fig. 31-36).

Double-outlet Right Ventricle

Double-outlet right ventricle is an anomaly in which more than 50% of both great vessels originate from the right ventricle. The aorta is positioned further to the right of the pulmonary artery and originates completely from the right ventricle, while the pulmonary artery may originate entirely from the right ventricle or have a biventricular origin (Taussig-Bing malformation). A VSD is always present, and other associated anomalies are frequent. The physiology of dou-

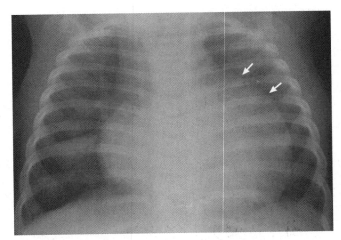

FIG. 31-36. Corrected transposition of great arteries (L-ventricular loop with I-TGA). There is a prominent elongated convexity of the upper left cardiac border. This is caused by the ascending aorta positioned to the left of the pulmonary artery and the inverted right ventricular outlet region.

ble-outlet right ventricle is determined to a great degree by the position of the VSD. A VSD oriented to the aortic valve (subaortic VSD) causes preferential flow from the left ventricle into the aorta and is frequently associated with significant pulmonic stenosis, resulting in physiology and radiographic appearance similar to tetralogy of Fallot. In the absence of pulmonic stenosis, preferential left ventricular to aortic flow may make cyanosis minimal. A VSD located beneath the pulmonic valve (Taussig-Bing malformation) causes preferential flow from the left ventricle into the pulmonary artery and consequently severe pulmonary arterial overcirculation. The right ventricular outflow is preferentially into the aorta; consequently, there is also cyanosis. Coarctation or interruption of the aortic arch is sometimes associated with the subpulmonic VSD. A large VSD may be situated beneath the origin of both great vessels (doubly committed VSD) or may be displaced away from both origins (noncommitted VSD). The great arteries tend to be side by side at the base of the heart, but either vessel can be located more anteriorly.

This is an admixture lesion that causes the combination of cyanosis (right-to-left shunt) and pulmonary arterial overcirculation (left-to-right shunt). The severity of pulmonic stenosis and the position of the VSD initially determine the relative severity of the two shunts.

Double-outlet left ventricle is an exceedingly rare anomaly in which both arteries originate from a morphologic left ventricle. The presentation and radiologic appearance are similar to double-outlet right ventricle (Tables 31-16 and 31-17; Fig. 31-37).

Tricuspid Atresia

Tricuspid atresia is the absence of a direct connection of the right atrium to the right ventricle. The atresia can be due to a membrane or a ridge of muscle between the cham-

TABLE 31-17. SALIENT RADIOGRAPHIC FEATURES OF DORV WITH PULMONIC STENOSIS

Decreased pulmonary vascularity
Normal or nearly normal cardiac size
Right ventricular prominence
Inconspicuous main pulmonary arterial segment
Right aortic arch in about 10%–15% of patients

bers. An atrial septal defect or patent foramen ovale is always present. Other associated lesions are frequent and are usually important in determining the physiology and clinical presentation. The most frequently associated lesions are TGA, VSD, and pulmonic stenosis. A classification of tricuspid atresia is based on the presence or absence of these associated lesions. Tricuspid atresia without TGA can be (1) with pulmonary atresia and no VSD; (2) with pulmonary stenosis and a small restrictive VSD; or (3) with no pulmonary stenosis and a large nonrestrictive VSD. Tricuspid atresia with TGA can be (1) with pulmonary atresia and a large VSD; (2) with pulmonary stenosis and a large VSD; or (3) with no pulmonary stenosis and a large VSD.

The most common form is tricuspid atresia with pulmonic stenosis and normally related great arteries and restrictive VSD. TGA is present in about 30% of patients with tricuspid atresia. It is usually associated with VSD and no pulmonic stenosis.

When the VSD is large and the pulmonary stenosis mild or nonexistent, there is pulmonary overcirculation. This is the situation both for normally related arteries and TGA. Restriction of pulmonary blood flow usually exists at pulmonic valvular and subvalvular levels or at a restrictive VSD. A small atrial septal communication also limits pulmonary

TABLE 31-16. SALIENT FEATURES OF DORV WITHOUT SIGNIFICANT PULMONIC STENOSIS

Pulmonary arterial overcirculation: It is one of the causes of cyanosis and pulmonary arterial overcirculation (see Fig. 31-37).
Cardiomegaly
Enlargement of left atrium, left ventricle, and right ventricle: Distinction between left and right ventricle enlargement during infancy is usually inconclusive.
Widened great artery pedicle due to side-by-side position of aorta and pulmonary artery (see Fig. 31-37): This is not always evident. It can be a distinguishing feature when compared to the appearance of d-TGA.
Prominent main pulmonary arterial segment: This can also be a distinguishing feature for DORV in comparison with d-TGA.
Signs of coarctation or interruption of the aortic arch

DORV, double-outlet right ventricle; TGA, transposition of the great arteries.

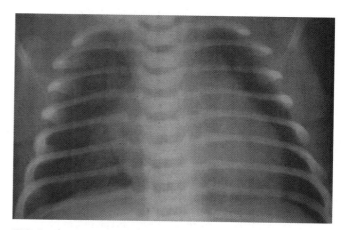

FIG. 31-37. Double-outlet right ventricle. Note pulmonary arterial overcirculation and cardiomegaly. Prominent great vessel region is shown in contradistinction to narrow great vessel region as seen in d-TGA.

TABLE 31-18. SALIENT RADIOGRAPHIC FEATURES OF TRICUSPID ATRESIA

With normally related great vessels, VSD, and pulmonic stenosis, the appearance is similar to tetralogy of Fallot (see Fig. 31-12). There is decreased pulmonary vascularity, small central pulmonary arteries, and normal or nearly normal heart size. A distinguishing feature from tetralogy, if discernible, is prominence of the left atrium and left ventricle and flat right atrial border (see Fig. 31-12).

With TGA, VSD without pulmonic stenosis, the typical feature of d-TGA, is present. There is pulmonary overcirculation, cardiomegaly, and a narrow vascular pedicle. A distinguishing feature may be the right atrial border. The right atrial border (right atrial enlargement) is frequently prominent in d-TGA, but it is not prominent or even flat in tricuspid atresia when the interatrial communication is large (see Figs. 31-12, 31-38, and 31-40).

With a small (restrictive) interatrial communication, the right atrium may enlarge considerably. The right atrium enlarges to the extent of causing considerable cardiomegaly as depicted on the frontal radiograph (see Fig. 31-39).

Tricuspid atresia with TGA is sometimes associated with left juxtaposition of the atrial appendages: the right atrial appendage extends posteriorly behind the great arteries and lies above the left atrial appendage. This causes a prominent upper left cardiac border and flattening of the right cardiac border (see Fig. 31-40).

VSD, ventricular septal defect; TGA, transposition of the great arteries.

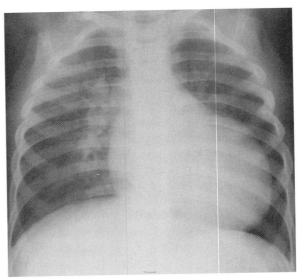

FIG. 31-38. Tricuspid atresia with transposition of great arteries. Radiograph shows the narrow base of the heart that is characteristic for transposition. Flat right atrial border is a feature of tricuspid atresia with nonrestrictive atrial septal defect.

flow and additionally causes the right atrium to enlarge. Despite obstruction to the right atrial outlet, the right atrium usually does not dilate since a large interatrial communication causes the right atrium to function as a venous conduit similar to the vena cavae (Table 31-18; Figs. 31-12 and 31-38 to 31-40).

Single Ventricle

Single ventricle consists of a predominant ventricle that receives both atrioventricular valves (double-inlet ventricle) and a tiny remnant portion of the other ventricle. A more specific term for most of the anomalies grouped under this title is *univentricular atrioventricular connections*. The great arteries can both originate from the dominant ventricle, or one may originate from the small ventricle. The dominant ventricle can be either the left or right.

Single ventricle is frequently associated with an abnormality of arterioventricular connection, such as TGA or double-outlet right ventricle. Normally related great vessels are uncommon with single ventricle. The left ventricular type of single ventricle is frequently associated with an inverted right ventricular outlet chamber and l-TGA. The dominant ventricle communicates with the outlet chamber through a "bulboventricular foramen."

The physiology is determined to a substantial degree by associated obstruction of the outflow to the pulmonary ar-

tery or aorta. There is an admixture of systemic and pulmonary venous blood in the dominant ventricle, so both cyanosis and pulmonary overcirculation occur. The presence and severity of the pulmonary overcirculation are regulated by pulmonary stenosis. If pulmonary stenosis is severe, the physiology and clinical presentation are similar to tetralogy of Fallot. If obstruction to pulmonary blood flow is not present, then the physiology and clinical presentation are similar to transposition. The physiology of the common ventricle is identical to a large VSD, which is really the

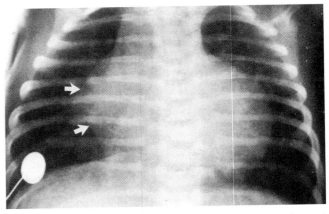

FIG. 31-39. Tricuspid atresia with small (restrictive) atrial septal defect and large ventricular septal defect. Small atrial septal defect is responsible for right atrial enlargement and thus cardiomegaly. Large ventricular septal defect results in pulmonary arterial overcirculation.

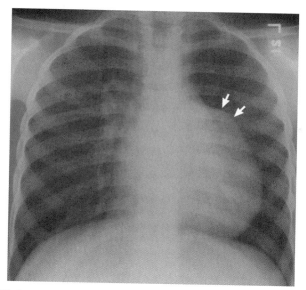

FIG. 31-40. Tricuspid atresia, transposition, and juxtaposition of atrial appendages. Prominent upper left cardiac border *(arrows)* is due to the abnormal position of the right atrial appendage on the left, above the left atrial appendage. The flat contour of the right atrium is also characteristic of this anomaly.

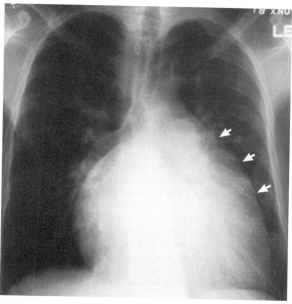

FIG. 31-41. Single ventricle with inverted outlet chamber (L-loop) and I-TGA. Prominent convexity of upper left cardiac border represents the inverted right ventricle outlet chamber *(arrows)* and the I-transposed ascending aorta.

proper designation for this lesion (Table 31-19; Fig. 31-41).

Truncus Arteriosus

Truncus arteriosus is a single trunk originating from the heart and supplying the pulmonary, systemic, and coronary arteries. The truncus straddles a large VSD. It is an admixture lesion, with both left-to-right and right-to-left shunts.

Two classification systems for truncus arteriosus are extant currently. The older and more familiar one was proposed by Collett and Edward in 1949. The types are grouped according to the site of origin of the pulmonary arteries from the truncus (Table 31-20; Fig. 31-42).

The truncal valve can have two to five cusps. The valves with numbers of cusps more or less than three are frequently incompetent, and truncal insufficiency can be severe. Hemitruncus is not infrequent; one pulmonary artery originates from the ascending aorta and the other arises directly from the right ventricle. Stenosis at the origin of the right and/or left pulmonary arteries is common, especially in types II

TABLE 31-19. SALIENT RADIOGRAPHIC APPEARANCE OF SINGLE VENTRICLE

With normally related arteries and no pulmonic stenosis, the appearance is like a VSD or d-TGA, depending on the preferential streaming in the ventricle. There is pulmonary overcirculation and cardiomegaly.

With significant pulmonic stenosis and normally related great arteries, the appearance is reduced pulmonary vascularity and normal or nearly normal heart size. The appearance is similar to tetralogy of Fallot.

With d-TGA, the appearance can be typical of d-TGA. Pulmonary blood flow may be increased or decreased.

With I-TGA, the appearance can be typical of I-TGA. Pulmonary blood flow may be increased or decreased. A notch along the upper left cardiac border may be due to the intersection of the contour of an inverted right ventricular outlet chamber with the dominant ventricle (see Fig. 31-41).

VSD, ventricular septal defect; TGA, transposition of the great arteries.

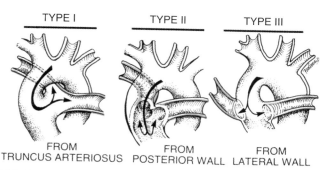

FIG. 31-42. The types of truncus arteriosus: type I, single origin of main pulmonary artery; type II, separate origins of left and right pulmonary arteries from dorsal aspect of the truncus; type III, separate origins of left and right pulmonary arteries from the left and right side of the truncus.

TABLE 31-20. TWO CLASSIFICATION SYSTEMS FOR TRUNCUS ARTERIOSUS

Type	Description
Grouped according to the site of origin of the pulmonary arteries from the truncus	
I	A main pulmonary artery originates from the proxima portion of the truncus, usually from the left posterolateral aspect
II	Right and left pulmonary arteries have individual origins from the posterior aspect of the truncus
III	One of both pulmonary arteries arises from the lateral aspect of the truncus
IV	No pulmonary arteries arise from the ascending truncus (aorta) but rather from the descending aorta. This type is not really a truncus arteriosus but rather pulmonary atresia with VSD and major pulmonary blood flow from bronchial and other systemic arteries originating from the descending aorta.
Classification of Van Pragh and Van Pragh	
I	Common pulmonary artery arises from truncus
II	Right and left pulmonary arteries arise separately from truncus
III	Absence of one pulmonary artery, other pulmonary artery arises from ductus
IV	Common pulmonary artery arises from truncus with arch interruption

TABLE 31-21. SALIENT RADIOGRAPHIC FEATURES OF TRUNCUS ARTERIOSUS

Pulmonary arterial overcirculation (see Fig. 31-4 and 31-17): Asymmetry of flow is not uncommon, even to the extent of plethora on one side and oligemia on the other.

Pulmonary venous hypertension or edema is frequent, especially in type I.

Cardiomegaly: The heart size is frequently but not always, proportionate to the pulmonary overcirculation. Cardiomegaly may also be related to truncal insufficiency.

Four chamber enlargement may be present.

Enlargement of left atrium and left ventricle is generally identified.

Prominent main pulmonary arterial segment (type I; see Fig. 31-4) or reduced main pulmonary arterial segment (type II or III): In type I, the left pulmonary artery has a higher position than usual, and a comma-shaped configuration ("hilar comma") as it curves upward and leftward (see Fig. 31-4).

Right aortic arch in about 35% of patients (see Figs. 31-4 and 31-17).

Dilated ascending aorta: There are two cyanotic lesions that are frequently associated with a large ascending aortic shadow: one causes decreased pulmonary vascularity (tetralogy of Fallot) and the other causes increased pulmonary vascularity (truncus arteriosus).

---

and III of Collett and Edwards. Consequently, asymmetry of blood flow occurs with this anomaly. A right aortic arch is common (Tables 31-21 and 31-22).

The physiology is characterized by excess pulmonary blood flow and frequently volume overload of especially left-sided chambers. This is one of the lesions causing pulmonary arterial overcirculation in a cyanotic patient. Congestive heart failure and pulmonary edema are common.

Total Anomalous Pulmonary Venous Connection

All pulmonary veins connect to a systemic venous structure or the right atrium directly in this anomaly. This is another admixture lesion. Generally, the pulmonary veins form a central confluence before entering the systemic venous site. Infrequently, they do not all join together and may drain to different sites. This anomaly is divided into three types based on the site of pulmonary venous drainage.

In the supracardiac type, connections are to the left innominate vein, right superior vena cava, or azygos vein. A left-sided vertical vein connects the pulmonary venous confluence to the left innominate vein. The cardiac type has connections to the right atrium or coronary sinus. In the infracardiac type, connection is below the diaphragm to the portal vein or one of its branches, ductus venosus,

or hepatic vein. In this type, a long vein courses from the pulmonary venous confluence and through the esophageal hiatus to its site of infradiaphragmatic connection. Pulmonary venous drainage is always obstructed with this type because of a variety of mechanisms, including narrowing or stenosis of the connecting vein at its site of connection with the systemic vein, or the systemic vein itself. The need for pulmonary venous blood to pass through the hepatic sinusoids has also been held to be an additional site of obstruction. However, portal venous pressure is not higher than pulmonary venous pressure in normal individuals. Infrequently, total anomalous pulmonary venous connection

TABLE 31-22. FREQUENCY OF RIGHT AORTIC ARCH IN CONGENITAL HEART DISEASE

Abnormality	Frequency (%)
Tetralogy of Fallot	20
Pulmonary atresia with ventricular septal defect	25
Truncus arteriosus	35
Double outlet right ventricle	12
Tricuspid atresia	10–15
Transposition of great arteries	5–8
Ventricular septal defect	2

TABLE 31-23. SALIENT RADIOGRAPHIC FEATURES OF TAPVC WITHOUT VENOUS OBSTRUCTION

Pulmonary arterial overcirculation (see Figs. 31-18 and 31-43). Pulmonary venous hypertension and edema may be present with extreme volume overload.

Cardiomegaly. This is usually proportionate to the pulmonary arterial overcirculation.

Enlargement of right atrium and right ventricle

The enlarged systemic vein into which drainage occurs or the anomalous connecting vein may be visible as the "snowman appearance" (see Figs. 31-18 and 31-43), dilated right superior vena cava, or dilated azygous vein or coronary sinus.

TAPVC, total anamalous pulmonary venous connections.

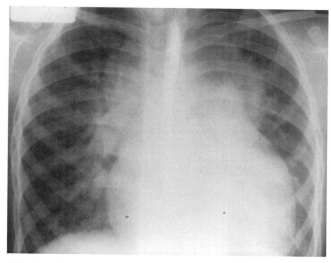

FIG. 31-43. Total anomalous pulmonary venous connection, supracardiac type (type I). Note pulmonary arterial overcirculation, cardiomegaly, and enlargement of superior mediastinum ("snowman" appearance). The snowman is caused by the dilated vertical vein connecting to the left innominate vein (left-sided enlargement) and the dilated superior vena cava (right-sided enlargement).

above the diaphragm is associated with pulmonary venous obstruction.

The physiology of total anomalous pulmonary venous connection depends on whether pulmonary venous obstruction exists. Mixing systemic and pulmonary venous blood occurs in the right atrium, and there is an obligatory right-to-left shunt of mixed venous blood through an interatrial connection. The size of the communication determines the volume of the flow to the left heart. Preferential flow from the right atrium is usually to the right ventricle and pulmonary artery, causing a large volume of recirculated blood. In total anomalous pulmonary venous connection above the diaphragm, the volume of pulmonary blood flow is very high and is the major feature, while cyanosis may be mild. The volume overload of the lungs may be so great that pulmonary edema occurs.

In total anomalous pulmonary venous connection with obstruction, the major feature is pulmonary venous hypertension and edema. The flow to the lungs is not very great. Because there is less pulmonary venous blood to mix with the desaturated systemic venous blood, cyanosis is conspicuous. Total anomalous pulmonary venous connection can occur in association with a number of other cardiac anomalies. It is a frequent lesion in patients with the asplenia syndrome (Tables 31-23 and 31-24; Fig. 31-43).

TABLE 31-24. SALIENT RADIOGRAPHIC FEATURES OF TAPVC WITH VENOUS OBSTRUCTION

Pulmonary edema (see Fig. 31-21)

Normal heart size

Prominence of right atrium and less frequently, right ventricle

Infrequently the connecting vein can be identified on the lateral view in a position behind the heart. A barium swallow may show an anterior impression on the esophagus.

TAPVC, total anamalous pulmonary venous connections.

Ebstein's Anomaly

Ebstein's anomaly is a deformity of the tricuspid valve in which one or more leaflets are displaced into the inflow portion of the right ventricle. The leaflets have lines of attachment to the right ventricle of varying length. The displacement into the right ventricle and the deformity of the valve cause tricuspid regurgitation, and the mural attachments in the right ventricle may cause obstruction to pulmonary blood flow. The septal and posterior leaflets are involved, while the anterior leaflet usually has a normal attachment to the atrioventricular ring. A small to substantial portion of the inflow region of the right ventricle has a thin wall and lacks ventricular myocardium (atrialization of the right ventricle). A patent foramen ovale or secundum atrial septal defect is present in about 80% of cases.

The physiologic consequence of the lesion is nearly always tricuspid regurgitation and usually a small-volume right-to-left shunt. Cyanosis may be absent or very mild. Occasionally the major effect is tricuspid obstruction, due to limitation of the atrioventricular inlet to only narrow slits in the displaced leaflets of the valve. In this circumstance the right-to-left shunt is more severe. In the 20% or so of patients without an interatrial communication, cyanosis is not present (Table 31-25).

Pulmonary Atresia With Intact Ventricular Septum

Pulmonary atresia with intact ventricular septum exists in two forms: hypoplasia of the right ventricle and tricuspid

TABLE 31-25. SALIENT RADIOGRAPHIC FEATURES OF EBSTEIN'S ANOMALY

Decreased pulmonary vascularity (see Figs. 31-3 and 31-14)
Cardiomegaly (see Figs. 31-3 and 31-14)
Enlarged right atrium: The right heart border is elongated, with a prominent convexity.
Enlargement of right ventricle. The right ventricle is less conspicuous than the atrium.
Main pulmonary arterial segment and hilar segments are small. However, the right ventricular outflow tract may produce a prominent bulge just caudal to the pulmonary arterial segment on the frontal view.
Small thoracic aorta

valve with little or no tricuspid regurgitation (type I) or a normal or enlarged right ventricle with significant tricuspid regurgitation (type II). This entity is distinct from pulmonary atresia with VSD (extreme form of tetralogy of Fallot).

The physiology of this lesion is reduced pulmonary blood flow, so that the volume of fully oxygenated blood entering the left atrium is small. The shunting of nearly all systemic venous blood occurs through the interatrial communication. There is admixture of desaturated and oxygenated blood in the left atrium. Because the volume of pulmonary venous blood is reduced, cyanosis is severe. Blood reaches the lung by a PDA and/or bronchial arteries (Tables 31-26 and 31-27).

Pulmonic Stenosis

Pulmonary valvular stenosis exists in two distinct syndromes. The most frequent type presents in an innocuous manner with mild symptoms, a systolic murmur, and a slightly abnormal thoracic radiograph. Infrequently, infants present with severe symptoms and marked cardiomegaly. The severity of the valvular stenosis is so great that the right ventricle dilates markedly and right ventricular failure ensues. Because of the elevated right-sided diastolic pressure,

TABLE 31-26. SALIENT RADIOGRAPHIC FEATURES OF TYPE I PULMONARY ATRESIA

Decreased pulmonary vascularity
Normal cardiac size or only slight cardiomegaly
Concave main pulmonary arterial segment and small hilar pulmonary arteries
Uplifted apex: This appearance may be due to left ventricular enlargement in the presence of a diminutive right ventricle.
Thoracic aorta can be enlarged.

TABLE 31-27. SALIENT RADIOGRAPHIC FEATURES OF TYPE II PULMONARY ATRESIA

Decreased pulmonary vascularity (see Fig. 31-13)
Cardiomegaly (see Fig. 31-13)
Right atrial and right ventricular enlargement
Small pulmonary arterial segment
Thoracic aorta may be enlarged.

there is considerable right-to-left shunting across a secundum atrial septal defect or stretched foramen ovale. When the stenosis is so severe that right ventricular failure occurs, the entity is called critical pulmonary stenosis (Tables 31-28 and 31-29; Fig. 31-44).

TABLE 31-28. SALIENT FEATURES OF COMPENSATED VALVULAR PULMONIC STENOSIS

Normal pulmonary vascularity
Normal cardiac size
Right ventricular enlargement or prominence: This is usually detected initially on the lateral view as a prominent convexity of the anterior cardiac border or filling of the retrosternal space.
Poststenotic dilatation of main pulmonary arterial segment (see Fig. 31-44)
Dilated and usually laterally displaced left pulmonary artery (see Fig. 31-44)

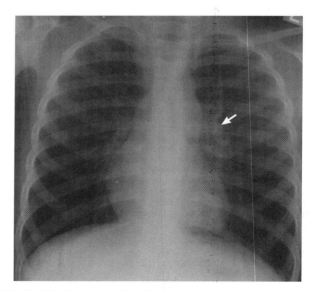

FIG. 31-44. Valvular pulmonic stenosis. Radiograph shows enlargement of the main and left pulmonary arterial *(arrow)* segments. The descending branch of the left pulmonary artery is frequently very prominent.

TABLE 31-29. SALIENT RADIOGRAPHIC FEATURES OF CRITICAL PULMONIC STENOSIS

Decreased pulmonary vascularity
Cardiomegaly
Enlargement of right atrium and ventricle
Enlarged main pulmonary arterial segment

Hypoplastic Left Heart

This lesion consists of several or all of the following features: hypoplastic ascending aorta, severe aortic stenosis or atresia, hypoplastic left ventricle (thick wall and diminutive cavity), and mitral atresia. The coronary arteries are perfused by right-to-left flow across a PDA and retrograde into the ascending aorta. An atrial septal communication is present so that admixture of pulmonary and systemic venous blood occurs in the right atrium. Consequently, there is volume overload of the right-sided chambers and excess pulmonary blood flow. The usual clinical presentation is severe congestive heart failure in the first few days of life (Table 31-30; see Fig. 31-22).

Coarctation of the Aorta

Coarctation of the aorta is a narrowing of the distal aortic arch and/or proximal descending aorta due to a discrete fibromuscular ring or a long- or short-segment tunnel narrowing of the aortic isthmus. There may also be hypoplasia of the posterior portion of the aortic arch. The coarctation usually occurs adjacent to the site of attachment of the ligamentum arteriosus and distal to the left subclavian artery. The coarctation is infrequently proximal to the origin of the left subclavian artery. The coarctation can extend into the origin of the left subclavian artery, causing stenosis of this artery. Both of these situations cause lower arterial pressure in the left compared to the right pulmonary artery. Anomalous origin of the right subclavian artery (retroesophageal right subclavian artery) from a site distal to the coarctation causes lower arterial pressure in the right arm.

TABLE 31-30. SALIENT RADIOGRAPHIC FEATURES OF HYPOPLASTIC LEFT HEART

Pulmonary arterial overcirculation and/or pulmonary edema (see Fig. 31-22)
Cardiomegaly (see Fig. 31-22)
Prominent right-sided chambers, especially the right atrium (see Fig. 31-22)
Because of the patent ductus, the aortic arch may be prominent (see Fig. 31-22).

Coarctation may be associated with a wide variety of congenital lesions, but two occur with noticeable frequency: PDA and VSD. The triad of coarctation, VSD, and PDA has been called the coarctation syndrome and is especially frequent when the lesion presents in early infancy. A bicuspid aortic valve occurs in a high percentage of patients.

The physiology is hypertension in arteries originating proximal to the site of coarctation and reduced blood flow to arteries arising below the coarctation. If the coarctation occurs proximal to the site of origin of one of the subclavian arteries, then there is hypertension in only one arm and rib notching on only the side with hypertension. The numerous causes of rib notching are listed in Table 31-31. The fourth to eighth ribs are the ones usually notched; the third and ninth ribs are less frequently notched. The notching consists of scalloped regions on the undersurface of the posterior portion of the ribs. The posterior upper surface is infrequently involved. Sclerosis may outline the scalloped sites. Rib notching is unusual in patients younger than 5 years of age. Rib notching depends on the origin of the ipsilateral subclavian artery proximal to the site of the coarctation. Coarctation proximal to the left subclavian arterial origin causes right-sided rib notching only, while an anomalous origin of the right subclavian artery from a site below the coarctation produces unilateral left-sided notching.

Hypertension usually causes left ventricular hypertrophy

TABLE 31-31. CAUSE OF RIB NOTCHING

Aortic obstruction
  Coarctation of the aorta
  Interruption of the aorta
  Acquired obstruction of the aorta: Takayasu's aortitis, atherosclerotic obstruction, etc.
  Unusual causes of coarctation: neurofibromatosis, Williams' syndrome, rubella syndrome
Subclavian arterial obstruction
  Blalock-Taussig shunt (upper two ribs)
  Takayasu's arteritis (usually unilateral)
  Atherosclerosis
Severely reduced pulmonary blood flow
  Tetralogy of Fallot
  Pulmonary atresia
  Tricuspid atresia
  Unilateral absence or atresia of a pulmonary artery
  Pulmonary emphysema
  Chronic pulmonary thromboembolic disease
Superior vena canal obstruction
Vascular shunts
  Pulmonary arteriovenous shunt
  Intercostal arteriovenous shunt
  Intercostal to pulmonary arterial shunt
Intercostal neuroma
Poliomyelitis (upper margin)
Hyperparathyroidism

(Modified from Felson B. Chest Roentgenology. Philadelphia: WB Saunders, 1973.)

TABLE 31-32. SALIENT RADIOGRAPHIC FEATURES IN COMPENSATED COARCTATION

Rib notching (see Fig. 31-45)

Retrosternal undulating soft tissue due to dilated tortuous internal mammary arteries (site of collateral flow)

Abnormal appearance of the aortic arch (see Fig. 31-45)

A notch on the proximal descending aorta followed by poststenotic dilatation causes a figure-3 sign on the aorta (see Fig. 31-45) and a reverse figure-3 sign on the barium-filled esophagus.

Left ventricular prominence

Prominent ascending aorta

A duplicated aortic "knob" may be caused by tortuosity of the posterior arch and proximal descending aorta causing kinking of the aorta: This is called pseudocoarctation of the aorta when no pressure gradient exists.

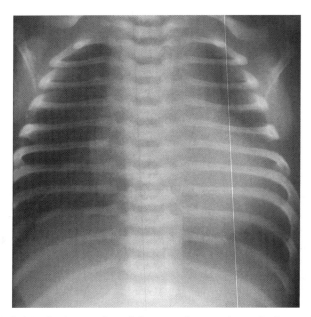

FIG. 31-46. Coarctation of the aorta in a newborn. Radiograph shows severe cardiomegaly without pulmonary arterial overcirculation. This is characteristic of a group V lesion, of which coarctation is the most frequent cause after 1 week of age.

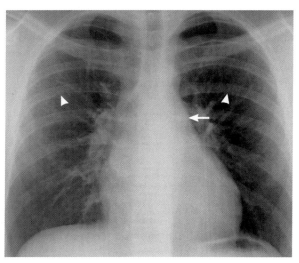

FIG. 31-45. Coarctation of the aorta. Abnormal contour of arch and proximal descending aorta. The duplicated aortic knob is due to poststenotic dilatation *(arrow)* in the proximal descending aorta. There is outward displacement of the lateral margin of the descending aorta. A figure-3 configuration is caused by the notch at the site of the coarctation with poststenotic dilatation. Rib notching is present *(arrowheads)*.

but may induce left ventricular dilatation and failure if extremely severe. Left ventricular dilatation, myocardial failure, and pulmonary edema are most likely to occur in early infancy (Tables 31-32 and 31-33; Figs. 31-45 and 31-46).

Interruption of Aortic Arch

The arch can be interrupted at any of three sites: beyond the left subclavian artery (type A); between the left subclavian and left common carotid arteries (type B); and between the innominate artery and left carotid artery (type C). Types A and B occur with approximately equal frequency; type C is rare. The right subclavian artery sometimes originates

TABLE 31-33. SALIENT RADIOGRAPHIC FEATURES IN DECOMPENSATED COARCTATION

Pulmonary venous hypertension or edema

Cardiomegaly (see Fig. 31-46)

Left ventricular enlargement

Pulmonary arterial overcirculation is present, with associated ventricular septal defect and patent ductus arteriosus.

Rib notching is not present during infancy.

The aortic knob is usually not characteristic during infancy. The only sign may be lateral displacement of the descending aortic stripe.

TABLE 31-34. SALIENT RADIOGRAPHIC FEATURES OF INTERRUPTION OF AORTIC ARCH

Isolated variety has the appearance as described for coarctation.

Interruption with ventricular septal defect and patent ductus arteriosus causes pulmonary arterial overcirculation and usually severe pulmonary edema with cardiomegaly (see Fig. 31-47).

The trachea is sometimes identified to lie exactly in the midline, and there is no indentation on the trachea (see Figs. 31-47 and 31-48).

If a patent ductus arteriosus is present, the posterior arch may be prominent yet the trachea, not indented, lies exactly in the midline (see Fig. 31-47).

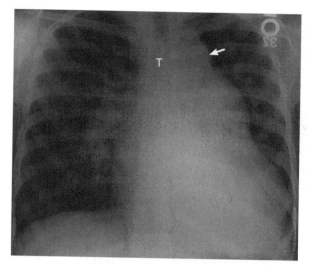

FIG. 31-47. Interruption of aortic arch with ventricular septal defect and patent ductus arteriosus. Radiograph shows pulmonary arterial overcirculation, cardiomegaly due to left ventricular enlargement, and enlargement of main pulmonary arterial and aortic arch segments. Despite the enlarged aortic arch segment *(arrow)*, the trachea *(T)* is situated directly in the midline.

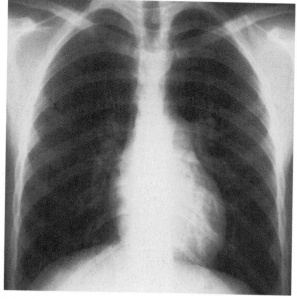

FIG. 31-49. Supravalvular aortic stenosis. Concavity is seen in the region occupied by the ascending aorta.

ectopically as a fourth aortic branch in this anomaly, which is called a type B2 interruption. In this circumstance, hypertension is confined to the carotid arteries.

This lesion can exist in an isolated form but usually is associated with VSD and PDA. There is an association with double-outlet right ventricle with subpulmonic VSD (Taussig-Bing malformation; Table 31-34; Figs. 31-47 and 31-48).

TABLE 31-35. SALIENT RADIOGRAPHIC FEATURES IN UNCOMPLICATED AORTIC STENOSIS

Normal heart size
Enlargement of ascending aorta: This occurs in valvular stenosis and about half of patients with discrete membranous subvalvular stenosis.
Ascending aorta is small in supravalvular form (see Fig. 31-49).

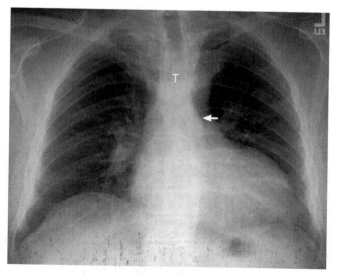

FIG. 31-48. Interruption of the aortic arch as an isolated anomaly. Radiographs show midline trachea and dilated proximal descending aorta *(arrow)* below the narrow site of interruption.

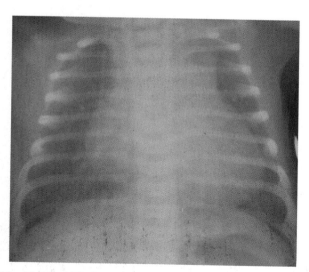

FIG. 31-50. Critical aortic stenosis. Radiograph in an infant shows pulmonary edema and cardiomegaly.

TABLE 31-36. SALIENT RADIOGRAPHIC FEATURES OF CRITICAL AORTIC STENOSIS

Pulmonary venous hypertension or edema (see Fig. 31-50)
Cardiomegaly (see Fig. 31-50)
Left ventricular enlargement

Aortic Stenosis

Congenital aortic stenosis is caused by a bicuspid aortic valve, unicuspid and unicommissural, or dysplastic valves.

It may be so severe as to induce intractable left ventricular failure in the neonate (critical aortic stenosis). Stenosis also occurs at the subvalvular (discrete membranous or tunnel forms) and supravalvular sites (Tables 31-35 and 31-36; Figs. 31-49 and 31-50; see also Table 32-1 in Chapter 32).

SELECTED READING

Elliott LB. Cardiac Imaging in Infants, Children, and Adults. Philadelphia: JB Lippincott, 1991.

Higgins CB. Radiography of congenital heart disease. In: Essentials of Cardiac Radiology and Imaging. Philadelphia: JB Lippincott, 1992:49.

32

VALVULAR HEART DISEASE

CHARLES B. HIGGINS

The goals of imaging in valvular heart disease are as follows:

1. Identification of stenosis or insufficiency of one or more valves
2. Estimation of the pressure gradient (or valve orifice area) and severity or volume of regurgitation
3. Quantification of ventricular volume, mass, and function
4. Sequential monitoring of ventricular volume, mass and function. Determination of response to therapy
5. Exclusion of significant coronary artery disease, especially prior to surgery.

Echocardiography is the most commonly used technique for the evaluation of valvular disease. For the most part, it has replaced cardiac catheterization for definitive diagnoses and assessment of severity of valvular dysfunction. The echocardiographic aspects of valvular heart disease are the topic of a number of chapters in other textbooks. The current role of angiography is the exclusion of significant coronary artery disease before surgery or as a contributing factor for heart failure in these patients. In the future, noninvasive imaging of coronary arteries by MR or multidetector CT may suffice for these purposes.

All valvular lesions exert a stress on the supporting ventricle. Valvular stenosis exerts a pressure overload, which involves the compensatory mechanism of myocardial hypertrophy. Regurgitation exerts a volume overload, which involves chamber dilatation. Eventually these compensatory mechanisms are dissipated, and in the end stage of valvular heart disease, myocardial failure and low cardiac output state ensue.

AORTIC STENOSIS

Aortic stenosis usually is described at three anatomic levels: supravalvular, valvular, and subvalvular. The classification of the types of aortic stenosis is presented in Table 32-1.

Supravalvular stenosis nearly always is a congenital anomaly, either as an isolated lesion or as part of the Williams syndrome. The supravalvular narrowing has roughly three configurations: focal constriction at the sinotubular junction (hourglass configuration) with poststenotic dilation of the mid and distal ascending aorta; focal membrane at the sinotubular junction; and tubular narrowing from the sinotubular junction to just below the origin of the innominate artery. The Williams syndrome is characterized by hypercalcemia, elfin facies, variable mental retardation and characteristic personality ("cocktail party personality"), hypertension, and additional peripheral arterial stenoses.

Concomitant cardiovascular lesions variably associated with supravalvular aortic stenosis include (1) aortic and pulmonary valvular stenoses, (2) peripheral pulmonary arterial stenoses, (3) diffuse hypoplasia of the aorta, (4) discrete stenoses of branches of the aortic arch and abdominal aorta, and (5) stenoses at region of the coronary arteries.

However, the coronary arteries usually are ectatic because they originate below the obstruction at the sinotubular junction and are thereby subjected to elevated pressure.

Valvular aortic stenosis may have either a congenital or acquired etiology. The congenital cause most often is a bicuspid aortic valve. A less common cause is a unicuspid valve; this type of valve causes more severe stenosis, usually presenting in the first year of life. A rare pathology is the primitive valve, usually consisting of a hypoplastic annulus containing a ring of gelatinous tissue. This lesion also presents most often during infancy. Rheumatic valvular aortic stenosis commonly occurs in association with mitral stenosis or regurgitation. Degenerative aortic stenosis is now the most frequent cause of calcific aortic stenosis in the adult. Although degenerative aortic stenosis once was considered to be a result of premature fibrosis and calcification of a bicuspid aortic valve, it is now recognized as degeneration of tricuspid aortic valves in elderly patients. The bicuspid aortic valve degenerates into hemodynamically significant aortic stenosis in the fourth and fifth decade; the tricuspid aortic valve degenerates into hemodynamically significant stenosis usually after the sixth decade. With the aging of the population, this type of aortic stenosis is becoming the most commonly encountered type. All types of acquired aortic stenosis are characterized by heavy calcification (calcific aortic stenosis).

TABLE 32-1. CLASSIFICATION OF AORTIC STENOSIS

Supravalvular
Congenital
  Hourglass shape
  Membranes or fibrous diaphragm
  Diffuse
Valvular
Congenital
  Bicuspid
  Unicuspid
  Primitive
  Annular hypoplasia
Acquired
  Rheumatic
  Degenerative
Subvalvular
Congenital
  Discrete
  Membranous
  Fibromuscular tunnel
  Extra mitral valve tissue
  Idiopathic hypertrophic subaortic stenosis (hypertrophic cardiomyopathy—asymmetric type)

Subvalvular aortic stenosis. Congenital subvalvular stenosis is caused most commonly by a thin membrane situated within 1 cm beneath the aortic cusps. Other types consist of a discrete fibromuscular ring or tunnel-like narrowing of the left ventricular (LV) outlet region. Redundant gelatinous tissue attached to the anterior mitral valve leaflet also may rarely cause subvalvular stenoses, either alone or as part of an endocardial cushion anomaly. Muscular subaortic stenosis is caused by the asymmetric form of hypertrophic cardiomyopathy.

Radiography

The findings on chest x-ray in **valvular aortic stenosis** depend on the severity and level of the obstruction and the age at presentation (see Table 30-6 in Chapter 30). The x-ray image in infants presenting with symptoms of heart failure is characterized by pulmonary edema and cardiomegaly. Cardiomegaly without pulmonary edema also may occur. On the other hand, x-rays in older children and adults may display only enlargement of the ascending aorta. In the presence of severe LV hypertrophy (reduced ventricular compliance) or with the onset of myocardial failure, pulmonary venous hypertension or edema may become evident. This usually occurs late in the natural history of uncomplicated valvular aortic stenosis. The extent and density of aortic valvular calcification roughly parallel the severity of the stenosis in adults before the seventh decade. On the other hand, ascending aortic dilation does not correlate

with severity of stenosis and may be substantial with a nonobstructive bicuspid valve.

Supravalvular aortic stenosis may cause a narrow base of the heart with inconspicuous ascending aortic region (right superior mediastinum; see Chapter 31). With **subvalvular aortic stenosis,** enlargement of the ascending aorta, often is not evident on the chest x-ray. Ascending aortic enlargement is discernible in about 50% of patients with the membranous type of subvalvular stenosis.

Magnetic Resonance Imaging

Magnetic resonance imaging (MRI) can be used to identify valvular dysfunction and to assess the effect of the lesion on ventricular volumes, mass, and function. In addition to identifying stenosis and regurgitation, the gradient across stenotic valves and volume of valvular regurgitation can be quantified. Sequential MR studies can be used for monitoring the severity of the valvular lesion and ventricular function over time and in response to therapy.

Identification of Aortic Stenosis

Aortic stenosis is identified using cine MR images. Cine MR imaging consists of multiple gradient echo (GRE) images in which the blood under normal flow conditions has bright (white) signal intensity. High-velocity jet flow, such as occurs with the flow across a valvular stenosis or the retrograde flow across a regurgitant orifice, produces a signal void (low-signal region within the bright signal of the blood pool). Identification of valvular stenosis on GRE images is based on the typical appearance of the downstream chamber or great artery. The signal void of a dysfunctional valve appears as an area of diminished or absent signal persisting for most of systole or diastole. Aortic stenosis is detected readily on images in coronal, axial, and vertical long-axis planes, which display an area of signal loss distal to the valve during ventricular systole (Fig. 32-1).

Recognition of the signal void on cine MR images is critically dependent on the TE value employed. The signal void diminishes in area with decreasing TE value. Indeed, the signal void may not be discernible with TE values of less than 6 msec. For depiction of the signal void, a TE value of 12 or greater is generally used.

Estimation of Valve Gradient

The valve gradient is estimated using velocity-encoded (VEC; phase contrast) cine MRI. VEC cine MRI measures the phase shifts that accumulate as hydrogen nuclei move through a magnetic field gradient. The net phase shifts of protons within various voxels are displayed in gray levels, in proportion to the degree of phase shift. Because phase shift is basically proportional to motion over time, VEC

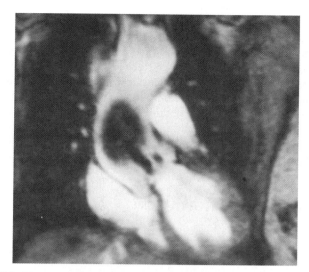

FIG. 32-1. Cine (gradient echo) MR image in the coronal plane during systole demonstrates a signal void emanating from the aortic valve in a patient with valvular aortic stenosis.

cine MRI can be used to measure flow velocity. Reconstruction of VEC data provides a magnitude image (anatomic information) and a phase image (velocity information in selected direction; Fig. 32-2). The velocity-encoding direction can be selected in any orientation or in all three dimensions. The cross-sectional area of the vessel can be measured by drawing a region of interest on the magnitude (amplitude) image. The same region of interest is then applied on the corresponding phase image, where spatial mean velocity is measured. The product of area and spatial mean velocity

provides the instantaneous flow volume for a specific time frame of the cardiac cycle. Integration of all instantaneous flow volumes throughout the cardiac cycle (usually 16 or higher) gives volume flow per heartbeat (see Fig. 32-2B). This technique has been validated in vitro with flow phantoms and in vivo by comparing flow measurements in the pulmonary artery and the aorta with left and right stroke volumes measured by cine GRE in healthy volunteers.

Although the signal void on cine GRE caused by turbulence allows identification of stenosis or regurgitation, signal loss potentially can vitiate quantification of velocity at such sites. It has been shown, however, that the reduction of echo time to 3.6 msec or less minimizes the problem of signal loss and that jet velocities up to 6.0 m/sec can be measured accurately in a flow phantom by phase-contrast MR imaging. Peak systolic jet velocities over 5.0 m/sec have been measured with this technique in patients with aortic stenosis. These values determined by phase-shift GRE have correlated with Doppler flow and catheter measurements. Using the measurement of peak velocity by VEC MR imaging, the pressure gradient can be estimated by the modified Bernoulli equation as $\Delta P = 4V^2$, where ΔP = pressure drop across the stenosis (mmHg) and V = peak velocity (msec). An example of the use of VEC to estimate the gradient across valvular aortic stenosis as derived from VEC measurement of a peak velocity of 4 meters per second looks like this:

$$\Delta P = 4V^2$$

$$\Delta P = 4(4)^2$$

$$\Delta P = 64 \text{ mmHg}$$

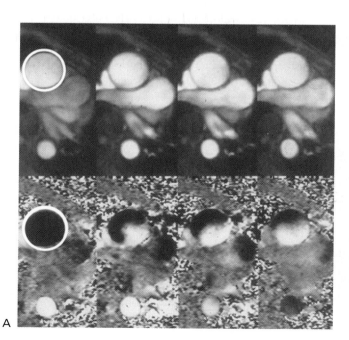

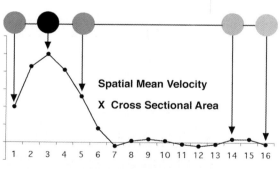

FIG. 32-2. **A.** Four magnitude (**top**) and phase (**bottom**) images acquired during the cardiac cycle to measure blood flow in the aorta. Regions of interest are drawn around the aorta on magnitude images to measure cross-sectional area and around phase images to measure spatial average velocity. Volumetric flow is the product of cross-sectional area and spatial average velocity. **B.** Schematic diagram of aortic blood flow versus time curve during an average cardiac cycle. Each point on the curve is derived from a pair of images acquired at 16 time points during a cardiac cycle.

However, it should be noted that this measurement by VEC has limitations. The number of images reconstructed for a cardiac cycle may lack temporal resolution for capturing the exact instant when peak velocity occurs. The direction of flow encoding may differ from the flow direction of the jet. These limitations can be minimized by using three-dimensional flow encoding, but this further reduces temporal resolution.

Quantification of Left Ventricular Volume, Mass, and Function

Ventricular mass and function can be measured precisely from a three-dimensional set of cine MR images that can be acquired in any plane. In contrast to echocardiography and cineangiocardiography, MR imaging does not rely on geometric assumptions or calculations based on partial sampling of the cardiac volume. Typically, a set of contiguous tomograms encompassing the entire heart from the apex to the bifurcation of the pulmonary artery is acquired. Cine MR images typically are acquired at 16 phases of the cardiac cycle. These images can be laced together and displayed in a cinematic format. When viewed in the cinematic format, it is possible to assess global right ventricular (RV) and LV function and to assess wall thickening and motion to define regional myocardial function. Breathhold cine MR imaging is possible by acquiring multiple lines of k-space within one R-R interval. Typical parameter settings (TR = 9 ms, TE = 2.8 ms, matrix = 256 × 128 pixels, 8 lines of k-space collected in every R-R interval) permit acquisition of 128 phase-encoding steps in only 16 heartbeats or within one breathhold period. In recent years, hybrid echo planar and balanced steady-state free precession sequences have been developed that provide more images (frames) per cardiac cycle and substantially reduce image acquisition time. The optimal technique for maximizing contrast between blood and myocardium is the use of balanced steady-state free precession sequences—true fast imaging with steady precession (FISP), balanced fast-field echo (FFE), and (FIESTA) (Fig. 32-3).

Ventricular cavity volumes are simply calculated as the sum of the cavity area times the slice thickness. Interobserver variabilities for LV end-diastolic volume and LV end-systolic volume have been shown to be less than 5% and 10%, respectively. Mass measurements are highly accurate, with excellent interstudy and interobserver variabilities for LV mass of less than 5%. Because interstudy variabilities of ventricular volumetric and mass measurements by cine MR imaging are small, this technique is ideal for monitoring the effectiveness of therapy in patients with aortic stenosis.

AORTIC REGURGITATION

Aortic regurgitation imposes a volume overload on the left ventricle as a consequence of retrograde flow across the aortic valve during diastole. Because of the excessive diastolic volume, the left ventricle becomes dilated. Regurgitation may be caused by lack of coaptation of the valvular cusps, annular dilatation, or ascending aortic dilatation. Aortic regurgitation has a number of possible causes (Table 32-2); moreover, it may be a component of several systemic diseases and inherited syndromes (Table 32-3). With some causes, there may be abnormalities at more than one site (e.g., Marfan's syndrome, aortoannular ectasia, and relapsing polychondritis).

Radiography

Findings on the chest x-ray are governed by the severity and chronicity of aortic regurgitation and whether there is associated pathology of the ascending aorta (see Table 30-13 in Chapter 30). The typical features of chronic regurgitation are (1) absence of pulmonary venous hypertension or edema, (2) cardiomegaly due to LV enlargement, and (3) ascending aortic and arch enlargement. Pulmonary venous hypertension and edema usually occur late in the natural history of chronic aortic regurgitation and signify the onset of myocardial failure. On the other hand, acute regurgita-

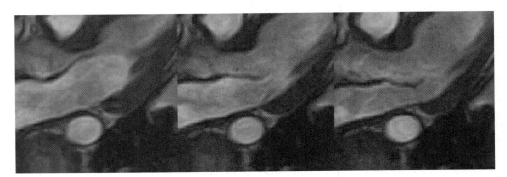

FIG. 32-3. Magnified views of cine MR images (balanced steady-state free precession) in the left ventricular outflow plane depict opening and closing of aortic and mitral valves. Images show three time points: diastole (**left**), near end-diastole (**center**), and systole (**right**).

TABLE 32-2. ETIOLOGY OF AORTIC REGURGITATION

Aortic cusps abnormality
  Bicuspid aortic valve
  Rheumatic disease
  Infective endocarditis
  Supracristal ventricular septal defect
  Syphilis
Aortic annulus abnormality
  Aortoannular ectasia
  Systemic hypertension
  Marfan's syndrome
  Aortic dissection (type A)
  Ankylosing spondylitis
  Relapsing polychondritis
Ascending aorta abnormality
  Aortoannular ectasia
  Marfan's syndrome
  Ehlers-Danlos syndrome
  Aortic dissection (type A)
  Relapsing polychondritis
  Ascending aortic aneurysm

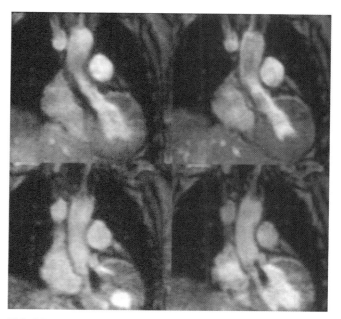

FIG. 32-4. Coronal cine MR images in systole (**top**) and diastole (**bottom**). The signal void emanating from the closed aortic valve in diastole indicates aortic regurgitation.

tion such as occurs with infective endocarditis may produce severe pulmonary edema even with normal cardiac size. Severe enlargement of the ascending aorta may reflect specific pathologies such as aortoannular ectasia, Marfan's syndrome, or ascending aortic aneurysm.

Magnetic Resonance Imaging

MRI is used to identify the presence and quantify the volume of aortic regurgitation. It also is used to monitor the effect of regurgitation on LV volumes, mass, and function.

TABLE 32-3. SYSTEMIC DISEASES OR INHERITED SYNDROMES ASSOCIATED WITH AORTIC REGURGITATION

Inherited syndromes
Marfan's syndrome
Ehler-Danlos syndrome
Osteogenesis imperfecta
Pseudoxanthoma elasticum
Systemic diseases
Rheumatoid arthritis
Rheumatoid variants
  Ankylosing spondylitis
  Psoriatic arthritis
  Reiter's syndrome
Relapsing polychondritis
Giant cell aortitis
Syphilis (luetic aortitis)

Identification of Aortic Regurgitation

Cine GRE imaging demonstrates the regurgitant jet as a signal void. This signal void emanates from the closed aortic valve and projects into the left ventricle during most or all of the diastolic period (Figs. 32-4 to 32-6). The area and volume of the signal void correspond roughly to the severity of regurgitation and thus serve as a semiquantitative estimate of aortic regurgitation. However, the size of the signal void depends on the TE value used and may not be evident with reduction of the TE below 6 msec. Additionally, the size of the signal void can be influenced by regurgitant orifice, LV diastolic pressure and function, aortic pressure, and orientation of the imaging plane to the direction of the regurgitant jet.

Acceleration of flow proximal to the regurgitant orifice (proximal convergence zone) produces a second flow void in the aorta just above the valve. The area of this signal void also provides an estimate of the severity of regurgitation. However, this measurement is not employed in clinical practice.

Quantification of Regurgitant Volume

Cine MR imaging also can be used for assessment of regurgitant volume by determining RV and LV stroke volumes. In the normal subject, RV stroke volume is nearly equivalent to LV stroke volume. Stroke volumes are calculated from a stack of MR images as the difference between end-diastolic and end-systolic volumes of each ventricle. The regurgitant

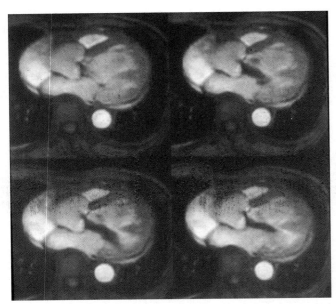

FIG. 32-5. Axial cine MR images starting at end-systole (**top left**) and in early, mid, and late diastole (**bottom right**). A signal void emanates from the aorta valve in diastole, indicating aortic regurgitation.

volume can be calculated by the difference between RV and LV stroke volumes. These calculations are valid only for patients with a single regurgitant valve. In patients with combined aortic and mitral regurgitation, this method assesses the total regurgitant volume of the left side of the heart.

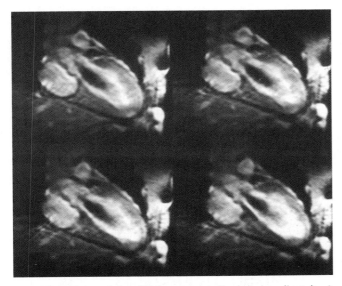

FIG. 32-6. Coronal cine MR images acquired during diastole. A signal void starts at the aortic valve and is projected into the LV chamber, indicating aortic regurgitation.

Another method for quantification of regurgitation is VEC cine MRI. With this technique, regurgitant volume can be calculated in two different ways. First, the regurgitant volume can be assessed by the difference between the systolic flow in the ascending aorta (LV stroke volume) and the systolic flow in the main pulmonary artery (RV stroke volume). The two stroke volumes are calculated from time-integrated measurements of flow volumes during systole on imaging perpendicular to the proximal ascending and another perpendicular to the main pulmonary.

VEC cine MRI can discriminate between antegrade and retrograde flow during the cardiac cycle, enabling retrograde flow to be measured directly to quantify regurgitation. For example, bright voxels in the ascending aorta during systole indicate antegrade flow, whereas dark voxels in diastole represent retrograde flow caused by aortic regurgitation (Fig. 32-7A). High accuracy and interstudy reproducibility ($r = 0.97$) of VEC MRI measurement of retrograde diastolic flow in the ascending aorta have been found in patients with chronic aortic regurgitation. Diastolic retrograde aortic flow equals aortic regurgitant volume (see Fig. 32-7B). The measurements of regurgitant volume and fraction by this method correlate closely with volumetric cine MRI measurements ($r > 0.97$). Measurement of regurgitant volume by this method in a group of patients evaluated at two separate occasions demonstrated high interstudy reproducibility ($r > 0.97$). This suggests that this approach is useful for follow-up and monitoring response to therapy in patients with aortic regurgitation.

Quantification of Left Ventricular Volumes, Mass, and Function

As discussed earlier in the section on aortic stenosis, cine MRI provides a highly accurate and reproducible measurement of ventricular volumes, mass, and function. The high interstudy reproducibility of these measurements makes it attractive for monitoring these parameters over time in patients with aortic regurgitation in order to document response to pharmacologic therapy and to recognize the appropriate time for valve replacement.

Cine MRI has disclosed the typical effect of aortic regurgitation on the left ventricle. According to the severity of regurgitation, there is an increase in LV end-diastolic and end-systolic volumes. Although LV wall thickness may be within the normal range (less than 12 mm at end diastole), the total LV mass may be increased substantially because of the increase in end-diastolic volume (mass = mean wall thickness × end-diastolic volume). Cine MRI demonstrates elevated LV stroke volume. The total stroke volume consists of the effective stroke volume and regurgitant volume. During the compensated phase of aortic regurgitation, the effective stroke volume remains in the normal range.

The following formulas are relevant for aortic regurgitation:

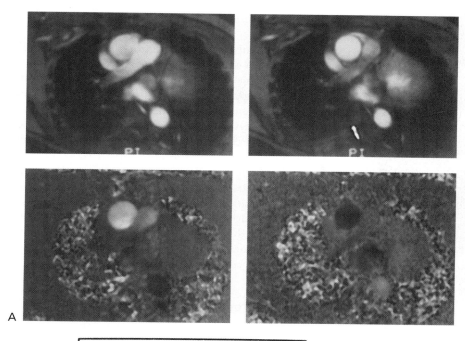

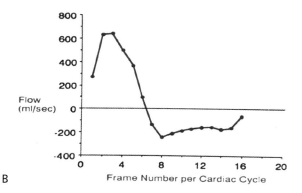

FIG. 32-7. **A.** Velocity-encoded cine MR images in the axial plane in aortic regurgitation. Magnitude (**top**) and phase (**bottom**) images in systole (**left**) and diastole (**right**). Note that on the phase images antegrade flow in systole is represented by bright voxels, whereas retrograde flow (aortic regurgitation) in diastole is represented by dark voxels in the ascending aorta. **B.** A flow-versus-time curve derived from image pairs at 16 phases of the cardiac cycle shows negative values (retrograde flow) in diastole. The area under the curve with negative values is the volume of aortic regurgitation.

Total LV stroke volume = effective stroke volume + regurgitant volume

Regurgitant volume = LV stroke volume − RV stroke volume

Regurgitant fraction = regurgitant volume/total LV stroke volume

MITRAL STENOSIS

Mitral stenosis usually is acquired and nearly always is caused by rheumatic fever. It is the salient lesion of rheumatic heart disease. Other etiologies are rare; these include congenital valvular, subvalvular (parachute mitral valve), or supravalvular stenosis; left atrial myxoma; and exuberant mitral annular calcification. Mitral stenosis often is accompanied by a variable degree of mitral regurgitation.

Mitral stenosis causes elevated left atrial pressure throughout diastole, and pulmonary venous hypertension produces pulmonary arterial hypertension. In long-standing mitral stenosis, pulmonary arterial hypertension may be severe, and pulmonary regurgitation eventually ensues across a dilated pulmonary annulus. The right ventricle eventually dilates, causing tricuspid regurgitation from a dilated annulus.

Radiography

The chest x-ray provides good insight into the severity of mitral stenosis by showing the relative severity of pulmonary

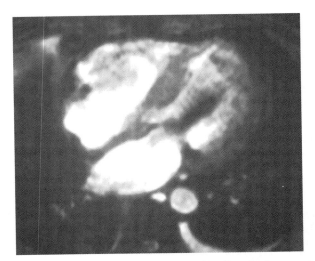

FIG. 32-8. Axial cine MR image acquired in diastole shows a signal void arising at the opened mitral valve leaflets. This is caused by mitral stenosis.

venous hypertension (see Table 30-8 in Chapter 30). In mild disease there may be only equalization or reversal of the diameter of upper and lower lobe pulmonary vessels (cephalization). In more severe disease or with an imposed hypervolemic state, interstitial pulmonary edema or alveolar pulmonary edema becomes evident. Interlobular septal thickening (Kerley B lines) usually are a sign of interstitial edema but may become permanent as a consequence of fibrosis or deposition of hemosiderin after multiple episodes of pulmonary edema. Rarely, high-density nodules (ossific nodules) in the lower lobes may be a consequence

of multiple episodes of alveolar pulmonary edema and hemorrhage.

In compensated mitral stenosis, only mild cardiomegaly or normal heart size is seen. The left atrium invariably is enlarged, causing a right retrocardiac double density. A convexity on the upper left cardiac border in the frontal view indicates enlargement of the left atrial appendage. This finding nearly always is evident in rheumatic mitral stenosis. Enlargement of the pulmonary arterial segment and right heart indicates pulmonary arterial hypertension. Enlargement of the right heart in the absence of pulmonary arterial enlargement usually indicates concomitant rheumatic tricuspid regurgitation.

The ascending aorta and aortic arch are characteristically small in isolated mitral valve disease. Even slight prominence of the thoracic aorta should raise suspicion of associated rheumatic aortic valve disease.

Magnetic Resonance Imaging

Magnetic resonance imaging can be used to identify mitral valvular stenosis and any associated mitral regurgitation; estimate the gradient across the valve; and quantify ventricular volume, mass, and function.

Identification of Mitral Stenosis

Cine MR images, using a TE greater than 6 msec, demonstrates a signal void emanating from the opened mitral valve in diastole and projected into the left ventricle (Fig. 32-8). This signal void is depicted well on images acquired in the axial or horizontal long-axis planes. Associated mitral regur-

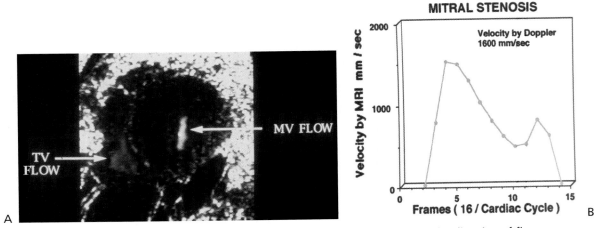

FIG. 32-9. A. Phase (velocity) image acquired in a plane perpendicular to the direction of flow across a stenotic mitral valve. The high-intensity elliptically shaped area is the flow channel of the stenotic mitral valve *(MV)*. This area is interrogated for the peak velocity during diastole to estimate the pressure gradient using the modified Bernoulli equation (peak gradient = 4 × peak velocity^2. **B.** Velocity versus time curve in mitral stenosis. The peak velocity in early diastole is slightly lower than the peak velocity measured by Doppler echocardiography.

gitation appears as a signal void projected into the left atrium during systole. Likewise, signal voids may be recognized in right-sided cardiac chambers if there is any associated pulmonary or tricuspid regurgitation.

Estimation of Valve Gradient

VEC (phase contrast) cine MRI is acquired in planes perpendicular or parallel to the stenotic jet (flow void) to sample the peak velocity of the jet (as discussed earlier in the section on aortic stenosis). The diastolic phase image containing the highest velocities can be selected. Then, the voxels with peak velocity on that phase image can be sought (Fig. 32-9). Using the measurement of peak velocity, the pressure gradient can be estimated by the modified Bernoulli equation as $\Delta P = 4V^2$, where ΔP = peak pressure gradient of mitral stenosis and V = peak diastolic velocity across the mitral valve. In general, the MR method is expected to underestimate the pressure gradient compared with Doppler echocardiography because it has a lesser sampling rate. Comparative studies have shown a good correlation between the two techniques, but the MR method has tended to underestimate the gradient.

Quantification of Left Ventricular Volumes, Mass, and Function

Some version of cine MR images is performed for quantification of LV volumes, mass, and function. As discussed earlier, cine MR is a highly accurate and reproducible method of monitoring LV function. Isolated mitral stenosis usually is associated with smaller than average LV volumes and normal ejection fraction.

MITRAL REGURGITATION

Mitral regurgitation may be caused by an abnormality of any portion of the mitral apparatus or by LV dilatation. The dysfunction may involve one or more of several components: leaflets, chordae, anterior and posterior papillary muscles, or annulus. The etiologies of mitral regurgitation are presented in Table 32-4.

Chronic mitral regurgitation produces left atrial and LV enlargement. Pulmonary venous hypertension or edema usually is less severe than with mitral stenosis. Pulmonary arterial hypertension is less common and less severe than with stenosis.

Acute onset of mitral regurgitation such as might occur with chordal or papillary muscle rupture imposes sudden onset of pulmonary venous hypertension with no time for compensating mechanisms to become operative. Severe pulmonary edema may ensue as a result. In this event, the left atrium and ventricle are normal in size. It has been noted

---

TABLE 32-4. ETIOLOGY OF MITRAL REGURGITATION

Leaflet distortion or perforation
  Rheumatic carditis
  Myxomatous degeneration (mitral valve prolapse)
  Bacterial endocarditis
  Asymmetric form of hypertrophic cardiomyopathy
  Left atrial tumor (myxoma)
  Congenital (parachute mitral valve; cleft mitral valve)
  Systemic lupus erythematosus
Chordae
  Myxomatous degeneration (spontaneous chordal rupture)
  Traumatic (weight lifting, etc.)
  Bacterial endocarditis
Papillary muscle
  Rupture from acute infarction
  Dysfunction during myocardial ischemia
  Congenital (parachute mitral valve)
Annulus
  Annular dilation with left ventricular enlargement
  Annular (periannular) calcification
  Myxomatous degeneration

---

that rupture of the posterior papillary muscle or chordae supported by it causes pulmonary edema confined to or more severe in the right upper lobe.

Mitral annular calcification occasionally is the sole cause of regurgitation. The cause of the calcification usually is unknown, but such calcification occurs more often in hypertension, aortic stenosis, hypertrophic cardiomyopathy, hyperlipidemia, and hypercalcemia. It is easy to distinguish mitral valve prolapse from flail. **Prolapse** is ballooning of the middle of the valve beyond the annulus during systole; the tips of the leaflets to which the chordae attach do not pass beyond the annulus. **Flail** is indicated by passage of the tips of the mitral leaflets beyond the annulus and into the left atrium during systole.

Radiography

The radiographic features of mitral regurgitation are regulated by the duration and severity of the lesion and associated lesions of the mitral and other valves (see Table 30-14 in Chapter 30). Isolated chronic mitral regurgitation is a volume overload lesion that causes left atrial and LV enlargement. In the absence of myocardial failure, the degree of cardiomegaly bears a rough relation to the severity of regurgitation. Signs of pulmonary venous and arterial hypertension are less prominent than with mitral stenosis. Nonrheumatic causes of mitral regurgitation usually do not cause radiographically discernible enlargement of the left atrial appendage.

Acute onset of mitral regurgitation is characterized by pulmonary edema with normal heart size. Rupture of the posterior papillary muscle or associated chordae may cause focal or more severe pulmonary edema of the right upper lobe.

Mitral Valve Prolapse

Mitral valve prolapse is observed on about 5% of left ventriculograms. Pathologically, it is caused by myxomatous degeneration of the mitral valve leaflets and chordae tendineae. Some patients with prolapse have mitral regurgitation, which often is mild. However, one complication that may occur—rupture of a chordae tendineae—can induce severe regurgitation. Other complications include supraventricular and ventricular arrhythmias, bacterial endocarditis, and cerebral emboli. Abnormal contraction of segments of the left ventricle and abnormal shape of the left ventricle have been observed in some patients with mitral valve prolapse.

Magnetic Resonance Imaging

MRI can be used to identify mitral regurgitation, quantify the regurgitant volume, and measure LV volumes, mass, and function.

Identification of Mitral Regurgitation

Cine MR in the axial, horizontal long axis (four-chamber), or vertical long axis can be employed to demonstrate the signal void caused by the jet flow of mitral regurgitation. The signal void originates at the closed valve in systole and is directed into the left atrium (Figs. 32-10 and 32-11). Demonstration of the signal void usually requires the use of a TE greater than 8 msec. The signal void prominence and size increase with increasing TE. The signal void ap-

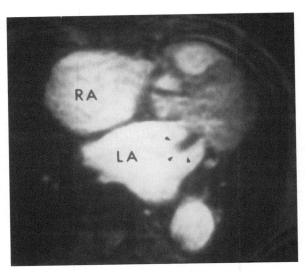

FIG. 32-11. Axial cine MR image in systole shows a flow void *(arrows)* projected into the left atrium *(LA)*, indicating mitral regurgitation. *RA*, right atrium.

pears through most or all of systole. The size of the signal void using contrast TE is related to the severity of mitral regurgitation. Transient signal voids may be evident adjacent to the normal mitral valve as it closes.

Quantification of Mitral Regurgitation

Mitral regurgitation is quantified using VEC cine MRI acquired in a plane parallel to and near the mitral annulus. One approach is to measure the retrograde flow across the valve (into the left atrium) during the systolic phase. This has proved to be complicated, however, because the flow jets occur in multiple orientations in any individual. Another and more robust approach has involved measuring LV diastolic inflow across the mitral annulus and systolic outflow in the proximal ascending aorta (Fig. 32-12). In normal subjects, these values are equivalent, and each represents a measurement of stroke volume (Fig. 32-13). In mitral regurgitation the diastolic mitral inflow exceeds the systolic aortic outflow; the difference represents the regurgitant volume (see Fig. 32-13). Any concomitant aortic regurgitation invalidates this approach.

As discussed earlier, a volumetric method also may be used to estimate the volume of mitral regurgitation. Using cine MR images (short-axis plane) encompassing the length of the ventricles, the area of the left and right ventricles are measured on end-diastolic and end-systolic images at each anatomic level to provide end-diastolic volume and end-systolic volume. The stroke volume of the left ventricle exceeds the stroke volume of the right ventricle by a volume equal to the mitral regurgitant volume. This method is valid only for isolated mitral regurgitation; it does not apply in

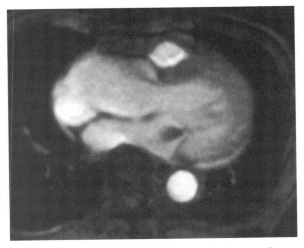

FIG. 32-10. Axial cine MR image in systole shows a flow void emanating from the closed mitral valve and projected into the left atrium. This is caused by mitral regurgitation.

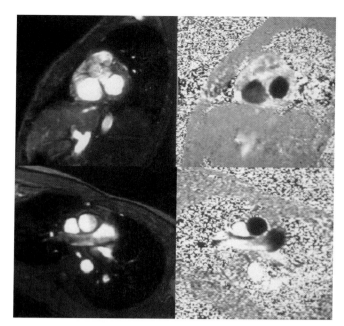

FIG. 32-12. Magnitude (**left**) and phase (**right**) images at the mitral annulus (**top**) and at the proximal ascending aorta (**bottom**). These are used to measure inflow and outflow of the left ventricle. Inflow exceeds outflow volume by the mitral regurgitant volumes (see Fig. 32-13).

the presence of a regurgitant lesion of the right ventricle or aortic regurgitation.

The following formulae are relevant to calculations in mitral regurgitation:

Stroke volume = end-diastolic volume − end-systolic volume (volumetric method)

Mitral regurgitant volume = LV stoke volume − RV stroke volume (volumetric method)

Mitral regurgitant fraction = regurgitant volume/LV stroke volume (volumetric method)

Mitral regurgitant volume = mitral inflow − aortic outflow (VEC method)

Mitral regurgitant fraction = regurgitant volume/mitral inflow (VEC method)

Quantification of Left Ventricular Volume, Mass, and Function

Cine MR images encompassing the left ventricle are used for assessing the LV volume, mass, and function. Because of the precision and reproducibility of LV volumetry using cine MR, this technique is optimal for monitoring LV volumes and function to assess therapy or to define criteria for surgical intervention.

PULMONARY STENOSIS

Pulmonary stenosis results when egress of blood from the right ventricle is obstructed. It can be divided into four types, depending on the level of obstruction: valvular, supravalvular, subvalvular, and midventricular. Pulmonary valvular stenosis usually is a congenital anomaly.

Pulmonary stenosis rarely is caused by rheumatic disease. The etiology of pulmonary stenosis is given in Table 32-5.

Radiography

The typical feature of valvular pulmonic stenosis is enlargement of the main and left pulmonary arterial segments. In

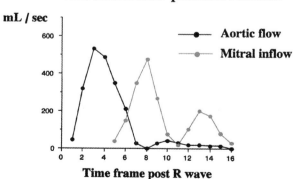

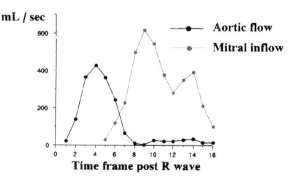

FIG. 32-13. Flow-versus-time curve for proximal aorta (left ventricular outflow) and mitral valve (left ventricular inflow) in normal subject and patient with mitral regurgitation. The area under the inflow curve is considerably greater than the area under the outflow curve in the patient with mitral regurgitation.

TABLE 32-5. ETIOLOGY OF PULMONARY STENOSIS

Valvular stenosis
Congenital
  Central perforated diaphragm
  Biscupid valve
  Dysplastic valve
  Acquired
  Tetralogy of Fallot
Acquired
  Rheumatic carditis
  Carcinoid syndrome
Supravalvular
Congenital
  Williams' syndrome
  Tetralogy of Fallot
Acquired
  Surgical (banding, etc.)
  Carcinoid syndrome
  Rubella syndrome
  Behçet's disease
  Takayasu's arteritis
Subvalvular
Congenital
  Isolated infundibular narrowing
  Tetralogy of Fallot
Acquired
  Infundibular hypertrophy (hypertrophic cardiomyopathy)
  Tumor
Midventricular
Anomalous muscle bundles (double-chamber right ventricle)

the absence of an associated intracardiac defect there is no oligemia. Obstruction at any level may cause RV enlargement. The radiographic features of congenital pulmonic stenosis are discussed in Chapter 31.

Magnetic Resonance Imaging

Cine MRI demonstrates the signal void caused by the jet flow of pulmonic stenosis. The site of origin of the signal void indicates the level of obstruction. A signal originating at the valve and projecting into the pulmonary artery indicates valvular pulmonic stenosis. MRI can be used to exclude rare causes of stenosis such as tumors or hypertrophic cardiomyopathy.

VEC cine MRI can be used to estimate the gradient across the stenotic valve. Cine MR is the most accurate technique for quantifying RV volumes and mass. Mass is calculated as the mass of the RV free wall (the septum is assigned to the left ventricle by convention).

PULMONARY REGURGITATION

Pulmonary regurgitation most often is caused by pulmonary arterial hypertension. It can occur in a congenital anomaly in which the pulmonary valve is absent. It nearly always occurs after pulmonary valvuloplasty and surgical correction of tetralogy of Fallot. Pulmonary regurgitation can be severe after repair of tetralogy, and over many years can cause severe RV dilatation and failure. Many patients with pulmonary regurgitation also have tricuspid regurgitation as a result of RV dilatation.

Radiography

The major feature of pulmonary regurgitation is enlargement of the main pulmonary arterial segment, central pulmonary arteries, and right ventricle.

Magnetic Resonance Imaging

Cine MRI demonstrates a diastolic signal void emanating from the pulmonary valve and projecting into the right ventricle (see Chapter 35). VEC cine MRI can be used to quantify the volume of regurgitation. Currently, it is used to monitor the regurgitant volume of patients after repair of tetralogy of Fallot. The total regurgitant volume of valvular regurgitation on the right side of the heart (pulmonary and tricuspid regurgitation) can be measured as the difference between RV and LV stroke volumes employing volumetric measurements of a stack of short-axis cine MR images that encompass the length of the heart. If the volume of pulmonary regurgitation is measured directly by VEC cine MRI in a plane perpendicular to the main pulmonary artery, tricuspid regurgitant volume can be assigned as the difference between the regurgitant volume measured by the two techniques. The volumetric technique gives total right-sided regurgitant volume; VEC cine MRI measurement in the pulmonary artery gives pulmonary regurgitant volume only.

Cine MR can be used to quantify RV volume, mass, and function. It has demonstrated substantial increases in RV volumes and mass and generalized hypokinesis in patients with severe pulmonary regurgitation after repair of tetralogy of Fallot.

TRICUSPID STENOSIS

Acquired **tricuspid stenosis** is uncommon in comparison with stenosis of left-sided valves. Congenital tricuspid stenosis is rare in comparison with congenital pulmonary stenosis. Other causes of tricuspid stenosis are rare (Table 32-6).

Radiography

The major feature on radiography is isolated right atrial enlargement. Enlargement of the right atrium may be difficult to discern on the chest x-ray. The superior vena cava and azygos vein may be dilated.

TABLE 32-6. ETIOLOGY OF TRICUSPID STENOSIS

Congenital
Pulmonary arterial hypertension
Rheumatic carditis
Carcinoid syndrome
Right ventricular or atrial tumors
Pericardial and paracardiac tumors (compression of tricuspid annulus)
Focal constrictive pericarditis (constriction of the tricuspid annulus)
Tricuspid annular (periannular) calcification

Magnetic Resonance Imaging

Cine MRI demonstrates the signal void across the stenotic tricuspid valve in diastole. VEC (phase-contrast) cine MR may be used to measure the peak velocity and thereby estimate the peak pressure gradient.

TRICUSPID REGURGITATION

Radiography

Tricuspid regurgitation produces cardiomegaly with right atrial and RV enlargement (see Table 30-15 in Chapter 30).

The most remarkable degree of cardiomegaly may occur with chronic severe tricuspid regurgitation. A cardiac silhouette extending from one lateral chest wall to the other ("wall to wall") usually is due to severe tricuspid regurgitation. This lesion does not produce pulmonary venous hypertension or edema. In severe cases, the pulmonary vascularity may appear attenuated.

Magnetic Resonance Imaging

Cine MR demonstrates a systolic signal void into the right atrium emanating from the tricuspid valve. Cine MR also is used to quantify RV volumes, mass, and function. With isolated tricuspid regurgitation, the stroke volume of the right ventricle exceeds that of the left ventricle by a volume equal to that of the tricuspid regurgitant volume.

SELECTED READING

Armstrong WF, Feigenbaum H. Echocardiography. In Braunwald E, Libby P, Zipes D (eds). Heart Disease, 6th ed. Philadelphia: WB Saunders, 2001:160.

Braunwald E. Valvular heart disease. In Braunwald E, Libby P, Zipes D (eds). Heart Disease, 6th ed. Philadelphia: WB Saunders, 2001: 1643.

Sondergaard L, Stahlberg F, Thomsen C. Valvular heart disease. In Higgins CB, de Roos A (eds). MRI and MRA of the Cardiovascular System. Philadelphia: Lippincott Williams & Wilkins, 2003: 155.

33

MYOCARDIAL AND PERICARDIAL DISEASES

CHARLES B. HIGGINS AND GABRIELE A. KROMBACH

Magnetic resonance imaging (MRI) is highly effective for the morphologic and functional evaluation of cardiomyopathies. It is used much less frequently than echocardiography, however, for the diagnosis and monitoring of cardiomyopathies. In comparison with echocardiography, the three-dimensional (3D) data set available with MRI provides a more precise and reproducible method for qualifying ventricular volumes, mass, and function. ECG-referenced multidetector CT (MDCT) and electron-beam CT also provide 3D data and consequently should have similar capabilities.

Both MRI and CT can display the pericardium. Consequently, these techniques are very effective for the diagnosis of constrictive pericarditis and other pericardial diseases.

This chapter will discuss the application of MRI in myocardial and pericardial disease. Multidetector and electron-beam CT can be used for many of the same applications.

TECHNIQUES

The ECG-gated spin-echo (SE) acquisitions in the axial and coronal planes are customarily used to demonstrate the morphology of the ventricles and pericardium. Sharp demarcation of the endocardium is achieved on single- or multiple-slice breath-hold turbo SE images with preparatory double-inversion recovery pulses applied to vitiate the signal of the blood pool (Fig. 33-1). Contrast-enhanced T1-weighted SE images may be applied to demonstrate regional or focal differential (hyper-) enhancement at sites of inflammation, ischemic injury, or fibrosis associated with some myocardial diseases.

Cine MR images are acquired for the purpose of quantifying ventricular volumes, mass, and global function. Cine MR images are obtained with standard gradient-echo, interleaved gradient-echo, or interleaved echo-planar sequences. A set of these images at multiple levels encompassing the heart provides a volumetric data set for the direct measurement of the end-diastolic, end-systolic, and stroke volumes, mass, and ejection fraction of both the left ventricle and right ventricles. The blood pool is bright on gradient-echo images. Contrast between bright blood and ventricular myocardium is high with newer rapid gradient-echo sequences. These balanced steady-state free precision techniques represented by true FISP and balanced fast field echo (bFFE) sequences provide a homogeneous bright signal of the blood pool throughout the cardiac cycle and relatively high temporal resolution in a short acquisition period (Fig. 33-2). Cine MRI sequences are usually acquired in the cardiac short axis encompassing both ventricles from base to apex and in one or more long-axis planes for the quantification of ventricular volumes and function (Fig. 33-3). On cine MR images, valvular regurgitation associated with cardiomyopathies or subvalvular stenosis accompanying some forms of hypertrophic cardiomyopathy may be recognized by a signal void (high-velocity jet flow). Recognition of the signal void depends on the use of a echo time (TE) value greater than 6 msec.

Velocity-encoded (VEC; phase contrast) cine MRI can be used to measure blood flow into the aorta or pulmonary artery to quantify the left ventricular (LV) or right ventricular (RV) stroke volume, respectively. It has also been used for direct measurement of the volume of valvular regurgitation, which may accompany some cardiomyopathies.

CLASSIFICATION OF CARDIOMYOPATHIES

According to the consensus of the World Health Organization and the International Society and Federation for Cardiology, cardiomyopathies are defined as diseases of the myocardium associated with cardiac dysfunction. Based on pathophysiologic features, they have been divided into four main categories: dilated, hypertrophic, restrictive, and arrhythmogenic RV cardiomyopathy. In addition, diseases of the myocardium that are associated with specific cardiac or systemic disorders are termed *specific cardiomyopathies*.

Dilated cardiomyopathy is characterized by dilation and diminished contractile function of the left ventricle or

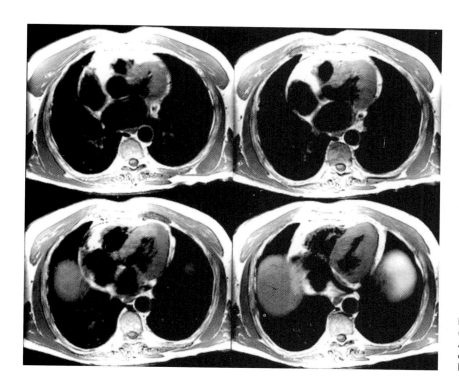

FIG. 33-1. Double-inversion turbo spin-echo (black blood) images in the transaxial plane in a patient with the apical form of hypertrophic cardiomyopathy. Images are arranged from base (**top left**) to apex (**bottom right**).

both ventricles. End-systolic and end-diastolic volumes are increased, whereas stroke volume and ejection fraction are decreased (Fig. 33-4). Mild to moderate mitral regurgitation and tricuspid regurgitation are frequently associated with the ventricular enlargement. The wall thickness of the left

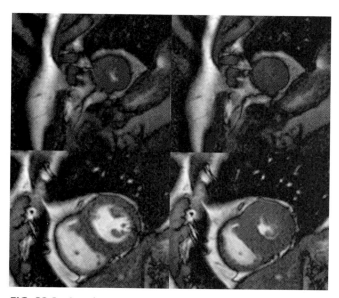

FIG. 33-2. Steady-state free precession (balanced FFE) cine images in a patient with the apical form of hypertrophic cardiomyopathy (same patient as in Fig. 33-1) at two anatomic levels in diastole (**top**) and systole (**bottom**).

ventricle is usually within the normal range, so that an overall increase in LV mass results. The most common cause of dilated cardiomyopathy is myocardial ischemia secondary to coronary artery disease in which the degree of myocardial dysfunction is frequently not explained by the obvious extent of myocardial infarction. Hypertension, viral diseases, alcoholism, diabetes, obesity, several toxins, and hereditary factors also lead to dilated cardiomyopathy. The most common clinical feature of dilated cardiomyopathy is LV failure. Mural thrombus may form in the dilated left ventricle, leading to risk from systemic embolization; mural thrombus can be readily demonstrated on cine MR images.

In **hypertrophic cardiomyopathy**, a variety of distribution patterns of inappropriate myocardial hypertrophy develop in the absence of an obvious hemodynamic stress (increased afterload), such as aortic stenosis or systemic hypertension. The disease is genetically transmitted in about half of the cases and follows an autosomal dominant inheritance pattern with variable penetrance. Possible manifestations are symmetric involvement of the entire left ventricle or both ventricles or asymmetric hypertrophy of the upper septum, midportion of the ventricular septum, or apex. Nonobstructive and obstructive hypertrophic cardiomyopathy can be distinguished by the associated hemodynamic alterations. Asymmetric septal hypertrophic cardiomyopathy can cause obstruction of the LV outflow tract. The hallmark is dynamic subvalvular aortic stenosis. During diastole, the LV outflow tract appears normal or slightly narrowed because of the presence of upper septal hypertro-

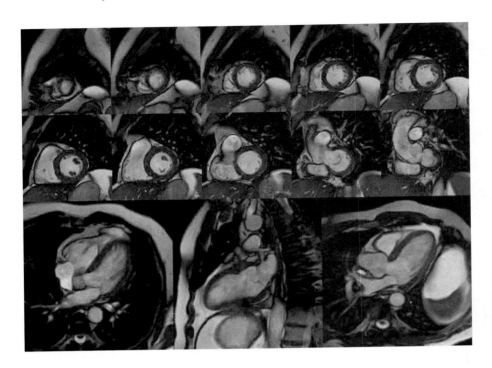

FIG. 33-3. Top and center. Series of cine MR (balanced FFE) images in the cardiac short axis plane from apex (**top left**) to base (**bottom right**). **Bottom.** Images in the horizontal long axis (**left**), vertical long axis (**middle**), and left ventricular outflow planes (**right**).

phy. Increasing stenosis develops during systole as the anterior leaflet of the mitral valve moves in an anterior direction toward the septum, thereby narrowing the outflow tract. Although uncommon in the Western world, apical hypertrophy is prevalent in Japan. This type of hypertrophic car-

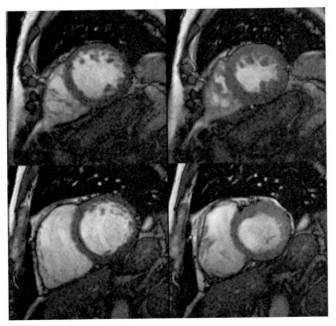

FIG. 33-4. Cine MR images at two levels at end diastole (**left**) and end systole (**right**) in a patient with dilated cardiomyopathy.

diomyopathy does not cause obstruction of the outflow tract. Symmetric hypertrophic cardiomyopathy is also recognized and may be a particularly severe form. Involvement of the right ventricle is a feature of the disease in infants and children.

Restrictive cardiomyopathy is characterized by hampered ventricular filling secondary to myocardial stiffness. Flow into the ventricles is rapid during early diastole; it then plateaus, and little filling takes place in late diastole. End-diastolic pressure is elevated in both ventricles, whereas systolic function is normal or only slightly reduced. Endomyocardial fibrosis and Loeffler endocarditis are now classified as types of restrictive cardiomyopathy. Loeffler endocarditis is associated with hypereosinophilia. Degranulation of endomyocardial eosinophils is suspected to be responsible for focal necrosis and subsequent fibrosis and for the formation of mural thrombus. Increased stiffness of the ventricular walls and reduction of the cavity by organized thrombus contribute to the restrictive filling pattern. Endomyocardial fibrosis, a different entity with a peak geographic distribution in equatorial Africa, is not associated with hypereosinophilia. In this disease, fibrosis of the apex and subvalvular regions leads to restrictive cardiomyopathy. Glycogen storage diseases, radiation fibrosis, and certain infiltrative diseases, such as amyloidosis and sarcoidosis, can also cause restrictive cardiomyopathy. Many cases of restrictive cardiomyopathy are idiopathic.

Specific cardiomyopathies are myocardial diseases that are associated with a specific cardiac or systemic disease. Hemochromatosis, sarcoidosis, amyloidosis, and hypertensive or metabolic cardiomyopathy are examples of specific cardiomyopathies. Dilated cardiomyopathy may be the result of inflammation (myocarditis). Idiopathic, infectious, or autoimmune forms of inflammatory cardiomyopathy have been distinguished.

Several classifications also consider infiltrative cardiomyopathy as an additional category. The definition of infiltrative cardiomyopathy refers solely to the histopathologic mechanism of infiltration of myocardial tissue, and the diseases in this group may cause either restrictive or dilated cardiomyopathy. Hemochromatosis is an example of an infiltrative cardiomyopathy in which the cardiomyopathy is of the dilated type, whereas amyloidosis and sarcoidosis usually cause a restrictive pattern.

IMAGING FEATURES

Dilated Cardiomyopathy

The morphologic characteristics of dilated cardiomyopathy are clearly depicted on ECG-gated SE MRI or cine MRI. Morphologic changes include enlargement of the left ventricle (see Fig. 33-4) and sometimes the right ventricle and atria. The thickness of the LV wall usually remains normal. The MRI features in dilated cardiomyopathy are frequently nonspecific, so that the various underlying causes cannot be distinguished. However, it is usually possible to distinguish between ischemic and nonischemic forms of dilated cardiomyopathy. In most cases of nonischemic dilated cardiomyopathy, the wall thickness of the left ventricle is uniform; no regional wall thinning is recognized (see Fig. 33-4). If the cardiac dilation is caused by myocardial ischemia, usually one or more regional areas of severe wall thinning with or without ventricular aneurysm are seen. MRI may demonstrate localized ventricular dilation after occlusion of a major coronary artery rather than global dilation, which is characteristic of dilated cardiomyopathy. Delayed contrast-enhanced MRI may be used to demonstrate regional hyperenhancement 10 to 15 minutes after an intravenous dose of gadolinium chelate at the site of prior myocardial infarction to distinguish patients with ischemic cardiomyopathy.

Ventricular mass, ventricular thickness, and ventricular volumes can be quantified with cine MRI to determine the severity of dilated cardiomyopathy. Cine MRI measurements of LV volumes, mass, and ejection fraction in dilated cardiomyopathy have been shown to be highly reproducible between studies. The 3D data set with MRI is especially useful for monitoring LV dimension and function over time. Because of its high degree of accuracy and reproducibility, MRI can be used to monitor the effect of treatment in individual patients and in clinical studies to assess the efficacy of new therapeutic interventions. For example, significant decreases in LV systolic volume, wall stress, and mass and an increase in ejection fraction have been shown

in dilated cardiomyopathy after angiotensin-converting enzyme inhibitor treatment and other therapies.

Although the right ventricle is usually less dilated and its systolic function is less severely depressed, RV diastolic abnormalities, such as an increased time to peak filling rate, have been detected using cine MRI and VEC (phase contrast) cine MRI. The profile of diastolic inflow velocity measured in the region of the tricuspid valve is flattened in comparison with that in healthy volunteers. It is suspected that the altered morphology and function of the left ventricle causes functional changes in RV filling.

The signal intensity on SE and gradient-echo images has not been found to be consistently altered in dilated cardiomyopathy, except in cardiomyopathy associated with hemochromatosis (Fig. 33-5). Shortening of relaxation rates has been shown on SE and gradient-echo images of myocardium overloaded with iron. In some patients with dilated cardiomyopathy caused by myocarditis, Gd-DTPA (gadolinium diethylenetriamine pentaacetic acid) produces hyperenhancement of regional myocardium on T1-weighted images. However, hyperenhancement is a nonspecific finding that can be caused by ischemia, fibrosis, inflammatory infiltration, edema, and other changes. In a patient with dilated cardiomyopathy, regional hyperenhancement is usually indicative of ischemic cardiomyopathy.

Hypertrophic Cardiomyopathy

The initial diagnosis of hypertrophic cardiomyopathy is nearly always established by echocardiography. The typical diagnostic feature on any imaging modality is a ratio of the end-diastolic thickness of the septum to the posterolateral wall greater than 1.3. Because not all patients have asymmetric hypertrophy, an additional criterion is concentric hypertrophy (end-diastolic wall thickness greater than 1.2 cm) in

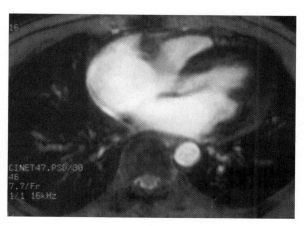

FIG. 33-5. Cine MR image in a patient with hemochromatosis. Note the low signal of the myocardium caused by iron deposition.

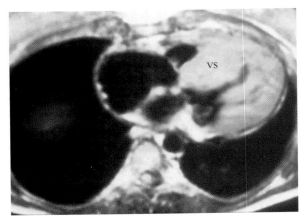

FIG. 33-6. ECG-gated spin-echo transaxial image of patient with the asymmetric form of hypertrophic cardiomyopathy. Note asymmetric thickening of ventricular septum *(VS)*.

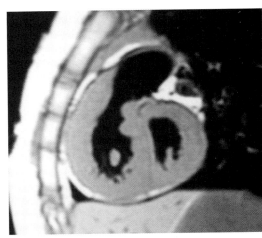

FIG. 33-8. ECG-gated spin-echo sagittal image of a young child with the concentric form of hypertrophic cardiomyopathy that more severely affects the right ventricle.

the absence of a cause for hypertrophy, such as hypertension, aortic stenosis, or extreme isometric exercise. MRI enables a precise delineation of the location and extent of hypertrophic myocardium in persons with hypertrophic cardiomyopathy (see Figs. 33-1, 33-2, and 33-6 to 33-10). MRI visualizes possible sites of hypertrophy (see Figs. 33-1, 33-2, and 33-8) with equal fidelity. The major clinical role of MRI is to evaluate unusual forms of hypertrophy that are difficult to assess with echocardiography. Another indication for MRI is sequential monitoring of the LV mass.

A comprehensive examination, which also addresses the functional impact of the hypertrophy, includes measurement of the LV mass, volume, and ejection fraction by cine MRI. In hypertropic cardiomyopathy, the end-systolic and end-diastolic wall thicknesses are increased (see Fig. 33-2).

The mean ratio of septal thickness to free-wall thickness has been shown on MR to be 1.5 ± 0.8 in the asymmetric septal type of hypertrophic cardiomyopathy, compared with 0.9 ± 0.3 in healthy volunteers and 0.8 ± 0.2 in concentric LV hypertrophy. A ratio of end-diastolic septal thickness to free-wall thickness of greater than 1:3:1 is considered highly suggestive of septal hypertrophic cardiomyopathy (see Fig. 33-6). The total LV mass is substantially increased in hypertrophic cardiomyopathy.

In addition to defining the location and severity of hypertrophy, MRI can differentiate between obstructive and nonobstructive hypertrophic cardiomyopathy. In the obstructive form, a jet flow in the narrowed outflow tract causes a signal void on gradient-echo images. A possible outflow tract gradient can be quantified by velocity mapping at sites proximal and distal to the stenosis. Additionally, mitral re-

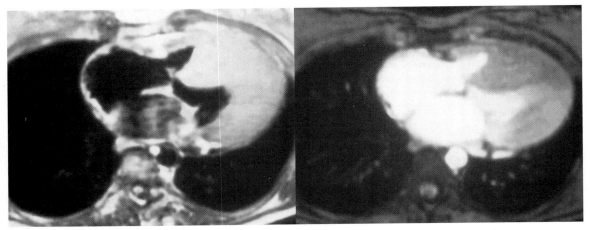

FIG. 33-7. ECG-gated spin echo (**left**) and cine MR transaxial images (**right**) in a patient with the symmetric form of hypertrophic cardiomyopathy.

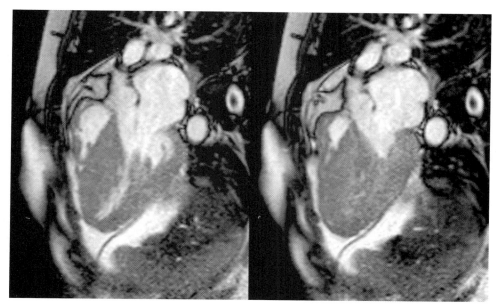

FIG. 33-9. Sagittal cine MR images in diastole (**left**) and systole (**right**) in the obstructive form of hypertrophic cardiomyopathy. Note severe septal hypertrophy in diastole and cavity obliteration in systole. (Courtesy of Scott Flamm, Houston, TX.)

gurgitation, which is frequent in hypertrophic cardiomyopathy, can be detected by cine MRI. It causes a signal void that projects into the left atrium during systole on cine MR images. The volume of mitral regurgitation can be quantified either by calculating the difference in stroke volumes of the ventricles or by measuring the difference in the inflow and outflow volumes of the left ventricle by means of VEC (phase contrast) cine MRI.

Myocardial-tagged cine MRI has shown a profound disturbance of the regional contraction pattern of the left ventricle in hypertrophic cardiomyopathy. Wall motion in the hypertrophic septum and cardiac rotation in the posterior

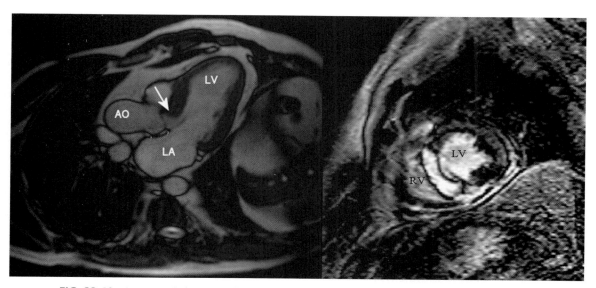

FIG. 33-10. Asymmetric hypertrophic cardiomyopathy. **Left.** The left ventricular outflow plane shows septal hypertrophy *(arrow)*. **Right.** After septal ablation (alcoholic injection into septal artery), an inversion recovery gradient-echo short axis image taken 10 minutes after administration of gadolinium chelate shows delayed enhancement of the induced septal infarction. *AO,* aorta; *LA,* left atrium; *LV,* left ventricle; *RV,* right ventricle.

region of the left ventricle are markedly reduced. Longitudinal and circumferential shortening of the ventricles is also reduced. At the same time, ventricular torsion is increased and thickening of the myocardium is more heterogeneous than in healthy volunteers.

Because of its high accuracy and reproducibility in quantifying LV mass, MRI has the potential to monitor the response to therapy in hypertrophic cardiomyopathy. Septal ablation has been used in patients with obstructive hypertrophic cardiomyopathy to cause infarction of the hypertrophic tissue and thereby reduce the gradient in the LV outflow tract (see Fig. 33-10). MRI has defined the size of the infarction and demonstrated a continuous improvement in the size of the outflow tract area during follow-up.

Delayed regional hyperenhancement after gadolinium contrast administration has been shown in some patients with hypertrophic cardiomyopathy. Signal enhancement has been found to be significantly greater in the most hypertrophic regions than in other regions of the ventricle. A characteristic site of hyperenhancement is the ventricular septum near its junction with the anterior ventricular wall. The increased signal intensity is most likely caused by regional myocardial ischemic injury, fibrosis, or both.

VEC cine MRI has demonstrated a decrease in blood flow per unit of myocardium at rest and in response to a vasodilator (dipyridamole) in patients with hypertrophic cardiomyopathy. Coronary blood flow to the LV myocardium was measured in the coronary sinus by VEC cine MRI and normalized by the ventricular mass to express flow as milliliters per minute per gram of LV myocardium. The ratio of vasodilator-induced to rest coronary flow (coronary flow reserve) was 1.72 ± 0.49 in hypertrophic cardiomyopathy and 3.01 ± 0.75 ($p < 0.01$) in normal subjects.

Restrictive Cardiomyopathy

The main purpose of MRI and CT in patients with restrictive cardiomyopathy is to differentiate this entity from constrictive pericarditis, which presents with the same clinical picture. Because the hemodynamic features of both diseases are similar, distinction solely on clinical grounds or by hemodynamics measured at cardiac catheterization is problematic. However, the differential diagnosis is essential because constrictive pericarditis can be treated effectively with surgical resection of the pericardium, whereas restrictive cardiomyopathy is usually fatal. In constrictive pericarditis, the pericardium is nearly always thickened, whereas restrictive cardiomyopathy does not have this feature.

MRI and CT can demonstrate pericardial thickening reliably. CT can also disclose calcification of the pericardium, a feature that is highly suggestive of constrictive pericarditis. The diagnostic accuracy of MRI for differentiating between these two diseases was 93% in a series of symptomatic patients.

The MRI features of restrictive cardiomyopathy, which

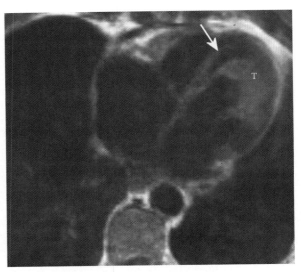

FIG. 33-11. ECG-gated spin-echo transaxial image in a patient with Loeffler's eosinophilic endomyocardial fibrous. Note the low signal intensity of the subendocardial myocardium (subendocardial fibrosis; *arrow*) in the anteroapical and anteroseptal regions and the adjacent high signal mass in the chamber caused by mural thrombus *(T).*

are characteristic but nonspecific, are caused by impaired diastolic filling of the ventricles. Impaired diastolic expansion of the ventricles causes dilation of the atria, inferior and superior vena cavae, and hepatic veins. Furthermore, stasis of blood in the atria leads to a high signal intensity in the atrial cavities on SE images. The restrictive filling pattern of the ventricles can be quantified and monitored during therapy by measuring the diastolic flow across the mitral and tricuspid valves with VEC cine MRI. Evaluation of possible atrioventricular valve regurgitation is also important in patients with restrictive cardiomyopathy and can be performed with cine MRI or VEC cine MRI.

In endomyocardial fibrosis, areas of circumscribed myocardial fibrosis have been detected as areas of low signal intensity on T1- and T2-weighted images. The ventricular walls may be severely thickened by the deposition of subendocardial fibrotic tissue, which causes a narrowing of the cavities and contributes further to the decreased diastolic ventricular filling. Mural thrombus adjacent to the subendocardial fibrous is a characteristic feature; both may be displayed on SE or cine MR images (Fig. 33-11).

Several specific cardiomyopathies can result in a restrictive filling pattern, the most common of which is cardiac amyloidosis.

SPECIFIC CARDIOMYOPATHIES

Amyloidosis

Interstitial deposition of amyloid fibrils causes thickening of the atrial and ventricular walls and the atrioventricular

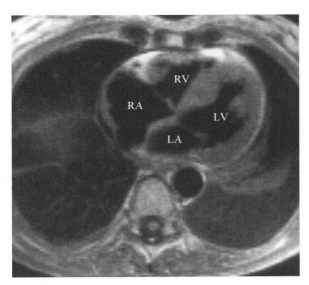

FIG. 33-12. ECG-gated spin-echo transaxial image of a patient with amyloid heart disease. Amyloid deposition has caused thickening of the ventricular septum (asymmetrical septal thickening), atrial septum, wall of the right atrium *(RA)*, and atrioventricular values. *LA,* left atrium; *LV,* left ventricle; *RV,* right ventricle.

valve leaflets (Fig. 33-12). Severe amyloid deposition in the ventricular myocardium may produce morphologic features simulating those of hypertrophic cardiomyopathy. However, these two entities can be differentiated by divergent ventricular contraction. In contrast to the hyperdynamic ventricular contraction seen in hypertrophic cardiomyopathy, the systolic contraction is diminished in amyloidosis. The ejection fraction and systolic wall thickening are depressed. Amyloidosis most commonly leads to restrictive cardiomyopathy with dilated atria. Alterations in the T1 and T2 relaxation rates of the myocardium may be detectable. The signal intensity of the myocardium has been found to be reduced on T1- and T2-weighted images in patients with amyloidosis in comparison with that in healthy volunteers and in patients with hypertrophic cardiomyopathy.

Sarcoidosis

Sarcoidosis can be manifested in the myocardium with typical granulomas and can cause restrictive cardiomyopathy. Only 5% of patients with systemic sarcoidosis have clinical evidence of cardiac involvement, but it is found at autopsy in 20% to 30% of such patients. Cardiac symptoms are highly suggestive of myocardial involvement in patients with systemic sarcoidosis. In patients with clinical manifestations of myocardial sarcoidosis who do not have systemic disease, however, the diagnosis is challenging, and myocardial biopsy is usually required for confirmation. Because distribution of the infiltration is patchy, nondirected biopsy is associated with false-negative results. MRI has displayed

sarcoid granulomas as nodules of high signal intensity on T2-weighted images and as focal areas of hyperenhancement on T1-weighted images after the administration of Gd-DTPA. These findings are not specific and can be observed in other inflammatory diseases. However, they can aid in guiding myocardial biopsies and have been used to monitor the response to steroid therapy. After the granulomas have regressed, postinflammatory scars may persist. These can be delineated as regions of diminished or absent wall thickening or as regions of diastolic wall thinning.

Hemochromatosis

Hemochromatosis may be primary or secondary. Primary hemochromatosis is an inherited autosomal recessive disease. Secondary hemochromatosis develops mainly when repeated blood transfusions are required to treat thalassemia and hemolytic anemias. Other common causes are chronic alcohol abuse and long-term hemodialysis. In primary hemochromatosis, iron is deposited in the liver and pancreas but the spleen remains normal. This characteristic distinguishes primary from secondary hemochromatosis, in which iron is also deposited in the spleen. Increased iron deposition in the cardiac myocytes in hemochromatosis causes diastolic and systolic cardiac dysfunction. After an initial asymptomatic period, cardiopathy caused by iron overload initially presents as diastolic dysfunction with a restrictive filling pattern. When the iron overload reaches a critical level, systolic functional abnormalities occur, and the disease takes the form of a dilated cardiomyopathy.

Iron reduces the T1 and T2 relaxation rates by introducing local magnetic field inhomogeneities, causing myocardial signal intensity to be reduced, especially on cine MR images (see Fig. 33-5). The amount of signal decrease on T2-weighted images correlates with the iron level in tissue but not with serum iron levels. MRI is a valuable tool for noninvasively estimating the iron concentration in the heart and for monitoring therapy.

Arrhythmogenic Right Ventricular Cardiomyopathy

Arrhythmogenic right ventricular cardiomyopathy (ARCV) may have characteristic features on SE and cine MRI. Typical findings are transmural fatty deposition in the RV free wall as displayed on T1-weighted SE images (Figs. 33-13 and 33-14). T1-weighted SE images may also demonstrate the focal deposition of fat in the myocardial wall as bright spots surrounded by the medium signal intensity of myocardium. Another feature is regional bulging or thinning of the RV free wall (Fig. 33-15). Thinning of the RV free wall is difficult to interpret because the thickness of the free wall varies among normal persons. Additional morphologic features include focal sacculations, aneurysms, and enlargement of the right ventricle. Cine MRI can demonstrate re-

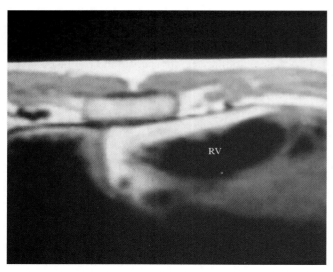

FIG. 33-13. ECG-gated spin-echo image shows transmural fat in the right ventricular *(RV)* free wall in a patient with arrhythmogenic RV dysplasia.

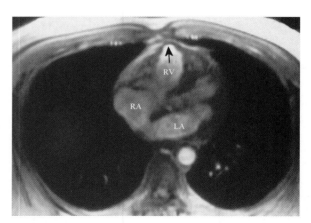

FIG. 33-15. Cine MR image shows regional dyskinesis *(arrow)* of the right ventricle in a patient with arrhythmogenic right ventricular dysplasia. *LA,* left atrium; *RA,* right atrium; *RV,* right ventricle.

gional or global RV contractile dysfunction (Fig. 33-16). It has also demonstrated regional dyskinesis and aneurysms. In advanced cases, severe RV dilation and tricuspid regurgitation may be present. For a definite diagnosis of ARVC, regional or global contraction abnormality should be identifiable on cine MRI.

Findings on MRI suggesting the diagnosis of ARVC now constitute a major criterion for establishing this diagnosis. The diagnosis is not definitely established by MR findings alone; the MR features are used in association with clinical

and electrophysiologic findings to establish the diagnosis. Moreover, MR studies may be equivocal for the diagnosis, and MRI cannot be relied upon to exclude early stages of this disease.

MYOCARDITIS

In the early stages of myocarditis, the clinical symptoms are often dominated by nonspecific complaints such as fatigue, weakness, and palpitations. Chest pain in the absence of myocardial ischemia is a more suggestive symptom of pericarditis or myocarditis. Profound dysfunction of the ventricles can be ascertained at later stages of the disease, after acute myocarditis has resulted in dilated cardiomyopathy. Most cases of myocarditis are caused by viral infections; the agents are cytomegalovirus in 45% and coxsackievirus B in 30% of cases. Currently, a tentative diagnosis of myocarditis is confirmed by endomyocardial biopsy, which typically shows intersitial edema, lymphocyte infiltration, and necrosis of myocytes. MRI has been proposed as a noninvasive test for diagnosing myocarditis and monitoring the response to therapy. Because of the intersitial edema, the T2 relaxation time is increased, so that the signal may be increased on T2-weighted images. Although this characteristic has been demonstrated in small series of patients, conventional T2-weighted sequences are frequently of poor quality and prone to motion artifacts. The advent of fast imaging sequences that are performed during a breath-hold has substantially improved image quality, and recent evaluations of such sequences in patients with myocarditis have shown promising results.

Another approach to the evaluation of myocardial inflammation is the demonstration of delayed regional or diffuse myocardial enhancement on T1-weighted images after the administration of Gd-DTPA. Delayed contrast-

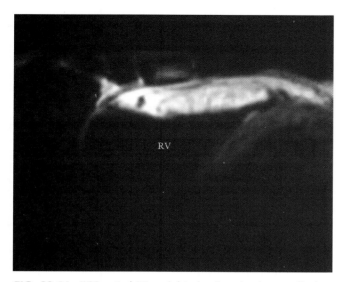

FIG. 33-14. ECG-gated T1-weighted spin-echo image displays transmural fat in the right ventricular *(RV)* wall in a patient with arrhythmogenic RV dysplasia.

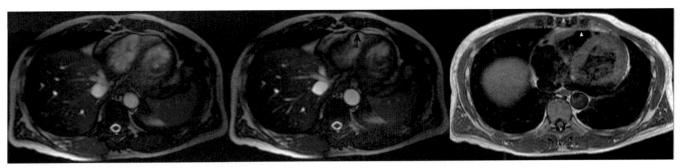

FIG. 33-16. Cine MR images in diastole (**left**) and systole (**center**) show regional dyskinesis *(arrow)* of the anteroapical portion of the right ventricle. Spin-echo image (**right**) shows regional wall thinning *(arrowhead)*.

enhanced T1-weighted SE imaging has shown hyperenhancement of the myocardium early after the onset of symptoms. There may be either focal or diffuse hyperenhancement of LV myocardium. The extent of myocardial hyperenhancement has roughly correlated with LV dysfunction and with the clinical functional status. However, contrast enhancement of the myocardium and an increased T2 relaxation rate are nonspecific findings that can also be encountered in idiopathic dilated and hypertrophic cardiomyopathy, sarcoidosis, and myocardial infarction. When a patient with a presumptive diagnosis of myocarditis is assessed, the imaging findings must be interpreted in relation to the clinical situation.

In Lyme disease, which is caused by the spirochete *Borrelia burgdorferi,* MRI demonstrates signs of myopericarditis. Characteristic features are ventricular wall thickening coupled with regional or global hypokinesis, areas of increased signal intensity in the ventricular wall, and pericardial effusion. The changes of the ventricular wall are located predominantly in the anterolateral wall and the apical region of the septum.

Chagas disease is caused by the protozoan *Trypanosoma cruzi.* This infection is characterized by acute, intermediate, and chronic phases. In chronic Chagas disease, the heart is the most frequently affected organ, and lymphocytic infiltration can be observed. Regions of focal inflammation have been shown to enhance strongly on T1-weighted images after the administration of Gd-DTPA. Apical aneurysm of the left ventricle is a characteristic of chronic Chagas disease.

HEART TRANSPLANTATION AND TRANSPLANT REJECTION

Measuring the ventricular volume, myocardial mass, and ejection fraction with cine MRI can be used to monitor the morphology and function of a newly transplanted heart. In a recent study, at 2 months after successful transplantation, MRI demonstrated an increase of the LV mass coupled with a decrease in the ratio of end-systolic wall stress to volume in comparison with normal volunteers. These changes were interpreted as a sign of early remodeling of the left ventricle.

Acute rejection is one of the main causes of death during the first year after transplantation. Currently, RV endomyocardial biopsy represents the gold standard for evaluating this condition. To reduce the need for biopsy, a modality that could replace this invasive test or efficiently guide its timing would be desirable. MRI as a noninvasive imaging modality has been considered for this purpose, and three different approaches have been assessed: (1) tissue characterization by evaluation of T2 relaxivity, (2) evaluation of changes in signal intensity after administration of contrast (gadolinium chelate), and (3) evaluation of changes in myocardial wall thickness.

The transplanted heart not only is at risk for rejection but also is subjected to the side effects of immunosuppressive drug therapy. For example, ventricular hypertrophy can be caused by cyclosporine. Therefore, if overall long-term success rates are to improve, not only the regular follow-up of individual transplant recipients but also the evaluation of new therapeutic approaches will be necessary. For this purpose, MRI is preferable to other imaging modalities because of its accuracy and interstudy reproducibility in quantifying ventricular volume and mass. For instance, felodipine, a calcium channel blocker, was shown to be capable of reversing cyclosporine-induced hypertrophy as assessed by cine MRI.

PERICARDIAL DISEASE

Normal Pericardium

The pericardium is composed of fibrous tissue and appears dark on T1- and T2-weighted SE images. In the area of the right ventricle, it is located between the bright mediastinal and subepicardial fat, which provides a natural high level of contrast, so that the sensitivity for visualization of the pericardium in this region is 100%. In regions adjacent to the lung, the natural contrast is lower, so that the sensitivity for visualization in the area of the lateral wall of the left ventricle is lower. The average thickness of the pericardium on MR images ranges from 1 to 2 mm. Anatomic studies have shown the thickness of the pericardium to be in the range of 0.4 to 1 mm. The overestimation on MRI has been presumed to result from motion-induced signal loss of the normal pericardial fluid, which cannot be readily distinguished from the pericardium itself. Pericardial thickness depends also on the anatomic level and increases toward the diaphragm. This effect results from the ligamentous insertion of the pericardium into the diaphragm and from its tangential direction to the imaging plane. Consequently, the measurement of pericardial thickness is most reliable at the midventricular level. The pericardium extends approximately to the level of the mid-ascending aorta and the bifurcation of the pulmonary artery. It forms a tube that encloses both great arteries. A second, more posterior pericardial tube surrounds the superior vena cava. Both compartments are connected by the transverse sinus, which is visible on MRI in 80% of cases. Fluid is nearly always seen in the superior pericardial recesses on MR images. The most frequently seen superior recesses are behind the ascending aorta and between the aorta and pulmonary artery.

Pericardial Effusion

MRI is very sensitive for the detection of generalized or loculated pericardial effusions. Pericardial effusion consisting of simple fluid has low signal on T1-weighted SE images and high signal on gradient-echo images (Fig. 33-17). The pericardial space normally contains 10 to 50 mL of fluid. MRI can detect a pericardial effusion as small as 30 mL, and in most normal subjects, fluid can be seen in the superior pericardial recess. MRI provides information on the location of a pericardial effusion and is especially effective for dem-

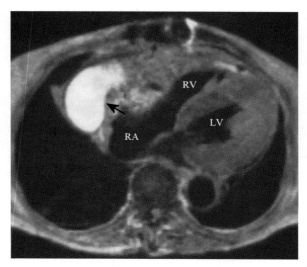

FIG. 33-18. T1-weighted spin-echo image shows a loculated hemorrhagic effusion *(arrow)*. High signal on this sequence is characteristic of hemorrhagic effusion. *LV*, left ventricle; *RA*, right atrium; *RV*, right ventricle.

onstrating loculated effusions (Fig. 33-18). Because of this uneven distribution, the total fluid volume cannot be calculated from the width of the pericardial space by applying a simple formula. However, a semiquantitative estimation can be obtained by measuring the width of the pericardial space in front of the right ventricle. A moderate effusion is associated with a width of more than 5 mm. Loculated effusion occurs when fluid is trapped by adhesions between the parietal and visceral pericardium. MRI is more sensitive than echocardiography in detecting loculated effusion because of its wide field of view.

Hemorrhagic effusion can be distinguished from nonhemorrhagic effusion by its characteristic signal intensity. Hemorrhagic effusion (hemopericardium) appears bright

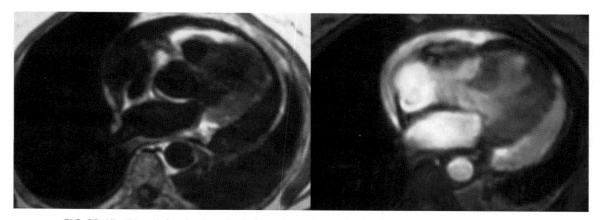

FIG. 33-17. T1-weighted spin-echo (**left**) and gradient-echo (cine MR; **right**) images of pericardial effusion. There is low signal on the spin-echo image and high signal on the gradient-echo image.

on T1-weighted SE images (see Fig. 33-18). Nonhemorrhagic effusions have low signal intensity on T1-weighted images (see Fig. 33-17). Further differentiation of nonhemorrhagic effusion as either transudative or exudative is not reliable by differences in signal intensity. Movement of the fluid during the cardiac cycle introduces flow-void effects that make an accurate assessment of the signal intensity problematic. Nonhemorrhagic pericardial effusion produces high signal on cine MR images (see Fig. 33-17).

Pericardial Thickening and Acute Pericarditis

Pericardial thickening is defined as an increase in the pericardial thickness to 4 mm or more. It appears as a widening of the low-signal pericardial line if it is caused by an increase of fibrous tissue. It may be difficult to distinguish thickening from a small rim of pericardial effusion by its signal intensity on T1-weighted SE images. However, the distribution of pericardial effusion differs considerably from the pattern of pericardial thickening. The accumulation of fluid is typically posterolateral to the left ventricle or in the superior recess, as mentioned earlier. If the fluid is not trapped by pericardial adhesions, its distribution changes during the cardiac cycle.

In acute pericarditis, fibrinous exudates and edema rather than an increase of fibrous tissue cause pericardial thickening (Fig. 33-19). There is invariably a pericardial effusion as well as thickened pericardium. After administration of gadolinium contrast, there is prominent enhancement of the thickened pericardium.

Constrictive Pericarditis

Constrictive pericarditis is associated with progressive pericardial fibrosis, which causes the pericardium to shrink and so limit diastolic ventricular expansion. It is a nonspecific reaction to various conditions, such as infectious pericarditis, connective tissue disease, neoplasm, trauma, long-term renal dialysis, cardiac surgery, and radiation therapy. Currently, constrictive pericarditis is most often a sequela of cardiac surgery in Europe and North America. However, tuberculous pericarditis remains a leading cause of constrictive pericarditis in Third World countries. The diagnostic features of constrictive pericarditis are a thickened pericardium (Fig. 33-20) coupled with signs of impaired diastolic filling of the right ventricle, such as dilation of the inferior vena cavae, hepatic veins, and right atrium. The volume of the right ventricle is frequently normal or reduced. Sometimes the right ventricle is elongated and narrowed so that it appears tubular, and the ventricular septum may have a sigmoid shape. Thickening of the pericardium is sometimes localized (Fig. 33-21). The diagnostic accuracy of MRI as well as CT in constrictive pericarditis exceeds 90%. As mentioned above, MRI effectively distinguishes between constrictive pericarditis and restrictive cardiomyopathy. Localized forms of constrictive pericarditis may cause unusual anatomic and functional abnormalities. Pericardial constriction of the right atrioventricular groove has appeared on MRI as pericardial thickening limited to this region, along with right atrial enlargement and a normal or small right ventricle (see Fig. 33-21). On cine MR, there is frequently early diastolic bowing of the ventricular system toward the left ventricle (diastolic septal bounce).

Absence of Pericardium

Congenital absence of the pericardium results from abnormalities of the vascular supply to the developing pericardium during embryogenesis. It is relatively rare and usually remains asymptomatic. However, partial absence of the pericardium may present with chest pain caused by herniation of the base of the left ventricle through the defect with compression of the left coronary arterial branches by the rim of the defect. Attachment of the pericardium to the sternum and diaphragm stabilizes the position of the heart

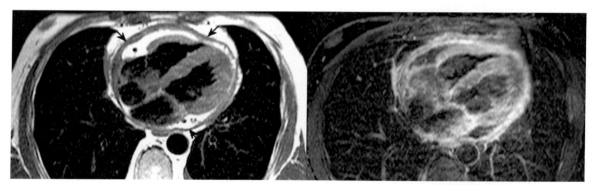

FIG. 33-19. Acute pericarditis; T1-weighted spin-echo images before **(left)** and after *(right)* gadolinium chelate administration. Thickened pericardium *(arrows)* is markedly enhanced by the contrast.

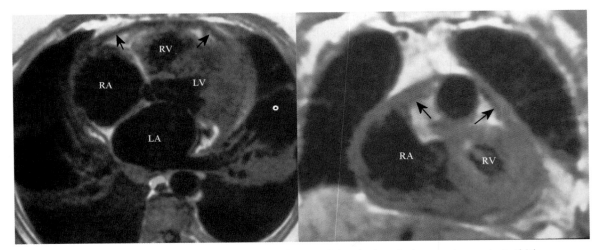

FIG. 33-20. Coronal (**right**) and transaxial (**left**) T1-weighted spin-echo images demonstrate thickened pericardium *(arrows)*. Coronal image shows thickened pericardium *(arrows)* extending over the pulmonary artery *(PA)*. *LA,* left atrium; *LV,* left ventricle; *RV,* right ventricle; *RA,* right atrium.

within the thorax. Consequently, complete absence of the pericardium on the left side is associated with leftward displacement of the heart because this stabilizing structure is missing (Fig. 33-22). A characteristic finding on transaxial CT or MR images is an interposition of lung parenchyma between the aortic knob and the main pulmonary artery. Absence of the low-signal pericardial line is an additional characteristic finding. In partial left-sided absence, MRI discloses herniation of a left atrial appendage routinely, but also the base of the left ventricle in some cases. The latter observation is extremely important since this is a potentially lethal complication.

Pericardial Cysts and Diverticula

Pericardial cysts are caused by developmental abnormalities and are alleged to occur when a small portion of the pericar-

dium is pinched off during embryonic development. Pseudocyst of the pericardium may develop after surgical pericardiotomy. Ninety percent of pericardial cysts are located in the cardiophrenic angles (70% on the right and 20% on the left side). However, they can occur anywhere in the pericardium, and a pericardial cyst at an unusual location sometimes cannot be distinguished from a thymic or bronchogenic cyst. Pericardial cysts usually do not communicate with the pericardial cavity. A cyst filled with simple fluid (low protein content) appears dark on T1-weighted images and homogeneously bright on T2-weighted images (Fig. 33-23). The cyst does not enhance after the administration of gadolinium chelate. If the cyst is filled with blood or proteinaceous fluid, it is bright on T1-weighted images. The pericardial rim is visible with the characteristic low signal intensity of the pericardium.

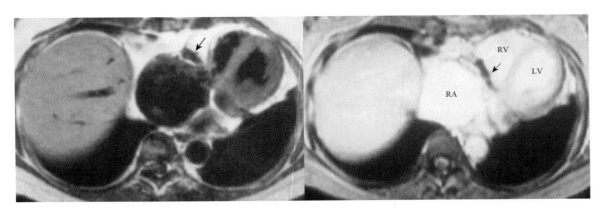

FIG. 33-21. Focal constrictive pericarditis. T1-weighted spin-echo (**left**) and cine MR (**right**) images demonstrate focal pericardial thickening in the right atrioventricular grove *(arrow)*. There is severe narrowing of the tricuspid annulus by the thickened constricting pericardium. *LV,* left ventricle; *RA,* right atrium; *RV,* right ventricle.

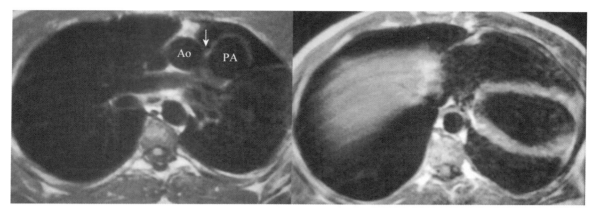

FIG. 33-22. Absence of pericardium. ECG-gated transaxial spin-echo images at the level of the great arteries (**left**) and the ventricles (**right**) demonstrate lung *(arrow)* interposed between the ascending aorta *(AO)* and the pulmonary artery *(PA)*. The heart is shifted into the left hemithorax.

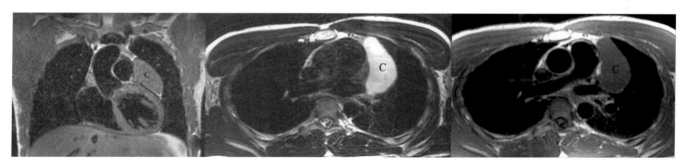

FIG. 33-23. Pericardial cyst. T1-weighted coronal (**left**) and T2-weighted transaxial (**middle**) spin-echo images and T1-weighted axial image after gadolinium chelate administration (**right**) demonstrate pericardial mass (cyst; *C*) with low intensity on T1-weighted images and homogeneous high signal on T2-weighted images but no contrast enhancement.

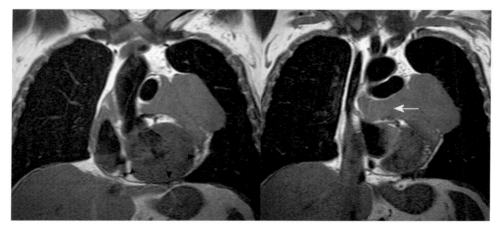

FIG. 33-24. ECG-gated spin-echo coronal images at the level of the right pulmonary artery (**left**) and 1 cm further ventral (**right**) show an extensive pericardial sarcoma. The tumor infiltrates throughout the left side of the pericardial cavity and the superior recesses *(arrow)*. The tumor is located between the left ventricle and the pericardium *(arrowhead)*, with an additional component that extends outside the pericardium.

In contrast to pericardial cysts, diverticula communicate with the pericardial cavity. They correspond to a congenital or acquired defect in the parietal pericardium. MRI may demonstrate variations in the size of a diverticulum during changes in body position.

Pericardial Tumors

Primary pericardial tumors occur less frequently than secondary tumors. Mesothelioma is the most common primary malignant tumor of the pericardium. Fibrosarcoma, angiosarcoma, and teratoma also occur in the pericardium. Characterization of the tumor entity is possible only for dermoids, lipoma, and low-grade liposarcoma, which show high signal intensity on T1-weighted images. However, the extent of the lesions, their relation to the cardiac structures and great vessels, and their effects on the cardiac function can be evaluated (Fig. 33-24). A pericardial mass containing discrete vascular structures may suggest angiosarcoma of the pericardium.

Secondary tumors occur either by extension from mediastinal or lung tumors or by metastasis. Pericardial metastases have been found in 22% of patients with cancer at autopsy. They are most frequently caused by lung and breast carcinoma, leukemia, and lymphoma. Metastases often cause hemorrhagic effusion. In such cases, it may be difficult to distinguish the tumor itself from the surrounding fluid because of the high signal intensity of the hemorrhagic fluid. Visualization of metastatic deposits can be improved by hyperenhancement after the administration of gadolinium contrast, while the pericardial fluid does not enhance.

MRI can be used to assess tumor infiltration of the pericardium. Interruption of the pericardial line can be used to distinguish a mass that infiltrates the pericardium from a lesion that reaches the pericardium but has not transgressed this boundary. If the pericardium is visible adjacent to a mass, pericardial invasion is unlikely.

SELECTED READING

Boxt LM, Rozenshtein A. Right ventricular dysplasia and outflow tract tachycardia. In: Higgins CB, de Roos A (eds). Cardiovascular MRI and MRA. Philadelphia: Lippincott Williams & Wilkins, 2003:122.

Frank H, Globits S. Magnetic resonance imaging of myocardial and pericardial diseases. JMRI 1999; 10:617.

Friedrich MG, Strohm O, Schulz-Menger J, et al. Contrast media-enhanced MR imaging visualizes myocardial changes in the course of viral myocarditis. Circulation 1998; 97:1802.

Kawada N, Sakuma H, Yamakado T, et al. Hypertrophic cardiomyopathy: magnetic resonance measurements of coronary blood flow and vasodilator flow reserve in patients and healthy subjects. Radiology 1999; 211:129.

Masui T, Finck S, Higgins CB. Constrictive pericarditis and restrictive cardiomyopathy: evaluation with MR imaging. Radiology 1992; 182–369.

34

CARDIAC AND PARACARDIAC MASSES

CHARLES B. HIGGINS AND GABRIELE A. KROMBACH

The term *mass* is used rather than *tumor* in this chapter because the most frequent mass within a cardiac chamber is thrombus rather than tumor. Primary tumors are rare. Secondary tumors, either metastatic or representing direct extension of primary tumors of another organ, are about 40 times more frequent than primary cardiac tumors.

Computed tomography (CT) and magnetic resonance imaging (MRI) can help determine the presence and extent of cardiac and paracardiac tumors. These modalities, especially MRI, can also sometimes characterize the mass. Although CT may be adequate for the evaluation of cardiac and paracardiac mass, MRI is usually employed for this purpose. Consequently, this chapter focuses on the findings on MRI.

Because of a wide field of view that encompasses the cardiovascular structures, mediastinum, and adjacent lung simultaneously, CT and MRI can display the intracardiac and extracardiac extent of tumors. In addition, the ability to image in multiple planes makes MRI especially suited for the demarcation of the spatial relationship of a mass to the various cardiac and mediastinal structures. The multiplanar approach overcomes the volume-averaging problem at the diaphragmatic interface encountered with a solely transaxial imaging technique such as CT. These features permit a clear delineation of the possible infiltration of a mass lesion into cardiac and adjacent mediastinal structures. In addition, MRI allows the assessment of functional parameters such as ventricular wall thickening, ejection fraction, or flow velocity in adjacent vessels. Therefore, the impact of a tumor on cardiac function can be evaluated.

In clinical practice, MRI is most often used to verify or exclude a possible mass suggested initially by echocardiography. Echocardiography clearly depicts cardiac morphology and provides an assessment of functional parameters. The effectiveness of transthoracic echocardiography is limited by the acoustic window, however, which varies considerably with patient habitus. Image quality of echocardiography may be severely decreased by obesity or chronic obstructive pulmonary disease. Transesophageal echocardiography overcomes this problem but adds invasiveness. The soft tissue contrast achieved with echocardiography remains limited in comparison with that obtained with MRI. Usually, pericardial involvement and infiltration of the myocardium can be better visualized with MRI.

Tissue characterization based on specific T1 and T2 relaxation times is possible to a limited degree. Nevertheless, definitive differentiation between benign and malignant tumors is usually not feasible. Most cardiac tumors have low to intermediate signal intensity on T1-weighted images and high signal intensity on T2-weighted images. However, the combination of imaging characteristics of a cardiac mass, such as location, signal intensity on T1- and T2-weighted images, possible hyperenhancement after the administration of paramagnetic contrast agents, and possible suppression of signal with the application of a fat-saturation technique, may render a specific tissue diagnosis highly probably in some cases.

TECHNIQUES

Computed Tomography

Multislice or spiral single-slice CT scans in the axial plane after contrast enhancement are used to identify and determine the extent of masses. For this evaluation, electron beam CT or retrospectively ECG-gated multislice CT acquisitions are not necessary. Collimation is usually 5 mm. Retrospective reconstruction of volumetric data in the sagittal or coronal plane may be useful.

Magnetic Resonance Imaging

ECG-gated transaxial T1-weighted spin-echo (SE) images of the entire thorax are initially acquired for the evaluation of suspected cardiac or paracardiac masses. In addition, such images are frequently acquired in the sagittal or coronal plane to delineate the regions that are displayed suboptimally in the transaxial plane, such as the diaphragmatic

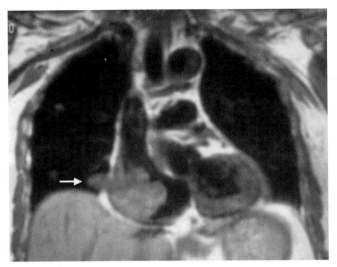

FIG. 34-1. Angiosarcoma. ECG-gated spin-echo image in the coronal plane shows a large tumor in the right atrium extending through the atrial wall *(arrow)*. The wide field of view of the coronal plane demonstrates the extent of this angiosarcoma.

enhanced T1-weighted images. Transaxial T2-weighted SE images are acquired to enhance the contrast between myocardium and tumor tissue, which usually has a longer T2 relaxation time, and to delineate possible cystic or necrotic components of a mass. The comparison of signal intensities of a mass lesion on T1-weighted and T2-weighted images may to a certain degree allow for tissue characterization. For example, lipomas have relatively high signal intensity on T1-weighted images and moderate signal intensity on T2-weighted images. Cystic lesions (filled with simple fluid) have low signal intensity on T1-weighted images and high signal intensity on T2-weighted images (Fig. 34-3). The administration of Gd-DTPA (gadolinium diethylenetriamine pentaacetic acid) usually improves the contrast between tumor tissue and myocardium on T1-weighted images and may facilitate tissue characterization. Hyperenhancement of tumor tissue with MR contrast agents indicates either an enlarged extracellular space of tumor tissue in comparison with normal myocardium (Fig. 34-4) or a high degree of vascularization of the mass. Application of

surface of the heart. Coronal images facilitate the evaluation of masses involving the aortopulmonary window and pulmonary hili, and mediastinal masses that extend through the cervicothoracic junction. The wide field of view afforded by sagittal and coronal images can readily display the extent of tumors (Figs. 34-1 and 34-2). Contrast between intramural tumor and normal myocardium may be low on non-

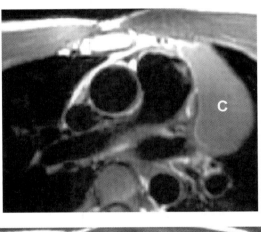

A

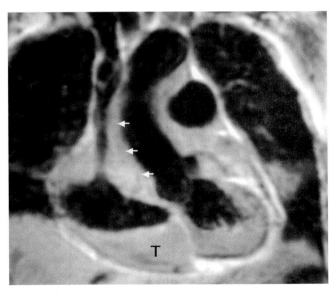

FIG. 34-2. Angiosarcoma. ECG-gated spin-echo image in the coronal plane demonstrates a tumor *(T)* infiltrating through the right atrial cavity and extending around the superior vena cava *(arrows)*.

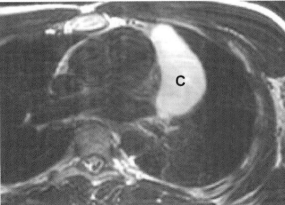

B

FIG. 34-3. Pericardial cyst. ECG-gated spin-echo T1-weighted (**A**) and T2-weighted (**B**) images of a pericardial cyst *(C)*. The simple fluid in the cyst has typical low signal on T1-weighted and homogeneous high signal on T2-weighted images.

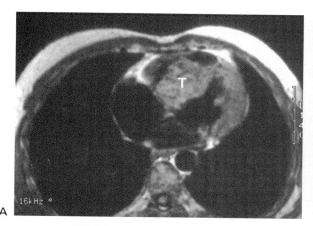
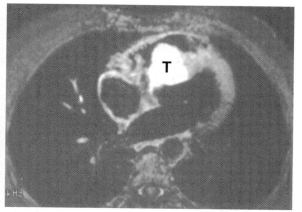

FIG. 34-4. Angiosarcoma. ECG-gated spin-echo T1-weighted images before (**A**) and after (**B**) gadolinium chelate administration demonstrates hyperenhancement of the tumor *(T)* compared with the septal myocardium. The postcontrast image uses fat saturation.

a fat-saturation sequence, which vitiates the bright signal of fat, is effective for the tissue characterization of lipomas (Fig. 34-5).

In patients with cardiac tumors, cine MRI provides valuable information regarding the movement of the cardiac mass relative to cardiovascular structures. Because cine MR images are acquired with gradient-echo sequences, a different contrast is obtained than with the SE technique. On SE images, flowing blood appears with low signal intensity, whereas gradient-echo images display the blood pool with high signal intensity. As a gradient-echo technique, cine MRI is prone to susceptibility effects, which occur in the presence of paramagnetic substances that cause local magnetic field inhomogeneities. Subacute and chronic thrombi contain substances that induce a magnetic susceptibility effect, which lowers the signal intensity on gradient-echo images. This feature can facilitate the delineation of these intraluminal masses, which have low signal intensity in contrast to the bright signal of intracavitary blood. Rarely, tumors that contain abundant iron or calcium may have low signal intensity and are delineated optimally on cine gradient-echo sequences. Masses depicted on tomographic images can be described in location as intracavitary, intramural, intrapericardial, or paracardiac (Fig. 34-6).

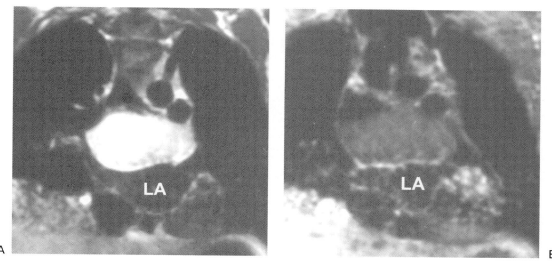

FIG. 34-5. Lipoma. ECG-gated spin-echo images in coronal plane, before (**A**) and after (**B**) fat saturation, of a mass situated above the left atrium *(LA)*. Signal of the mass is suppressed with fat saturation.

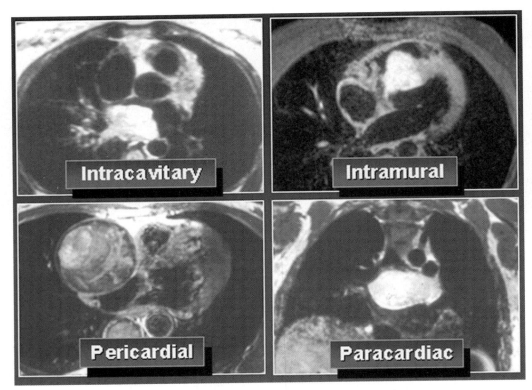

FIG. 34-6. Location of masses on tomographic imaging.

BENIGN PRIMARY CARDIAC TUMORS

About 80% of primary cardiac tumors are benign. Although these tumors do not metastasize or invade locally, they may lead to significant morbidity and mortality by causing arrhythmias, valvular obstruction, or embolism. An intramyocardial location can interfere with normal conduction pathways and produce arrhythmias, obstruct coronary blood flow, or diminish compliance or contractility through replacement of myocardium.

Myxoma

Myxoma, the most common benign cardiac tumor, accounts for 25% of primary cardiac masses. It is located in the left atrium in 75% of cases and in the right atrium in 20% of cases. This tumor is usually spherical, but the shape may vary during the cardiac cycle because of its gelatinous consistency. Left atrial myxomas are typically attached by a narrow pedicle to the area of the fossa ovalis (Fig. 34-7, left). Infrequently, myxomas have a wide base of attachment to the atrial septum (see Fig. 34-7, right). However, a wide mural attachment is more frequently encountered with malignant tumors. The extent of attachment may be difficult to assess for large tumors, which fill nearly the entire cavity so that they are compressed against the septum. As a result,

the tumor appears to have broad contact with atrial septum on static MR images. Myxomas can grow through a patent foramen ovale and extend into both atria, a condition that has been described as a "dumbbell" appearance. Cine MRI permits an evaluation of tumor motion and may help to identify the site and length of attachment of the tumor to the wall or walls of the cardiac chambers. With this technique, myxomas have been shown to prolapse through the funnel of the atrioventricular valve (Fig. 34-8) or into the corresponding ventricle during diastole.

Usually, myxomas display intermediate signal intensity (isointense to the myocardium) on T1-weighted SE images. On T2-weighted SE images, myxomas usually have higher signal intensity than myocardium. However, myxomas with very low signal intensity have also been observed. Fibrous stroma, calcification, and the deposition of paramagnetic iron following interstitial hemorrhage can reduce the signal intensity of the tumor on T2-weighted SE images. Rarely, myxomas have been reported to be invisible on SE images because of a lack of contrast with the dark blood pool. Such tumors can be delineated with cine MRI, on which they appear with high contrast against the surrounding bright blood. Most myxomas show increased signal intensity after the administration of Gd-DTPA on T1-weighted images (Fig. 34-9), which is probably secondary to an increased interstitial space and therefore a larger distribution volume of the contrast agent within the tumor than in normal tissue.

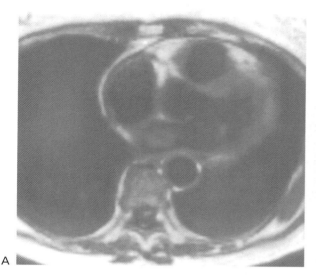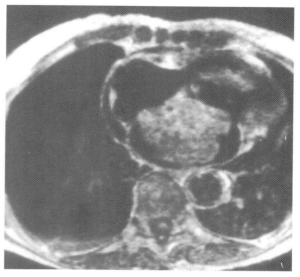

FIG. 34-7. Myxomas. ECG-gated spin-echo images display two left atrial myxomas with a narrow point of attachment (pedicle; **A**) and a wide point of attachment (**B**) to the left side of the atrial septum.

Lipoma and Lipomatous Hypertrophy of the Atrial Septum

Lipomas are reported to be the second most common benign cardiac tumor in adults but may actually be the most common. They may occur at any age but are encountered most frequently in middle-aged and elderly adults. Lipomas consist of encapsulated mature adipose cells and fetal fat cells. The tumor consistency is soft, and lipomas may grow to a large size without causing symptoms. Lipomas are typically located in the right atrium (Fig. 34-10) or atrial septum. They arise from the endocardial surface and have a broad base of attachment. Lipomas have the same signal intensity as subcutaneous and epicardial fat on all MRI sequences. Because fat has a short T1 relaxation time, lipomas have high signal intensity on T1-weighted images, which can be suppressed with fat-saturating pulse sequences (see Fig. 34-10). Usually, they appear with homogeneous signal intensity but may have a few thin septations. They do not enhance after the administration of contrast. On T2-weighted images, lipomas have intermediate signal intensity.

Lipomatous hypertrophy of the atrial septum is considered to be an entity distinct from intracavitary lipoma. Lipomatous hypertrophy of the atrial septum is more common and is alleged to be a cause of supraventricular arrhythmias. Lipomatous hypertrophy is defined as a deposition of fat

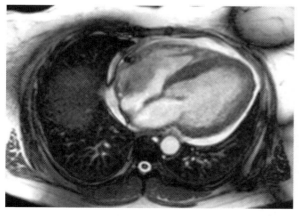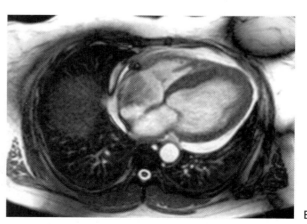

FIG. 34-8. Myxoma. Cine MR images (balanced steady-state free precession) in the axial plane display a right atrial myxoma in diastole (**A**) and systole (**B**). The motion of the tumor is evident with movement into the tricuspid valve during diastole.

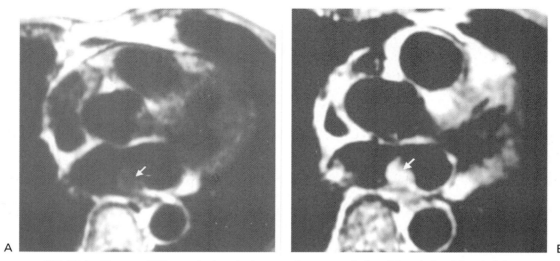

FIG. 34-9. Myxoma. ECG-gated spin-echo images of a myxoma before (**A**) and after (**B**) gadolinium chelate administration. Tumor *(arrows)* increases substantially in signal intensity.

in the atrial septum around the fossa ovalis that exceeds 2 cm in transverse diameter. It spares the fossa ovalis, a characteristic feature that is clearly delineated with T1-weighted SE images (Fig. 34-11). Lipomatous hypertrophy has the same cellular composition as lipoma but is not encapsulated and infiltrates through the tissue of the atrial septum. It is not a true neoplasm. Fatty tissue may extend from the septum into both atria to a considerable degree. Signal intensity on MRI is similar to that of lipomas.

Papillary Fibroelastoma

Papillary fibroelastomas constitute about 10% of benign primary cardiac tumors. These tumors consist of avascular fronds of connective tissue lined by endothelium. Papillary fibroelastomas are attached to the valves by a short pedicle in approximately 90% of cases. They usually do not exceed 1 cm in diameter. Papillary fibroelastomas have been found on the aortic (29%), mitral (2%), pulmonary (13%), and tricuspid (17%) valves. Right-sided tumors usually remain asymptomatic. Symptoms associated with fibroelastoma are related to embolization of thrombi, which may accumulate on the tumor. Because of their high content of fibrous tissue, they have low signal intensity on T2-weighted images. The diagnosis of these valvular tumors is challenging because of their small size, low contrast relative to the blood pool on SE images, and location on the rapidly moving valves. With recent advances in fast cine MR sequences and improved

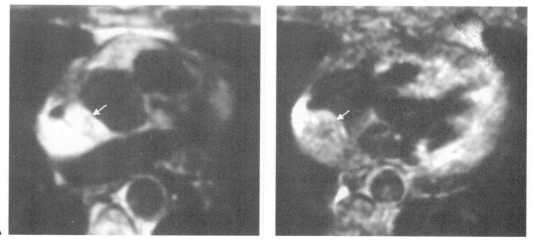

FIG. 34-10. Lipoma. ECG-gated spin-echo images of a lipoma *(arrows)* of the right atrium without (**A**) and with (**B**) fat saturation prepulse sequence. With fat saturation, signal is depleted from the right atrial mass.

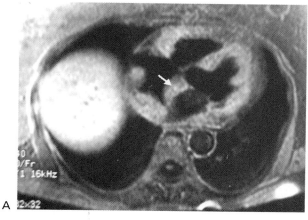

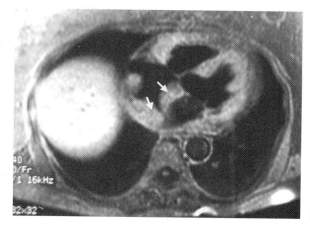

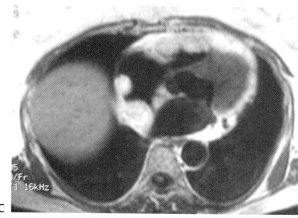

FIG. 34-11. Lipomatous hypertrophy (infiltration) of the atrial septum. ECG-gated T1-weighted spin-echo images before (**A** and **B**) and after (**C**) fat saturation show the atrial septum thickened by fatty infiltration. Signal of the fat is decreased on the fat-saturation image.

homogeneity of the bright blood pool signal, however, the visualization of valve motion during the cardiac cycle has become possible. Small masses attached to valves have been accurately depicted with MRI. In many cases, such lesions can be assessed only with cine MRI. In these cases, signal intensity characteristics after the administration of Gd-DTPA cannot be evaluated, and the differential diagnosis between thrombus and tumor may not be feasible. Cine MRI can be used to assess the effect of valvular tumors on valve function; it demonstrates jet flow caused by either obstruction or regurgitation.

Rhabdomyoma

Rhabdomyomas are the most common cardiac tumors in children, representing 40% of all cardiac tumors in this age group. Thirty to 50% of rhabdomyomas occur in patients with tuberous sclerosis. Rhabdomyomas may vary in size and are frequently multiple. They are characterized by an intramural location and involve equally the left and right ventricles. Small, entirely intramural tumors may be difficult to identify. Larger tumors distort the shape of the myocardial wall or may bulge into the cavity. Larger tumors can

also distort the epicardial contour of the heart. Rhabdomyomas may have a signal intensity similar to that of normal myocardium on SE images and may display hyperenhancement after the administration of gadolinium contrast.

Fibroma

Fibroma is the second most common benign cardiac tumor in children. It is a connective tissue tumor that is composed of fibroblasts interspersed among collagen fibers. It arises within the myocardial walls. Unlike most other primary cardiac tumors, fibromas usually do not display cystic changes, hemorrhage, or focal necrosis, but dystrophic calcification is common. Fibromas may cause arrhythmias and have been reported to be associated with sudden death. Approximately 30% of these tumors remain asymptomatic and may be discovered incidentally because of heart murmurs, ECG changes, or abnormalities on chest roentgenography. Fibromas occur most often within the septum or anterior wall of the RV and can reach a large diameter (Figs. 34-12 and 34-13). On T2-weighted MR images, they are characteristically hypointense to the surrounding myocardium, which is compatible with the short T2 relaxation time of

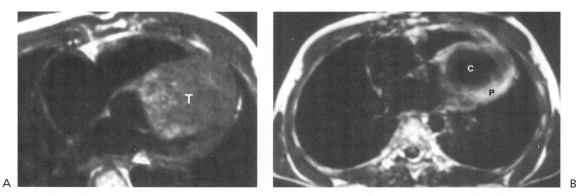

FIG. 34-12. Fibroma. ECG-gated T1-weighted spin-echo images before (**A**) and after (**B**) gadolinium chelate administration show a fibroma *(arrow)* of the ventricular septum in a young child. There is hyperenhancement of the periphery of the mass but no enhancement of the center.

fibrous tissue. On T1-weighted images, fibromas may appear isointense to the myocardium. Fibromas show delayed hyperenhancement of the periphery of the tumor early after the administration of Gd-DTPA. Administration of Gd-DTPA has been effective for demarcating these intramural tumors more clearly from normal myocardium (see Figs. 34-12 and 34-13). Hyperenhancement of compressed myocardium at the margin of the tumor facilitates delineation of the borders of the nonenhancing tumor. Delayed (15 to 20 minutes after administration) hyperenhancement of the entire mass has also been observed.

The differential diagnosis for intramural masses in children is rhabdomyoma versus fibroma. If the tumor is solitary and has low signal intensity on T2-weighted images, fibroma is more likely. If multiple tumors are present with

high intensity on T2-weighted images, rhabdomyomas are the likely diagnosis.

Pheochromocytoma

Pheochromocytomas arise from neuroendocrine cells clustered in the visceral paraganglia in the posterior wall of the left atrium, roof of the right atrium, atrial septum, behind the ascending aorta, and along the coronary arteries. Pheochromocytomas can be found at each of these locations but are predominantly encountered in and around the left atrium (Figs. 34-14 and 34-15). Most are located outside of the cardiac chamber. They usually have a broad interface with the heart. Hypertension, the most common symptom, is related to catecholamine overproduction by the mass. The

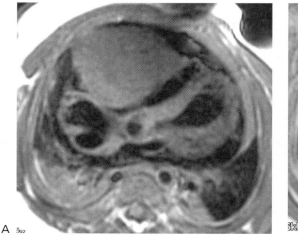
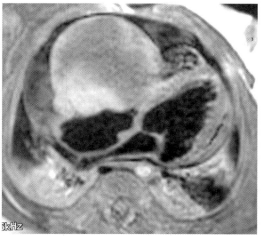

FIG. 34-13. Fibroma. ECG-gated T1-weighted spin-echo transaxial images before (**A**) and after (**B**) gadolinium chelate administration in an infant. The periphery of the huge mass shows hyperenhancement. The center of the mass shows low intensity on the cine MR image. The mass bulges off the free wall of the right ventricle.

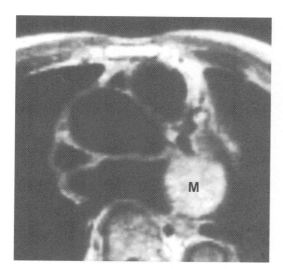

FIG. 34-14. Pheochromocytoma. ECG-gated T1-weighted spin-echo images show a mass of high signal intensity *(M)* adjacent to the left atrium.

average age at diagnosis is 30 to 50 years. Cardiac pheochromocytomas are usually benign. Pheochromocytomas are generally highly vascularized. The average size ranges from 3 to 8 cm at diagnosis. Pheochromocytomas are hyperintense to the myocardium on T2-weighted images and isointense or hyperintense on T1-weighted images (see Figs. 34-14 and 34-15). After Gd-DTPA administration, they show strong signal enhancement because of their high vascularity. Enhancement may be heterogeneous, with central nonenhancing areas, related to tumor necrosis. The combination of imaging findings, clinical symptoms, and biochemical

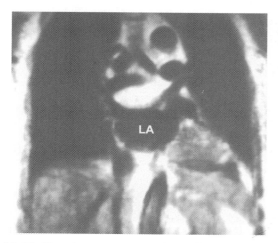

FIG. 34-15. Pheochromocytoma. ECG-gated T1-weighted image in coronal plane. The mass *(M)* originates from the aortic body and is situated above the roof of the left atrium *(LA)*. It has high signal intensity on T1-weighted images.

evidence of catecholamine overproduction usually permits a confident diagnosis.

Hemangioma

Cardiac hemangiomas are composed of endothelial cells that line interconnecting vascular channels. These vascular cavities are separated by connective tissue. According to the size of the vascular channels, hemangiomas are divided into capillary, cavernous, or venous types. Calcification, which can easily be identified on CT, is often present in these tumors. Hemangiomas may involve the endocardium, myocardium, or epicardium. They have been found in all chambers and also the pericardium. On T2-weighted images, hemangiomas are hyperintense. On T1-weighted images, they are of intermediate signal intensity but can have higher intensity than myocardium (Fig. 34-16). Because of interspersed calcifications and possible flow voids at areas of blood flow in the channels of hemangiomas, they may have inhomogeneous signal intensity. They usually show intense enhancement after the administration of gadolinium contrast because of their rich vascularity.

MALIGNANT PRIMARY CARDIAC TUMORS

One fourth of primary cardiac tumors are malignant; sarcomas represent the largest number, followed by primary cardiac lymphomas. The features of malignant cardiac tumors are the following: involvement of more than one cardiac chamber; extension into pulmonary veins, pulmonary arteries, or vena cavae; wide point of attachment to the wall of a chamber or chambers; necrosis within the tumor; extension outside the heart; and hemorrhagic pericardial effusion. A combined intramural and intracavitary location is another suggestive feature of malignant tumors (Fig. 34-17). MRI is effective for demonstrating invasion of the pericardium and extension into the pericardial fat (Figs. 34-1 and 34-18). Pericardial infiltration is displayed on MRI as a disruption, thickening, or nodularity of the pericardium, often combined with pericardial effusion. Cardiac tamponade as a consequence of hemorrhagic pericardial effusion may be demonstrated as diastolic indentation of the right atrial free wall.

Extension into the mediastinum and metastasis are also clear signs of malignancy. The organs most frequently involved are the lungs, pleurae, mediastinal lymph nodes, and liver. The rapid growth of malignant cardiac tumors may cause focal necrosis in the central part of the tumor. Necrotic areas are delineated as regions of lower signal intensity within a hyperenhancing mass after the administration of Gd-DTPA (Fig. 34-19).

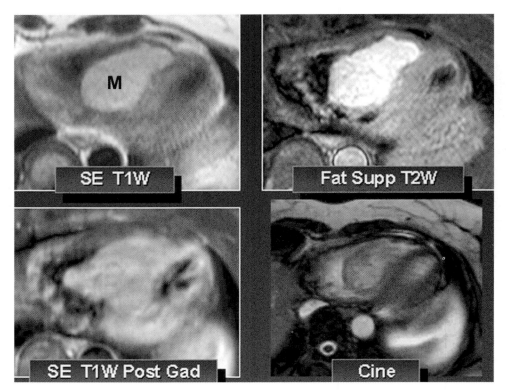

FIG. 34-16. Hemangioma. T1-weighted (**top left**), T2-weighted fat-saturation (**top right**), and T1-weighted after gadolinium chelate administration (**bottom left**) spin-echo images and a gradient-echo cine MR image (**bottom right**) demonstrate a large mass *(M)* originating in the septum and bulging into the right ventricular cavity. The mass has high signal on all sequences.

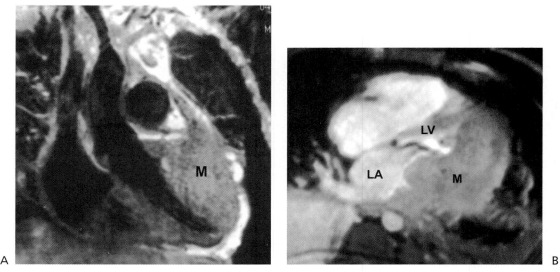

FIG. 34-17. Lymphoma. Coronal spin-echo (**A**) and gradient-echo (cine MR; **B**) images demonstrate a large mass *(M)*, which involves the lateral wall of the left ventricle and extends into the left ventricular *(LV)* and atrial *(LA)* cavities.

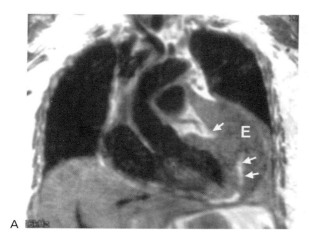
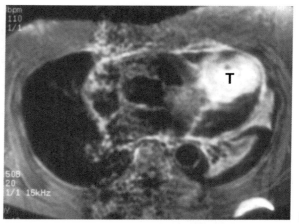

FIG. 34-18. Rhabdomyosarcoma. Coronal (**A**) and transaxial after gadolinium chelate administration (**B**) spin-echo images. Coronal images show a loculated pericardial effusion *(E)* with high intensity on T1-weighted imaging (hemorrhagic effusion). The epicardial fat line *(arrows)* is disrupted by the tumor extending into the pericardial space. Transaxial image after contrast administration shows the tumor *(T)* demonstrated by the marked enhancement, whereas the pericardial fluid is not enhanced.

Angiosarcoma

Angiosarcomas are the most common malignant cardiac tumors in adults and constitute one third of malignant cardiac tumors (Figs. 34-1, 34-2, 34-4, 34-20, and 34-21). They occur predominantly in men between 20 and 50 years of age. This entity has been divided into two clinicopathologic forms. Most frequently, angiosarcomas are found in the right atrium (see Figs. 34-1, 34-2, 34-20, and 34-21). In this form, no evidence of Kaposi sarcoma is found. Another form is characterized by involvement of the epicardium or pericardium in the presence of Kaposi sarcoma. These lesions are usually small, localized, and asymptomatic. This form is associated with the acquired immunodeficiency syndrome. Angiosarcomas consist of ill-defined anastomotic vascular spaces that are lined by endothelial cells and avascular clusters of moderately pleomorphic spindle cells surrounded by collagen stroma. T1-weighted SE imaging usu-

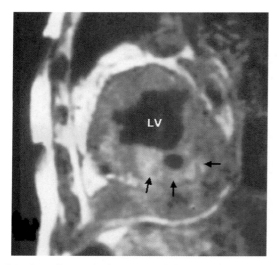

FIG. 34-19. Left ventricular myocardial sarcoma. Sagittal image after gadolinium chelate administration demonstrates enhancement of the mass *(arrows)* involving the diaphragmatic wall of the left ventricle *(LV)*. The central necrotic region does not enhance. There is a large loculated pericardial effusion below the diaphragmatic wall.

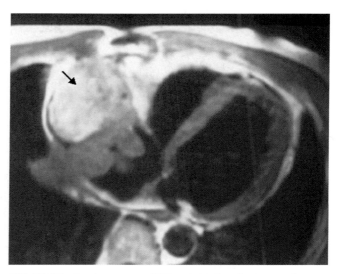

FIG. 34-20. Angiosarcoma. ECG-gated spin-echo image demonstrates a mass filling most of the right atrium and extending through the atrial wall. The tumor has heterogenous intensity on this T1-weighted image. High signal region *(arrow)* represents intratumoral hemorrhage.

ally demonstrates heterogeneous signal intensity of the tumor with focal areas of high signal intensity, which presumably represent hemorrhage (see Fig. 34-20). However, angiosarcomas can also have homogeneous signal intensity. After contrast administration, angiosarcomas show hyperenhancement. Some of the tumors show regions of low signal intensity on both T1- and T2-weighted images. These central regions have high signal intensity on cine gradient-echo images and represent vascular channels (see Fig. 34-21). This finding is often described as a "cauliflower" appearance. Cases with diffuse pericardial infiltration have been found to show linear hyperenhancement along vascular spaces.

Rhabdomyosarcoma

Rhabdomyosarcomas are the most common malignant cardiac tumors in children. They can arise anywhere in the myocardium and are often multiple. Their signal intensity on MRI is variable. Rhabdomyosarcomas may be isointense to the myocardium on T1- and T2-weighted images, but areas of necrosis can exhibit heterogeneous signal intensity and patchy hyperenhancement after Gd-DTPA administration (see Fig. 34-18). Extracardiac extension into the pulmonary arteries and descending aorta has been clearly delineated with MRI.

Other Sarcomas (Fibrosarcoma, Osteosarcoma, Leiomyosarcoma, Liposarcoma)

Other possible primary sarcomas are fibrosarcomas, osteosarcomas, leiomyosarcomas, and liposarcomas. These all are rare tumors, representing approximately 4% of primary cardiac masses. The signal intensity characteristics of these entities are nonspecific. Most of these tumors show signal intensity isointense to normal myocardium on T1-weighted images and hyperintense on T2-weighted images. Most of these tumors show increased signal intensity on T1-weighted images after Gd-DTPA administration, so that the lesions are more conspicuous and the delineation of the tumor margins is increased.

Lymphoma

Primary cardiac lymphoma is less common than secondary lymphoma involving the heart, which usually represents the spread of non-Hodgkin's lymphoma. Primary lymphoma of the heart most often occurs in immunocompromised patients and is highly aggressive. Almost all primary cardiac lymphomas are B-cell lymphomas. Although primary cardiac lymphoma is rare, it is mandatory to consider this entity in the diagnosis of malignant cardiac tumors because early chemotherapy is usually effective. These tumors arise most often on the right side of the heart, especially in the right atrium, but have also been found in the other chambers (see Fig. 34-17). A large pericardial effusion is frequently present. Variable morphology of the masses has been described; both circumscribed polypoid and ill-defined infiltrative lesions have been reported. Lymphomas may appear hypointense to the myocardium on T1-weighted images and hyperintense on T2-weighted images. After Gd-DTPA administration, homogeneous or heterogeneous enhancement of the tumor, depending on the presence of necrosis, may be seen. Some lymphomas consist of a large extracardiac mediastinal mass as well as an invasive mass of the cardiac chambers (Fig. 34-22).

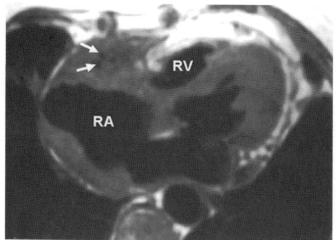
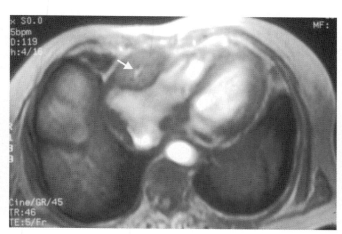

FIG. 34-21. Angiosarcoma. T1-weighted spin-echo (**A**) and gradient-echo (**B**) images show components of the mass along the posterior right atrial wall and in the pericardial cavity. Note the sinuous regions in the pericardial mass, which represent vascular channels. These channels have high signal because of blood flow on the gradient-echo images *(arrows)*. RA, right atrium; RV, right ventricle.

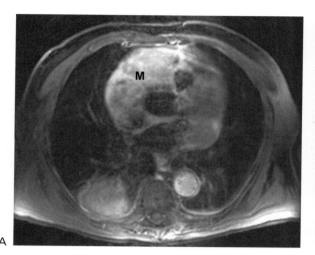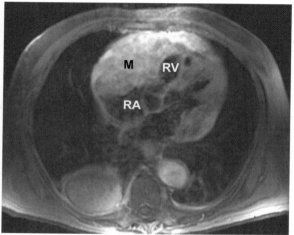

FIG. 34-22. Lymphoma. T1-weighted spin-echo image with fat saturation after gadolinium chelate administration at the level of the right atrium (**A**) and the right ventricle (**B**). A mass (*M*) invades the right atrial cavity and right ventricular wall. RA, right atrium; RV, right ventricle.

SECONDARY CARDIAC TUMORS

Secondary tumors of the heart and pericardium are about 40-fold more frequent than primary tumors. Three routes of spread to the heart can be discerned: (1) direct extension from intrathoracic tumors (mediastinum and lungs); (2) extension of abdominal malignancies through the inferior vena cava into the right atrium (renal, adrenal, and hepatic carcinomas); (3) metastasis.

Direct Extension From Adjacent Tumors

Tumors of the lung and mediastinum can infiltrate the pericardium and heart directly (Figs. 34-23 and 34-24). It is important to recognize invasion of the heart because such a tumor is usually nonresectable. In mediastinal lymphoma, possible invasion of the pericardium can change the staging of the tumor. MRI is especially suited for delineating paracardiac tumors and possible extension into the heart because of its wide field of view. MRI clearly shows extension of these tumors to the cardiac structures and possible evidence of hemorrhagic or nonhemorrhagic pericardial effusion. MRI is effective in demonstrating invasion of the pericardium and myocardium in advanced lung cancer.

Metastasis

Melanomas, leukemias, and lymphomas (see Fig. 34-22) are the tumors that most frequently metastasize to the heart,

FIG. 34-23. Mediastinal tumor (*T*) invading the pericardium and atrial walls. LA, left atrium; RA, right atrium.

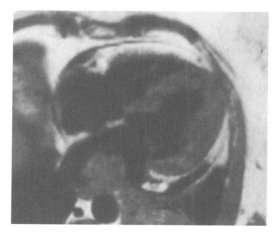

FIG. 34-24. Extension of lung cancer through left atrial wall.

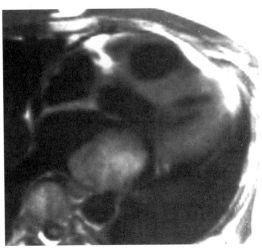

FIG. 34-25. Metastasis to the left atrium. ECG-gated T1-weighted spin-echo transaxial images.

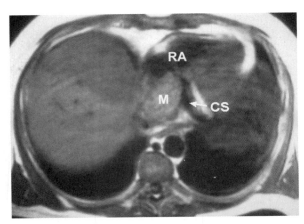

FIG. 34-27. Renal cell carcinoma. Direct extension of mass *(M)* into the right atrium via inferior vena cava. CS, coronary sinus; RA, right atrium.

but cardiac metastases can arise from almost any malignant tumor in the body. Melanomas have the highest frequency of seeding into the heart and are frequently found in the heart at autopsy. The mechanism of metastatic spread of tumors to the heart is direct seeding to the endocardium, passage of tumor emboli through the coronary arteries, or retrograde lymphatic spread through bronchomediastinal lymphatic channels. MRI is highly effective for delineating the location and extent of metastatic tumors in cardiac chambers (Figs. 34-25 and 34-26) and assessing potential respectability.

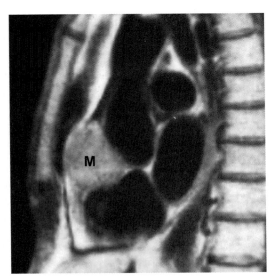

FIG. 34-26. Metastasis to right atrial appendage. ECG-gated T1-weighted spin-echo sagittal image shows a large mass *(M)* filling and expanding the right atrial appendage.

Transvenous Extension Into the Heart

Another site for the entry of secondary tumors into the heart is tumor extension through the large veins connecting with cardiac chambers. Tumor thrombus arising from carcinoma of the kidney, liver, or adrenal gland can extend through the inferior vena cava into the right atrium (Fig. 34-27), and primary carcinoma of the thymus can extend through the superior vena cava. The evaluation of the possible attachment of such tumors to the atrial wall is mandatory for surgical planning. If the atrial walls are not infiltrated, complete resection of the tumor may still be possible.

INTRACARDIAC THROMBUS

Thrombus is the most common intracardiac mass, involving most frequently the LV or left atrium. Atrial thrombus is encountered in patients with mitral valve disease or atrial fibrillation. LV mural thrombus is associated with akinetic or dyskinetic regions of the ventricle. It is most often located in the LV at the site of myocardial infarction (Fig. 34-28) or in dilated cardiomyopathy. However, any region of the ventricular cavity with static blood is prone to thrombus formation. MRI is especially advantageous for detecting thrombus in the left atrial appendage, which may be difficult to assess using transthoracic echocardiography (Fig. 34-29).

On SE images, the signal intensity of thrombus can vary from low to high depending on age-related changes in the composition of the thrombus. The signal intensity of thrombus can with time be influenced by paramagnetic hemoglobin breakdown products, such as intracellular methemoglobin and hemosiderin, or superparamagnetic substances, such as ferritin. Fresh thrombus usually shows high signal intensity on T1- and T2-weighted SE images, whereas older thrombus has low signal intensity on T1- and T2-

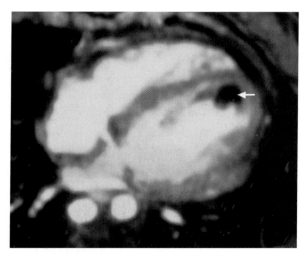

FIG. 34-28. Left ventricular thrombus after myocardial infarction. Transaxial gradient-echo (cine MR) image shows a low-intensity intracavitary mass *(arrow)*.

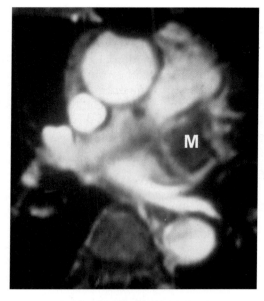

A

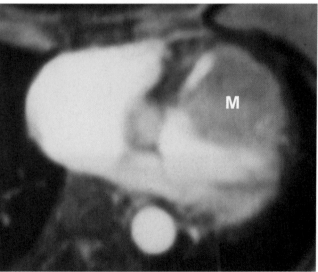

B

FIG. 34-29. Left atrial appendage thrombus **(A)** and metastatic tumor of the right ventricle **(B)**. Transaxial gradient echo (cine MR) image shows a mass *(M)* filling the left atrial appendage with low intensity. The mass *(M)* in the right ventricle has intermediate signal intensity.

weighted images. Intracavitary high signal on SE images caused by slowly flowing blood may be difficult to distinguish from thrombus. However, this problem can be overcome either by using the SE sequences after inversion recovery pulses to null intracavitary signal or by using cine MRI.

DIFFERENTIATION BETWEEN TUMOR AND BLOOD CLOT

The distinction between clot and tumor is more reliably made with gradient-echo sequences. The gradient-echo technique is more sensitive to susceptibility and T2* effects than is the SE technique. As the various blood degeneration products pass through the different stages of magnetic susceptibility, they continue to cause shortening of T2* relaxivity; the result is low signal intensity of the thrombus on gradient-echo images (see Figs. 34-28 and 34-29). An exception to this generalization is fresh thrombus, which can have high signal intensity. Tumor tissue usually is hyperintense in comparison with myocardium and skeletal muscle on T2-weighted SE images and cine MR images. However, some myxomas containing substantial iron produce low signal and so mimic thrombus. Another method for differentiating between tumor and clot is to use Gd-DTPA-enhanced T1-weighted images. Thrombus does not enhance after the administration of Gd-DTPA, whereas tumors show enhancement (see Fig. 34-9). Tumor can usually be differentiated from thrombus by using gradient-echo images and T1-weighted SE images after Gd-DTPA administration.

DIFERENTIATION OF CARDIAC MASSES FROM NORMAL ANATOMIC VARIANTS

A potential pitfall in the evaluation of intracardiac masses may arise from the misdiagnosis of normal anatomic variants, such as a prominent crista terminalis, eustachian valve, or Chiari network. The crista terminalis, a fibromuscular band extending between the ostia of the superior and inferior vena cavae on the posterior right atrial wall, represents a residuum of the septum spurium where the sinus venosus was incorporated into the right atrial wall. The Chiari network, a reticulum situated in the right atrium, is attached to the region of the crista terminalis and extends to the valves of the inferior vena cava and coronary sinus, or sometimes to the floor of the right atrium near the ostium of the coronary sinus. The Chiari network is derived from the valvulae venosi. These structures regress to variable degrees, and a nodule-like residue in the right atrium is visible on MRI in some patients. Awareness of these variants can prevent misinterpretation as mass lesions.

SELECTED READING

Araoz PA, Eklund HE, Welch TJ, et al. CT and MR imaging of primary cardiac malignancies. Radiographics 1999; 19:1421.

Araoz PA, Mulvagh SL, Tazlaar HD, et al. CT and MR imaging of benign primary cardiac neoplasms with echocardiographic correlation. Radiographics 2000; 20:1303.

Barakos JA, Brown JJ, Higgins CB. MR imaging of secondary cardiac and pericardiac lesions. AJR Am J Roentgenol 1989; 153:47–50.

Fujita N, Caputo GR, Higgins CB. Diagnosis and characterization of intracardial masses by magnetic resonance imaging. Am J Cardiol Imaging 1994; 8:69.

Mader MT, Poulton TB, White RD. Malignant tumors of the heart and great vessels: MR imaging appearance. Radiographics 1997; 17:145.

Schvartzman PR, White RD. Imaging of cardiac and paracardiac masses. J Thorac Imaging 2000; 15:265.

Siripornpitak S, Higgins CB. MRI of primary malignant cardiovascular tumors. J Comput Assist Tomogr 1997; 21:462.

35

MAGNETIC RESONANCE IMAGING OF CONGENITAL HEART DISEASE

CHARLES B. HIGGINS AND GAUTHAM P. REDDY

The overall objectives of imaging in congenital heart disease are the precise delineation of cardiovascular anatomy and the quantitative assessment of function. The evaluation of congenital heart disease was one of the first applications of cardiac magnetic resonance imaging (MRI) and continues to be one of its most important indications. MRI has significant advantages over other modalities, including echocardiography and angiography, for the definitive assessment of congenital cardiovascular anomalies. MRI does not require the use of a contrast agent or ionizing radiation. The absence of ionizing radiation is a major advantage of MRI in children, who in the past have been exposed to large does of radiation during cine angiography for initial diagnosis and postoperative monitoring.

The role of MRI has been greatly influenced by the perceived success of echocardiography as the primary noninvasive imaging technique in congenital heart disease. The major applications have been for lesions incompletely evaluated by echocardiography. However, substantial technological improvements, especially fast gradient-echo imaging (steady-state free precession [SSFP]) and contrast-enhanced magnetic resonance angiography (MRA), make MRI at least equal to echocardiography in the diagnosis of all types of congenital heart disease in children and adults. Echocardiography is still considered to be the more effective and easily applicable modality for infants. On the other hand, MRI is becoming recognized as more effective in adolescent and adult congenital heart disease.

At present, the major indications for MRI in congenital heart disease are as follows:

1. Thoracic aortic anomalies, such as coarctation and arch anomalies
2. Pulmonary arterial anomalies and pulmonary atresia
3. Complex cyanotic disease, such as atresia of atrioventricular valves and double-inlet ventricles
4. Abnormalities of pulmonary venous connections
5. Postoperative evaluation of complex procedures
6. Coronary arterial anomalies
7. Adolescent and adult congenital heart disease

TECHNIQUES

MRI studies are directed toward precise display of the cardiovascular anatomy and quantification of ventricular function and blood flow. An advantage of MRI in congenital heart disease is measurement of right ventricular volumes and function.

For children younger than 8 to 10 years and children unwilling or unable to remain immobile and cooperative during imaging, light anesthesia without intubation is used. This is usually under the control of an anesthesiologist. The favored drug is intravenous propofol. Blood pressure, heart rate, and oxygen saturation are monitored during the procedure.

Anatomy

Assessment of anatomy is done with one or more of the following techniques: ECG-gated multislice spin-echo (black-blood images); breath-hold single-slice or multislice turbo spin-echo (black blood); balanced SSFP (white blood); and contrast-enhanced three-dimensional (3D) MRA. The latter technique is usually applied for the evaluation of anomalies of the great arteries, pulmonary veins, and surgical shunts.

Function

The techniques used in the evaluation of right and left ventricular function are the gradient-echo techniques that are generically called cine MRI. There are a multitude of cine MRI sequences; the most frequently applied are standard cine MRI; interleaved (breath-hold) cine MRI; balanced SSFP; and real-time cine MRI. Because of optimized homogeneous contrast between cavitary blood and myocardium, balanced SSFP sequences (balanced FFE; true FISP; FIESTA) are now preferred. The so-called real-time sequence may be advantageous in infants and young children who cannot hold their breath.

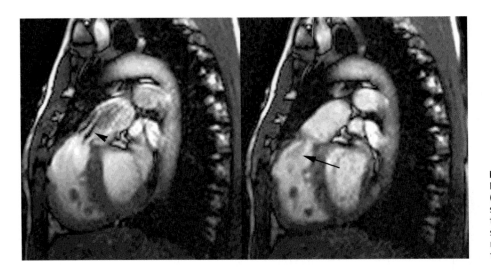

FIG. 35-1. Postoperative tetralogy of Fallot. Sagittal cine MR images in systole (**left**) and diastole (**right**) demonstrate a signal void *(arrowhead)* projected into the pulmonary artery (pulmonary stenosis) and a signal void *(arrow)* into the right ventricle (pulmonary regurgitation).

Cine MR images are used to quantify ventricular volumes and function. Right and left ventricular volumes are indexed to body surface areas (EDV/m^2 and ESV/m^2). A distinct advantage of MRI compared to echocardiography is its precision and reproducibility for quantifying right ventricular volume and function. For ventricular volumetrics, images are acquired in the cardiac short-axis plane.

Cine MR images are also used to evaluate valvular function. Planes approximately parallel to the valve leaflet or cusps can demonstrate valve motion, such as the horizontal long-axis plane for assessing mitral valve motion. The high-velocity jet caused by valvular stenosis and regurgitation may be identified on cine MR images as a flow void (Fig. 35-1). However, flow voids may not be discernible if the echo time (TE) is less than 6 msec, and visible flow voids become smaller with decreasing TE value.

Volume and Velocity of Blood Flow

Quantification of blood flow is done using velocity-encoded (VEC; phase contrast) MRI. In phase contrast imaging, the signal intensity signifies the velocity of blood at each pixel. ECG-gated phase contrast images can be produced in which each image shows the velocity at a different time in the cardiac cycle. Because these are cine-images, they can be referred to as VEC cine MRI. A region of interest drawn around a blood vessel will give the mean velocity within the vessel at that point in the cardiac cycle. The cross-sectional area of the vessel can be multiplied by the spatial mean velocity to obtain the flow in the blood vessel.

VEC cine MRI is used to measure valvular regurgitant volume (Fig. 35-2); differential flow in central pulmonary arteries; systemic to pulmonary shunt flow; flow through conduits (Rastelli and Fontan conduits); and collateral flow in coarctation.

ACYANOTIC LESIONS

Left-to-Right Shunts

Echocardiography provides essential diagnostic information in most left-to-right shunts. MRI is used for a few specific purposes. The major indications are for the following suspected lesions: sinus venosus atrial septal defect (ASD), partial anomalous pulmonary venous connection, and supracristal ventricular septal defect (VSD). VEC cine MRI may also be employed to measure the systemic to pulmonary flow ratio.

Atrial Septal Defect

Spin-echo and cine MR images in the transaxial or four-chamber planes demonstrate the site of the ASD (Fig. 35-3). MR clearly depicts the defect in the portion of the septum separating the superior vena cava from the left atrium, which is diagnostic of a sinus venosus ASD (Fig. 35-4). It also shows the anomalous connection of the right upper lobe pulmonary vein to the superior vena cava adjacent to the septal defect. On spin-echo MR images, the thin fossa ovalis can be mistaken for an ASD. To avoid this error, the defect should be evident at two adjacent anatomic levels or confirmed by a flow jet (void) across the defect on cine MRI.

VEC cine MRI measurement in the main pulmonary artery and proximal ascending aorta can be used to calculate pulmonary to systemic flow ratio (Qp/Qs) (Fig. 35-5). The imaging planes are placed perpendicular to the direction of blood flow in each artery using sagittal images to site their planes. Good correlations have been found for Qp/Qs, measured by VEC cine MR and oximetric samples acquired at cardiac catheterization.

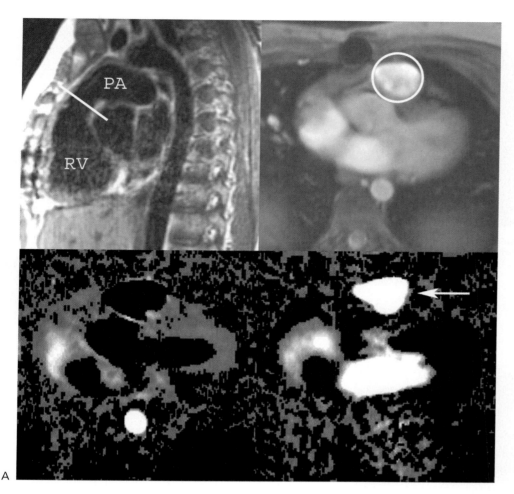

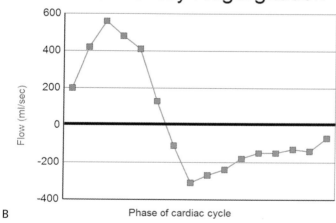

FIG. 35-2. A. Postoperative tetralogy of Fallot. Sagittal spin-echo image (**top left**), axial magnitude image (**top right**), and phase images in systole (**bottom left**) and diastole (**bottom right**). Phase contrast images show forward flow in systole (dark voxels) and retrograde flow in diastole (bright voxels; *arrow*). Region of interest for flow measurements is shown on the pulmonary artery. **B.** Flow versus time curve displays the forward and retrograde flow in the pulmonary artery. Area under negative component of the curve yields a direct quantification of the volume of regurgitation.

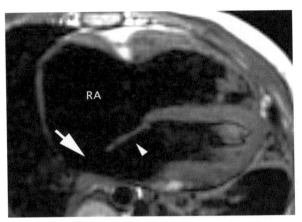

FIG. 35-3. Secundum atrial septal defect. ECG-gated transaxial spin-echo image shows the defect *(arrow)* in the atrial septum *(arrowhead). RA,* right atrium.

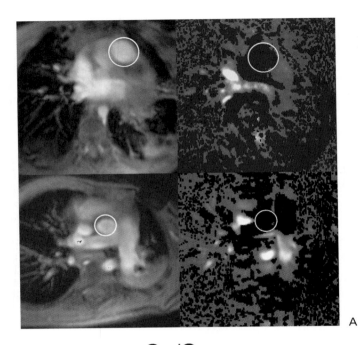

A

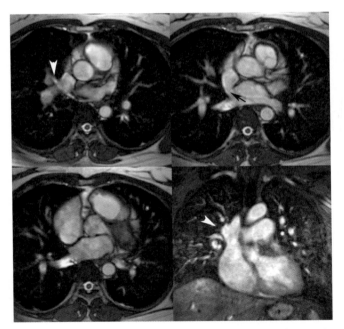

FIG. 35-4. Sinus venosus atrial septal defect. Cine MR images in three axial planes (**top row and bottom left**) and the coronal plane (**bottom right**) show the defect *(arrow)* in the portion of the atrial septum between the superior vena cava and the left atrium. The right upper lobe pulmonary vein *(arrowhead)* connecting at the junction of the superior vena cava *(SVC)* with the right atrium is associated with the sinus venosus defect. Coronal image shows the dilatation of the SVC at the site of connection of the anomalous pulmonary vein.

Qp/Qs

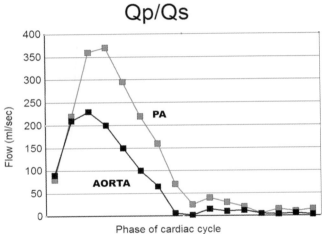

B

FIG. 35-5. A. Atrial septal defect. Magnitude (**left**) and phase (**right**) images from VEC cine MR in planes perpendicular to the long axis of the pulmonary artery (**top**) and the proximal ascending aorta (below). Regions of interest surround the aorta and pulmonary artery. **B.** Flow versus time curves for the aorta and pulmonary artery. Because of the left-to-right shunt, the area under the pulmonary artery curve is greater. The area under each curve provides a direct measurement of the pulmonary to systemic flow ratio (2.1:1).

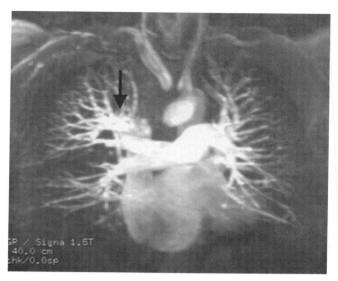

FIG. 35-6. Partial anomalous pulmonary venous connection. Contrast-enhanced 3D MRA shows anomalous connection of the right upper pulmonary vein *(arrow)* to the superior vena cava.

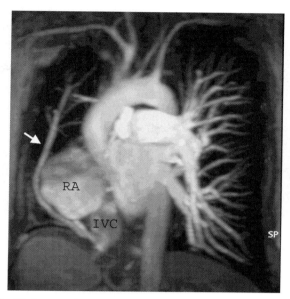

FIG. 35-8. Partial anomalous pulmonary vena connection in scimitar syndrome. Contrast-enhanced 3D MRA shows the scimitar vein *(arrow)* connecting with the inferior vena cava, hypoplastic right pulmonary artery, and dextroposition of the heart. *IVC,* inferior vena cava; *RA,* right atrium. (Courtesy of Gus Bis, Detroit, MI.)

Partial Anomalous Pulmonary Venous Connection

MRI and MRA are the procedures of choice for identifying the presence and connections of this anomaly. MRA is crucial in this regard (Figs. 35-6 and 35-7). The connection of the right-sided pulmonary veins to a common vein that

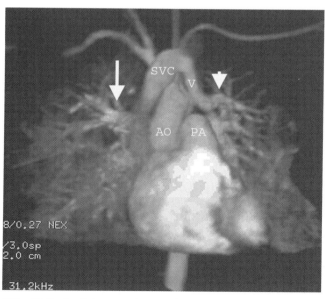

FIG. 35-7. Partial anomalous pulmonary venous connection. Contrast-enhanced 3D MRA shows anomalous connection of the left upper vein *(arrowhead)* to a vertical vein and the right upper vein *(arrow)* to the superior vena cava. *AO,* ascending aorta; *PA,* pulmonary artery; *SVC,* superior vena cava; *V,* vertical vein.

courses to the inferior vena cava can be displayed in the scimitar syndrome (Fig. 35-8).

Ventricular Septal Defect

MRI in the transaxial, horizontal long axis or four-chamber plane can precisely demonstrate the site of single or multiple VSDs (Fig. 35-9). The supracristal VSD is characterized by a defect that lies between the right ventricular outlet and the base of the aorta (Fig. 35-10). On cine MR, a flow void apparently passes from the base of the aorta (it actually passes from just below the aortic valve) to the right ventricular outlet region and into the proximal pulmonary artery (see Fig. 35-10). VEC cine MRI can be used to calculate Qp/Qs for VSDs.

Aorta to Right-sided Shunts

MRI is rarely used to demonstrate patent ductus arteriosus or aorticopulmonary window (Fig. 35-11). With recent improvements in coronary MRA, it may be effective for demonstrating the presence and sites of emptying of coronary arteriovenous fistulas. MRI and MRA are very effective for demonstrating sinus of Valsalva aneurysms and fistulas.

Atrioventricular Septal Defect/ Atrioventricular Canal (Endocardial Cushion Defect)

These terms denote a spectrum of abnormalities that have in common an abnormal septation between the atria and

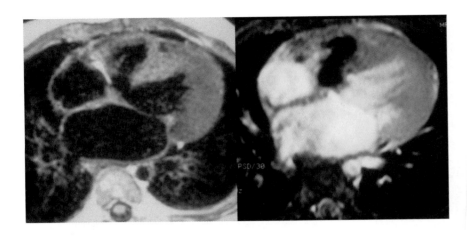

FIG. 35-9. Ventricular septal defect. Spin-echo (**left**) and gradient-echo (**right**) axial images show a defect in the perimembranous ventricular septum. A signal void at the defect is projected into the right ventricle.

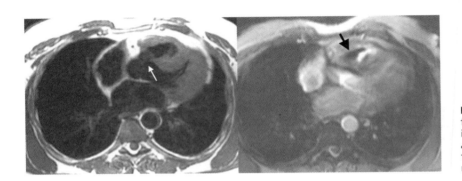

FIG. 35-10. Supracristal ventricular septal defect. Spin-echo (**left**) and cine MR (**right**) images in the axial plane demonstrate a defect *(white arrow)* in the outlet portion of the septum. A flow void *(black arrow)* projects into the upper region of the right ventricular outflow region.

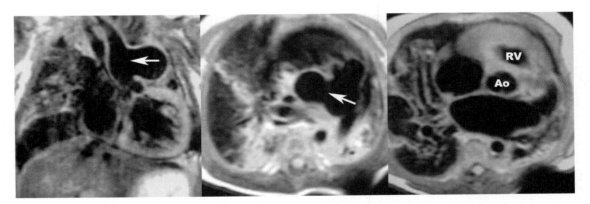

FIG. 35-11. Aorticopulmonary window. Coronal (**left**) and axial (**center and right**) spin-echo images demonstrate a defect *(arrow)* between the proximal ascending aorta and the pulmonary artery. *Ao,* aorta; *RV,* right ventricular outlet region.

ventricles. They are also called endocardial cushion defects because the defects are considered to be abnormalities of the embryologic endocardial cushions, which grow together in the center of the heart and divide the atria from the ventricles.

In the normal heart, the atrioventricular septum separates the right atrium from the left ventricle. The atrioventricular septum lies between the more apically located normal tricuspid valve and mitral valve (Fig. 35-12). In all cases of atrioventricular septal defect, the tricuspid and mitral valves lie at the same level, and the atrioventricular septum is defective. This abnormal relationship can be shown on MRI in the transaxial or four-chamber plane. In the mildest form of atrioventricular septal defect, the shunt is from the left ventricle to the right atrium, which can be evident on cine MRI. In other cases, the atrial septum adjacent to the atrioventricular valve orifice may also be absent, resulting in an **ostium primum ASD**. Some patients have an inlet VSD, usually located in the same axial image as the atrioventricular valve or valves. In the most severe cases, both the atrial and ventricular portions of the septum around the valve origins are absent, a condition referred to as **complete atrioventricular canal**. This creates a common atrioventricular valve orifice with continuous, common atrioventricular valve leaflets (Fig. 35-13).

Coarctation of the Aorta

MRI is the procedure of choice for definitive diagnosis and assessment of the severity of coarctation. MRI has been shown to be effective for preoperative assessment of coarctation and for postoperative evaluation of recurrent or persistent hypertension. To evaluate coarctation, spin-echo se-

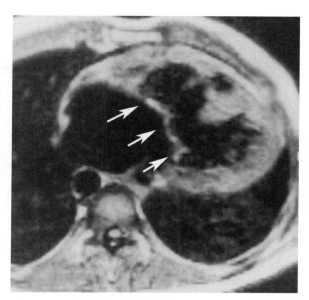

FIG. 35-13. Atrioventricular canal (endocardial cushion) defect. Axial spin-echo image shows a large defect in the inlet portion of the ventricular septum. A single atrioventricular valve *(arrows)* spans the inlet of both ventricles.

quences are obtained in the axial, sagittal, and oblique sagittal planes. The diameter of the narrowing can be precisely measured with MRI, especially with the use of thin (3-mm) sections through the center of the stenosis. Thin oblique sagittal images through the long-axis plane of the aorta show the diameter of the stenosis and provide an accurate measurement of its length (Fig. 35-14).

The oblique sagittal images also display the dimension of aortic isthmus (region between the left subclavian artery and the ligamentum arteriosum and the aortic arch). In some cases, a single 3-mm slice in this plane may not display the coarctation and arch because of tortuosity of the arch and proximal descending aorta, but the assessment can be done from adjacent images. Gadolinium-enhanced 3D MRA can display the entire thoracic aorta on a single image with the use of maximum intensity projection or volume-rendering reconstruction techniques (Fig. 35-15). Gadolinium-enhanced MRA is also effective for demonstrating collateral vessels (Fig. 35-16).

VEC cine MRI can be applied to demonstrate the presence of and estimate the volume of collateral circulation to the descending aorta below the coarctation site (Fig. 35-17). This is accomplished by using two imaging planes perpendicular to the aorta; one is about 2 cm beyond the coarctation and the other at the level of the diaphragm. In the normal aorta, volume flow is greater (about 5% to 7% higher) at the proximal site. On the other hand, in a hemodynamically significant coarctation, volume flow is greater at the diaphragm because of flow through the intercostal and mammary arteries and other collaterals into the distal aorta. The presence of greater volume flow at the diaphrag-

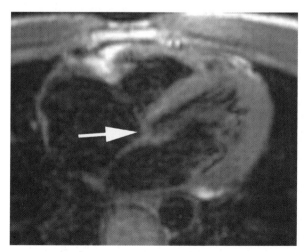

FIG. 35-12. Atrioventricular septum. Axial spin-echo image shows the small portion *(arrow)* of ventricular septum separating the left ventricle and the right atrium. Note the more ventral position of the tricuspid valve relative to the mitral valve.

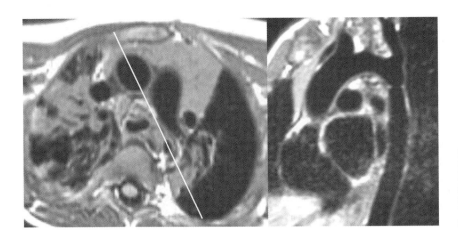

FIG. 35-14. Coarctation of aorta. Axial **(left)** and oblique sagittal **(right)** spin-echo images. A line bisecting the ascending and descending aorta at the coarctation prescribes the oblique sagittal plane (long-axis plane of thoracic aorta). This latter image displays the coarctation site along with the arch.

matic level is considered a functional indicator of hemodynamic significance of the coarctation. There is a rough linear relationship between the percentage of stenosis and the volume of collateral circulation. After stenting of the coarctation, VEC cine MRI has demonstrated reversal of the collateral flow, since volume flow at the proximal site becomes greater than at the distal one. Theoretically, VEC cine MRI can also be used to estimate the gradient across the coarctation. Using a plane perpendicular to the coarctation, peak velocity of flow can be estimated. Applying the modified Bernoulli formula (peak pressure gradient $= 4 \times$ peak velocity^2), the peak gradient is estimated.

Arch Anomalies

There are numerous types of arch anomalies resulting from abnormal resorption of the anterior or posterior segments of the embryonic double-arch configuration. However, the only ones encountered with any frequency are complete (patent) double arch, double arch with atretic posterior component of the left arch (Fig. 35-18), right arch with aberrant (retroesophageal) left subclavian artery (Fig. 35-19), and left arch with aberrant right subclavian artery. The first three produce complete vascular rings that narrow the trachea and esophagus. Compression of the trachea is by the aortic component situated between the vertebral body and the esophagus. The vascular ring with right arch and

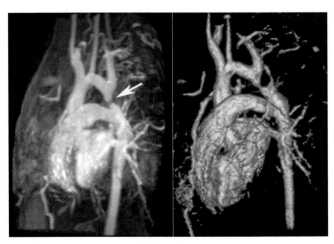

FIG. 35-15. Coarctation of aorta. Contrast-enhanced 3D MRA in the sagittal plane shows a discrete juxtaductal coarctation *(arrow)* on the maximum intensity projection **(left)** and the volume-rendered 3D reconstruction **(right)**.

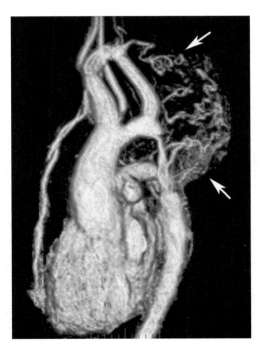

FIG. 35-16. Coarctation of aorta. Contrast-enhanced 3D MRA in the sagittal plane shows long-segment coarctation caused by Takayasu's arteritis. Note the abundant collateral arterial connections *(arrows)*.

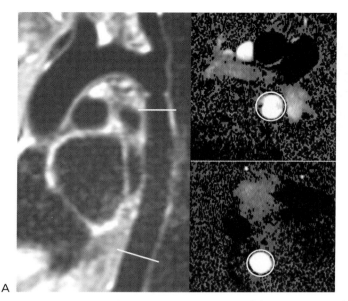

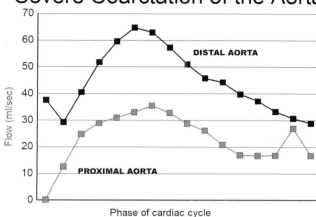

A   B

FIG. 35-17. A. Coarctation of the aorta. Sites of planes for magnitude and phase images in the proximal (**top**) and distal aorta (**bottom**) used to estimate the volume of collateral flow. **B.** Flow versus time curves for the proximal and distal descending aorta show a larger flow volume in the distal compared with the proximal aorta caused by retrograde flow in aortic branches below the coarctation. The volume of collateral flow is estimated as the difference in flow volumes (areas under the curves) at the two sites.

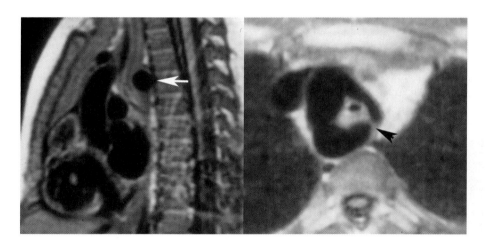

FIG. 35-18. Double aortic arch. Spin-echo images in sagittal (**left**) and axial (**right**) planes display posterior compression of the trachea by a retroesophageal component *(arrow)* of a double arch. The axial plane shows that the right arch is the larger of the two and also shows a short atretic posterior segment *(arrowhead)* of the left arch.

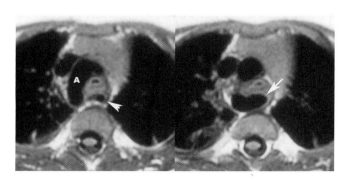

FIG. 35-19. Right aortic arch with aberrant left subclavian artery. Spin-echo axial images (**left**) show the right arch *(A)* and aberrant left subclavian artery *(arrowhead)*. Another axial image shows the diverticulum *(arrow)* of the descending arch, which is the site of origin of the left subclavian artery.

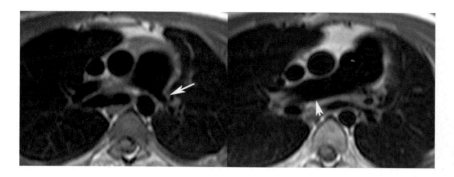

FIG. 35-20. Branch pulmonary artery stenoses. Transaxial spin-echo images display stenosis *(arrow)* of the left pulmonary artery. Note the size of the right pulmonary artery *(arrowhead)* for comparison.

aberrant left subclavian artery is completed by the posterior component that is tethered anteriorly by a left-sided ligamentum arteriosum. With mirror-image right aortic arch, the ligamentum courses between the left innominate artery and the proximal left pulmonary artery. On the other hand, with non–mirror-image right aortic arch, the ligamentum courses between the descending aorta and the proximal left pulmonary artery. At the site of attachment of the ligamentum, there is an enlargement or diverticulum of the descending aorta. This localized dilatation tethered anteriorly by the left-sided ligamentum is the structure that compresses the trachea and esophagus rather than the left subclavian artery itself. These anatomic arrangements can be readily discerned on MR images in the transaxial plane.

For the evaluation of arch anomalies, spin-echo images are acquired in sagittal (5-mm slice thickness) and transaxial (3-mm slice thickness) planes (see Fig. 35-18). These images display the aortic anomaly and verify that the anomalous component produces airway compression. Cine MR images may be used to display the pulsatile nature of the airway obstruction. In some cases, the site of maximal airway compression is at the carina or even involves a proximal bronchus.

Contrast-enhanced 3D MRA may be used to demonstrate the arch anomaly. The MRA acquisition is usually done in the sagittal plane.

Pulmonary Arterial Anomalies

Pulmonary arterial anomalies are evaluated using spin-echo MRI (Fig. 35-20) and contrast-enhanced 3D MRA (Fig. 35-21) for depicting morphology and VEC (phase contrast) MRI for measuring blood flow. Spin-echo images are acquired in the transaxial plane followed by images along the long axis of the right (oblique coronal plane) and left (oblique sagittal plane) pulmonary arteries. Contrast-enhanced 3D MRA is usually acquired in the coronal plane; a short acquisition period is optimal to depict the pulmonary arteries before enhancement of the left heart and aorta. VEC cine sequence is obtained perpendicular to the long axis of the right, left, and main pulmonary arterial segments.

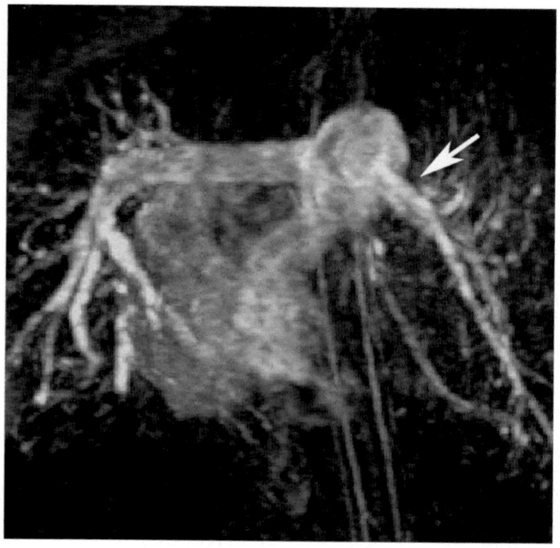

FIG. 35-21. Branch pulmonary artery stenosis. Contrast-enhanced 3D MRA in the coronal plane shows stenosis *(arrow)* of the left pulmonary artery.

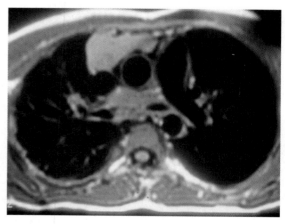

FIG. 35-22. Absent pulmonary artery. Spin-echo axial image shows absence of the right pulmonary artery. There is no pulmonary artery coursing between the ascending aorta and the right bronchus.

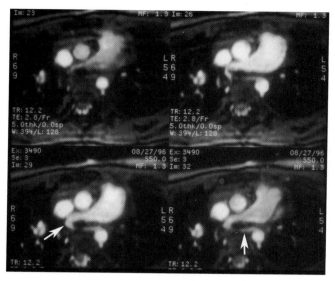

FIG. 35-23. Pulmonary artery sling. Gradient-echo images in the axial plane arranged from cranial (**top left**) to caudal (**bottom right**) demonstrate the origin of the left pulmonary artery *(arrows)* from the proximal right pulmonary artery. The left pulmonary artery curves around and posterior to the right bronchus.

Compared to echocardiography, MRI is more useful for examining the right and left pulmonary arteries, as well as the lobar and segmental arteries. MRI is especially useful for demonstrating central and peripheral pulmonary artery stenoses (see Figs. 35-20 and 35-21), absent pulmonary artery (Fig. 35-22), and pulmonary artery sling (Fig. 35-23). MRI and MRA are the preferred techniques for the evaluation of residual pulmonary arterial stenoses after repair of tetralogy of Fallot (Fig. 35-24).

The hemodynamic significance of pulmonary arterial stenoses is assessed by VEC cine MRI measurement of blood flow separately for each pulmonary artery (Fig. 35-25). Since flow is also measured for the main pulmonary artery,

the values can be expressed as the percentage of total pulmonary blood flow to each lung. The measurement can be done before and after angioplasty to document therapeutic benefit, although such measurements may not be possible in the presence of stainless steel stents.

Congenital Aortic Stenosis

MRI is not used to evaluate aortic stenosis; this is done with echocardiography. The major role of MRI is to evaluate the severity of poststenotic dilatation of the ascending aorta. Severe aortoannular ectasia of the proximal ascending aorta in association with aortic stenoses can occur in childhood (Fig. 35-26). MRI and MRA in the sagittal plane are optimal for demonstrating the dimensions of the aorta. VEC cine MRI may be used to quantify concomitant aortic regurgitation.

Coronary Artery Anomalies

Coronary MRA has now become recognized as the most reliable technique for demonstrating anomalies of the origin and course of the coronary arteries. Coronary anomalies may occur as isolated lesions or in association with other congenital cardiac anomalies, especially tetralogy of Fallot.

Coronary artery anomalies can be classified as major (origin of a coronary artery from the pulmonary artery) or minor (ectopic origin from the aorta). Ectopic aortic origin may be innocuous or potentially lethal. The potentially lethal anomalies have a proximal course between the base of the aorta and the right ventricular outlet region (interarterial course). With innocuous ectopic origin, the proximal course of the anomalous artery passes ventral to the right ventricular outlet region or behind the aorta (retroaortic course). While selective (x-ray) coronary arteriography can demonstrate ectopic origin, it usually cannot confidently and precisely define the proximal course of the artery.

The current approach to coronary MRA employs a respi-

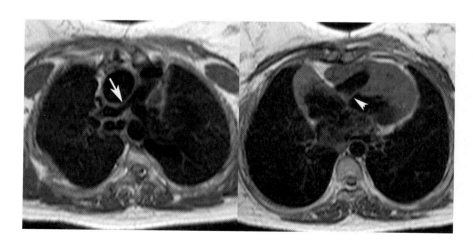

FIG. 35-24. Right pulmonary arterial stenosis *(arrow)* after repair of tetralogy of Fallot. Note the patch *(arrowhead)* at the site of ventricular septal defect.

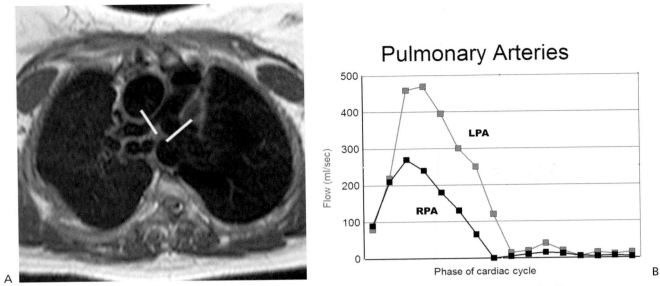

FIG. 35-25. A. Sites of acquisition of velocity-encoded (phase contrast) cine MR sequence for the right and left pulmonary arteries. **B.** Flow versus time curves for the right and left pulmonary arteries demonstrate drastically impaired flow in the right pulmonary artery.

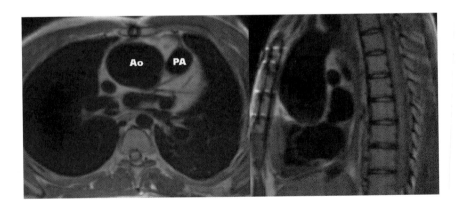

FIG. 35-26. Poststenotic dilatation of the ascending aorta. Axial and sagittal spin-echo images show aneurysmal dilatation of the sinus of Valsalva and the ascending aorta. *Ao*, aorta; *PA*, pulmonary artery.

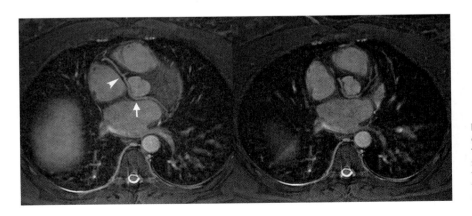

FIG. 35-27. Anomalous origin of the left coronary artery from the right coronary artery with a retroaortic course. Two adjacent sections from coronary MRA display the ectopic origin of the left coronary artery from the right coronary *(arrowhead)* and passage of the left artery behind the aorta *(arrow)*.

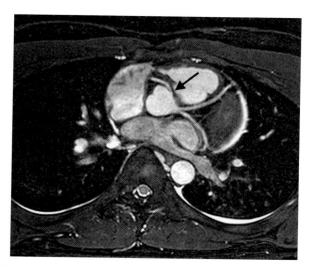

FIG. 35-28. Ectopic origin of the right coronary artery with an interarterial course. Coronary MRA shows the origin of the right coronary artery *(arrow)* from the right end of the left sinus of Valsalva in a position where the proximal portion of the artery is compressed between the aorta and the right ventricular outlet region.

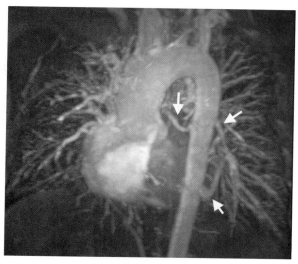

FIG. 35-30. Pulmonary atresia with ventricular septal defect. Contrast-enhanced 3D MRA in the coronal plane display several large systemic to pulmonary artery collaterals *(arrows)* arising from the descending aorta.

ratory navigator-compensated 3D free-breathing technique. This technique displays clearly the origin of the coronary artery from the sinus of Valsalva and its proximal course. A single coronary artery may arise from either the right or left sinus of Valsalva, or both coronary arteries may arise individually from one sinus of Valsalva (Fig. 35-27). In a child with chest pain or syncope during exercise or aborted sudden death, coronary MRA must exclude a proximal interarterial course (Fig. 35-28).

CYANOTIC LESIONS

Tetralogy of Fallot

Tetralogy of Fallot consists of obstruction to the right ventricular outlet region (usually multilevel), malalignment outlet VSD, enlarged aorta overriding the VSD, and a hypertrabeculated, hypertrophied right ventricle. These features are clearly defined on spin-echo MR images in the transaxial (Fig. 35-29) and sagittal planes. Transaxial images demonstrate the VSD and the position of the aorta overriding the defect. Sagittal and transaxial images are used to assess the size of the main and central pulmonary arteries and to display focal stenoses. Imaging oriented in a plane parallel to the long axis of the right (oblique coronal plane) and left (oblique sagittal plane) pulmonary arteries is used to assess the severity of central pulmonary arterial stenoses, which are common in this anomaly. Contrast-enhanced 3D MRA is also employed to demonstrate pulmonary arterial stenoses and the systemic source of collateral flow to the lungs (Fig. 35-30). VEC cine MRI can be used to define differential blood flow to the two lungs.

Tetralogy of Fallot is usually repaired by relieving the

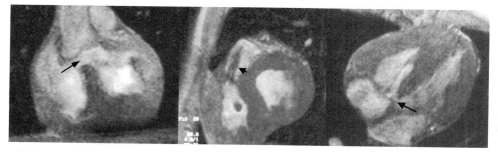

FIG. 35-29. Tetralogy of Fallot. Oblique coronal **(left)**, sagittal **(center)**, and axial **(right)** cine MR images show ventricular septal defect *(arrows)*, aorta overriding the defect, and pulmonic stenosis *(arrowhead* on flow void).

pulmonic stenosis and closing the VSD. Stenosis of the main or branch arteries, the size of the right ventricle outflow tract, and the size of the right ventricle are important to assess in preoperative planning and are well delineated by MRI. Coronary anomalies may occur in patients with tetralogy of Fallot. The most important is the origin of the left anterior descending coronary artery from the right coronary artery with anomalous artery passing anterior to the right ventricle outflow tract. Adequate sizes of the central pulmonary arteries and the presence of a central confluence may signify that the patient is a candidate for a Rastelli procedure connecting the right ventricle to the pulmonary artery.

Pulmonary Atresia

Pulmonary atresia with VSD is an extreme form of tetralogy of Fallot in which a direct connection from the right ventricle to the pulmonary arteries is lacking. On axial MRI, a solid layer of muscle in the region of the right ventricle outflow tract indicates an infundibulum with a blind end. No connection between the right ventricle and the pulmonary artery confluence (if present) is evident on sequential images (Fig. 35-31). The atresia can be focal, limited to the valve level, or more extensive. The length of the atresia can be determined by inspecting sequential axial tomograms. Focal membranous pulmonary atresia may be indistinguishable from severe stenosis on axial MR images because of partial volume averaging. The use of 3-mm-thick spin-echo images reduces partial volume effects. Cine MRI in the axial or sagittal planes can establish the presence or absence of flow across the valve. A markedly enlarged aorta is seen

overriding a perimembranous VSD (see Fig. 35-31). Blood is usually delivered to the lungs via systemic to pulmonary collateral channels, which can be seen as abnormal vessels originating from the descending aorta and traveling toward the lungs or connecting with the pulmonary arteries (see Fig. 35-31). These are shown best on contrast-enhanced 3D MRA (see Fig. 35-30).

The surgical correction of pulmonary atresia with VSD usually consists of placing a conduit from the right ventricle to the central pulmonary arteries (if present) or to a surgically created confluence of pulmonary arteries and larger systemic to pulmonary collateral vessels (unifocalization procedure). Therefore, it is important for the surgeon to know whether a native confluence of the pulmonary arteries is present, its size, and the number and size of collateral vessels. Axial spin-echo MRI is excellent for defining the main pulmonary arteries. The collateral channels are especially well seen on contrast-enhanced MRA (see Fig. 35-30).

It is important to assess the sizes of the central pulmonary arteries in patients who have tetralogy of Fallot with severe stenosis or pulmonary atresia. Thin (3-mm) transaxial MR images can readily depict the sizes of the main, right, and left pulmonary arteries. The right pulmonary artery is observed on the image that contains the right main bronchus, coursing in front of the right bronchus, and the left pulmonary artery passes over the left main bronchus and is seen on the image containing the left bronchus or on the one just above. The identification of central pulmonary arteries and of a central confluence of the right and left pulmonary arteries is a unique capability of MRI, since opacification of the vessels with contrast is not required. The pulmonary

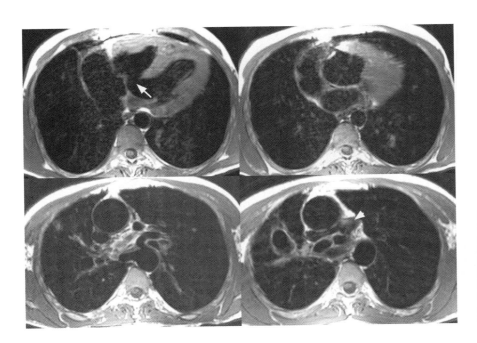

FIG. 35-31. Pulmonary atresia with ventricular septal defect. Spin-echo axial images arranged from caudal (**top left**) to cranial (**bottom right**) demonstrate a single large artery (aorta) at the base of the heart, which overlies the ventricular septal defect *(arrow)*. Right ventricular wall is hypertrophied. Note the central confluence *(arrowhead)* of the right and left pulmonary arteries distal to the atretic segment.

arteries are frequently hypoplastic, or the central or peripheral arteries may contain one or more stenoses.

Cine MRI can be used to identify the blood supply to the lungs. Pulmonary and bronchial arteries have bright signal on cine MRI. On transaxial images at the level of the carina, pulmonary arteries can be differentiated from bronchial arteries. Bronchial arteries or systemic to pulmonary artery collaterals arise from the aorta or its branches and are usually located dorsal to the bronchi, whereas pulmonary arteries are ventral to the bronchi. On occasion, a bronchial artery originating from a subclavian artery is seen ventral to the bronchi.

Pulmonary Atresia With Intact Ventricular Septum

A VSD is not identified in this form of pulmonary atresia with intact ventricular septum. In this variety of pulmonary atresia, MRI is effective for demonstrating the size of the RV, which varies from markedly hypoplastic to dilated. The pulmonary arteries are usually normal or nearly normal in size and do not contain stenoses.

Cine MR images can be acquired in the short-axis plane to quantify the volumes of the right and left ventricles. The size of the right ventricle is critical for determination of the surgical approach. A right ventricle of adequate size is necessary to consider treatment with a conduit from the right ventricle to the pulmonary arteries.

Exit of blood from the right ventricle in this anomaly is by tricuspid regurgitation or retrograde flow through myocardial sinusoid and coronary arteries into the aorta. Cine MR can demonstrate and give some insight into the severity of tricuspid regurgitation.

Abnormalities of Ventriculoarterial Connections

These abnormalities consist of complete transposition of the great arteries (TGA), corrected transposition of the great arteries (CTGA), double-outlet right ventricle (DORV), and double-outlet left ventricle. The last anomaly is exceedingly rare. Truncus arteriosus will also be considered under this heading.

A critical step in evaluating these anomalies is determining the morphology of the ventricles. This is readily accomplished using transaxial images that show the characteristics of a right ventricle: infundibulum (tunnel of myocardium) separating the atrioventricular and semilunar valves; moderator band; and corrugated surface of the right ventricular aspect of the septum (Fig. 35-32). The left ventricle shows direct fibrous continuity between the two valves, the papillary muscles, and the smooth surface of the left ventricular aspect of the septum.

Ventriculoarterial connections can be concordant or discordant. Concordant connections are right ventricle to pulmonary artery and left ventricle to aorta. Discordant connections occur in a diverse group of anomalies in which the great arteries are inverted (transposition). Both great arteries arise predominantly from one of the ventricles (double-outlet ventricle). The ventriculoarterial connections and the arterial relationships are depicted on coronal and transverse MR images.

A great artery is considered connected to a ventricle if more than half of its orifice arises from that ventricle. A series of transaxial images extending from the aortic arch to the diaphragm demonstrates these connections. The initial determination is to identify the aorta unequivocally by following one of the great arteries to the arch. If this great artery (aorta) connects to the right ventricle and the pulmonary artery to the left ventricle, then the diagnosis of complete TGA is established (Fig. 35-33). At the base of the heart, the aorta is anterior and to the right of the pulmonary artery in most cases and is called d-TGA. The transaxial images also demonstrate the position of the ventricles in relation to each other and their connections to the atria (atrioventricular connections). Typically, in the presence of situs solitus, the images show the right ventricle situated to the right of the left ventricle and connected to the right atrium (D-ventricular loop). If the ventricles are inverted, the right ventricle is to the left of the left ventricle and

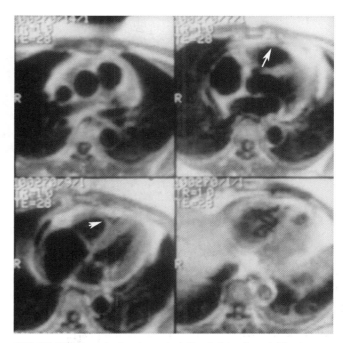

FIG. 35-32. Ventricular characteristics. Spin-echo axial images arranged from cranial (**top left**) to caudal (**bottom right**) show a conus (complete tunnel of myocardium; *arrow*) separating the pulmonary and tricuspid valves. This is a distinguishing feature of the right ventricle. The right ventricle also has a moderator band (*arrowhead*) and the tricuspid valve is positioned more ventral than the mitral valve.

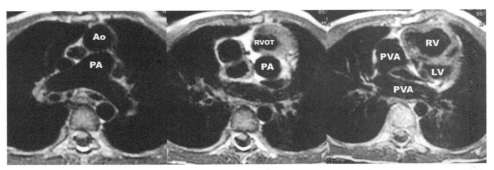

FIG. 35-33. d-Transposition of great arteries. Spin-echo images arranged from cranial (**left**) to caudal (**right**) show the aorta *(Ao)* ventral and slightly to the right of the pulmonary artery *(PA).* The aorta is shown connecting to the right ventricle *(RV)* and the pulmonary artery to the left ventricle *(LV).* There is a baffle (Mustard procedure) in the atrium, separating the mitral valve from the pulmonary venous atrium *(PVA).* RVOT, right ventricular outflow track.

connected to the left atrium (L-ventricular loop). The most frequent types of TGA are complete TGA (situs solitus, D-ventricular loop, d-TGA; see Fig. 35-33) and corrected TGA (situs solitus, L-ventricular loop, l-TGA; Fig. 35-34). The latter anomaly is considered to be corrected (corrected transposition) in terms of blood flow in the central circulation since systemic venous blood flows from the right atrium into the left ventricle and out to the pulmonary artery for normal oxygenation, precluding obligatory cyanosis. Transaxial MR images also demonstrate anomalies frequently associated with complete and corrected transposition, such as ASD, VSD, subvalvular and valvular pulmonic stenosis, tricuspid atresia, and Ebstein anomaly.

Transaxial MR images demonstrate connection of both great arteries to the right ventricle in DORV (Fig. 35-35). Rarely, both great arteries connect to the anatomic left ventricle, indicating double-outlet left ventricle. Transaxial images are very effective for demonstrating the relationship of

the obligatory VSD to the great arteries in DORV. The defect may be just below the aortic orifice (subaortic VSD) or pulmonary artery orifice (subpulmonary VSD); beneath both orifices (doubly committed VSD); or removed some distance from both (noncommitted VSD; Table 35-1).

Truncus Arteriosus

Truncus arteriosus was classified by Collet and Edwards based on the origin of the pulmonary artery from the common arterial trunk. In type I, a septum divides the origin of the aorta and pulmonary trunk. In type II, the right and left pulmonary arteries are close to each other but arise separately from the pulmonary trunk. In type III, right and left pulmonary arteries arise further laterally. The lesion labeled type IV truncus is in fact pulmonary atresia with VSD rather than truncus arteriosus.

Axial, sagittal, and coronal MR images at the base of the

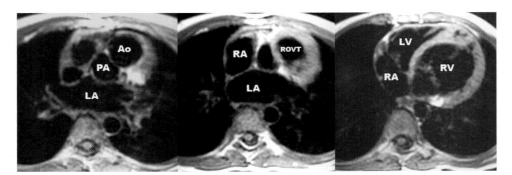

FIG. 35-34. l-Transposition of great arteries. Spin-echo axial images arranged from cranial (**left**) to caudal (**right**) demonstrate the aorta *(Ao)* ventral and to the left of the pulmonary artery. It is connected to the morphologic right ventricle *(RV),* which lies to the left of the left ventricle *(LV).* The right ventricle is connected to the left atrium. The pulmonary artery *(PA)* is connected to the left ventricle, which is connected to the right atrium. *RVOT,* right ventricular outflow track.

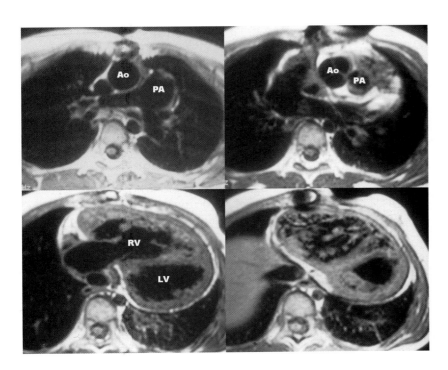

FIG. 35-35. Double-outlet right ventricle. Spin-echo axial images arranged from cranial (**top left**) to caudal (**bottom right**). At the base of the heart the aorta *(Ao)* and pulmonary artery *(PA)* lie side by side. Both great arteries are connected to the right ventricle *(RV)* There are coni beneath both great arteries, and trabeculation of the right ventricular side of the ventricular septum. *LV,* left ventricle.

heart can show the truncus arteriosus aligned over the VSD (Fig. 35-36). The origins of the main pulmonary artery from the truncus in type I can be delineated with MRI. Axial images can show the relative sizes of the ventricles. Because it can demonstrate a small infundibular chamber in pulmonary atresia, MRI can be used to distinguish truncus arteriosus from pulmonary atresia.

The relative sizes and confluence of the pulmonary arteries are useful pieces of information because surgical treatment involves excision of the pulmonary arteries from the common trunk and the creation of a conduit from the right ventricle to the pulmonary arteries (Rastelli procedure). Also important in the evaluation is the demonstration of a right aortic arch (35%) and other arch anomalies. Cine MRI and VEC cine MRI can be employed to identify and quantify the severity of truncal regurgitation. Cine MRI can also be used to quantify the volume and mass of the two ventricles.

TABLE 35-1. SUMMARY OF ANATOMY OF VENTRICULOARTERIAL CONNECTION ABNORMALITIES

Complete transposition
Situs solitus (right atrium on right side of chest)
D-ventricular loop (right ventricle to the right of left ventricle)
d-TGA (aorta anterior and to right of pulmonary artery)
Corrected transposition
Situs solitus
L-ventricular loop (right ventricle to the left of left ventricle)
l-TGA (aorta anterior and to the left of pulmonary artery)
Double-outlet right ventricle
Aorta orifice >50% overlies the right ventricle
Pulmonary orifice >50% overlies the right ventricle
Subaortic, subpulmonary, doubly committed or noncommitted VSD
Double-outlet left ventricle
Aorta orifice >50% overlies the left ventricle
Pulmonary orifice >50% overlies the left ventricle
Truncus arteriosus
One enlarged great artery (truncus) overlies both ventricles
VSD immediately beneath orifice of truncus

TGA, transposition of the great arteries; VSD, ventricular septal defect.

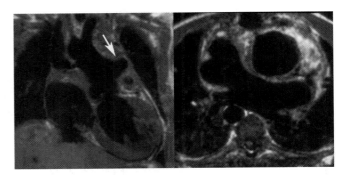

FIG. 35-36. Truncus arteriosus, type I. Spin-echo images in the coronal (**left**) and axial (**right**) planes demonstrate a large single artery arising from the heart. The pulmonary artery *(arrow)* arises from the left side of the truncus, and the aortic arch is right-sided.

ANALYSIS OF COMPLEX CONGENITAL HEART DISEASE USING MRI: SEGMENTAL APPROACH

The analysis of complex congenital heart disease requires a systematic approach. The approach most widely used today is the segmental one, in which the heart is partitioned into three main segments (atria, ventricles, and great vessels) and the connections between them (atrioventricular and ventriculoarterial connections). Transaxial images from the aortic arch to the upper abdomen clearly demonstrate the segmental cardiovascular anatomy and connections of one segment to the other (atrioventricular connections and ventriculoarterial connections) and the types of situs.

Visceroatrial Situs

The right atria and left atria are described by their morphologic structure and not necessarily their position. An atrium with the morphologic features of a left atrium, which may rarely be located to the right of midline, is called a morphologic left atrium. Transaxial MR images can clearly depict the characteristic morphologic features of the atria.

The most definite features of the atria are the appendages. On an axial MR image, the right atrial appendage appears as a triangular structure with a broad-based opening into the right atrium. This is in distinction to the left atrial appendage, a long, narrow, finger-like projection with a narrow orifice. The atrial appendages are the most constant part of the atria, even in complex abnormalities. If the atrial appendages are difficult to identify, the next most reliable structure is the drainage of the inferior vena cava (IVC). The atrium connection to the IVC is considered the morphologic right atrium. Superior vena caval and pulmonary venous drainage is variable and is not used to identify atrial morphology.

Ventricular Loop

The normal rightward bending of the primitive cardiac tube places the morphologic right ventricle on the right side of the heart. This rightward bending is called D-looping (D for dextro, right). If the primitive heart tube bends to the left, the result is called L-looping (L for levo, left), in which the morphologic right ventricle is placed on the left side of the heart. A heart with the morphologic right ventricle on the left side has an L-ventricular loop. In situs solitus, a D-loop is normal. In situs inversus, an L-loop is normal.

Atrioventricular connections can be concordant or discordant. In normal, concordant atrioventricular connections, the right atrium is connected to the right ventricle and the left atrium to the left ventricle. The atrioventricular valves remain with their respective ventricles, regardless of the type of ventricular loop. The mitral valve resides with the left ventricle and the tricuspid valve is part of the right

ventricle, except in patients with double-inlet ventricle. Identification of ventricular morphology indicates the type of atrioventricular valve within the ventricle.

Discordant atrioventricular connections are right atrium to left ventricle and left atrium to right ventricle. Congenitally corrected TGA is an example of an anomaly with atrioventricular discordance.

Great Artery Relationships

Transaxial images at the base of the heart clearly define the normal relationship of the pulmonary artery anterior and to the left of the aorta. Such images also identify concordant (aorta connected to left ventricle and pulmonary artery connected to right ventricle) and discordant (aorta connected to right ventricle and pulmonary artery connected to left ventricle) ventriculoarterial connections.

Complete TGA is an example of atrioventricular concordance and ventriculoarterial discordance. Corrected TGA is an example of atrioventricular and ventriculoarterial discordance. Double discordance results in blood flowing in a normal pattern serially through the pulmonary and systemic circulation.

Abnormalities of Atrioventricular Connections

Discordant Atrioventricular Connections

The right atrium connects with the left ventricle and the left atrium connects with the right ventricle, constituting discordant connections, in corrected transposition (see Figs. 35-34 and 35-37). One of the most frequent anomalies in patients with situs inversus is corrected transposition. In this anomaly, the anatomic right atrium (situated left of midline) connects discordantly to the left ventricle and the anatomic left atrium (situated right of midline) connects to the right ventricle. Mirror-image dextrocardia occurs with situs inversion. In contrast, isolated dextrocardia consists of situs solitus with a right-sided cardiac apex (see Fig. 35-37).

Double-inlet Ventricle (Single Ventricle; Univentricular Heart)

This complex anomaly consists of one adequate-size ventricle and one rudimentary ventricle. The most frequent type is double-inlet left ventricle: both atrioventricular valves connect to the morphologic left ventricle. The enlarged left ventricle is attached to a rudimentary right ventricular outlet via a bulboventricular foramina (Fig. 35-38). In many instances, l-TGA is an associated anomaly.

Cine MRI can provide a set of end-diastolic and end-systole images encompassing the entire heart; consequently, it is the optimal method for quantifying the volumes, mass, and function of the dominant and rudimentary ventricle.

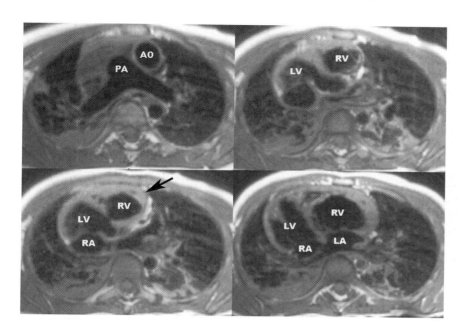

FIG. 35-37. Situs solitus with corrected transposition and isolated dextrocardia. Spin-echo axial images arranged from cranial (**top left**) to caudal (**bottom right**). The right atrium *(RA)* is right-sided and the left atrium *(LA)* is left-sided, indicating situs solitus. The right ventricle *(RV)* is positioned to the left of the left ventricle *(LV)*. The aorta *(Ao)* is anterior and leftward to the pulmonary artery *(PA)*. Note the conus *(arrow)* and moderator band on the left-sided ventricle, indicating it is a morphologic right ventricle in an L-ventricular loop. Thus, this arrangement of connections is situs solitus, L ventricular loop, l-transposition, which constitutes corrected TGA. The cardiac apex is right-sided, which indicates isolated dextrocardia.

Volumetric data may be essential for surgical planning (Fontan procedure versus two-ventricle repair).

Atresia of Atrioventricular Valve

Either the tricuspid or mitral valves can be atresic; tricuspid atresia is more frequent. Tricuspid atresia is associated with

d-TGA in nearly 50% of patients. It is also frequently associated with valvular or subvalvular pulmonary stenosis or atresia. The right ventricle is invariably hypoplastic. Transaxial MR images demonstrate a bar of muscle and fat across the atrioventricular inlet of the right ventricle (Fig. 35-39). Both spin-echo and cine MR images display the degree of right ventricle hypoplasia, interatrial communication, VSD, and

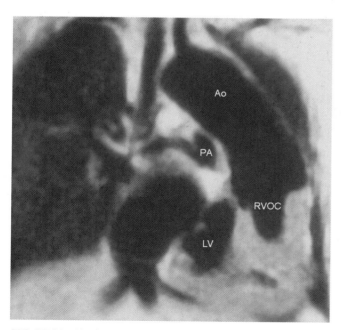

FIG. 35-38. Single ventricle (double-inlet left ventricle; *LV*) with a small right ventricular outlet chamber *(RVOC)*. Note that the aorta *(Ao)* is left-sided, indicating l-TGA. There is pulmonary atresia with distal reconstitution of the pulmonary artery *(PA)*.

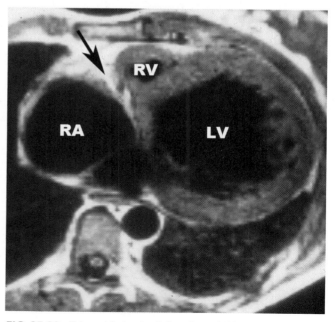

FIG. 35-39. Tricuspid atresia. Spin-echo axial image shows a bar of fat and muscle *(arrow)* separating the right atrium *(RA)* from the hypoplastic right ventricle *(RV)*. The left ventricle *(LV)* is enlarged.

ventriculoarterial connections. In a few cases, a think membrane separates the right atrium and right ventricle (imperforate tricuspid valve). The atrial and ventricular septal openings permit systemic venous blood to flow into the ventricles.

MR is frequently used to evaluate tricuspid atresia after various stages of surgical correction. Spin-echo MR images and 3D contrast-enhanced MRA are effective for displaying the anatomy of the Glenn anastomosis (Fig. 35-40) and the Fontan procedure and the status of the central pulmonary arteries (Fig. 35-41). VEC cine MR may be employed to quantify blood flow in the Glenn shunt (superior vena cava), Fontan conduit (inferior vena cava to pulmonary artery conduit), and pulmonary arteries.

Ebstein Malformation

Ebstein malformation is a primary abnormality of the tricuspid valve in which the septal and anterior leaflets of the valve adhere to the right ventricle wall. The leaflets become free at a variable distance, at a location more apical than usual, so that the tricuspid valve orifice is displaced toward the apex. The right atrioventricular ring still defines the border of the anatomic right ventricle; however, because the valve orifice is more apical than usual, the functional part of the right ventricle is truncated. The portion of the right ventricle that is basal to the valve orifice becomes "atri-

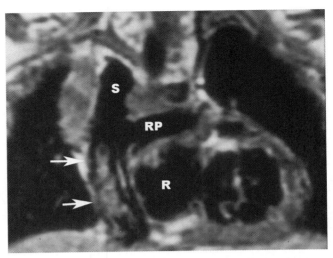

FIG. 35-41. Fontan procedure, extra-atrial type. Spin-echo coronal image shows the conduit *(arrows)* between the inferior vena cava and the right pulmonary artery *(RP)*. The superior vena cava *(S)* is connected to the top of the right pulmonary artery (Glenn anastomosis). The conduit is located lateral to the right atrium *(R)*, thus the connotation extra-atrial Fontan.

alized," meaning that it functions as part of the atrium rather than as part of the right ventricle. The atrialized portion of the right ventricle is thin-walled and nontrabeculated, and it may become dilated. Ebstein anomaly is frequently associated with an ASD.

MRI can demonstrate the position of tricuspid valve (Fig. 35-42), and cine MRI can be used to quantify chamber size and the ejection fraction of the functional right ventricle. Cine MR also demonstrates the systolic signal void projected into the right atrium, indicating tricuspid regurgitation, which is invariably present with this anomaly.

Hypoplastic Left Heart Syndrome

The term *hypoplastic left heart syndrome* refers to several different anomalies, all of which lead to underdevelopment of the left ventricle. It is usually caused by aortic stenosis or atresia, mitral stenosis or atresia, or both. As in tricuspid atresia, the degree of ventricular hypoplasia varies, depending on the location and severity of the obstruction. For example, in mitral atresia without a large ASD and VSD, the left ventricle may be a small mass of muscle with no visible lumen (Fig. 35-43). On the other hand, if the mitral valve is patent and the problem is primarily one of aortic valvular hypoplasia, the left ventricle may be normal in size and hypertrophied. In all cases, the right atrium tends to be enlarged and the right ventricle to be dilated and hypertrophied. Axial MRI can readily depict the chamber enlargement and ventricular hypertrophy.

In most cases of hypoplastic left heart syndrome, little blood flows through the ascending aorta. Blood tends to

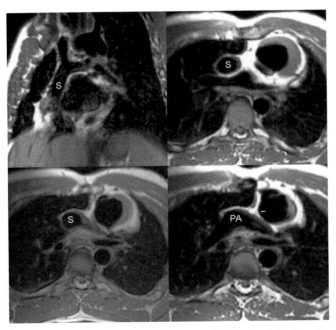

FIG. 35-40. Glenn shunt. Coronal (**upper left**) and axial spin-echo images from cranial (**top right**) to caudal (**bottom right**). The superior vena cava *(S)* is attached to the right pulmonary artery, with flow to both pulmonary arteries (bidirectional Glenn shunt).

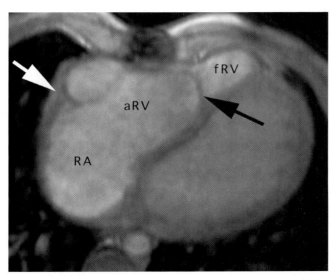

FIG. 35-42. Ebstein anomaly. Gradient-echo axial image shows that the attachments of the septal leaflets *(black arrow)* of the tricuspid valve are displaced into the right ventricle. The level of the tricuspid annulus *(white arrow)* is the normal site of attachment. Right-sided chambers are enlarged due to tricuspid regurgitation. *RA,* right atrium; *ARV,* atrialized right ventricle; *fRV,* functional right ventricle.

flow from the pulmonary artery through the ductus arteriosus into the aorta, then in retrograde fashion to the aortic root to supply the coronary arteries. As a result, the ascending aorta is usually very small and the main pulmonary artery, which receives most of the cardiac output, is very large. The diameters of the great arteries are clearly defined on axial MR images.

Hypoplastic left heart syndrome is treated by the Norwood procedure, in which the large right ventricle is made to pump blood to the systemic circulation. This is accomplished by severing the main pulmonary artery and anastomosing the proximal pulmonary stump to the ascending

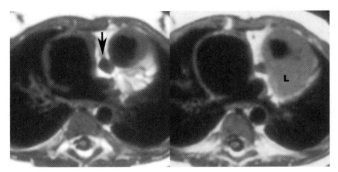

FIG. 35-43. Hypoplastic left heart syndrome. Spin-echo axial images demonstrate the severely hypoplastic ascending aorta *(arrow)* and lack of cavitation of the left ventricle *(L)* at the level displayed.

aorta. The pulmonary circulation is reestablished by routing systemic blood into the pulmonary circulation, initially with a systemic to pulmonary shunt and later with a Fontan procedure. An important role for MRI in hypoplastic left heart syndrome has been the evaluation of the morphology and function of the various stages of the Norwood procedure.

Total Anomalous Pulmonary Venous Connection

In the embryo, the pulmonary veins grow from the lung buds and come together to form a confluence, which normally is incorporated into the posterior wall of the left atrium. However, if this confluence joins the circulatory system elsewhere, a situation is created in which the entire pulmonary venous return is anomalous: total anomalous pulmonary venous connection (TAPVC). TAPVC is usually classified according to the location of the venous insertion. It may be supracardiac (type I), in which the pulmonary venous confluence usually drains into the superior vena cava or an anomalous left-sided "vertical vein," which in turn drains into the left brachiocephalic vein. TAPVC at the cardiac level (type II) usually drains into the right atrium. In type III TAPVC, the pulmonary venous confluence drains below the diaphragm into the inferior vena cava or the portal venous system. As the pulmonary veins pass below the diaphragm, obstruction to flow frequently results in pulmonary venous hypertension.

MRI has been shown to be highly accurate for the diagnosis of anomalous pulmonary venous connection. TAPVC can be diagnosed when MRI demonstrates that no pulmonary veins drain into the left atrium. Transaxial MRI and gadolinium-enhanced MRA can demonstrate the location of the anomalous connection along with enlargement of the superior vena cava or coronary sinus, or the presence of a common pulmonary vein posterior to or above the left atrium.

Situs Abnormalities

The right-sided abdominal and thoracic structures are usually on the same side as the morphologic right atrium; likewise, the left-sided organs are usually on the same side as the morphologic left atrium. In a developmental anomaly in which both atria have morphologic features of a right atrium (RA isomerism), the visceral and thoracic structures tend to be right-sided. Likewise, bilateral left atria (LA isomerism) are associated with bilateral left-sided visceral and thoracic structures.

The bronchi and pulmonary arteries have a characteristic relationship in isomerism syndromes. In RA isomerism, both lungs usually have three lobes and both bronchi have the pattern of a right bronchus—that is, the pulmonary artery runs in front of and beneath the main bronchus

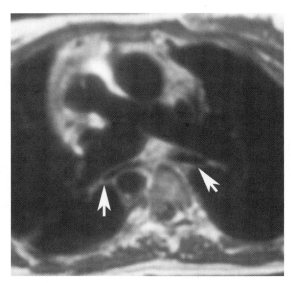

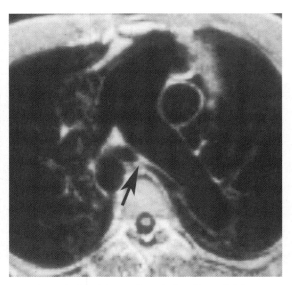

FIG. 35-44. Right-sided isomerism. Spin-echo axial image at the level of the main bronchi *(arrows)* shows that both pulmonary arteries are situated ventral to the bronchi.

FIG. 35-45. Left-sided isomerism. Spin-echo axial image at the level of the carina *(arrow)*. Both pulmonary arteries course above the main bronchi.

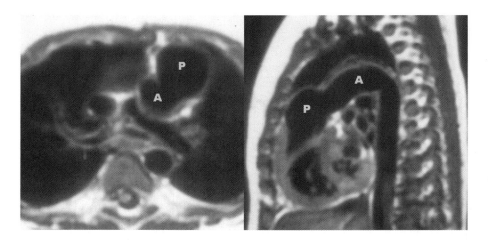

FIG. 35-46. Norwood procedure. Spin-echo axial **(left)** and sagittal **(right)** images show the anastomosis of the proximal pulmonary artery *(P)* to the ascending aorta *(A)*. Sagittal view shows the pulmonary artery *(P)* connected to a reconstructed distal ascending aorta *(A)* and arch. Blood flow to the distal pulmonary artery is reconstituted with a central shunt (not shown).

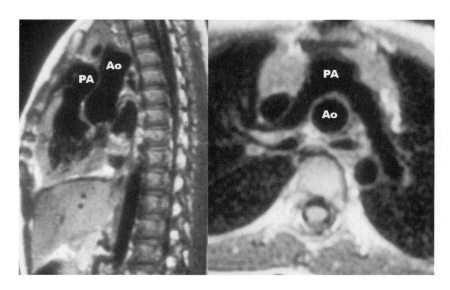

FIG. 35-47. Jatene procedure. Spin-echo images in the sagittal **(left)** and axial **(right)** planes show the arterial correction. The aorta *(Ao)* above the anastomosis is situated between the right and left pulmonary arteries. This position can cause narrowing of the branch pulmonary arteries. *PA,* pulmonary artery.

(a type of bronchus known as an eparterial bronchus) (Fig. 35-44). Right-sided isomerism is often associated with asplenia syndrome. The liver is large and crosses the midline, and the spleen is often absent.

In left-sided isomerism, both lungs have two lobes and both the right and left pulmonary arteries pass over their respective bronchi. This type of bronchial pattern is known as hyparterial because the bronchus passes below the pulmonary artery (Fig. 35-45). Left-sided isomerism is associated with polysplenia syndrome, characterized by multiple spleens. The inferior vena cava is frequently interrupted, with azygous continuation.

Coronal and transaxial MR images are very effective for showing the anatomy of the pulmonary arteries in order to establish the diagnosis of isomerism. MRI also clearly defines the systemic, pulmonary venous anatomy and the morphology of the atrial appendages.

Postoperative Evaluation

MRI is excellent for the postoperative evaluation of congenital heart disease. The wide field of view permits effective depiction of complex repairs used to correct complex lesions.

Contrast-enhanced 3D MRA and tomographic images demonstrate surgical anastomoses, conduits, and shunts. Moreover, the 3D data set available from contiguous cine MR images at multiple phases in the cardiac cycle permits precise quantification of left and right ventricular volumes, mass, and function. Since cine MRI has high interstudy reproducibility, it is the best technique available for serial monitoring of ventricular volumes, mass, and function after surgery.

Spin-echo MRI and 3D contrast-enhanced MRA have demonstrated the anatomy of complex repairs such as the Norwood procedure for hypoplastic left heart (Fig. 35-46); the Jatene procedure (arterial switch) for TGA (Fig. 35-47); the Fontan procedure for functional single ventricle (see Fig. 35-41); the Rastelli procedure for pulmonary atresia (Fig. 35-48); and various repairs of tetralogy of Fallot (see Figs. 35-1 and 35-48).

VEC cine MRI is employed for quantification of the volume and fraction of pulmonary regurgitation (see Fig. 35-2), volume flow through various components of the Fontan repair, and differential flow in the central pulmonary arteries (see Fig. 35-25). After various surgical procedures

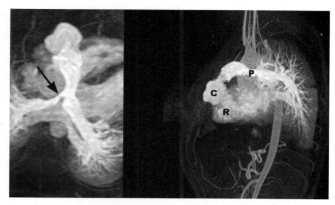

FIG. 35-48. Rastelli procedure. Contrast-enhanced 3D MRA in oblique axial **(left)** and sagittal **(right)** planes shows a conduit *(C)* between the right ventricle *(R)* and the pulmonary artery *(P)*. The oblique axial plane depicts a stenosis *(arrow)* of the right pulmonary artery.

in cyanotic congenital heart disease, residual stenosis of the central pulmonary arteries is frequent. VEC cine MRI can be used to demonstrate disparity in flow between the right and left pulmonary arteries and changes after angioplasty.

SELECTED READING

Araoz PA, Reddy GP, Higgins CB. Congenital heart disease: morphology and function. In: Higgins CB, de Roos A (eds). MRI and MRA of Cardiovascular System. Philadelphia: Lippincott Williams & Wilkins, 2002:302.

Donnelly LF, Higgins CB. MR imaging of conotruncal abnormalities. AJR Am J Roentgenol 1996; 166:925–928.

Fogel MA, Hubbard AM, Fellows KE, et al. MRI for physiology and function in congenital heart disease; functional assessment of the heart preoperatively and postoperatively. Semin Roentgenol 1998; 33:239.

Higgins CB, Silverman NH, Kersting-Sommerhof BA, Schmidt K. Congenital Heart Disease: Echocardiography and Magnetic Resonance Imaging. New York: Raven Press, 1990.

Kilner PJ. Adult congenital heart disease. In: Higgins CB, de Roos A, eds. MRI and MRA of Cardiovascular System. Philadelphia: Lippincott Williams & Wilkins, 2002:353.

Reddy GP, Higgins CB. Congenital heart disease: measuring physiology with MRI. Semin Roentgenol 1998; 33:228.

Roest AAW, Helbing WA, van der Wall EE, de Roos A. Postoperative functional evaluation of congenital heart disease. In: Higgins CB, de Roos A (eds). MRI and MRA of Cardiovascular System. Philadelphia: Lippincott Williams & Wilkins, 2002:339.

36

MAGNETIC RESONANCE IMAGING OF ISCHEMIC HEART DISEASE

CHARLES B. HIGGINS

The evaluation of ischemic heart disease by noninvasive imaging techniques has usually involved nuclear imaging and echocardiography for initial diagnosis, monitoring, and assessment of severity. Coronary angiography has been employed for precise definition of coronary arterial stenoses and to guide therapeutic interventions. In the first two decades of cardiovascular magnetic resonance imaging (MRI), its application in ischemic heart disease was meager. With the introduction of MR imagers adapted for cardiovascular imaging, however, the capability for the comprehensive evaluation of ischemic heart disease has been demonstrated.

The comprehensive evaluation of ischemic heart disease requires the following steps:

1. Detect and assess the severity of ischemic heart disease
2. Define the coronary anatomy
3. Evaluate and monitor myocardial revascularization
4. Determine myocardial viability
5. Demonstrate complications of myocardial infarction

The role of MRI in accomplishing each of these tasks will be addressed. The evaluation of ischemic heart disease by MRI remains technically complex because of the multitude of acquisition sequences used to accomplish a comprehensive evaluation. The various sequences will be described briefly in relation to the specific tasks.

DETECTION OF ISCHEMIC HEART DISEASE

Stress Function

Pharmacologic stress is employed to induce a regional contraction abnormality as a functional indicator of a hemodynamically significant coronary arterial stenosis. This is the method used to identify ischemic heart disease by echocardiography. The pharmacologic stressor is usually an infusion of dobutamine. The dose is gradually increased to simulate intermediate stress (20 μg/kg/min) and then peak stress (40 μg/kg/min). The maximum level of stress should achieve a heart rate equal to 85% of the maximum heart rate predicted for age. Atropine can be administered to achieve this heart rate.

Cine MRI is performed in the short-axis plane at multiple levels and one of the long-axis planes in the baseline state, at intermediate stress, and at peak stress using a balanced steady-state free precession sequence (variably named by the manufacturers as balanced fast field echo [balanced FFE], true FISP, or FIESTA). With these sequences, cine MR images consisting of 16 to 40 phases can be acquired at three anatomic locations in a breath-hold of 10 to 20 seconds (Fig. 36-1).

For the analysis, the left ventricle as displayed on the multiple short-axis images and a vertical long-axis image is divided into 17 segments according to the consensus protocol of the American Heart Association. Left ventricular dysfunction during stress is indicated by a segmental decrease in wall thickening, wall motion, or both (Fig. 36-2). The sensitivity and specificity for detecting a hemodynamically significant stenosis (greater than 50% reduction in luminal diameter) of the coronary artery subserving the dysfunctional segment are about 85%. This level of diagnostic accuracy is equivalent to stress echocardiography.

Stress Perfusion

Pharmacologic stress is used to evoke a perfusion deficit in the myocardium supplied by a coronary artery with a hemodynamically significant stenosis. The pharmacologic agents used are dipyridamole and adenosine. MR images are acquired in the short-axis plane at three to five anatomic levels during the first passage of intravenously injected gadolinium chelate (0.03 to 0.05 mmol/kg; Fig. 36-3). A saturation recovery or inversion recovery fast gradient-echo sequence is used to diminish the signal of myocardium before the arrival of the contrast. The images at each anatomic level are acquired at a rate of about 1 per second for about 30 seconds. A regional perfusion deficit is usually visible (see Figs. 36-3 and 36-4). The defect may be subendocardial or nearly transmural. Quantitative analysis of the regional intensity–time curve during initial passage of the contrast

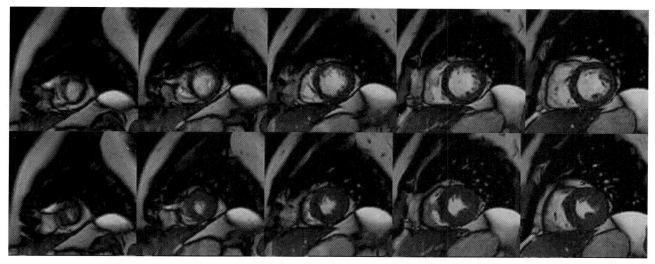

FIG. 36-1. End-diastolic (**top**) and end-systolic (**bottom**) cine MR images in the short axis extending from apex (**left**) to base (**right**) of the ventricles.

can improve the diagnostic accuracy. The prime discriminatory parameter is the maximum upslope of the curve.

The sensitivity and specificity for identifying a hemodynamically significant stenosis are about 85%. The diagnostic accuracy of MR perfusion imaging has been found to be equal or better than single photon emission tomography and positron emission tomography. However, there has been limited experience with MR perfusion imaging, so comparisons with simple photon computed tomography and positron emission tomography should be considered still tenta-

END-DIASTOLIC

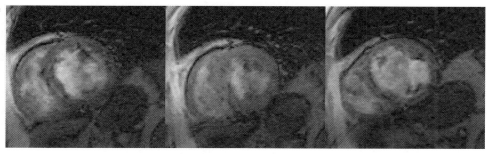

END-SYSTOLIC

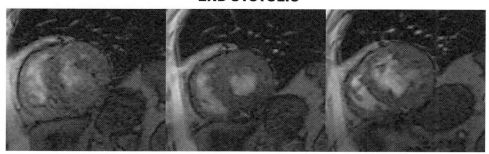

FIG. 36-2. End-diastolic and end-systolic images at a single anatomic level at basal state (**left**) and during intermediate (**center**) and peak (**right**) stress induced by infusion of dobutamine. At peak stress, there is severe reduction in wall thickening and wall motion in the anteroseptal region of the left ventricle. (Courtesy of Gregory Hundley, M.D., Winston-Salem, NC.)

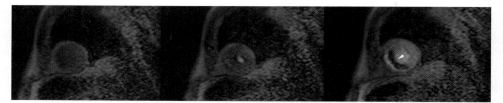

FIG. 36-3. Inversion recovery short-axis images before **(left)** and after the arrival of gadolinium chelate in the left ventricular cavity **(center)** and myocardium **(right)** demonstrate a large transmural perfusion deficit in the ventricular septum *(arrowhead).*

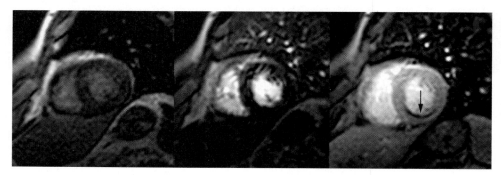

FIG. 36-4. Inversion recovery short-axis images at several time frames after administration of gadolinium chelate demonstrate a subendocardial perfusion deficit *(arrow)* in the posterior wall of the left ventricle. (Courtesy of Scott Flamm, M.D., Houston, TX.)

tive. An expected advantage of MR perfusion imaging is greater sensitivity in detecting small subendocardial perfusion deficits (see Fig. 36-4) and for demonstrating triple-vessel disease with diffuse myocardial ischemia (Fig. 36-5).

Coronary Flow Reserve

Velocity-encoded (VEC; phase contrast) cine MR can be used to measure the flow velocity and flow volume of individual major coronary arteries. This is usually done using a breath-hold version of this sequence. This sequence provides a pair of images at approximately 12 to 16 phases of the cardiac cycle. The pair consists of magnitude and phase images acquired perpendicular to the direction of blood flow (Fig. 36-6). A set of images is acquired in the basal state and in the vasodilated state induced by dipyridamole or adenosine. From these images, peak velocity of flow can be calculated in each state (see Fig. 36-6). Coronary flow reserve is the ratio of maximal flow to basal flow. A normal value is designated as a ratio greater than 2.3 to 2.5. In the presence of a hemodynamically significant stenosis (more than 50% reduction in luminal diameter), it is lower than 2.3.

This technique can be used to demonstrate a hemodynamic stenosis before treatment. After stent placement, measurement of coronary flow reserve with MR can be used

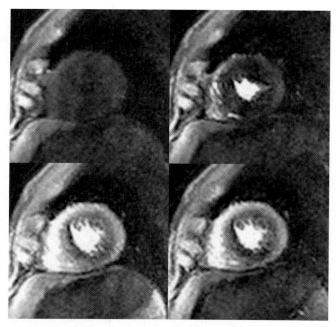

FIG. 36-5. Inversion recovery short-axis images before and at three time intervals after arrival of gadolinium chelate in the left ventricle show perfusion deficits around the entire circumference of the myocardium, indicating the likelihood of triple-vessel disease. (Courtesy of Hajime Sakuma, M.D., Mie, Japan.)

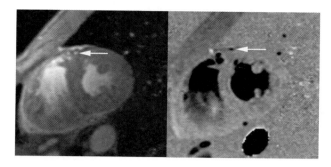

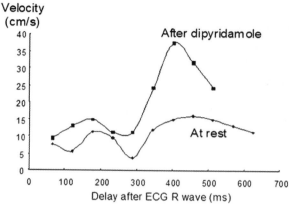

Blood flow velocity curve

FIG. 36-6.   Top. Velocity-encoded cine MR in the short-axis plane consisting of magnitude **(left)** and phase **(right)** images. These images, acquired at 16 phases of the cardiac cycle, can be used to interrogate flow and flow velocity in the left anterior descending coronary artery *(arrow)*. **Bottom.** Graph shows the velocity versus time curves for left anterior descending coronary artery flow velocity in the basal and vasodilated state provoked by dipyridamole.

to monitor the coronary functional status in order to detect recurrence of stenosis.

Abnormal coronary flow and flow reserve may occur in myocardial and vascular diseases in the absence of a stenosis of the epicardial coronary arteries. VEC cine MR may be

used to measure the average flow to the left ventricular myocardium by interrogating the flow in the coronary sinus. The coronary sinus conducts about 90% of the left ventricular myocardial flow. Since total coronary flow is proportional to left ventricular mass, total coronary flow is normalized to left ventricular mass to express the flow in ml/min/g myocardium. Left ventricular mass is measured from a stack of cine MR images encompassing the entire left ventricle. The VEC images are acquired in the basal and vasodilated states to calculate coronary flow reserve. Abnormally low coronary flow reserve has been elicited by this method in patients with heart transplants, hypertrophic cardiomyopathy, and dilated cardiomyopathy.

CORONARY ANATOMY

A number of MRI techniques have been explored for displaying coronary artery anatomy. These have included two- and three-dimensional acquisition techniques; breath-hold and free-breathing techniques; and white blood and black blood MR sequences. No technique has proved totally suitable, so experimentation continues with several imaging techniques. At present, 3D, free-breathing techniques with respiratory compensation seem to be most effective. The 3D data used to reconstruct the coronary arteries are restricted to a short period of the cardiac cycle (about 50 msec) when there is little respiratory motion. Diaphragmatic motion is monitored (navigator echo) to minimize the effect of respiratory excursion of the heart. Data are used from only about the shallowest 10% of diaphragmatic motion. Conspicuity of the coronary arteries is augmented by applying various prepulses that reduce the signal of the surrounding fat and myocardial tissue.

Under optimized circumstances, impressive images of the coronary arteries can be produced using selected restricted volumes along the predicted course of the major coronary arteries or more recently using whole-heart coronary MRA (Fig. 36-7). However, the sensitivity and specificity for demonstrating hemodynamically significant stenoses (more than

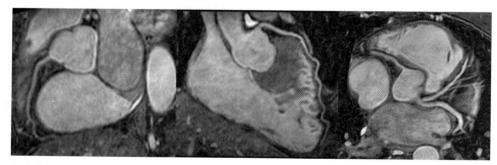

FIG. 36-7. MRA of right and left coronary arteries using a balanced FFE sequence encompassing the whole heart. (Courtesy of Oliver Weber, PhD San Francisco, CA.)

50% luminal narrowing) remain marginal for routine clinical application. The sensitivities and specificities of MRA for this purpose are about 90% and 50%, respectively. However, coronary MRA has a good diagnostic accuracy for identifying left main stenosis and triple vessel disease. Importantly, a normal coronary MRA has nearly 100% negative predictive value for left main and triple-vessel disease.

EVALUATION OF MYOCARDIAL REVASCULARIZATION

MR techniques can be used to demonstrate the morphology and blood flow in revascularization conduits and internal mammary arterial and saphenous vein grafts. Contrast-enhanced 3D MRA during breath-holding can depict stenoses in the conduit. The hemodynamic significance of the stenoses can be assessed using VEC (phase contrast) cine MR with the acquisition in a plane perpendicular to the long axis (flow direction) of the conduit. Revascularization conduits without stenoses, similar to normal coronary arteries, can be shown to have higher peak diastolic flow compared with systolic flow (diastole flow/systolic flow is greater than 1). Conduits with stenoses have higher systolic flow (diastolic flow/systolic flow less than 1), or essentially non-pulsatile flow patterns. Basal flow and coronary flow reserve have also been found to be lower in conduits with significant stenoses. However, basal flow is importantly influenced by the status of the myocardial vascular bed subserved by a bypass conduit and number of distal anastomoses. Frequently, coronary flow reserve is lower than 2.0 even in conduits without stenoses, since the distal native coronary arteries are not normal.

MYOCARDIAL VIABILITY

There are two approaches for determining regional myocardial viability after ischemic injury using MR. One approach probes the contractile reserve of a dysfunctional segment of the left ventricle using a low dose of a beta-adrenergic agonist, dobutamine (5 to 10 μg/kg/min). Cine MR performed in the basal state displays left ventricular segments with contractile dysfunction, usually severe hypokinesis or akinesis, which raises the question of residual viability in the segments. Under stimulation with a low dose of dobutamine, segments composed of mostly viable myocardium demonstrate improvement in wall motion and wall thickening (more than 2 mm) during systole. An additional sign of a segment with residual viability is end-diastolic wall thickness greater than 5.5 mm.

Another approach to viability assessment is delayed contrast enhancement. This approach employs an inversion recovery gradient-echo sequence with an inversion time set to attenuate the signal of normal myocardium at 10 to 15

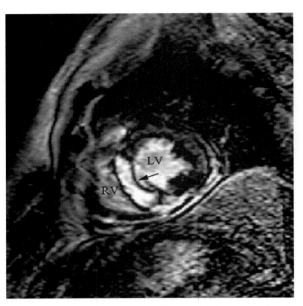

FIG. 36-8. Inversion recovery gradient-echo image in the short-axis plane using an inversion time, which attenuates the signal of normal myocardium. The image was acquired 15 minutes after intravenous administration of gadolinium chelate (0.2 mmol/kg). There is delayed (persistent) contrast enhancement of a septal myocardial infarction *(arrow)*. *LV,* left ventricle; *RV,* right ventricle.

minutes after contrast medium administration. At 10 to 15 minutes after intravenous administration of 0.2 mmol/kg gadolinium chelate, the MR sequence is done. At this time, the contrast is substantially cleared from viable myocardium, but nonviable myocardium (necrotic or fibrotic) shows delayed contrast enhancement (Fig. 36-8).

Determination of regional myocardial viability has clini-

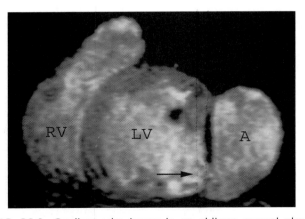

FIG. 36-9. Gradient-echo image in an oblique coronal plane shows a large false aneurysm of the posterolateral wall of the left ventricle. A narrow ostium *(arrow)* connects the aneurysm with the left ventricular chamber. *A,* pseudoaneurysm; *LV,* left ventricle; *RV,* right ventricle.

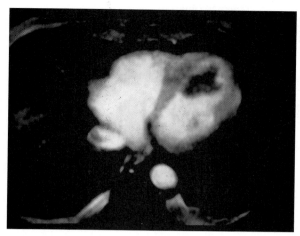

FIG. 36-10. Cine MR image in a transaxial plane shows a mural thrombus at the site of an anteroapical myocardial infarction.

cal importance, since segments determined to be nonviable do not benefit from revascularization. On the other hand, those determined to be viable demonstrate improved regional function after revascularization.

COMPLICATIONS OF MYOCARDIAL INFARCTION

Cine MR or electrocardiogram-gated spin-echo images can demonstrate the complications that may be caused by myocardial infarction, such as true and false left ventricular aneurysms (Fig. 36-9), mural thrombus (Fig. 36-10), and mitral regurgitation due to papillary muscle dysfunction or rupture. MR is particularly effective for demonstrating the

narrowing ostium between the left ventricular chamber and false aneurysm (see Fig. 36-9).

SELECTED READING

Baer FM, Theissen P, Scheider CA, et al. Dobutamine magnetic resonance imaging predicts contractile recovery of chronically dysfunctional myocardium after successful revascularization. J Am Coll Cardiol 1998; 31:1040.

Gerber BL, Garot J, Bluemke DA, et al. Accuracy of contrast-enhanced magnetic resonance imaging in predicting improvement of regional myocardial function in patients after acute myocardial infarction. Circulation 2002; 106:1083.

Hundley WG, Hamilton CA, Thomas MS, et al. Utility of fast cine magnetic resonance imaging and display for the detection of myocardial ischemia in patients not well suited for second harmonic stress echocardiography. Circulation 1999; 100:1697.

Kim WY, Danias PG, Stuber M, et al. Coronary magnetic resonance angiography for the detection of coronary stenosis. N Engl J Med 2001; 345:1863.

Nagel E, Klein C, Paetsch I, et al. Magnetic resonance perfusion measurements for the noninvasive detection of coronary artery disease. Circulation 2003; 108:432.

Ramani K, Judd RM, Holy TA, et al. Contrast magnetic resonance imaging in the assessment of myocardial viability in patients with stable coronary artery disease and left ventricular dysfunction. Circulation 1998; 98:2687.

Sakuma H, Higgins CB. Coronary blood flow measurements. In: Higgins CB, de Roos A, eds. MRI and MRA of the Cardiovascular System. Philadelphia: Lippincott Williams & Wilkins, 2003:284.

Sechtem U, Baer FM, Voth E, et al. Stress functional MRI: detection of ischemic heart disease and myocardial viability. J Magn Res Imag 1999; 10:667.

Stuber M, Botnar RM, Kissinger KV, Manning WJ. Coronary MRA: technical approaches. In: Higgins CB, de Roos A, eds. MRI and MRA of the Cardiovascular System. Philadelphia: Lippincott Williams & Wilkins, 2003:252.

Watzinger N, Saeed M, Wendland MF, et al. Myocardial viability: magnetic resonance assessment of functional reserve and tissue characterization. J Cardiol Magn Reson 2001; 3:195.

37

COMPUTED TOMOGRAPHY OF ISCHEMIC HEART DISEASE

GARY R. CAPUTO AND DOUGLAS P. BOYD

Coronary heart disease caused 515,204 deaths in the United States in 2000 and is the single leading cause of death in this country today. Some 12,900,000 Americans—about 6.3 million males and 6.6 million females—alive today have a history of heart attack, angina pectoris, or both. It is estimated that this year 1.1 million Americans will experience either a first or recurrent coronary attack. About 515,000 of these people will die, 250,000 of them without being hospitalized. Most of these are sudden deaths caused by cardiac arrest, usually resulting from ventricular fibrillation.

About 7.6 million Americans age 20 and older have survived a heart attack, and about 6.6 million Americans have angina pectoris. The estimated age-adjusted prevalence of angina is greater in women than in men. From 1990 to 2000 the death rate from coronary heart disease declined by 25%, but the actual number of deaths declined only 7.6%.

THE COST OF CARDIOVASCULAR DISEASE

It is estimated that the cost, both direct and indirect, of cardiovascular diseases and stroke will be $351.8 billion in 2003, according to the American Heart Association and the National Heart Lung and Blood Institute (NHLBI). The cost of physicians and other professionals, hospital and nursing home services, medications, home health care, and other medical durables are the direct costs. Indirect costs include the lost productivity that results from illness and death. This is only the economic cost; the true cost in human terms of suffering and lost lives is incalculable.

Coronary artery disease often remains silent until a major catastrophic event occurs. Therefore, markers such as coronary calcification, which can indicate that a person is in the process of developing coronary atherosclerosis, have gained importance in recent years. This chapter reviews the significance and pathophysiology of coronary calcification, the current imaging methods available for its detection, vulnerable plaque characterization using CT, and recent developments in CT coronary angiography.

Complex coronary artery intimal plaques often become calcified, and the presence of calcium has been recognized for many years as a marker of coronary atherosclerosis. More than 50 years ago, Blankenhorn found in a necropsy series of 89 patients that in each instance coronary calcification was associated with intimal plaque. Although calcification is a reliable marker of the atherosclerotic process, its presence does not necessarily signify the presence of site-specific significant stenosis. Plaques that narrow the coronary arterial lumen only minimally or moderately may be vulnerable, and may rupture, producing thrombotic occlusion.

Fatty streaks, the earliest detectable atherosclerotic lesions, may occur in the first decade of life and are found increasingly by the second decade. Atherosclerotic plaques are composed of lipid masses covered by a fibrous cap that can thin and rupture, exposing the blood within the vessel lumen to collagen, lipids, and smooth muscle cells in the vessel wall, leading to platelet deposition and coagulation cascade system activation, with resultant thrombus formation. The thrombi can cause vessel occlusion and infarction, or can undergo vessel wall incorporation as complex plaque, causing gradual vessel lumen narrowing. Calcification usually is associated with complex plaque formation. Calcium deposition usually is most prominent in the proximal coronary artery segments, with deposition in distal portions rarely occurring in the absence of proximal involvement (Fig. 37-1).

Some investigators have argued that because the prevalence of coronary calcification increases with age, it is merely a sign of the aging process. Nevertheless, a direct relation between the severity of coronary atherosclerosis and the extent of coronary calcification has been shown by several quantitative pathologic studies.

CORONARY ARTERY CALCIFICATION DETECTION

Plain radiography of the chest, fluoroscopy, single-detector helical CT, multidetector CT, and electron beam CT

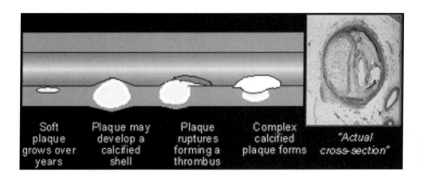

FIG. 37-1. The typical progression of the atherosclerotic process, with soft plaque maturing into complex calcified plaque.

(EBCT) have been used to detect coronary artery calcification. Coronary artery calcification is not easily detected on chest radiography, with an accuracy of only 42% compared with fluoroscopy, and is useful only when extensive coronary calcification is present. In the past, fluoroscopy has been used more widely for the detection of coronary artery calcification. Its sensitivity in detecting coronary calcification as an indicator of a hemodynamically significant stenosis (diameter reduction of 50% or more) is 40% to 79%, with a specificity of 52% to 95% when compared to angiography. The sensitivity of digital subtraction fluoroscopy was somewhat better (92% vs. 63%). The disadvantages of fluoroscopy include its sensitivity, which is only moderate; its dependence on the operator's skill and experience; the duration of the study; and the number of views required. It is further limited by patient body habitus, overlying anatomic structures, and variations in imaging equipment. Quantification of calcium is not possible with fluoroscopy, intraobserver and interobserver variability has not been measured, and filming is not often obtained.

Because calcium causes attenuation of the x-ray beam, computed tomography (CT) is extremely sensitive in detecting calcification. Until recent years, conventional CT has been limited because of poor temporal resolution, motion artifacts, volume averaging, breathing misregistration artifacts, and inability to quantify the extent of the plaque. Preliminary studies performed in the late 1980s compared the detection of calcification on older-generation, single-slice, conventional CT scans against the detection of stenosis of 70% or greater on angiograms. Detection of extensive calcification demonstrated a high positive predictive value for significant coronary artery disease. Angiograms showed some stenosis in 88% of calcified vessels and 57% of non-calcified vessels detected on CT scans. Of those vessels without luminal stenosis, 33% still showed some evidence of calcification. Among vessels with any degree of stenosis, 69% showed some calcification. Sections 10 mm thick were used in this study, and the scan times were not reported, which may have resulted in smaller calcifications being missed. In general, older-generation conventional CT was

found to be superior to fluoroscopy for detecting calcification in coronary arteries and to angiography in detecting calcification in significant coronary artery disease.

EBCT was found to have significant advantages over older-generation, single-slice, conventional CT scanners in the detection of coronary artery calcification because of its rapid imaging and high spatial resolution. Sections 3 mm thick can be scanned in 100 msec, without utilizing contrast material, at a dose of radiation of less than 1.1 cGy, with pixel sizes of 0.25 to 0.5 mm^2, which enable the detection of small amounts of calcium with considerable accuracy. Since no specific Hounsfield unit (HU) value is indicative of the presence of calcification in a lesion, some investigators chose an arbitrary level of +130 HU. This level was chosen because the attenuation of soft tissues is about +50 HU, and +130 HU was thought to be a large enough increase that any structures registering +130 HU probably would contain calcium. A density area of 2 mm^2 or greater is considered a calcific lesion, whereas an area of less than 2 mm^2 is considered noise. The entire coronary arterial tree can be imaged during one breathhold using the 100-msec speed that minimizes cardiac motion. Using the Agatston analysis method, Hounsfield unit weights of 1 for 130 to 200 HU, 2 for 201 to 299 HU, 3 for 300 to 399 HU, and 4 for 400 HU and above are assigned and multiplied by the area of each lesion to obtain an individual lesion score. These individual lesion scores are summed throughout the coronary arterial tree to obtain the total coronary calcium score. CT scanner or dedicated workstation software enable the operator to quantify the calcification area, which is important in monitoring the progression or possible regression of disease. Three-dimensional reconstruction is afforded by acquiring contiguous scans. Intra- and interobserver reproducibility determinations have correlation coefficients of 0.99. Some investigators have considered that densities between +115 and +130 HU indicate precursors of calcification formation (Figs. 37-2 and 37-3).

The use of EBCT for detecting calcific deposits was first reported by Tanenbaum et al. and Janowitz et al. The former study used 50-msec scan times and 1.5 mm^2 of spatial

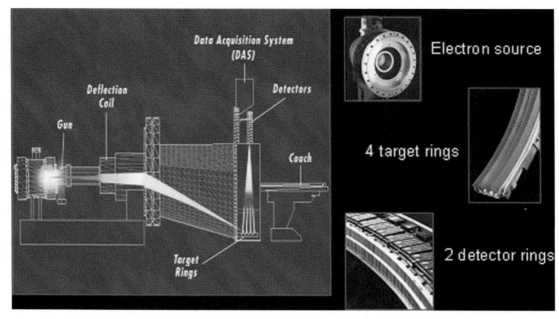

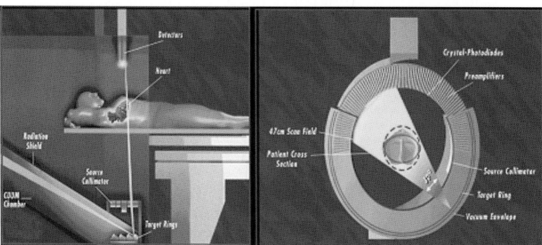

FIG. 37-2. Electron beam computed tomographic (EBCT) scanner configuration. The electron beam is generated by an electron source and then focused onto one of four tungsten target rings lying in a gantry beneath the patient. Each 210-degree sweep of the electron beam on the target ring produces a 30-degree fan beam of x-rays that pass through the patient to detectors above, producing a cross-sectional image.

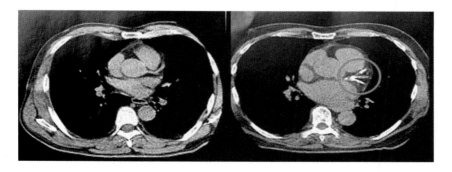

FIG. 37-3. EBCT coronary calcification screening examinations. **Left.** The left main and proximal left anterior descending coronary artery depicted without evidence of calcification. **Right.** Dense calcification in the left main, proximal left anterior descending, ramus intermedius, and proximal circumflex coronary arteries *(circle)*.

resolution and coronary angiography to examine 54 patients, and a luminal diameter reduction of 50% of the left main coronary artery and 70% for all other coronary arteries was considered significant. Coronary angiography showed significant coronary artery disease in 43 patients, and 88% of these had detectable calcium in at least one coronary artery, with a specificity of 100%. The first large series, in which EBCT was used to detect calcification of the coronary arteries in 584 consecutive subjects, 30 to 69 years old, with and without histories of coronary artery disease, was done by Agatston et al., and employed 100-msec, 3-mm-thick scans. One hundred nine patients had a history of coronary artery disease—either a history of myocardial infarction (22 patients) or angiographic evidence of more than 50% diameter narrowing of coronary arteries (87 patients)—and 475 did not, with a mean age for all subjects of 48 years. Significant differences ($p = 0.0001$) were found between the two groups, with sensitivities of 71% to 74% and specificities of 70% to 91%. The negative predictive value of a zero calcification score was 94% to 100%. EBCT showed calcium in 90% and fluoroscopy in 52% of the 50 patients who underwent both procedures. The study showed that the mean total calcium score increased with age. EBCT appeared to be an excellent technique for detecting and quantifying calcification of coronary arteries. The prevalence of coronary calcification in the 30- to 39-year-old group was 25% in individuals without a history of coronary artery disease versus 100% in individuals with a history of coronary artery disease. The prevalence of calcification in individuals without coronary artery disease increased to 39% at ages 40 to 59, 73% at ages 50 to 59, and 74% at ages 60 to 69. Comparable figures for individuals with coronary artery disease were 88% (ages 40 to 49), 96% (ages 50 to 59), and 100% (ages 60 to 69), with $p < 0.0001$ between all groups. The authors concluded that the total calcium score and the number of lesions increased with age, and calcification was significantly greater in those patients with a history of coronary artery disease than in those without (Fig. 37-4).

Stanford et al., in a group of 150 patients undergoing coronary angiography from two institutions, determined that absence of calcium on EBCT scans appeared to be a significant indicator of the absence of coronary artery disease. Only one patient had significant stenosis in the absence of calcification. EBCT has proven to be a noninvasive method for detecting calcification and demonstrates evidence of coronary atherosclerosis when the disease is in its nonobstructive, preclinical stage. Because the presence of coronary calcification is an independent risk factor for coronary artery disease, EBCT is superior to conventional risk-factor analysis in the detection of nonobstructive disease for prediction of future cardiac events. Generally, it is thought than calcium in the coronary arteries is associated with atherosclerosis and that its quantity reflects the overall extent of the atherosclerotic process. Some investigators have sug-

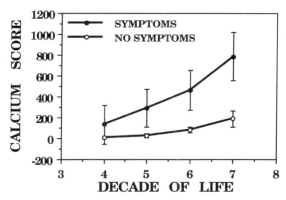

FIG. 37-4. Comparison of patients from the EBCT study of Agatston et al. with a history of symptomatic coronary artery disease *(upper curve)* versus those without symptoms *(lower curve)*. The authors concluded that the total calcium score and the number of lesions increased with age, and calcification was significantly greater in those patients with a history of coronary artery disease than in those without. Error bars depict two standard deviations around the mean.

gested that a coronary artery calcification study that shows no calcium significantly diminishes the need for further testing.

COMPLEMENTARY ROLE OF EBCT AND NUCLEAR CARDIOLOGY TECHNIQUES

Both EBCT and nuclear cardiology techniques are valuable and complementary in the noninvasive assessment of patients with suspected coronary artery disease. However, they provide different information about the patient. Berman and colleagues have been proponents of the concept that EBCT provides anatomic information on coronary atherosclerosis, in contrast to myocardial perfusion single-photon emission CT (SPECT) which assesses the physiologic significance of a coronary stenosis, making these two techniques highly complementary. In selecting one of these diagnostic tests, it is important to consider the issues being raised in an individual patient. EBCT is best suited to assess the risk in an individual patient of developing clinical coronary artery disease. The level of risk will determine who needs aggressive medical management. EBCT testing and clinical assessment alone usually is sufficient; in some cases nuclear testing can be of additional value. Another issue in a patient with suspected coronary artery disease is the risk of cardiac death. Determining the level of risk may lead to considerations of coronary revascularization. EBCT and nuclear cardiology studies appear to operate in a complementary fashion to address this issue.

In patients with known coronary atherosclerosis, another important issue is the risk of subsequent cardiac events, especially in asymptomatic patients in whom revascularization might be inappropriate unless substantial risk of cardiac death is present. EBCT and SPECT are likely to be complementary in this setting. Studies have demonstrated that patients with low EBCT scores are at low risk for cardiac death and usually do not need further testing. A clinical question that is still under discussion is whether patients with abnormal EBCT require further risk assessment testing. Although study reports vary somewhat, it has been documented that the risk ratio for patients with an abnormal EBCT is greater than 1. The early prognostic data from the small populations studied with EBCT to date are promising, but only preliminary information is available on the risk of cardiac death with EBCT. In contrast, multiple nuclear cardiology studies considering risk stratification in tens of thousands of patients have been performed. Large populations have been studied with nuclear cardiology techniques for prediction of cardiac death. The extent and severity of stress myocardial perfusion defects is a strong predictor of cardiac death, with the death rate increasing in proportion to the degree of abnormality on stress SPECT studies. The combination of perfusion and function, as measured by gated myocardial perfusion SPECT, provides even more information for the prediction of cardiac death than is provided by stress perfusion measurements alone.

Clearly, it would not be cost-effective for all patients with abnormal EBCTs to go on to more costly SPECT testing, and a paradigm will have to be developed. He et al. evaluated the frequency of stress-induced ischemia by myocardial perfusion SPECT in 292 men and 78 women undergoing both myocardial perfusion SPECT and EBCT for coronary calcification. The patients were categorized as having no (coronary calcium score 0), minimal (coronary calcium score 1 to 10), mild (coronary calcium score 11 to 100), moderate (coronary calcium score 101 to 399), and extensive (coronary calcium score above 400) coronary calcification. These investigators found that only one patient who demonstrated coronary calcium scores of 100 or less had an abnormal myocardial perfusion SPECT. Overall, 12% of patients with moderate coronary calcium scores had abnormal myocardial perfusion SPECT, and 47% of patients with extensive coronary calcium scores had abnormal myocardial perfusion SPECT. Recent data from Miranda et al. have confirmed these findings. In 233 consecutive patients with no history of coronary artery disease who had EBCT and myocardial perfusion SPECT, no patients with coronary calcium scores below 100 had abnormal myocardial perfusion SPECTs. In the moderate coronary calcium score category, 4.1% of patients demonstrated abnormal myocardial perfusion SPECT, and of those with coronary calcium scores above 400, 15% demonstrated abnormal myocardial perfusion SPECT. These investigators demonstrated that in this population the optimal cutpoint for predicting the abnormal myocardial perfusion SPECT occurred at a coronary calcium score of 399, providing confirmation that this limit indicates extensive coronary

atherosclerosis, as originally proposed by Rumberger et al. With this cutpoint, the sensitivity and specificity for predicting an abnormal myocardial perfusion SPECT study using EBCT were 82% and 62%, respectively. These data validated previously established criteria for extensive coronary atherosclerosis and previous findings on the relation between SPECT and EBCT studies. However, their findings also suggest that the frequency of abnormal scans in patients with a coronary calcium score above 400 may be lower than previously suggested.

Miranda et al. have developed a paradigm for the use of EBCT and SPECT in coronary artery disease assessment and risk stratification. Patients with a very low likelihood of coronary artery disease probably would not warrant testing. Patients with a low-to-intermediate likelihood of coronary artery disease, as often is observed in asymptomatic patients with coronary disease risk factors, would undergo an EBCT study. If the EBCT study is abnormal, and the coronary calcium score is less than 400, medical management would be indicated. How aggressive the medical management should be is determined by the degree of risk factors and the level of abnormality found on EBCT. If the EBCT score is over 400, patients would generally be considered appropriate candidates for SPECT. Patients with a coronary event risk of greater than 1% per year by SPECT (and clinical assessment) would be appropriate candidates for coronary angiography. Patients with an intermediate-to-high likelihood of coronary artery disease might be appropriate candidates to proceed directly to SPECT. Those patients considered to be at even higher risk might proceed directly to catheterization. In these intermediate-to-high-likelihood patients, EBCT might be appropriate, if the SPECT scans are found to be normal, to evaluate the extent of atherosclerosis and to help guide medical management. EBCT also might help motivate these patients to comply with medical management of their coronary artery disease.

EBCT EVALUATION OF CORONARY ARTERY DISEASE PROGRESSION AND REGRESSION

Multiple trials of cholesterol reduction with statins have demonstrated a positive mortality benefit in primary and secondary prevention. The ability to track the progression or regression of atherosclerosis noninvasively might provide clinicians with effective tools to evaluate therapies directed at the possible prevention or treatment of coronary artery disease. Coronary artery calcium, identified by EBCT, is closely correlated with the atherosclerotic plaque burden, which has been shown to be a powerful predictor of future cardiac events. Recent studies have demonstrated the ability of EBCT to monitor the progression of coronary plaque burden and to document an individual's response to risk factor modification and medical intervention. Preliminary studies have demonstrated slowing progression of coronary artery calcium build-up in response to lipid-lowering therapy, which has been shown to reduce cardiovascular morbidity and mortality. Slowing the expansion of the atherosclerotic burden, as in reducing the continued accumulation of coronary artery calcium, ultimately may be shown to reduce the risk of death and myocardial infarction.

EBCT can be used to assess changes of coronary atherosclerosis in response to therapy noninvasively by interval quantification of coronary artery calcium. Janowitz et al. demonstrated that the score progression was more marked in patients with obstructive coronary artery disease compared with patients who had no clinically manifest disease (27% vs. 18%). Maher et al., in a preliminary study (n = 81), demonstrated an increase in the coronary artery calcium score by 24% each year after baseline. Budoff et al., in a larger study (n = 299), with an average 2.2-year follow-up period, demonstrated that coronary artery calcium scores increased a mean of 33% per year, predicting that the coronary artery calcium score will more than double every 2.5 years on average. Mitchell et al. observed 347 patients for 1.4 years, demonstrating an annual average increase in coronary artery calcium scores of 21% in men and 18% in women. Goodman et al., in a small study of young patients with end-stage renal disease, demonstrated a mean calcium score increase of 59% per year, with a doubling of score by 20 months. Callister et al., using EBCT in a 1-year observational study, demonstrated the effect of statin therapy on 149 asymptomatic persons with high levels of cholesterol. There was a significant net increase in mean calcium volume score among individuals not treated with cholesterol-reducing medications (mean change, 52 ± 36%; $p < 0.001$). At the follow-up visit, a net reduction in the calcium volume score was observed only in the 65 statin-treated patients whose final low-density lipoprotein cholesterol (LDL-C) levels were below 120 mg/dl (mean score change, 27 ± 23%; $p = 0.01$ for comparison with untreated subjects). Individuals treated less aggressively and with an average LDL-C level higher than 120 mg/dl showed a calcium volume score increase of 25 ± 22% ($p < 0.001$ for comparison with aggressively treated subjects).

Budoff et al. performed an observational study in 123 persons with hypercholesterolemia. Participants reporting use of a statin (n = 60) had a 15% annual rate of progression of their EBCT scores compared with a 39% annual increase for the 62 persons in the non-treatment group ($p < 0.001$). This represented a 61% reduction in the rate of progression obtained with statin therapy.

Preliminary results of an ongoing study of 160 persons with established coronary artery disease have demonstrated a slowing of the atherosclerotic process resulting from treatment of patients with severe hypercholesterolemia. Combination treatment with simvastatin, niacin, and vitamin E resulted in an annual calcium score progression of 20% as compared with a median of 40% progression measured in the untreated group.

Two studies have reported the outcome of patients observed serially for evidence of coronary calcium progression. In one study, Raggi et al. observed 269 asymptomatic subjects for an average of 2.5 years. Of the 22 cardiovascular events recorded at the end of the follow-up period (death, myocardial infarction, and revascularizations), 20 events occurred in patients with continued expansion of coronary calcium volume score. Only two events (one myocardial infarction and one coronary angioplasty) occurred in patients with evidence of stabilization of disease ($p < 0.001$ for test on proportions). In a second study, Shah et al. evaluated 225 moderate- to high-risk asymptomatic individuals with EBCT scores above 20 at baseline (81% male, mean age 60 ± 9 years). All subjects underwent sequential EBCT scanning at a minimum interval of 1 year and were interviewed at the time of the follow-up visit. The time between scans averaged 3 years, with a range of 1 to 7 years. A total of 30 events occurred in 23 patients: 8 myocardial infarctions, 4 strokes, 13 coronary angioplasties, and 5 bypass surgeries. In the patients who did experience events, the mean coronary artery calcium score (Agatston method) increase was 35% per year. This was significantly greater than the change in coronary artery calcium measured in patients who did not have cardiac events (mean annual change: 22%, $p = 0.04$). Of the 23 patients who sustained events, 78% demonstrated significant coronary artery calcium score progression (defined as >20% per year), whereas only 37% of the patients without follow-up events showed this degree of progression ($p < 0.001$ for test on proportions). No individual who had a coronary event exhibited regression or lack of progression of coronary artery calcium. An annual event rate of 6.45% was observed in patients with significant progression (coronary artery calcium >20% per year), which was significantly greater than the 1.5% annual event rate in individuals with progression of 1% to 20%, or 0% for those with regression (lower calcium score on follow-up visit), or lack of progression. The relative risk of a cardiac event for those experiencing progression was 17.7-fold greater (95% confidence intervals 13–38, $p < 0.001$) than those without significant progression (coronary artery calcium change <20% per year), using multivariate analysis. The only other factor that was independently predictive was age (odds ratio 6.7, $p = 0.008$). Hypertension, diabetes, hypercholesterolemia, tobacco use, family history of premature coronary artery disease, and gender failed to predict events. In these two studies, cardiovascular events were strongly associated with rapid progression of atherosclerotic plaque, as assessed by EBCT coronary calcium.

CORONARY CALCIFICATION SCREENING USING MULTIDETECTOR COMPUTED TOMOGRAPHY

Multidetector CT (MDCT) scanners have undergone significant improvements in their ability to perform cardiac imaging. Previously limited by artifacts caused by cardiac motion and slow acquisition speeds, the latest-generation scanners are able to obtain multiple slices with a temporal resolution of less than 100 msec, in an attempt to minimize motion artifacts. This is done using prospective and retrospective electrocardiographic gating, multislice detectors, and partial and segmented reconstruction algorithms. The major CT manufacturers have committed significant resources to protocol optimization and cardiac applications development in pursuit of the potential large cardiac imaging market, including coronary calcium quantification, coronary CT angiography, and functional analysis. Given the large commitment of resources, the current higher in-plane and z-axis spatial resolution, and superior signal-to-noise ratio of multidetector scanners (albeit at the cost of higher radiation burden), it appears that they will be capable of performing cardiac imaging with a quality approaching or possibly surpassing that of older-generation EBCT scanners.

Few studies have been published on detection of coronary artery calcification with single-slice helical CT, and even fewer on its detection with MDCT. This is not surprising, in light of the fact that single-slice helical CT and MDCT scanners capable of cardiac imaging have only recently become available. Several studies have been performed comparing EBCT and single-slice helical CT in the same patients. Carr et al., in a study of 36 patients, found a correlation coefficient of 0.98 for calcium scoring. Becker et al. studied a group of 100 patients with similar results. Although the number of patients in these studies is small and the large spread of calcium scores tends to produce high correlation coefficients, it appears that the scores are similar, if not identical (Fig. 37-5).

Some EBCT investigators have stated that the data developed with EBCT studies and based on age- and gender-based calcium score percentiles and risk profiles should not be applied to calcium scores obtained by single-slice helical CT and MDCT scanners. Currently, no data support the position that calcium scores from different CT manufacturers are comparable or that serial studies done to compare disease progression or regression can be done using different scanners. With EBCT, however, most centers are using similar or identical protocols.

Reproducibility of calcium scores by single-slice helical or MDCT is another issue that must be addressed. In limited studies, reproducibility of single slice helical CT-derived calcium scores appears to be comparable to that of EBCT, if not better. The improved signal-to-noise ratio and better spatial resolution of single-slice helical CT may be an advantage in reproducibility. Some data suggest that volume scores from single-slice helical CT may be more reproducible than Agatston scores. Until additional, larger studies examining whether single-slice helical and MDCT-derived calcium scores are equivalent have been completed, it remains prudent to apply single-slice helical and MDCT scores clinically with care when EBCT databases are used. It is hoped that in the future manufacturer-specific databases will be developed for single-slice helical and MDCT calcium scores. However, given the relatively large variation in EBCT reproducibility, it is unlikely that significant clinical errors will occur when using the general guidelines developed from EBCT data to risk-stratify asymptomatic subjects by single-slice helical or MDCT scores. This may not be the case in symptomatic individuals, when the absence of calcium (calcium score of 0) is being used to rule out coronary artery disease. EBCT studies have shown a high accuracy rate in ruling out coronary artery disease in patients presenting to the emergency room with chest pain when the calcium score is 0. Comparable studies still are needed with single-slice helical and MDCT scanners to show similar accuracy, especially when older-generation, single-slice scanners are used.

CORONARY ARTERY VULNERABLE PLAQUE CHARACTERIZATION

Prospective studies have demonstrated that in patients presenting to the emergency department with chest pain and no initial objective signs of myocardial ischemia, a negative electron beam CT for coronary calcium indicated an excel-

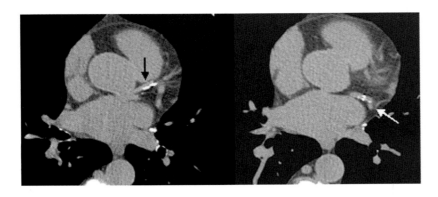

FIG. 37-5. Prospectively gated MDCT images, 2.5-mm slice thickness, demonstrating calcification in the proximal left anterior descending *(black arrow)* and circumflex coronary arteries *(white arrow).*

lent prognosis with regard to major cardiac events over the subsequent 1 to 4 months. EBCT yielded negative predictive values in the range of 98% to 100%. In symptomatic patients undergoing coronary angiography, increased amounts of coronary calcium detected by electron beam CT were highly predictive of subsequent events over 30 months. Coronary calcium is associated very closely with coronary atherosclerotic plaque development. The use of EBCT for accurate quantitative measurements has led to an increased interest in understanding the clinical importance of coronary calcium, particularly in terms of the ability to identify unstable coronary plaques that underlie the clinical acute coronary syndromes. Histopathologic studies have demonstrated that calcium is a frequent feature of ruptured plaques, but the presence or absence of calcium alone does not permit reliable distinction between unstable versus stable plaques.

The risk of acute coronary syndromes caused by plaque disruption and thrombosis depends on the composition of the plaque rather than the severity of the stenosis. Thus, the reliable noninvasive assessment of plaque configuration would constitute an important step forward for risk stratification in patients with known or suspected coronary artery disease. Rupture-prone plaques in the coronary arteries, the so-called vulnerable plaques, tend to have a thin fibrous cap (cap thickness of 65 to 150 mm) and a large lipid core. Acute coronary syndromes often result from rupture of a modestly stenotic vulnerable plaque, not visible by x-ray angiography.

Coronary lesions in varying phases of development may be present in the same artery, and in areas of calcification, other adjacent areas of the artery probably will contain lipid-laden plaque. CT voxel attenuation distribution data (in HU) vary from negative (lipid-laden) to highly positive (calcium-laden).

Teichholz et al. studied the potential of EBCT to assess lipid-laden plaque and inhomogeneity quantitatively at sites having no apparent calcification in proximal segments of the left anterior descending coronary artery using voxel attenuation distribution differences. These investigators found that the mean voxel attenuation in the coronary atherosclerotic group was significantly less than that for the normal group (25.4 ± 2.8 vs. 36.3 ± 2.1 HU, $p < 0.005$). This suggests that there was more lipid-laden plaque in the region of interest within a coronary artery for the coronary atherosclerotic group than in a similar region of interest in the normal group. The percentage of voxels with attenuation less than 0 HU was significantly greater in the coronary atherosclerotic group than in the normal group ($22.9 \pm 2.3\%$ vs. $7.3 \pm 1.0\%$, $p < 0.00001$). This also is consistent with the notion that there is more lipid-laden plaque in the left anterior descending coronary artery in patients with abnormal calcium scores. The standard deviation of the voxel attenuations for the coronary atherosclerosis group

was significantly greater than that for the normal group (31.8 ± 1.0 vs. 23.9 ± 0.7 HU, $p < 0.00001$). This suggests more inhomogeneity in a region of interest within a coronary artery in the coronary atherosclerotic group than in the normal group. Similar analyses were performed using a subset of 20 patients from the coronary atherosclerosis group with overall calcium scores below 300. The results were not significantly different from those for the entire atherosclerotic population. Their results suggest that electron beam CT voxel attenuation distribution data are useful in quantitatively assessing lipid-laden plaque and inhomogeneity associated with the atherosclerotic process.

Schroeder et al. conducted a study designed to evaluate the accuracy of determining coronary lesion configuration by MDCT. The results were compared with the findings of intracoronary ultrasound. The intracoronary ultrasound and multislice CT scans (Somatom Volume Zoom, Siemens, Forchheim, Germany) were performed in 15 patients. Plaque composition was analyzed according to intracoronary ultrasound (plaque echodensity: soft, intermediate, calcified) and MDCT criteria (plaque density expressed in HU). Thirty-four plaques were analyzed. With intracoronary ultrasound, the plaques were classified as soft (n = 12), intermediate (n = 5), and calcified (n = 17). Using MDCT, soft plaques had a density of 14 ± 26 HU (range, -42 to $+47$ HU), intermediate plaques of 91 ± 21 HU (61 to 112 HU) and calcified plaques of 419 ± 194 HU (126 to 736 HU). Significant differences of plaque density were noted among the three groups ($p < 0.0001$). These investigators' results indicate that the configuration of coronary lesions might be differentiated correctly by MDCT.

These preliminary studies suggest that rupture-prone soft plaques may be detected by electron beam and MDCT, and these noninvasive CT methods might become an important diagnostic tool for risk stratification in the future (Figs. 37-6 and 37-7).

CLINICAL VALUE OF CORONARY CALCIFICATION DETECTION

Although mortality rates have declined during the past decade, widespread cardiovascular morbidity persists, as does the need for improved detection and prevention programs to affect the natural history of the disease. Conventional risk factors alone are not always helpful in the complete estimation of cardiovascular risk in an individual patient. Individual patient information regarding the development and extent of the atherosclerotic process in the coronary arteries may permit treatment interventions that could reduce an individual's cardiovascular morbidity and possibly mortality. For decades, clinicians have concerned themselves with the diagnosis and care of obstructive coronary artery disease, and have been preoccupied with its quantifi-

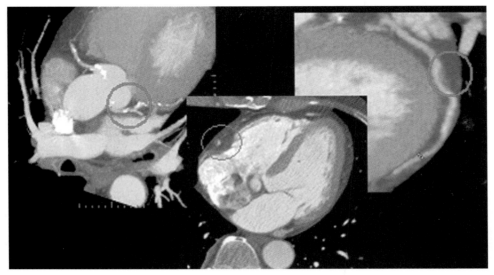

FIG. 37-6. MDCT coronary angiogram demonstrating both calcified and noncalcified plaque *(circles).*

cation. However, it now appears that the total burden of atherosclerotic disease rather than the severity of the focal stenosis may be a more significant prognostic indicator of subsequent cardiac events. Therefore, noninvasive imaging technologies directed at detection of atherosclerotic disease rather than quantification of luminal stenosis have gained the attention of clinicians. It is expected that these techniques may improve risk stratification in the individual patient, when the information derived from these techniques is added to conventional risk factors for atherosclerosis.

Coronary artery calcification is an atherosclerosis marker indicating intimal atheromata, often before the atheromata reduce the luminal diameter by 50%, after which point they become detectable by stress electrocardiography or SPECT. The amount of calcification increases with age and with multiple vessel involvement, but does not equate with a site-specific stenosis. Coronary artery calcification may not always predict vessel-specific future cardiac events: it has been shown repeatedly that thrombotic occlusions with infarction can occur in areas of noncalcified plaque. However, most patients having coronary events will have detectable calcification somewhere within their coronary arterial tree. Rapid progression of atherosclerotic plaque as assessed by coronary calcium detected using EBCT has been associated strongly with cardiovascular events. CT appears to be the most useful technique for detecting coronary artery calcification. The significantly faster scan times of EBCT, coupled with high-resolution images, provide advantages over other techniques. Single-slice helical and MDCT are other techniques currently being evaluated for the accurate

detection of calcification, and preliminary results are very promising.

At this time, coronary artery calcification detection has utility in (1) early detection of calcification in asymptomatic persons in whom risk-factor modification may be indicated; (2) evaluation of the progression or possible regression of calcification as an indicator of the activity of the atherosclerotic process; and (3) demonstration of the absence of calcification, since in all but a very small percentage of persons (less than 5%), this appears to rule out significant stenosis.

ELECTRON BEAM CORONARY ANGIOGRAPHY

Selective coronary angiography has been the reference standard for defining the presence, site, and severity of coronary artery disease for many years. More than one million coronary angiographic procedures, at a cost of several billion dollars, are performed annually in the United States. Coronary angiographic procedures are invasive, expensive (over $5000), and labor intensive; they often require a short hospital stay for monitoring; and they have well-established morbidity (1.5%) and mortality (0.15%). Pathology studies have demonstrated that the severity of coronary arteries stenoses often are underestimated during coronary angiography, possibly because of limitations in fluoroscopic image resolution and the inherent projectional imaging. The development of a less invasive and less expensive test (about $2000) for imaging the coronary arteries has been long

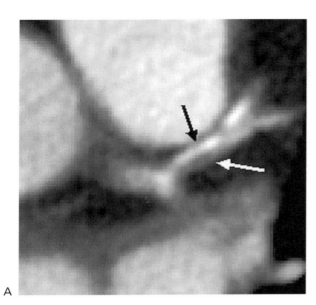

FIG. 37-7. A. EBCT (C-150) proximal left anterior descending coronary artery demonstrating complex hard *(black arrow)* and soft *(white arrow)* plaque. **B.** EBCT (C-150) histogram analysis demonstrating HU ranges: light gray, 0 to 113; white, 114 to 254; black, 255 to 343; and darker gray, 344 or greater. If a threshold of 130 HU is used for calcium, soft plaque would be contained in the light gray regions and calcified complex plaque would be contained in the white, black and darker gray regions.

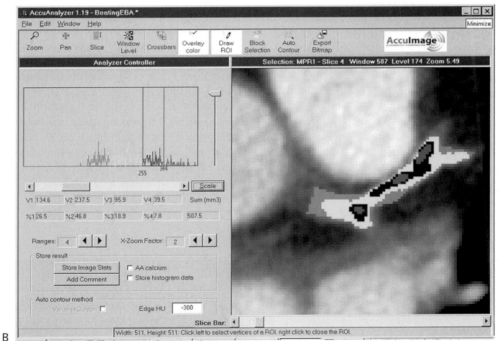

awaited, but many attempts to image the coronary arteries noninvasively have failed. Rapid motion during the cardiac cycle, superimposed respiratory motion, and small vessel diameters have remained daunting obstacles for noninvasive visualization of the coronary arteries. Because coronary artery disease remains a major cardiac disease affecting adults, and it is the single major cause of death in America, the noninvasive depiction of coronary artery pathoanatomy remains the Holy Grail for cardiac imaging investigators.

In recent years, EBCT, developed by Boyd at the University of California San Francisco in the 1980s, has emerged as a technology with the potential for performing noninvasive coronary angiography, with a radiation exposure estimated to be one third of that of a diagnostic conventional coronary angiogram.

CLINICAL VALUE OF NONINVASIVE CORONARY ANGIOGRAPHY

It is important to keep in mind that within the foreseeable future noninvasive tomographic imaging modalities for coronary artery disease will not reach the same level of image quality as can be obtained using invasive, selective coronary angiography, nor will it provide a means for interventional treatment. However, these methods may find their clinical niche in the work-up of coronary artery disease, if it is found that they can reliably rule out the presence of significant coronary stenoses that would be a potential target for revascularization therapy. The noninvasive methods for coronary visualization should be evaluated in the context of trying to avoid "negative" invasive coronary angiograms (i.e., those that are not followed by revascularization therapy). If noninvasive methods for coronary visualization can be applied carefully and knowledgeably in selected patients, they may be effectively integrated into the spectrum of diagnostic tools available to the cardiologist for use in patients with established or suspected coronary artery disease.

Budoff et al. have stated the clinical indications for electron beam coronary angiography as follows:

1. After bypass surgery to evaluate graft patency
2. Postangioplasty or poststenting to evaluate patency
3. After stress testing (or stress imaging) when the clinical results are equivocal
4. Follow-up of persons with previous angiography to define certain known lesions
5. Evaluation of persons with fear of traditional angiography to define their coronary anatomy
6. Annual follow-up of patients after cardiac transplantation
7. As a potential alternative to noninvasive testing to evaluate obstructive disease

Projected and evolving indications include the following:

1. Low to intermediate probability of hemodynamic, significant coronary stenosis (SPECT summed stress score)
2. Assessment of atypical symptoms in patients after coronary artery bypass grafting or percutaneous transluminal coronary angioplasty
3. Assessment of congenital coronary anomalies

Future indications might include noninvasive assessment of myocardial muscle bridging, patients with cardiomyopathy, and pharmacologic stress coronary flow analysis. Clinical contraindications are similar to those for conventional coronary angiography, and the patients who are included are as follows:

1. Those with chronic renal insufficiency (creatinine above 2.0 mg/dl)
2. Those with severe contrast medium allergy
3. Those with high-risk anatomy (as defined by history or noninvasive testing), and who will most likely require subsequent revascularization
4. Those with extensive coronary calcification (total coronary calcification score above 1500), which potentially can obscure hemodynamically significant coronary stenoses

PATIENT PREPARATION AND SCAN ACQUISITION

The three modes of the EBCT scanner provide the ability to acquire information that is similar to that provided by a conventional coronary angiogram (Fig. 37-8).

An intravenous line is started in the right or left antecubital fossa. A standard 3-mm slice thickness, noncontrast, coronary calcium examination is performed with deep breathhold in single-slice mode. With the patient in the fasting state, a resting multislice mode, dynamic flow study is performed with administration of approximately 25 ml of nonionic contrast at 3 to 4 cc/sec. When earlier-model EBCT scanners (e.g., C-150, C-300) are employed, following appropriate timing selection, 4 L/min of nasal oxygen, 0.4 mg of nitroglycerin spray, and infusion of about 125 ml of contrast medium at 3 to 4 ml/sec is given with single-slice mode acquisition of 3×2 axial images with 100-msec images acquired with ECG gating, beginning at 40% of R-to-R interval during a single breathhold. Finally, using the same contrast bolus, a resting dynamic ECG gated wall motion study of the heart is then performed using the multislice cine mode. When the latest model EBCT (e-Speed) is used, contiguous 1.5-mm slice thickness, 50-msec images are acquired during six to eight time frames, acquiring coronary anatomy and ventricular wall motion in one acquisition. The contrast images are then reconstructed using four-dimensional imaging software on an imaging workstation. Nasal oxygen greatly enhances the patient's ability to hold their breath. Nitroglycerin is optional but dilates the coronary arteries, which assists in defining the coronary anatomy (Figs. 37-9 to 37-11).

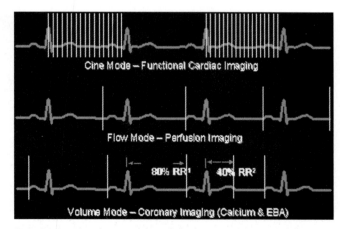

FIG. 37-8. The three modes of the EBCT scanner used for a CT coronary angiographic study. The multislice flow mode is employed for the first-pass study used for bolus timing and qualitative myocardial perfusion. The multislice cine mode is used for cardiac volumes and ventricular ejection fraction determination. The single-slice volume mode is employed for the coronary calcification and angiographic portions of the examination.

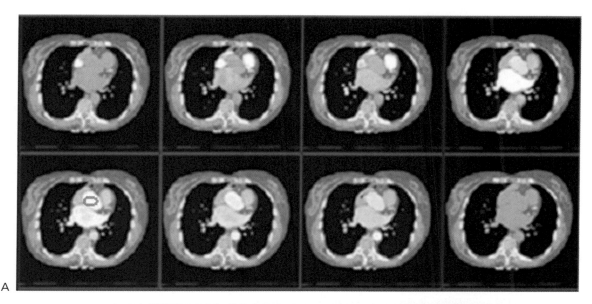

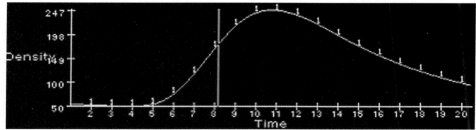

FIG. 37-9. A. Multislice-mode, ECG-gated, dynamic flow study at the base of the heart demonstrating contrast passing from the right-sided cardiac chambers *(upper left)* to the left sided cardiac chambers *(lower right)*. These images are used for bolus timing by placing a region of interest in the root of the aorta *(circle at lower left)* and myocardial regions of interest at lower cardiac levels for qualitative myocardial perfusion. The region of interest placed in the root of the aorta in the upper panel is used to create a time-density curve from the dynamic flow images. **B.** The optimal time for performing the coronary angiographic acquisition is determined as the delay between starting injection and scanning plus the time to achieve 50% to 65% of the peak density, as indicated by the vertical line. In this example, a 6-second delay is added to 8 seconds to obtain a 14-second delay to be employed for the coronary angiographic acquisition.

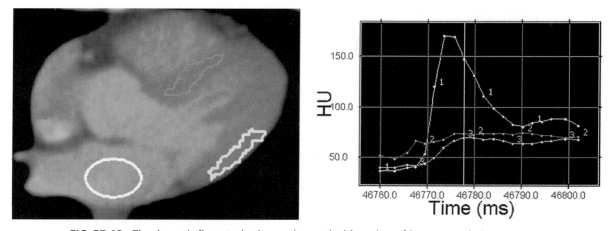

FIG. 37-10. The dynamic flow study also can be used with region-of-interest analysis to compare qualitative flow in the septum and posterior wall of the left ventricle to the left atrium at rest (*1*, aorta; *2*, septum; *3*, posterior wall). Studies are ongoing evaluating adenosine pharmacologic stress/rest imaging for the evaluation of the hemodynamic significance of coronary stenoses.

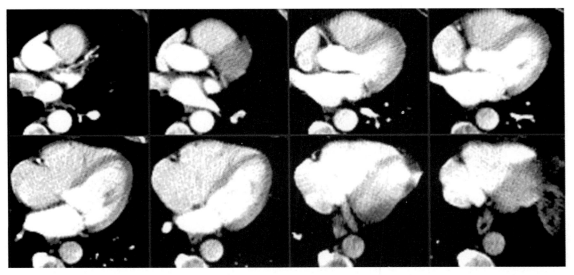

FIG. 37-11. Multislice-mode, ECG-gated, dynamic cine study. These images are used for cardiac volumes and ventricular ejection fraction determination.

A three-dimensional data set is obtained by stacking many two-dimensional CT tomograms together. Multiplanar, tomographic reformatting along the axes of the coronary arteries can be accomplished during one to three time frames during the cardiac cycle (and, more recently, one to six time frames using e-Speed) with dynamic movie display. Three-dimensional reconstructions are made using a shaded surface rendering or a volume rendering technique (Fig. 37-12).

The use of EBCT to detect the patency of aortocoronary bypass grafts was reported as early as 1986. Subsequent investigations using transaxial tomograms showed a very high accuracy, sensitivity, and specificity for detecting whether bypass grafts were occluded or patent. In a study of 56 patients, Achenbach et al. reported a sensitivity and specificity of 100% for bypass graft occlusion, and a sensitivity of 100% and specificity of 97% for bypass graft stenosis, with 84% of graft segments evaluable. Recently introduced three-dimensional curvilinear rendering techniques are able to reconstruct the graft completely, and thus allow assessment of nonoccluding obstructions with high diagnostic accuracy, sensitivity, and specificity.

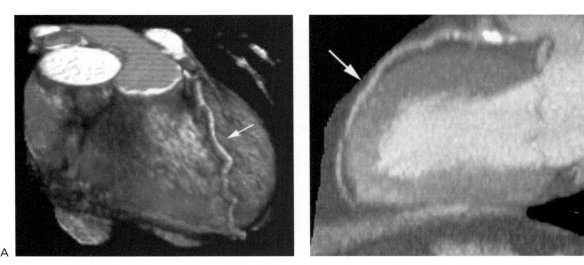

FIG. 37-12. A 66-year-old man with rapidly progressive coronary artery calcification scores. EBCT (C-150) volume-rendered view (**A**) and curvilinear projection view (**B**) of the left anterior descending coronary artery *(arrows)*.

Multiple studies comparing EBCT with conventional coronary angiography for visualization of native coronary artery stenoses and studies in healthy volunteers have been published. The image quality was sufficient to allow reliable evaluation of the coronary arteries with relatively high sensitivity and specificity for the detection of significant stenoses in a high percentage of cases.

Diagnostic accuracy can be reduced by cardiac motion artifacts (particularly in the case of the right and circumflex coronary arteries), respiratory motion, overlapping anatomic structures, ECG triggering problems due to irregular heart rhythm, and problems in assessing the lumen in the presence of heavy overlying calcifications (Fig. 37-13; Table 37-1).

Research and clinical EBCT coronary angiography stud-

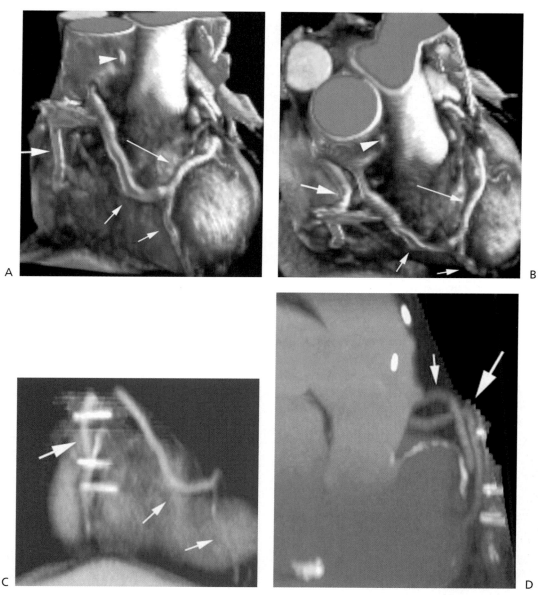

FIG. 37-13. EBCT (C-150) volume-rendered and projection views. A 72-year-old woman who refused interval invasive coronary angiography, status post–four vessel coronary artery bypass grafting with three saphenous vein bypass grafts. **A.** Skip graft *(long arrow)* to the mid portion of the left anterior descending coronary artery *(short arrows at bottom center)* and its poorly visualized, small, diagonal branch, obtuse marginal branch of the circumflex, occluded with stump *(arrowhead)*, and right coronary artery graft *(large arrow at left)* with its undersurface attached to the sternum. **C** and **D.** The proximal portion of the skip graft demonstrates moderate narrowing. **B** and **D.** The distal left anterior descending coronary artery is severely diseased and fills poorly. **D.** The right coronary artery is heavily calcified.

TABLE 37-1. MULTIPLE STUDIES COMPARING EBCT CORONARY ANGIOGRAPHY WITH CONVENTIONAL CORONARY ANGIOGRAPHY

Study[a]	Patients	Nonevaluated Segments[b] (%)	Sensitivity[c] (%)	Specificity (%)
Nakanish, 1997	37	—	74	95
Schermend, 1998	28	12	82	88
Reddy, 1988	23	10	88	79
Rensing, 1998	37	19	77	94
Achenbach, 1998	125	25	92	94
Budoff, 1999	52	11	78	71
Achenbach, 2000	36	20	92	91
Leber, 2001	87	24	78	93
Ropers, 2002	118	24	90	66
Nikolaou, 2002	20	11	85	77

[a] These studies all employed the older detector technology employed on the earlier generation electron beam CT scanners (C100/C150/C300), which are inferior to the new technology employed by the e⁻Speed scanner. The e⁻Speed's faster speed, higher resolution, and cine capability will increase the evaluable segments and improve sensitivity and specificity.
[b] Coronary segments that could not be evaluated due to motion artifacts, calcification, or nonvisualization.
[c] In evaluable segments.
(From Achenbach S, Moshage W, Ropers D, et al. Noninvasive, three-dimensional visualization of coronary artery bypass grafts by electron beam tomography. Am J Cardiol 1997; 79:856–861.)

ies currently are in progress at several prominent academic medical centers in the United States and abroad. The negative predictive value of an electron beam coronary angiogram for the presence of a hemodynamically significant stenosis is probably on the order of 95% to 98%, with further clinical studies ongoing (Figs. 37-14 to 37-16).

In a study of 50 patients, Achenbach et al. reported a sensitivity of 94% and specificity of 82% for detection of high-grade restenosis using contrast-enhanced electron beam coronary angiography after percutaneous transluminal angioplasty with 88% of coronary segments evaluable (Fig. 37-17).

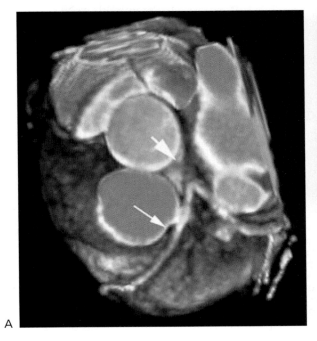

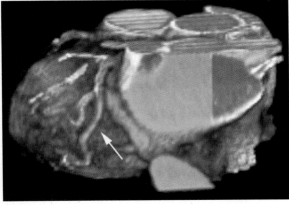

FIG. 37-14. A 71-year-old man has been referred to rule out the presence of coronary artery disease. **A.** Cranially angulated volume-rendered view of the left main coronary artery *(large arrow)*, left anterior descending coronary artery *(small arrow)*, and circumflex coronary artery. **B.** Circumflex coronary artery and its obtuse marginal branch *(arrow)*.

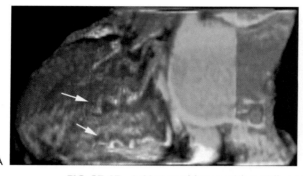
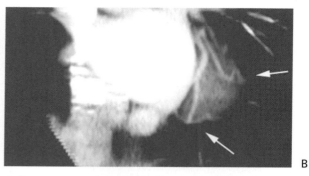

FIG. 37-15. A 66-year-old man with rapidly progressive coronary artery calcification scores. Volume-rendered **(A)** and projection **(B)** views of the circumflex coronary artery and its obtuse marginal branch *(small white arrows)*.

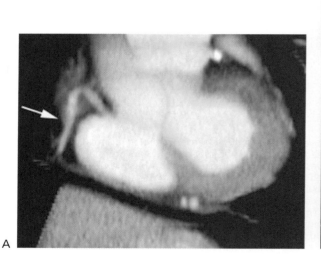
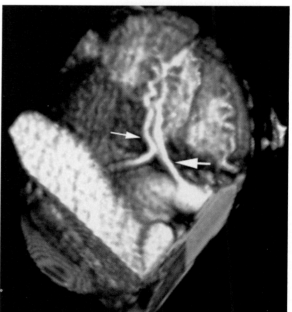

FIG. 37-16. A 66-year-old man with rapidly progressive coronary artery calcification scores. **A.** EBCT (C-150) projection view of the proximal and mid portion of the right coronary artery *(small white arrow)*. **B.** Volume-rendered caudal view of the posterior descending coronary artery *(small arrow)* and middle cardiac vein *(large arrow)*, both running in the posterior interventricular groove.

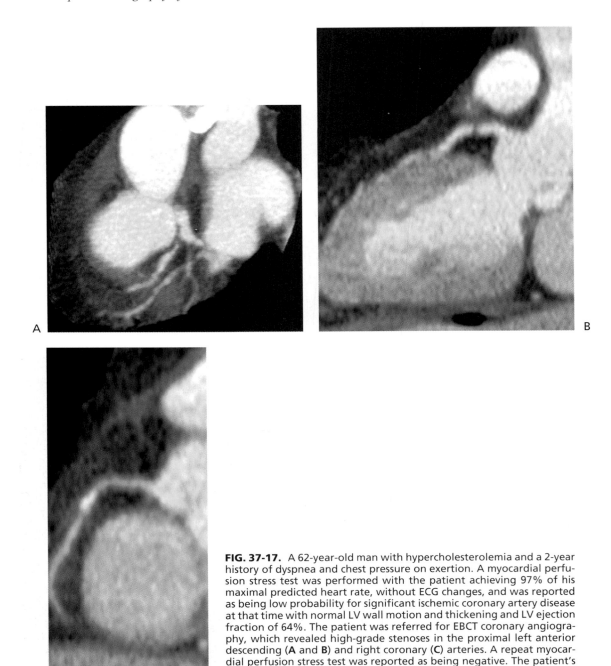

FIG. 37-17. A 62-year-old man with hypercholesterolemia and a 2-year history of dyspnea and chest pressure on exertion. A myocardial perfusion stress test was performed with the patient achieving 97% of his maximal predicted heart rate, without ECG changes, and was reported as being low probability for significant ischemic coronary artery disease at that time with normal LV wall motion and thickening and LV ejection fraction of 64%. The patient was referred for EBCT coronary angiography, which revealed high-grade stenoses in the proximal left anterior descending (**A** and **B**) and right coronary (**C**) arteries. A repeat myocardial perfusion stress test was reported as being negative. The patient's symptoms persisted, and a conventional coronary angiogram was performed and confirmed the findings of the high-grade stenoses demonstrated by the EBCT coronary angiogram.

CHARACTERIZATION OF CORONARY ANOMALIES

Coronary artery anomalies are observed in about 1% of patients undergoing diagnostic coronary angiography and are detected in about 1% of routine autopsy examinations. Although most of these anomalies lack hemodynamic significance, possible consequences include myocardial ischemia and sudden death. The ability to identify coronary artery anomalies reliably and to define their anatomic course exactly, therefore, is a prerequisite for any modality that attempts noninvasive coronary artery imaging. Currently, the diagnostic method of choice for detecting coronary anomalies is invasive coronary angiography. However, misinterpretations are common. Contrast-enhanced electron beam coronary angiography permits not only visualization of the

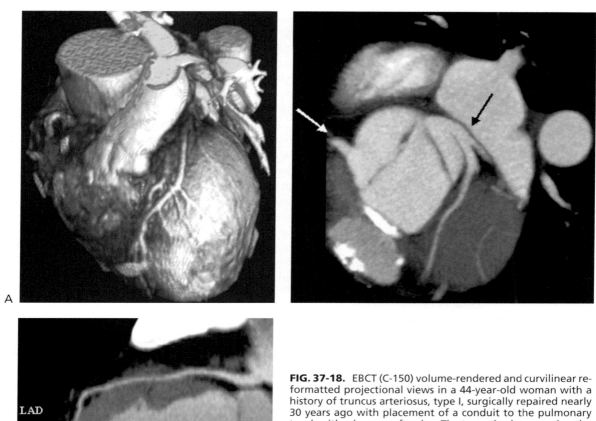

FIG. 37-18. EBCT (C-150) volume-rendered and curvilinear reformatted projectional views in a 44-year-old woman with a history of truncus arteriosus, type I, surgically repaired nearly 30 years ago with placement of a conduit to the pulmonary trunk with a homograft valve. The truncal valve served as the aortic valve. Both valves began failing with development of aortic regurgitation and pulmonary regurgitation. The patient was referred for electron beam coronary angiography to assess for the presence of congenital coronary anomalies associated with truncus arteriosus. The left coronary artery is seen to originate abnormally from the posterior sinus of Valsalva *(black arrow in* **B***)*, while the right coronary artery originates normally from the right sinus of Valsalva *(white arrow in* **B***)* LAD, left anterior descending coronary artery.

coronary arteries and detection of significant stenoses but also characterization of the course of anomalous coronary arteries. The use of invasive angiography as the gold standard to define the course of anomalous coronary arteries, therefore, may no longer be justified, and CT coronary angiographic techniques may become the method of choice to evaluate congenital coronary anomalies (Figs. 37-18 to 37-20).

MULTIDETECTOR CT CORONARY ANGIOGRAPHY

Conventional CT has been revolutionized in the past several years by the availability of multislice CT detector systems. When first introduced, these detectors were able to acquire 4 simultaneous slices, but systems now available can acquire

8, 16, or more slices simultaneously. In addition to gantry rotation speeds of 500 msec, partial reconstruction algorithms, and retrospective or prospective electrocardiographic gating, image-acquisition times of approximately 300 msec can be obtained. If a patient's heart rate is 60 to 70 beats/min or less, images of acceptable quality with little cardiac motion can be created when images are reconstructed during the time of least cardiac motion in the cardiac cycle (at heart rates <70 to 80 beats/min). At faster heart rates, motion artifact can result in images that are uninterpretable. This problem has been alleviated, in part, by the use of segmental reconstruction algorithms, which use data from different heartbeats and different detector rings to reconstruct images with temporal resolutions equal to the minimum reconstruction time divided by the number of heartbeats used—approximately 70 msec in the case of four heartbeats and gantry rotation speeds of 500 msec. The technique assumes that the heart is always in the same phase

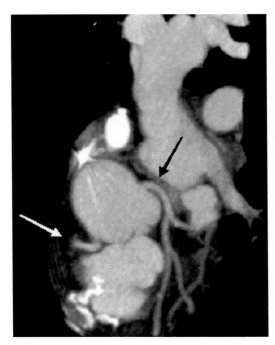

FIG. 37-19. A 52-year-old man was diagnosed as having tetralogy of Fallot at the age of 5 years and underwent repair of his ventricular septal defect and a pulmonary valvotomy at that time. The patient was referred for electron beam coronary angiography to define his coronary anatomy. He was found to have abnormal origin of the left coronary artery *(black arrow)* from the posterior sinus of Valsalva and normal origin of the right coronary artery *(white arrow)* from the right sinus of Valsalva.

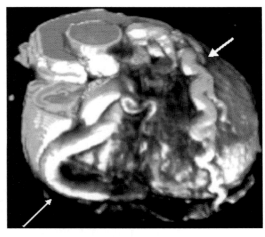

FIG. 37-20. This adult male patient was noted to have a continuous murmur. EBCT (C-150) volume-rendered view coronary angiogram demonstrates massively dilated right *(small arrow)* and left *(large arrow)* coronary arteries secondary to a coronary arteriovenous fistula.

and position as the previous acquisition, which may be a faulty assumption. The use of data from several heartbeats introduces the possibility of errors from data averaging or misregistration from changes in heart rate. This technique has been used in other cardiac imaging modalities, most notably magnetic resonance and nuclear techniques, for depicting cardiac wall motion.

MDCT acquisition employing segmented reconstruction algorithms attempts to improve temporal resolution, but can complicate the data acquisition and may require further refinement before MDCT will be reliable for all patients. A complex relation exists between the patient's heart rate and the data acquisition from multiple detector rings. Varying the table pitch or gantry rotation speed has been suggested as an approach to this problem. Pharmacologic agents such as beta-blockers (metoprolol) or diltiazem may be required to improve image quality by reducing heart rates to 60 beats/min or less (Fig. 37-21).

With initial implementations, there is an incumbent increase in radiation exposure in MDCT compared with EBCT. Radiation exposure from prospectively gated studies is inherently less than that from retrospectively gated studies. The tube currents employed generally are higher with MDCT, which increases radiation exposure, with a resultant increase in image quality. Lower tube currents can be used with MDCT, bringing the signal-to-noise ratio, image quality, and radiation exposure to levels comparable to that of EBCT. However, these reductions often prove unacceptable to imaging clinicians. There has been significant disagreement among health physicists as to the actual increase in dose with MDCT compared with EBCT, with estimates ranging as high as 20 to 30 times the exposure, depending on which protocol is used for MDCT. Protocols are being optimized to reduce radiation exposure, such as modulating the x-ray beam only during 180 degrees of scanning, and using ECG gating for the diastolic phase of the cardiac cycle. Clearly, the differences in radiation exposure will change as these MDCT strategies are implemented. Recent data suggest that radiation exposure with MDCT is similar to that of EBCT at comparable spatial resolution. It may be reasonable to accept the higher radiation doses of MDCT if it results in increased image quality and improved diagnostic accuracy. This would be particularly significant in the area of coronary CT angiography, where an accurate study would eliminate the need for conventional coronary angiography. However, further studies comparing MDCT with conventional coronary angiography are needed to evaluate its diagnostic accuracy. In the case of coronary calcium scoring, the added resolution most likely will not be important, and the increased radiation exposures may not be justified. Reduction in MDCT technique may be required to decrease radiation exposure.

The newest-generation multi-row detector CT scanners, with revolution times of 500 msec, offer the possibility of sampling enough projections to perform retrospective ECG

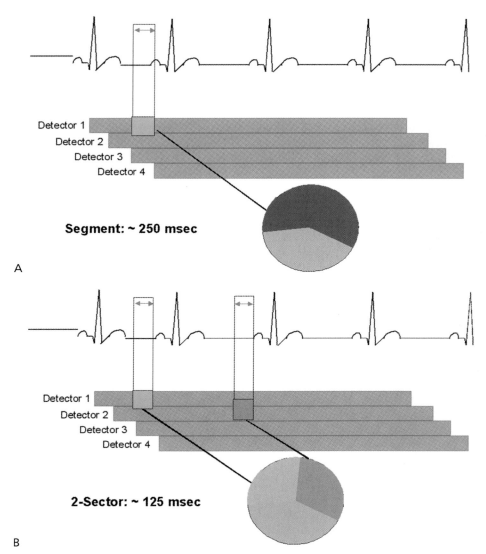

Segment: ~ 250 msec

A

2-Sector: ~ 125 msec

B

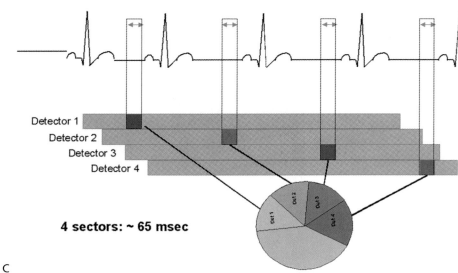

4 sectors: ~ 65 msec

C

FIG. 37-21. The technique used for segmented reconstruction of retrospectively gated MDCT. **A.** The inherent 250-msec temporal resolution when data is acquired from a single heartbeat using a 500-msec gantry rotation speed and a single detector. **B.** When two different heart beats and two different detector rings are used, 125-msec segments are generated corresponding to the same point in the cardiac cycle, generating images with an effective temporal resolution of 125 msec. **C.** When four different heartbeats and four different detector rings are used, 65-msec segments are generated, corresponding to the same point in the cardiac cycle, generating images with an effective temporal resolution of 65 msec. Gantry rotation speed and table pitch must be adjusted to the patient's heart rate. (Courtesy of GE Medical Systems.)

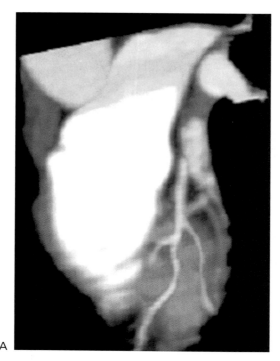

A

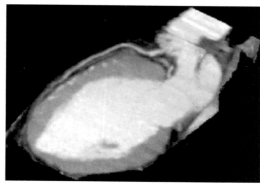

B

FIG. 37-22. A. Projection view from a CT coronary angiogram performed using a four-slice MDCT scanner depicting the left anterior descending coronary artery, a septal perforating branch, and diagonal branch. **B.** Projection view from another CT coronary angiogram performed using a four-slice MDCT scanner depicting the left anterior descending coronary artery.

heart rate. Most manufacturers' protocols recommend or require that the patient's heart rate be between 60 and 70 beats/min or even lower. This mandate necessitates the use of beta-blockers such as metoprolol given either orally (100 mg the night prior to the study and a second 100 mg administered 2 hours before) or intravenously (5 mg IV followed by a maximum of two additional 5-mg IV doses, for a total of 15 mg, over 15 minutes) just prior to the study. Using beta-blockers will make this technique inappropriate for patients with a history of asthma or borderline low blood pressures.

Although EBCT has been the reference standard for coronary artery calcium measurement, CT coronary angiography will be measured against contrast angiography, and both EBCT and MDCT will have to prove themselves against this standard. Currently there is more experience with EBCT angiography in clinical practice, with studies showing a high negative predictive value for normal studies and somewhat less accuracy for obstructive disease. Overall accuracy has been in the range of 85% for proximal disease. Until recently, single-slice helical CT and MDCT coronary angiography have demonstrated very impressive images in selected cases, but have had few data published in prospective clinical trials. Future studies will elucidate the accuracy, sensitivity, and specificity of MDCT scanners for the detection of coronary artery stenoses (Figs. 37-22 to 37-26; Table 37-2).

Other factors that must be considered include the residual motion in the CT acquisition window. Because the goal of CT coronary angiography most often is the detection of stenosis, the need for images free of blurring is of critical importance. Residual cardiac motion within the acquisition window, and not the spatial resolution of the EBCT technique itself, ultimately will limit the actual resolution of EBCT coronary angiograms. Earlier investigators have suggested that for artifact-free cardiac imaging, acquisition times should be less than 50 msec. Image acquisition times

gating of a spiral CT data set, or, preferably, 4, 8, or 16 slices acquired simultaneously with prospective ECG gating and partial scan reconstruction with view sharing, achieving higher temporal resolution. This latter approach most closely approximates the 100-msec data acquisition performed using EBCT, and avoids any reconstruction artifacts caused by helical acquisition. Few clinical studies have been published to date comparing CT and conventional coronary angiography using the newest-generation multi-row detector CT scanners. However, a limitation of multi-row detector CT coronary angiography, which may, in many circumstances, be significant, is its dependence on the patient's

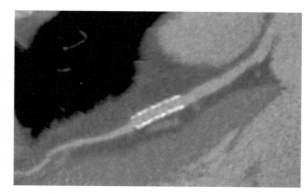

FIG. 37-23. MDCT coronary angiogram of a patent stent in the left anterior descending coronary artery. There is no evidence of stent restenosis.

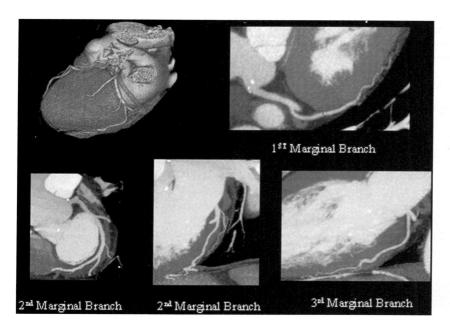

FIG. 37-24. Sixteen-slice MDCT coronary angiogram of the circumflex coronary artery and its obtuse marginal branches.

TABLE 37-2. STUDIES COMPARING MULTIROW DETECTOR CT CORONARY ANGIOGRAPHY WITH CONVENTIONAL CORONARY ANGIOGRAPHY

Study	Patients	Nonevaluated Segments[a] (%)	Sensitivity (%)	Specificity (%)
Knez, 2001	44	6	75	98
Achenbach, 2001	64	32	85	76
Niemen, 2001	35	27	81	97

[a] A relatively large percentage of coronary segments could not be evaluated, possibly related to heart rate control.

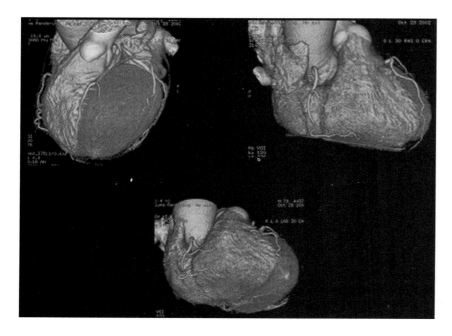

FIG. 37-25. MDCT coronary angiogram. Left anterior oblique *(upper left)*, right anterior oblique *(upper right)*, and caudal *(lower)* 3D volume-rendered views generated to simulate angled views obtained in the cardiac catheterization laboratory.

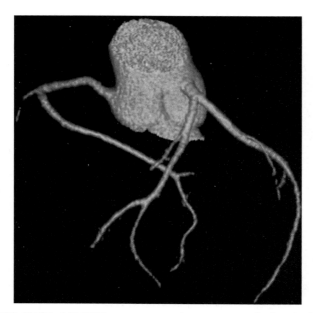

FIG. 37-26. MDCT 3D coronary vessel tree generated using single seeding in the root of the aorta and automated cardiac chamber removal.

of 19.1 and 10.0 msec have been proposed to completely eliminate coronary motion (Figs. 37-27 and 37-28).

e⁻ SPEED EBCT CORONARY ANGIOGRAPHY

The right coronary artery travels at about 50 mm/sec, and the left coronary artery travels at approximately 25 mm/sec during the cardiac cycle. If the average coronary artery diameter is 3 mm, this means that the right coronary artery will travel an entire diameter during a 50-msec CT acquisition window, which is discouraging. To address the problem of residual motion in the acquisition window, the manufacturer of the electron beam CT undertook a project that endeavored initially to double both its temporal and spatial resolution (50-msec acquisition window, 1.5-mm slice thickness). The purpose of this project was to determine if a new 50- to 100-msec multiphase diastolic EBCT coronary angiographic imaging protocol, referred to as cine EBA, could improve upon the image quality of single phase EBCT coronary angiograms. Cine EBA was performed using six cardiac phases, with end-systole defined by a heart rate–adjusted delay approximating 40% of the R-R interval.

Multiphase cine EBA provides good visualization of a very high percentage of proximal and most coronary segments, over a wide range of heart rates, and significantly improved visualization compared to single-phase EBA. The

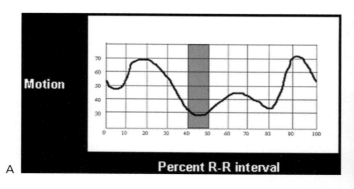

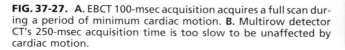

A

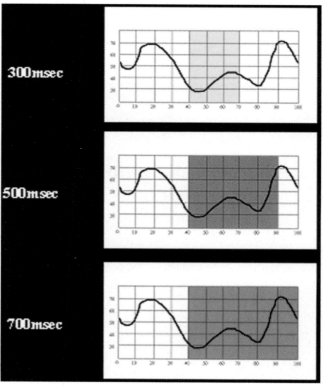

B

FIG. 37-27. A. EBCT 100-msec acquisition acquires a full scan during a period of minimum cardiac motion. **B.** Multirow detector CT's 250-msec acquisition time is too slow to be unaffected by cardiac motion.

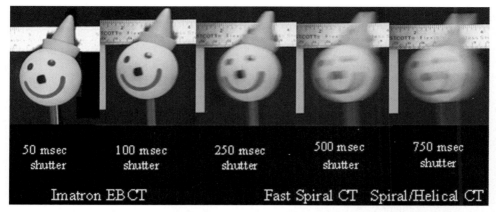

FIG. 37-28. The problem of residual motion in the acquisition window is depicted photographically. The clown head is atop a dowel that is oscillating back and forth like a pendulum at a frequency that would approximate a heart beating at 70 beats/min. Note the progressive degradation in image quality as the camera's shutter speed increases from 50 to 100 (EBCT temporal resolution) to 250 (MDCT temporal resolution) to 500 to 750 msec. This is the same effect that can be seen in a CT coronary angiogram with slower acquisition speeds and longer acquisition windows.

cine EBA 100-msec acquisition did not provide sufficient temporal resolution to completely eliminate coronary motion, however.

By comparison, the 50-msec acquisition provides significantly improved visualization of the coronary segments, apparently due to reduction in residual cardiac motion and blurring. This finding supported the suggestion of earlier investigators, that acquisition times should be less than 50 msec, to reduce artifacts in cardiac imaging. This "proof of principle" prototype, dubbed "cheetah" (the fastest land animal, able to travel at speeds greater than 70 mph) has resulted in the development of the fastest commercially available cardiac CT scanner (e-Speed, GE Imatron, South San Francisco, CA), capable of 33-msec acquisition speeds with a 1.5-mm slice thickness, generating images at the same frame rate as the cardiac catheterization laboratory (30 frames/sec). There appears to be no technical barrier that would prevent the reduction of the acquisition time even further. Cine EBA may prove to be a suitable replacement for, or adjunct to, more invasive diagnostic coronary angiography once it has been developed further (Figs. 37-29 and 37-30).

Although current applications of cardiac CT were developed and pioneered by users of the EBCT, the capabilities of MDCT are approaching that of EBCT and may be superior to electron beam CT in spatial resolution. The eventual role of MDCT in cardiac applications is uncertain at present, but given the current state of the art and expected near-term improvements in technology, it appears that MDCT will play an increasing role, challenging the dominance that EBCT has had thus far, due, at least in part, to its wider availability. The recent rapid advances in MDCT technology are bringing the quality of data produced by that technology close to, and, in some instances, superior to the quality of that provided by earlier-model EBCT scanners. As clinicians take advantage of the wide availability of MDCT multi-row detector CT compared with EBCT, cardiac CT will move more easily into the mainstream of medical practice. We can also look forward to significant improvements in EBCT technology that are needed to maintain a competitive advantage, including development of even faster scanners with improved spatial resolution and multi-slice capability.

CT CORONARY ANGIOSCOPY

Virtual reality techniques have been applied to CT coronary imaging, and a new technique, virtual coronary angioscopy, has been developed. Van Ooijen et al. presented initial results on coronary artery fly-through imaging recently using EBCT. More recently, Schroeder et al. presented their initial results using MDCT coronary angioscopy.

When performing coronary angioscopy, the image data are transferred into three-dimensional voxels, each of which contains a certain density value, expressed in HU. Voxels with different HU can be visualized using different colors. To make the vessel lumen visible, contrast medium–enhanced blood within the coronary arteries is made transparent by excluding the voxels within the lumen (level of 100 to 200 HU) from the endoscopic image. The vessel wall is well-defined, because it has a significantly lower density than the contrast-enhanced lumen (level of 80 to 100 HU). Calcifications can be visualized when they are denser than the contrast medium (level over 250 HU). The simultaneous display of three-dimensional volume-rendered models,

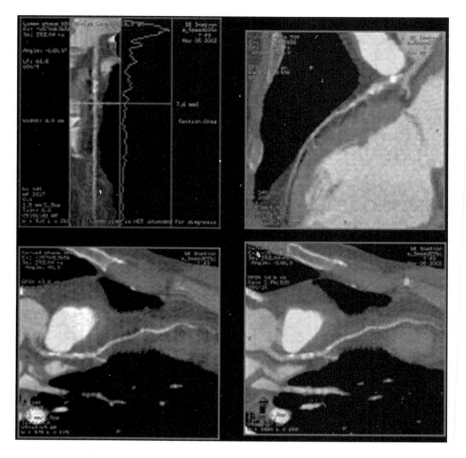

FIG. 37-29. Curvilinear reformatted projection views of the left coronary artery imaged using an e-Speed electron beam CT scanner.

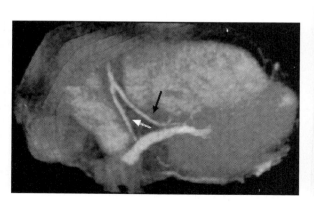

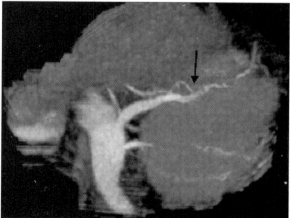

FIG. 37-30. e⁻Speed electron beam coronary angiograms of the distal right coronary artery, the posterior descending coronary artery *(black arrows),* and the posterolateral branch *(white arrow).*

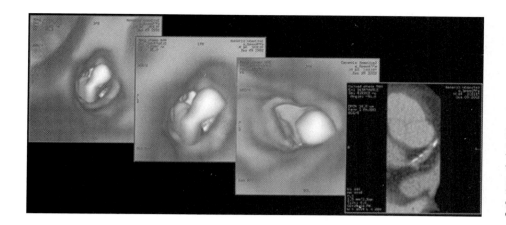

FIG. 37-31. Navigator view performed on a GE Advantage Windows workstation. **Right to left.** Transaxial view through the left main and calcified proximal left anterior descending coronary artery, and three rendered angioscopic navigator views of these calcifications.

multiplanar reformatted or axial slice images, and endoscopic views allows accurate interactive navigation of the viewpoint. Key frames are selected in a path through the vessel with software interpolation of frames between key frames to create a fly-through movie. The scan starts with the navigator positioned at the region of interest; automatic path definition then allows one to find the accurate way from one target point to another, creating the illusion of a moving-catheter angioscopic view through the vessel lumen of the coronary arteries. A fly-through of coronary arteries, venous bypass grafts, and stents is feasible in clinical practice and ultimately may develop into a diagnostic technique that will allow comprehensive three-dimensional delineation of the vessel lumen (Fig. 37-31).

THE FUTURE OF CT CORONARY IMAGING

Currently implemented technical improvements in EBCT and those under development, such as multiplying the number of detector elements and reducing the tomogram acquisition time from 100 msec to less than 50 msec, will allow EBCT to approach the spatial and temporal resolution of cine fluoroscopy.

EBCT coronary imaging has a very bright future, because calcium quantification provides information on the plaque burden of the coronary arteries, and contrast-enhanced CT will determine the severity of obstructive disease reliably. Vulnerable plaque characterization also may be possible. The combination of single-slice and multislice cine EBCT acquisition permits assessment of the degree of coronary calcification, presence, site, and severity of coronary artery stenoses, relative myocardial perfusion, and ventricular function, affording a comprehensive cardiac evaluation during a 30-minute examination. Future studies will be ongoing, evaluating the accuracy, sensitivity, and specificity of MDCT scanners for the detection of coronary artery calcium and stenoses. Initial results are promising. The recent

developments in EBCT and MDCT coronary imaging have finally placed the Holy Grail within our grasp.

SELECTED READING

Achenbach S, Moshage W, Ropers D, et al. Noninvasive, three-dimensional visualization of coronary artery bypass grafts by electron beam tomography. Am J Cardiol 1997; 79:856–861.

Agatston AS, Janowitz WR, Hildner FJ, et al. Quantification of coronary artery calcium using ultrafast computed tomography. J Am Coll Cardiol 1990; 15:827–832.

Becker CR, Kleffel T, Crispin A, et al. Coronary artery calcium measurement: agreement of multirow detector and electron beam CT. AJR Am J Roentgenol 2001; 176:1295–1298.

Budoff MJ, Lane KL, Bakhsheshi H, et al. Rates of progression of coronary calcification by electron beam computed tomography. Am J Cardiol 2000; 86:8–11.

Callister TQ, Raggi P, Cooil B, et al. Effect of HMG-CoA reductase inhibitors on coronary artery disease as assessed by electron-beam computed tomography. N Engl J Med 1998; 339:1972–1978.

Carr JJ, Crouse JR, Goff DC, et al. Evaluation of subsecond gated helical CT for quantification of coronary artery calcium and comparison with electron beam CT. AJR Am J Roentgenol 2000; 174: 915–921.

Goodman WG, Goldin J, Kuizon BD, et al. Coronary-artery calcification in young adults with end-stage renal disease who are undergoing dialysis. N Engl J Med 2000; 342:1478–1483.

Hachamovitch R, Berman DS, Shaw LJ, et al. Incremental prognostic value of myocardial perfusion single photon emission computed tomography for the prediction of cardiac death: differential stratification for risk of cardiac death and myocardial infarction. Circulation 1998; 97:535–543.

He ZX, Hedrick TD, Pratt CM, et al. Severity of coronary artery calcification by electron beam computed tomography predicts silent myocardial ischemia. Circulation 2000; 101:244–251.

Janowitz WR, Agatston AS, Viamonte M. Comparison of serial quantitative evaluation of calcified coronary artery plaque by ultrafast computed tomography in persons with and without obstructive coronary artery disease. Am J Cardiol 1991; 68:1–6.

Maher JE, Bielak LF, Raz JA, et al. Progression of coronary artery calcification: a pilot study. Mayo Clin Proc 1999; 74:347–355.

Miranda R, Schisterman E, Gallagher A, et al. The extent of coronary calcium by electron beam computed tomography discriminates the likelihood of abnormal myocardial perfusion SPECT [abstract]. Circulation 2000; 102:II-543.

Mitchell TL, Pippin JJ, Wei M, et al. Progression of volume of coronary artery calcification [abstract]. In: Advances of Electron Beam Computed Tomography. Iowa City: University of Iowa Press, 1998:29.

Raggi P, Callister TQ, Nicholas J, et al. Cardiac events in patients with progression of coronary calcification on electron beam computed tomography [abstract]. Radiology 1999; 213:351.

Rumberger JA, Behrenbeck T, Breen JF, Sheedy PF II. Coronary calcification by electron beam computed tomography and obstructive coronary artery disease: a model for costs and effectiveness of diagnosis as compared with conventional cardiac testing methods. J Am Coll Cardiol 1999; 33:453–462.

Schroeder S, Kopp AF, Baumbach A, et al. Noninvasive detection and evaluation of atherosclerotic coronary plaques with multislice computed tomography. J Am Coll Cardiol 2001; 37:1430–1435.

Shah AS, Sorochinsky B, Mao SS, et al. Cardiac events and progression of coronary calcium score using electron beam tomography [abstract]. Circulation 2000; 102:II-604.

Stanford W, Breen J, Thompson B, et al. Can the absence of coronary calcification on ultrafast CT be used to rule out nonsignificant coronary artery stenosis? J Am Coll Cardiol 1992; 19:189A.

Tanenbaum SR, Kondos GT, Veselik KE, et al. Detection of calcific deposits in coronary arteries by ultrafast computed tomography and correlation with angiography. Am J Cardiol 1989; 63:870.

Teichholz LE, Petrillo S, Larson AJ, Klig V. Quantitative assessment of atherosclerosis by electron beam tomography. Am J Cardiol 2002; 90:1416–1419.

Van Ooijen PM, Oudkerk M, van Geuns RJ, et al. Coronary artery fly through using electron beam computed tomography. Circulation 2000; 102:E6–E10.

Index

Note: Page numbers followed by *f* indicate an illustration; page numbers followed by *t* indicate a table.